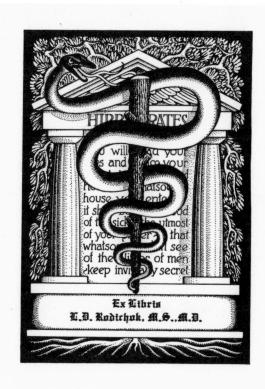

Greenfield's Neuropathology

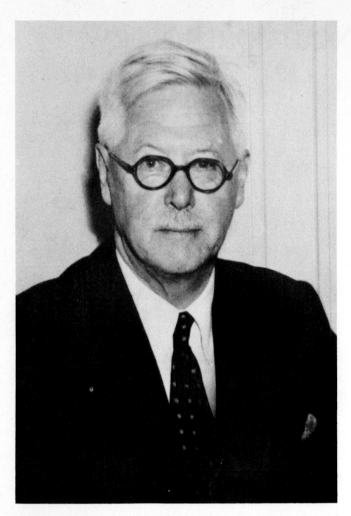

Joseph Godwin Greenfield 1884-1958

Greenfield's Neuropathology

Edited by

W. Blackwood MB, FRCP(Ed), FRCS(Ed), FRCPath

Professor of Neuropathology, Institute of Neurology, The National Hospital, Queen Square, London

J. A. N. Corsellis FRCP, FRCPath, FRCPsych

Consultant Neuropathologist, Runwell Hospital, Wickford, Essex
Honorary Lecturer in Neuropathology at the Institute of Psychiatry, London

With a Foreword by

W. H. McMenemey DM, FRCP, FRCPath, FRCPsych

Emeritus Professor of Pathology, University of London; formerly of the Institute of Neurology
Honorary Consultant Pathologist, National Hospitals for Nervous Diseases

AN EDWARD ARNOLD PUBLICATION
Distributed by
YEAR BOOK MEDICAL PUBLISHERS, INC.
35 E. Wacker Drive, Chicago

© Edward Arnold (Publishers) Ltd. 1976

First published 1958 by
Edward Arnold (Publishers) Ltd.
25 Hill Street, London W1X 8LL

Reprinted 1960
Second edition 1963
Reprinted 1965, 1967, 1969, 1971
Third edition 1976

Distributed in the United States of America, South and Central America,
Puerto Rico and the Philippines by
YEAR BOOK MEDICAL PUBLISHERS, INC.

ISBN: 0-8151-0840-0

by arrangement with
Edward Arnold (Publishers) Ltd.

Library of Congress Catalog Card Number: 75-44533

Printed in Great Britain by
T. and A. Constable Ltd.
Hopetoun Street, Edinburgh

Contributors

Adams, J. Hume, PhD, MB, MRCP, FRCPath
Professor of Neuropathology
Institute of Neurological Sciences
Southern General Hospital, Glasgow

Blackwood, W., MB, FRCP(Ed), FRCS(Ed), FRCPath
Professor of Neuropathology
Institute of Neurology
The National Hospital, Queen Square, London

Brierley, J. B., MD, FRCPath, FRCPsych
MRC Laboratories
Woodmansterne Road, Carshalton, Surrey

Corsellis, J. A. N., FRCP, FRCPath, FRCPsych
Consultant Neuropathologist
Runwell Hospital, Wickford, Essex
Honorary Lecturer in Neuropathology
Institute of Psychiatry, London

Crome, L., MC, FRCP(Ed), FRCPath
Formerly Consultant Neuropathologist
Queen Mary's Hospital for Children
Carshalton, Surrey

Daniel, P. M., DM, DSc, FRCP, FRCS, FRCPath, FRCPsych
Professor of Neuropathology
Institute of Psychiatry, London

Harriman, D. G. F., MD, FRCP, FRCPath
Senior Lecturer in Neuropathology
University of Leeds
Honorary Consultant Neuropathologist
The General Infirmary, Leeds

Hughes, J. Trevor, MA, DPhil, MD, FRCP(Ed), MRCPath
Clinical Lecturer in Neuropathology
University of Oxford
Consultant Neuropathologist
The Radcliffe Infirmary, Oxford

Meldrum, B. S., PhD, MB, BChir
Senior Lecturer
Institute of Psychiatry, London

Oppenheimer, D. R., MA, DM, MRCPath
University Lecturer in Neuropathology
University of Oxford
Honorary Consultant in Neuropathology
The Radcliffe Infirmary, Oxford
Fellow of Trinity College, Oxford

Smith, W. Thomas, MD, FRCP, FRCPath
Professor of Neuropathology, University of Birmingham
Consultant Neuropathologist, West Midlands RHA
Consultant Pathologist, Central Birmingham Health District (T)

Stern, J., PhD
Clinical Biochemist
Queen Mary's Hospital for Children
Carshalton, Surrey

Strich, S. J., DM, MRCP, MRCPath, MRCPsych
Formerly Reader in Neuropathology
Institute of Psychiatry, London

Treip, C. S., MA, MD, PhD, FRCPath
Lecturer in Pathology, University of Cambridge
Honorary Consultant Neuropathologist, Addenbrookes Hospital
Cambridge

Urich, H., MD, FRCP, FRCPath
Professor of Neuropathology
Institute of Pathology, The London Hospital

Yates, P. O., MD, FRCPath
Professor of Neuropathology
University of Manchester

Foreword

by W. H. McMenemey

Joseph Godwin Greenfield died at Bethesda, Maryland, on 2nd March 1958, where latterly he had been working after his retirement from The National Hospital, Queen Square, London. He did not live to see the publication of the first edition of the book which he planned, supervised and produced, with the cooperation of four colleagues from England. Florence, his wife, who almost single-handed had prepared the final typescript, was busy on the index at the time of his sudden decease.

Dr Greenfield was the son of a medical graduate of University College London, William Smith Greenfield, who had migrated to Edinburgh to hold with distinction the chair of clinical medicine and pathology from 1881 until his retirement in 1912. Godwin was born in 1884 and qualified in Edinburgh in 1908. His first appointment at The National Hospital was in June 1910 as junior house physician. In January 1914, after gaining experience in Leeds, he returned to become the first whole-time pathologist, succeeding a line of eminent neurologists who, since 1889, had made time to study pathological material in the hospital's laboratory; they included Frederick Batten, James Collier, (Sir) Farquhar Buzzard, (Sir) Gordon Holmes and S. A. Kinnier Wilson. With Dr Farquhar Buzzard, he was co-author of *Pathology of the Nervous System* (London, 1921), a classic which to read gives pleasure, and with Dr E. A. Carmichael he published another classic, *The Cerebrospinal Fluid in Clinical Diagnosis* (London, 1925). Although primarily a pathologist, he never lost sight of his clinical training and it was probably with some reluctance that he decided to abandon manometry and clinical pathology in order to concentrate on the histopathology of the nervous system. So he encouraged a loyal and talented assistant pathologist in the person of the late Professor John Cumings to develop the clinical laboratory: in time there was to emerge from this a separate department of chemical pathology headed by the latter, who was already engaged on joint studies with Dr Greenfield's successor, Dr William Blackwood.

As a neuropathologist, Dr Greenfield deservedly enjoyed a world-wide reputation. His humble premises in Queen Square, formerly Victor Horsley's operating theatre, were approached through a pipe-lined basement corridor and were well known to discerning students of neurology who came from many countries to study his methods. In 1938 his department was transferred into a new Rockefeller building in the hospital but there was scarcely time to settle in before preparations for war disturbed long-term plans for research. Then came orders for the transfer of in-patients and services from Queen Square to Enfield. Back in London on the conclusion of hostilities he again set to work, but in 1949 he reached the age of retirement as had been laid down in the National Health Service Act (1946).

Dr Greenfield was fortunate to work at a time when techniques were relatively simple and opportunities were great. But he had to contend with a very limited budget and with material from the patients in his hospital only, although as his reputation grew, more and more specimens were sent to him from other parts of the country. His experience therefore was wide and varied, even if initially he lacked the opportunities offered to those who work in a general, as distinct from a neurological, hospital. He was a superb technician and liked nothing better than to work with his hands. He had few reagents but he used them with great effect. He cherished the razors on the microtome and was severely critical of those who misused them. His photographic equipment was simple, indeed almost primitive, but he used it with ingenuity and efficiency. An accomplished carpenter also, he was indeed a true artisan of the laboratory. But those of us who were privileged to enjoy his company and benefit from his experience will remember the man for what he was. If, to the newcomer, his presence was somewhat commanding and even stern, he was invariably courteous and attentive. A smile would soon appear and often a reassuring chuckle. He was, in fact, a shy man. He could be stubborn and would sometimes initiate a debate to test one's confidence in an opinion: one was vindicated if he gave in gracefully with his customary smile. Above all he was modest both in his wants and his claims. The fact that he invited others to share with him in the production of his book is a measure both of his modesty and of his generosity since he had the experience and the ability to complete it alone. His technical staff consisted of the versatile and somewhat assertive John Anderson, author of a useful technical handbook, and sometimes a boy. His reports and correspondence were invariably in his very legible handwriting. No secretary guarded the door of his small, somewhat dreary office which adjoined that historic theatre: the door, in fact, was almost always open and as often as not he was at the microscope demonstrating to a visitor who sought his opinion. He wrote well and, as an editor, boldly and with relish eradicated the chaff from the germ with his customary good humour.

The National Hospital, which in 1948 had been linked with Maida Vale Hospital as The National Hospitals for Nervous Diseases, was not affiliated through its postgraduate medical schools with the University of London until 1950, so Dr Greenfield was never eligible for the professorial status he so richly deserved, but he was dean of The National Hospital's own medical school during twenty formative years beginning with 1923. His influence on the smooth and steady development of the embryonic Institute of Neurology (founded in 1950 as a result of the amalgamation of the two postgraduate medical schools) can be seen in retrospect to have been important.

Dr Greenfield's years of 'retirement' were remarkable. For five years he held a research post in the Institute of Neurology and then in June 1954 he accepted an invitation as visiting professor in Bethesda at the National Institute of Neurological Diseases and Blindness. During those busy nine years he set his mind to new problems and to planning and writing his chapters in *Neuropathology*. He attended the meeting in Paris concerned with the organization of the 1st International Congress of Neuropathology, and in September 1952 led the party from the United Kingdom to Rome for that highly successful inaugural gathering of persons interested in the specialty. In 1950 he founded the Neuropathological Club which in 1962 adopted the title of the British Neuropathological Society. It still retains that friendly and informal atmosphere wherein he delighted to meet his colleagues. At the 2nd International Congress of Neuropathology held in London in 1955 he was president and he returned again from Washington in 1957 to attend the 1st International Congress of Neurological Sciences at Brussels, of which the 3rd International Congress of Neuropathology was an integral part. In the previous summer the University of Edinburgh had honoured its distinguished son with the LL.D., as they had his father in 1913.

Dr Greenfield was a little above average height, of athletic build and he carried himself well. He played golf and tennis and was fond of gardening. In the year 1947, Godwin and Florence Greenfield moved from Hampstead to the village of Westcott in Surrey. Garden Hill, their new home, was a cottage with behind it a hillside garden and arboretum. In this sylvan setting he would steer his guests along grassy walks debating the diagnosis of some tree with unusual leaf pattern, as if it was a wayward astrocyte of uncertain lineage. As his hair whitened with age an arthritis of the right hip became increasingly incapacitating and painful, but of this he never complained. This then was the contented teacher, whom so many of us remember with affection.

When the time came to consider a second edition of *Neuropathology*, the remaining contributors accorded it the eponymous title which it clearly merited. Mrs Greenfield was closely associated with us in its production and, with the help of Professor Dorothy Russell who had readily agreed to revise the important chapter on head injuries, she again prepared the index.

Dr Ronald Norman agreed to act as editor. His professional life had been primarily concerned with the clinical care of the mentally handicapped but in his latter years he had been given charge of a laboratory largely devoted to the histological and chemical study of mental disease, which for many years had been his main interest. He had often turned, as others had done, to Dr Greenfield for advice and instruction. A cultured man with wide interests, editorial experience and with a critical judgement valued by all who knew him, he was well qualified for the task and he saw to it that as much as possible of Dr Greenfield's original writing should be retained, having due regard to the advances in knowledge which had accrued over a period of five years. The second edition was published in 1963. Regrettably Dr Norman died on 20th August 1968 and so the surviving contributors, two of whom had retired and another was due to retire soon, decided that a recruitment of authors was necessary, especially in view of the rapid progress of, and specialism in, neuropathology. There was no lack of candidates because 'the Club' which Dr Greenfield founded had grown into a lively and sizeable scientific forum. In the autumn of 1972 Mrs Greenfield died but she had lived to see planned and well advanced this third edition of the book to which she had devoted so much of her time.

Recent advances in neuropathology have depended in part on new knowledge acquired in neuro-biology, virology and cytochemistry, for which new techniques, often complicated and expensive, have been evolved. Much has been learned with the aid of the electron microscope and this machine is now regarded as an important investigating medium. But the purpose of this book remains as it was in the first and second editions, namely, to help those who wish to be able to recognize the gross and micro-scopical features of disease of the central nervous system. The working tool of the neuropathologist is still the light microscope.

W. H. McM.
London

Preface to third edition

The second edition of *Greenfield's Neuropathology* maintained the popularity of the first and after some years it became clear that a third would be needed. Dr Norman, however, had died in 1968 and Professor Meyer and Professor Russell felt that the preparation of a new version should be passed to the next generation of British neuropathologists guided by Dr Greenfield's colleagues and successors at the National Hospitals, Professor McMenemey and Professor Blackwood. A new team of contributors was therefore selected, all of whom had known well the authors of the original book and had been deeply influenced by their teaching. The fundamental approach of the present volume has, therefore, remained that of Greenfield and his contemporaries; it is the subject-matter that has changed, for so much has happened in the neurosciences during the last ten years that extensive revision, and indeed rewriting, of many chapters has become inevitable. Thus Professor William Blackwood has revised the important introductory chapter while Professor Peter Yates has taken over that on vascular disease. Dr James Brierley has extended the chapter on the experimental and human aspects of hypoxia. The chapters on intoxications, poisons and nutritional disorders have been rewritten by Professor Walter Smith. Dr Dennis Harriman has revised the chapter on bacterial infections while Professor Hume Adams has been responsible for those on parasitic, fungal and viral infections. Dr Sabina Strich has contributed the chapter on cerebral trauma. Professor Henry Urich has expanded Dr Norman's chapter on malformations and the para-natal disorders, and has also contributed a largely new chapter on peripheral nerves. Demyelinating diseases and the system disorders of the basal ganglia and the cerebellum have been the responsibility of Dr David Oppenheimer, while Dr Trevor Hughes has written the chapter on the diseases of the spine and spinal cord. Together with Dr Brian Meldrum, Dr Nicholas Corsellis has dealt with the subject of the epilepsies and he has recast the two chapters: one on ageing and the dementias and the other on the psychoses of obscure origin. Lastly, because of Professor McMenemey's much regretted retirement, Dr Corsellis has joined Professor Blackwood to assist in editing the present volume.

The new topics introduced include a chapter on the diseases of muscle by Dr Denis Harriman, and on the diseases of the pituitary and the hypothalamus by Professor Peter Daniel and Dr Cecil Treip. The previous sections on the neuronal storage diseases and the leuco-dystrophies have been combined and expanded by Dr Len Crome and Dr Jan Stern into a new chapter on inborn lysosomal enzyme deficiencies.

In spite of the omission of certain sections, the present edition is considerably larger than the previous two. It is nevertheless still contained within a single volume.

The list of contributors to this edition testify to the growth of the speciality of neuropathology in the years since the book first appeared. It was Dr Greenfield who was one of those most responsible for this expansion in the United Kingdom and it seems fitting, at the time of publication of this third edition, to pay a special tribute to him. Professor William McMenemey, therefore, who knew him so well and for so long, has included the appreciation of him in the Foreword.

Acknowledgements

A book of this kind depends greatly on the efforts and kindness of many more people than the editors can thank individually. We are particularly indebted to Dr Magda Erdohazi, Dr B. D. Lake and Dr K. Suzuki for their assistance with Chapter 12 and to the Muscular Dystrophy Group of Great Britain for a grant which helped greatly towards the writing of Chapter 19. The support of the Medical Research Council to individual contributors has been invaluable. We would like to thank Mr James Mills for the new photographs in Chapter 1 and Mr Norman Le Page for many in Chapter 12. We are also indebted to numerous authors and editors for allowing us to borrow illustrations, the sources of which are acknowledged in the legends. We are most grateful to the Librarians and to the staff of the Institute of Neurology, Queen Square, and to those at the Royal Society of Medicine. We would particularly like to thank our secretaries Miss Diane Johnston, Miss Mary Symon, Mrs Roma Abbott and Mrs Linda Dove for their lasting co-operation and help. Each contributor has advised on the items to be incorporated in the index and we have been fortunate in having the devoted skill of Mrs Muriel Castell who has integrated this raw material into a structure which should prove of great practical use to the reader. The editorial work has been much lightened by the expert assistance of Mr J. Rivers. Finally, we offer our sincere thanks to the publishers, Edward Arnold, and particularly to Mr P. J. Price and to Miss Barbara Koster. Their encouragement and forbearance during the years of preparation, coupled with their determination towards the end, helped us greatly to overcome the many problems which beset the production of works of this nature.

W. B.
J. A. N. C.
London

Contents

1

Normal Structure and General Pathology of the Nerve Cell and Neuroglia

Revised by W. Blackwood

The most important elements in the nervous system are the cell bodies and processes of neurons. Great importance is therefore attached to the various ways by which neurons undergo degeneration and death. But since neurons are fed by blood vessels and bound together by neuroglia and collagenous connective tissues, the neuropathologist must take account of changes in these tissues, and also in the meningeal coverings of the brain and spinal cord. These may be more obvious than the changes in the neurons. Cellular proliferation may hide or mask the changes in the neurons, which can only react by degeneration or death. It is true that in certain diseases the degenerative changes which neurons undergo may be quite unusual and almost pathognomonic. But these changes are usually less evident than the 'inflammatory' and cellular proliferation and may need special staining methods for their demonstration. In many degenerative diseases the overgrowth of astrocytes and proliferation of their fibres may be more striking than the disappearance of nerve cells or their axons. For this reason the term 'sclerosis' with various descriptive adjectives such as 'cortical' or 'lobar' has been given to processes in which the primary event is degeneration of certain neurons as a whole, and with the prefixes 'multiple', 'disseminated' or 'diffuse' to degenerations in which the myelin sheath is most affected. Non-neoplastic proliferation of neuroglial cells is considered to be almost always a reaction to the degeneration of neurons or myelin, or a concomitant reaction to the noxa to which this is due. The reactions of the vascular and supporting tissues are important in that they may help towards our understanding of the pathogenesis of nervous diseases. Nevertheless the most impor-

tant study is that of the changes in the cell bodies and/or processes of the neurons themselves since it is to these that the symptoms of disease are due.

From the beginning, neuropathology has had two chief objectives, first the topography of the lesion and secondly its nature. The relative importance of these two objectives varies in different conditions, but in most diseases the two objectives are complementary and both are essential. In the early days of neuropathology the great French and German schools were distinguished by the emphasis laid on one or the other of these objectives.

The French genius for anatomy was reflected in the School of Charcot for which the distribution of the lesions in relation to nuclei and tracts had special importance. When the lesion was focal, or confined to a special system or related group of systems, it could be correlated with the symptoms observed during life. Their clinicopathological studies, during the late nineteenth and earlier part of the twentieth centuries, contributed information on the sensory tracts and nuclei and on various aspects of mental activity, especially aphasia and apraxia, which cannot, by their nature, be confirmed by animal experiment. The influence which studies of this kind have had on clinical neurology has been far reaching and profound.

On the other hand, the German school of Weigert, Nissl and Alzheimer and their pupils, especially Jakob and Spielmeyer, was specially interested in the alterations which the neurons and neuroglial cells underwent in disease and in the interpretation of these changes in relation to aetiology and pathogenesis. This method of study is fundamental to the understanding of diseases of the nervous system.

It is the object of present-day neuropathology to integrate these two disciplines. This twofold quest imposes a heavy task on those who undertake it, since they must be not only pathologists but also anatomists and to some extent clinical neurologists and psychiatrists. A neuropathologist must know the history and details of the patient's illness before he makes his examination, otherwise he may often fail to examine some part of the nervous system. This applies most obviously to such outlying parts as the optic nerves and retina, the internal ear, and the dorsal root ganglia and peripheral nerves, but it happens too often that no examination is made of the spinal cord even in cases with signs of paraplegia or ataxia.

This combined aim of modern neuropathology has resulted in techniques which are far removed from the simpler methods in everyday use for the other tissues of the body. In general, paraffin embedding is not so suitable for nervous tissues as either celloidin or frozen sections, owing to the greater shrinkage of the tissues and more complete removal of lipids during the process of embedding. Post mordanting with mercury or chrome salts may reduce these disadvantages, but restricts the choice of staining methods. Very large paraffin sections are also less easily handled than celloidin sections of similar size. In some laboratories skill in dealing with large frozen sections has made their use the method of choice for many techniques, but the use of smaller frozen sections is more general both as a preliminary to further examination and for special staining methods such as fat stains and silver impregnation. Celloidin embedding remains the most ideal routine method. Its relative freedom from shrinkage and other artefacts, the greater retention of lipids, even without post mordanting, and the wide range of staining processes available for celloidin sections offset the disadvantages of slowness and expense.

Special techniques in neuropathology are used, for the most part, to make more obvious what can be seen only faintly with more ordinary staining methods, rather than to discover structures or changes which are otherwise invisible. In many cases, however, their use is obligatory. The extent and degree of demyelination, or of fibrous gliosis, of damage to axons, neurofibrils, or nerve cells can only be judged by the use of special techniques. Such structures as neurofibrillary tangles in nerve cells and senile plaques are difficult to see without the use of silver impregnations. In this way some techniques come into routine use while others are reserved for special cases.

Neuropathology has always been concerned with the changes which occur in the living body in response to disease. These can be studied by looking at tissues removed after death or at operation. Disease processes, often similar to those seen in the human, can be studied in animals where they may occur naturally or may be induced experimentally. Immunofluorescent microscopy is increasingly applied to the elucidation of pathological processes, particularly to viral infections (see p. 313). Tissue culture is used in an attempt to study reactions in living tissues. The pathologist has been aware for a long time that his aim was to explore structure to its ultimate limit and here he is being helped by the electron microscope (Hirano 1971). He is also aware of the importance of biochemistry in respect of structure and living processes. He is demonstrating the various enzymes and their location by the techniques of histochemistry and ultrastructural histochemistry. In a sense, the old-established techniques of neuropathology have always been histochemical, although often based more on empiricism than on scientific principles. Weigert's use of haematoxylin to stain myelin is not very different from Baker's stain for phosphatides, and the osmic acid techniques are based upon the reducing power of unsaturated fatty acids on osmium tetroxide. On the other hand, the various staining methods for glial fibres have been developed almost entirely from empirical observations by such masters as Carl Weigert and Frank B. Mallory. A similar empiricism appears to have guided the Spanish school as well as Golgi and Bielschowsky in their use of silver stains. Modern histochemical techniques aim less at staining structural elements than at localizing and making biochemical activities visible within the cells and their organelles. Numerous methods have been developed to visualize the activities of enzymes such as the cytochrome oxidases, dehydrogenases, specific and unspecific phosphatases, and cholinesterases (Adams 1969).

The neuron

Normal histology

The neuron, the most complex cell in the body, may undergo alterations in disease which are of comparable complexity. These are revealed microscopically by alterations in shape, staining reactions and structure, which cannot be interpreted without a more detailed knowledge of the neuronal composition than we possess at present. Certain typical neuronal alterations have, however, long been recognized as the results of certain forms of lesion or disease, and the metabolic changes which lead to some of these histological changes are beginning to be understood. These are essentially problems in histochemistry which may soon be clarified by the rapid advances which are taking place in that subject.

The cerebral and cerebellar cortex contains several layers of neuronal bodies and a dense mass of their dendrites with an underlying white matter which contains only nerve fibres. The cerebrum also contains large central nuclei of grey matter or 'basal ganglia'. The cerebellum also has basal nuclei in which its efferent fibres are relayed. In the spinal cord the grey matter containing the nerve cells forms a central H-shaped column which is surrounded by white matter. In the brainstem grey and white matter are less readily separable. Some nuclei, such as the nuclei in the floor of the 4th ventricle, consist chiefly of grey matter; other nuclei, such as the nuclei pontis, contain a larger admixture of myelinated fibres and in the reticular formation the nerve cells are rather loosely scattered among the myelinated fibres.

It has been calculated that the cerebrum contains more than 20,000 million neurons. These are of varied form and size. The larger cells in the cerebral cortex and corpus striatum and those which give rise to the motor nerves in the brainstem and spinal cord are pyramidal in shape with their axons arising from the base of the cell. This shape is characteristic of efferent cells. The cells of the dorsal root ganglia and those of the mesencephalic root of the trigeminal nerve are spherical in shape; in the second sensory nuclei of the brainstem and spinal cord and the thalamus a more or less oval shape is the rule. Other nerve cells vary between these two extremes, some being more multipolar, others having more rounded outlines.

Bipolar cells are found in the cochlear and vestibular ganglia, the olfactory organ and the retina. The fusiform cells described by Cajal in the auditory cortex are a special form. The flask shape of the Purkinje cells of the cerebellar cortex is also unusual. Their spherical cell bodies give off at one pole an axon and at the other a thicker process which breaks up into a frond of dendrites which spreads out across the lamella at right angles to its length.

The size of nerve cells varies from very large to very small. The largest cells, the Betz cells in the 5th layer of the motor cortex, the large anterior horn cells in the cervical and lumbo-sacral enlargements of the spinal cord and the cells in the dorsal root ganglia, may measure 80 μm in the greatest diameter of the cell body. The smallest neurons, the granule cells in the cerebellar cortex, and those in the retina and olfactory bulb, consist of little more than a rounded darkly staining nucleus, about 5 μm in diameter, and an axon which runs for a comparatively short distance among neighbouring cells. In the brainstem particularly there are cells of all sizes, the axons of which run for very varied distances from the perikarya. According to Hyden (1947), in the larger neurons the axon may have 1000 times the bulk of the cell body, and the nutrition of this large process must make great demands on the metabolism of the cell.

Constitution and structure

The nerve cell is one of the very few cell types in the human body which cannot be replaced if destroyed as it does not undergo cell division after the first few weeks of infancy. At the same time it has great metabolic activity, requiring a constant supply of oxygen and glucose. The large nucleus and nucleolus of a nerve cell resemble those seen in an embryonic or neoplastic cell and are indicative of abundant protein production. No nerve cell in the central nervous system can tolerate anoxia for much more than 15 minutes at normal body temperature, and the more susceptible cells in the cerebral cortex cannot survive more than 5 minutes of complete circulatory arrest. When the metabolic needs of cortical neurons are reduced by lowering the body temperature these times can be considerably exceeded. Similarly, if the level of blood sugar falls to 20 mg per 100 ml consciousness is lost and hypoglycaemia of this level for several hours usually entails the death of many neurons in the cerebral cortex.

The cell body and processes of a neuron contain various structures. The changes which they may undergo in disease form the basis of neuropathology. As these changes can only be understood by comparison with the normal, the various constituents of the nerve cell must first be shortly described.

Nucleus and nucleolus

The nucleus varies considerably in different types of nerve cell and in the same cell type in different mammalian species. The vesicular nucleus with a large central nucleolus seen in larger cells may appear distinctive (Fig. 1.1), but all nuclei contain the same chemical elements although in different proportions. These are: (1) nucleoplasm composed of weakly acidophilic protein. (2) Chromatin or deoxyribonucleic acid (DNA) in granules of varying size and fine threads. These stain with basic aniline dyes and are Feulgen positive.

The nucleolus, which is spherical and more or less central, is composed of a mixture of ribonucleic acid (RNA) and a basic (acidophilic) protein, which are in the form of electron dense granules and fine filaments. It is amphophilic and Feulgen negative. The nucleolus often contains one or more 'vacuoles'.

The proportions of nuclear chromatin and of nucleolus vary considerably in neurons of different types, especially in relation to their size. In the large nerve cells the nucleolus is large and the chromatin is present in small amount, being confined to very fine granules under the nuclear membrane and one or two larger paranucleolar granules. At the other extreme the cerebellar granule cells have a small central nucleolus which is covered and partly obscured by abundant chromatin granules. In general, as Olszewski (1947) points out, there is a positive correlation in man between the amount of Nissl substance and the size of nucleolus, and a negative correlation between the amounts of Nissl substance and nuclear chromatin. Most nerve cells have only one nucleolus, although two or more have been described in developing neurons.

In some of the larger cells the chromatin, in addition to fine granules, may form a rounded

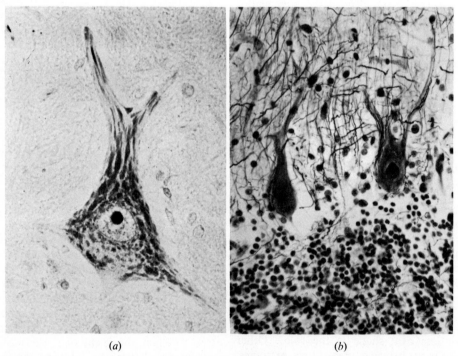

(a)   (b)

Fig. 1.1 Normal nerve cells. (*a*) Cell from ventral horn of lumbar cord; note absence of Nissl granules in axon hillock. Nissl. × 550. (*b*) Purkinje cells, cerebellar cortex. Basket fibres surround the cells and pass up the dendrites. Bielschowsky. × 400.

or oval mass, 0·5 to 2 μm in diameter, which usually lies close to or in contact with the nucleolus, but sometimes it lies free in the nucleoplasm or in contact with the nuclear membrane. This nucleolar satellite or sex chromatin was shown by Barr and Bertram (1949) to be larger in the female than in the male in many nerve cells; in the human this sex difference can be well seen in the sympathetic ganglia and cerebral cortex but it is not so distinct in Purkinje cells.

Cajal (1909) described an argyrophilic dot in the nucleoplasm of large nerve cells under the name of accessory body. This has no relation to chromatin and its nature is not known (Lindsay and Barr 1955).

As Marinesco (1909) pointed out, the cells of the substantia nigra and locus ceruleus may normally contain, in the nucleoplasm, acidophilic bodies which become larger, more sharply defined and more numerous in old people. These bodies may be mistaken for intranuclear inclusions, the earlier stages of which they closely resemble, but they do not displace the nucleolus. Although usually single, two or three such bodies may be seen lying close to the nucleolus.

By electron microscopy the nucleus is seen to be surrounded by what appear to be two membranes. In places the space between the membranes is continuous with the cisternae of the endoplasmic reticulum of the cytoplasm. The surface of the nucleus is interrupted by regularly spaced, imperforate nuclear pores, where the two membranes merge (Peters, Palay and Webster 1970).

Nissl granules or Nissl substance—(endoplasmic reticulum)

These names are used for the flakes of basophilic material in the cytoplasm of nerve cells and dendrites which were described by Nissl in 1894.

It is necessary to distinguish the changes which may have resulted from the mode of death or post-mortem autolysis from those which are related to a chronic or subacute nervous disease. Certain well-defined changes in the Nissl substances, such as central or peripheral chromatolysis, fortunately require some little time to develop and are never the result of agonal or post-mortem changes.

The electron microscope shows the Nissl substance to be composed of aggregations of rough or granular endoplasmic reticulum. This is a delicate laminated system of cisternae (Fig. 1.2),

the outer surfaces of which are studded with small particles called ribosomes. Clusters or rosettes of free ribosomes are present between the cisternae and elsewhere in the cytoplasm. Ribosomes are composed chiefly of ribonucleic acid and are responsible for the basophilia of the Nissl substance. In the living cell proteins, both enzymatic and structural, are synthesized in relation to these ribosomes. Nissl substance is absent from the axon hillock but is visible at the base of the dendrites. The electron microscope reveals that rough endoplasmic reticulum is present in dendrites and to a lesser degree in axons.

Relationship of Nissl substance to nucleus

It is noticeable that, when a previously damaged and chromatolytic nerve cell is recovering, the nucleolus enlarges and Nissl substance appears first at the periphery of the nucleus. The similarity in chemical composition of Nissl granules to most of the nucleoproteins of the nucleus led Einarson (1933) to consider that they might be derived from the nucleus, either during ontogenesis only, or both in the developing and adult nerve cell. Studying the response of motor nerve cells to prolonged electrical stimulation or to section of the axon, he found that, after the loss of Nissl granules which resulted from these procedures, there followed an increase in the amount of nucleoprotein round the nucleolus. This migrated to the periphery of the nucleus, especially in the region of the nuclear cap which became more prominent and was in these early stages partly intra- and partly extranuclear. Later it became entirely extranuclear and there was an accumulation of fine Nissl granules in its neighbourhood. As the Nissl substance increased, the nuclear cap became less evident. These observations suggest that the Nissl substance is reformed after chromatolysis from the ribose nucleoprotein of the nucleolus.

Artefact appearances of nerve cells

In experimental work on the lower mammals some nerve cells appear rather pale and rounded (hypochromic) and others darker and more polygonal (hyperchromic). These appearances may sometimes be seen in human material, especially in biopsies. In the past there was considerable discussion as to whether these cells were to be interpreted as being diseased or abnormal or whether the appearances were due to artefact.

The problem was investigated by Koenig and Koenig (1952) and appears to have been resolved by Cammermeyer (1961) in the experimental animal, where immediate perfusion of the brain *in situ* and a subsequent delay of several hours

Mitochondria

Mitochondria are small ovoid bodies 0·3 to 1·0 μm wide and up to 5 μm long; electron microscopy shows them to be contained by a double membrane, the inner layer of which is enfolded

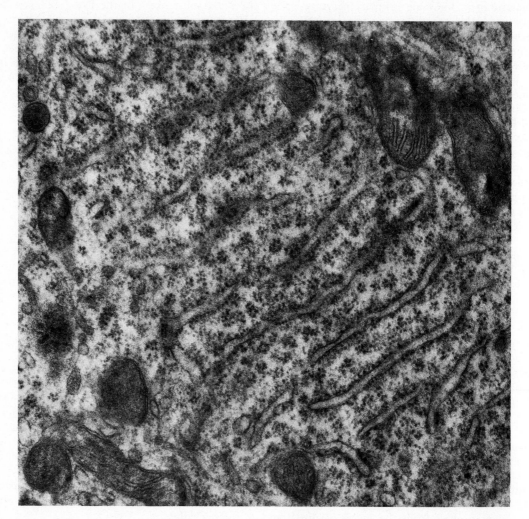

Fig. 1.2 Purkinje cell in the rat cerebellus showing a Nissl body with mitochondria of varying size, the channels of the endoplasmic reticulum and the dense granules covering the membranes and lying in clusters between. × 44,000. (Reproduced from the 1972 edition of Maximow and Bloom's *Textbook of Histology*, Saunders, Philadelphia, by kindness of Professor S. L. Palay.)

before autopsy produced material free of 'dark' neurons, while removal of the unfixed brain at necropsy with subsequent fixation produced many dark neurons. Gonatas (1966) considered that pallor of neurons in human biopsies should be interpreted as due to artefact.

into cristae (Fig. 1.2). They occur randomly throughout the cytoplasm of the neuron and its processes. In the cell body they are found at the periphery of Nissl substance; they are numerous near pre-synaptic membranes (Peters *et al.* 1970). Mitochondria are the principal site at which glucose is finally oxidized in the tricarboxylic cycle. One of their chief functions is the production of the energy-rich phosphate compounds (ATP) for the rest of the cell (Davison 1974, personal communication).

The Golgi apparatus

Smooth or agranular endoplasmic reticulum, without ribosomes and therefore not staining with thionin, is present in the cytoplasm. It is especially prominent in the Golgi apparatus, which is present in the form of a twisted network close to the nucleus. Seen under the electron microscope, it is composed of five to seven layers of broad flattened cisternae and a number of small vesicles. The exact function of the Golgi apparatus in the neuron is not known, but it is probably concerned with the formation of primary lysosomes and the biosynthesis of glycoprotein. The vesicles may be coated vesicles or lysosomes or multivesicular bodies.

Lysosomes

Lysosomes are spherical bodies bounded by a single membrane which is separated by an electron-lucid rim from the electron dense matrix. They contain hydrolytic enzymes such as acid phosphatase. In their original state they are called primary lysosomes. They interact with unwanted material in the cytoplasm which they degrade and are then called secondary lysosomes. Such is a multivesicular body, where small, presumably fluid-filled vacuoles are present within the lysosome. Lipid material in lysosomes often assumes a myelin-like pattern. At the end stage, when the content of hydrolytic enzyme is small, they may be called residual bodies (see also p. 505).

Lipochrome or lipofuscin

In many nerve cells, but more noticeably in large nerve cells, with the exception of Purkinje cells, part of the nerve cell body is occupied by a mass of yellow or orange lipid granules. They are not present under the age of seven and increase with age. They are acid fast, PAS positive and stain strongly with Sudan black. When viewed under the electron microscope the granules are seen to be lobulated, membrane bound and electron dense. They contain particulate and lamellar material and are usually vesiculated. They are thought to develop from lysosomes.

Accumulation of lipochrome or lipofuscin is common in ageing neurons and may also occur in wasting diseases. Neurons of different types and different systems have different tendencies to accumulate pigment. For example, the larger pyramidal cells of the cerebral cortex and the motor nerve cells of the ventral horns of the spinal cord very commonly contain a collection of lipochrome granules near the axon hillock, and the olivary and dentate nucleus and the external geniculate body in the adult always contain large accumulations of these granules, which may occupy about half the cell body. Pathological accumulations of lipochrome are therefore not always easily distinguished from the normal, especially in the cerebral cortex. In certain forms of dementia many of the cortical nerve cells appear to consist of little except lipochrome granules, but this may be due rather to shrinkage and atrophy of the other cell constituents leaving the relatively resistant lipochrome in possession.

Neurofibrils

By silver impregnation it is possible to demonstrate fibrils passing smoothly through the cytoplasm of the neuron and along the dendrites and axon. In light microscopy these are called neurofibrils. On electron-microscopy neurofilaments and microtubules are found in neurons and presumably form the basis of the neurofibrils. Microtubules, which are found in the cells of many tissues, are long tubular structures, 20 to 26 nm in diameter, which on transverse section show an electron dense wall, about 6 nm thick, surrounding a lighter core, in which is a centrally placed dense dot. Neurofilaments are thinner, 10 nm in diameter, and on transverse section show an electron dense wall, 3 nm thick, surrounding a lighter core. They occur in bundles (Peters et al. 1970). The neurofibrils in the cell body appear to be rather more resistant to many forms of injury than the Nissl granules and are often preserved when the latter have disappeared. See also Bray (1974).

Surface membrane

The cell body and processes of nerve cells are enclosed by a clearly defined membrane which can be seen electron-microscopically to have three layers, two external electron dense layers separated by a less dense layer. The plasma membrane is modified at synaptic junctions (Peters et al. 1970).

Processes of nerve cells—the axon

From that region of the cell body, which in large neurons contains the least Nissl substance, a solitary process called the axon is given off. The axon, when seen by electron-microscopy, contains microtubules, many neurofilaments, mitochondria, agranular endoplasmic reticulum, vesicles and multivesicular bodies. On leaving the cell body the axon is at first unmyelinated for a short distance.

The contents of the axon are under pressure and the experiments of Weiss (1943) and Weiss and Hiscoe (1948) first suggested that material was transported along the axon to the nerve ending. This was confirmed autoradiographically by Droz and Leblond (1963) and has since received increasing interest (Weiss 1967; Barondes 1969; Weiss and Mayr 1971). Some material is transported at a fast (100 to 500 mm/day) and some at a slow rate (0·4 to 3·0 mm/day). Most of it moves towards the nerve endings but some moves towards the cell body (Lasek 1970; Bradley, Murchison and Day 1971).

Dendrites

All nerve cells within the central nervous system have one or more dendritic processes. The number of dendrites varies greatly. Anterior horn cells in the spinal cord have from 3 to 20 (Chu 1954) and cortical pyramids also have many. Their length may be 20 times the width of the cell body, and they branch freely. The dendrites of Purkinje cells arise as one or two thick processes at the pole of the cell opposite to the axon, and these branch fanwise in a plane at right angles to the long axis of the folium. Cortical neurons have very few or no dendrites at birth, and the increase in the number and length of these is part of the process of maturation which takes place during the first few months of extra-uterine life (Conel 1939-59).

Dendrites contain microtubules throughout their length and Nissl granules at least in their more proximal parts, although the endoplasmic reticulum extends further towards the periphery. Cajal described numerous fine club-shaped spicules, known also as thorns, globules and gemmules, which stand out from the dendrite throughout its length, except near its base. They are stained both by Ehrlich's methylene blue and Golgi's silver chromate techniques. They are best seen in cortical pyramidal cells and in Purkinje cells. Cajal considered the late appearance of these projections to indicate the maturity of the neurone, and that they may help to collect nervous impulses (i.e. to act as postsynaptic structures). Conel also observed their increase in calibre and number during early postnatal development. Gray (1961) described and illustrated the electron-microscopic appearance of dendritic spines: these can be seen arising from dendrites, and to all appearances are postsynaptic structures. They consist of two sacks which may be intercommunicating, with a band of considerable electronic density between them. Microtubules do not continue into the spine.

Nerve endings

In the central nervous system it is common to find that the larger axons, for example those arising from the pyramidal cells of the cerebral cortex and the Purkinje cells of the cerebellar cortex, give off one or more collateral fibres soon after leaving their cell of origin. Similarly the large axons which enter the spinal cord by the dorsal roots branch as soon as they enter the cord. Thereafter the fibres may run for long distances, either in the fibre tracts of the central nervous system or in peripheral nerves, without giving off any branches. Near their termination they divide into a greater or smaller number of branches and as these approach their termination they lose their myelin sheath and may break up into a number of fine terminal twigs, which enter the peripheral end-organ or make synaptic connection with the cell bodies or dendrites of other neurons.

In the central nervous system many axons make contact of this kind by means of ring-like endings which are usually called *boutons terminaux*. These can be stained by the more specific silver impregnations for axons. On the large nerve cells of the ventral horns of the spinal cord many such endings are seen both on the cell body and the dendrites. The pyramidal cells of the cerebral cortex have fewer, and the neurons of the corpus geniculatum externum may have only one small ring applied to the cell body (Glees and le Gros Clark 1941). With other nerve cells, for example those of the nucleus caudatus (Glees 1944), synaptic contact may be made by fine axonal ramifications without boutons. The ring endings degenerate when the axon which terminates in them is cut (Hoff and Hoff 1934; Foerster and

Gagel 1934; Fedorow 1935). They are therefore dependent for their nutrition on the nerve cell from which the axon arises.

De Robertis (1956, 1958), Wickoff and Young (1956), Palay (1956, 1958), Gray (1961), among others, have shown electron microscopically that presynaptic and postsynaptic areas are well defined in especially dense clusters near the densest, and probably most active parts, of the synaptic membranes. They are spherical or oval in shape with a limiting membrane 4 to 5 nm thick and a size varying between 20 to 65 nm. It has been suggested that they represent the quantal unit of transmitter substance. They have, in fact, been

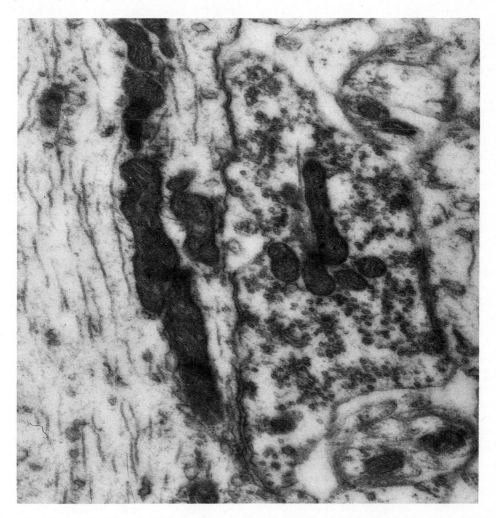

Fig. 1.3 Abducens nucleus of the rat. A terminal bouton (centre) containing mitochondria and numerous microvesicles separated by a double membrane from dendrite (left) which shows mitochondria and microtubules. × 40,000. (Reproduced from *J. Biophys. Biochem. Cytol.* 1956, **2** (suppl.), 193, fig. 2, by kindness of Professor S. L. Palay.)

by membranes and are also separated by an intersynaptic space (Fig. 1.3). Presynaptic terminals (for example boutons terminaux) contain microvesicles together with numerous mitochondria; microvesicles are absent, however, in the postsynaptic area. Microvesicles were first described by De Robertis and Bennett (1954). They occur observed to increase both in number and in size after electrical stimulation and to disappear when the terminal degenerates (de Robertis 1958).

Myelin sheath

According to Duncan (1934), all axons with a diameter greater than 1 μm in the central and peripheral nervous systems of vertebrates are surrounded by a myelin sheath. The thickness of this sheath varies and does not always bear the same relation to the thickness of the axon. De Renyi (1929) found that in the average peripheral nerve fibre the axon was 7 times the thickness of the myelin sheath. Arnell (1936) in unfixed peripheral nerves found the relative areas of myelin sheath to axon to average 1 : 3·5 with variations from 1 : 1 to 1 : 6. In other words, the relation of the diameter of the axon to the thickness of the myelin sheath varies from 5 : 1 to 25 : 1. This ratio is fairly well preserved when nervous tissue is fixed directly in osmic acid, but with slower fixatives the myelin sheath swells at the expense of the axon. In formalin fixed tissue, therefore, the myelin sheath looks thicker than it should.

The lipid of the myelin sheath is a complex substance containing cerebrosides, phospholipids and cholesterol. According to observations in polarized light (Schmidt 1936) and small angle X-ray diffraction (Schmitt, Bear and Clark 1935), the lipid molecules are orientated radially in double concentric layers separated by a layer of denatured protein between each pair. This protein has long been identified with neurokeratin, but Le Baron and Folch-Pi (1956) and Folch-Pi, Casals, Pope, Meath, Le Baron and Lees (1959) have suggested that it is a trypsin resistant protein fraction. The total thickness of these three layers has been calculated to be about 17 to 18·6 nm which would allow over 100 such repeating periods in a myelin sheath of 2 μm thickness. X-ray diffraction studies have added more detail to the concept of this fundamental repeating unit, and both Finean (1961) and Robertson (1961) have correlated these findings with those observed on the electronic screen.

Myelin is anisotropic. In cross-sections of nerve fibres, under crossed Nicol prisms, the sheath is interrupted along the line of polarization and at right angles to this. The appearance of a thick myelin sheath or a globule of myelin under these optical conditions therefore resembles a bright Maltese cross. Thinner sheaths form a bright circle broken into four quadrants. In longitudinal sections the sheath is anisotropic in the plan of polarization.

Sperry and Waelsch (1950) have produced evidence that myelin, and even the unsaponifiable lipids which it contains, are synthesized in the brain and not carried there in a preformed state by the blood stream. In the newborn infant myelin is almost entirely absent in the cerebrum, but increases gradually during the first months and more rapidly between the third and thirteenth month of extra-uterine life. Thereafter there is a constant increase of myelin in relation to the lipids contained in the nerve cells and axons, until the brain reaches its full adult size at the age of 10 to 12 years when the proportion becomes the same as in the adult brain (Brante 1949). This increase in amount of the white matter in relation to the grey is the characteristic pattern of growth of the brain during childhood.

The myelin sheath begins shortly after the axon leaves the cell body and is continued up to the terminal branches, which may carry a fine myelin sheath for part of their extent but are thereafter unmyelinated. Both in the peripheral and central nervous systems it is broken at intervals by constrictions or nodes. In peripheral nerves these have long been known as the nodes of Ranvier, which occur at regular intervals along the nerve fibre. Cajal (1909) described similar nodes on the nerve fibres of the central nervous system and these have been confirmed by Bielschowsky (1928) and more recently by numerous authors. Collateral branches are given off only at these nodes, and in the cortex of the mouse, the axons and the branches may be naked for a considerable distance at these points (Chang 1952). The electron microscope shows that the myelin sheath of the central nervous system is essentially similar to that of the peripheral nervous system, except that the cytoplasm on the external surface of the myelin lamellae is a longitudinally orientated narrow ridge, rather than a complete layer as in the peripheral nervous system.

In the peripheral nervous system the plasma membrane of a Schwann cell is spirally arranged around a segment of an axon to form the myelin lamellae: in the central nervous system the plasma membrane of an oligodendroglial cell is spirally arranged around a segment of one or more axons (Peters *et al.* 1970).

Pathology of the neuron

Basic reactions of the neuron to injury

Injury to the axon

Injury to the axon produces rather different reactions in the cell body in different types of nerve cell. In general the larger motor and sensory neurons react to section of the axon by attempted regrowth. This is associated with changes in the cell body which are described under the name of *central chromatolysis* or *axonal reaction* (Fig. 1.4a). This reaction, which is seen in typical form in the cells of the motor nuclei of the cranial nerves, was used by the pioneers of neuroanatomy to map out the nuclei which give rise to different nerves or to different parts of such nerves as the oculomotor and vagoglossopharyngeal. Nerve cells which give rise to tracts which begin and end within the central nervous system often go on from this stage of reaction to atrophy and eventual disappearance (*Gudden's atrophy*). This biphasic reaction is well seen in the dorsomedial nucleus of the thalamus after frontal lobectomy or leucotomy (Meyer, Beck and McLardy 1947), in the corpus geniculatum externum after lesions of the optic radiations or calcarine cortex (Putnam and Putnam 1926), and in the inferior olives after lesions of the cerebellar cortex (Stewart and Holmes 1908; Brodal 1940). As in each of these instances the nerve cells which react are those from which the damaged fibres originate, an area-to-area relationship can be mapped out between the cerebral or cerebellar cortex and the nuclei which project to them. *Gudden's atrophy* is associated with shrinkage of the cell body, loss of Nissl granules, and dedifferentiation in the nucleus. Some nerve cells, such as those of the retina, show no stage of reaction to injury of their axons, but undergo atrophy from the first.

Central chromatolysis

This reaction of the nerve cell to a lesion of its axon is best seen in neurons whose axons are partially contained within the peripheral nervous system—cells which regenerate their peripherally directed axons after injury, such as the large motor cells of the ventral horns of the spinal cord and the motor nuclei of the brainstem. It is most severe when the axon is severed near to its cell of origin. It begins within 48 hours after division of the nerve and reaches its maximum after 15 to 20 days. During this period the cell body becomes more rounded and swells and the Nissl granules close to the nucleus become smaller and powdery and eventually are not visible. The nucleus also swells and moves away from the axon hillock, often coming to lie against the margin of the cell. In the later stages it may become oval or reniform. The typical appearances in the later stages are shown in Fig. 1.4b. At this stage the rounded and somewhat enlarged cell with its enlarged and eccentric nucleus has only a peripheral zone of rather small Nissl granules. From this stage the cell may either degenerate and disappear, or may gradually recover. If the latter, the Nissl substance is gradually re-formed, probably by the nucleus, and may eventually be present in larger amounts than normal (stage of hyperchromasia). The cell body shrinks, its outline between the dendrites again becomes concave, and the nucleus returns to its original situation. This is a slow process which may take as much as 80 days. Thus after section of a motor nerve close to the brain stem or spinal cord the process of reaction in the cell body covers a period of 100 days or more. The early change, as seen by the electron microscope, consists of reversible swelling of mitochondria and the cisternae of the rough endoplasmic reticulum. Nissl aggregates then disperse to the periphery of the cell and the cisternae fragment, though the number of ribosomes remains apparently unchanged. Some mitochondria become large, show a compact array of cristae and numerous granules. The nucleolus enlarges. Later, with recovery, the smooth endoplasmic reticulum increases and numerous dense bodies appear (Mackey, Spiro and Wiener 1964).

Examination by light-microscopy alone suggested that the appearances of the early stages of central chromatolysis represented a loss of RNA from the cell body. Chemical and autoradiographic studies have however shown that the RNA and protein content and anabolism are increased and not decreased at this stage. This apparent contradiction may be explained as follows. The cell increases in volume and the ribosomes, though increased in number, are no longer aggregated in localized and therefore darkly staining Nissl bodies, but are separated and dispersed throughout a greater volume and are therefore no longer visible under the light microscope (Lieberman 1971).

The cells of the dorsal root ganglia react in a similar manner to lesions of the peripheral nerves, but show much slighter changes after section of the proximal process. Section of the dorsal roots may cause some reaction in a few cells, but lesions of the cord involving the dorsal columns produce no change in these cells. No alteration of shape can be seen in these spherical cells, but the disappearance of Nissl granules from the central zone of the cell, the more powdery appearance in the peripheral granules and the eccentricity of

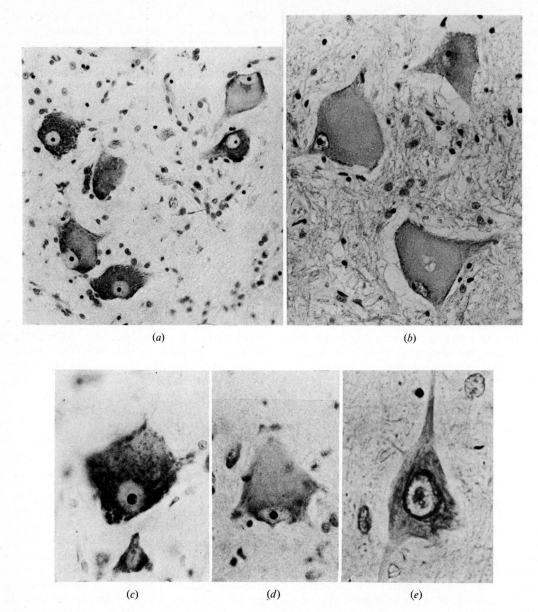

(a)   (b)

(c)   (d)   (e)

Fig. 1.4 Central and peripheral chromatolysis. (a) Axonal reaction in ventral horn cells of lumbar cord in a macaque 7 days after lesion of cauda equina. (b) Severe central chromatolysis in ventral horn cells of lumbar cord from venous stagnation due to angioma. (c) Slight, and (d) severe central chromatolysis in cortical pyramidal cells in pellagra. (e) Peripheral chromatolysis in a case dying in severe epileptic attack. (Reproduced by the kindness of Professor L. Einarson.) a, b, c, d, Thionin; e, Gallocyanin chromalum.

the nucleus are similar to those seen in motor cells.

A similar reaction to section or injury of the axon is seen in the cells of origin of certain intrinsic tracts in the brainstem and spinal cord. It has been most studied in the Betz cells of the motor cortex and in the cells of Clarke's column. However, in these situations recovery does not usually occur, and after a time the cells degenerate further and disappear. Meyer, Beck and McLardy (1947) found that some of the cells which remained in the dorsomedial nucleus of the thalamus 4 months after prefrontal leucotomy were shrunken and deeply stained; this may represent a stage of partial recovery in these cells.

Axonal reaction, similar to that seen in the cells of the dorsal root ganglia, is also seen in the autonomic system. Section of the cervical sympathetic nerve produces swelling, chromatolysis and eccentricity of the nucleus in cervical sympathetic ganglia below it, and resection of the hypogastric plexus may cause typical chromatolysis in the cells of the intermediolateral column in the lumbosacral segments of the cord.

It is doubtful whether prolonged partial deprivation of blood produces a similar reaction in the cell body. It is so characteristic of lesions of the axon that Adolf Meyer (1901) called the reaction of the pyramidal cells of the cerebral cortex in pellagra *central neuritis* (Fig. 1.4c and d). In general it is an unusual finding in neuropathology and one which in most cases suggests an axonal lesion rather than direct damage to the nerve cell. It may, however, be found in typical form in certain virus infections of the nervous system such as poliomyelitis (Einarson 1949) and subacute inclusion body encephalitis (Brain, Greenfield and Russell 1948). In poliomyelitis it may appear as early as 3 days after the onset of paralysis. In these diseases it may go on to complete destruction of the nerve cell or, according to Bodian (1949), may be a reversible change.

Wallerian degeneration (secondary degeneration) in the central nervous system

Wallerian degeneration is the name given to the process of disintegration which affects an axon and its myelin sheath after its connection with its cell body has been interrupted. Waller (1850) described the process after cutting the hypoglossal or glossopharyngeal nerves in frogs, i.e. in the peripheral nervous system, but the same term is used for nerve fibres in the central nervous system. Nerve fibres within the central nervous system undergo Wallerian degeneration, according to Cajal, at a rate which is proportional to their thickness. In young animals, in which he studied the phenomena, the largest axons show varicosities as early as 30 hours from the time of severance from the nerve cell body. In 4 to 8 days they become broken up into shorter oval or spherical fragments. In medium-sized myelinated fibres the axon is still in the varicose or beaded state at the end of a week and breaks up from

the 14th to the 15th day onwards. In fine fibres the process is even slower, and many show little change during the first 10 days. Changes in the myelin sheath occur along with these changes in the axon. As the latter becomes varicose, irregular fusiform swellings also appear along the course of the myelin sheath, which soon breaks at the constrictions and forms a series of ellipsoids enclosing fragments of axon. These are again broken or shrink into even smaller structures. Breakdown of the myelin into simpler lipids occurs at the same time, and, according to Jakob, lipids which stain by Marchi's method begin to appear about the 4th day. Lorrain-Smith and Mair (1909), using a modified myelin stain, also found the earliest evidence of myelin katabolism on the 4th day. Daniel and Strich (1969) found Marchi positive material at 48 hours in the baboon. In man the process is a slow one, much slower than in peripheral nerves. It is unusual to find much evidence of Marchi degeneration before the 20th day, and ovoids and spherules of unchanged myelin may be present 6 weeks after a necrotic lesion affecting the proximal part of the nerve fibre. At this stage considerable free cholesterol is present as well as phosphatides, cerebrosides, fatty acids and neutral fat (Hurst 1925). By 3 months most or all of the myelin has broken down into simpler lipids and neutral fat, and some is in process of removal by phagocytic cells. After 6 months most of the lipid has become neutral fat. Disappearance of myelin from a tract, as seen by the Weigert method, is not very evident in less than 2 months from the time of the lesion. Smith (1956) has shown that, for ten weeks after a lesion, the Marchi positive material, resulting from degeneration of nerve fibres, is extracellular. It then becomes progressively intracellular, in phagocytes, until by twelve months it is all intracellular. Fifteen months after the original lesion, Marchi positive material can still be present in large amount in a degenerate tract. The demonstration of Marchi positive material is affected by the period of fixation of the tissue in formalin. Extracellular Marchi positive material will not stain if fixation has been prolonged. Intracellular material in its early stages is similar, but later formed intracellular material will stain positively even after prolonged fixation (Smith, Strich and Sharp 1956).

The process of myelin katabolism is more easily followed by the use of Sudan IV on frozen sections, combined with a polarizing microscope.

The normal chrome or terracotta staining of myelin, associated with a Maltese-cross anisotropism, may still be seen in ovoids and balls of myelin for several weeks after Wallerian degeneration has begun in the tract or fibre system; cholesterol esters do not take up the dye and when viewed under crossed Nicol prisms appear as colourless anisotropic crystals; the other lipids assume an increasingly red colour as their composition approaches that of neutral fat, and at the same time they lose their anisotropic character.

Because the process of Wallerian degeneration in the central nervous system is relatively slow, it is possible to trace degenerating axons and their synaptic endings for several weeks after the injury (Kuypers 1958). Modifications of Bielschowsky's technique by Glees, Nauta, Gygax, Fink and Heimer, elaborated by anatomists for experimental animals, are applicable to man, and are reviewed by Bowsker, Brodal and Walberg (1960) and by Heimer (1967).

The cellular reaction to Wallerian degeneration in the central nervous system

The first reacting cells in Wallerian degeneration were called myeloclasts by Jakob, who considered them to be derived from microglia. Cramer and Alpers (1932) derive them from oligodendroglia, Daniel and Strich (1969) prefer to call them neuroglia and point out that they may be considered as axonophages rather than myeloclasts. These are small cells with rather ragged cell bodies and small irregularly rounded nuclei. They appear after the 4th day, both between fibres and also, very characteristically, in the spaces within distended myelin sheaths (Fig. 1.26g). They increase in numbers during the next two weeks and their cytoplasm becomes more granular, containing fine fatty droplets. They appear to be transitory and their nuclei are often pyknotic or have undergone karyorrhexis. As the myelin slowly breaks down into simpler lipids, phagocytes appear, derived presumably from microglia. They engulf the lipid granules and eventually migrate with them to the walls of the blood vessels where they are seen from 3 months onwards filling the adventitial or Virchow–Robin spaces. The electron-microscopic features of these phagocytes, in the cat, are discussed by Bignami and Ralston (1969). They observed that, at first, the phagocytes take up degenerating myelin and that later this is broken down to form lipid droplets.

The astrocytes also react to the breakdown of

the nerve fibre and myelin sheath by enlargement of both cell body and nucleus. This appears at a rather later stage than the first of the reactions already described and proceeds at a slow tempo. Although fine lipid droplets may be seen along their margins it is unlikely that they take any active part in the katabolism of myelin. Glial fibres are laid down parallel to the degenerated nerve fibres.

Trans-synaptic degeneration

In certain nuclei, an atrophy of nerve cells similar to that seen in Gudden's atrophy may follow damage to the axons which make synaptic connection with them. Foix, Chavany and Hillemand (1926) called this *trans-synaptic atrophy or degeneration*. It is best known in the nerve cells of the corpus geniculatum externum after lesions of the retina, optic nerves or optic tracts (Fig. 1.5) and in the inferior olives after lesions of the central tegmental tract. In the former case the cells undergo simple atrophy similar to the later stages of their reaction to lesions of the optic radiations. The neurons of the inferior olive, on the other hand, undergo an initial irregular hypertrophy, often associated with vacuolation of their cytoplasm, during the first few months after the lesion (Fig. 1.6). Later the nerve cells atrophy and disappear (Gautier and Blackwood 1961). This trans-synaptic degeneration seems to occur most commonly after lesions of tracts which form the chief, or the only, afferent link to the neurons in question. It probably also occurs, although much more slowly, in nerve cells which make synaptic or other functional connections with neurons which have degenerated or been destroyed. For example, degeneration has been observed in the optic nerves and tracts after long-standing lesions of the optic radiations or calcarine cortex (von Meyendorf 1934). A 'retrograde' trans-synaptic degeneration of this character is the most reasonable explanation for the degeneration of the inferior olives which follows destruction of the Purkinje cells by heat stroke and has also been accepted by many authors as the explanation of the olivary degeneration which accompanies cerebellar cortical degeneration of the familial type described by Holmes (1907) as well as in similar cases of isolated character (Marie, Foix and Alajouanine 1922).

Peripheral chromatolysis

Peripheral chromatolysis is, in some respects, the antithesis of central chromatolysis. It is most often seen in human pathology as a change affecting the motor nerve cells in the anterior horns of the spinal cord in cases of progressive muscular atrophy. In such cases it appears to be a stage in the degenerative process, or, perhaps more accurately, in the fight for survival. Nerve cells showing peripheral chromatolysis are usually

of peripheral chromatolysis are found in normal dorsal root ganglia and especially in sympathetic ganglia, in which their numbers increase on mild stimulation, but diminish with progressively longer stimulation giving place to cells showing central chromatolysis. In the dorsal root ganglion cells, peripheral chromatolysis is not uncommonly seen

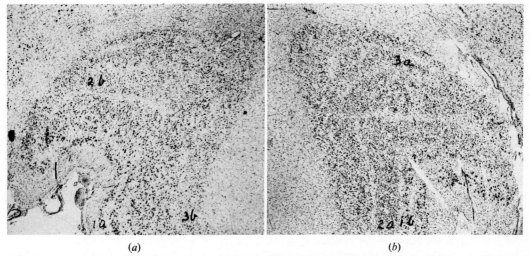

(a)   (b)

Fig. 1.5 Trans-synaptic atrophy of external geniculate body resulting from the loss of the right eye. (a) Left side. Atrophy of layers 1a, 2b and 3b. (b) Right side. Atrophy of layers 1b, 2a and 3a.

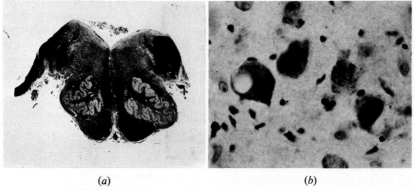

(a)   (b)

Fig. 1.6 Swelling of the inferior olive and vacuolar degeneration of its neurons resulting from a lesion of the olivocerebellar fibres in the cerebellum. The appearances are similar to those seen after a lesion of the central tegmental tract.

smaller and more rounded than normal. The dendrites and the peripheral zone of the cell contain no Nissl granules, but a darkly staining mass of these is collected round the nucleus, which is usually in or near the centre of the cell and contains rather more chromatin than normal. Einarson (1945) and Einarson and Lorentzen (1946) have shown that cells showing some degree

as a late stage of reaction to lesions or section of the peripheral nerves. According to Einarson, peripheral chromatolysis, when seen as an early reaction to noxious agents, is a stage towards cell death, but when it occurs as a late reaction it appears to be a stage in the process of recovery, and indicates an active restoration of Nissl substance from the nucleus (Fig. 1.4e).

Simple atrophy

Simple atrophy seems to be the best term to describe the effects of those metabolic disturbances of the neuron which lead to its gradual degeneration and death. Simple atrophy appears to be the basis of many systemic degenerations, both when hereditary, as in Friedreich's ataxia, or isolated, as in amyotrophic lateral sclerosis and some cases of olivopontocerebellar degeneration. Many forms of peripheral neuropathy, especially those due to vitamin deficiency (Aring, Bean, Roseman, Rosenbaum and Spies 1941), show a similar pathogenesis. These have been studied experimentally by many workers, among whom Bertrand, Liber and Randoin (1934), Swank (1940) and Swank and Prados (1942) have given full histological descriptions. Triorthocresyl phosphate, which in man and domestic fowls causes degeneration both of the long tracts of the spinal cord and the peripheral nerves, seems to affect nerve fibres in a similar manner (Cavanagh 1954).

Simple atrophy has certain definite characteristics: fibres of larger diameter are affected before those of medium and smaller size; the nerve fibre is affected more at its periphery than near the nerve cell body, and the cell body often shrinks and becomes sclerotic without showing the chromatolysis of axonal reaction. Cavanagh (1964) has called this the 'dying-back' process.

In hereditary and other systemic atrophies it has long been known that the distal part of the nerve fibre suffers before the proximal part, especially in olivoponto-cerebellar degeneration. It is easily demonstrable in the more acute cerebellar degenerations in which the long tracts of the spinal cord also undergo degeneration. In such cases the pyramidal tracts at the level of the medulla may show no evidence of myelin katabolism, but on passing down the spinal cord they contain progressively more sudanophilic and Marchi-staining lipids (Greenfield 1934). When the atrophic process is slow and the patient dies many years after the onset of symptoms, there may be little or no evidence of the katabolic processes which the nerve fibres have undergone. The tempo of degeneration is so slow that the products of the breakdown of myelin and axon are removed almost as quickly as they are formed and sudanophilic lipids are very scanty. In such cases one does not see the beaded or fusiform swellings of the myelin sheath which are a very characteristic appearance in the early stages of Wallerian degeneration in the central nervous system. However, when Purkinje cells undergo simple atrophy their axons often end, in the granular layer, in a globular or fusiform swelling to which the name *torpedo* is usually given. This end-swelling is often seen to lie just distal to a recurrent collateral branch, and it appears to have the characters of a retraction bulb. In the more chronic and slighter forms of simple atrophy in peripheral nerves, such as those seen in pellagra, the evidence that the nerve fibres are damaged is given more by the disappearance of the larger axons and myelin sheaths than by obvious katabolic changes in them (Aring *et al*. 1941). However, in other more acute cases of peripheral neuropathy, katabolic changes may be seen, especially in the more distal parts of the nerves, similar to those described in Wallerian degeneration. When the process is severe and continues for some weeks it may result in death of the whole neuron. In peripheral neuropathy this is associated especially with loss of nerve cells in the dorsal root ganglia and secondary degeneration of the dorsal columns of the cord. Less often there is destruction of the motor neurons of the ventral horns.

Nissl's types of degeneration of the cell body

While central and peripheral chromatolysis and simple atrophy are characteristic reactions of the perikaryon to physiological stresses such as overwork, loss of function, or interference with metabolism owing to absence of vitamins, a number of other forms of degeneration were recognized in classical neuropathology and were considered to be the result of abnormal environmental conditions such as anoxia, high temperature and endogenous or exogenous toxins or chemical poisons.

Perfusion fixation and delayed removal of the brain from hypoxic animals (see p. 45) have shown that some of the changes described by Nissl and Spielmeyer in human brains, which had necessarily been removed and fixed by ordinary methods, must be considered as artefacts.

It is convenient to group Nissl's cell changes as follows:

Degeneration with swelling of the cell body
  (a) Nissl's acute cell disease (Spielmeyer's acute swelling)
  (b) Nissl's severe cell disease (Spielmeyer's liquefaction).

Because these terms are now seldom used by neuropathologists they will not be considered further. For details the reader should refer to the previous editions of this book or to Spielmeyer (1922).

Degeneration with shrinkage of the cell body
    (c) Ischaemic change (incrustation of the Golgi network. See pp. 46-51.
    (d) Homogenizing cell change. See p. 51.
    (e) Nissl's chronic cell degeneration.

Types of neuronal degeneration related to certain forms of organic disease of the nervous system. Certain types of degeneration in nerve cells are recognized as occurring so constantly and characteristically in special forms of organic nervous disease as to be useful for diagnostic purposes. They will be dealt with later in this book.
    Alzheimer's fibrillary degeneration. See p. 804.
    Neuroaxonal dystrophy. See p. 180.
    Granulovacuolar degeneration. See p. 808.
    Swelling and argyrophilic inclusions in Pick's disease. See p. 819.
    Lewy bodies. See p. 612.
    Lafora bodies. See p. 788.
    Neurolipidosis. See Chapter 12.

Other changes related to neurons

Haematin pigment in nerve cells
In haemorrhagic areas in the cortex, and less commonly elsewhere in the central nervous system, neurons containing small granules, or rods or black or dark-brown quadrangular crystals, are often seen. In some cases the neurons are the only cells in a haemorrhagic area to show these inclusions. In other cases they are seen also in microglial and endothelial cells and in polymorphonuclear leucocytes. These crystals resemble melanin in bleaching with hydrogen peroxide, but they may be distinguished from melanin both in being easily dissolved in alkalis, and in being brightly anisotropic (Fig. 1.7). They are identical in composition with formol haemoglobin pigment, and with the pigment granules of malarial parasites. It is not known in what form this pigment exists during life, as up to the present they have only been seen when formalin has been used in the fixing fluid. They may result from an alteration by formalin of haemoglobin which has been absorbed from the neighbouring haemorrhage by the nerve cells in the vicinity. Rand and

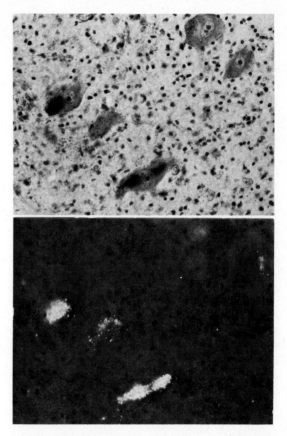

Fig. 1.7 Haematin pigment in nerve cells. An area of the cerebral cortex near small haemorrhages. The dark haematin granules in (a) appear bright under crossed Nicol prisms in (b).

Courville (1946) found this pigment in neurons in contused areas of cortex in patients who died within a few hours to $3\frac{1}{2}$ days after head injury and considered that the nerve cells take up haemoglobin during life and that this is then agglutinated into smaller collections in the cytoplasm of the neuron. In a case dying 14 days after a head injury they found golden-yellow inclusion particles in the nerve cells in the neighbourhood of a cortical contusion and considered that the processes of disintegration of haemoglobin might be continued within the cytoplasm of the nerve cells. Greenfield had noticed the early appearance of this pigment in nerve cells in cases of cortical contusion, but he had not seen crystals or granules corresponding to later breakdown products of haemoglobin.

Rand and Courville's observation, however, suggests that the intravital absorption of haemoglobin from neighbouring haemorrhage may be the forerunner of the iron-incrustation or ferrugination of nerve cells which is commonly seen in old areas of infarction. They consider that not all nerve cells which contained pigment granules of this nature were degenerated, although some showed obvious changes and some were ghost cells. In Greenfield's experience some degree of ischaemic change is the rule in neurons containing haematin granules.

Ferrugination or iron incrustation of nerve cells

Haematoxophilic granules replacing dead nerve cells are commonly seen in areas of old infarction. These granules may only depict the triangular shape of the cell body, or they may extend as thin strands for considerable distances in the lines of the dendrites. Usually there is no visible protoplasm in relation to these granules, and they can only be considered as nerve cells in the sense that the position previously occupied by the neuron is now occupied more or less completely by haematoxophilic granules (Fig. 1.8). With Prussian blue staining they are seen to consist largely of iron. It is uncertain whether they also contain calcium. Why nerve cells dying from ischaemia are sometimes, but by no means always,

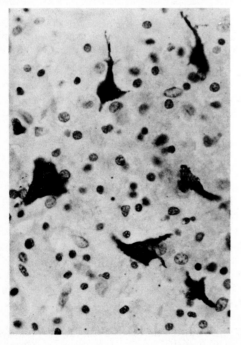

Fig. 1.8 Incrustation (ferrugination) or nerve cells in an old ischaemic area of cortex. Haematoxylin van Gieson.

replaced by these granules is quite unknown. The iron in them is too abundant to be accounted for by that present in their Nissl granules, and the suggestion that this appearance may result when neurons have absorbed haemoglobin from a neighbouring haemorrhage has at least this measure of support.

Selective necrosis of the granular layer of the cerebellar cortex

From time to time, in routine examination of the cerebellum, in cases without clinical evidence of cerebellar dysfunction, there is, in stained sections, an extensive and striking pallor of the whole width of the granular layer, contrasting with a well-stained Purkinje cell layer (Fig. 1.9*a*). The nuclei of the granule cells stain faintly and have blurred outlines, while some are deformed and some disintegrated (Fig. 1.9*b*). The cytoplasm appears to merge with that of adjacent cells. There is no glial or cellular response and the remainder of the cerebellar structures are unaffected (Olsen 1959). The cause of this change is unknown, but most authors consider that it is agonal. Ikuta, Hirano and Zimmermann (1963), however, incubated post-mortem slices of cerebellum in cerebrospinal fluid and found, that while there was no significant change at 60° and 4°, there was selective necrosis of granule cells within 48 hours at 37° and 45°.

Separation of Purkinje cell layer from the granular layer of the cerebellum

An occasional appearance in the cerebellum, after immersion fixation, is separation of the Purkinje cell layer from the granular cell layer (Fig. 1.10). This should be considered as artefact (Cammermeyer 1972).

Mucocytes (Grynfeltt or Buscaino bodies)

It is not uncommon to find basophilic, metachromatic, structureless looking, rounded, oval or lobulated masses, averaging 100 μm diameter, usually in the white matter, of both normal and abnormal brains, both in man and animals (Fig. 1.11). In formalin fixed tissue, they are more likely to appear if, at some later stage in preparation, immersion in alcohol is prolonged (Ferraro 1928). Sometimes further processing of the tissue dissolves out the metachromatic material, leaving vacuoles in the white matter (Fig. 1.11).

Ferraro considered that the bodies were derived from myelin, with alcohol acting as a 'special

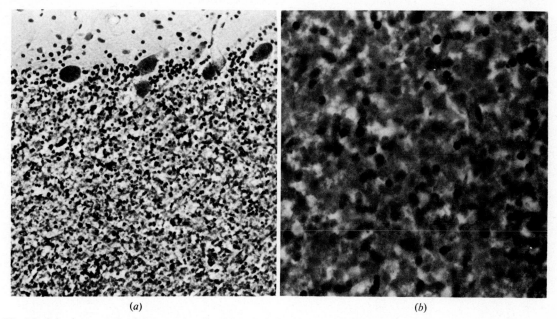

(a)   (b)

Fig. 1.9 Selective necrosis of the granule cells of the cerebellar cortex. (a) Celloidin; haematoxylin van Gieson. × 210.
(b) × 600.

sensitizer of otherwise undemonstrable lesions'. Smith (1949) considered that they were derived from myelin, or the ground substance of brain and that there was 'no evidence to show that they are entirely artefacts, but a pathological agent or pathophysiological process leading to their appearance has not been found.' Cammermeyer (1972) was of the opinion that there was strong circumstantial evidence of post-mortem trauma as a causal factor.

Ibrahim and Levine (1967) found histochemically that in the rat they contained cerebroside and sulphatide and possibly also an acidic mucopolysaccharide. They considered that the bodies were caused by the solution and subsequent precipitation of some myelin component by the fixative. Aparicio and Lumsden (1970) concluded that, in the guinea-pig, they contained some acidic lipids (certainly sulphatide and possibly ganglioside), also neutral cerebrosides as well as possibly protein and found electron microscopically that they were extracellular and in immediate contiguity with the myelin sheaths. Adornato, O'Brien, Lampert, Roe and Neustein (1972) showed electron microscopically that they were composed of irregularly curved, lamellar structures which were derived from myelin.

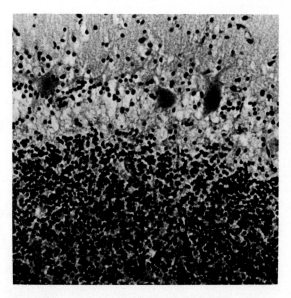

Fig. 1.10 Separation of the Purkinje layer from the granular layer of the cerebellum. Celloidin; haematoxylin van Gieson. × 210.

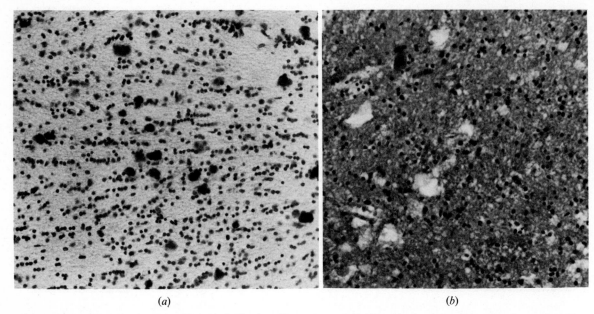

(a)   (b)

Fig. 1.11 Mucocytes. (a) Metachromatic bodies in white matter. Celloidin; thionin mounted in Mersol.   × 210.   (b) White matter, same case as (a).   The mucocytic material has been dissolved.   Celloidin; haematoxylin van Gieson mounted xylene balsam.   × 210.

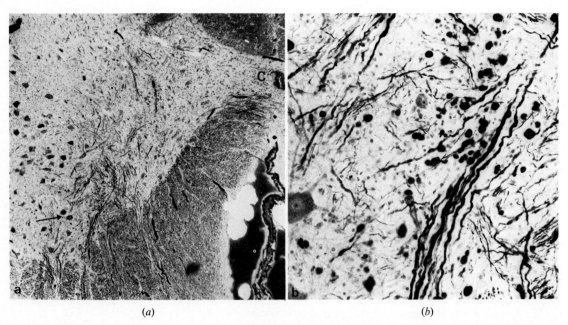

(a)   (b)

Fig. 1.12 Argyrophile bodies. (a) Anterior horn spinal cord.   Arrow points to nerve cell and to the bodies beyond. C, central canal.   Celloidin; Gross Nissl.   × 48.   (b) Higher power of (a), to right of arrow.   × 240.

Argyrophile bodies in the human spinal cord

In the anterior horns of the lumbosacral segments of the adult spinal cord, numerous rounded 5 to 30 μm diameter argyrophile bodies are to be found (Fig. 1.12). Most of them lie in a definite group in the anterior part of the anterior horns. They lie among axons and some appear to be attached to axons. They stain in the same way as axons. Smith (1955) found that they were constantly present in adult cords and were not restricted to any age group or pathological process. They bear a resemblance to 'retraction balls', but she did not consider that they were pathological in nature, or at least that they were not consequent upon any specific pathological process.

Neuroglia and microglia

The spongioblasts of the developing nervous system differentiate into three main types of cell, *astrocytes*, *oligodendroglia* and *ependymal* cells. It seems unlikely that mature cells of one type undergo metaplasia to another type of glial cell except in neoplasms.

In addition to these essentially neuroectodermal forms of supporting and lining tissue it will be convenient to describe here the *microglia*, which were for long confused with the true neuroglia but are now considered as histiocytic in origin and function.

Astrocytes

Astrocytes are divided into *protoplasmic* and *fibrous* forms (Fig. 1.13). The fibrous is distinguished from the protoplasmic form under the light microscope chiefly by the presence, in the cell body and processes, of fine firm-looking fibres, although with the electron microscope fibres are also seen to be present in the protoplasmic form. In both types, small rounded or oval argyrophilic dots called gliosomes lie near the surface of the cell body and processes, and the electron microscope shows these structures to be mitochondria (Mugnaini and Walberg 1964) lying deep to the cell membrane. In fixed preparations they appear to be raised above the surface of the processes (Fig. 1.13) but this is an artefact. The shrinkage artefacts which fixation can produce in glial cells, as compared to cells in tissue culture, were well shown by Pomerat (1952). Astrocytes have large rounded nuclei with only a moderate content of chromatin. Under the electron microscope (Fig. 1.14) the nuclei of protoplasmic astrocytes are round or ovoid and smoothly outlined: those of fibrous astrocytes are irregular in shape with indentations. The outlines of the cell bodies and processes have the opposite appearance, those of the fibrous astrocytes being smooth and those of the protoplasmic astrocytes being irregular, as if distorted by surrounding structures. The cytoplasm of both forms is of low electron density with a few elongated mitochondria, a small amount of rough endoplasmic reticulum and a Golgi complex. Homogeneous and heterologous dense bodies (probably lysosomes) are visible and also small dense granules (20 to 40 nm diameter) of glycogen. Fibres are present in both, being few in the protoplasmic form (Peters *et al.* 1970). The processes of astrocytes run for a considerable distance into the surrounding tissues, branching freely. In fibrous astrocytes they are longer and branching is less frequent and takes place at a more acute angle than in protoplasmic astrocytes, in which the numerous branches, coming off at a wide angle, give a mossy appearance to the tissue. These differences help to distinguish fibrous from protoplasmic astrocytes in sections stained by gold-mercury or silver impregnation (Fig. 1.15). With ordinary cell stains, such as haematoxylin and eosin, the processes of normal astrocytes cannot be distinguished from the background of nervous tissue. They may be impregnated differentially by Cajal's gold mercuric chloride or del Rio Hortega's silver carbonate techniques. One or more of the processes, usually thicker than the others, make contact with the wall of a blood vessel by means of a conical *foot-plate*. This is most easily seen in the cerebral cortex round the smaller blood vessels. The capillaries in the brain and cord are almost completely covered by astrocytic foot-plates which are attached to the basement membranes of the external surfaces of the endothelial cells. Similar, more elongated, foot-plates are seen attached to the pia mater both in the brain and cerebellum.

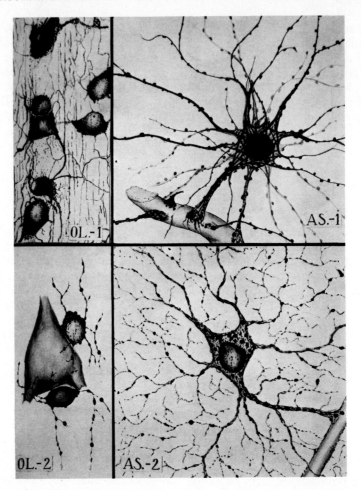

Fig. 1.13 Types of neuroglial cell. AS.-1. Fibrous astrocyte. AS.-2. Protoplasmic astrocyte. OL.-1. Inter-fascicular oligodendroglia. OL.-2. Satellite oligodendrocytes. (Reproduced by the kindness of Dr Wilder Penfield.)

Fibrous astrocytes are present throughout the central nervous system, except in certain regions of grey matter in which the protoplasmic type of astrocyte is normally found to predominate. In such regions a few fibrous astrocytes are found around the larger vessels. These regions are the 3rd, 4th and 5th layers of the cerebral cortex, the nucleus caudatus except under the ependyma, the putamen and the substantia gelatinosa Rolandi. The globus pallidus contains fibrous astrocytes in the bundles of myelinated nerve fibres which traverse it and round the large vessels. There is a thick feltwork of neuroglial fibres in the sub-ependymal tissue, especially round the iter of Sylvius, the 4th ventricle and the central canal of the spinal cord. A thinner, but fairly dense, layer of tangential fibres is also present in the subpial layer of the brain and spinal cord, and

round larger blood vessels within the brain. These neuroglial fibres tend to become thicker in the senile nervous system. Throughout the brain-stem and especially in the medulla, neuroglial fibres form a closer network than in the white matter of the brain and cerebellum. These may be associated with the movements and alterations of alignment which take place in the medulla. In the inferior olives the neuroglial feltwork is normally more dense than in any other part of the brainstem except under the floor of the 4th ventricle (Weigert 1895). For this reason apparent neuroglial sclerosis of these nuclei cannot be accepted as pathological unless associated with degeneration of its cells and fibres.

The cerebellar astrocytes deserve special mention. As in other parts of the brain those in the white matter are of the fibrous type, but in

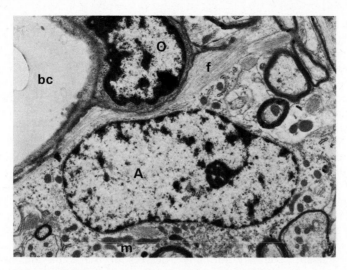

Fig. 1.14 Fibrous astrocyte, cat, spinal cord. Note the numerous fibrils (f), mitochondria (m), blood capillary (bc), nucleus of astrocyte (A), nucleus of oligodendrocyte (o). ×9000. (Reproduced by courtesy of Dr L. S. Illis, Wessex University Centre, Southampton University Hospitals.)

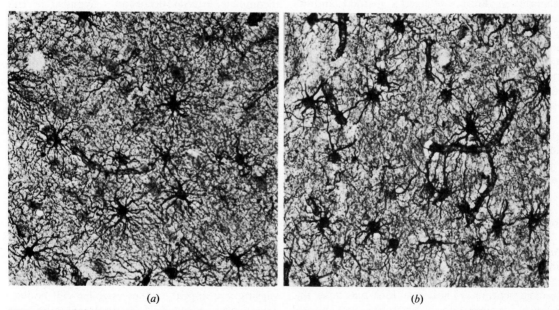

(a)   (b)

Fig. 1.15 Normal astrocytes. (a) Protoplasmic, (b) fibrous astrocytes in the cortex. Cajal's gold sublimate. ×280.

the granular layer only protoplasmic astrocytes can be found. In the molecular layer two types of astrocyte have been described, (1) *Bergmann's cells* or *Golgi's epithelial cells* and (2) *Feathered cells of Fañanas*. It is doubtful whether there is any real difference between these. Their nuclei, which resemble those of other astrocyte types, usually lie either in the same zone as the Purkinje cells, or immediately superficial to this. From the Bergmann's cells, a single process arises on the superficial side of the cell body and very soon branches, giving off a few fine parallel fibres which run straight to the pial surface. They make contact with the pia mater by fine foot-plates. A few turn at right angles under the pia and run for a short distance parallel to the surface forming a rudimentary subpial layer. The astro-cytes of the molecular layer, as well as the proto-plasmic astrocytes of the granular layer, readily form fibres under pathological conditions. In most cases of cerebellar cortical sclerosis the majority of the neuroglial fibres in the molecular layer remain orientated perpendicular to the surface, but in congenital syphilis there is often a more disorderly arrangement.

Neuroglial fibres readily undergo autolysis *post mortem* and it is often difficult to stain them when the necropsy has been delayed for more than twenty-four hours after death. Indeed for good demonstration of these fibres the brain should be well fixed as early as possible.

Under the light microscope their outline is straight and sharply defined. They are normally extremely fine and are only visible with high magnification. Their high refractility makes them visible when unstained under phase-contrast illumination. They have much the same staining reactions as fibrin. Weigert's method and its derivatives (Holzer, Victoria blue) stain the fibres but not the cytoplasm of the astrocytes. Mallory's phosphotungstic acid haematoxylin also stains them differentially but it stains myelin a similar purple colour. With Mallory's connective tissue stain and its derivatives (Masson's tri-chrome, Heidenhain's Azan) after suitable fixation, they stain red against the blue of the cytoplasm. With Mallory's methods and in good silver impregna-tions the fibres can be seen to lie in the proto-plasm of the processes and cell body, sweeping past the nucleus from one process to another.

Reactions of astrocytes to disease or injury

Astrocytes are less vulnerable than nerve cells and fibres, but are much more easily damaged than connective tissue. They react to all noxae which damage neurons. These reactions may take the form of degeneration, hypertrophy and hyper-plasia or fibre formation. Transition stages in which astrocytes remain for a considerable time without either undergoing dissolution or forming fibres are also recognized, at least in protoplasmic astrocytes. Apart from this the reactions of fibrous and protoplasmic astrocytes are to a great extent similar, since protoplasmic astrocytes in their progressive reactions tend to develop fibres, at least in some of their expansions.

Investigations have been made into the stimuli which cause astrocytes to react. The experiments of Penfield (1927) and Penfield and Buckley (1928) indicated that the presence of necrotic brain tissue stimulated the formation both of fibrous tissue and of neuroglial fibres. Rand and Courville (1932), from the study of brain injuries, considered that gliosis occurs only as the result of tissue destruction and that 'the intensity of the glial reaction in the zone of proliferation is in direct proportion to the proximity of the reacting cells to the injury'. The neuroglial sclerosis, which follows degeneration of a tract or the demyelination of a plaque of disseminated sclero-sis, is well explained by this theory. But there is evidence that neuroglial hyperplasia may be stimulated by other factors. Oedema and minor degrees of ischaemia are constantly associated with swelling of the cell bodies of astrocytes, which goes on to the formation of new neuroglial fibres. This begins quite early. The swelling of the cell body often appears within a week of an incomplete arterial occlusion. Syphilis, in the forms of general paralysis and chronic meningo-vascular syphilis, is associated with the out-growth of pads of neuroglial fibres, through breaks in the ependyma and pia mater, into the ventricular and subarachnoid spaces. Some forms of virus encephalitis, especially subacute sclerosing panencephalitis, are associated with a marked pro-liferation of astrocytes, both in the cortex and white matter, which appears to be out of propor-tion to the amount of neuronal destruction.

Degenerative changes are seen in astrocytes which have been damaged beyond recovery. The cell body swells and becomes visible at one side of the nucleus. Its outline is at first rounded but later becomes irregular. The processes break off and disintegrate into granules which Alzheimer (1910) called 'filling bodies'. To this loss of pro-cesses Cajal gave the name *clasmatodendrosis* (breaking up of branches). Lipid granules of varying size appear in these swollen cell bodies. The nucleus meanwhile becomes pyknotic and irregular and eventually disappears and the cyto-plasm undergoes dissolution. If these changes take place rapidly there is little swelling of the cell body, but if more slowly, as in the neighbour-hood of a septic focus, it continues to enlarge for a time. Under conditions which are not so severe astrocytes may undergo *hypertrophy and hyperplasia* (Fig. 1.16a and b). In these the cell body enlarges without losing its processes. The nucleus also enlarges, stains more darkly and often divides, giving rise either to two daughter cells or to a large binucleated cell (Fig. 1.17*a*).

Mitotic division in astrocytes. In previous editions Greenfield stated that small astrocytes in mitosis, or the later phases of mitosis in swollen nuclei, but no mitotic figures. This was considered to be evidence in favour of amitotic division in protoplasmic astrocytes. Cavanagh and Lewis (1969) and Cavanagh (1970) made wounds in the brains of adult rats and found

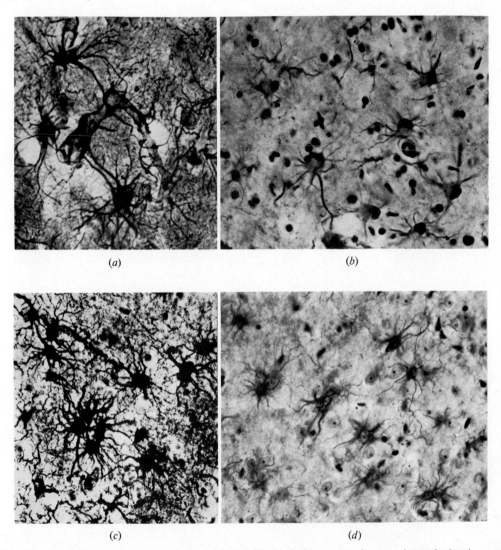

(*a*)   (*b*)

(*c*)   (*d*)

Fig. 1.16 Reactions of protoplasmic astrocytes. (*a*) and (*b*) Cortical astrocytes in general paresis showing moderate hypertrophy. (*a*) Cajal's gold sublimate. ×450. (*b*) Silver carbonate. ×350. (*c*) Cortical astrocytes in subacute encephalitis showing division into 4 daughter cells. Cajal's gold sublimate. (*d*) Astrocytes in putamen in presenile chorea showing formation of fibres. Mallory's phosphotungstic acid haematoxylin.

astrocytes, are never seen and that it is probable that astrocytes do not undergo mitosis except when neoplastic. Lapham (1962), examining reactive protoplasmic astrocytes in human necropsy material, found an increase in the number of nuclei and a build up of DNA in some swollen many mitoses in nearby astrocytes during the following days. The greatest activity was 2 to 3 days after wounding. They found that the number of mitoses, around the wound and also in the intact subependymal plate, was noticeably affected by the delay between death and fixation.

A delay of less than 5 minutes reduced the number by about 50% and a delay of 30 minutes by about 75%. This was due to the short time taken for mitosis to proceed to completion. Although, in the human, this period is likely to be longer, the chance of finding mitotic figures is almost certainly reduced by any delay in fixation. It is therefore possible that mitoses are seldom seen in regions of astrocytic hyperplasia in the human because of the short period of time during which the nucleus is in mitosis and the usually long period between death and fixation of the

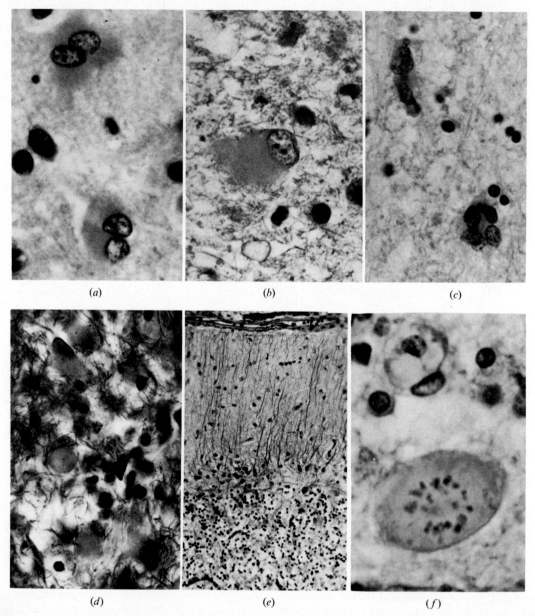

(a)   (b)   (c)

(d)   (e)   (f)

Fig. 1.17 Astrocytic reactions. (a) Binucleated swollen-bodied cortical astrocytes. (b) Large fibre-forming astrocyte in white matter. Mallory's phosphotungstic acid haematoxylin. (c) Irregular multinucleation of astrocytes in white matter in area of oedema round a cerebral abscess. (d) Swelling of astrocytes and fibre formation in diffuse sclerosis PTAH. (e) Isomorphous gliosis in cerebellar cortex in carcinomatous cerebellar degeneration. PTAH. (f) Abnormal glial cell close to an infective necrotic process. Phagocyte at foot of picture.

tissue. Examination of rapidly fixed biopsies, taken a few days after a brain wound in a human, should provide evidence on the problem, as suggested by Lapham (1962).

Under moderately unfavourable conditions such as in ischaemia or subacute encephalitis, and in the oedematous white matter surrounding cerebral tumours, less severe *hypertrophy* of the cell bodies of the astrocytes is commonly seen. It is characteristic of this hypertrophy that it affects all the astrocytes in most of the area in almost equal degree. It results in irregularly rounded cells with angular projections from which the processes arise (Fig. 1.17*b*). The cytoplasm is usually

of the term protoplasmic as a general description of cells which have undergone this change.

The amount of astrocytic swelling may vary greatly. In the slightest and earliest stages a small rounded or irregular cell body no larger than the nucleus may appear at one side of this. Enlargement to diameters of 15 μm are common and are often accompanied by the formation of new fibres. From this stage, under favourable circumstances, the cell body gradually shrinks. At the same time, either by the extension of new processes from the cell body or by more frequent branching, new fibrous expansions are formed and increase the density of the

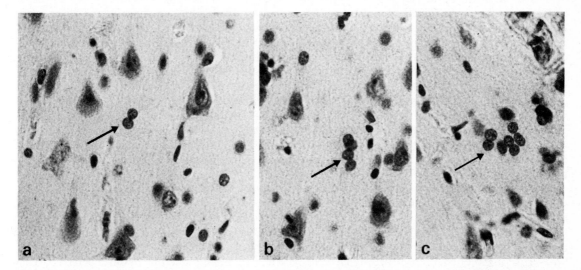

Fig. 1.18 Cerebral cortex, case of subacute encephalitis, from a region where loss of nerve cells was not obvious nor was there perivascular cuffing. In (*a*) there are 2, in (*b*) 4 and in (*c*) a pair and 5 astrocyte nuclei close together. This is evidence of astrocyte multiplication or hyperplasia. Celloidin; haematoxylin van Gieson.   × 440.

homogeneous, but may contain a few granules or vacuoles near its margin. Its outline is more clearly defined than in cells undergoing clasmatodendrosis. Swollen cells arising from fibrous astrocytes do not usually contain any fibres in their cell body, though these usually remain intact in the processes. The nucleus, which may be slightly enlarged, lies on one side of the cell, usually on that furthest from the chief processes. Occasionally two nuclei are present at opposite poles of the cell but mitoses are not seen. The names *swollen-bodied* and *plump astrocytes* are given to these cells. Although swollen-bodied cells may arise from protoplasmic as well as from fibrous astrocytes, the absence of fibres from the cell body in both cases does not justify the use

glial feltwork. This process of gliosis after the formation of swollen-bodied astrocytes is usually associated with a moderate increase in astrocyte nuclei, but this is much less evident than the increase of neuroglial fibres.

The protoplasmic astrocytes of the cortex often show more nuclear division than formation of new fibres (Fig. 1.16*c*). This is especially seen in some cases of subacute encephalitis and in the earlier stages of cortical atrophy. In these conditions pairs of nuclei are frequently seen, groups of four nuclei are not uncommon, and even larger groups may be seen (Fig. 1.18). In dividing, astrocytes appear to share the expansions and if two foot-plate processes are present one goes to each cell. In this way the nuclei come to be near the inner, apposed margins of the cells and the expansions to come off from their outer margins (Fig. 1.16c). A group of two or more closely apposed astrocytic nuclei is an easily recognized histological clue to previous death of a neuron (Fig. 1.18).

When *mildly unfavourable conditions persist for some time*, as for example in an area of oedema round a cerebral abscess, the cell body may continue to enlarge up to 25 μm or more in diameter. Large reniform or irregular nuclei may be seen in such cells. At this stage the cell body may lose its processes and become rounded and the nucleus may break up into fragments, probably heralding the death of the cell (Fig. 1.17f). The appearance of some such cells suggests an early stage in mitotic division, but mitotic division of proven astrocytes in human post-mortem material does not seem to have been recorded. The above changes may, however, be followed by recovery, with the formation of new fibre-containing processes. It seems probable that the giant astrocytes which are often seen in the scars of slowly progressive lesions, such as diffuse sclerosis of the white matter, or in the neighbourhood of a tuberculoma, result from a long-continued reaction of this kind.

The pattern of the newly formed feltwork of astrocytic fibres varies with environmental factors. In regions where there is preservation of some nerve fibres or axons, as for example in the plaques of disseminated sclerosis, the intact nerve fibres govern the orientation of neuroglial fibres. The name *isomorphous gliosis* is given to this pattern in which the previous arrangement of neuroglial fibres is preserved. On the other hand, when a tract is uniformly degenerated, or when there is gradual replacement of degenerating white matter by neuroglial tissue, the arrangement is more random. Neuroglial fibres which are attached to the connective tissue of meninges or blood vessels run perpendicularly to them but elsewhere the pattern is quite irregular (*anisomorphous gliosis*). Whorls of glial fibres are not uncommon in long-standing degenerations in the dorsal columns in tabes and Friedreich's ataxia. Penfield (1927) and del Rio Hortega and Penfield (1928) showed that, when collagenous tissue is formed in wounds of the brain, the neighbouring astrocytes become attached to it by strong processes, which appear to be pulled on by the later contraction of the collagen. In this way elongated or *piloid astrocytes* (Penfield 1932) may be

formed. It is not uncommon in cortical scars to see a number of such cells lying parallel to one another in palisade arrangement above a layer of connective tissue.

Alzheimer types of neuroglial cell (see page 171)

Rosenthal fibres

These are elongated, tapering, rod-like to club-shaped bodies, about 5 to 8 μm in diameter and up to 40 μm long, rather opaque, hyaline, PTAH-positive structures. By electron-microscopy they prove to be intracellular and are found exclusively in the cell bodies and processes of astrocytes. They consist of rounded or elongated dense masses of finely granular osmophilic material surrounded by or attached to glial filaments. They are found occasionally in regions of long-standing but intense fibrillary gliosis, as in multiple sclerosis or syringomyelia, frequently in astrocytomata of the optic nerve or cerebellum and invariably in Alexander's disease. Herndon et al. (1970) suggest that in multiple sclerosis there is a latent metabolic abnormality affecting the astrocytes which leads to the accumulation of abnormal intracellular products of degradation.

Corpora amylacea

Corpora amylacea (Fig. 1.19), are spherical bodies, average diameter 15 μm, which are often found in the grey matter close to the pia, or around blood vessels in the white matter of the brain and cord. They are more numerous in older persons. They contain an amorphous basiphilic material, sometimes with a deeper staining central core. They stain positively with iodine, methyl violet, PAS, and with Best's stain for glycogen. They are metachromatic with toluidine blue. Ramsay (1965) has shown electron microscopically that they are intracytoplasmic bodies, forming swellings in the processes of fibrous astrocytes. They represent a non-specific degenerative change and contain a glycogen-like substance to which phosphate and sulphate groups are bound (Stam and Roukema 1973).

Oligodendroglia

Oligodendroglia have small round dark nuclei. They appear as *perineuronal satellites* in the grey matter and as *interfascicular glia* in the white matter. A few occur as *perivascular satellites*. In all three types the nucleus is small, of the same size and appearance as that of a lymphocyte, with abundant closely set chromatin granules. The cell body, which is small and irregularly rounded or oblong, in silver preparations gives off a few protoplasmic expansions. In the satellite cells, some expansions wrap themselves round the cell body of a neuron while others end freely. In the interfascicular cells they pass, often for considerable distances, along the surface of myelinated fibres. These expansions branch less often and less regularly than those of astrocytes and do not join connective tissue by footplates, but like astrocytes they contain gliosomes

cortex and the large cells of the basal ganglia. They are rare round the large motor cells of the anterior horns of the cord, of the motor nuclei of the brainstem and of the precentral gyrus. They are not seen in relation to Purkinje cells. It seems probable that they multiply in many forms of neuronal degeneration and the term *satellitosis of nerve cells* is often used, but it is difficult to tell whether the satellites round a particular neuron are in excess. Certainly six or more such cells are not infrequently seen round a single neuron under what appear to be normal conditions.

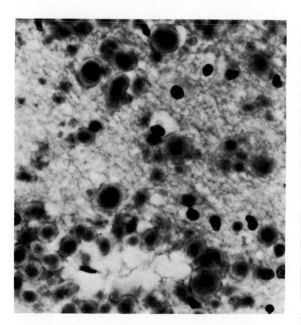

Fig. 1.19 Corpora amylacea. Celloidin; haematoxylin and eosin. × 630.

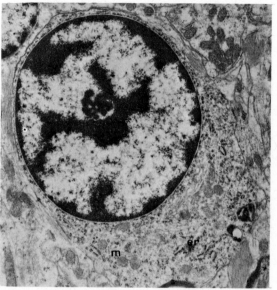

Fig. 1.20 Oligodendrocyte, cat, spinal cord. Note rough endoplasmic reticulum (er), mitochondria (m). × 9000. (Reproduced by courtesy of Dr L. S. Illis).

i.e. mitochondria (Fig. 1.13). Under the electron microscope (Fig. 1.20) the oligodendrocyte appears relatively electron dense, both the rounded, ovoid or irregularly shaped nucleus and the cytoplasm, where many small pale granules take up most of the space between the rough endoplasmic reticulum, the rosettes of free ribosomes, the mitochondria and the Golgi apparatus. Microtubules are present, especially in the processes, which can seldom be seen leaving the cell body. Cytoplasmic fibrils and glycogen granules are very few (Peters *et al.* 1970).

Perineuronal satellites. They are common round the medium-sized pyramidal cells of the

The interfascicular oligodendroglia are by far the most numerous cells in the white matter where they lie in rows of closely apposed nuclei between the myelinated fibres.

Del Rio Hortega (1928) and Penfield considered that the interfascicular oligodendroglia held a relationship to myelin in the central nervous system similar to that of the Schwann cells in peripheral nerves (Fig. 1.21). After the discovery that the myelin of peripheral nerves was formed by the spirally arranged cell membrane of the Schwann cell and that there was an inner and an outer collar of Schwann cell cytoplasm enclosing the myelin, evidence was sought for a similar

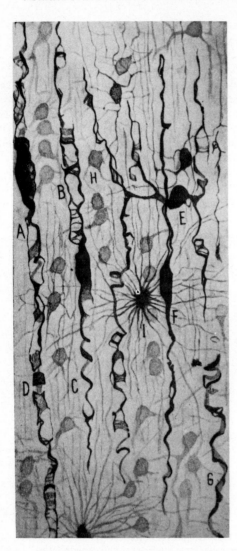

Fig. 1.21 Glial cells in the white matter of the medulla of the cat. Cells labelled AD, BC, F, G (type 4 oligodendrocytes) and E (type 3 oligodendrocyte) are related to underlying myelin sheaths (not stained in this preparation). Type 4 cell is related to single myelinated fibres, type 3 to several myelin segments. Type 2 oligodendrocytes are labelled H and an astrocyte I. (From Del Rio-Hortega (1928), *Mem. Real Soc. Espan. Hist. Nat*, **14**, 5. Reproduced by courtesy of Dr R. P. Bunge.)

relationship between central myelin and the oligodendrocyte. The evidence eluded the electron microscopists until 1960 when Maturana, Peters and Bunge showed that the myelin of the central nervous system is formed from the coiled cell membrane of the oligodendrocyte, that oligodendroglial cytoplasm is to be found internal to and external to the myelin and that there is a

tongue-shaped connection of this cytoplasm with the cell body of an oligodendrocyte. Sometimes a single oligodendrocyte is connected to segments of myelin around more than one nerve fibre (Figs. 1.22 and 1.23). The fascinating story of this discovery should be read in Bunge (1968).

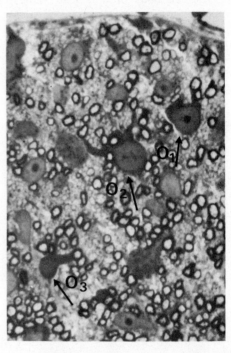

Fig. 1.22 Microphotograph of a portion of spinal cord of a 5-day-old kitten, with the pia appearing at the top. Myelin sheaths are visible throughout this area. Three myelin-related cells (oligodendrocytes o_1, o_2, o_3,) are shown, each displaying two processes that appear to become related to at least two different myelinated axons. A 1 μm section of OsO_4-fixed and Epon-embedded tissue. Toluidine blue. $\times 1200$. (Reproduced by courtesy of Dr R. P. Bunge.)

Ependyma

The ventricles, iter of Sylvius and central canal of the cord, except at the area postrema of the 4th ventricle, are covered by ependymal cells which normally lie side by side in palisade formation. Their nuclei, which are oval and rather longer and more darkly stained than astrocyte nuclei, are arranged in a regular line. The inner, or ventricular, part of the cell body is cylindrical, ending on a flat surface to which cilia are attached. Under these is a line of very small oval bodies named *blepharoplasts* (Greek for 'eyelash fixatives'), which are oriented in the long axis of

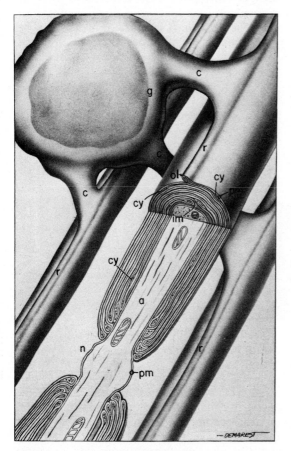

Fig. 1.23 Diagram illustrating both the known and the hypothetical aspects of the mature myelin sheath and its relationship to glial cells. The unit or plasma membrane (pm) is here designated by two lines separated by a space except in the mitochondrion where it is represented by a single line. The inner mesaxon (im), formed as a glial process completes the inital turn around an axon (a) and starts a second, is retained after myelin formation is completed. Some cytoplasm of the glial process is present here. Cytoplasm is trapped occasionally at cy. On the fully formed sheath exterior a piece of glial cytoplasm is also retained. In transverse sections this cytoplasm is confined to a loop (ol) of plasma membrane (pm), but along the internode length it forms a ridge (r) which is continuous with a glial cell body (g) at c. When viewed transversely, the sheath components are oriented in a spiral, only the innermost and outermost layers ending in loops; in the longitudinal plane every myelin unit terminates in a separate loop near a node (n). Within these loops glial cytoplasm is also retained. (Reproduced by courtesy of Dr R. P. Bunge.)

the cells; they are stained by phosphotungstic acid haematoxylin after Zenker fixation. The outer part of the cell consists of one, two or more tapering processes containing fine fibrils which pass into and merge with the underlying nervous tissues.

Ependymal cells have a limited reaction to disease processes. They gradually lose their cilia with age. Those which line the ventricles and iter of Sylvius remain as an unbroken line. The central canal of the cord is usually encroached on, often during childhood, by ingrowth of neuroglial fibres. These fibres separate the lining ependymal cells into irregular groups of oval, darkly staining nuclei. These have been interpreted as proliferations in response to disease, but the great variation in the normal makes any such interpretation open to question.

The most common reaction of the ependymal surfaces to inflammation or irritation is *granular ependymitis*. In general paresis this is found in the floor of the 4th ventricle, near the foramen of Monro and, in severe cases, also in the walls of the frontal horns of the lateral ventricles. It may also follow any inflammation of the ventricles, especially mild attacks of meningococcal meningitis. The appearance, which is best seen on oblique illumination, has been likened to coarse ground glass, but is usually more obviously granular than this. Under the microscope the granulations appear as small hillocks of neuroglial fibres, which may be partly or entirely covered by ependymal cells, or may have a broken line of ependymal nuclei at their base and one or two similar nuclei at higher levels (Fig. 1.24a). There is usually little evidence of proliferation or reaction by the ependymal cells and the name is therefore more applicable to the naked eye than to microscopic appearances. A slight degree of granular ependymitis in the roof of the 4th ventricle near its upper end is so common that it cannot be considered abnormal.

A different appearance in seen in chronic meningovascular syphilis when the whole of the ependyma on the floor of the 4th ventricle is often covered with a pad of neuroglial fibres (Fig. 1.24b). In this case, instead of being smooth and glistening, the ventricular surface has a dull matt appearance and the median raphe is less clearly marked than normal.

In hydrocephalus the continuity of the line of ependymal cells on the inner aspect of the ventricles is broken by the stretching of their walls.

Usually rows of ependymal cells alternate with gaps in which none is seen. In subacute and chronic cases these gaps are filled by neuroglial fibres which form cushions elevated slightly above the line of the ependymal cells. There is no evidence that the ependyma proliferates in an attempt to cover these bared areas.

Del Rio Hortega found that microglial cells invaded the central nervous system from the meninges during the later stages of embryonic development. At this time large numbers of small cells with short irregular processes can be seen in those areas of white matter which are in contact with the meninges, especially at the base

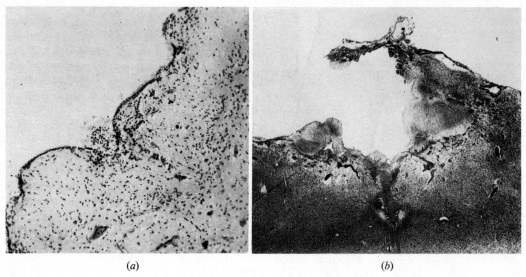

(a)   (b)

Fig. 1.24 Ependymitis. (*a*) Granular ependymitis in the 4th ventricle in a case of general paresis. (*b*) Neuroglial out-growth filling the V of the 4th ventricle in chronic cerebrospinal syphilis.

Microglia

The separation by del Rio Hortega (1919) of the microglia from the group of small cells in the central nervous system, which Cajal (1913) had called the *third element*, was an important turning point in the history of neuropathology. His demonstration that the microglia, although normally present in the tissues of the central nervous system, were of mesoblastic origin and had many of the characters and potentialities of histiocytes elsewhere in the body, provided a simple answer to the question of the origin of the phagocytes in the central nervous system. This answer was challenged by Konigsmark and Sidman (1963), who labelled the monocytes of the blood of mice with tritiated thymidine, made occipital stab wounds and concluded that about 65% of the resulting phagocytes were of haematogenous origin. Their conclusions were contrary to the experiments conducted by Hain (1963) and were adversely criticized by Feigin (1969). Cammermeyer (1970) concluded that microglia possess the power to proliferate.

of the brain and round the brainstem. From these foci the microglia migrate throughout the central nervous system and eventually become most abundant in the grey matter. In their resting stage they develop two or more thin processes with fine lateral projections which can be stained by special silver impregnation techniques but are not visible with ordinary tissue stains. In the grey matter they may lie free as bipolar or multipolar cells or may be perineuronal or perivascular satellites. In the white matter most of them occur round the vessels. The nucleus remains small and hyperchromic, and its shape is related to the number of cell processes; in bipolar cells it is elongated, when three or more processes are present it may be irregularly triangular or polyhedral. Only rarely is it as evenly spherical as the nucleus of an oligodendrocyte and it is rather more hyperchromic. These characteristics usually make it possible to distinguish microglial from oligodendroglial nuclei with general tissue stains. Microglia are not easily identified by electron microscopy (Fig. 1.25). In the cytoplasm of the rat's microglia, ribosomes and endoplasmic reticulum are sparse, in contrast to oligodendroglia. They do not contain the glycogen granules and parallel filaments of astrocytes. Golgi apparatus is present and numerous dense bodies, some of them showing the halos characteristic of lysosomes, are a special feature (Mori and Leblond 1969).

Therefore, although they are very characteristic of the response to virus infection, they are not always evidence of inflammation. In typhus fever the characteristic perivascular nodules are, in the central nervous system, formed largely of microglial cells, although histiocytes from the vessel walls also take part in the process. It is often

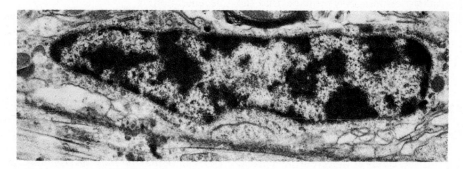

Fig. 1.25 Microglial cell, cat, spinal cord. Note scanty cytoplasm and dense nucleus. × 9000. (Reproduced by courtesy of Dr L. S. Illis.)

Microglial cells react rapidly to noxious stimuli by hyperplasia and multiplication by mitosis (Cammermeyer 1970). They are actively phagocytic. As they are less vulnerable than neuroglial cells, they may remain active in areas where both the neurons and neuroglia have undergone necrosis and they are often seen, laden with lipid granules, in and around such partially necrotic areas. The reactions of the microglia may be classified as (a) *hyperplasia*, (b) *hypertrophy*, (c) *phagocytosis of lipid*, (d) *neuronophagy*, (e) *calcification*.

(a) *Hyperplasia* of microglia is seen in many forms of acute and subacute encephalitis, as well as in the neighbourhood of softenings. It may be diffuse in an area, giving an appearance of increased cellularity, but where the reaction is less intense it may be quite focal. In this way clumps of microglial cells or *glial stars* may be formed. These often contain 10 to 20 small closely set microglial nuclei. These *glial stars* or *knots* are common in encephalomyelitis. They occur chiefly in the grey matter, but may also be seen in the white matter both in the brain and spinal cord. While it is impossible to be certain that some of those in the grey matter are not related to dead nerve cells this is less likely in the white matter. Small glial knots may also be seen in the white columns of the cord in what appear to be purely degenerative conditions.

difficult or impossible to be certain whether cells which proliferate in the immediate neighbourhood of vessels, for example in post-infectious encephalomyelitis, are of microglial or vascular origin. In some the nuclei are too large to be characteristic of microglia, whereas in others hyperchromic nuclei of irregular shape may belong to either type of cell.

(b) *Hypertrophy* of microglia is seen most characteristically in the cerebral cortex in general paralysis (paretic dementia) but is also found in other forms of subacute encephalitis. The processes enlarge both in length and to a less extent in width. They may lose some of their lateral spines but do not otherwise change their form. The nucleus also enlarges. A very characteristic appearance is given by the bipolar microglial cells which normally lie radially orientated in the cerebral cortex. In these cells the nucleus becomes more elongated and the processes may become stainable by Nissl's method for some distance from its poles. With silver technique they may be seen to run for long distances perpendicular to the surface with little branching (Fig. 1.26a). To cells of this kind Nissl gave the name *rod cells* (Stäbchenzellen). In general paralysis their processes may contain fine granules which give the Prussian blue and Turnbull's blue reactions for iron. When the multipolar cells hypertrophy, their nuclei become more lobulated and may assume very irregular shapes, though the lobules are never so separate as in polymorphonuclear leucocytes (Fig. 1.26b). Asteroid or long curved, sometimes horseshoe shaped, nuclei are not uncommon. This process of simple hypertrophy is often associated with some increase in number, but this is not so evident as in more acutely destructive lesions. It is probable that the hypertrophied cells may revert to a more normal size, since rod cells and other hypertrophic forms may not be present in the cortex in treated cases of general paralysis.

(c) When microglial cells take on the *phagocytosis of lipids* the cell body enlarges and the processes become shorter and thicker. This process may go on until the cell becomes spherical, but in the earlier stages, or when degenerating myelin is less abundant as in the cerebral or cerebellar cortex, phagocytosis of lipid may occur in processes which still extend some distance from the cell body (Fig. 1.26c and d). Indeed, fine lipid droplets may be found in typical rod cells. The reaction of microglia to the breakdown of nervous tissue is fairly rapid. Rand and Courville (1932), in cases of cerebral trauma, found reacting forms of microglia within a few hours of the accident and rounded lipid phagocytes after 3 or 4 days. They noted that only amitotic division was seen during the first 2 or 3 days after an injury, but mitotic division was present in later stages. Even cells which are already charged with lipid granules may undergo mitosis during the first few days of a necrotic lesion.

The migratory activity of microglial cells was emphasized by del Rio Hortega (1932), who saw the accumulation of phagocytes in an area of necrosis as partly a multiplication of the cells already in the area and partly an invasion from outside. Their powers of migration are probably comparable to those of histiocytes in other tissues of the body. After ingestion of lipid they appear to become inert and remain in the same area for many weeks in most cases. Eventually they find their way, either by slow migration or owing to the flow of tissue fluids, to the walls of the blood vessels, where macrophages accumulate both round and within the perivascular (Virchow–Robin) spaces (Fig. 1.26f). These cells may not be the same as those which undertook the earlier stages of lipid katabolism. There may well be, as earlier German studies suggested, relays of lipid phagocytes. The histiocytic cells in the

Virchow–Robin spaces may undertake the last stages of the process. Nuclei of macrophages of microglial origin tend to retain the same shape as in the original cell (Fig. 1.26e). Thus elongated or triangular nuclei are common in rounded macrophages, especially in the earlier stages, and should not be considered as evidence of pyknotic degeneration.

The *nomenclature of lipid phagocytes* in the central nervous system has never been satisfactory. There are many objections to the old term *compound granular corpuscle*, the word 'compound' being meaningless. The term *fat granule cell* is applicable to the later stages of myelin katabolism, but may be misleading in the earlier stages. *Foamy cell*, which is used in general pathology, is perhaps rather too indefinite, and *lattice cell*, though a literal translation of the German *Gitterzell* has no obvious meaning to the uninitiated. Greenfield preferred the term *lipid phagocyte* but we propose to use the term *macrophage*.

(d) *Neuronophagy*. When nerve cells undergo rapid death it is common to find their cell bodies and proximal dendrites invaded by phagocytic cells. When the necrotic process is very acute, as in the anterior horn cells in poliomyelitis, the earliest invading cells may be polymorphonuclear leucocytes, but in later stages the great majority of the phagocytes appear to be derived from the microglia. When necrosis of nerve cells is less acute than in poliomyelitis the phagocytic cells are less numerous and often form a ring round the cell body or invade it at a few places only. For this process the term *neuronophagy*, which was given by classical writers, is apt and descriptive. True neuronophagy by microglial cells must be distinguished from satellitosis, which is mainly a reaction of oligodendroglia. In the former case the nerve cell is undergoing dissolution, while in the latter case it shows much less evidence of degeneration.

Neuronophagy is specially common in all forms of encephalomyelitis which affect the grey matter, and it may be that the manner of death of the neuron has a special chemotactic attraction for microglial cells. It is less common when neurons die as the result of anoxia or direct trauma, although it may be seen in both these conditions. For example, in the anoxaemic condition of the lower spinal cord called *subacute necrotic myelitis* by Foix and Alajouanine (1926) neuronophagy

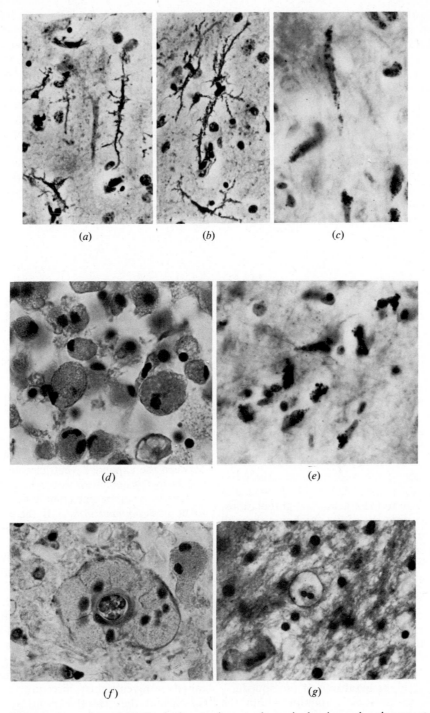

Fig. 1.26 Microglial reactions. (*a*) and (*b*) Cerebral cortex in general paresis showing early enlargement of microglia; (*a*) rod cell, (*b*) triradiate cell.   Silver carbonate.   × 400.   (*c*) and (*d*) Cerebral cortex in subacute encephalitis; (*c*) rod cell filled with small lipid granules, (*d*) thickening and shortening of processes as lipid granules are absorbed.   Scharlach R haemalum.   (*e*) and (*f*) Focus of softening in spinal cord; (*e*) macrophages, (*f*) collection of macrophages in Virchow–Robin space of small vessel.   Iron haematoxylin van Gieson.   × 550.   (*g*) Myeloclast (axonophage) in swollen myelin sheath in oedematous area of subcortical white matter.

of anterior horn cells is not uncommon. A very characteristic appearance may be seen in the neuronophagy of Purkinje cells. Here the microglial phagocytes are grouped not only round the cell body but also along the dendrites in the molecular layer where the normal paucity of nuclei makes their increase very obvious. A shrub-like arrangement of cell bodies and short processes is thus formed, to which Spielmeyer gave the name *Gliastrauchwerk* (glial shrub formation). This was first described in typhus fever, but is also seen, affecting few or many Purkinje cells, in some forms of virus encephalitis and also in non-inflammatory processes, for example in the cerebellar degeneration associated with carcinoma.

(e) *Calcification*. Microglia may calcify in conditions such as the Sturge–Weber syndrome, Fahr's disease and certain forms of encephalitis (Alexander and Norman 1960). In the Sturge–Weber syndrome these calcified cells are frequently found in or near areas of cortical neuronal destruction and below areas of massive calcification and they may stand out with the clarity of silver impregnation. Other microglial cells are seen to be more coarsely incrusted and their branches to be ending in small balls of calcified material. These may be precursors of 'free' concretions. In contrast, neurons rarely calcify in the Sturge–Weber syndrome.

Hydrocephalus

About 750 ml of cerebrospinal fluid are secreted daily by the choroid plexuses of the lateral and fourth ventricles (Davson 1967). The fluid passes out of the fourth ventricle through the lateral apertures (foramina of Luschka) and the usually patent median aperture (foramen of Magendie) on to the external surface of the brainstem, cerebellum and spinal cord, where it is contained within the meshwork of the pia-arachnoid and passes into the nervous tissue along the Virchow–Robin spaces. The fluid passes upwards, over the external surface of the midbrain, into the basal cisterns and thence it follows the fissures and sulci of the brain to the arachnoidal granulations. These are invaginations of the arachnoid through the walls of the venous sinuses, chiefly the superior sagittal venous sinus. Here the fluid passes into the venous blood stream.

An abnormal amount of cerebrospinal fluid is called *hydrocephalus*. Hydrocephalus can result from:

(1) an overproduction of cerebrospinal fluid by a papilloma of the choroid plexus, but Milhorat (1972) considered this not proved,

(2) an obstruction to the flow of cerebrospinal fluid, as by atresia of the aqueduct, or the presence of a tumour within the ventricles or aqueduct, or compression of the pathway by an externally situated tumour, or obliteration of the subarachnoid space by an organizing inflammatory exudate or blood,

(3) failure of absorption, by exudate or blood blocking the arachnoidal granulations. Whether venous sinus thrombosis extending into the lateral lacunae can cause failure of absorption is not certain.

Various qualifying terms may be applied to the word hydrocephalus. According to its position, it is called *internal* if within the ventricles, or *external* if situated on the surface of the brain and cord. If clinically there is a communication between the expanded ventricles and the lumbar sac the hydrocephalus is said to be *communicating*; if there is no apparent communication it is said to be *non-communicating*. If the hydrocephalus results from a loss of brain substance (as in senile dementia) it is called *compensatory*. If it results from an obstruction to the flow of fluid (as from a glioma of the thalamus obliterating the cavity of the 3rd ventricle) it is called *obstructive*. Obstructive hydrocephalus is associated with a raised pressure in the cerebrospinal fluid proximal to the obstruction. This results in enlargement of the ventricles, and a loss of white matter from around the ventricles and from the corpus callosum. Since the brain tissue is incompressible, the raised intraventricular pressure is transmitted throughout the central nervous system. If obstructive hydrocephalus occurs before the fusion of the cranial bones, the skull enlarges. If it occurs after fusion of the bones, they will become thinned. This will be most noticeable at the base of the skull in respect of the orbital roofs, the posterior clinoid processes, the floor of the middle fossa and the tegmen tympani. The ependymal lining of the ventricles is often focally deficient, with proliferation of the sub-ependymal glia, sometimes with the production of ependymal granulations. The choroid plexuses become atrophic. Experimentally induced obstructive hydrocephalus in animals has revealed many aspects of hydrocephalus in its early stages. Using adult cats, Ogata, Hochwald, Cravioto and Ransohoff (1972) showed that at 7 days there was a marked rise in intraventricular pressure, a moderate increase in intraventricular volume and a minimal amount of transventricular absorption of cerebrospinal fluid. The ependymal cells were flattened and stretched. At 21 days there was partial multifocal separation and destruction of ependymal cells, an increased extracellular space in the adjacent white matter and a greater transventricular absorption of cerebrospinal fluid. The ventricles were greatly dilated, but the intraventricular pressure was lower than in the acute stage.

Weller, Wisniewski and Shulman (1971) in puppies, 20 to 40 days after obstruction, found that the ependyma was either disrupted or completely absent, with replacement by loosely packed astrocytic processes. There was damage to the periventricular white matter, the extracellular spaces were distended with fluid and there was degeneration of nerve fibres. It appeared that it was in this early oedematous phase, when the ependyma was damaged, that the severe tissue damage occurred. After this, in puppies, the cerebrospinal fluid pressure returned to normal, a modified ependyma was reconstituted and there was little or no extracellular fluid. Widespread loss of nerve fibres and widespread astrocytic fibre formation were visible. Similar changes were seen by Weller and Shulman (1972) in the brains of human infants in both the early oedematous and the later reparative phase.

Adams and his co-workers (Adams, Fisher, Hakim, Ojemann and Sweet 1965; Adams 1966) described certain rare cases of *normal pressure hydrocephalus*, where the ventricles may be considerably enlarged and yet the intraventricular pressure is not raised above that formerly considered as being within normal limits. Such patients show dementia, ataxia and urinary incontinence. They may derive some benefit if the intraventricular fluid is drained through a non-return valve into the superior vena cava. The condition may follow subarachnoid haemorrhage (either from trauma or from a ruptured aneurysm) or there may not be any evidence of an antecedent illness. Several of their patients were believed to have had a raised intracranial pressure early in the course of the illness, but, at the time of the ventricular decompression, the lumbar puncture pressures were 140 to 180 mm water. As yet there is no satisfactory explanation for the above findings. Adams suggests that normal sized ventricles do not enlarge under normal pressures of cerebrospinal fluid, but if they have once been enlarged, they behave differently and will dilate further even under normal pressures of cerebrospinal fluid.

References

Adams, C. W. M. (1969) Enzyme histochemistry applications and pitfalls, in *Handbook of Neurochemistry* (Ed. Lajtha, A.), Vol. 2, Chapter 22, Plenum Press, New York.

Adams, R. D., Fisher, C. M., Hakim, S., Ojemann, R. G. & Sweet, W. H. (1965) Symptomatic occult hydrocephalus with 'normal' cerebrospinal-fluid pressure. A treatable syndrome. *New England Journal of Medicine*, **273**, 117-126.

Adams, R. D. (1966) Further observations on normal pressure hydrocephalus. *Proceedings of the Royal Society of Medicine*, **59**, 1135-1140.

Adornato, B. T., O'Brien, J. S., Lampert, P. W., Roe, T. F. & Neustein, H. B. (1972) Cerebral spongy degeneration of infancy: A biochemical and ultrastructural study of affected twins. *Neurology (Minneapolis)*, **22**, 202-210.

Alexander, G. L. & Norman, R. H. (1960) *The Sturge-Weber Syndrome*, John Wright, Bristol.

Alzheimer, A. (1910) Nissl/Alzheimer Arbeiten. *Beiträge zur Kenntnis der pathologischen Neuroglia und ihrer Beziehungen zu den Abbauvorgangen im Nervengewebe*, **3**, 401-554.

Aparicio, S. R. & Lumsden, C. E. (1970) Significance of metachromatic bodies in nervous tissue in *Proceedings of VIth International Congress of Neuropathology*, pp. 1091-1092, Masson, Paris.

Aring, C. D., Bean, W. B., Roseman, E., Rosenbaum, M. & Spies, T. D. (1941) The peripheral nerves in cases of nutritional deficiency. *Archives of Neurology and Psychiatry (Chicago)*, **45**, 772-787.

Arnell, N. (1936) Untersuchung über die Dicke des Achsenzylinders und der Markscheide in nicht fixierten

Spinalnerven des Menschen und des Hundes sowie über den Einfluss von Formalin Fixierung, Paraffinein-bettung und AG-Imprägnierung auf dieselbe. *Acta Psychiatrica Neurologica*, **11**, 5-47.

Le Baron, F. N. & Folch-Pi, J. (1956) The isolation from brain tissue of a trypsin-resistant protein fraction containing combined inositol, and its relation to Neurokeratin. *Journal of Neurochemistry*, **1**, 101-108.

Barondes, S. H. (1969) Axoplasmic transport in *Handbook of Neurochemistry* (Ed. Lajtha, A.), Vol. 2, Chap. 18, p. 435, Plenum Press, New York.

Barr, M. L. & Bertram, L. F. (1949) A morphological distinction between neurones of the male and female and the behaviour of the nucleolar satellite during accelerated nucleoprotein synthesis. *Nature (London)*, **163**, 676-677.

Bertrand, I., Liber, A. F. & Randoin, L. (1934) Altérations anatomiques du système nerveux au cours de l'avitaminose expérimentale. *Archives d'anatomie microscopique*, **30**, 297-380.

Bielschowsky, M. (1928) Zentrale Nervenfasern in *Handbuch der mikroskopischen Anatomie des Menschen* (Ed. von Möllendorff, W.), Vol. 4, pp. 97-107, Springer Verlag, Berlin.

Bignami, A. & Ralston, H. J. (1969) The cellular reaction to Wallerian degeneration in the central nervous system of the cat. *Brain Research*, **13**, 444-461.

Bodian, D. (1949) *Poliomyelitis: Pathogenesis of Early Stage, Pathologic Anatomy*, pp. 62-84, Pitman Medical, London.

Bowsker, D., Brodal, A. & Walberg, F. (1960) The related values of the Marchi method and some silver impregnation techniques—a critical survey. *Brain*, **83**, 150-160.

Bradley, W. G., Murchison, D. & Day, M. J. (1971) The range of velocities of axoplasmic flow. A new approach and its application to mice with genetically inherited spinal muscular atrophy. *Brain Research*, **35**, 185-197.

Brain, W. R., Greenfield, J. G. & Russell, D. S. (1948) Subacute inclusion encephalitis (Dawson type). *Brain*, **71**, 365-385.

Brante, G. (1949) Studies on lipids in nervous system with special reference to quantitative chemical determination and topical distribution. *Acta Physiologica Scandinavica*, **18**, Suppl. 63, 1-18.

Bray, D. (1974) The fibrillar proteins of nerve cells. *Endeavour*, **33**, 131-136.

Brodal, A. (1940) Experimentelle Untersuchungen uber die olivocerebellare Lokalisation. *Neurology and Psychiatry*, **169**, 1-153.

Bunge, R. P. (1968) Glial cells and the central myelin sheath. *Physiological Reviews*, **48**, 197-251.

Cajal, S. R. y. (1909) *Histologie du Système Nerveux de l'Homme et des Vertèbres*, Maloine, Paris.

Cajal, S. R. y. (1913) Contribucion al conocimiento de la neuroglia del cerebro humano. *Trabajos del Laboratorio de Investigaciones Biologicas, Madrid*, **11**, 254-315.

Cammermeyer, J. (1961) The importance of avoiding 'dark' neurons in experimental neuropathology. *Acta Neuropathologica (Berlin)*, **1**, 245-270.

Cammermeyer, J. (1970) The life history of the microglial cell: a light microscopic study in *Neurosciences Research* (Ed. Ehrenpreis, S. and Solnitzky, O. C.), Vol. 3, pp. 44-129, Academic Press, New York.

Cammermeyer, J. (1972) Nonspecific changes of the central nervous system in normal and experimental material in *The Structure and Function of Nervous Tissue*, Vol. 6, pp. 131-251, Academic Press, New York.

Cavanagh, J. B. (1954) The toxic effects of tri-ortho-cresyl phosphate on the nervous system. An experimental study in hens. *Journal of Neurology Neurosurgery and Psychiatry*, **17**, 163-172.

Cavanagh, J. B. (1964) The significance of the 'dying back' process in experimental and human neurological disease. *International Reviews of Experimental Pathology*, **3**, 219-267.

Cavanagh, J. B. (1970) The proliferation of astrocytes around a needle wound in the rat's brain. *Journal of Anatomy*, **106**, 471-487.

Cavanagh, J. B. & Lewis, P. D. (1969) Perfusion-fixation, colchicine and mitotic activity in the adult rat brain. *Journal of Anatomy*, **104**, 341-350.

Chang, H. T. (1952) Cortical and spinal neurons: Cortical neurons with particular reference to the apical dendrites. *Cold Spring Harbor Symposia on Quantitative Biology*, **17**, 189-202.

Chu, L. W. (1954) A cytological study of anterior horn cells isolated from human spinal cord. *Journal of Comparative Neurology*, **100**, 381-413.

Conel, J. R. (1939-59) *The Postnatal Development of the Human Cerebral Cortex*, 6 Vols., Harvard University Press, Cambridge, Mass.

Cramer, F. & Alpers, B. J. (1932) The function of the glia in secondary degeneration of the spinal cord. (The oligodendroglia as phagocytes.) *Archives of Pathology*, **13**, 23-55.

Daniel, P. M. & Strich, S. (1969) Histological observations on Wallerian degeneration in the spinal cord of the baboon. *Acta Neuropathologica*, **12**, 314-328

Davson, H. (1967) *Physiology of the Cerebrospinal Fluid*, Churchill, London.

Droz, B. & Leblond, C. P.   (1963) Axonal migration of proteins in the central nervous system and peripheral nerves as shown by autoradiography. *Journal of Comparative Neurology*, **121**, 325-346.

Duncan, D.   (1934) A relation between axone diameter and myelination determined by measurement of myelinated spinal root fibres. *Journal of Comparative Neurology*, **60**, 437-471.

Einarson, L.   (1933) Notes on morphology of chromophil material of nerve cells and its relation to nuclear substances. *American Journal of Anatomy*, **53**, 141.

Einarson, L.   (1945) Struktur og deres histologiske tilstandsae ndringer ved experimentel fremkaldte pinktroneue Aktivitetsstader. *Acta Jutlandica*, **17**, 1-150.

Einarson L. & Lorentzen, K. A.   (1946) Om nervecellerues indre struktur og deres tilstandsae ndringer under irritation, inaktivitet og degeneration. *Acta Jutlandica*, **18**, 1-116.

Einarson, L.   (1949) On the internal structure of the motor cells of the anterior horns and its changes in poliomyelitis. *Acta Orthopaedica Scandinavica*, **19**, 27-54.

Federow, E. G.   (1935) Essai de l'étude intravitale des cellulis nerveuses et des connexions inter-neuronales dans le système nerveux autonome. *Trabajos del Laboratorio de Investigaciones Biologicas, Madrid*, **30**, 403-434.

Feigin, I.   (1969) Mesenchymal tissues of the nervous system. *Journal of Neuropathology and Experimental Neurology*, **28**, 6-24.

Ferraro, A.   (1928) Acute swelling of the oligodendroglia and grapelike areas of disintegration. *Archives of Neurology and Psychiatry*, **20**, 1065-1079.

Finean, J. B.   (1961) X-Ray diffraction—electron microscopic studies of nerve myelin in *Electron Microscopy in Anatomy* (Ed. Boyd, J. D. *et al.*) (Anatomical Society Symposium), pp. 114-122, Arnold, London.

Foerster, O. & Gagel, O.   (1934) Die tigrolytische Reaktion der Ganglionzelle. *Mikro-anatomische Forschung*, **36**, 567-575.

Foix, C., Chavany, J. A. & Hillemand, P.   (1926) Le syndrome myoclonique de la calotte. Etude anatomounique du nystagmus du voile et des myoclonies rythmiques associats oculaires, faciales, etc. *Revue Neurologique*, **1**, 942-957.

Foix, C. & Alajouanine, T.   (1926) La myélite nécrotique sabaigue. *Revue Neurologique*, **2**, 1-42.

Folchi-Pi, J., Casals, J., Pope, A., Meath, J. A., Le Baron, F. N. & Lees, M.   (1959) Chemistry of myelin development in *Biology of Myelin* (Ed. Korey, S. R.), pp. 122-137 (Progress in Neurobiology, Vol. IV), Hoeber-Harper, New York.

Gautier, J. C. & Blackwood, W.   (1961) Enlargement of the inferior olivary nucleus in association with lesions of the central tegmental tract or dentate nucleus. *Brain*, **84**, 349-361.

Glees, P. & Le Gros Clark, W. E.   (1941) The termination of optic fibres in the lateral geniculate body of the monkey. *Journal of Anatomy*, **75**, 295-308.

Glees, P.   (1944) The anatomical basis of cortico-striate connexions. *Journal of Anatomy*, **78**, 47-51.

Gonatas, N. K.   (1966) The significance of 'pale' neurons in human cortical biopsies. *Journal of Neuropathology and Experimental Neurology*, **25**, 637-645.

Gray, E. G.   (1961) Ultrastructure of synapses of the cerebral cortex and of certain specialisation of neuroglial membranes in *Electron Microscopy in Anatomy* (Ed. Boyd, J. D. *et al.*) (Anatomical Society Symposium), pp. 54-73, Arnold, London.

Greenfield, J. G.   (1934) Subacute spino-cerebellar degeneration occurring in elderly patients. *Brain*, **57**, 161-176.

Hain, R. F.   (1963) Discussion on Konigsmark and Sidman's paper on origin of gitter cells in mouse brain. *Journal of Neuropathology and Experimental Neurology*, **22**, 327-328.

Heimer, L.   (1967) Silver impregnation of terminal degeneration in some forebrain fibre systems; A comparative evaluation of current methods. *Brain Research*, **5**, 86-108.

Herndon, R. M., Rubinstein, L. J., Freeman, J. M. & Mathieson, G.   (1970) Light and electron microscopic observations on Rosenthal fibres in Alexander's disease and in multiple sclerosis. *Journal of Neuropathology and Experimental Neurology*, **29**, 524-551.

Hirano, A.   (1971) Electron microscopy in neuropathology in *Progress in Neuropathology* (Ed. Zimmerman, H. M.), Vol. 1, pp. 1-61, Heinemann Medical, London.

Hoff, E. C. & Hoff, H. E.   (1934) Spinal terminations of the projection fibres from the motor cortex of primates. *Brain*, **57**, 454-474.

Holmes, G.   (1907) A form of familial degeneration of the cerebellum. *Brain*, **30**, 466-489.

Hurst, I. W.   (1925) A study of the lipoids in neuronic degeneration and in amaurotic family idiocy. *Brain*, **48**, 1-42.

Hyden, H.   (1947) The nucleoproteins in virus reproduction. *Cold Spring Harbor Symposia on Quantitative Biology*, **12**, 104-114.

Ibrahim, M. Z. M. & Levine, S.   (1967) Effect of cyanide intoxication on the metachromatic material found in the central nervous system. *Journal of Neurology, Neurosurgery and Psychiatry*, **30**, 545-555.

Ikuta, F., Hirano, A. & Zimmerman, H. M.   (1963) An experimental study of post mortem alterations in the granular layer of the cerebellar cortex. *Journal of Neuropathology and Experimental Neurology*, **22**, 581-593.

Koenig, R. S. & Koenig, H.   (1952) An experimental study of post mortem alterations in neurons of the central nervous system. *Journal of Neuropathology and Experimental Neurology*, **11**, 69-78.

Konigsmark, B. W. & Sidman, R. L.   (1963) Origin of brain macrophages in the mouse. *Journal of Neuropathology and Experimental Neurology*, **22**, 643-676.

Kuypers, H. G. J. M.   (1958) Cortico-bulbar connexions to the pons and the lower brain stem in man. *Brain*, **81**, 364-388.

Lapham, L. W.   (1962) Cytological and cytochemical studies of neuroglia I.   A study of the problem of amitosis in reactive protoplasmic astrocytes. *American Journal of Pathology*, **41**, 1-21.

Lasek, R. J.   (1970) Protein transport in neurons. *International Review of Neurobiology*, **13**, 289-324.

Lieberman, A. R.   (1971) The axon reaction: a review of the principal features of perikaryal responses to axon injury. *International Review of Neurobiology*, **14**, 50-124.

Lindsay, H. A. & Barr, M. L.   (1955) Further observations on the behaviour of nuclear structures during depletion and restoration of Nissl material. *Journal of Anatomy*, **89**, 47-62.

Lorrain-Smith, J. & Mair, W.   (1909) An investigation of the principles underlying Weigert's method of staining medullated nerve. *Journal of Pathology and Bacteriology*, **13**, 14-27.

Mackey, E. A., Spiro, D. & Wiener, J.   (1964) Chromatolysis in dorsal root ganglia. *Journal of Neuropathology and Experimental Neurology*, **23**, 508-526.

Marie, P., Foix, C. & Alajouanine, T.   (1922) De L'Atrophie cérébelleuse Tardive.   A Prédominance Corticale. (Atrophie parenchymateuse primitive des lamelles du cervelet, atrophie paleocérébelleuse primitive.) *Revue Neurologique*, **2**, 849-885, 1082-1111.

Marinesco, G.   (1909) *La Cellule Nerveuse*, Doin, Paris.

Meyer, Adolph.   (1901) On parenchymatous systemic degenerations mainly in the central nervous system. *Brain*, 47-115.

Meyer, A., Beck, E. & McLardy, T.   (1947) Prefrontal leucotomy: A neuro-anatomical report. *Brain*, **70**, 18-49.

Milhorat, T. H.   (1972) *Hydrocephalus and the Cerebrospinal Fluid*, Williams & Wilkins, Baltimore.

Mori, S. & Leblond, C. P.   (1969) Identification of microglia by light and electron microscopy. *Journal of Comparative Neurology*, **135**, 57-80.

Mugnaini, E. & Walberg, F.   (1964) Ultrastructure of neuroglia. Ergebnisse der Anatomie und der Entwicklungsgeschichte, **37**, 194-236.

Niessl von Mayendorf, M.   (1934) Communication—Sur une nouvelle conception du neurone. *Revue Neurologique*, **1**, 1024-1026.

Nissl, F.   (1894) Ueber eine neue Untersuchungsmethode des Centralorgans speciell zur Festellung der Localisation der Nervenzellen. *Zentralblatt für Nervenheilkunde*, **17**, 337-398.

Ogata, J., Hochwald, G. M., Cravioto, A. & Ransohoff, J.   (1972) Light and electron microscopic studies of experimental hydrocephalus. *Acta Neuropathologica (Berlin)*, **21**, 213-223.

Olsen, S.   (1959) Acute selective necrosis of the granular layer of the cerebral cortex. *Journal of Neuropathology and Experimental Neurology*, **18**, 609-619.

Olszewski, J.   (1947) Zur Morphologie und Entwicklung des Arbeitskerns unter besonderer Berücksichtigung des nervenzellkerns. *Biologisches Zentralblatt*, **66**, 265-304.

Palay, S. L.   (1956) Synapses in the central nervous system. *Journal of Biophysics, Biochemistry and Cytology*, **2**, Suppl. 193-202.

Palay, S. L.   (1958) The morphology of synapses in the central nervous system. *Experimental Cell Research Suppl.*, **5**, 275-276.

Penfield, W.   (1927) The mechanism of cicatricial contraction in the brain. *Brain*, **50**, 499-517.

Penfield, W. & Buckley, W.   (1928) Punctures of the brain. The factors concerned in gliosis and in cicatricial contraction. *Archives of Neurology and Psychiatry (Chicago)*, **20**, 1-13.

Penfield, W.   (1932) Neuroglia: normal and pathological in *Penfield's Cytology and Cellular Pathology of the Nervous System*, Vol. 2, pp. 423-479, Hoeber, New York.

Peters, A., Palay, S. L. & Webster, H. de F.   (1970) *The Fine Structure of the Nervous System*, Harper and Row, New York.

Pomerat, C. M.   (1952) Dynamic neurogliology. *Texas Reports in Biology and Medicine*, **10**, 885-913.

Putnam, T. J. & Putnam, I. K.   (1926) Studies on the central visual system. 1. The anatomic projection of the retinal quadrants on the striate cortex of the rabbit. *Archives of Neurology and Psychiatry (Chicago)*, **16**, 1-20.

Ramsay, H. J. (1965) Ultrastructure of corpora amylacea. *Journal of Neuropathology and Experimental Neurology*, **24**, 25-39.

Rand, C. W. & Courville, C. B. (1932) Histologic changes in the brain in cases of fatal injury to the head. III. Reaction of microglia and oligodendroglia. *Archives of Neurology and Psychiatry (Chicago)*, **27**, 605-644.

Rand, C. W. & Courville, C. B. (1946) Histological changes in the brain in cases of fatal injury to the head. VII. Alterations in nerve cells. *Archives of Neurology and Psychiatry (Chicago)*, **55**, 79-110.

de Renyi, G. St. (1929) The structure of cells in tissues as revealed by microdissection. II. The physical properties of the living axis cylinder in the myelinated fibres of the frog (*Journal of Comparative Neurology*, **47**, 405-425). III. Observations on the sheaths of myelinated nerve fibres in the frog (**48**, 293-310). IV. Observations on neurofibrils in the living nervous tissue of the lobster (*Homanis Americanus*) (**48**, 441-457).

del Rio-Hortega, P. (1919) El tercer elemento de los centros nerviosos. I. La microglia. II. Intervencion de la microglia en los procesos patologicas. III. Naturaleza probable de la microglia. *Boletin de la Sociedad Espanola de Biologia*, **9**, 69-120.

del Rio-Hortega, P. & Penfield, W. (1928) Cerebral cicatrix: the reaction of neuroglia to brain wounds. *Archives of Neurology and Psychiatry (Chicago)*, **19**, 180-181.

del Rio-Hortega, P. (1932) Microglia in *Penfield's Cytology and Cellular Pathology of the Nervous System*, Vol. 2, pp. 483-534, Hoeber, New York.

de Robertis, E. & Bennett, H. S. D. (1954) Submicroscopic vesicular component in the synapse. *Federation Proceedings*, **13**, 35.

de Robertis, E. (1956) Submicroscopic changes of the synapse after nerve section in the acoustic ganglion of the guinea pig. An electron microscope study. *Journal of Biophysics, Biochemistry and Cytology*, **2**, 503-512.

de Robertis, E. (1958) Submicroscopic morphology and function of the synapse. *Experimental Cell Research*, Suppl. **5**, 347-369.

Robertson, J. D. (1961) The unit membrane in *Electron Microscopy in Anatomy* (Ed. Boyd, J. D. *et al.*) (Anatomical Society Symposium), pp. 74-99, Arnold, London.

Schmitt, F. O., Bear, R. S. & Clark, G. L. (1935) X-ray diffraction studies on nerve. *Radiology*, **25**, 131-151.

Schmidt, W. J. (1936) Doppelbrechung und Feinbau der Markscheide der Nervenfasern. *Zeitschrift für Zellforschung und mikroskopische Anatomie*, **23**, 657-676.

Smith, M. C. (1949) Metachromatic bodies in the brain. *Journal of Neurology, Neurosurgery and Psychiatry*, **12**, 100-110.

Smith, M. C. (1955) Argyrophile bodies in the human spinal cord. *Journal of Neurology, Neurosurgery and Psychiatry*, **18**, 13-16.

Smith, M. C. (1956) Observations on the extended use of the Marchi method. *Journal of Neurology, Neurosurgery and Psychiatry*, **19**, 67-78.

Smith, M. C., Strich, S. J. & Sharp, P. (1956) The value of the Marchi method for staining tissue stored in formalin for prolonged periods. *Journal of Neurology, Neurosurgery and Psychiatry*, **19**, 62-64.

Sperry, W. M. & Waelsch, H. (1950) Chemistry of myelination and demyelination. Multiple sclerosis and the demyelinating diseases. *Proceedings of the Association for Research in Nervous and Mental Disorders*, **18**, 255-267.

Spielmeyer, W. (1922) *Histopathologie des Nervensystems*, Springer Verlag, Berlin.

Stam, F. C. & Roukema, P. A. (1973) Histochemical and biochemical aspects of Corpora Amylacea. *Acta Neuropathologica (Berlin)*, **25**, 95-102.

Stewart, T. G. & Holmes, G. (1908) On the connection of the inferior olives with the cerebellum in man. *Brain*, **31**, 125-137.

Swank, R. L. (1940) Avian thiamine deficiency; correlation of pathology and clinical behaviour. *Journal of Experimental Medicine*, **71**, 683-702.

Swank, R. L. & Prados, M. (1942) Avian thiamine deficiency. II. Pathologic changes in the brain and cranial nerves (especially the vestibular) and their relation to the clinical behaviour. *Archives of Neurology and Psychiatry (Chicago)*, **47**, 97-131.

Waller, A. (1850) Experiments on the section of the glossopharyngeal and hypoglossal nerves of the frog, and observations of the alterations produced thereby in the structure of their primitive fibres. *Philosophical Transactions*, **140**, 423-429.

Weigert, C. (1895) Festschrift zum fünfzigjährigen Jubiläum des ärztlichen Vereins zu Frankfürt am Main.

Weiss, P. (1943) Nerve regeneration in rats following tubular splicing of second nerves. *Archives of Surgery*, **46**, 525-547.

Weiss, P. & Hiscoe, H. B.   (1948) Experiments on mechanism of nerve growth.   *Journal of Experimental Zoology*, **107**, 315-395.

Weiss, P.   (1967) Neuronal dynamics.   *Neurosciences Research Progress Bulletin*, **5**, 371-400.

Weiss, P. & Mayr, R.   (1971).   Neuronal organelles in neuroplasmic ('axonal') flow.   I. Mitochondria. II. Neurotubules.   *Acta Neuropathologica* (*Berlin*), Suppl. **5**, 187-206.

Weller, R. O., Wisniewski, H. & Shulman, K.   (1971) Experimental hydrocephalus in young dogs: histological and ultrastructural study of the brain tissue damage.   *Journal of Neuropathology and Experimental Neurology*, **30**, 613-627.

Weller, R. O. & Shulman, K.   (1972) Infantile hydrocephalus: clinical histological and ultrastructural study of brain damage.   *Journal of Neurosurgery*, **36**, 255-265.

Wickoff, R. G. W. & Young, J. Z.   (1956) Motorneuron surface.   *Proceedings of the Royal Society of London, Series B*, **144**, 440-450.

2

Cerebral Hypoxia

J. B. Brierley

The energy requirements of the brain demand adequate supplies of oxygen and glucose as well as certain amino acids, hormones and vitamins. All these are provided by the functions of respiration and circulation.

Respiration

At sea level the atmospheric pressure is 760 mm Hg, of which the partial pressure of oxygen is 149 mm Hg. The stream of oxygen from the atmosphere to the neuronal mitochondria can be envisaged as a cascade over five successive steps (Luft and Finkelstein 1968) (Fig. 2.1). Within the pulmonary alveoli the oxygen tension is reduced to 105 mm Hg because of the presence of carbon dioxide and water vapour. The small difference between the oxygen tensions in alveoli (105 mm Hg) and arterial blood (96 mm Hg) is not due to restricted diffusion from one to the other, but to venous admixture from bronchopulmonary veins and to a few pulmonary arteriovenous shunts. Within the vascular bed of the brain, oxygen tension falls to about 34 mm Hg in the veins and venous sinuses. This fall in oxygen tension takes place largely within the capillary bed.

Circulation

The normal adult brain receives about 15% of the cardiac output although the brain accounts for only 2·5% of the body weight. Expressed in other terms, the overall blood flow is about 45 ml/100 g/minute in the adult and about twice as high in children aged 6 years because of a higher respiratory rate (McIlwain 1966).

The oxygen content of blood falls from 19·6 ml/100 ml to 12·9 ml/100 ml while passing through the brain so that 6·7 ml of oxygen/100 ml blood

are used to meet the requirements of brain oxidative metabolism. The carbon dioxide content rises from 48·2 ml/100 ml in arterial blood to 54·8 ml/100 ml in the internal jugular vein, indicating a production by the brain of 6·6 ml CO_2/100 ml blood. Thus the respiratory quotient (CO_2/O_2) of the brain is almost unity, implying that glucose is the most likely source of energy by oxidation.

The maintenance of normal overall brain blood flow ('volume flow') is dependent upon cardiac output, systemic blood pressure and peripheral vascular resistance. Thus the supply of oxygen and substrate to the brain may be compromised by impairment of the action of the heart, by stenosis in the carotid and vertebral arteries in the neck, in the circle of Willis and its branches up to the arteriolar level and by any rise in central venous pressure. It must be emphasized, however, that at normal blood pressure the internal cross-sectional area of an artery must be reduced by up to 90% before blood flow is impaired (Tindall, Odom, Cupp and Dillon 1962; Fiddian, Byar and Edwards 1964). On the other hand a considerably smaller degree of stenosis can lead to a reduction in blood flow if the blood pressure falls. There is also evidence from angiographic studies (Kuhn 1962) that the 'velocity flow' of the blood in the vertebrobasilar arterial system is less than that in the carotid system, an observation which may be relevant to the greater involvement of the posterior portions of the cerebral hemispheres in most types of brain hypoxia.

Where the 'oxygen cascade' from atmosphere to venous blood is concerned, an impairment of circulation will be manifest as some reduction in brain venous oxygen tension and a widening of the brain arteriovenous oxygen difference (Fig.

2.1). While more oxygen is being removed from the slowly moving blood, carbon dioxide accumulates in the tissues. This partly compensates for the reduced amount of oxygen reaching the tissue by facilitating the dissociation of oxyhaemoglobin and ensuring maximal vasodilatation.

in blood flow. *Consumptive hypoxia* occurs when the oxygen requirements of hyperactive neurons exceed the available supply. *Asphyxia*, although meaning literally a pulseless state is seldom used in that sense, but is usually taken to mean suffocation (Van Liere and Stickney 1963). They

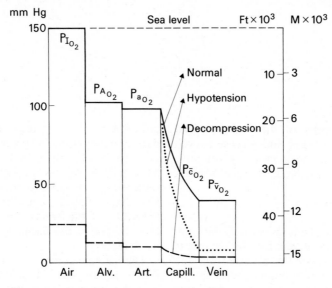

Fig. 2.1 The decrease in oxygen tension from inspired air to venous blood ('oxygen cascade', modified from Luft and Finkelstein 1968). Ordinate = P_{O_2} (mm Hg) and corresponding altitudes (feet and metres). Hypotension—venous oxygen tension is low as a result of reduced flow through capillary bed. Decompression—oxygen tension is reduced at each step from inspired air to venous blood.

The dependence of the brain upon glucose as its main oxidizable substrate contrasts with other body organs. Muscle oxidizes substances other than glucose when glucose is lacking; the brain has only a limited ability to do so. This is why cerebral function fails in hypoglycaemia rather than, for example, muscular function: coma ensues with the heart still beating (McIlwain 1966). The correspondence between the neuronal alterations due to hypoglycaemia and those due to hypoxia in all its forms, justifies the consideration of the former in this chapter on Brain Hypoxia.

Terminology
Anoxia implies an absence of oxygen in the inspired air or a total cessation of respiration. In *hypoxia* alveolar oxygen tension is reduced to some extent leading to a corresponding hypoxaemia. *Ischaemia* implies an arrest of flow within the whole or some part of the cerebral circulation and *oligaemia* implies some reduction

consider that the term asphyxia should be employed only when '. . . there is not only a hypoxia but also an increased carbon dioxide tension in the blood and tissues. Used in this sense, asphyxia is often a frequent consequence of hypoxia.'

The categories of brain hypoxia
These must be based upon the physiological considerations outlined above and are therefore similar to those of Barcroft (1925). These referred to the body as a whole and its literal application to the nervous system has limited justification. Thus, in the intact human subject or experimental animal, brain damage does not result from either uncomplicated hypoxic hypoxia or uncomplicated anaemic hypoxia (with the exception of carbon monoxide poisoning). Commonly, at least two of the several physiological factors upon which the classification is based are involved in any one case. Since 1925, other categories of brain hypoxia such as those due to the poisoning of

brain respiratory enzymes (histotoxic hypoxia) and the lack of the chief metabolic substrate, glucose, i.e. hypoglycaemia or oxyachrestic hypoxia have been added. Thus the following classification of brain hypoxia takes account of the views of Van Liere and Stickney (1963), Luft (1965) and Brierley (1972).

I. *Stagnant* (ischaemic and oligaemic)

A. Ischaemic—the brain or some portion of it is deprived of its blood supply.

B. Oligaemic—the brain or some portion of it receives a reduced supply of blood.

II. *Anoxic and hypoxic*

A. Anoxia—in the absence of oxygen in the pulmonary alveoli, there is anoxaemia and a little later anoxia in brain tissue.

B. Hypoxia—a reduced oxygen tension in the alveoli leads to brain tissue hypoxia through the medium of hypoxaemia.

III. *Anaemic*

As a result of a reduced haemoglobin content, the oxygen content of the blood is reduced while oxygen saturation and tension may be normal. This situation may be brought about by blood loss, and by iron-deficient or haemolytic anaemias. There is no evidence that uncomplicated anaemic hypoxia due to the above factors can lead to brain damage. Reports of such damage as a consequence of severe haemorrhage (Erbslöh 1958) usually include reference to pallidal necrosis, but are not documented in respect of the predictable fall in systemic blood pressure.

Carbon monoxide poisoning, by reducing the amount of circulating haemoglobin available to combine with oxygen, is the only example of anaemic hypoxia apparently capable of producing ischaemic alterations in grey and white matter.

IV. *Histotoxic* (Peters and Van Slyke 1932)

The oxygen tension and content of arterial blood are normal while those in brain venous blood are raised because the poisoning of brain respiratory enzymes results in a failure to utilize oxygen.

V. *Hypoglycaemia*

In spite of a normal arterial oxygen tension the brain is unable to utilize oxygen because of a deficiency of glucose (oxyachrestia; Lawrence, Meyer and Nevin 1942).

The neuronal alterations resulting from hypoxia

The identification of the neuronal alterations unequivocally attributable to hypoxia is critically dependent upon satisfactory fixation. This is because certain stages in the time course of hypoxic neuronal damage can be and often are confused with certain types of artefact. In the human brain, histological artefact is due partly to the autolysis that takes place between death and autopsy, partly to the slow penetration of the fixative in which the brain is immersed and partly to shortcomings in the processing of the tissue. While cytological appearances are virtually identical in optimally prepared celloidin and paraffin sections, artefact will occur particularly in the latter if dehydration is hurried, and will be most conspicuous in the infant brain because of its high water content (McIlwain 1966).

In experimental animals artefact arises most commonly from removal of the brain immediately after death and its immersion in a fixative. This procedure inevitably gives rise to neuronal hyperchromasia ('dark cells' Fig. 2.2) hydropic cell change ('water change' Fig. 2.3) perineuronal and perivascular spaces, (Scharrer 1938; Koenig and Koenig 1952; Cammermeyer 1961). All these artefacts are absent when the brain of a normal animal is fixed by intravascular perfusion *in vivo* and its removal is delayed according to the fixative used.

The use of perfusion-fixation has permitted the identification, with the light microscope, of unequivocal neuronal alterations in the primate brain 20 minutes after an episode of controlled hypoxia. For this reason, evidence from experimental primates is combined with that from the human brain in the following descriptions of the neuronal alterations due to hypoxia.

It must be recognized, however, that while immersion-fixation of the brain of a human subject of any age will obscure the earliest stages of hypoxic/ischaemic neuronal alterations because of histological artefact, it will not hinder the recognition of the later stages of the same process (after a survival of days or weeks) when they are characterized initially by a loss of nerve cells and eventually by a gliomesodermal reaction.

While the neuronal alterations in the several types of hypoxia are relatively stereotyped, there is great variation in their distribution, so that certain characteristic patterns can be recognized. This implies that, for the accurate delineation of the consequences of hypoxia in any one brain, the neuropathological examination should be based on a considerable number of large blocks which include neuro-anatomical features such as arterial boundary zones in the neocortex; the hippocampus at at least two levels; the major anatomical divisions of the basal ganglia; the brainstem (usually four or five levels) and spinal cord (at three or four levels) both cerebellar hemispheres and the vermis. The choice of embedding medium will be made according to personal experience and the available technical skills. Embedding in celloidin is slow but has the merits of ease of section-cutting and staining and also provides thick sections (15 to 30 μm) which permit the assessment of those minor reductions in neuronal populations which may escape recognition in thinner paraffin sections.

Ischaemic cell change
This term is applied to a process that begins with early and subtle alterations and ends with the disappearance of the neuron. Studies in experimental primates and in selected human material have shown that the time course of this alteration is constant for neurons according to their site (neocortex, hippocampus, cerebellum, etc.) and their size (e.g. small versus large pyramidal cells).

Thus in the absence of clinical information but given a histological preparation of good quality, the interval between a hypoxic episode and death can be predicted with reasonable accuracy in the brain of an experimental animal. In the human brain, however, the corresponding prediction will be less accurate.

The earliest stage of ischaemic cell change is *microvacuolation*, a term introduced by Brown and Brierley (1966) to describe neuronal alterations in the rat brain when unilateral interruption of blood flow in one common carotid artery was followed by intermittent exposure to nitrogen (Levine 1960).

Microvacuolation has also been observed in the primate brain after profound arterial hypotension, hypoglycaemia (Brierley, Brown and Meldrum 1971*a*, *b*) and periods of status epilepticus (Meldrum and Brierley 1973); and also in the brains of human subjects dying 1 hour after cardiac arrest and 3 to 4 hours after open-heart surgery (Brierley, unpublished cases).

The contour of the nerve cell is unaltered and the dimensions and staining properties of the nucleus and nucleolus are normal. Small, apparently empty spherical bodies or microvacuoles (diameter 0·16 to 2·5 μm) are present in the cytoplasm and in the proximal portions of the axon and dendrites (Fig. 2·4*a* and *b*). The cytoplasm either stains normally with all dyes or exhibits some increased staining with cresyl violet, slight eosinophilia and a pale blue or mauve colour with Luxol fast blue.

In general, microvacuolation can be seen earlier and persists for a shorter time in small neurons than in large in which it can be seen up to about 4 hours. Microvacuolation has been seen in the Purkinje cells up to 2 hours after a period of hypoxia in experimental primates and in a human subject surviving one hour after cardiac arrest.

Electron-microscopic studies have shown that most microvacuoles are expanded mitochondria which, while retaining their double limiting membrane, show considerable disorganization of the cristae (Fig. 2.5). A few microvacuoles correspond to dilated tubules and cisternae of the endoplasmic reticulum (McGee-Russell, Brown and Brierley 1970; Brown and Brierley 1971).

The stage of simple *ischaemic cell change* (Fig. 2.6) follows that of microvacuolation and has been described and illustrated by Spielmeyer (1922) and Greenfield and Meyer (1963). In a pyramidal neuron the cell body is shrunken and, together with the proximal portions of the axon and dendrites, stains darkly with aniline dyes,

Fig. 2.2 Normal rat. Brain removed immediately after death and immersed in formalin. Hippocampus showing 'dark cells'. Paraffin; cresyl violet. × 300.

Fig. 2.3 *M. mulatta*. Incomplete perfusion fixation. Cerebral cortex showing 'hydropic cell change' with peripheral vacuolation of cytoplasm. Paraffin; cresyl violet and Luxol fast blue. × 500.

Fig. 2.4 Rat. (*a*) Perfusion fixation ½ hour after 40 minutes' intermittent exposure to nitrogen with interruption of one common carotid artery. Ipsilateral hippocampus showing microvacuolation of neuronal cytoplasm and normal nuclei. Paraffin; cresyl violet. × 500.

(*b*) Perfusion fixation with glutaraldehyde immediately after 15 minutes' intermittent exposure to nitrogen. Microvacuolation in pyramidal neurons of hippocampus. Epon; toluidine blue. × 1500.

Fig. 2.5 Rat preparation as in Fig. 2.4*b*. Perfusion fixation with glutaraldehyde 1 hour after 40 minutes' intermittent exposure to nitrogen. Electronmicrograph of hippocampal pyramidal neuron. Expanded mitochondria with disorganised cristae lie within a perikaryon that shows some increase in matrix density. There is dilatation of both smooth and granular endoplasmic reticulum. The nucleus shows irregular shrinkage and some increase in electron density. × 5000.

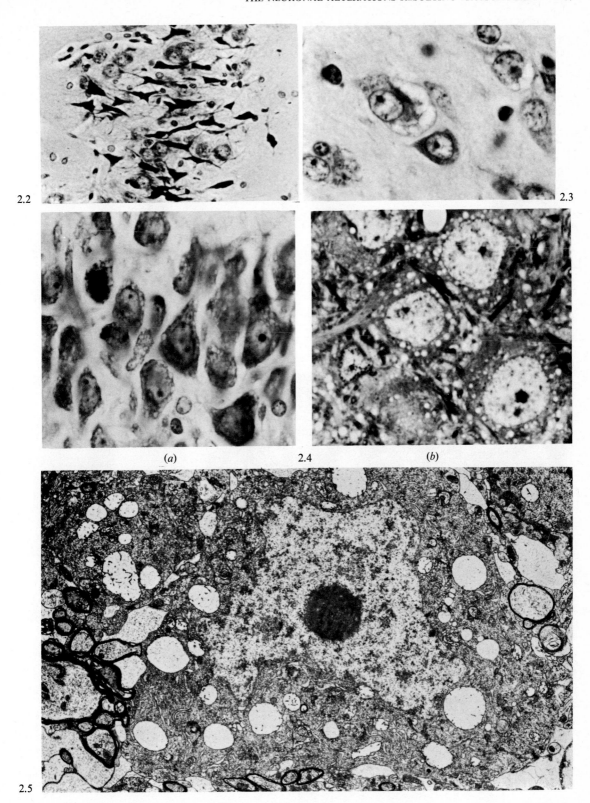

2.2

2.3

(a)   2.4   (b)

2.5

and the Nissl substance is dispersed and finely granular. The presence of microvacuoles indicates a transitional stage from that of microvacuolation (Fig. 2.7). The cytoplasm usually stains a vivid pink with eosin and from bright blue to dark mauve with Luxol fast blue. The nucleus is triangular, it stains more or less intensively with aniline dyes (so that the nucleolus may be almost invisible), and a dark blue with Luxol fast blue (Fig. 2.6). It should be noted that blue-staining of the nucleus may precede any alterations in the cytoplasm. At this stage the nucleolus may be swollen.

Simple ischaemic cell change can be identified in the brains of experimental primates from 30 minutes to 4 hours after a hypoxic episode and it

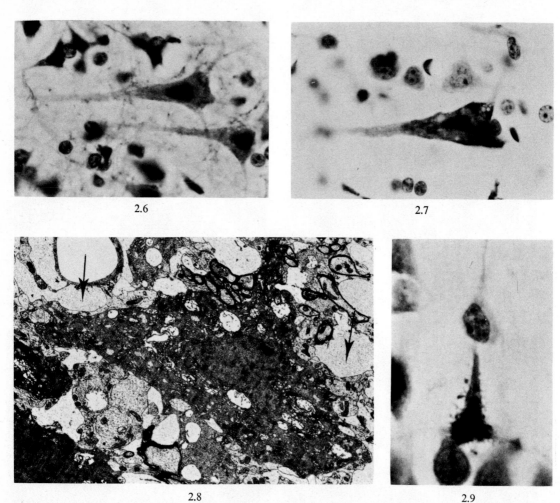

2.6   2.7

2.8   2.9

Fig. 2.6 *M. mulatta.* Perfusion fixation 2 hours after hypotensive episode. Ischaemic cell change in pyramidal neuron of cerebral cortex. Within the slightly shrunken soma, there is loss of Nissl substance and the nucleus is triangular and darkly stained. Paraffin; cresyl violet and Luxol fast blue. × 800.

Fig. 2.7 *M. mulatta.* Perfusion fixation 1½ hours after hypotensive episode. Ischaemic cell change in pyramidal neuron of cerebral cortex. A few microvacuoles can be seen in the cytoplasm. Paraffin; cresyl violet. × 800.

Fig. 2.8 Rat preparation as in Fig. 2.4*b*. Survival 1 hour after 40 minutes' intermittent exposure to nitrogen. Electron-micrograph of hippocampal pyramidal neuron showing marked increase in electron density of nucleus and perikaryon. There are some swollen mitochondria and some expansion of the cisternae and vesicles of the Golgi complex. This is the equivalent of ischaemic cell change. Note the expanded astrocytic processes (arrows) around the neuron and a blood vessel. × 3700.

Fig. 2.9 *Papio papio.* Perfusion fixation 3 hours after status epilepticus. Ischaemic cell change with incrustations in small pyramidal neuron of cerebral cortex. Paraffin; cresyl violet and Luxol fast blue. × 275.

evolves more rapidly in small than in large neurons: In the human brain this stage persists for at least 6 hours.

The electron-micrographic appearances of ischaemic cell change consist of an increased electron density of the cytoplasm which may contain a small number of expanded mitochondria (residual microvacuoles) within which the remnants of cristae can be identified. There is also variable aggregation of free ribosomes and of ribosomal rosettes. The cisternae of the granular endoplasmic reticulum are swollen and the Golgi complex is also dilated (Fig. 2.8). As in the previous stage, the perineuronal and peri-vascular spaces correspond to expanded astrocytic processes.

The succeeding stage of *ischaemic cell change with incrustations* is characterized by further shrinkage of the neuronal cytoplasm while some degree of pink staining with eosin and blue staining with Luxol fast blue remains. Typical incrustations are spherical or irregular bodies lying on or close to the surface of the cell body and the apical dendrite (Fig. 2.9). At this stage in the smaller stellate and polymorphic neurons the cytoplasm is greatly reduced or even absent and the shrunken dark-staining nucleus may persist for three or four days. The incrustations

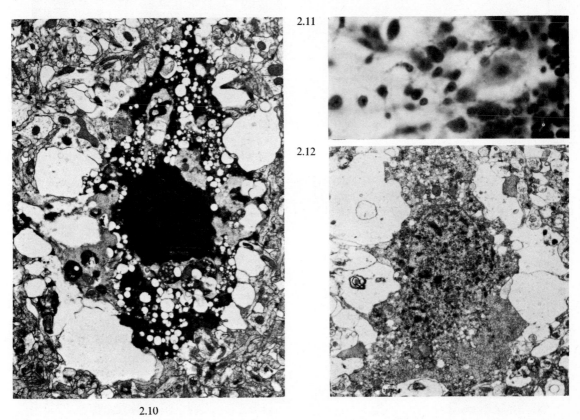

2.11

2.12

2.10

Fig. 2.10 Rat preparation as in Fig. 2.4*b*. Survival 2 hours after 40 minutes' intermittent exposure to nitrogen. Electron-micrograph of neocortical pyramidal neuron. Around the nucleus the vacuolated electron-dense cytoplasm contrasts with less dense membrane-limited areas. Some of the electron-dense portions of the perikaryon and dendrites correspond to the incrustations of the light microscope. The neuron is surrounded by swollen astrocytic processes.   × 5800.

Fig. 2.11 Male aged 60 years dying 48 hours after hypotensive episode during anaesthesia. Cerebellum, showing homogenizing change in a Purkinje cell. The cell is shrunken and lacks Nissl substance. The nucleus is shrunken and dark-staining. Celloidin; cresyl violet.   × 300.

Fig. 2.12 Rat preparation as in Fig. 2.4*b*. Survival 24 hours after 40 minutes' intermittent exposure to nitrogen. Electron-micrograph of neocortical pyramidal neuron showing that the electron density of nucleus and perikaryon is less than at the 'incrusted' stage (Fig. 2.10). Normal organelles are not recognisable and the origin of the various spaces cannot be decided. The greater part of the cytoplasm is occupied by granular material of moderate electron density. This is the equivalent of homogenizing cell change.   × 4200.

usually persist longer than the remnants of the cytoplasm.

The salient fine structural feature of the incrusted nerve cell is marked electron density of the nucleus within which the nucleolus is often indistinguishable. The cytoplasm is usually of comparable electron density and is invaginated by the swollen processes of astrocytes. Dense areas of cytoplasm occurring in the periphery of the perikaryon and in the cell processes are the counterparts of the incrustations seen with the light microscope (Fig. 2.10). Vacuoles of various sizes probably represent dilated cisternae and vesicles of smooth and granular endoplasmic reticulum and the remains of swollen mitochondria. Axosomatic synaptic contacts are

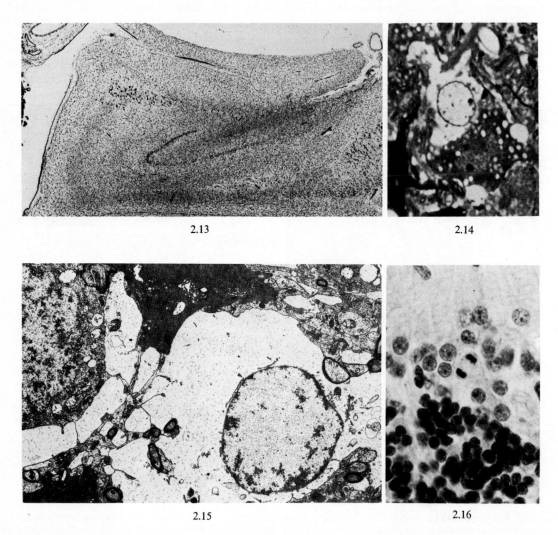

2.13

2.14

2.15

2.16

Fig. 2.13 Sclerosis of the hippocampus in a life-long epileptic. The structure is reduced in size, intensely gliosed and neurons remain only in h_2. Celloidin; cresyl violet. ×18.

Fig. 2.14 Rat preparation as in Fig. 2.4b. Survival 1 hour after 40 minutes' intermittent exposure to nitrogen. Hippocampus showing an astrocyte with vesicular nucleus and expanded clear cytoplasm and processes adjacent to a pyramidal neuron showing microvacuolation. Epon; cresyl violet. ×1150.

Fig. 2.15 Rat preparation as in Fig. 2.4b. Survival 1 hour after 40 minutes' intermittent exposure to nitrogen. Electromicrograph showing an astrocyte with normal nucleus but expanded and watery cytoplasm adjacent to neurons showing ischaemic change. ×3700.

Fig. 2.16 *M. mulatta*. Perfusion fixation 5 days after subatmospheric decompression. Mitotic figure in Bergmann astrocyte. Celloidin; cresyl violet. ×550.

usually recognizable and may be normal apart from the great density of the post-synaptic membrane. In some there may be depletion and dissolution of synaptic vesicles or other evidence of degeneration.

At the next stage the nerve cell, with a uniformly eosinophilic cytoplasm and a shrunken triangular nucleus exhibits *homogenizing cell change* which is well seen in the Purkinje cells of the cerebellum (Fig. 2.11).

In electron micrographs homogenizing cell change is characterized by a decreased electron density of nucleus and cytoplasm (Fig. 2.12). The two nuclear membranes may be separated by finely granular material which can escape into the cytoplasm when the outer membrane ruptures. Dense mitochondria recognizable in the cytoplasm consist of heterogeneous debris embedded in a granular matrix. Other areas of cytoplasm have a more homogeneous character. The periphery of the perikaryon is invaginated by swollen astrocytic processes.

The associated glial and mesodermal reactions

While the time course of the neuronal alterations following a critical period of hypoxia of any type is rapid, the greater part of the macroglial and the whole of the microglial and mesodermal reactions take place after neurons have been irreversibly damaged (i.e. after the stage of microvacuolation) and may continue for days, weeks or even months. These reactions are more or less proportional to the extent of neuronal destruction, so that a particular population of neurons having suffered up to total destruction is replaced by a slowly shrinking volume of glial and mesodermal elements.

After an ill-defined period of time a region of selective neuronal destruction is slowly transformed into one of sclerosis as in certain laminae of the neocortex, in the hippocampus (Fig. 2.13) and in the basolateral portions of the amygdaloid nuclei. Infarction of nervous tissue after a period of hypoxia other than ischaemic is relatively rare.

As neuronal microvacuolation (MV) proceeds, some affected neurones may be partly surrounded by apparently empty spaces and so may nearby blood vessels. In well fixed material these perineuronal and perivascular spaces are subdivided by fine trabeculae (Fig. 2.14). Electron-microscope studies in the brains of rats and monkeys have shown that these spaces are the expanded and

electronlucent processes of *astrocytes* within which the mitochondria are usually normal (Brown and Brierley 1971, 1972, 1973) (Fig. 2.15).

Some increase in the diameter of astrocytic nuclei close to damaged neurons can be seen with the light microscope 2 to 12 hours after a period of hypoxia and proliferation of astrocytes by mitotic division attains a maximum frequency after 4 to 6 days in most vulnerable regions. In the cerebellum mitotic figures are particularly conspicuous among the Bergmann astrocytes (Fig. 2.16). In each region the products of astrocytic mitotic division are of fibrous type, and after 10 to 15 days the mitotic division of astrocytes is rarely seen.

While the extent of neuronal destruction and that of astrocytic proliferation are usually proportional, it must be borne in mind that, when hypoxic damage attains the level of infarction with total destruction of neurons, glia and even blood vessels, the associated astrocytic proliferation is then restricted to the periphery of the necrotic region (Fig. 2.17). When the damage is of lesser degree, fibrous astrocytes proliferate and their processes, together with collagen and reticulin fibres derived from mesodermal sources, contribute to the formation of a glio-mesodermal network within which occasional neurons may survive.

Alterations in the *oligodendrocytes* within a region of hypoxic damage are slight and seldom more than the 'acute swelling' described in this and in many other situations by Penfield and Cone (1926). However, this type of cell change is not only non-specific but may also be artefactual, if only because it is hardly ever seen in comparable regions of hypoxic damage in the brains of experimental primates fixed by perfusion *in vivo*.

The intrinsic or indigenous *microglia*, where hypoxic damage is purely neuronal, are transformed into rod cells (Stäbchenzellen) which are characteristically orientated at right angles to the pial surface of the neocortex, radially within the hippocampus (Fig. 2.18) and in the molecular layer of the cerebellum and more or less haphazardly in the basal ganglia and brainstem. After a survival of two or three days, fine lipid droplets may be seen in the cytoplasm and a little later division by mitosis takes place (Fig. 2.19a and b). The daughter cells develop into typical lipid phagocytes (Fig. 2.20) which may have no obvious relationship to nerve cells and are probably involved in the removal of myelin debris. Others lying close to the surfaces of dead neurons divide mitotically so that the original contour of the nerve cell becomes outlined by a capsule of microglial cells and lipid phagocytes—the stage of neuronophagy (Fig. 2.21).

When hypoxic damage is restricted to nerve

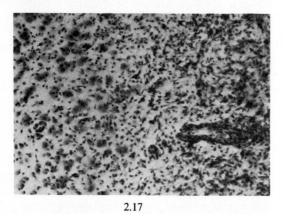

2.17

sole source of lipid phagocytes (Figs. 2.22, 2.23). Similar lipid phagocytes are also derived from the pia mater.

Whatever their origin, there is little evidence to show that lipid phagocytes migrate actively from the sites of their formation. Thus their number and the pattern of their distribution after protracted survivals mirror the original destruction of tissue. If the latter was virtually restricted to a neocortical lamina, the distribution of lipid phagocytes will be correspondingly laminar (Fig. 2.24). If the initial hypoxic damage attained the level of infarction, lipid phagocytes will not reflect any particular pattern.

Associated alterations in white matter

When hypoxic damage is restricted to a small proportion of a vulnerable neuronal population there is only a limited destruction of the intrinsic nerve fibres and no primary alteration in the surrounding white matter. With increasing

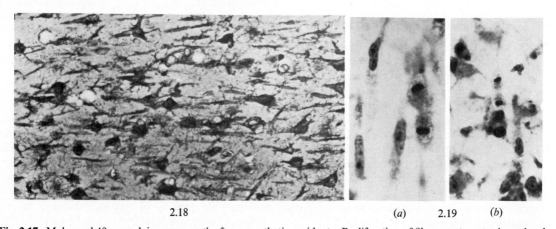

2.18   (a)   2.19   (b)

Fig. 2.17 Male aged 40 years dying one month after anaesthetic accident. Proliferation of fibrous astrocytes in molecular layer of cortex. Intense gliomesodermal reaction in deeper layers. Celloidin; cresyl violet. × 120.
Fig. 2.18 *M. Mulatta.* Perfusion fixation 7 days after subatmospheric decompression. Hippocampus showing radially arranged rod cells between pyramidal neurons. Paraffin; silver impregnation. × 450.
Fig. 2.19 (*a* and *b*) Same animal as Fig. 2.18. Hippocampus showing mitotic figures in rod cells. Paraffin; cresyl violet. × 650.

cells, the blood vessels may appear entirely normal and there is no evidence of escape of any haematogenous element into the tissue.

However, the intrinsic microglial cells are not the only source of lipid phagocytes in a region of hypoxic damage. When this attains the level of infarction only the peripheral arteries may be preserved. It is then evident that certain elements in the adventitia of the latter can be the

neuronal destruction some pallor of myelin staining becomes apparent in the adjacent white matter. After a survival of a week or more, lipid phagocytes can be identified and in the extreme situation of subtotal cortical destruction (a rare sequel of circulatory arrest) virtually the whole of each centrum semiovale may be occupied by lipid phagocytes showing some accumulation around blood vessels (Fig. 2.25). Myelin stains

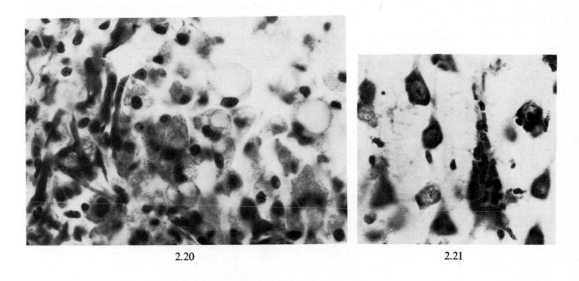

2.20   2.21

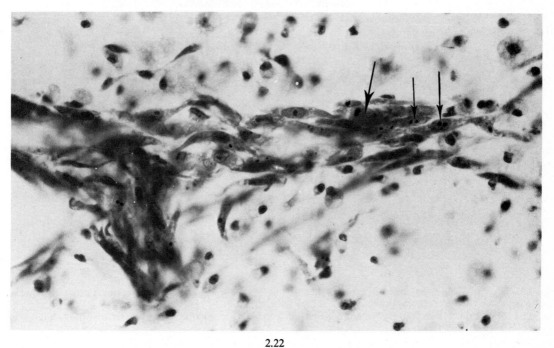

2.22

Fig. 2.20 *M. mulatta*. Perfusion fixation 7 days after severe hypotension. Lipid phagocytes in a cortical boundary zone lesion. The cytoplasm is variably foamy and vacuolated. Celloidin; cresyl violet and Luxol fast blue. × 900.

Fig. 2.21 *M. mulatta*. Perfusion fixation 7 days after subatmospheric decompression. A hippocampal pyramidal neuron is virtually surrounded by microglial nuclei, the process of neuronophagy. Celloidin; cresyl violet. × 1100.

Fig. 2.22 *M. mulatta*. Perfusion fixation 7 days after severe hypotension. Boundary zone lesion showing proliferation of fusiform cells derived from vascular adventitia. The nuclei contain two centrosomes (small arrows). Mitotic division (large arrow) gives rise to lipid phagocytes. Celloidin; cresyl violet and Luxol fast blue. × 1300.

may show only a moderate degree of pallor while fat is readily demonstrable and the Holzer method will reveal the associated dense isomorphic fibrous gliosis. In the corpus callosum myelin destruction is usually greater in the posterior half or third. After survivals of weeks or months Wallerian degeneration may be seen in the corticospinal

after cardiac arrest, hypoglycaemia, neonatal hypoxaemia and carbon disulphide and sodium nitrite intoxication.

Primary hypoxic alterations in white matter may be either diffuse or focal. In the diffuse form there is demyelination in each centrum semiovale, spreading from the periventricular region out into

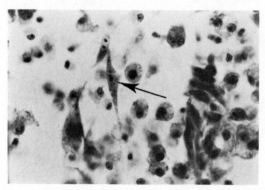

2.23

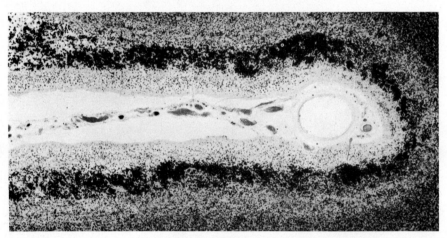

2.24

Fig. 2.23 Same animal as Fig. 2.22. The foamy cytoplasm of the adventitial cell (arrow) resembles that of the nearby lipid phagocytes. Celloidin; cresyl violet and Luxol fast blue. × 1200.

Fig. 2.24 Male, aged 17 years, dying 9 months after cardiac arrest. Occipital lobe showing laminar disposition of lipid phagocytes. Celloidin; Marchi. × 15.

tracts as a consequence of neuronal destruction in the precentral gyri (Fig. 2.26).

While the primary damage to myelinated fibres which is often seen after carbon monoxide and cyanide intoxications will be described under those headings, it is important to emphasize that such damage is not specific. Brucher (1967) pointed out that major white matter damage may be seen

the digital white matter of the convolutions but usually sparing the subcortical U-fibres. The corpus callosum, anterior commissure and white matter of the cerebellum may also be involved. Sometimes there is a relative preservation of myelin around blood vessels giving an overall speckled or 'thrush breast' appearance. After survival of only a few days, the region of myelin destruction presents a spongy and often finely cystic texture and, in cases with longer survival, the small cysts may become confluent to form larger ones, which may be visible to the naked eye in the brain slice.

Focal demyelination is seen as fairly circumscribed areas of demyelination of various sizes within which destruction of myelin is virtually complete and the lesion is eventually filled with lipid phagocytes.

Although figures are not available, major involvement of the white matter as a direct sentative sample. Another is that neurons differ widely in their susceptibility to hypoxia. Those that are susceptible are found within a general pattern of structures some or all of which are involved in all categories of hypoxia. Relatively subtle variations within this general pattern of selectively vulnerable regions represent the neuropathology of each category.

Although differences between nerve cells in their susceptibility to a lack of oxygen were appreciated by the end of the last century, the elaboration of the concept of selective vulnera-

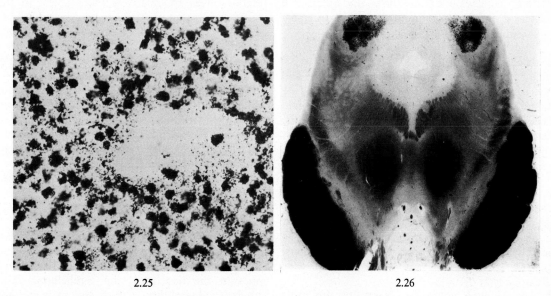

2.25   2.26

Fig. 2.25 Male, aged 42 years, dying 8 months after severe hypotension. Perivascular accumulation of lipid phagocytes in white matter. Celloidin; Marchi. × 450.
Fig. 2.26 Male, aged 17 years, dying 9 months after cardiac arrest. Midbrain. Marchi positive staining in cerebral peduncles indicates Wallerian degeneration in tracts descending from neurons destroyed at higher levels. Celloidin; Marchi.

sequel of circulatory arrest, systemic hypotension and hypoglycaemia is unusual.

'Selective vulnerability' within the brain—morphological aspects

The neuropathological consequences of hypoxia in any one case are a function of the number of cellular elements damaged or destroyed and also of the survival time. A correct assessment of the alterations in the brain as a whole can only be derived from the study of many regions. The great complexity of brain anatomy is one reason why there can be no such thing as a fully repre-

bility to hypoxia has been due, in particular to Spielmeyer (1925), Scholz (1953, 1963) and Meyer (1936, 1956, 1963).

There is also an order of vulnerability to hypoxia within the several cytological elements of the nervous system. 'In general the nerve cells are the most sensitive elements in a state of oxygen deficiency. They are followed by oligodendroglia and astrocytes while the microglia and the cellular elements of the vessels are the least vulnerable' (Jacob 1963).

Where neurons are concerned the phylogenetically older portions of the nervous system are more resistant than the newer. Thus the grey matter of the spinal cord and the greater part of that in the brainstem may be undamaged in the presence of almost total destruction of the cerebral cortex.

The pattern of 'selective vulnerability'
The neocortex
Damage is usually greater in the parietal and occipital lobes and decreases towards the temporal and frontal poles. Within any lobe hypoxic damage is commonly greater around sulci than over the crests of gyri. Among the cortical layers the third is most vulnerable, the fifth and sixth are somewhat less and the second and fourth (external and internal granular) layers are most resistant.

Allocortex (3 layers)
The convexities of the *para-hippocampal gyri* and the islets of Calleja on their dorsal surfaces are remarkably resistant to hypoxia. The entorhinal region, interposed between the islets and the Sommer sector (h. 1) of the hippocampus, is often involved in continuity with ischaemic damage in the latter.

Within the hippocampus (Ammon's horn or cornu ammonis) the Sommer sector (h. 1) and the endfolium (h. 3 to 5) are the most vulnerable, while h. 2 is often referred to as the 'resistant zone'. The fascia dentata (dentate gyrus) is the least vulnerable component of the hippocampus.

Basal ganglia
In the *striatum* ischaemic alterations are most frequent within the outer halves of the head and body of the caudate nucleus and in the outer half of the putamen. In each, the small polymorphic cells are more vulnerable than the larger pyramidal elements. In addition to the special case of carbon monoxide intoxication (see below) damage in the *pallidum* may occur in all types of hypoxia. There is no evidence for an intrinsic difference between the vulnerabilities of the two segments. Primary hypoxic damage in the *thalamus* is commonest in the anterior nuclear complexes, followed closely by the dorsomedial nuclei (parvocellular portions) and the lateral angles of the ventrolateral nuclei. Involvement of the centromedian nuclei is infrequent and the sensory relay nuclei, together with the midline and intralaminar nuclei, may be regarded as the most resistant in the thalamus. Alterations in the geniculate bodies are also unusual and when

present usually involve the lateral. In the *amygdaloid nucleus* the more superficial or corticomedial portion is resistant and the deeper or basolateral portion is relatively vulnerable; damage in the latter is usually associated with severe ischaemic alterations in the hippocampus.

The supraoptic, paraventricular and lateral nuclei of the *hypothalamus* are very rarely affected by hypoxia. Alterations in the mamillary bodies are rare in adults but frequent in infants and young children.

In the adult *brainstem* the reticular zones of the substantia nigrae, the inferior colliculi and the inferior olives are relatively vulnerable. In the infant and young child there may be additional ischaemic alterations in the oculomotor, the spinal nuclei of the fifth nerves, the cochlear and vestibular nuclei, the nuclei ambiguii and the nuclei gracili and cuneati in the lower medulla.

Among the neuronal constituents of the three layers of the *cerebellar cortex* the Purkinje and basket cells are most vulnerable to the effects of hypoxia. They are followed by the granule cells while the Golgi cells are the most resistant. Alterations in the dentate nuclei and in the roof nuclei are usually considerably less than those in the Purkinje cells.

Arterial boundary zones
As a consequence of a rapid and considerable reduction in cerebral perfusion pressure ischaemic alterations may be seen along the arterial boundary zones in the neocortex and cerebellum. The apparent vulnerability of these regions is due not to any peculiarity of architecture or blood supply but to a local haemodynamic disturbance (see p. 62).

Stagnant hypoxia

Ischaemic hypoxia in the central nervous system as a whole
The sequence of events following abrupt and total interruption of the human cerebral circulation was described by Rossen, Kabat and Anderson (1943). Five seconds after inflation of a pneumatic pressure cuff around the neck, the eyes became fixed in the midline, the visual fields narrowed sometimes to the point of blindness and consciousness was lost at the 6th second. From the start of nitrogen over-breathing (anoxic anoxia) consciousness is lost at 17 to 20 seconds.

The period of 6 seconds represents the oxygen reserve of the tissue while the additional 11 to 14 seconds is made up of the circulation time between heart and brain and the time required for the blood to become desaturated.

In the clinical situation a cessation of brain circulation occurs only in the event of systemic circulatory arrest. If not deliberate, as in open heart surgery under hypothermia, this is usually due to cardiac asystole or ventricular fibrillation and is most commonly a complication of surgery under general anaesthesia at normal body temperature. Cardiac arrest accounted for 212 deaths in the series of 517,151 anaesthetics (i.e. 1 in 2384) surveyed by Stephenson, Reid and Hinton (1953) and for 199 deaths in the series of 600,000 (i.e. 1 in 3018) reported by Beecher and Todd (1954), both series coming from the USA. Corresponding figures for the United Kingdom are not available as such cases are registered only as 'anaesthetic deaths'. Milstein (1956) has estimated that cardiac arrest related to surgery is the cause of about 300 deaths a year in Great Britain. The incidence is slightly higher in males than in females (6 : 4) and 20% of all cases occur during the first decade of life. While the nature of the anaesthetic agent may influence the frequency of cardiac arrest there is no convincing evidence that any one anaesthetic is associated with a specific neuropathological picture.

The great majority of cases, 87% according to Stephenson *et al.* (1953), die within 24 hours of the cardiac arrest and in their series of 1200 cases only 8 endured protracted survival in a 'decerebrate state'.

In the human subject, cardiac arrest is usually an unexpected emergency so that its precise duration is seldom known and serial records of even heart rate and blood pressure before and after the event are virtually non-existent. Cardiac arrest may be preceded and is often initiated by a period of hypoxaemia which may reduce cardiac output and cerebral blood flow. Eventually, sinus rhythm is restored either spontaneously, after defibrillation or after some period of internal or external cardiac massage. Even then some time may elapse before cardiac output returns to a normal level. Thus, in any one case there will be a varying proportion between the period of true circulatory arrest and that comprising the preceding and the succeeding periods of reduced brain blood flow. The ultimate neuropathological picture will reflect this proportion.

If circulatory arrest was of abrupt onset and termination and lasted more than 3 to 4 minutes at normal body temperatures the brain damage will be generalized within neocortex and cerebellum but variable in the basal ganglia. On the other hand, if a shorter period of circulatory arrest was preceded and/or followed by appreciable periods of reduced cerebral blood flow, the neuropathological alterations within at least the neocortex and cerebellum will show accentuation along the arterial boundary zones. Such accentuation is a feature characteristic of the brain damage due to severe arterial hypotension (see p. 62).

Macroscopic appearances of the brain
These depend on the extent of the initial neuronal destruction and on the survival time.

Within the first few days the brain may appear normal externally and also after cutting. In a minority of cases there may be some evidence of brain swelling, such as flattening of the neocortical gyri, prominence of the unci and slight herniation of the parahippocampal gyri and of the cerebellar tonsils. Haemorrhage in the brainstem has not been reported and infarction of the calcarine cortex is rare (seen in 1 out of 30 personal cases). The ventricular system may be narrowed.

When survival is for 36 hours or more it may be possible to discern laminar or patchy cortical discoloration around sulci, particularly in the parietal and occipital lobes.

With survival for longer periods there may be an appreciable reduction in the weight of the brain, some milky opacity of the leptomeninges and evidence of atrophy of the cortical gyri and cerebellar folia, all of which may present a more or less granular surface. In coronal slices ventricular enlargement is slight after survival for a few weeks but may be considerable when it is months or years (Fig. 2.27). There is a parallel reduction in the width of the cortical ribbon with increasing survival times and this is most marked in the parietal and occipital lobes. An intracortical band of necrosis of variable width is often visible. It may appear grey and gelatinous or take the form of an apparently empty slit separating the outer and inner layers of the cortex or all the cortical layers from the white matter (Fig. 2.28). While the parahippocampal gyri are usually relatively well preserved, the hippocampi present various degrees of shrinkage and a cres-

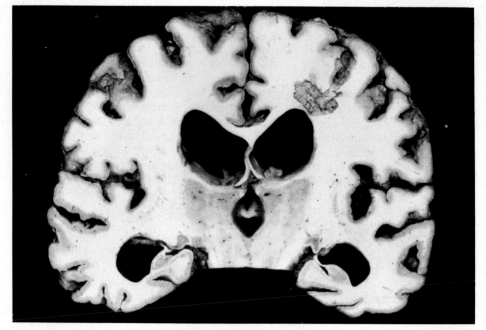

2.27

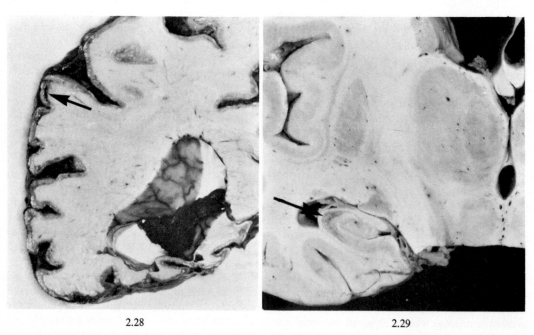

2.28   2.29

Fig. 2.27 Male, aged 48 years, dying 5 months after cardiac arrest. Brain slice showing cortical necrosis and enlargement of third and lateral ventricles.

Fig. 2.28 Male, aged 58 years, dying 5 months after cardiac arrest. Brain slice showing slit (arrow) at cortex-white matter junction.

Fig. 2.29 Same case as Fig. 2.28. The Sommer sector (arrow) of the hippocampus appears as a crescent of spongy tissue.

centic slit may be seen within each Sommer sector (h. 1) (Fig. 2.29).

Macroscopic alterations in the basal ganglia are unusual if survival is for less than 36 hours. Thereafter there may be patchy discoloration in the outer half of the head and body of the caudate nucleus and in the upper third of the putamen. There may be some orange-brown discoloration of the globus pallidus.

Even when neocortical destruction is severe the thalami may appear grossly normal when survival is for only a few weeks. Sometimes patchy discoloration may be seen in the anterior nuclear complexes, the dorsomedial nuclei and in the upper halves of the ventrolateral nuclei. With increasing survival times there is a gradual shrinkage of the thalami and in particular each pulvinar may become narrow and wedge-shaped. Neocortical destruction may eventually add an element of retrograde neuronal degeneration in the corresponding thalamic association nuclei.

In the amygdaloid nuclei, the corticomedial portions usually appear normal while the basolateral portions may show variable shrinkage and sometimes focal discoloration.

In the adult brainstem, after protracted survival, there may be some flattening of the ventral aspect of the pons, narrowing of the medullary pyramids and variable shrinkage of the inferior olives. In the infant and young child it may be possible to detect shrinkage and discoloration in the inferior colliculi, the spinal nuclei of the fifth nerves and in the nuclei gracili and cuneati.

Macroscopic alterations in the cerebellum may be recognizable after survival for 4 to 10 days and take the form of softening of the deeper folia over the dorsal aspects and posterior borders of the hemispheres and vermis. After survival for weeks or months the damaged folia are sclerotic, the central white matter is reduced in volume and the dentate nuclei appear shrunken and grey-brown in colour.

Microscopic appearances
The involvement of the 'selectively vulnerable' regions of the brain can be seen to its fullest extent in certain instances of circulatory arrest. The neuropathological changes after a few hours' to several months' survival have been presented by Desmarest and L'Hermitte (1939), Weinberger, Gibbon and Gibbon (1940), Courville (1954), Neubuerger (1954), Mandel and Berry (1959),

Lapresle and Milhaud (1962), Brierley (1965), Brierley, Adams, Graham and Simpson (1971), Amann, Gerstenbrand and Jellinger (1971).

When survival is from a few hours to a few days, microscopic alterations contrast with the macroscopic normality of the brain before and after slicing. They consist of ischaemic cell change and the earliest stages of glial and mesodermal reactions.

The *cerebral cortex* examined at low magnification may appear normal. At higher magnification some stage of ischaemic cell change is recognizable. Microvacuolation (p. 46) has been seen in small and large pyramidal neurons after survival for 1 hour (personal case). After survival for 4 to 12 hours, typical ischaemic cell change, with and without incrustations, and also early homogenizing change are readily identifiable. Damage is usually greatest in the parietal and occipital lobes and decreases towards the temporal and frontal poles (Fig. 2.30a and b).

With increasing length of survival, the loss of neurons is accompanied by a gliomesodermal reaction, the picture ranging from minor necrosis within a single lamina up to almost total cortical destruction. In the latter situation, some neurons in the second and fourth layers may survive and there is usually a marked proliferation of fibrous astrocytes in the molecular layer. Attention must be drawn to those exceptional cases in which a total destruction of the 5th and 6th cortical layers results in a virtual isolation of the outer neocortical layers from the subjacent white matter. In spite of the apparent normality of the neurons in these layers, the EEG is universally isoelectric (Amann *et al.* 1971; Brierley, Adams *et al.* 1971; Ingvar and Brun 1972).

The hippocampus. This structure may show any stage and degree of ischaemic damage (Fig. 2.31) but total infarction of the Sommer sector (h. 1) and of the endfolium (h. 3 to 5) is rare. The gliomesodermal reaction is, as elsewhere, proportional to the extent of neuronal destruction. When the latter is minor, a few lipid phagocytes lie within a loose network of glial fibres which are particularly well developed in the endfolium (h. 3 to 5).

The amygdaloid nucleus. Ischaemic alterations most frequently involve the basolateral portion and when they are severe and survival is long, this portion may be considerably reduced in size with a corresponding expansion of the tip of the inferior horn of the ventricle.

Caudate nucleus and putamen. Involvement of these structures is common but by no means invariable. It ranges from a destruction of some of the smaller neurons along the upper borders (Fig. 2.32) to total necrosis with cyst formation after long survival.

Globus pallidus. Here also ischaemic damage is inconstant and may affect either segment or both up to the level of infarction.

Thalamus. The anterior, dorsomedial and ventrolateral nuclei are most commonly damaged. Ischaemic alterations are usually uniform in the anterior and dorsomedial nuclei but limited to the upper third or half of the ventrolateral nucleus. Even when ischaemic damage is severe and extensive in the cortex, alterations in the thalami are only moderate and infarction of thalamic nuclei has not been described. Neocortical damage, in cases of long survival, will add some element of retrograde degeneration in the thalamic association nuclei.

Subthalamic nucleus. Damage in this structure is quite common and the ensuing gliomesodermal reaction contrasts sharply with the surrounding white matter (Fig. 2.33).

Hypothalamus. Ischaemic alterations are seen occasionally in the mamillary bodies of adults and frequently in those of infants and young children.

Brainstem. The influence of age on the pattern of the ischaemic alterations due to circulatory arrest can be seen most clearly in the brainstem. In the adult, alterations are usually restricted to the reticular zone of the substantia nigra, the inferior colliculi and the medullary olives.

In infants and young children there is often the additional involvement of the nucleus of the third nerve, the superior olive, the motor and the spinal nuclei of the fifth nerve, the vestibular nuclear complex, nucleus solitarius, nucleus cuneatus and nucleus gracilis (Fig. 2.34). This pattern of damage in the nuclei of the brainstem corresponds more or less closely to that observed in the infant monkey after neonatal asphyxia (Ranck and Windle 1959).

Involvement of the same brainstem nuclei has sometimes been seen in the adult after circulatory arrest (Neuberger 1954; Lindenberg 1963; Gilles 1963; Brierley, Adams *et al.* 1971).

Cerebellum. Involvement of Purkinje cells may be restricted to a few in the floors of some sulci or may be very widespread and associated with some thinning of the granule layers. The dorsal aspects of the hemispheres and the superior vermis are more affected than the ventral aspects of the hemispheres and the inferior vermis.

Attempts to arrest the cerebral circulation in normothermic experimental animals have been numerous and the literature was reviewed by Hoff, Grenell and Fulton (1945), who emphasized the role of the collateral circulation in deciding the completeness of circulatory arrest in any one species. The principal methods used to arrest cerebral blood flow are: (i) arrest of the heart using electric shock or potassium chloride, (ii) inflation of a cuff around the neck, with or without earlier ligature of the vertebral arteries, (iii) ligature of the pulmonary artery, (iv) ligature of the carotid and vertebral arteries with or without ligature of sources of collateral circulation such as internal mammary and intercostal arteries, (v) ligature of the ascending aorta together with the superior and inferior venae cavae, (vi) elevation of the pressure of the cerebrospinal fluid above that of the systolic blood pressure and (vii) replacement of the animal's heart by a heart-lung machine which can be stopped and restarted to give a desired period of circulatory arrest.

In the majority of studies the presence or absence of brain damage in survivors has been inferred from clinical evidence and not from neuropathological examination. When the latter has been carried out, survival was rarely for less than 2 days, the 'on/off' nature of circulatory arrest seldom proved and fixation of the brain by *in vivo* perfusion was seldom employed.

Fig. 2.30 Male, aged 17 years, dying 9 months after cardiac arrest. (*a*) Frontal cortex showing relative preservation of cytoarchitecture over crest of gyrus. Celloidin; cresyl violet. × 11. (*b*) Occipital lobe showing gross narrowing of cortex and marked gliomesodermal proliferation in layer 3. Celloidin; cresyl violet. × 11.

Fig. 2.31 Male, aged 49 years, dying 7 months after cardiac arrest. Hippocampus showing almost total loss of neurons in h. 1 and relative preservation in h. 2 and in h. 3 to 5. Celloidin; cresyl violet. × 9.

Fig. 2.32 Female, aged 56 years, dying 2 weeks after cardiac arrest. Basal ganglia. There is patchy neuronal loss with gliomesodermal proliferation in the putamen. Celloidin; cresyl violet. × 18.

Fig. 2.33 Male, aged 2½ years, dying 30 days after cardiac arrest, Subthalamic nucleus showing marked gliomesodermal proliferation. Celloidin; cresyl violet. × 9.

Fig. 2.34 Same case as Fig. 2.33. Lower medulla showing discrete necrosis in each nucleus gracilis. Celloidin: Heidenhain. × 11.

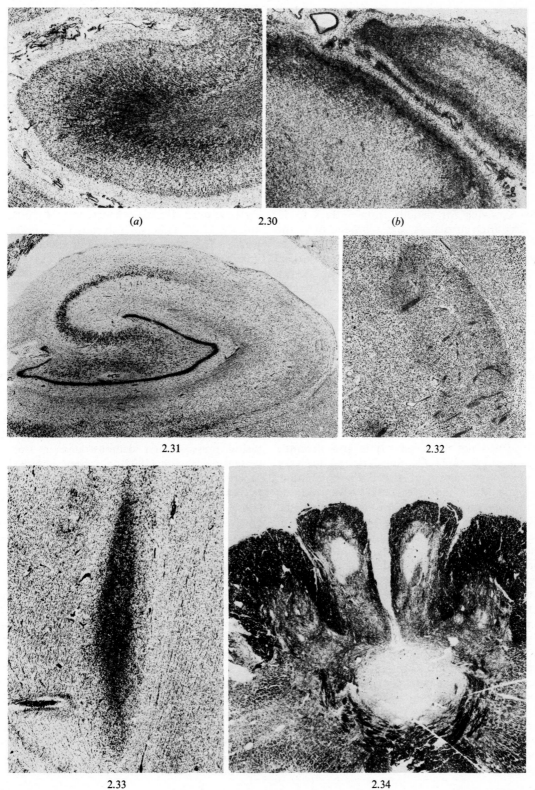

(a) 2.30 (b)

2.31 2.32

2.33 2.34

Weinberger *et al.* (1940) obtained circulatory arrest in cats by clamping the pulmonary artery, survival times ranged from 2 days to 6 weeks and the brains were fixed by immersion in formalin after immediate removal. Neuropathological alterations, seen when circulatory arrest exceeded $3\frac{1}{4}$ minutes, were localized in the cortex within a pattern suggestive of arterial boundary zones and they were patchy in the basal ganglia. Cortical and cerebellar damage became generalized only when the period of arrest was from $7\frac{1}{2}$ to $7\frac{3}{4}$ minutes. No mention was made of the hippocampi.

Grenell (1946) described the brain damage in dogs surviving for periods from 7 days to 11 months after circulatory arrest produced by the inflation of a pressure cuff around the neck at the level of a laminectomy performed earlier. Fixation was by perfusion after bleeding. It was noted that small neurons were more vulnerable than large and regional vulnerability decreased from the cerebral cortex through the hippocampus and cerebellum to the brainstem and spinal cord. Neuropathological studies of the effects of circulatory arrest on the primate brain are few. Hill and Mott (1906) ligatured the four major brain arteries of monkeys. Cytological alterations seen in the immersion-fixed brains from 10 minutes onwards included chromatolysis and 'coagulation necrosis'. Ischaemic cell change was not described. It is now accepted that interruption of the four arteries does not produce total arrest of the brain circulation. Recently, Miller and Myers (1972) have produced circulatory arrest in the brains of juvenile and adult rhesus monkeys by temporary occlusion of the ascending aorta and the superior and inferior venae cavae, thus leaving the pulmonary and coronary vessels unobstructed. If there were no subsequent cardiopulmonary complications, brain damage was restricted to the brainstem, globus pallidus and occasionally the hippocampus. The considerable generalized involvement of the cerebral cortex and cerebellum constantly seen after circulatory arrest in man was not reproduced. If systemic hypotension occurred after the arrest there was cortical damage along arterial boundary zones. The concentration of alterations in the brainstem is a known consequence of hypoxic stresses in the immature subject. As the ages and weights of the animals showing brainstem damage were not stated the role of age cannot be excluded.

Oligaemic hypoxia

Global oligaemia implies some reduction in the overall flow of blood through the brain. Subsequent neuropathological alterations, if any, are determined by the oxygenation of the blood, the rate at which blood flow was reduced, the lowest level of flow attained and its duration and also by the rate at which normal brain blood flow was restored.

Overall brain blood flow is a function of the perfusion pressure (mean arterial blood pressure minus venous sinus or intracranial pressure) and the cerebrovascular resistance. The latter is determined by the intracranial pressure (a minor factor at normal levels), the viscosity of the blood and the tone of the smooth muscle in the vessel walls. This muscle tone is influenced by the intraluminal pressure, the tensions of oxygen and carbon dioxide in the blood and also its pH.

It has been observed in experimental animals and in man that cerebral blood flow is unaltered if the systemic blood pressure is slowly reduced by a third to one-half. Within this range, the constancy of flow (autoregulation), in spite of a falling blood pressure, is due to the progressive reduction in cerebrovascular resistance resulting from vasodilatation. The smooth muscle of brain arterioles relaxes as the perfusion pressure falls and contracts as the pressure rises. This relationship between vascular calibre and perfusion pressure first demonstrated in isolated vessels by Bayliss (1902) has been observed in superficial brain vessels through cranial windows by Forbes, Nason and Wortman (1937) and Fog (1938). Vasodilatation has been shown to be greatest in the anastomotic vessels along the arterial boundary zones (Brierley, Brown, Excell and Meldrum 1969). Once vasodilatation is maximal, autoregulation ceases, overall blood flow falls parallel to the perfusion pressure but the boundary zones are the first regions in which flow is reduced to a critical level (Fig. 2.35). In any one case brain damage will conform to one of the three patterns described by Adams, Brierley, Connor and Treip (1966).

(i) Ischaemic alterations are concentrated along the boundary zones between the arterial territories in the cerebral cortex, and in the cerebellum (Fig. 2.35) and are variable in the basal ganglia.

The boundary zone pattern of ischaemic brain damage is usually seen after a conscious subject has collapsed as a result of some sudden reduction in cardiac output or when an episode of anoxaemia or hypoxaemia has led to a secondary depression of the myocardium (see pp. 66 and 67).

J. E. Meyer (1953) first reported that localized necrosis of grey and white matter at the boundary zones ('watersheds') between major arterial territories, could be the consequence of a sudden fall in blood pressure. However, Wolf and Siris (1937) had illustrated symmetrical necrosis in the boundary zones between anterior and middle cerebral arteries (although these were not recognized as such) in four patients submitted to neurosurgical procedures in the sitting position.

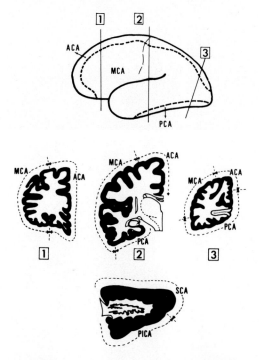

Fig. 2.35 The arterial territories of the human cerebrum and cerebellum. ACA, Anterior cerebral artery; MCA, Middle cerebral artery; PCA, Posterior cerebral artery; SCA, Superior cerebellar artery; PICA, Posterior inferior cerebellar artery.

Serial estimations of blood pressure gave evidence of abrupt arterial hypotension. These observations have been confirmed and extended by Zülch (1953), Zülch and Behrend (1961) and Romanul and Abramowicz (1964). Experimental verification of the hypothesis that a sudden and major reduction in brain perfusion pressure (uncomplicated by hypoxaemia) was the critical factor in the production of boundary zone lesions was provided by the studies of Brierley and Excell

(1966), Brierley *et al.* (1969) and Meldrum and Brierley (1969), in *M. mulatta*.

The neocortex around the parieto-occipital sulci, representing the junction between the territories of the anterior, middle and posterior cerebral arteries, is the most vulnerable portion of the boundary zones as it is most remote from the origin of each major artery (Zülch 1953; Zülch and Behrend 1961). Minimal boundary zone lesions are most likely to occur in this region while larger lesions spread anteriorly along the anterior/middle cerebral artery and/or the middle/posterior cerebral artery boundary zones. In the former, involvement of the pre- and postcentral gyri is not unusual, but extension around the frontal pole on to the orbital surface is exceptional.

The middle/posterior cerebral artery boundary zone passing forwards and downwards into the temporal lobe is rarely involved to its full extent.

Neocortical boundary zone lesions vary widely in their morphology from case to case and often within one brain. A minor lesion may appear as a crescent of ischaemic nerve cells or gliomesodermal reaction in the third and/or fifth and sixth layers in the floor of a sulcus or over the crest of a gyrus (Fig. 2.36) or as one or more perivascular foci of similar nature. Larger lesions may take the form of typical laminar necrosis (Fig. 2.37) within which islands of normal neurons may be preserved. Major lesions may involve all layers over a wide area (Fig. 2.38). Alternatively, the damage may be quite irregular and islands of preserved nerve cells may occur at random within the lesion (Fig. 2.39). Boundary zone lesions may or may not be haemorrhagic (Fig. 2.40).

Involvement of the white matter is unusual and when present is usually associated with large irregular cortical lesions. In the coronal plane the damaged white matter takes the form of a wedge with its apex directed towards the lateral ventricles.

Although Coceani and Gloor (1966) stated that, in *Macaca mulatta* '. . . the hippocampus definitely lies on the watershed between the carotid and vertebrobasilar arterial territories . . .' it is surprising that it is so rarely involved in this species or in man when major lesions are present in the arterial boundary zones of cerebrum and cerebellum.

Ischaemic alterations in the basal ganglia cannot be regarded as boundary zone lesions if only because there are virtually no anastomoses of importance between the several arterial terri-

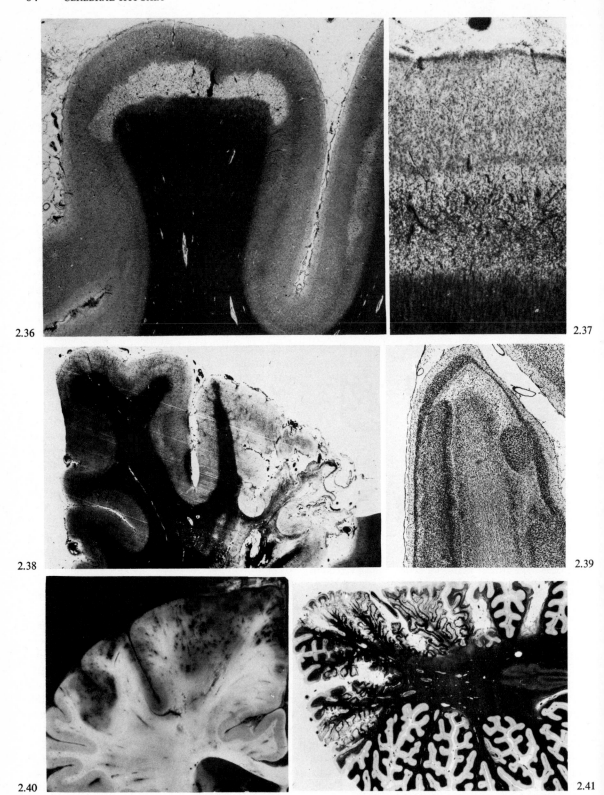

2.36

2.37

2.38

2.39

2.40

2.41

tories (Vander Eecken 1959). Such lesions must be attributed to a critical reduction in blood flow through the capillary bed.

While neocortical boundary zone lesions may occur in the absence of ischaemic lesions in the basal ganglia, the converse is very rare. In the caudate nucleus the sites of predilection are the outer border and the inferomedial portions of the head. The outer border of the body may show patchy damage while the tail is rarely involved.

Damage in the putamen is usually in the upper part of the anterior third and less in the posterior two-thirds. The outer and the inner segments of the globus pallidus are equally involved. Alterations in thalamus and amygdaloid nucleus are rare.

In the cerebellum the minimal lesion in the boundary zone between the territories supplied by the superior and the posterior inferior cerebellar arteries (Fig. 2.35) occurs in the depths of the cortex adjacent to the central white matter. Larger lesions are triangular in vertical section with their apices at this point and their bases at the posterior border (Fig. 2.41).

Within the brainstem of experimental primates the reticular zone of the substantia nigra often shows damage when there are lesions in the arterial boundary zones of cerebrum and cerebellum (Nicholson, Freeland and Brierley 1970) but such involvement is unusual in man. Ischaemic alterations may also be seen occasionally in the inferior colliculi, the medial vestibular nuclei, the dorsal nuclei of the vagi, the spinal nuclei of the trigeminal nerves and nuclei gracili and cuneati.

(ii) Ischaemic alterations are generalized in the cortex of cerebrum and cerebellum, minor or absent in the hippocampi and often severe in the thalami. The number of reported instances showing this pattern of damage is small and they have usually been patients under anaesthesia. The limited information available from the reported cases suggests that the generalized brain damage is due to hypotension (sometimes postural) of relatively slow onset and of long duration. Probably a slowly falling perfusion pressure within a fully dilated vascular bed reduces flow to a critical level in the brain as a whole and not just in the boundary zones.

In the first reported case showing this distribution of ischaemic alterations (Brierley and Cooper 1962) neuronal loss in the cortex was laminar or pseudo-laminar (Fig. 2.42) and decreased from the occipital lobes forwards. It was minor in the hippocampi, absent in the caudate and lentiform nuclei but considerable in the thalami. Loss of neurons was slight and patchy in the reticular zone of the substantia nigra and in the olives but considerable among the Purkinje cells in the cerebellum. Similar neuropathological findings were reported in four additional cases by Adams *et al.* (1966).

(iii) Ischaemic alterations are generalized in the cortex of cerebrum and cerebellum but with variable accentuation along the arterial boundary zones. The hippocampi are usually spared and there is patchy damage in the basal ganglia. This pattern is seen when a conscious subject collapses after brief cardiac arrest (followed by cardiac massage) or some post-operative hypotension. It was also seen as a consequence of sub-atmospheric decompression in the cats of Altmann and Schubothe (1942) and the two baboons of Brierley and Nicholson (1969). It has not been produced in experimental primates as a consequence of hypotension uncomplicated by hypoxaemia. The precise physiological basis for this pattern of brain damage remains undefined but an initial abrupt reduction in blood flow followed by a reduced overall flow of hypoxaemic blood is probable.

As the neuropathology of this group of cases includes the features of groups (i) and (ii) in varying proportion a separate description is not merited. Descriptions of five typical cases have

Fig. 2.36 Male, aged 46 years, dying 5 weeks after a severe hypotensive episode. Second frontal gyrus showing necrosis of deeper cortical layers. Celloidin; Heidenhain. × 9.

Fig. 2.37 Male, aged 45 years, dying 4 weeks after severe hypotensive episode. Frontal cortex showing gliomesodermal reaction in layers 5 and 6. Celloidin; PTAH. × 13.

Fig. 2.38 Female, aged 58 years, dying 3 months after severe hypotensive episode. There is irregular necrosis of the cortex in the second and third frontal gyri and patchy subcortical demyelination. Celloidin; Heidenhain. × 1·5.

Fig. 2.39 *M. mulatta.* Subatmospheric decompression with secondary hypotension. Occipital lobe showing irregular loss of cortical neurons with preservation of islands of normal cells. Celloidin; cresyl violet. × 10.

Fig. 2.40 Male, aged 48 years, dying 4 days after severe hypotensive episode. Brain slice showing haemorrhage within cortex and white matter along boundary zone between anterior and middle cerebral arteries.

Fig. 2.41 Male, aged 61 years, dying 7 months after severe hypotensive episode. Cerebellum showing necrotic foliae at boundary zone between superior and posterior inferior cerebellar arteries. Celloidin; PTAH. × 1·25.

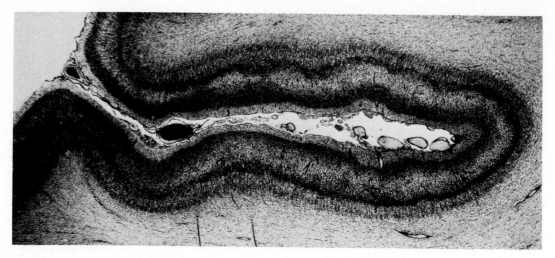

Fig. 2.42 Female, aged 24 years dying 8 days after period of sustained moderate hypotension.   Occipital lobe showing neuronal loss and gliomesodermal proliferation in third layer.   Celloidin; cresyl violet.   × 11.

been presented by Adams *et al.* (1966), and a single case by Brierley and Miller (1966).

Anoxia and hypoxic hypoxia

Anoxia

This term implies that the blood leaving the lungs is devoid of oxygen.   This occurs if atmospheric pressure falls to zero when pressurization fails in the vehicle of an astronaut orbiting in space or within his space suit while he is outside the vehicle, if there is complete obstruction of the respiratory tract above the tracheal bifurcation, if respiration is arrested after disease or injury to the spinal cord, after crush injuries of the thorax and after the arrest of alveolar oxygen exchange due to the inhalation of inert gases or to drowning.

The physiological events in each of these situations have not been documented, but the anoxia due to the inhalation of pure nitrogen by conscious volunteers has been studied by Gastaut, Bostem, Fernandez-Guardiola, Naquet and Gibson (1961), Gastaut, Fischgold and Meyer (1961) and Ernsting (1963).   After 15 to 16 seconds of nitrogen overventilation (which induced anoxaemia rapidly), Ernsting (1963) observed that the EEG showed low-voltage activity at 11 to 13 cycles per second and consciousness was lost at 17 to 20 seconds.   The subsequent course of events has been provided by studies in experimental animals.   Thus Swann and Brucer (1949) exposed

dogs to pure nitrogen and observed hyperventilation, cyanosis and convulsions within the first minute.   Bradycardia was recorded later as the heart began to fail and the blood pressure to fall.   Apnoea occurred at the third minute and the blood pressure was 5 to 20 mm Hg at the fifth minute.   Survival after 5½ minutes was only possible if administration of oxygen was combined with external cardiac massage.   If resuscitation was delayed until 6½ minutes, brain damage was evident.

It is well known that circulation through the brain must be arrested for 4 to 5 minutes before there is irreversible damage.   It is evident that in the human subject or experimental animal a pure anoxaemia will be complicated by some degree of circulatory failure within that period of time and therefore cannot, *per se*, give rise to brain damage.   If resuscitation is successful and brain damage is eventually proved, this must be ascribed to a combination of anoxaemia and some reduction in cerebral blood flow.   This combination, for reasons already elaborated (pp. 62-65), is likely to lead to ischaemic alterations along the arterial boundary zones.

Accidental or suicidal hanging is an apparent example of anoxic anoxia, yet published reports are not surprisingly devoid of information relating to immediate and subsequent cardiovascular function.   From the reviews of Hoff *et al.* (1945) and Jacob (1957) it is evident that ischaemic alterations are usually seen in the cortex of cerebrum and cerebellum, the hippocampi and the basal ganglia, but their precise distribution, particularly where arterial boundary zones are concerned, has not been defined. Thus there is, as yet, no justification for the delineation of purely anoxic brain damage.

Hypoxic hypoxia
This term implies some reduction in the oxygen tension of arterial blood as a consequence of a lowered oxygen content of the inspired air (high altitudes, failure of pressurization in aircraft, inhalation of air admixed with inert gases including anaesthetics) or any impairment of pulmonary function.

Many attempts have been made to define a 'critical' level of blood oxygenation below which brain damage will occur. In this sense Campbell (1965) considered 30 mm Hg to be the critical oxygen tension for arterial blood while the corresponding level in brain venous blood was 17 to 19 mm Hg according to Luft (1965) and 12 mm Hg according to Cohen (1966). However, the observations of Gray and Horner (1970) in human subjects do not endorse such values for critical oxygen tensions. They showed that oxygen tensions as low as 7·5 mm Hg in arterial and 2·0 mm Hg in venous blood were compatible with survival without clinical evidence of brain damage. Further, Lübbers (1966) has stressed that venous oxygen tension is not a reliable index of brain tissue hypoxia and that local tissue oxygen tensions of 1·0 mm Hg or less can be recorded by appropriate electrodes on the brain of a normal experimental animal.

The concept of a particular oxygen tension 'critical' for the production of brain damage also assumes that in the human subject or experimental animal such a level can be sustained without any alteration in brain blood flow, long enough to be the sole cause of irreversible neuronal damage. In the literature of so-called hypoxic brain damage in the human brain virtually all reports are devoid of data concerning blood pressure and heart rate during the period of hypoxaemia. Nevertheless Scholz (1952, 1957) and Buchner (1957) considered that oligaemia resulted in alterations in the cortex of cerebrum and cerebellum and in the hippocampus while damage in the striatum, globus pallidus and subthalamic nucleus was considered to be the consequence of hypoxaemia. While the existence of these two patterns of ischaemic brain damage is

indisputable, their correlation with equally unequivocal physiological situations in man remains unsupported by the appropriate physiological data.

Recent studies in experimental primates have provided answers to the questions (i) can uncomplicated hypoxaemia produce brain damage, and (ii) are the 'cortical' and 'basal ganglia' patterns of brain damage regularly associated with oligaemia and hypoxaemia respectively?

(i) The exposure of primates to subatmospheric decompression in a decompression chamber provides a model for hypoxic hypoxia (Nicholson and Ernsting 1967; Brierley and Nicholson 1969; Nicholson et al. 1970; Brierley 1971; Blagbrough, Brierley and Nicholson 1973). Using this model it has been shown that, in the brains of baboons and rhesus monkeys, damage in the cortex of cerebrum and cerebellum was concentrated along arterial boundary zones but was inconstant and variable in the basal ganglia. The involvement of the boundary zones was in itself a clear indication that some reduction in cerebral perfusion followed the initial hypoxaemia. It was observed that bradycardia occurred towards the end of the decompression when respiration was greatly slowed. Thus the observed brain damage could not be attributed to an uncomplicated hypoxaemia (Fig. 2.1).

(ii) The distribution of brain damage after decompression included 'cortical' as well as 'basal ganglia' patterns as described by Scholz (1952, 1957) and Buchner (1957). In the physiologically different situation of systemic hypotension with normal arterial oxygenation (oligaemic hypoxia) the same two patterns of damage were observed (Brierley et al. 1969). These experimental studies have shown that hypoxic and oligaemic hypoxia can each lead to the 'cortical' and 'basal ganglia' distributions of ischaemic alterations and it is probable that the two patterns will have an anatomical rather than a physiological explanation. This conclusion was underlined by a single animal submitted to decompression in which brain damage was entirely cortical in one hemisphere and restricted to the basal ganglia in the other.

The critical contribution of a secondary oligaemia to hypoxaemia in the production of brain damage was supported by the observations of Brown and Brierley (1968) in rats exposed intermittently to nitrogen. Ischaemic brain damage occurred only when a considerable bradycardia occurred towards the end of each period of hypoxia. The evidence now available from many experimental studies is in line with the conclusion of Schneider (1961) that 'ischaemia is the last common path of all forms of hypoxia'. Thus the neuropathology of hypoxic hypoxia is that of oligaemic hypoxia (pp. 62-66).

Anaemic hypoxia

Carbon monoxide intoxication

Carbon monoxide gives rise to anaemic hypoxia by virtue of an affinity for the ferrous heme of haemoglobin that is about 250 times greater than that of oxygen. The remaining functional haemoglobin is normally saturated with oxygen, the blood oxygen tension is normal but the oxygen content is reduced. Further, the dissociation curve of oxyhaemoglobin is shifted to the left so that less oxygen is available to the tissues at a particular oxygen tension. The affinity of carbon monoxide for the iron of cytochrome oxidase implies the possibility of an additional histotoxic hypoxia. According to Warburg (1926), such enzymatic inhibition only occurs at a concentration of CO that would be lethal because of the disruption of oxygen transport by the blood. Nevertheless a relatively low level of circulating carboxyhaemoglobin may lead to significant local enzymatic inhibition in regions such as the globus pallidus and reticular zone of the substantia nigra which have a high iron content.

According to Bour, Tutin and Pasquier (1967), carbon monoxide poisoning is a consequence of accidental or suicidal exposures in about equal proportions. Most accidental cases are due to escape of illuminating gas in a domestic setting. Carbon monoxide is also a component of the fumes from solid-fuel heaters and the exhaust gases of internal-combustion engines. Examples from industry are fewer and include accidents in blast furnaces and in mines. In the latter, explosions due to the ignition of coal dust and of fire damp are the usual sources of carbon monoxide.

In a non-anaemic subject 15 to 20% of haemoglobin may combine with carbon monoxide before symptoms appear and these are an expression of the inability of the remaining oxyhaemoglobin to meet tissue oxygen requirements. When the level of carboxyhaemoglobin exceeds 20% there is dyspnoea on exertion and slight headache. At a level of 30% there is severe headache, fatigue

and impaired judgement. Consciousness is lost at a level of 60 to 70% and a concentration of 70% or more is rapidly fatal.

The clinical symptomatology of carbon monoxide intoxication may take one of two forms:

(i) Monophasic, in which survival may range from hours to years but without remission of symptoms.

(ii) Biphasic, in which a period of coma or unconsciousness is followed by an interval of apparent normality lasting 2 to 30 days. This, in turn is succeeded by some combination of a considerable variety of neuropsychiatric symptoms. While this biphasic pattern of symptoms has often been regarded as a specific feature of carbon monoxide intoxication, Plum, Posner and Hain (1962) showed that it could also be the sequel of quite different types of hypoxia such as cardiac arrest and exposure to nitrogen.

Garland and Pearce (1967) described four personal cases and also presented a comprehensive review of the neurological complications of CO poisoning. Among these, the more important were epileptic seizures, visual failure (cortical), object and finger agnosia, apraxias, dysphasia, transient deafness, Parkinsonism, incontinence, degrees of mental impairment, amnestic syndromes and a wide variety of psychotic states. These authors drew attention to the rarity of clinical evidence of permanent brain damage among the numerous survivors of exposure to CO. They also made the important observation that no combination of neurological and psychiatric symptoms can be regarded as the specific consequence of exposure to CO as all such combinations may be encountered after cardiac arrest, hypoglycaemia, closed head injury, air embolism and hepatic encephalopathy.

When death occurs within a few hours after poisoning, the blood, brain, muscles, skin and viscera display the pink-red colour characteristic of carboxyhaemoglobin. The brain and meninges are usually congested. Haemorrhages are frequent and may be either petechial, with a predilection for white matter and the corpus callosum in particular, or large and without preferential sites. Alterations in the basal ganglia, unless haemorrhagic, are seldom recognizable if survival is for less than 24 hours.

When death is delayed there is the usual relationship between survival time and macroscopic alterations. Thus reduction in brain weight with evidence of cortical atrophy will be evident after survival for weeks or months but absent if survival was for only a few days. When survival is for 48 hours or more, brain weight may be increased as a result of oedema and/or vascular congestion. Macroscopic inspection of the brain may then show petechial haemorrhages and early necrosis in the globus pallidus, hippocampus and sometimes in the reticular zone of the substantia nigra. This latter finding was first described by Hiller (1924) and a microscopic description was subsequently provided by Meyer (1926). Meyer (1963) pointed out that ischaemic pallidal necrosis could also be the sequel of cyanide intoxication

and upper portion of the inner segment of the globus pallidus. It often extends upwards to involve the internal capsule and the external segment and sometimes downwards into the sublentiform region. When survival is long, haemosiderin may be seen in lipid phagocytes and deposits of pseudo-calcium around the larger blood vessels.

The minimal pallidal lesion may be no more than an irregular slit at the junction between the inner segment and the internal capsule. Lapresle and Fardeau (1967) have pointed out that this can be missed if serial sections are not studied.

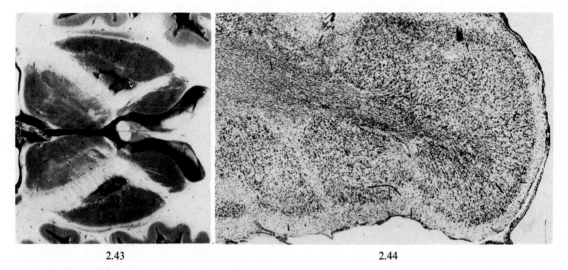

2.43   2.44

Fig. 2.43 Male 48 years dying 9 months after carbon monoxide intoxication. Horizontal brain slice showing irregular necrosis with cyst formation in each globus pallidus.
Fig. 2.44 CO poisoning, 16 years' survival. Focal loss of nerve cells with subsequent gliosis in cerebral cortex and white matter. Nissl. × 20.

and of anaesthetic accidents. Further, after carbon monoxide intoxication the globus pallidus may be normal (Meyer 1928; Hsü and Ch'eng 1938; Lapresle and Fardeau 1967; Brierley, two unpublished cases).

Macroscopic examination usually shows that the typical pallidal lesion attains the level of a well-circumscribed infarct after a survival of 48 hours or even less (Fig. 2.43). The lesions are not always symmetrical. Thereafter there is the usual proliferation of lipid phagocytes, fibrous astrocytes and blood vessels in the central zone and the formation of a well-defined peripheral capsule of gliomesodermal elements within which the products of tissue breakdown are encysted. The lesion is more commonly seen in the anterior

Ischaemic necrosis may also be seen in the cerebral cortex. It may be focal and often perivascular or it may appear as a continuous laminar process involving the third and sometimes the second layers or alternatively only the fifth and sixth layers. Similar alterations may be seen in the hippocampus (particularly h. 1 and h. 3 to 5) and also in the Purkinje cells of the cerebellum. In a case with survival for 16 years (Meyer 1926) the cerebral hemispheres, particularly in the frontal and occipital lobes, presented the picture of granular atrophy. In Nissl preparations, the cortex showed irregular focal loss of neurons with gliosis and retraction of the surface (Fig. 2.44). A similar case with survival for 15 years was described by Raskin and Mullaney (1940).

The report of Poursines, Alliez and Toga (1956) is important because it indicates that systemic circulatory factors may supplement the anaemic hypoxia due to carbon monoxide. A woman aged 33 years lived 26 days after a suicidal attempt by exposure to illuminating gas. There was typical necrosis in each globus pallidus and also in the subthalamic nuclei. In the neocortex, ischaemic necrosis was focal and there was also a marked concentration of alterations along the boundary zones between the anterior and middle cerebral arteries and a lesser concentration along the boundaries between the middle and posterior cerebral arteries. The cerebellum and brainstem were not described. The distribution of lesions along arterial boundary zones suggests some reduction in brain perfusion pressure (see p. 62) but evidence relating to cardiac and respiratory functions was lacking. The observation of Neubuerger and Clarke (1945) that patchy infarction of the myocardium was seen in a case surviving for 13 days after carbon monoxide poisoning suggests that while the level of circulating carboxyhaemoglobin may be insufficient *per se* to produce brain damage, it may be brought about if there is additional hypoxaemia or reduction in cerebral blood flow.

Alterations in the white matter are a common and often conspicuous neuropathological consequence of carbon monoxide intoxication. However, their extent is not necessarily proportional to damage in grey matter and the latter may even appear normal in the presence of extensive demyelination. White matter damage usually takes one or more of three forms:

(i) Discrete and usually perivascular foci of myelin destruction occur throughout the centra semiovale, in the corpus callosum (particularly in its anterior half), in the internal and external capsules and in the optic tracts. Similar foci may be seen beneath the ependyma around the cerebral ventricular system and some of these foci may be haemorrhagic. Within each focal lesion the breakdown of myelin and of axis cylinders is followed by the proliferation of lipid phagocytes and of fibrous astrocytes.

(ii) Destruction of myelinated fibres is diffuse and widespread. It may extend from the frontal to the temporal and occipital poles with more or less concentration around the ventricular system. Involvement of the corpus callosum leads to a butterfly-like distribution of myelin damage in the coronal plane. Usually there is sparing of the subcortical U-fibres and of a narrow subependymal zone. Within the centra semiovale there is a progressive gliomesodermal reaction with a peripheral concentration which provides a sharp demarcation between normal and abnormal tissue.

(iii) A pallor of myelin staining or frank demyelination takes the form of plaques which may or may not be confluent. The plaques occur in the more posterior and deeper parts of the central white matter and are unusual in the commissures. They also tend to spare the subcortical U-fibres, the internal and external capsules and the optic pathway. Microscopically the plaques show a more or less spongy texture, a relative sparing of myelin sheaths around blood vessels and sometimes a concentric demyelination similar to that described by Balò (1928). In comparison with the breakdown of myelin there is a relative preservation of the axis cylinders. Eventually the accumulation of Marchi positive material within lipid phagocytes is associated with the proliferation of fibrous astrocytes which are more numerous around the periphery of the plaque than within its centre.

Lapresle and Fardeau (1966) analysed white matter damage in 16 cases. In a well-illustrated report they suggested that alterations of type (i) occurred in cases that were comatose from the outset and died within one week. Lesions of type (ii) were usually seen in cases with an unremitting coma terminating in death after 9 to 140 days. Other instances of this type have been described by Neubuerger and Clarke (1945), Kubik (1949), Seitelberger and Jellinger (1960) and Brucher (1967).

Lesions of type (iii) were first described by Grinker (1925) and are usually associated with the biphasic clinical picture. Jacob (1939) was the first to suggest that degeneration in white rather than in grey matter was the neuropathological substrate in those cases in which neuropsychiatric symptoms followed the initial intoxication after some period of apparent normality. Other examples of this relationship are the two cases of Hsü and Ch'eng (1938), the single case of Eros and Priestman (1942), the four cases of Lehoczky (1949) in one of which demyelination was of the concentric type described by Balò (1928), the six cases of Lapresle and Fardeau (1966) and the two cases of Vuia (1967).

One of the first experimental investigations of CO poisoning was that of Ferraro and Morrison

(1928), who exposed rabbits repeatedly to illuminating gas rather than pure CO. Neuronal alterations were more frequent in the hippocampus than in the globus pallidus. Meyer (1928) observed pallidal softenings in all nine cats exposed to CO but the hippocampus was involved in only one. In a comparative study, Meyer (1932) showed that exposure to CO resulted in a purely pallidal necrosis in the dog while in the rabbit and guinea-pig the involvement of the pallidum was similar to that of the cerebral cortex, hippocampus and cerebellum.

Yant, Chronyak, Schrenk, Patty and Sayers (1934) studied the effects in the dog of rapid asphyxiation by CO (death at the end of an exposure of 20 to 30 minutes) and slow CO asphyxiation (with death at 16 to 165 days). In the first group of animals the diverse neuronal alterations are probably attributable to histological artefact (brains were fixed by immersion). In animals surviving days and weeks there was loss of neurons and a corresponding gliomesodermal reaction in the cerebral cortex and the corpus striatum. There was also a diffuse demyelination in animals surviving more than a few days.

Lewey and Drabkin (1944) exposed dogs to CO for $5\frac{1}{2}$ hours a day, for 6 days a week and for 11 weeks. Abnormal electrocardiograms were noted in some and after survival for 3 months small foci of necrosis were seen in the cerebral cortex, globus pallidus, white matter and brainstem.

Ehrich, Bellet and Lewey (1944) in a neglected paper reviewed the evidence for abnormal electrocardiograms and for myocardial ischaemic lesions after exposure to CO. They described the electrocardiograms in the dogs of Lewey and Drabkin (1944) and also described and illustrated the focal haemorrhagic and necrotic lesions seen in the myocardia of those animals in which the level of CO Hb exceeded 75% for 1 hour or more. This single experimental study endorsed earlier observations and also drew attention to the fact that CO might damage heart muscle and thereby add an element of oligaemia to hypoxia of anaemic type.

There have been three studies of the effects of acute exposures to CO on the primate nervous system. Meyer (1933) subjected five rhesus monkeys to repeated exposures to CO up to the point of respiratory arrest without producing any alterations in their brains. Van Bogaert, Dallemagne and Wégria (1938) studied chronic CO intoxication in the rhesus monkey during a period of 6 months and also acute intoxication during periods of 3 and 12 hours. Pathological examination of body organs and the central nervous system revealed no abnormality.

Ginsberg, Myers and McDonagh (1974) exposed 19 juvenile rhesus monkeys to gas mixtures containing 0·2 or 0·3% CO plus normal amounts of oxygen for periods of 60 to 325 minutes. Arterial blood pressure, respiratory rate electrocardiogram and EEG were recorded continuously. Arterial and jugular blood samples were taken at intervals for measurement of gas tensions and pH. A carboxyhaemoglobin level of 72 to 77% was maintained throughout the exposure. Some degree of hypotension occurred in all animals, respiration was not depressed and cardiac arrhythmias were common. The EEG was slowed progressively and intermittent isoelectric periods were seen in 12 animals.

Fourteen animals survived the exposure for from 2 weeks to 5 months. Three showed severe neurological disabilities, three mild disabilities and eight appeared normal.

In the brains of all animals white matter damage was the salient feature. This was usually symmetrical and more marked anteriorly. The demyelination was either diffuse or in the form of plaques. The cerebral cortex, cerebellum, brainstem and spinal cord were stated to be normal and alterations in the globus pallidus and hippocampus were seen in less than one-fifth of the brains. It was concluded that the predominantly white matter damage was related to hypotension and metabolic acidosis rather than to the anaemic hypoxia. This conclusion is surprising in view of the fact that the damage due to sufficient hypotension is found in grey matter and rarely in white. While this study has again underlined the importance of systemic circulatory factors, the concentration of damage in white matter may be due to the cytotoxic effect of CO together with a moderate reduction in blood flow and perhaps an additional acidosis.

Histotoxic hypoxia

Cyanide

The histotoxic effects of the cyanide ion are due to the inhibition of cytochrome oxidase, the terminal enzyme in the respiratory electron transport chain which utilizes the oxygen derived from the dissociation of oxyhaemoglobin. Cyanide probably combines reversibly with the iron (ferric heme) of cytochrome oxidase. It does not combine with circulating haemoglobin but only with methaemoglobin. The latter may be formed *in vivo* when sodium nitrite is given in the treatment of cyanide intoxication and *post mortem* as a breakdown product of haemoglobin.

There is no essential difference between the neuropathological effects of sodium and potassium cyanide, hydrocyanic acid and cyanogen chloride (CNCl).

In acute intoxication death ensues rapidly as a result of respiratory failure and is often preceded by convulsions. In such cases the brain shows no more than hyperaemia and, occasionally, petechial subarachnoid and subdural haemorrhages; there are no significant microscopic alterations.

Only a few human cases with delayed death have been described. That of Lambert (1919) was a man aged 40 dying 16 days after the accidental inhalation of hydrocyanic acid gas. There was coma for the first three days with frequent convulsions. Macroscopically there were small haemorrhages in the white matter of cerebrum and cerebellum. Microscopically there was a conspicuous loss of Purkinje cells in the cerebellum and regressive changes with gliosis in the cerebral cortex. Haymaker, Ginzler and Ferguson (1952) have suggested that a single case may have been reported first by Schmorl (1920) and subsequently by Edelman (1921). This was a man aged 43 years dying 36 hours after accidental exposure to hydrocyanic acid. Gross inspection showed general hyperaemia and a symmetrical haemorrhagic softening, the size of a cherry, in each globus pallidus. Microscopically the latter structures showed ring haemorrhages, hyaline thrombi in vessels and regressive changes in nerve cells.

Experimental studies have considerably amplified the limited human observations to show that cyanide can damage both neurons and myelin sheaths after administration by any route.

The first experimental study was that of Meyer (1933), who gave from one to seven subcutaneous injections of potassium cyanide during a period of 3 to 9 days to four dogs and two rabbits. The alterations observed, similar to those described after carbon monoxide poisoning, included ischaemic necrosis of the cerebral cortex, symmetrical and selective necrosis of the globus pallidus and the reticular zone of the substantia nigra, necrosis of the Sommer sector of the hippo-campus, loss of cerebellar Purkinje cells and early softening of the white matter, particularly the corpus callosum. This remains the only experimental investigation in which ischaemic cell change, with and without incrustations, was described and illustrated.

The report of Ferraro (1933) is the first in which the demyelination due to cyanide was considered to resemble that observed in multiple sclerosis. Fourteen cats and four monkeys received increasing subcutaneous injections of potassium cyanide. Convulsions were common and ranged from a single seizure to status epilepticus lasting 24 hours or more. The survival times, the method of fixation and the techniques of fixation and staining were not stated. In the cerebral hemispheres, demyelination, patchy and sometimes concentric, tended to spare the subcortical U-fibres and to involve the periventricular white matter, the corpus callosum and the optic pathway. Nissl's 'acute cell change' was seen in cerebral cortex and spinal cord, the only regions mentioned.

The apparent similarity between the demyelination due to cyanide poisoning and multiple sclerosis led to numerous experimental studies of cyanide intoxication and may explain why neuronal alterations received less attention. Hurst (1940), using monkeys, injected potassium cyanide in divided intramuscular doses over 17 to 103 days. Survival ranged from 2 hours to 13 days after the last injection. Neuronal alterations of a nonspecific nature were seen in 13 animals and involved, in decreasing order of frequency, the globus pallidus, caudate nucleus, cerebellum, putamen, cerebral cortex and substantia nigra. The hippocampus was spared in all. Damage in white matter ranged from partial demyelination to necrosis, the latter being seen after survivals of several days.

Hicks (1950a) injected successive doses of sodium cyanide into rats intraperitoneally. Convulsions began within a minute of each injection but there was no significant cardiac or respiratory depression. Ischaemic necrosis occurred in decreasing order of frequency in the corpus striatum, cerebral cortex, substantia nigra, hippocampus and cerebellum. Demyelination in the corpus callosum was seen in about a quarter of the animals.

Haymaker *et al.* (1952) studied in the dog the effects of cyanogen chloride (CNCl) and hydrocyanic acid (HCN) by inhalation and sodium cyanide and CNCl by the intravenous route. Animals exposed singly to any one compound survived for from a few minutes to 14 days. The pathological changes and their distribution in the central nervous system were essentially the same regardless of the form of cyanide employed and the method of its administration. After a survival of 2 to 3 hours, cortical neurons and Purkinje cells showed eosinophilia of the cytoplasm. Cell loss and gliomesodermal reaction increased with survival time particularly in the 4th, 5th and 6th cortical layers around sulci in the frontal and parietal lobes and in the striatum, pallidum and substantia nigra and less frequently in the thalamus and cerebellum. They were rare in the hippocampal formation. Demyelination was also unusual and always associated with alterations in nearby grey matter. In this study respiratory and circulatory functions were not monitored.

In the rat brain, damage in grey and white matter resulted from a single controlled exposure to hydrocyanic acid gas (HCN) (Levine and Stypulkowski 1959a) and also from a single intravenous injection of potassium cyanide (Levine and Wenk 1959). The former became the model for many subsequent studies with the light and electron microscopes of the alterations in white matter after exposure to cyanide.

Levine and Stypulkowski (1959b) examined the brain damage due to cyanide after unilateral ligature of a common carotid artery in rats. The animals were killed 2 to 4 days later and their brains were fixed by immersion. In grey matter, alterations restricted to the side of carotid ligature were greater in small than in large animals. On the other hand, damage in white matter, greater in larger animals, was always symmetrical in the corpus callosum and its radiations and was also seen in the hippocampal and anterior commissures. It was concluded that, in a normal animal exposed to cyanide, the involvement of grey matter, usually a concomitant of deep intoxication, was most probably due to the accompanying ischaemia and/or hypoxic hypoxia. The symmetry of white matter damage in the presence of unilateral ischaemia was attributed to symmetrical maximal metabolic depression. The role of vascular factors in determining the topography of white matter damage was stressed by Levine (1967), who suggested that concentration in the splenium of the corpus callosum was due to its remoteness from the origin of the anterior cerebral artery and sparing of the peripheral portion was due to the greater vascularity of the nearby grey matter.

The important study of Hirano, Levine and Zimmermann (1967), also in the rat, showed that the earliest alteration (after 1 to 2 hours) in the fine structure of white matter was swelling of axis cylinders within which mitochondria were expanded and their cristae more or less disorganized. At this stage, myelin sheaths, glial elements and extracellular space all appeared normal. Damage to myelin was only appreciable during a later or reactive phase.

When sodium cyanide was given by slow intravenous infusion to lightly anaesthetized Rhesus monkeys with physiological monitoring, it was shown (Brierley 1975) that an initial hyperventilation was followed sooner or later by failing respiration, cardiac arrhythmia and some fall in blood pressure. Grey matter damage consisting of ischaemic cell change was seen in only one animal and was restricted to the striatum. It was attributed to a combination of moderate systemic hypotension and raised central venous pressure while the histotoxic effects of cyanide were maximal. Apparently cyanide can only damage brain neurons in the presence of its secondary effects on respiration and circulation so that the entity of pure histotoxic brain damage in the intact animal may not exist.

Azides

Sodium azide (NaN$_3$) inhibits the action of cytochrome oxidase and its ability to depress the respiration of brain cortex has been demonstrated in vitro. The experimental studies of Hurst (1942) in the monkey and of Hicks (1950b) and Környey (1963) in the rat showed that myelinated fibres could be damaged as well as nerve cells. An important systemic effect of the administration of sodium azide, organic azides and diazides by oral and intravenous routes is a rapid lowering of systemic blood pressure. For this reason they have been used in the treatment of hypertension in man.

While there are no neuropathological reports of azide intoxication in man, Mettler and Sax (1972) have described cerebellar damage as a consequence of the intravenous injection of sodium azide in rhesus monkeys. A single injection produced hyperventilation, pupillary dilatation, a fall in blood pressure to about 25 mm Hg and a convulsion. Animals that recovered exhibited ataxia and subsequent neuro-pathological examination showed that alterations, confined to the cerebellum, ranged from almost complete decortication to minor cortical damage in the depths of sulci around the horizontal fissures. As this region is an arterial boundary zone it was recognized that any cytotoxic specificity of azide for cerebellar neural elements could not be separated from its considerable hypotensive effect.

Hypoglycaemia

Hypoglycaemia may lead to damage in the human brain when the associated coma is irreversible. i.e. it does not respond to the administration of glucose. Where brain damage was concerned, Meyer (1963) stated that 'the findings in the literature show some variation, but there is no doubt that they closely resemble those which occur in other types of anoxia'. It is well known, however, that hypoglycaemic coma may be accompanied or followed by some depression of cardiovascular or respiratory functions, epileptic seizures or raised intracranial pressure, each of which may contribute to the brain damage ultimately observed. The ability of uncomplicated hypoglycaemia to produce typical ischaemic alterations in the brains of experimental primates has been demonstrated only recently (see below).

The situations in which hypoglycaemia may occur are diverse and have been classified on the bases of aetiology and of clinical presentation by Marks and Rose (1965).

Neuropathological descriptions of the brain damage attributed to hypoglycaemia in man have been derived from (i) patients dying after insulin shock therapy for psychoses, (ii) diabetic patients developing irreversible coma after treatment with insulin, (iii) rare instances of islet cell tumours of the pancreas (insulinoma), (iv) very rare instances of attempted suicide by injection of insulin, (v) examples of idiopathic hypoglycaemia in infants and (vi) occasional instances of 'white liver' disease in infants with proved hypoglycaemia (as in two of the 12 cases of Cullity and Kakulas (1970) and a single personal case).

The intact and sliced brain may appear normal. Brain swelling is unusual and was present and of only slight degree in one of the six cases of Lawrence et al. (1942); it was also slight in one of the eight cases of Brierley (1965) and absent in the three cases of Vital, Picard, Arné, Aubertin,

Fenelon and Mouton (1967). Enlargement of the ventricular system, cortical atrophy and shrinkage of the hippocampi are marked only when survival is for more than a few months. In a personal case (attempted suicide by the injection of insulin) survival was for 16 years and the brain weighed 700 g. In addition to general cortical atrophy the first, second and third temporal gyri on each side were reduced to paper-thin membranes while the parahippocampal gyri were intact and the hippocampi showed only moderate sclerosis.

Microscopic alterations are almost invariable in the cerebral cortex and consist of some stage in the ischaemic neuronal process up to and beyond cell loss. References in the literature to Nissl's 'severe cell change' must be treated with caution if only because this has not been reported in the brains of optimally fixed experimental primates after controlled hypoglycaemia.

In the cerebral cortex ischaemic cell change is sometimes focal but more usually laminar (Fig. 2.45) with an emphasis on the third and fifth layers. Occasionally necrosis of all layers may be seen, particularly in the posterior half of the brain but usually with a relative preservation of the visual cortex. Demyelination, diffuse rather than focal, may accompany the cortical damage as described by Richardson and Russell (1952). Also, normal myelin staining may be associated with widespread fibrillary gliosis in the white matter as in two of the six cases of Lawrence et al. (1942).

The hippocampi are almost invariably involved in a typical hypoxic necrosis (Fig. 2.46) which sometimes approaches the level of infarction. Among subcortical structures the almost total necrosis of the striatum seen in the third case of Lawrence et al. (1942) is probably exceptional. These structures were normal in the three cases of Vital et al. (1967) and showed minor or moderate damage in six of the eight cases of Brierley (1965). There is general agreement that involvement of the globus pallidus is unusual. In the thalamus, neuronal alterations are not severe and when present usually involve the anterior, dorsomedial and ventrolateral nuclei. Where the cerebellum is concerned the view of Meyer (1963) that damage to Purkinje cells is appreciably less than in other types of hypoxia must be endorsed. In the brainstem neuronal alterations are slight in the inferior colliculi and inferior olives.

2.45

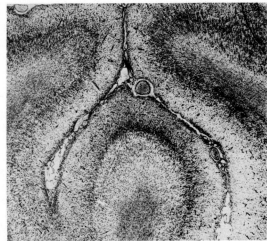

Fig. 2.45 Female, aged 29 years, dying 3 weeks after hypoglycaemia induced for treatment of schizophrenia. Occipital cortex showing neuronal destruction and glio-mesodermal proliferation, largely in the outer layers. Celloidin; cresyl violet. × 6.5.

Fig. 2.46 Same case as Fig. 2.45. Hippocampus, showing almost total neuronal destruction in h. 1 (Sommer sector) and h. 3 to 5 (endfolium), with relative preservation of h. 2. Celloidin; cresyl violet. × 10.

2.46

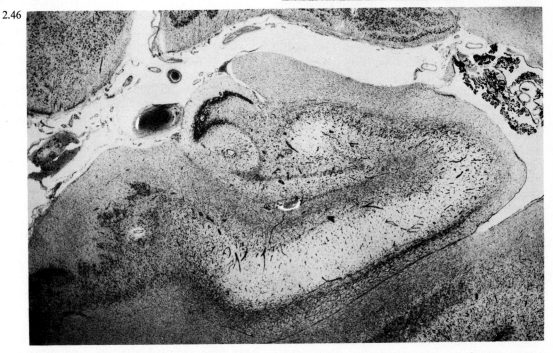

Studies of the neuropathological sequelae of hypoglycaemia in experimental animals are numerous. Most were carried out in subprimates, the brain was removed with minimal delay and fixed by immersion so that histological artefacts most probably account for the very diverse neuronal alterations that have been reported. So far there have been only three studies of hypoglycaemia in experimental primates. Finley and Brenner (1941) in *M. mulatta* produced hypoglycaemia by the intramuscular injection of insulin. After immersion, fixation ischaemic cell change was described only after survival for 9 hours and blood pressure, blood oxygenation and respiration were not monitored.

The long-term neurological and neuropathological effects of uncomplicated insulin-induced hypoglycaemia in the rhesus monkey were studied by Kahn and Myers (1971) and Myers and Kahn (1971). Blood pressure, gas tensions, pH, acid-base status and glucose were monitored as well as the electrocardiogram. Normal blood oxygenation was maintained by mechanical ventilation if required. Blood glucose fell to 20 mg/100 ml after $1\frac{1}{2}$ to 3 hours, this level of hypoglycaemia lasted from 4 to 10 hours in eleven animals and was terminated by the intravenous injection of glucose. In the seven animals with persisting neurological impairment, convulsions occurred in five during the recovery phase. Neuropathological alterations consisted of nerve cell loss and gliomesodermal reaction in the striatum, neocortex and hippocampus in decreasing order of frequency.

In an attempt to define the early stages of the neuronal alterations due to uncomplicated hypoglycaemia in *M. mulatta* under light pentobarbitone anaesthesia, Meldrum, Horton and Brierley (1971) monitored brain arterial and venous blood gas tensions, pH and glucose. The electrocardiogram, EEG and somato-sensory evoked potentials were also recorded. Hypoglycaemia was induced by the intravenous injection of insulin during periods of 2 to 7 hours and was terminated after 2 to 8 hours by the injection of glucose. The brains were fixed by *in vivo* perfusion after survival for 30 minutes to 15 hours.

The neuropathological alterations observed in eight of the fifteen animals (Brierley *et al.* 1971*a*, *b*) consisted of ischaemic cell change at the stage of microvacuolation after survival for half an hour and then of typical ischaemic cell change without and later with incrustations. In seven animals there was a diffuse involvement of the neocortex but with some concentration in the occipital and parietal regions. The hippocampi, corpora striata and the cerebellar Purkinje cells were each involved in one animal. In these animals blood glucose was below 20 mg/100 ml for more than 2 hours, there was no epileptic activity, blood pressure and oxygenation were well maintained, there was no rise in intracranial pressure and there was no post-mortem evidence of brain swelling. In the eighth animal ischaemic alterations were concentrated along the cortical arterial boundary zones. The cerebral perfusion pressure had fallen to 28 to 32 mm Hg for 30 minutes while the blood glucose did not fall below 34 mg/100 ml. Neither this degree of hypoglycaemia nor the hypotension *per se* would have resulted in brain damage. Evidently one factor can potentiate the effects of the other. This conclusion is also supported by the experiments of Meyer and Portnoy (1958) in the cat. After occlusion of the middle cerebral artery, localized neurological signs could be obtained by inducing hypoglycaemia and abolished by the administration of glucose. While the experiments of Kahn and Myers and of Meldrum *et al.* indicate that blood glucose must fall to 20 mg/100 ml if uncomplicated hypoglycaemia is to produce brain damage, a higher level of blood sugar if combined with some hypotension, hypoxaemia or epileptic activity may have the same outcome.

It is now apparent that ischaemic cell change is the consequence of each type of hypoxia as well as hypoglycaemia. While the term is physiologically inappropriate in the latter situation it is appropriate where the neuronal alteration is concerned. The microvacuoles characteristic of its earliest stage have been shown to be expanded mitochondria (McGee-Russell *et al.* 1970; Brown and Brierley 1972, 1973). Thus mitochondrial swelling and eventual internal disorganization is a critical change in both hypoxia and hypoglycaemia.

The report of Anderson, Milner and Strich (1967) described a very different neuropathological picture as the apparent consequence of hypoglycaemia in the human infant. Neuronal alterations were generalized, including chromatolysis with cytoplasmic vacuolation in some and fragmentation of nuclear chromatin in others, with no suggestion of the pattern of 'selective vulnerability' seen in the adult brain. In view of the similarity between some of the reported neuronal alterations and autolytic changes these findings must be treated with reserve until confirmed by others.

Peripheral neuropathy is a rare complication of spontaneous hypoglycaemia, only 24 cases having been reported (Danta 1969). The clinical picture is that of a distal sensorimotor neuropathy. No pathological studies are available and electrophysiological examinations showed only slight reduction in conduction velocity.

Mild peripheral neuropathies, mainly sensory, have been reported after insulin-induced hypoglycaemia (Wauchope 1933; Stern, Dancey and McNaughton 1942); Ziegler (1954) and Williams (1955) described amyotrophy as a consequence of hypoglycaemia.

Selective vulnerability
Anatomical, physiological and metabolic aspects

Those regions of the central nervous system that are vulnerable to hypoxia in its widest sense have already been enumerated (p. 56). From the subsequent descriptions of the neuropathological changes characterizing each of the major categories of brain hypoxia it will now be apparent that only global brain ischaemia (exemplified by cardiac arrest) can lead to ischaemic alterations in a majority of the vulnerable regions in a majority of cases. An overall reduction in brain blood flow, with or without an element of hypoxaemia, results in a concentration of ischaemic alterations along arterial boundary zones. Obviously, these zones must also be regarded as regions of selective vulnerability. They are involved, not because of any intrinsic peculiarities of neuronal metabolism, structure or arrangement, but solely because of the haemodynamic disturbances that follow a reduction in perfusion pressure within the system of arterial anastomoses from which their blood supply is derived.

Experimental studies in primates have shown that hypotension (global oligaemia) and sub-atmospheric decompression (hypoxic hypoxia) can result in cerebral and cerebellar cortical boundary zone lesions of major to minor degree. In the basal ganglia alterations may range from major necrosis to complete normality. Such wide variations in the site and extent of the ischaemic alterations after a relatively uniform stress are most likely to be due to peculiarities in vascular anatomy at any level from the arterial trunk to the microcirculation.

The wide variations in the damage observed in arterial boundary zones, the basal ganglia and the hippocampi also imply that only some fraction of all selectively vulnerable regions is involved in any one case. On the other hand, in the great majority of cases, there is sparing of the anterior horn cells of the spinal cord, the motor nuclei of the brainstem and the principal nuclei of the hypothalamus. While it is accepted that the higher and more recently evolved regions of the telencephalon are most vulnerable to hypoxia, it is important to stress that where the neocortex is concerned hypoxic damage is never complete. Even in instances of the 'apallic state' lamination is usually recognizable in the frontal lobes and within each lamina there may be large numbers of normal neurons.

Two major hypotheses have been advanced to explain the characteristic distribution of hypoxic brain damage. The one advanced by Spielmeyer (1925) and his school has come to be known as the 'vascular theory'. The other was C. and O. Vogt's (1937) concept of 'pathoclisis', which postulated particular physicochemical properties

as a basis for local vulnerability. The vascular theory invoked anatomical factors such as the length and tortuous course of a particular artery as well as physiological factors such as vaso-spasm and stasis. The arguments for and against the vascular theory have been reviewed by Scholz (1963) and Meyer (1963). Where the hippocampus is concerned the length and tortuous course of the artery supplying the Sommer sector (Uchimura 1928), the rake-like pattern of terminal hippocampal arterioles (Scharrer 1940) and the fact that '. . . the hippocampus definitely lies on the watershed between the carotid and vertebro-basilar territories' (Coceani and Gloor 1966) all suggest that the hippocampus will be particularly vulnerable if there is an overall reduction in the supply of blood and oxygen to the brain. However, the observation (p. 63) that after hypotension in man the hippocampus is usually normal, while major lesions may be present in the cortical boundary zones, implies that anatomical vascular factors alone cannot account for the sparing of the structure when blood flow is greatly reduced. Neither can they explain why typical hypoxic alterations occur when in addition to a normal or only slightly reduced blood flow there is some reduction in blood oxygen or glucose content as in carbon monoxide intoxication and hypoglycaemia respectively.

Scholz (1963, p. 259) demonstrated the inability of the vascular theory to explain the neuropathological changes seen in the cerebellum after protracted survival. '. . . the Purkinje cells are those most vulnerable to hypoxia, they are followed by the granular cells whereas the Golgi cells are the most resistant. This scale of vulnerability can hardly be explained by differences in vascularization as suggested by Uchimura. . . .' The same argument can be applied to the zones of the hippocampi, the layers of the neocortex, the subdivisions of the amygdaloid complex and of the lentiform nuclei. Apparent confirmation of the role of a vascular factor in the genesis of hypoxic brain damage was advanced by Lindenberg (1955, 1963) who claimed that the typical alterations in the selectively vulnerable regions could be attributed to compression of arteries by a presumably invariable post-hypoxic brain swelling. In order that intracranial pressure should exceed that within arteries it was stated that '. . . acute lowering of systemic arterial pressure is a pre-requisite for such compression . . .' (Lindenberg 1963). However, manometric evidence for such hypotension and the corresponding levels of intra-cranial pressure have not been published. This hypothesis ignores the fact that intracranial pressure is sustained by cerebral perfusion pressure and can only exceed it in rare agonal states. It is easy to demonstrate, in the experimental primate with a post-hypoxic rise in intracranial pressure, that a sudden hypotensive episode will produce an immediate and parallel fall in intracranial pressure (Brierley, Meldrum and Brown 1971). Scholz (1963) pointed out that vascular compression could not explain the vulnerability of special fields in a structure such as the hippocampus and Brierley (1961) and Brierley et al. (1971) have stressed that post-hypoxic brain swelling is by no means invariable and that typical ischaemic alterations in the vulnerable regions can develop in its absence. Further, when such swelling does occur, it does not give rise to the major internal herniations and brainstem haemorrhages so often seen in acute space-occupying or traumatic lesions.

The local physicochemical properties postulated by the theory of pathoclisis have proved hard to isolate and define and of those that have been investigated none has been proved to have a role in the genesis of hypoxic damage in a particular region. Thus the demonstration by Maske (1955) of a high concentration of zinc in the hippocampi of animals has been confirmed in human post-mortem material by Friede (1966) using the histo-chemical method of Timm (1958). The concentration of the metal is high in h. 2 and 3 and low in h. 1. McLardy (1962) has demonstrated that the zinc is concentrated not in the cell bodies of h. 2 and 3 but in the terminations of the mossy fibres derived from the cells of the dentate gyrus. A parallel distribution of lactic dehydrogenase in these regions led Friede (1966) to speculate that high levels of the enzyme may imply an improved capacity for anaerobic glycolysis and thus an increased ability to survive hypoxia.

Further evidence for metabolic differentiation within the hippocampus was provided by Cogges-hall and MacLean (1958), who found, in mice, that a single dose of 3-acetyl-pyridine, a nicotinic acid analogue, resulted in partial or complete loss of neurons in the zinc-rich zones h. 2 and 3. While there is increasing evidence to show that physicochemical differences do exist in the hippo-campus and that some are coincident with the distribution of ischaemic damage, it is not yet possible to, say which are causally related to the phenomenon of selective damage. Other bio-chemical factors of more critical importance may yet be discovered.

The development by Levine (1960) of a preparation in the rat (unilateral carotid artery ligature followed by exposure to nitrogen), in which uni-lateral anoxic–ischaemic damage occurred in 80% of animals, provided a model in which the results of histo- and cytochemical techniques could be compared with those of conventional neuro-histology. Such an approach seemed to offer the possibility of identifying the earliest alterations in the vulnerable regions in biochemical terms and thus of providing an explanation for their vulnerability. The first 5 years of such studies were reviewed by Spector (1965) and it is evident that all workers were in more or less close agreement with the view of Becker (1963) that, where anoxic-ischaemic damage is concerned, in standard preparations detectable abnormalities before 12 hours are rare. Invariably all such standard preparations were derived from material fixed by immersion immediately after death and without awareness of the histological artefact and the poor quality of tissue preservation inseparable from this procedure (p. 45). Inevitably, it was claimed that histochemical techniques could define a 'biochemical lesion' before any that could be identified by the conventional staining of such poorly preserved material (MacDonald and Spector 1963).

Using in vivo perfusion-fixation of the rat Levine preparation, Brown and Brierley (1966, 1968) showed that microvacuolation was the earliest stage of ischaemic cell change and could be recognized when animals were perfused immediately after 5 and 15 minutes intermittent exposure to nitrogen (Brown and Brierley 1973) (see p. 46). The conclusion is inescapable that if a 'biochemical lesion' does precede that revealed by the light microscope in optimally fixed material, it must be demonstrated not after a survival of hours when neuronal damage is far advanced and irreversible but within the first few minutes of survival. Until cytochemical studies employing light and electron microscopes have been deployed within this narrow interval of time the local metabolic factors underlying selective vulnerability will be elusive.

The respirator brain

This term is synonymous with 'Brain death' which '. . . occurs when irreversible damage to the cerebral hemispheres and brainstem is so severe that the nervous system can no longer maintain internal homeostasis, i.e. autonomous respiratory, circulatory and temperature-regulating functions' (Plum 1972). After the commencement of mechanical ventilation, systemic circulatory failure develops within a few days or occasionally a few weeks. The electroencephalogram is isoelectric throughout this period and although reflex responses may be obtainable at a spinal level, they are entirely absent within the brainstem. Such total arrest of brain function is usually brought about by an arrest of circulation within the cranial cavity, which is often confirmed by the failure to obtain an angiogram, as the contrast medium is halted at the entry foramina of the carotid and vertebral arteries (Heiskanen 1964).

The clinical situations terminating in intracranial circulatory arrest include cardiac arrest, status epilepticus, head injury and space-occupying lesions, when each is severe enough to produce brain swelling. However, internal herniae need not be present (Mitchell, de la Torre, Alexander and Davis 1962). In the post-hypoxic situation, experimental studies (Brierley, Meldrum and Brown 1971) have shown that, during mechanical ventilation, intracranial pressure may fall gradually to a normal level.

In the absence of circulation, the dead brain undergoes a process of *in vivo* autolysis so that, at autopsy, its consistency is semi-fluid, it hardens poorly or not at all in formalin and sections, if obtainable, usually show poorly stained nuclei exhibiting more or less karyorrhexis. The cytoplasm, if it can be identified, is reduced to poorly staining fine fragments. (For references giving details of all cytological appearances, see Matakas, Cervos-Navarro and Schneider 1973.) In practice, the neuropathologist confronted with a poorly stained and often unrecognizable preparation will be able to refer to the clinical evidence in order to confirm a diagnosis of brain death

References

Adams, J. H., Brierley, J. B., Connor, R. C. R. & Treip, C. S. (1966) The effects of systemic hypotension upon the human brain. Clinical and neuropathological observations in 11 cases. *Brain*, **89**, 235-268.

Altmann, H. W. & Schubothe, H. (1942) Funktionelle und organische Schädigungen des Zentral-nervensystems der Katze im Unterdruckexperiment. *Beiträge zur pathologischen Anatomie und allgemeinen Pathologie*, **107**, 3-116.

Amann, E., Gerstenbrand, F. & Jellinger, K. (1971) Schwerer Hirnschaden (apallisches Syndrom) nach Herzstillstand. *Pädiatrie und Pädologie*, **6**, 121-134.

Anderson, J. M., Milner, R. D. G. & Strich, S. J. (1967) Effects of neonatal hypoglycaemia on the nervous system: a pathological study. *Journal of Neurology, Neurosurgery and Psychiatry*, **30**, 295-310.

Balò, J. (1928) Encephalitis periaxialis concentrica. *Archives of Neurology and Psychiatry (Chicago)*, **19**, 242-264.

Barcroft, J. (1925) *The Respiratory Functions of the Blood*. Part I. *Lessons from High Altitudes*, Cambridge University Press, London.

Bayliss, W. M. (1902) On the local reaction of the arterial wall to changes of internal pressure. *Journal of Physiology (London)*, **28**, 220-232.

Becker, N. H. (1963) Cytochemical studies in cerebral hypoxia in *Selective Vulnerability of the Brain in Hypoxaemia* (Eds. Schadé, J. P. & McMenemey, W. H.), pp. 317-325, Blackwell Scientific, Oxford.

Beecher, H. K. & Todd, D. P. (1954) *A Study of the Deaths associated with Anesthesia and Surgery*. American Lecture Series No. 254, Thomas, Springfield, Illinois.

Blagbrough, Avril E., Brierley, J. B. & Nicholson, A. N. (1973) Behavioural and neurological disturbances associated with hypoxic brain damage. *Journal of the Neurological Sciences*, **18**, 475-488.

Bogaert, L. van, Dallemagne, M. J. & Wegria, R. (1938) Recherche sur le besoin d'oxygène chronique et aigu chez Macacus Rhesus. Absence de lésions expérimentales des centres nerveux après intoxication par l'oxyde de carbone, le nitrite de soude et l'appauvrissement de l'air en oxygène. *Archives Internationales de Médicine Expérimentale*, **13**, 335-378.

Bour, H., Tutin, N. & Pasquier, P. (1967) The central nervous system and carbon monoxide poisoning. I. Clinical data with reference to 20 fatal cases in *Carbon Monoxide Poisoning* (Eds. Bour, H. & Ledingham, I. McA.), pp. 1-30, Progress in Brain Research, Vol. 24, Elsevier, Amsterdam.

Brierley, J. B. (1961) Some neuropathological contributions to problems of hypoxia in *Cerebral Anoxia and the Electroencephalogram* (Eds. Gastaut, H. & Meyer, J. S.), pp. 164-171, Thomas, Springfield, Illinois.

Brierley, J. B. (1965) The influence of brain swelling, age and hypotension upon the pattern of cerebral damage in hypoxia in *Proceedings of the 5th International Congress of Neuropathology, Zürich*, pp. 21-28, in *Excerpta Medica International Congress* Series No. 100.

Brierley, J. B.   (1971) The neuropathological sequelae of profound hypoxia in *Brain Hypoxia* (Eds. Brierley, J. B. & Meldrum, B. S.), pp. 147-151, Clinics in Developmental Medicine 39/40, Spastics International Medical Publications, Heinemann Medical, London.

Brierley, J. B.   (1972) The neuropathology of brain hypoxia in *Scientific Foundations of Neurology* (Eds. Critchley, M., O'Leary, J. L. & Jennett, B.), Vol. 2, pp. 243-252, Heinemann Medical, London.

Brierley, J. B.   (1975) A comparison between the effects of profound hypotension, hypoxia and cyanide on the brain of *M. mulatta* in *Primate Models of Neurological Disorders* (Ed. Meldrum, B. S.), Raven Press, New York.

Brierley, J. B., Adams, J. H., Graham, D. I. & Simpson, J. A.   (1971) Neocortical death after cardiac arrest. *Lancet*, **2**, 560-565.

Brierley, J. B., Brown, A. W., Excell, Barbara J. & Meldrum, B. S.   (1969) Brain damage in the Rhesus monkey resulting from profound arterial hypotension.   I. Its nature, distribution and general physiological correlates.   *Brain Research* **13**, 68-100.

Brierley, J. B., Brown, A. W. & Meldrum, B. S.   (1971*a*) The nature and time course of the neuronal alterations resulting from oligaemia and hypoglycaemia in the brain of *Macaca mulatta*. *Brain Research*, **25**, 483-499.

Brierley, J. B., Brown, A. W. & Meldrum, B. S.   (1971*b*) The neuropathology of insulin-induced hypoglycaemia in a primate (*M. mulatta*); Topography and cellular nature in *Brain Hypoxia* (Eds. Brierley, J. B. & Meldrum, B. S.), Clinics in Developmental Medicine 39/40, pp. 225-229, Spastics International Medical Publications, Heinemann Medical, London.

Brierley, J. B. & Cooper, J. E.   (1962) Cerebral complications of hypotensive anaesthesia in a healthy adult. *Journal of Neurology, Neurosurgery and Psychiatry*, **25**, 24-30.

Brierley, J. B. & Excell, Barbara J.   (1966) The effects of profound systemic hypotension upon the brain of M. Rhesus.   Physiological and pathological observations.   *Brain*, **89**, 269-298.

Brierley, J. B., Meldrum, B. S. & Brown, A. W.   (1971) Post-hypoxic brain swelling: physiological and anatomical aspects in *Brain Hypoxia* (Eds. Brierley, J. B. & Meldrum, B. S.), Clinics in Developmental Medicine 39/40, pp. 136-143. Spastics International Medical Publications, Heinemann Medical, London.

Brierley, J. B. & Miller, A. A.   (1966) Fatal brain damage after dental anaesthesia.   Its nature, aetiology and prevention.   *Lancet*, **2**, 869-873.

Brierley, J. B. & Nicholson, A. N.   (1969) Neuropathological correlates of neurological impairment following prolonged decompression.   *Aerospace Medicine*, **40**, 148-152.

Brown, A. W. & Brierley, J. B.   (1966) Evidence for early anoxic-ischaemic cell damage in the rat brain. *Experientia*, **22**, 546-547.

Brown, A. W. & Brierley, J. B.   (1968) The nature, distribution and earliest stages of anoxic-ischaemic nerve cell damage in the rat brain as defined by the optical microscope.   *British Journal of Experimental Pathology*, **49**, 87-106.

Brown, A. W. & Brierley, J. B.   (1971) The nature and time course of anoxic-ischaemic cell change in the rat brain.   An optical and electron microscope study in *Brain Hypoxia* (Eds. Brierley, J. B. & Meldrum, B. S.), Clinics in Developmental Medicine 39/40, pp. 49-60, Spastics International Medical Publications, Heinemann Medical, London.

Brown, A. W. & Brierley, J. B.   (1972) Anoxic-ischaemic cell change in rat brain.   Light microscopic and fine-structural observations.   *Journal of the Neurological Sciences*, **16**, 59-84.

Brown, A. W. & Brierley, J. B.   (1973) The earliest alterations in rat neurones after anoxia-ischaemia.   *Acta neuropathologica (Berlin)*, **23**, 9-22.

Brucher, J. M.   (1967) Neuropathological problems posed by carbon monoxide poisoning and anoxia in *Carbon Monoxide Poisoning* (Eds. Bour, H. & Ledingham, I. McA.), Progress in Brain Research, Vol. 24, pp. 75-100, Elsevier, Amsterdam.

Buchner, F.   (1957) Die Pathologie der cellulären und geweblichen Oxydationen. *Handbuch der allgemeinen Pathologie*, Band 4/2, pp. 569-668, Springer Verlag, Berlin.

Cammermeyer, J.   (1961) The importance of avoiding 'dark' neurones in experimental neuropathology.   *Acta neuropathologica, (Berlin)* **1**, 245-270.

Campbell, E. J. M.   (1965) Respiratory failure.   *British Medical Journal*, **1**, 1451-1460.

Coceani, F. & Gloor, P.   (1966) The distribution of the internal carotid circulation in the brain of the Macaque monkey (Macaca mulatta).   *Journal of Comparative Neurology*, **128**, 419-428.

Coggeshall, R. E. & Maclean, P. D.   (1958) Hippocampal lesions following administration of 3-acetylpyridine. *Proceedings of the Society for Experimental Biology and Medicine*, **98**, 687-689.

Cohen, P. J.   (1966) The effects of decreased oxygen tension on cerebral circulation, metabolism and function in *Proceedings of the International Symposium on the Cardiovascular and Respiratory Effects of Hypoxia*, Kingston, Ontario (Eds. Hatcher, J. D. & Jennings, D. B.), pp. 81-104, Karger, Basel.

Courville, C. B.   (1954) Case studies in cerebral anoxia.   III. Structural changes in the brain after cardiac standstill during spinal anesthesia.   *Bulletin of the Los Angeles Neurological Society*, **19**, 142-150.

Cullity, G. J. & Kakulas, B. A.   (1970) Encephalopathy and fatty degeneration of the viscera: an evaluation.   *Brain*, **93**, 77-88.

Danta, G.   (1969) Hypoglycemic peripheral neuropathy.   *Archives of Neurology (Chicago)*, **21**, 121-132.

Desmarest, E. & L'Hermitte, J.   (1939) Étude anatomoclinique d'un cas de réanimation à la suite d'une syncope opératoire.   Interruption complète de la circulation, massage du coeur.   *Revue Neurologique*, **71**, 308-314.

Edelmann, F.   (1921) Ein Beitrag zur Vergiftung mit gasformiger Blausäure insbesondere zu den dabei auftretenden Gehirnveränderungen.   *Deutsche Zeitschrift für Nervenheilkunde*, **72**, 259-287.

Ehrich, W. E., Bellet, S. & Lewey, F. H.   (1944) Cardiac changes from CO poisoning.   *American Journal of Medical Science*, **208**, 511-523.

Erbslöh, F.   (1958) Das Zentralnervensystem bei Krankheiten des Herzens und der Lungen.   I. Die Hinveränderungen beim Herzstillstand und bei der akuten Herz-und Kreislauffinsuffizienz in *Henke-Lubarsch-Rössle Handbuch der Speziellen Pathologischen Anatomie und Histologie*, Band XIII, p. 1330, Springer, Heidelberg.

Ernsting. J.   (1963) Some effects of brief profound anoxia upon the central nervous system in *Selective Vulnerability of the Brain in Hypoxaemia* (Eds. Schadé, J. P. & McMenemey, W. M.), pp. 41-45, Blackwell Scientific, Oxford.

Eros, G. & Priestman, G.   (1942) Cerebral vascular changes in carbon monoxide poisoning.   *Journal of Neuropathology and Experimental Neurology*, **1**, 158-172.

Ferraro, A.   (1933) Experimental toxic encephalomyelopathy (Diffuse sclerosis following subcutaneous injections of potassium cyanide).   *Psychiatric Quarterly*, **7**, 267-283.

Ferraro, A. & Morrison, R.   (1928) Illuminating gas poisoning.   An experimental study of the lesions of the nervous system in acute and chronic stages.   *Psychiatric Quarterly*, **2**, 506-541.

Fiddian, R. V., Byar, D. & Edwards, E. A.   (1964) Factors affecting flow through a stenosed vessel.   *Archives of Surgery*, **88**, 83-89.

Finley, K. H. & Brenner, C.   (1941) Histologic evidence of damage to the brain in monkeys treated with metrazol and insulin.   *Archives of Neurology and Psychiatry (Chicago)*, **45**, 403-438.

Fog, M.   (1938) Relationship between blood pressure and tonic regulation of pial arteries.   *Journal of Neurology and Psychiatry*, **1**, 187-197.

Forbes, H. S., Nason, G. I. & Wortman, R. C.   (1937) Cerebral circulation: vasodilation in the pia following stimulation of the vagus, aortic and carotid sinus nerves.   *Archives of Neurology and Psychiatry (Chicago)*, **37**, 334-350.

Friede, R. L.   (1966) The histochemical architecture of the Ammons horn as related to its selective vulnerability.   *Acta neuropathologica (Berlin)*, **6**, 1-13.

Garland, H. & Pearce, J.   (1967) Neurological complications of carbon monoxide poisoning.   *Quarterly Journal of Medicine*, **36**, 445-455.

Gastaut, H., Bostem, F., Fernandez-Guardiola, A., Naquet, R. & Gibson, W.   (1961) Hypoxic activation of the EEG by nitrogen inhalation.   I. Preliminary observations in generalized epilepsy in *Cerebral Anoxia and the Encephalogram* (Eds. Gastaut, H. & Meyer, J. S.), pp. 343-354, Thomas, Springfield, Illinois.

Gastaut, H., Fischgold, H. & Meyer, J. S.   (1961) Conclusions of the International Colloquium on Anoxia and the EEG in *Cerebral Anoxia and the Electroencephalogram* (Eds. Gastaut, H. & Meyer, J. S.), pp. 599-617, Thomas, Springfield, Illinois.

Gilles, F. H.   (1963) Selective symmetrical neuronal necrosis of certain brain stem tegmental nuclei in temporary cardiac standstill.   *Journal of Neuropathology and Experimental Neurology*, **22**, 319.

Ginsberg, M. D., Myers, R. E. & McDonagh, B. F.   (1974) Experimental carbon monoxide encephalopathy in the primate.   II. Clinical aspects.   Neuropathology and physiologic correlation.   *Archives of Neurology*, **30**, 209-216.

Gray, F. D. & Horner, G. H.   (1970) Survival following extreme hypoxemia.   *Journal of the American Medical Association*, **211**, 1815-1817.

Greenfield, J. G. & Meyer, A.   (1963) General pathology of the nerve cell and neuroglia in *Greenfield's Neuropathology*, pp. 1-70, Arnold, London.

Grenell, R. G.   (1946) Central nervous system resistance: I. The effects of temporary arrest of cerebral circulation for periods of two to ten minutes.   *Journal of Neuropathology and Experimental Neurology*, **5**, 131-154.

Grinkler, R. R.   (1925) Über einen Fall von Leuchtgasvergiftung mit doppelseitiger Pallidumerweichung und schwerer Degeneration des tieferen Grosshirnmarklagers.   *Zeitschrift für die gesamte Neurologie und Psychiatrie*, **98**, 433-456.

Haymaker, W., Ginzler, A. M. & Ferguson, R. L. (1952) Residual neuropathological effects of cyanide poisoning. A study of the central nervous system of 23 dogs exposed to cyanide compounds. *Military Surgeon*, **111**, 231-246.

Heiskanen, O. (1964) Cerebral circulatory arrest caused by acute increase of intracranial pressure. A clinical and roentgenological study of 25 cases. *Acta Neurologica Scandinavica*, **40**, *Suppl. 17*, 1-57.

Hicks, S. P. (1950a) Brain metabolism *in vivo*. I. The distribution of lesions caused by cyanide poisoning, insulin hypoglycemia, asphyxia in nitrogen and fluoroacetate poisoning in rats. *Archives of Pathology*, **49**, 111-137.

Hicks, S. P. (1950b) Brain metabolism *in vivo*. II. The distribution of lesions caused by azide, malonitrile, plasmocid and dinitrophenol poisoning in rats. *Archives of Pathology*, **50**, 545-561.

Hill, L. & Mott, F. W. (1906) The neurofibrils of the larger ganglion cells of the motor cortex of animals in which the four arteries have been ligatured to produce cerebral anaemia. *Proceedings of the Physiological Society of London*, p. 4.

Hiller, F. (1924) Ueber die krankhaften Veränderungen in Zentralnervensystem nach Kohlenoxydvergiftung. *Zeitschrift für die gesamte Neurologie und Psychiatrie*, **93**, 594-646.

Hirano, A., Levine, S. & Zimmerman, H. M. (1967) Experimental cyanide encephalopathy. Electron microscopic observations of early lesions in white matter. *Journal of Neuropathology and Experimental Neurology*, **26**, 200-213.

Hoff, E. C., Grenell, R. G. & Fulton, J. F. (1945) Histopathology of the central nervous system after exposure to high altitudes, hypoglycemia and other conditions associated with central anoxia. *Medicine*, **24**, 161-217.

Hsü, Y. K. & Ch'eng, Y. L. (1938) Cerebral subcortical myelinopathy in carbon monoxide poisoning. *Brain*, **61**, 384-392.

Hurst, E. W. (1940) Experimental demyelination of the central nervous system. 1. The encephalopathy produced by potassium cyanide. *Australian Journal of Experimental Biology and Medical Science*, **18**, 201-223.

Hurst, E. W. (1942) Experimental demyelination of the central nervous system. 3. Poisoning with potassium cyanide, sodium azide, hydroxylamine, narcotics, carbon monoxide, etc. *Australian Journal of Experimental Biology and Medical Science*, **20**, 297-312.

Ingvar, D. & Brun, A. (1972) Das komplette apallische Syndrom. *Archiv für Psychiatrie und Nervenkrankheiten*, **215**, 219-239.

Jacob, H. (1939) Über die diffuse Hemisphärenmarkerkrankung nach Kohlenoxydvergiftung bei Fällen mit klinisch intervallärer Verlaufsform. *Zeitschrift für die gesamte Neurologie und Psychiatrie*, **167**, 161-179.

Jacob, H. (1957) Strangulation in *Henke-Lubarsch-Rössle Handbuch der Speziellen Pathologischen Anatomie und Histologie*, Band. XIII, pp. 1712-1731, Springer Verlag, Heidelberg.

Jacob, H. (1963) CNS tissue and cellular pathology in hypoxaemic states in *Selective Vulnerability of the Brain in Hypoxaemia* (Eds. Schadé, J. P. & McMenemey, W. H.), pp. 153-163, Blackwell Scientific, Oxford.

Kahn, K. J. & Myers, R. E. (1971) Insulin-induced hypoglycaemia in the non-human primate. I. Clinical consequences in *Brain Hypoxia* (Eds. Brierley, J. B. & Meldrum, B. S.), Clinics in Developmental Medicine 39/40, pp. 185-194, Spastics International Medical Publications, Heinemann Medical, London.

Koenig, R. S. & Koenig, H. (1952) An experimental study of post mortem alterations in neurons of the central nervous system. *Journal of Neuropathology and Experimental Neurology*, **11**, 69-78.

Környey, S. (1963) Patterns of CNS vulnerability to CO, cyanide and other poisoning in *Selective Vulnerability of the Brain in Hypoxaemia* (Eds. Schadé, J. P. & McMenemey, W. M.), pp. 165-176, Blackwell Scientific, Oxford.

Kubik, C. S. (1949) Pathological findings in five cases of carbon monoxide poisoning. *Journal of Neuropathology and Experimental Neurology*, **8**, 112-113.

Kuhn, R. A. (1962) The speed of cerebral circulation. *New England Journal of Medicine*, **267**, 689-695.

Lambert, S. W. (1919) Poisoning by hydrocyanic acid gas with especial reference to its effects upon the brain. *Neurology Bulletin*, **2**, 93-105.

Lapresle, J. & Fardeau, M. (1966) Les leucoencéphalopathies de l'intoxication oxycarbonée. Étude de seize observations anatomocliniques. *Acta Neuropathologica (Berlin)*, **6**, 327-348.

Lapresle, J. & Fardeau, M. (1967) The central nervous system and carbon monoxide poisoning. II. Anatomical study of brain lesions following intoxication with carbon monoxide (22 cases) in *Carbon Monoxide Poisoning* (Eds. Bour, H. & Ledingham, I. McA.), Progress in Brain Research, Vol. 24, pp. 31-74, Elsevier, Amsterdam.

Lapresle, J. & Milhaud, M. (1962) Lesions du système nerveux central après arrêt circulatoire. Étude de 10 cas. *La Presse Médicale*, **70**, 429-432.

Lawrence, R. D., Meyer, A. & Nevin, S. (1942) The pathological changes in the brain in fatal hypoglycemia. *Quarterly Journal of Medicine*, **11**, 181-202.

De Lehoczky, T. (1949) Du mécanisme physiopathologique des lésions centrales de l'intoxication oxycarbonée. *Acta neurologica Belgica*, **49**, 488-503.

Levine, S. (1960) Anoxic-ischaemic encephalopathy in rats. *American Journal of Pathology*, **36**, 1-17.

Levine, S. (1967) Experimental cyanide encephalopathy. Gradients of susceptibility in the corpus callosum. *Journal of Neuropathology and Experimental Neurology*, **26**, 214-222.

Levine, S. & Stypulkowski, W. (1959a) Experimental cyanide encephalopathy. *Archives of Pathology*, **67**, 303-323.

Levine, S. & Stypulkowski, W. (1959b) Effect of ischemia on cyanide encephalopathy. *Neurology (Minneapolis)*, **9**, 407-411.

Levine, S. & Wenk, E. J. (1959) Cyanide encephalopathy produced by intravenous route. *Journal of Nervous and Mental Disease*, **129**, 302-305.

Lewey, F. H. & Drabkin, D. L. (1944) Experimental chronic carbon monoxide poisoning of dogs. *American Journal of Medical Science*, **208**, 502-511.

Lindenberg, R. (1955) Compression of brain arteries as a pathogenetic factor for tissue necroses and their areas of predilection. *Journal of Neuropathology and Experimental Neurology*, **14**, 223-243.

Lindenberg, R. (1957) Die Gefässversorgung und ihre Bedeutung für Art und Ort von kreislaufbedingten Gewebsschäden und Gefässprozessen in *Henke-Lubarsch-Rössle. Handbch. spez. path. Anat.*, Band. XIII, pp. 1071-1110, Springer, Heidelberg.

Lindenberg, R. (1963) Patterns of CNS vulnerability in acute hypoxaemia, including anaesthesia accidents in *Selective Vulnerability of the Brain in Hypoxaemia* (Eds. Schadé, J. P. & McMenemey, W. H.), pp. 184-209, Blackwell Scientific, Oxford.

Lübbers, D. W. (1966) The oxygen pressure field of the brain and its significance for the normal and critical oxygen supply of the brain in *Oxygen Transport in Blood and Tissue* (Eds. Lübbers, D. W., Luft, U. C., Thews, G. & Witzleb, E.), pp. 124-139, Thieme, Stuttgart.

Luft, V. C. (1965) Aviation physiology—the effects of altitude in *Handbook of Physiology*, Section 3, Respiration, Vol. II, pp. 1099-1145, American Physiological Society, Washington, D.C.

Luft, V. C. & Finkelstein, S. (1968) Hypoxia: a clinical-physiological approach. *Aerospace Medicine*, **39**, 105-110.

Macdonald, M. & Spector, R. G. (1963) The influence of anoxia on respiratory enzymes in rat brain. *British Journal of Experimental Pathology*, **44**, 11-15.

McGee-Russell, S. M., Brown, A. W. & Brierley, J. B. (1970) A combined light and electron microscope study of early anoxic-ischaemic cell change in rat brain. *Brain Research*, **20**, 193-200.

McIlwain, H. (1966) *Biochemistry and the Central Nervous System*, 3rd Edn., Churchill, London.

McLardy, T. (1962) Zinc enzymes and the hippocampal mossy fibre system. *Nature (London)*, **194**, 300-302.

Mandel, M. M. & Berry, R. G. (1959) Human brain changes in cardiac arrest. *Surgery, Gynecology and Obstetrics*, **108**, 692-696.

Marks, V. & Rose, F. C. (1965) *Hypoglycaemia*, Blackwell Scientific, Oxford.

Maske, H. (1955) Über den topochemischen Nachweis von Zink in Ammonshorn verschiedenen Säugetiere. *Naturwissenschaften*, **42**, 424.

Matakas, F., Cervos-Navarro, J. & Schneider, H. (1973) Experimental brain death. I. Morphology and fine structure of the brain. *Journal of Neurology, Neurosurgery and Psychiatry*, **36**, 497-508.

Meldrum, B. S. & Brierley, J. B. (1969) Brain damage in the Rhesus monkey resulting from profound arterial hypotension. II. Changes in the spontaneous and evoked electrical activity of the neocortex. *Brain Research*, **13**, 101-118.

Meldrum, B. S. & Brierley, J. B. (1973) Prolonged epileptic seizures in primates. Ischemic cell change and its relation to ictal physiological events. *Archives of Neurology (Chicago)*, **28**, 8-17.

Meldrum, B. S., Horton, R. W. & Brierley, J. B. (1971) Insulin-induced hypoglycaemia in the primate: relationship between physiological changes and neuropathology in *Brain Hypoxia* (Eds. Brierley, J. B. & Meldrum, B. S.), Clinics in Developmental Medicine 39/40, pp. 207-224, Spastics International Medical Publications, Heinemann Medical, London.

Mettler, F. A. & Sax, D. S. (1972) Cerebellar cortical degeneration due to acute azide poisoning. *Brain*, **95**, 505-516.

Meyer, A. (1926) Ueber die Wirkung der Kohlenoxydvergiftung auf das Zentralnervensystem. *Zeitschrift für die gesamte Neurologie und Psychiatrie*, **100**, 201-247.

Meyer, A. (1928) Über das Verhalten des Hemisphärenmarks bei der menschlichen Kohlenoxydvergiftung. *Zeitschrift für die gesamte Neurologie und Psychiatrie*, **112**, 172-186.

Meyer, A.   (1932) Experimentelle Vergiftungsstudien.   II. Vergleichende phylogenetische Untersuchungen über Kohlenoxydvergiftung des Gehirns.   *Zeitschrift für die gesamte Neurologie und Psychiatrie*, **139**, 422-423.

Meyer, A.   (1933) Experimentelle Vergiftungsstudien.   III. Über Gehirnveränderungen bei experimenteller Blausäurevergiftung.   *Zeitschrift für die gesamte Neurologie und Psychiatrie*, **143**, 333-348.

Meyer, A.   (1936) The selective regional vulnerability of the brain and its relation to psychiatric problems.   *Proceedings of the Royal Society of Medicine*, **29**, 1175-1181.

Meyer, A.   (1956) Neuropathological aspects of anoxia.   *Proceedings of the Royal Society of Medicine*, **49**, 619-622.

Meyer, A.   (1963) Anoxic poisons and the problems of anoxia and selective vulnerability in *Greenfield's Neuropathology*, 2nd Edition, pp. 237-261, Arnold, London.

Meyer, J. E.   (1953) Über die Lokalisation frühkindlicher Hirnschäden in arteriellen Grenzgebieten.   *Archiv für Psychiatrie und Nervenkrankheiten*, **190**, 328-341.

Meyer, J. S. & Portnoy, H. D.   (1958) Localized cerebral hypoglycemia simulating stroke.   A clinical and experimental study.   *Neurology (Minneapolis)*, **8**, 601-614.

Miller, J. R. & Myers, R. E.   (1972) Neuropathology of systemic circulatory arrest in adult monkeys.   *Neurology (Minneapolis)*, **22**, 888-904.

Milstein, B. B.   (1956) Cardiac arrest and resuscitation.   *Annals of the Royal College of Surgeons of England*, **19**, 69-87.

Mitchell, O. C., de la Torre, R., Alexander, E. & Davis, C. H.   (1962) The non-filling phenomenon during angiography in acute intracranial hypertension.   Report of 5 cases and an experimental study.   *Journal of Neurosurgery*, **19**, 766-774.

Myers, R. E. & Kahn, K. J.   (1971) Insulin-induced hypoglycaemia in the non-human primate.   II. Long-term neuropathological consequences in *Brain Hypoxia* (Eds. Brierley, J. B. & Meldrum, B. S.), Clinics in Developmental Medicine 39/40, pp. 195-206, Spastics International Medical Publications, Heinemann Medical, London.

Neubuerger, K. T.   (1954) Lesions of the human brain following circulatory arrest.   *Journal of Neuropathology and Experimental Neurology*, **13**, 144-160.

Neubuerger, K. T. & Clarke, E. R.   (1945) Subacute carbon monoxide poisoning with cerebral myelinopathy and multiple myocardial necroses.   *Rocky Mountain Medical Journal*, **42**, 29-34.

Nicholson, A. N. & Ernsting, J.   (1967) Neurological sequelae of prolonged decompression.   *Aerospace Medicine*, **38**, 389-394.

Nicholson, A. N., Freeland, Susan A. & Brierley, J. B.   (1970) A behavioural and neuropathological study of the sequelae of profound hypoxia.   *Brain Research*, **22**, 327-345.

Penfield, W. & Cone, W.   (1926) Acute swelling of oligodendroglia.   A specific type of neuroglia change.   *Archives of Neurology and Psychiatry (Chicago)*, **16**, 131-153.

Peters, J. P. & Van Slyke, D. D.   (1932) Hemoglobin and Oxygen in *Quantitative Clinical Chemistry*, Vol. I, pp. 518-562, Williams and Wilkins, Baltimore.

Plum, F.   (1972) Organic disturbances of consciousness in *Scientific Foundations of Neurology* (Eds. Critchley, M., O'Leary, J. L. & Jennett, B.), Section VI, Vol. 3, pp. 193-201, Heinemann Medical, London.

Plum, F., Posner, J. B. & Hain, R. F.   (1962) Delayed neurological deterioration after anoxia.   *Archives of Internal Medicine*, **110**, 18-25.

Poursines, Y., Alliez, J. & Toga, M.   (1956) Étude des lésions corticales d'un cas d'intoxication oxycarbonée.   *Révue Neurologique*, **94**, 731-735.

Ranck, J. B. & Windle, W. F.   (1959) Brain damage in the monkey, *Macaca mulatta* by asphyxia neonatorum.   *Experimental Neurology*, **1**, 130-154.

Raskin, N. & Mullaney, O. C.   (1940) The mental and neurological sequelae of carbon monoxide asphyxia in a case observed for 15 years.   *Journal of Nervous and Mental Disease*, **92**, 640-659.

Richardson, J. E. & Russell, D. S.   (1952) Cerebral disease due to functioning islet-cell tumours, with pathological reports.   *Lancet*, **2**, 1054-1059.

Romanul, F. C. A. & Abramowicz, A.   (1964) Changes in brain and pial vessels in arterial border zones.   *Archives of Neurology (Chicago)*, **11**, 40-65.

Rossen, R., Kabat, H. & Anderson, J. P.   (1943) Acute arrest of cerebral circulation in man.   *Archives of Neurology and Psychiatry (Chicago)*, **50**, 510-528.

Scharrer, E.   (1938) On dark and light cells in the brain and the liver.   *Anatomical Record*, **72**, 53-65.

Scharrer, E.   (1940) Vascularization and vulnerability of the Cornu Ammonis in the opossum.   *Archives of Neurology and Psychiatry (Chicago)*, **44**, 483-506.

Schmorl. (1920) Demonstrationen 3. Gehirn bei Blausäurevergiftung. *Münchener Medizinische Wochenschrift*, 67, 913.

Schneider, M. (1961) Survival and revival of the brain in anoxia and ischaemia in *Cerebral Anoxia and the Electroencephalogram* (Eds. Gastaut, H. & Meyer, J. S.), pp. 134-143, Thomas, Springfield, Ill.

Scholz, W. (1952) Les nécroses parenchymateuses électives par hypoxémie et oligémie et leur expression topistique. *Proceedings of the First International Congress of Neuropathology (Rome)*, Vol. I, pp. 321-346.

Scholz, W. (1953) Selective neuronal necrosis and its topistic patterns in hypoxemia and oligemia. *Journal of Neuropathology and Experimental Neurology*, 12, 249-261.

Scholz, W. (1957) An nervösesystemegebundene (topistische) Kreislaufschäden in *Henke-Lubarsch-Rössle Hand. spez. path. Anat. Hist.*, XIII/1, Bandteil, B, pp. 1326-1383.

Scholz, W. (1963) Topistic lesion in *Selective Vulnerability of the Brain in Hypoxaemia* (Eds. Schadé, J. P. & McMenemey, W. M.), pp. 257-267, Blackwell Scientific, Oxford.

Seitelberger, F. & Jellinger, K. (1960) Zur Frage der CO-leucoencephalopathie. *Wiener klinische Wochenschrift*, 72, 422-429.

Spector, R. G. (1965) Enzyme chemistry of anoxic brain injury in *Neurohistochemistry* (Ed. Adams, C. W. M.), pp. 547-557, Elsevier, Amsterdam.

Spielmeyer, W. (1922) *Histopathologie des Nervensystems*, pp. 74-79, Springer Verlag, Berlin.

Spielmeyer, W. (1925) Zur Pathogenese örtlich elektiven Gehirnveränderungen. *Zeitschrift für die gesamte Neurologie und Psychiatrie*, 99, 756-776.

Stephenson, H. E., Reid, L. C. & Hinton, J. W. (1953) Some common denominators in 1200 cases of cardiac arrest. *Annals of Surgery*, 137, 731-744.

Stern, K., Dancey, T. E. & McNaughton, F. L. (1942) Sensory disturbances following insulin treatment of psychoses. *Journal of Nervous and Mental Disease*, 95, 183-191.

Swann, H. G. & Brucer, M. (1949) The cardiorespiratory and biochemical events during rapid hypoxic death. I. Fulminating hypoxia. *Texas Reports on Biology and Medicine*, 7, 511-538.

Timm, F. (1958) Zur Histochemie des Ammonshorngebietes. *Zeitschrift für Zellforschung*, 48, 548-555.

Tindall, G. T., Odom, G. L., Cupp, H. B. & Dillon, M. L. (1962) Studies on carotid artery flow and pressure: observations in 18 patients during graded occlusion of proximal carotid artery. *Journal of Neurosurgery*, 19, 917-923.

Uchimura, J. (1928) Zur Pathogenese der örtlich elektiven Ammonshornerkrankung. *Zeitschrift für die gesamte Neurologie und Psychiatrie*, 114, 567-601.

Vander Eecken, H. M. (1959) *The Anastomoses between the Leptomeningeal Arteries of the Brain*, Thomas, Springfield, Ill.

Van Liere, E. J. & Stickney, J. C. (1963) *Hypoxia*, University of Chicago Press, Chicago.

Vital, C. I., Picard, J., Arné, L., Aubertin, J., Fenelon, J. & Mouton, L. (1967) Étude anatomoclinique de 3 cas d'encephalopathie hypoglycémique (dont un après sulfamidotherapie). *Le Diabète*, 12F, 291-296.

Vogt, C. & Vogt, O. (1937) Sitz und Wesen der Krankheiten im Lichte der topistischen Hirnforschung und des Variierens der Tiere. *Journal für Psychologie und Neurologie (Leipzig)*, 47, 237-457.

Vuia, O. (1967) Leucoencéphalopathie souscorticale par intoxication au CO. *Acta neuropathologica (Berlin)*, 7, 305-314.

Warburg, O. (1926) Über die Wirkung des Kohlenoxyds auf den Stoffwechsel der Hefe. *Biochemische Zeitschrift*, 177, 471-486.

Wauchope, G. M. (1933) Hypoglycaemia: critical review. *Quarterly Journal of Medicine*, 26, 117-156.

Weinberger, L. M., Gibbon, M. H. & Gibbon, J. H. (1940) Temporary arrest of the circulation to the central nervous system. II. Pathologic effects. *Archives of Neurology and Psychiatry (Chicago)*, 43, 961-986.

Williams, C. J. (1955) Amyotrophy due to hypoglycaemia. *British Medical Journal*, 1, 707-708.

Wolf, A. & Siris, J. (1937) Acute non-traumatic encephalomalacia complicating neurosurgical operations in the sitting position. *Bulletin of the Neurological Institute of New York*, 6, 42-61.

Yant, W. P., Chornyak, J., Schrenk, H. H., Patty, F. A. & Sayers, R. R. (1934) Studies in asphyxia. *Public Health Bulletin (Washington)*, No. 211, 1-61.

Ziegler, D. K. (1954) Minor neurologic signs and symptoms following insulin coma therapy. *Journal of Nervous and Mental Disease*, 120, 75-78.

Zülch, K. J. (1953) Neue Befunde und Deutungen aus der Gefässpathologie des Hirns und Rückenmarks. *Zentralblatt für allgemeine Pathologie und Pathologische Anatomie*, 90, 402.

Zülch, K. J. & Behrend, R. C. H. (1961) The pathogenesis and topography of anoxia, hypoxia and ischemia of the brain in man in *Cerebral Anoxia and the Electroencephalogram* (Eds. Gastaut, H. & Meyer, J. S.), pp. 144-163, Thomas, Springfield, Ill.

3

Vascular Disease of the Central Nervous System

Revised by P. O. Yates

Applied anatomy and physiology

Arterial blood supply

The *brain* is supplied with blood through the internal carotid and vertebral arteries. These vessels anastomose at the base of the brain via the basilar artery and the circle of Willis, the potential efficiency of which can be judged from cases in which sufficient blood for survival reached the brain through one internal carotid or one vertebral artery, the other three vessels being closed by thromboatherosclerosis. In such cases additional blood supply is often found from the external carotids by retrograde flow along such branches of the upper internal carotid as the ophthalmic artery. Considerable variation occurs in the size and completeness of the component branches of the circle of Willis; perhaps only about 20% are of the standard pattern (Riggs and Rupp 1963).

From the circle of Willis the arterial distribution may be simplified by considering it to consist of (1) paramedian vessels perforating the base of the brain to supply structures near the midline, (2) short circumferential vessels supplying the thalamus, lentiform nuclei and other basal ganglia, and (3) long circumferential branches, the anterior, middle and posterior cerebral arteries, supplying principally the cortex and underlying white matter.

There is evidence of anastomosis between the anterior, middle and posterior cerebral arteries, at arterial level in the pia arachnoid (Vander Eecken and Adams 1953) and at capillary level within the cerebral tissue. Exceptionally, significant arterial anastomoses between the central and the peripheral system may be found near the angle of the lateral ventricle where the most lateral of the striate vessels contributes a sub-

stantial branch to the post-central gyrus in 4% of cases (Cole 1967).

Following obstruction of one of the main cerebral arteries or one of its major branches, the anastomosis may only be sufficient to take over part of the bed of supply of the obstructed artery. The amount taken over depends, *inter alia*, upon the blood pressure in the anastomosing vessels. When this is high a considerable amount of tissue, in the theoretical field of supply of the occluded artery, may survive. When, however, the diastolic pressure is low, as in ulcerative endocarditis, the region of necrosis will be considerably larger Such necrosis affects not only the cortex but also the underlying white matter. In the frontal and occipital lobes the region of necrosis is somewhat wedge-shaped and extends almost as far as the ventricular wall.

The brainstem and cerebellum are also supplied with blood on the basis of (1) paramedian branches from the basilar artery, (2) short circumferential branches and (3) long circumferential arteries such as the superior, anterior and posterior inferior cerebellar arteries. There are anastomoses between surface branches of these last three paired arteries across the midline and with each other; and also between branches of the superior cerebellar and posterior cerebral arteries. These surface anastomoses, although abundant, are however only occasionally sufficient to supply all the cerebellar cortex if one or more of the arteries, or pairs of arteries, is obstructed by disease. Atkinson (1949) found that coloured gelatin injected into the anterior inferior cerebellar artery always stained the cerebellar distribution of the artery, but did not spread into the territory of adjacent arteries. In the pons the paramedian arteries, which supply the ventromedial portion of the brainstem, do not anastomose significantly with each other across the midline, or with the other arteries supplying the brainstem.

The ventrolateral portions of midbrain and pons are supplied by the short circumferential arteries, but there is disagreement about the blood supply of the tegmentum, as revealed both by injection techniques and by infarction following vascular occlusion. Foix and Hillemand (1926) decided that the tegmentum of the midbrain is supplied by the superior cerebellar arteries and that the tegmentum of the pons is supplied by the short circumferential arteries. Kubik and Adams (1946) agreed that the tegmentum of the pons is supplied by the short circumferential arteries but considered that there is a varying contribution by the paramedian and long circumferential arteries. Atkinson (1949) found, however, that the lateral parts of the tegmentum of the pons are supplied by the anterior inferior cerebellar arteries while Biemond (1951) considered that the superior cerebellar arteries supply the tegmentum of both midbrain and pons.

Venous drainage

In contrast to the arteries, the surface veins of the brain have abundant anastomoses of large calibre. The ill effects of localized venous obstruction are therefore slight. Obstruction of portions of the superior sagittal sinus may cause only slight parasagittal infarction. Very much more serious is concomitant thrombosis of adjacent veins which obstructs the collateral circulation. The veins of the brain drain into the dural venous sinuses and through them into the internal jugular veins. The dural sinuses also communicate with the vascular channels in the diploe of the bones of the skull and these channels communicate with extracranial veins. Fracture of the skull can thus initiate retrograde thrombosis. In addition there are emissary veins which connect the dural venous sinuses with extracranial veins. The cavernous sinuses are connected via the ophthalmic veins with the facial veins, via emissary veins passing through foramen ovale and the carotid canal with the pterygoid and pharyngeal venous plexuses, and via the basilar venous sinuses with the spinal veins. The lateral venous sinuses are connected via mastoid emissary veins with the occipital veins, and the superior sagittal sinus is connected with extracranial posterior parietal veins via the parietal emissary veins. All these venous communications are potential pathways for the intracranial spread of extracranial pyogenic infection.

An important anastomotic series of venous channels connect those of the posterior fossa with the vertebral plexuses and thence to the veins of the rest of the body. It has been suggested by Batson (1957) that these represent an important route for the passage of metastatic tumour to the nervous system.

Histology

The capillaries of the central nervous system are similar histologically to those elsewhere in the body except that they have no envelope of reticulin fibres. They are lined by flattened, polygonal, endothelial cells joined together by cement substance and covered by the expanded footplates of the astrocytes. However, the endothelial cells appear to have more tight junctions than is usual in capillaries in the rest of the body (Fig. 3.1) and this fact together with the absence of potential gaps or fenestrae penetrating their cytoplasm and with possible differences in the basement membrane is thought to support the idea that a blood–brain barrier to some substances is present at this level (Reese and Karnovsky 1967). Such a barrier is not found in areas such as pars postrema and infundibular region where fenestrated endothelial cells are described

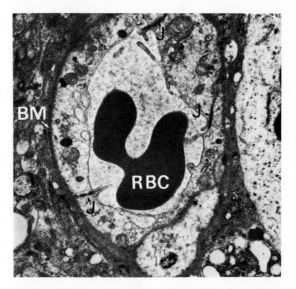

Fig. 3.1 Electromicrograph of a cerebral capillary showing three tight junctions (J) between endothelial cells, a well-defined basement membrane (BM) and a relative paucity of cytoplasmic spaces such as might constitute a fenestration system. Red blood cell (RBC) in lumen.

(Bodenheimer and Brightman 1968). The prolongations of the subarachnoid space, called the Virchow–Robin spaces, exist in relation to arteries and arterioles, veins and venules, but not to the capillaries.

The arterioles and *small arteries* are lined by endothelial cells surrounded by a well-developed internal elastic lamina. The media is composed of fibrous tissue and of plain muscle. The amount of muscle is much less than in vessels of similar calibre elsewhere in the body which reflects the situation of these vessels supported as they are by the almost closed intracranial location. These arteries do, however, hypertrophy in response to hypertension in a similar manner to vessels elsewhere in the body (Cook and Yates 1972).

The larger arteries (Fig. 3.30) also have walls which are thinner than those of arteries in the rest of the body. The internal elastic lamina is well developed but both the muscular coat and the adventitia are thin. There is no external elastic lamina. The surface arteries, unlike those within the brain tissue, have an extensive sympathetic and parasympathetic nerve supply; the functional significance of this remains in doubt in view of the fact that only local O_2 and CO_2 tensions seem to have any effect on vascular tone. It might be that a neural communication between veins and arteries from a particular territory is needed for such local autoregulation to be effective.

The venules and *veins* are lined by endothelial cells. The walls, which are thinner than those of most veins elsewhere in the body, are composed chiefly of fibrous tissue. Smooth muscle is not present and there is very little elastic tissue. There are no valves in the veins of the brain but they have been seen in relation to the spinal veins (Suh and Alexander 1939).

The walls of the *venous sinuses* are composed of dense fibrous tissue lined by endothelial cells.

Types of vascular disease

Clinically cerebrovascular disease may manifest in three main ways—as a major stroke, often resulting in death or very severe disability; as a minor stroke with relatively minor neurological disorder and often nearly full recovery; as a transient ischaemic attack which may involve any aspect of cerebral function but which is short lived with complete recovery and which may be repeated identically many times. This sort of classification which has no specific basis in pathological correlation offers little for the understanding of prognosis, therapy or prevention. All three types of event may be caused by obstruction of vessels or by rupture of vessels and there are several aetiological possibilities in either process.

A useful way of considering the pathology is to divide cerebrovascular diseases broadly into the *obstructive* leading to ischaemia and perhaps infarction and the *disruptive* allowing haemorrhage and tissue displacement. Even this separation is not clear cut for a vessel that has burst lacks the luminal pressure to maintain its distal flow and ischaemia will occur within its territory.

Epidemiology

There is increasing interest in potential clues that epidemiological studies may provide to the aeti-

ology of the various cerebrovascular diseases. However, the statistics on which hypotheses might be erected are based on mixtures of clinical and pathological diagnoses and the use of nonspecific terms such as stroke and apoplexy. Even the term cerebral thrombosis has been debased by common usage in cases where no diagnostic precision is implied.

Analysis of mortality figures for different countries, races, climates and dietary habits often show great differences (Kurtzke 1969); a very high rate of cerebral haemorrhage among the Japanese and the American Negroes; a mortality from all forms of cerebrovascular disease 20% greater for Scotland than for adjacent England and Wales; an apparently much lower than average figure for Belgium and for Mexico which in the latter country may simply reflect a very young population structure.

Attempts have been made to show a changing incidence with time in different types of cerebrovascular disease. In England and Wales during this century a decreasing death rate from cerebral haemorrhage and an increase in that from cerebral infarction has been shown (Yates 1964) although the latter increase was remarkably halted during the war years of 1940-45; reduced diet and cigarette consumption might both have had some effect (Fig. 3.2). A change in the relative significance of cerebral haemorrhage and cerebral infarction was also noted for Ontario (Anderson

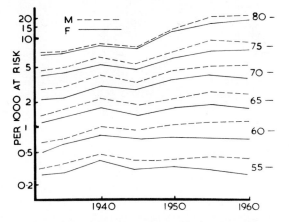

Fig. 3.2 Death rates for cerebral infarction from 1932 to 1960. Log scale. Note the dip in the curves over the war years, 1940-45, and that the male death rate is higher at all points.

and MacKay 1968). However, all such studies have been criticized (Kurtzke 1969) as merely noting changing fashions in diagnosis.

Because the different types of disease have their peak incidence at different ages, subarachnoid haemorrhage before hypertensive intracerebral haemorrhage and cerebral infarction latest, their relative importance as causes of morbidity and death will depend very much on the age structure of a particular population and only age-related statistics have any real significance. In fairly stable populations cerebrovascular disease as a whole accounts for about 15% of all deaths, subdivided approximately into 1·5% due to subarachnoid haemorrhage, 4·5% to intracerebral haemorrhage and 9% to cerebral infarction.

Both subarachnoid and intracerebral haemorrhage appear to occur about equally in male and female but cerebral infarction based mostly on atherothrombotic disease is, like coronary heart disease, predominantly a disease of men (Yates 1966).

Stenosis and occlusion of the internal carotid and vertebral systems

It has long been known, forgotten by the majority, and re-emphasized (Gowers 1893; Chiari 1905; Hunt 1914; Hultquist 1942; Fisher 1951) that ischaemic lesions of the brain, in particular infarction in the distribution of the middle cerebral artery, may be secondary to disease of the internal carotid arteries in the neck. For example, Hunt pointed out that the main artery of the neck should always come under suspicion when, at necropsy, such a focus of softening is found in association with a healthy-looking circle of Willis or with no demonstrable occlusion of the middle cerebral artery. Hutchinson and Yates (1956, 1957, 1961) have emphasized the importance of concomitant consideration and investigation of the vertebral arteries, in the neck as well as within the skull. When a disease process, such as atherosclerosis, affects one of these four main arteries it is likely to have affected the others to a varying degree. For purposes of discussion, stenosis and occlusion of the internal carotid system will be separated from stenosis and occlusion of the vertebral-basilar system, but they should not be so considered in relation to the patient.

Stenosis and occlusion of the internal carotid artery During recent years an increasing amount of attention has been paid to thrombosis of the internal carotid artery. In the living, diagnosis has been made much easier by arteriography; and at necropsy the relative frequency of atherosclerotic narrowing, pointed out by Chiari (1905), has been re-emphasized by Hultquist (1942) who, in 1300 unselected necropsies between 1938 and 1941, found macroscopical thrombosis of a carotid artery in 38 cases. It was twice as frequent in men as in women and, although found in young persons, was commonest in the age groups 50 to 70 (men), 60 to 80 (women).

In all cases of apparent embolism or thrombosis of the middle cerebral artery an examination of the internal carotid arteries should be carried out; for it is in relation to the middle cerebral artery that disease of the internal carotid artery is most likely to give rise to complications (Torvik and Jörgensen 1964).

Changes in the artery. Whilst giant-celled arteritis has been seen and thrombo-angiitis obliterans has been reported, the usual cause of obstruction of the internal carotid artery is atherosclerosis with superimposed thrombus (Figs. 3.3, 3.4 and 3.5). The thrombus is often partly organized. The narrowing frequently commences just distal to the origin of the artery or less often in the sigmoid portion of the artery. The obstruction is often incomplete and from the old thrombus a tongue of recent thrombus may extend cranially within the lumen of the artery. Sometimes the obstruction is complete. Then the proximal part of the thrombus, which is older, is partly red and partly grey in colour. It is a laminated thrombus, for it has formed in flowing blood. Distal to this level the artery often contains red thrombus, formed from stagnant blood, which frequently fills the lumen as far as the origin of a branch of the artery, where laminated thrombus may once

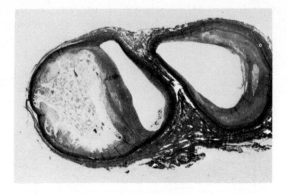

Fig. 3.3 Carotid bifurcation showing a large atheromatous mass distending the intima of the internal carotid sinus with thinning of the medial coat over it.

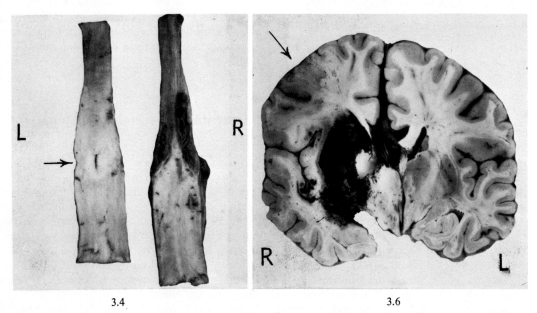

3.4   3.6

Fig. 3.4 Carotid arteries from the neck of a man aged 61. The common and internal carotid arteries have been opened up. The arrow indicates the site of origin of the internal carotid artery. Note that, on the left, there is atherosclerotic intimal thickening in this region, and that on the right antemortem thrombus is adherent to this region and extends up the internal carotid artery.

Fig. 3.6 Same case as Fig. 3.4 showing recent infarction of cortex and basal ganglia (the hole on the medial aspect is artefact). Small thrombi, probably embolic from the internal carotid, were found in adjacent arteries. The exact age of this infarct is not certain but clinically it was within 7 days of death. Older infarction (clinically 6 weeks) is visible in the region of the arrow. No history of previous cerebral disease. Same case as Figs. 3.13, 3.14, 3.19, 3.21, 3.22, 3.23.

more be found. This branch may be the ophthalmic artery, but in some cases the thrombus may extend as far as, or into, the commencement of the middle and anterior cerebral arteries. Carotid artery obstruction may occur bilaterally

(Frøvig 1946) but is commoner unilaterally, being as frequent on the left as on the right.

Changes in the brain (Figs. 3.6 and 3.7). The brain may show extensive softening, involving either the major part of the distribution of the

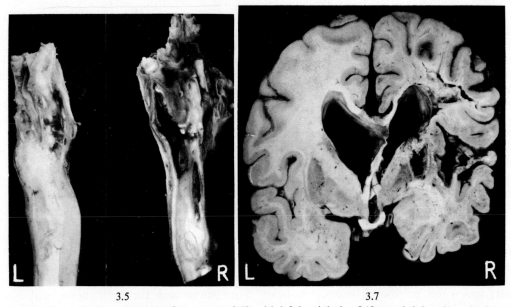

3.5   3.7

Fig. 3.5 Carotid arteries from the neck of a man, aged 62, with left hemiplegia of 18 months' duration. Both common carotid arteries showed a ring of calcification and atheroma at their points of bifurcation. On the left side the internal carotid, which has been opened up, is atheromatous with adherent thrombus. On the right side, about 2·5 cm above its origin, the internal carotid is almost completely occluded by old pale thrombus. Below this, recent reddish thrombus extends downwards into the lumen of the common carotid artery.

Fig. 3.7 Brain from same case as Fig. 3.5. On the right side there is old infarction, with cystic replacement of grey and white matter, including the putamen and internal capsule. The hemisphere is shrunken and the ventricles show compensatory dilatation.

middle cerebral artery or the peripheral portion of this territory, or small focal softenings particularly in the internal capsule. The softening is seldom of the same age in all regions, some being old and some recent: in the grey matter some portions are haemorrhagic, and others pale. In addition foci of softening are sometimes found in the distribution of the anterior or posterior cerebral arteries. Although the softenings are predominantly on the side of the thrombosed artery, they may be found on the opposite side, which has an apparently or relatively healthy carotid artery.

It may be possible to find obstructive lesions in the cerebral arteries related to the softenings. When the thrombosis extends into the middle cerebral artery the cause of the recent infarction is obvious. In some cases of long duration many branches of the middle cerebral artery are extensively occupied by old organized thrombus and appear pale, solid and threadlike (Fig. 3.17). But in other cases it may not be possible to find any macroscopical obstruction to the middle cerebral

artery or to its larger branches. It may even be difficult or impossible to find any microscopical obstruction, although it cannot be said with certainty whether there is any organic obstruction until the whole vascular tree has been examined in serial sections.

When an obstruction is found it may be partial, complete or recanalized, concentric or eccentric, recent or old. If recent it may take the form of a partly coiled, partly organized thrombus, with only slight attachment to the adjacent, otherwise healthy, vessel wall; an appearance compatible with an impacted embolus. The evidence of embolism is not, however, always definite and, especially when the obstruction is older and organized, it may not be possible to say whether it was originally embolic or locally thrombotic. In older lesions the internal elastic lamina and the media of the artery usually appear healthy, while the lumen is obstructed to a varying degree by cellular fibrous tissue in which, at some levels, long cholesterol crystals may be found. Sometimes, in the same microscopical section, healthy, patent, leptomeningeal arteries are found close to those with organic obstruction.

Clinically the condition may (1) be without symptoms or signs; (2) reveal itself by episodic attacks of transient motor or sensory impairment with considerable or complete recovery; (3) show gradual development of hemiplegia; (4) give rise to sudden permanent hemiplegia. Transient attacks of blindness are not uncommon. A full explanation of the clinical and arteriographic or post-mortem findings is not always easy. There is little doubt that some of the lesions are due to the spread of thrombus up into one or more of the branches of the circle of Willis. Some of the lesions appear to be embolic in nature, from detached portions of the thrombus in the internal carotid artery or its branches. Subsequent fragmentation and disimpaction of such emboli may explain the transitory character of some attacks. Pale friable emboli, probably composed mostly of platelets and a few polymorph leucocytes, have been seen with the ophthalmoscope passing along the retinal arteries during attacks of blindness (Fisher 1959; Russell 1961; McBrien, Bradley and Ashton 1963). Alternatively, such recurrent cerebrovascular episodes may be the result of failure of the collateral circulation (Symonds 1955; Denny-Brown 1960).

If only one internal carotid is completely occluded and no extension above the circle of Willis is present and the other extracranial arteries are well patent, then it is usual not to find any ischaemic damage in the appropriate hemisphere. However, in the process of narrowing and thrombosis emboli may have been formed and have caused a series of clinical episodes of minor or transient stroke which cease when final carotid occlusion occurs.

When one internal carotid artery is obstructed, the blood flow to the ipsilateral hemisphere is assisted or taken over by a collateral circulation originating in (1) the contralateral internal carotid artery, which sends its blood across the midline via the anterior communicating artery, and (2) the ipsilateral external carotid artery, which, through branches of the facial artery and the superficial temporal artery, anastomoses with the dorsal nasal, frontal and supra-orbital branches of the ophthalmic artery. The direction of the blood flow in the ophthalmic artery is reversed so that the blood enters rather than leaves the internal carotid artery distal to its sigmoid portion. A collateral circulation may also originate in (3) the

basilar artery from which the blood may pass anteriorly via the posterior communicating artery. These arteries have then to supply not only their original territory but also part or whole of the threatened cerebral hemisphere and possibly the optic nerve. Sometimes this collateral circulation is inadequate. This may be due to an incomplete circle of Willis or because of narrowness of calibre, from developmental causes or disease, of the arteries forming the circle. There will then be immediate irreversible ischaemic damage to the cerebral hemisphere. Often, however, the collateral circulation is, at first, adequate, or at least sufficient to prevent serious damage with permanent clinical symptoms and signs. With the passage of time, however, the diseased carotid artery will become further obstructed, the sources of collateral supply will themselves become narrowed by atherosclerosis, and the circulation through the vessels of the threatened cerebral hemisphere and the optic nerve will reach a precarious state. Such a circulation may easily be reduced below the critical level by such factors as a temporary fall in blood pressure or blood volume. This will produce temporary local ischaemia with reversible or irreversible clinical effects (Corday, Rothenberg and Putman 1953).

While it is true that collateral blood vessels hypertrophy in young humans when a major artery such as an internal carotid has been obstructed usually by trauma or ligation, there is little evidence that this occurs in the elderly patient. Experimental work in this field is usually done on young healthy animals (Lowe 1962) and is therefore irrelevant to the human situation.

The common and occasionally the internal carotid arteries may be the site of accidental trauma (Hughes and Brownell 1968) following road traffic accidents; their location closely in front of the vertebral transverse processes puts them at risk. A hemiplegia occurring some hours or days after an accident may not always be due to intracranial haemorrhage but rather to extension of thrombus from the site of trauma up to and including the middle cerebral artery.

Subclavian artery

'Steal' syndromes
Obstruction of the subclavian and innominate arteries obviously contributes to the whole picture of cerebrovascular insufficiency but its particular importance lies in the part that such an occlusion

may play in causing the 'subclavian steal syndrome' (Reivich, Holling, Roberts and Toole 1961). If the obstruction is proximal to the origin of a vertebral artery, the blood supply to the arm might depend largely on retrograde flow down this vessel thus 'stealing' blood from the basilar artery and the circle of Willis. Exercise of the arm muscles demanding a fourfold increase of blood flow might act to precipitate clinical evidence of cerebral ischaemia.

It will be readily appreciated that where collateral or anastomotic arteries of any size are concerned, similar reversed flow leaks from the cerebral vessels may be found. For example, occlusion of the origin of an external carotid may cause flow out of the skull via the ophthalmic artery and other such channels; if the common carotid is occluded, retrograde flow down the internal to fill the external carotid territory may be observed.

Within the skull similar 'internal steal' situations may occur between one major cerebral artery and another. It may also become a problem at the periphery of areas of cerebral infarction where local blood flow studies have shown an inappropriately rich arterial flow (Lassen 1966). It appears that loss of tone in these surviving vessels, by reducing peripheral resistance, causes a fall in the perfusion pressure elsewhere in the territory of the parent artery.

Stenosis and occlusion of the basilar-vertebral system

The basilar artery is formed inferiorly by the confluence of the two vertebral arteries. At its upper end it usually divides into two posterior cerebral arteries. All these arteries and their branches, including the extracranial portions of the vertebral arteries, should be considered or investigated in toto in any case where ischaemic lesions in the hind brain and occipital regions are suspected, or in cases where the contribution of this tree to the blood flow in the circle of Willis is under consideration (Hutchinson and Yates 1956).

Sometimes the narrowing or obstruction extends into, or is only noticed in, the intracranial portions of the tree, in particular in the basilar artery (Kubik and Adams 1946; Biemond 1951) but thromboatheroma more commonly affects the extracranial parts, especially the origins from the subclavian arteries. Small and large emboli of cardiac or aortic arch origin are not infrequent causes of transient or permanent clinical disability and it is clear that many of the transient attacks previously attributed to micro embolization of the carotid circulation are the result of similar obstruction in the hind brain circulation.

The cervical course of the vertebral arteries through the lateral parts of the cervical vertebrae is well protected from trauma in the young but is very vulnerable in the middle aged and elderly.

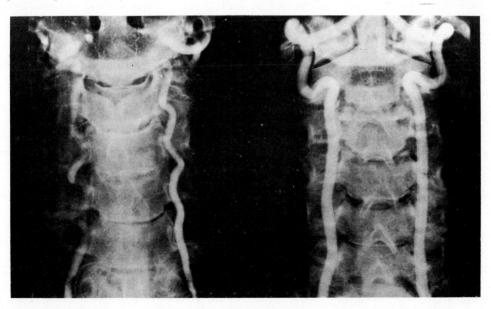

Fig. 3.8 Post-mortem angiography of vertebral arteries, right side normal, left showing distortion by osteoarthritic change and stenosis by atheroma.

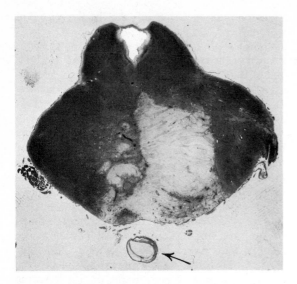

Fig. 3.9 Basilar artery occlusion of 7 weeks' duration. At this level of the pons the basilar artery (arrow) is athero-sclerotic and contains antemortem thrombus. Pale staining foci of coagulative necrosis, with · peripheral organization, are present in the distribution of the para-median arteries. On the right side their complete field appears to be involved. Note the midline watershed and the relative escape of the tegmentum. Celloidin; haema-toxylin van Gieson. × 2.

The distorting effect of osteoarthritic changes of the neurocentral joints may be considerable (Fig. 3.8) and together with atherosclerotic changes in the arteries may be sufficient to cause obstruction following certain movements of the neck (Hutchin-son and Yates 1956). Attacks of syncope, tinnitus, dizziness and ataxia in the elderly may often have such a pathological basis.

Attempts to treat arthritic changes in the neck by manipulative techniques may damage diseased and tortuous vertebral arteries producing throm-bosis and obstruction or a flood of microemboli (Pratt-Thomas and Berger 1947).

Ischaemic lesions are most often found in the distribution of the short paramedian branches of the basilar artery (Fig. 3.9). Such infarcts may, in part, be unilateral and they are pale. Infarcts may also be present in the cerebellar cortex, or in the distribution of the short circumferential arteries of the brainstem, or in the distribution of the posterior cerebral arteries. The tegmentum of the pons is very seldom involved and then usually only in part (see also p. 96).

The intimate relationship of the vertebral arteries is particularly disadvantageous in the process of birth. Assisted cephalic and breech presentations all involve twisting and pulling of the neck. Yates (1959) has reported a 42% occurrence of bruising and haemorrhagic dissec-tion of the vertebral arteries in 250 cases of neo-natal death. The significance of ischaemia of the hind brain in failure to initiate cardiorespiratory function is obvious but in those who may survive such events, poor suckling, extraocular palsies, inner ear deafness and other disabilities referable to damage in the territory of the vertebro-basilar system bring to mind a picture seen in many birth damaged children. It may be that some sudden 'infant cot deaths' are due to a failure of the damaged respiratory centre to respond to the increase of CO_2 which occurs during sleep.

Occlusion of certain intracranial arteries

The arteries of the central nervous system have a fairly constant anatomical distribution, and occlusion of an artery, or of one or more of its larger branches, produces a relatively constant disorder of function. Full consideration of the anatomical distribution of the arteries and of the clinicopathological correlation of the lesions is outside the scope of this book. For further information the literature referred to under each artery should be consulted. Additional ana-tomical publications are Beevor (1908), Stopford (1915, 1917), Abbie (1934). Adams (1943) gives a detailed list of the arterial distribution to the cerebellum. Critchley and Schuster (1933) and Atkinson (1949) describe the branches of the basilar artery. The clinical syndromes resulting from arterial occlusion have been reviewed by Tichy (1949) and by Kiloh (1953).

Usually the arterial occlusion has been secondary to atherosclerosis or to embolism, sometimes to syphilis, or to mechanical or surgical trauma. In patients with atherosclerosis or syphilis, which are generalized arterial diseases, the occlusion of the named artery is only the most obvious lesion: there are often many other small lesions elsewhere in the brain or spinal cord. Generalized arterial disease also modifies the opening up of collateral pathways. In cases due to embolism it is always possible that other emboli have occluded small vessels elsewhere, and in cases of mechanical trauma, or where the arteries have been clipped or cauterized by the surgeon, the ill effects of the arterial occlusion are seldom the only patho-logical process present. For all these reasons it is unlikely, in man, that the obvious arterial lesion is the only one present. It is therefore unwise to state that, in man, ischaemic destruction of a certain region is the cause of a certain disability of function. The study of a number of cases, however, reveals that there is a sufficiently close correlation between a major lesion in the distribution of a certain artery and certain clinical findings to make the investigation of this subject worth while. In patients who survive for an adequate length of time, a study of the secondary degenerations is of importance. Apart from surgical ablation or destruction of tissue, which in many parts of the brain is too dangerous or is not indicated, localized arterial obstruction is one of the few disease processes which has enabled us to make satisfactory observations on the course of fibre pathways, on secondary degenerations and on the anatomical basis of disordered functions.

Anterior cerebral artery

The principal field of supply of the anterior cerebral artery is the cortex and the underlying white matter (to a depth of about 25 mm) on the medial aspect, and a 25-mm broad strip on the superior part of the convexity of the frontal and parietal lobes as far back usually as the parieto-occipital fissure, also the genu and anterior four-fifths of the corpus callosum. Through the recurrent artery of Heubner, which leaves it early in its course and passes through the anterior perforated substance, it supplies the lower part of the head of the caudate, the lower part of the frontal pole of the putamen, the frontal pole of the globus pallidus and the portion of the anterior limb of the internal capsule lying between them.

The disturbance of function varies with the portion of the artery which is occluded. If the distal field of supply, which includes the paracentral lobule, is obstructed, there is crural monoplegia with sensory disturbance of a cortical type (Critchley 1930). In atheromatous cases this may be bilateral and cause spastic paraplegia.

Middle cerebral artery

The principal field of supply of this artery includes the lateral part of the orbital surface of the frontal lobe, the temporal pole, the insula and all the convexity of the cerebral hemisphere, except the strip supplied by the anterior cerebral artery and a part posteriorly, including the occipital pole, supplied by the posterior cerebral artery. It supplies the underlying white matter (which in-cludes the superior half of both limbs of the internal capsule and the optic radiation, where it lies lateral to the occipital horn of the lateral ventricle). In addition the middle cerebral artery supplies the caudate (except for the inferior portion of its head, and its tail), the putamen (except for the lower part of its frontal pole) and the lateral part of the globus pallidus.

Our records show that this artery is more often obstructed than any other cerebral artery, the obstruction being either of the main trunk or of some of its branches. If the main artery is suddenly obstructed, as it commonly is by embolism, the region of infarction may correspond closely to the principal field of supply. Associated with this lesion there is severe hemiplegia (most severe in the arm), sensory disturbance of the cortical type, profound aphasia (if the dominant hemisphere is involved), sometimes hemianopia which is not always complete (Foix and Levy 1927) and disturbance of vestibular function (Carmichael, Dix and Hallpike 1956).

Posterior cerebral artery

Although in the human, in the majority of cases, this artery is anatomically a branch of the basilar artery, it is morphologically a continuation of the posterior communicating artery and therefore a branch of the carotid artery (Abbie 1934, Williams 1936). The concept clarifies the distribution of the posterior communicating artery and the posterior cerebral artery to the basal ganglia.

The principal field of supply of the posterior cerebral artery is the inferior surface of the hemisphere behind the temporal pole, the medial surface of the occipital lobe, the lateral surface of the hemisphere in the region of the occipital pole, and the underlying white matter which, on the medial aspect of the occipital lobe, is narrow. It also supplies the mammillary body, the subthalamic nucleus, the posterior half of the thalamus including the geniculate bodies, the posterior two-thirds of the cerebral peduncle, the substantia nigra, red nucleus and the superior cerebellar peduncle.

Occlusion by atherosclerosis and thrombosis, or secondary to vertebral-basilar obstruction, or to pressure against the free edge of the tentorium cerebelli by a supratentorial space-occupying lesion, commonly obstructs the peripheral branches of the artery which supply the visual cortex. Occasionally the main stem of the artery is occluded, and this causes infarction in the major portion of its anatomical distribution. Because of the collateral circulation through the anterior choroidal artery, the subthalamic nucleus and the lateral geniculate body are not destroyed; because of the collateral circulation through the middle cerebral artery, the posterior portion of the calcarine cortex, where the macula is represented (Holmes 1934), is spared.

In association with the infarction there are numerous syndromes (Foix and Masson 1923) according to the portion of the artery which is occluded. If the whole artery is occluded there will be homonymous hemianopia with macular sparing, hemiparesis and disturbance of sensation. If the lesions are on the side of the dominant hemisphere there will be alexia.

Anterior choroidal artery

The principal field of supply of the anterior choroidal artery is the pyriform cortex, the posteromedial border of the anterior commissure, part of the head and most of the tail of the caudate nucleus, the posteromedial part of the amygdaloid nucleus, the medial part of the globus pallidus, the lateral part of the lateral geniculate body, the middle third of the cerebral peduncle, the subthalamic region, the posterior two-thirds of the posterior limb of the internal capsule, the beginning of the optic radiation, the antero-inferior parts of the fascia dentata and hippocampus (including the uncus) and the choroid plexus.

Proved cases of occlusion of the anterior choroidal artery are rare (Abbie 1933). The infarcts were found in the distal portion of the distribution of the artery, and caused constant destruction of the retrolenticular portion of the internal capsule, part of the optic radiation and part of the globus pallidus, with inconstant damage to the cerebral peduncle, lateral part of the lateral geniculate body, the head of the caudate, optic tract, anterior commissure and amygdaloid nucleus. In association with this infarction there were hemiplegia, hemianaesthesia and hemianopia.

Earle, Baldwin and Penfield (1953) have postulated that the sclerotic lesions of the uncus, hippocampus and inferior temporal gyrus, which are often found in people with temporal lobe epilepsy, are the result of compression, during birth, of arteries and their branches against the free edge of the tentorium cerebelli. Of these

they consider that the anterior choroidal artery and its branches are the most important.

Superior cerebellar artery

The principal field of supply of this artery is the dorsolateral portion of the upper part of the brainstem (midbrain and cranial part of the pons), the superior cerebellar peduncle, part of the dentate nucleus and part of the cortex of the superior part of the cerebellar hemisphere. Exactly how much of the tegmentum of the midbrain and pons is supplied by this artery remains uncertain.

Occlusion of this artery is rare. It has been reported with atherosclerosis by Guillain, Bertrand and Peron (1928) and by Russell (1931), with atherosclerosis and syphilis by Davison, Goodhart and Savitsky (1935) and as the result of an embolus by Freeman and Jaffe (1941).

The infarction may involve the dorsolateral midbrain and pons, including the caudal portion of the mesencephalic root of the 5th nerve, the central tegmental tract, the lateral part of the medial lemniscus, and the lateral lemniscus; the superior cerebellar peduncle, the roof nuclei of the 4th ventricle, part of the dentate nucleus and the adjacent part of the superior surface of the cerebellum. Secondary degeneration may be seen in the contralateral red nucleus and the ipsilateral inferior olivary nucleus. In association with the infarction there may be ipsilateral signs of cerebellar dysfunction, ipsilateral involuntary movements especially of the upper extremity, together with contralateral loss of appreciation of pain and temperature over the whole body.

Anterior inferior cerebellar artery

The principal field of supply of this artery is the lateral portion of the tegmentum of the middle portion of the brainstem (the caudal part of the pons and the cranial part of the medulla), the inferior part of the middle cerebellar peduncle, the inferior cerebellar peduncle, the flocculus and adjacent cerebellar hemisphere.

Damage to this artery is considered by Atkinson (1949) to be the principal cause of death following operative removal of an acoustic Schwannoma. Proven cases of occlusion of this artery, secondary to atherosclerosis, are extremely rare. Two cases have been published, one by Goodhart and Davison (1936, case 6) and one by Adams (1943). In Goodhart and Davison's case the infarction was confined to the cerebellar cortex. In Adams's case the flocculus, the biventral and the superior and inferior semilunar lobules of the cerebellum were infarcted, and in the brainstem the lesion extended from the level of the mid-pons to the middle of the inferior olive. The structures involved were the caudal portion of the middle cerebellar peduncle, the inferior cerebellar peduncle, the rostral part of the spinal nucleus and tract of the 5th nerve, the 7th nerve, the 8th nerve, the ventral and dorsal cochlear nuclei, the lateral portion of the spinal vestibular nucleus and the ventral spinocerebellar tract: most of the adjacent lateral spinothalamic tract was spared. There was secondary degeneration of nerve cells in the 7th nerve nucleus, contralateral pontile and inferior olivary nuclei. In association with the infarction the patient showed ipsilateral cerebellar dysfunction, loss of pain and temperature and diminished light touch sensibility over the face, paralysis of the muscles of the face, deafness, Horner's syndrome, together with contralateral incomplete loss of pain and temperature sensibility over the body.

Posterior inferior cerebellar artery

This artery supplies a wedge of tissue in the medulla which extends vertically from just above the level of the cuneate and gracile nuclei to the upper limit of the medulla. On the surface the wedge extends from just posterior to the inferior olivary nucleus dorsally to include the inferior cerebellar peduncle. Centrally the apex of the wedge reaches the tegmentum in its lateral part. The artery also supplies part of the inferior

surface of the cerebellar hemisphere, part of the dentate nucleus, and the roof nuclei of the 4th ventricle (Gillilan 1969).

Ischaemic lesions occur more frequently in the distribution of this artery than of any other cerebellar artery. These are usually the result of atheroma with superadded thrombotic occlusion, which often commences in the vertebral artery (Fisher, Karnes and Kubik 1961 (see also p. 93)). An infrequent cause is syphilis and embolism is rare. The principal lesion is a retro-olivary softening in the medulla. Infarction of the cerebellum is usually slight because of the free anastomosis with other cerebellar arteries. Spillane (1937) had a case with involvement of the dentate nucleus.

The lesion in the medulla has been described by Foix, Hillemand and Schalit (1925), Merritt and Finland (1930), Goodhart and Davison (1936), Smyth (1939) and Levine, Cheskin and Applebaum (1949). It consists of an infarct which involves almost all the field of supply with the exception of the tegmentum. The structures involved are the descending nucleus and tract of the 5th nerve, some of the internal arcuate fibres, the spinal vestibular nucleus and tract or fibres passing from it to the medial longitudinal fasciculus, the nucleus ambiguus and fibres emerging from the dorsal motor nucleus of the 9th and 10th nerves, autonomic fibre pathways, the lateral spinothalamic and spinocerebellar tracts, olivocerebellar fibres as they pass to the inferior cerebellar peduncle, and the ventral part of the inferior cerebellar peduncle. The facial nucleus is occasionally involved.

Significance of obstructive vascular disease

Among the principal functions associated with the blood vessels of the central nervous system are: (1) Conveyance of oxygen to the tissues and carrying away of carbon dioxide. This exchange takes place at capillary level. (2) Conveyance of glucose and other metabolites to the tissues. (3) Removal of waste products, both those soluble in tissue fluids and those carried by phagocytes. (4) Regulation of tissue fluids with regard to water and acid-base level. (5) Regulation of temperature. (6) Production and absorption of

cerebrospinal fluid. (7) Taking part in the work of the blood–brain barrier.

When considering vascular disease one may therefore consider:

(1) *Abnormalities of the circulating blood whereby these functions cannot be carried out.* The blood may be abnormal in respect of the quantity of haemoglobin or the ability of the haemoglobin to carry oxygen, as in the anaemias or in carbon monoxide poisoning. This is termed *anaemic hypoxaemia* or *anaemic anoxaemia* in relation to

the blood, and *anaemic hypoxia* or *anaemic anoxia* in relation to the oxygen available to the tissues. The haemoglobin may be sufficient but it may be unsaturated with oxygen as in drowning, asphyxia and in high-altitude sickness. The terms then used are *anoxic anoxaemia* and *anoxic anoxia*. The blood may be deficient in glucose as in hypoglycaemic coma; it may be too hot as in heat stroke. These abnormalities are dealt with in other sections of the book.

(2) *Disease processes whereby healthy blood does not circulate properly through the blood vessels* (ischaemia and stagnant anoxia). It is with such conditions that this chapter is largely concerned. The blood may not circulate through the whole central nervous system because of arrest or impairment of cardiac action; or part of the central nervous system because of embolism or thrombosis.

Interference with the supply of blood reaching a portion of the nervous system can be expected to cause damage which lies somewhere between the extremes of temporary impairment of function and death of the tissue.

The type of cell and tissue which dies and the extent of the necrosis depend largely upon the relative vulnerability of the cells and tissues, the rate of reduction of blood flow, and the type of vessel which is obstructed.

Relative vulnerability of cells and tissues

The questions of the relative ability of the various cells of the nervous system to survive ischaemia is still debated. There is little doubt that the metabolism and function of neurons cease within 5 to 10 minutes; such loss of cell function may persist for much longer periods so that survival of the organism without artificial aid may be impossible. Many experiments which purported to stop the circulation for precisely defined periods failed to take account of sludging and transient thrombosis of small vessels which might extend the period of ischaemia for several hours. There remains therefore considerable uncertainty about the true capacity of nerve cells to survive ischaemia. At the edges of infarcted brain tissue, astrocytes, microglia and capillaries can be readily found indicating greater resistance to cessation of blood flow.

The nerve cells of certain areas of the brain such as layers 3 and 4 of the cerebral cortex appear to show a selective vulnerability. Such

an interpretation may be incorrect, the real difficulty being in re-establishing the microcirculation to these territories.

The rate of reduction of blood flow below a critical level is most important in relation to the collateral or anastomotic circulation. If the blood flow through an artery is gradually reduced, as by atherosclerosis, there is often sufficient time for the anastomotic vessels to dilate and compensate. If, however, the obstruction is sudden, as by an embolus, much of the tissue dies before an adequate anastomotic circulation is established.

Type of vessel affected. The effects of vascular obstruction vary with the type of vessel which is principally involved. The obstruction may be in relation to a major artery or at arteriolar or capillary level or in relation to veins or dural venous sinuses.

The smallest cortical lesions, on the arterial side of the circulation, which are histologically recognizable, are those due to an impaired circulation through the smaller cortical arteries and arterioles. Sometimes the process is confined to the distribution of single arterioles, and the anoxia is of such a degree that the only cells which die are the nerve cells. In the early state the lesion is visible histologically (Fig. 3.10), in

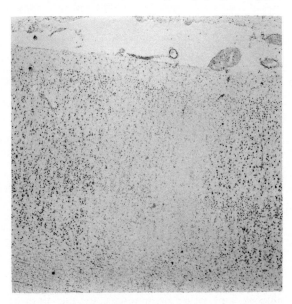

Fig. 3.10 Region of pallor in the cortex, situated near the temporal pole at the periphery of the distribution of the middle cerebral artery, in a patient with thombosis of the middle cerebral artery on the same side. Note that the pial vessels appear healthy at this level. Celloidin; Nissl. × 30.

Nissl preparations, as a perivascular *region of pallor* running down at right angles to the surface of the cortex (Spielmeyer's *Erbleichung*). The nerve cells are still present but they are smaller than normal, the cytoplasm stains poorly with basic dyes and the nuclei are small and darkly stained; in haematoxylin-eosin preparations the cytoplasm is eosinophilic. This picture soon changes to one of increased cellularity, due to the presence of numerous rod-shaped microglia. The final stage is one of tissue shrinkage and perivascular fibrous gliosis. Such regions of cortical pallor and scarring are found in patients with atherosclerosis and with hypertensive arteriosclerosis.

Granular atrophy of the cortex has a similar anatomical basis and probably results from more severe focal anoxia. At necropsy, after removal of the arachnoid, the affected surface of the brain resembles the surface of a kidney with 'granular atrophy' (Fig. 3.11). The condition, which is rare, is often bilaterally symmetrical. Pentschew (1933) found that it was usually limited to the middle frontal gyrus and to the parieto-occipital convolutions. Lindenberg and Spatz (1939), in one group of their cases of thrombo-angiitis obliterans, found a sickle-shaped zone of granular atrophy on the convexity of each cerebral hemisphere, stretching from the frontal pole upwards towards the vertex and then down to the occipital pole. Sometimes it was also present on the inferior surface of the hemisphere, running from the occipital to the temporal pole. Lindenberg pointed out that this distribution corresponds with the border zone between the cortical fields of the anterior, middle and posterior cerebral arteries. When the lesion is widespread and has this watershed distribution bilaterally it is often the result of severe general hypotensive vascular failure in cases of shock. If the watershed is unilateral it suggests proximal occlusion of perhaps the internal carotid with hypotension or inadequate collateral circulation allowing inadequate flow to the 'last fields of irrigation'.

Microscopically, the multiple depressions in the cortex correspond with regions of softening and coarse fibrous gliosis which run in at right angles to the cortex (Fig. 3.12). Hyaline degeneration may affect the small intracerebral arterioles, but the cause of the cortical lesions probably lies at

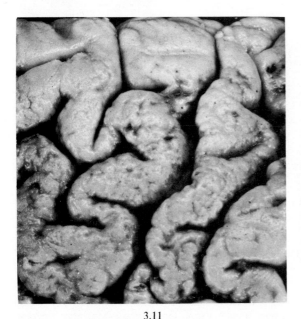

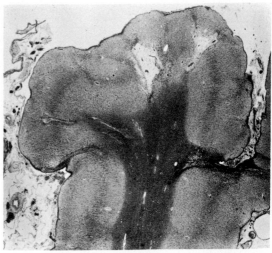

3.11   3.12

Fig. 3.11 Granular atrophy of the cortex. Lateral aspect of the left cerebral hemisphere after removal of the leptomeninges. Note the numerous depressions of the surface.

Fig. 3.12 Region of granular atrophy from the same case as Fig. 3.11; a man aged 37 with chronic endarteritis of uncertain type. Note the thickened and narrowed arteries in the leptomeninges and the numerous depressions in the cortex which are associated with the softenings and scars which run in at right angles to the surface. Celloidin; phosphotungstic acid haematoxylin. × 9.

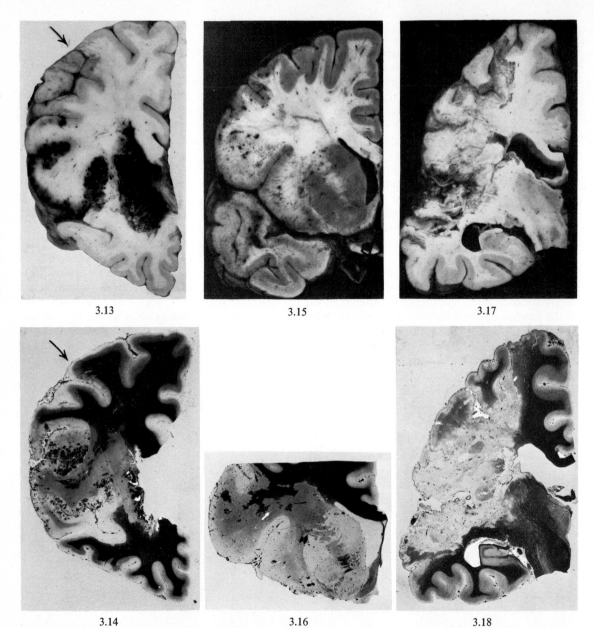

3.13   3.15   3.17

3.14   3.16   3.18

Fig. 3.13 Coronal section, frontal lobe, atherosclerotic carotid artery (same case as Figs. 3.26 and 3.27). In the lower part of the picture is recent, embolic, haemorrhagic infarction of the cortex. The underlying white matter is also necrotic, although this is not clearly visible. This part of the brain is swollen and the line of demarcation between cortex and white matter is ill-defined (see also Figs. 3.19 and 3.21). In the upper part of the picture (arrow) is an older lesion, of about 6 weeks' duration (see also Figs. 3.22 and 3.23).

Fig. 3.14 Myelin preparation of Fig. 3.13. Note the sharp edge to the necrotic white matter, which does not stain. In some places only the subcortical U-fibres are necrotic; in other places the deep white matter is damaged. Note the older lesions (arrow).

Fig. 3.15 Embolic occlusion of middle cerebral artery, of 3 weeks' duration. from thrombus overlying atherosclerotic myocardial infarct of left ventricle. The necrotic grey matter, which is friable, is not clearly defined from the white matter. In the centrum semi-ovale the edge of the necrotic white matter is clearly visible. The inferomedial half of the corpus striatum (supplied by the recurrent artery of Heubner) is not necrotic.

Fig. 3.16 Myelin preparation of middle part of Fig. 3.15. Note the sharp edge to the necrotic white matter.

Fig. 3.17 Old infarct (clinically 5 months) due to atherosclerotic carotid artery occlusion. The products of tissue destruction have been largely removed, leaving cystic spaces. Note that the edge of the infarct, which goes down to the ventricular wall, is clearly defined. The hemisphere is shrunken, the ventricle dilated. Middle cerebral artery distribution.

Fig. 3.18 Myelin preparation of Fig. 3.17 showing well-defined margin of the infarct corresponding to that seen in Fig. 3.17. Celloidin; Loyez.

a more proximal site in the arterial tree, at the level of the arterioles and small arteries in the pia arachnoid. Narrowing of these vessels by hypertensive arterio- and arteriolosclerosis, by syphilitic endarteritis, by atherosclerosis or by thrombo-angiitis obliterans has been reported in cases with granular atrophy. Pentschew found that it may occur as a sequel of carbon monoxide poisoning.

Granular atrophy of the brain is almost invariably associated with granular atrophy of the kidneys. Pentschew noted this association in 9 out of 11 cases, and Lindenberg and Spatz in all 7 of the cases in which the kidneys were examined.

Infarction

When a large artery, such as one of the named arteries of a cerebral hemisphere, is obstructed, especially if the obstruction is rapid as by an embolus, the region affected is usually an extensive zone of cortex and a considerable depth of the underlying white matter. The earliest change which is visible to the naked eye is one of swelling of both grey and white matter. Sometimes the extent of very early infarction can best be appreciated in a brain after fixation when the infarcted tissue remains 'softened'. The grey matter is congested, either diffusely or in a patchy fashion and it is often stippled with petechial haemorrhages. This is called *haemorrhagic infarction* (Figs. 3.13 and 3.14). The white matter looks pale and, in the early stages, may be difficult to distinguish from the normal. This appearance is called pale infarction or more accurately *ischaemic necrosis*. The swelling which accompanies these changes is considerable. In the case of a large infarct, it may constitute a 'space occupying lesion' and produce secondary vascular lesions in the region of the midbrain (see below).

Changes in the grey matter
In the early stages, microscopical examination of the infarcted grey matter reveals a state of widespread tissue damage. At the centre of a large infarct this may consist of coagulative necrosis of all elements. In small infarcts and at the periphery of large infarcts the damage is less severe and the appearances are those of disintegration of nerve cells, myelin sheaths and oligodendroglia, varying degrees of damage to astrocytes, survival of microglia and blood vessels, with pericapillary and perivenular haemorrhages. Often the small

blood vessels are filled by neutrophil polymorph leucocytes which can also be seen in the surrounding disintegrating parenchyma (Fig. 3.19), sometimes in large numbers. This is evidence that blood is flowing in this region. Many of these polymorphonuclear leucocytes pass, in the perivascular spaces, to the subarachnoid space and may be found in the cerebrospinal fluid on lumbar puncture (Cone and Barrera 1931).

After 4 or 5 days, under usual circumstances, the polymorph leucocytic infiltration is replaced by an infiltration of mononuclear phagocytes, many of which are already ingesting the sudanophilic and crystalline anisotropic products of neuronal and myelin disintegration. At this stage the endothelial cells of the capillaries show both hypertrophy and hyperplasia (Figs. 3.20 and 3.21); mitotic figures can sometimes be seen in them. The number of capillaries appears to be increased, although it is difficult to know whether this increase is real. The red blood corpuscles disintegrate and material staining positively with Prussian blue can be seen in phagocytes. To the naked eye, from about this stage onwards, a haemorrhagic infarct will look brown because of the blood pigments. At the margin of old haemorrhagic infarcts of the grey matter it is not uncommon to find small structures with the shape of shrunken nerve cells, which stain strongly with Prussian blue. These are called ferruginated nerve cells (see p. 18).

The process of tissue breakdown and phagocytosis and removal continues (Figs. 3.15, 3.22 and 3.23). Cystic spaces filled with fluid replace the parenchyma (Figs. 3.17 and 3.18). Repair is effected by the astrocytes at the margins of the lesion. They show both hypertrophy and hyperplasia and lay down astrocytic fibres. The bodies of many of the astrocytes are swollen with an abundance of hyaline eosinophilic cytoplasm; some are binucleated (Figs. 3.24 and 3.25). After some months the picture is one of large or small cystic spaces, containing fluid and variable numbers of fat phagocytes, bordered by astrocytes and astrocytic fibres. In many of the spaces run small healthy looking blood vessels. It is the blood vessels which first receive the benefit of the circulating blood after the opening up of the collateral circulation; their survival must be ascribed to this and perhaps to a relatively greater capacity to withstand anoxia.

The margin between an old infarct and the adjacent grey matter is sharply defined. The

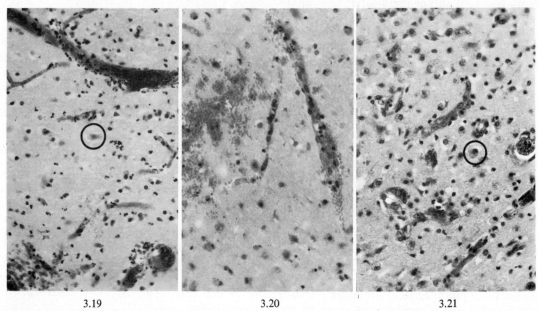

3.19   3.20   3.21

Figs. 3.19, 3.20 and **3.21**   Recent infarction of grey matter showing (3.19) polymorphonuclear leucocytes migrating from the dilated blood vessels into the necrotic parenchyma.   The circle encloses a dead nerve cell; (3.20) hyperplasia of the capillary endothelium and diapedetic haemorrhage; (3.21) at a later stage, capillary endothelial hyperplasia and the appearance of phagocytes distended with products of tissue disintegration (circle).   Celloidin; haematoxylin van Gieson. × 195.

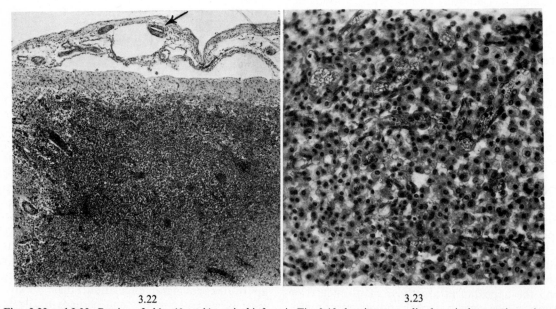

3.22   3.23

Figs. 3.22 and **3.23**   Portion of older (6 week) cortical infarct in Fig. 3.13 showing recanalized cortical artery (arrow) and disintegration of all but layer I of the cortex.   The necrotic tissue has broken down and has been replaced by innumerable distended phagocytes.   Blood appears to be circulating through the numerous capillaries which are dilated.   They still show endothelial hyperplasia.   Celloidin; haematoxylin van Gieson.   × 34 and × 195.

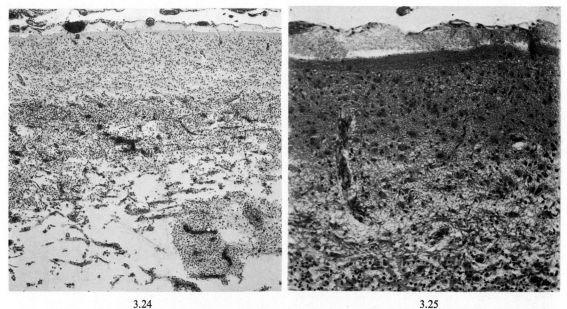

3.24   3.25

Fig. 3.24 Cerebral infarct, clinically 6 weeks' duration. The superficial layers of the cortex have survived. The rest of the cortex and the underlying white matter are largely replaced by spaces filled with fluid and traversed by blood vessels. Groups of phagocytes are also present. Celloidin; haematoxylin and eosin. × 30.

Fig. 3.25 Higher power of upper part of Fig. 3.24. Astrocytic hypertrophy and hyperplasia are visible in the superficial layers of the cortex. Some astrocytes are binucleated. Haematoxylin and eosin. × 150.

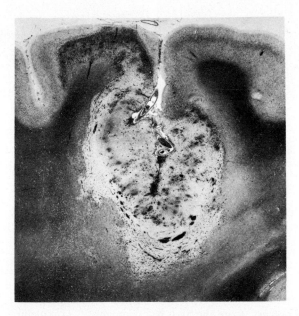

Fig. 3.26 Isolated embolic cerebral infarct, 3 weeks' duration, same case as Figs. 3.15 and 3.16. The central portion of the infarct shows coagulative necrosis. At the periphery there is cellular reaction, which is more marked in the grey matter. Organizing thrombus is visible in the cortical arteriole within the sulcus. Celloidin, haematoxylin van Gieson. × 4.

subpial margin of an infarct is usually composed of layer I of the cortex in which there is much astrocytic gliosis. Sometimes, however, the ischaemia has been so prolonged or severe that even this layer is absent. The wall is then formed of pia mater, from which a small number of delicate collagen fibrils pass towards the surviving blood vessels at the margin of the cyst.

In large infarcts some central portions of the grey matter may, from the first, show coagulative necrosis (Fig. 3.26). Even when the collateral circulation opens up, the blood does not circulate through the capillaries of this central portion and everything within this zone dies. Disintegration and phagocytosis of this dead material proceeds

infarction of the brainstem. In the first few days it may be very difficult to see a pale infarct with the naked eye (Figs. 3.13 and 3.14), but within about 24 hours it becomes visible in stained preparations by the poor staining of the myelin. The tissue swells, the nuclei of oligodendroglia and astrocytes disappear and Pickworth preparations show empty capillaries. Only at the periphery of the lesion is there any sign of reaction. Here the axons are swollen and the myelin sheaths are ballooned (Fig. 3.27). Between the thin rim of distended myelin and the axon there is a space which does not stain: presumably it contained fluid. The axons degenerate and disappear and then the distended myelin sheaths begin to dis-

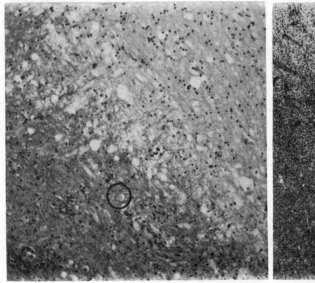 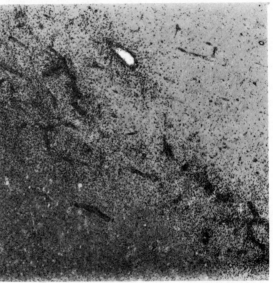

3.27   3.28

Figs. 3.27 and **3.28**   Edge of an infarct of the white matter.   Fig. 3.27 was clinically of 5 days' duration (same case as Fig. 3.20).   The infarcted white matter, upper right-hand side of the picture, shows coagulative necrosis and stains poorly. At the margin of the lesion the myelin sheaths are distended and sometimes contain a swollen axon (circle).   Fig. 3.28 was clinically of 3 weeks' duration (same case as Figs 3.15, 3.16 and 3.26).   The infarcted white matter, upper right-hand side of picture, shows coagulative necrosis and stains poorly.   At the margin of the lesion numerous phagocytes can be seen, particularly around the dilated blood vessels.   Celloidin; haematoxylin van Gieson.   × 100 and × 28.

from the periphery. Here the end stage is that of a large cavity filled only with clear fluid. This process, although it may occur in the cerebral cortex, is more commonly seen in the caudate and putamen (Fig. 3.7).

Changes in the white matter

In the white matter, the process, from the first, is one of coagulative necrosis without haemorrhage (so called pale infarct). In passing it should be mentioned that a similar process is found in

integrate. Occasional cells are seen within them, either small mononuclear cells with rounded hyperchromatic nuclei or compound granular corpuscles. Reactionary changes take place in the adjacent blood vessels. The larger vessels are distended with blood and the capillaries show endothelial hyperplasia. The myelin sheaths now disintegrate completely, sudanophilic lipid and anisotropic elongated crystalline material appear and are ingested by mononuclear phagocytes. Lymphocyte-like cells appear in the perivascular spaces. Gradually the phagocytes, distended with lipid, become less numerous in the parenchyma, more numerous in the perivascular spaces. Astrocytes show hypertrophy and hyperplasia and lay down astrocytic fibres.

The process of disintegration gradually spreads into the central zone of coagulative necrosis (Fig. 3.28) and the macroscopical appearance is one of a mass of slightly granular yellowish material separated by a narrow ragged cavity from the surrounding healthy looking nervous tissue. Blood never returns to this central zone; the capillaries and the astrocytes die, in addition to the nerve fibres and oligodendroglia, so that there are no local cells to multiply and effect repair. Astrocytes from the periphery do not grow into this region to any appreciable extent and the end result is a cystic space filled with clear fluid.

Explanation of morphological changes

The process which underlies haemorrhagic infarction of the grey matter is considered to be as follows. Immediately after obstruction of the artery, blood ceases to flow through its arterioles and capillaries. The tissue around its capillaries ceases to receive oxygen, katabolic products accumulate and cellular damage commences in nerve cells, oligodendroglia, astrocytes, microglia and capillary walls, in that order of vulnerability. The next event is an opening up of the anastomotic vessels at the periphery of the ischaemic zone, and there is experimental evidence (Meyer, Fang and Denny-Brown 1954) that this is dependent upon local metabolic factors, of which CO_2 appears to be relatively important. If the blood pressure in the surrounding arterial fields is not low, blood will flow in through the anastomotic vessels and there will be a return of the circulation of blood through the capillary network.

These capillaries are not, however, quite normal. Sometimes the duration of ischaemia has been so short that they are only unduly distensible, in which case the result will be one of marked congestion. More often, however, the duration of ischaemia has been such that, not only are the walls unduly distensible, but also they are so damaged that they are unduly permeable to plasma and red blood corpuscles. The result will be congestion, swelling of the tissue from leakage of plasma and also petechial haemorrhages from diapedesis of red blood corpuscles. This is red or haemorrhagic infarction.

A factor of great importance is the pressure of the blood in the arterial fields surrounding the ischaemic zone. It has been shown experimentally in the monkey (Meyer et al. 1954) that the anastomotic circulation does not become established if the systemic blood pressure falls below 60 mm Hg. The same factor appears to operate in the human. In one case the surgeon was forced, at operation for a suprasellar tumour, to ligate the anterior cerebral artery and the recurrent artery of Heubner. Following the operation the systemic blood pressure remained low. At post mortem examination, 10 days later, the infarction in the grey matter in the distribution of the clipped arteries was pale, an indication that blood had not entered in any appreciable quantity through the anastomotic circulation.

The pallor, congestion or haemorrhagic nature of the infarct in the grey matter will be directly related to the amount of blood re-entering parts or the whole of the devitalized capillary bed. This blood may enter at various places, in varying amounts, through the anastomotic circulation. It may however also re-enter through the original artery if the obstruction is relieved, as by disintegration of the original embolus, the particles of which pass onwards to block only some of the branches of the original artery. Fisher and Adams (1951) consider that this is the main factor in the production of the mottled pale and haemorrhagic infarcts which are so commonly seen in the grey matter in cerebral embolism. They suggest that blockage of an artery by an embolus causes pale infarction in the tissues supplied by that artery. Later, due to fragmentation of the embolic material, and possibly to relaxation of local vascular spasm, the embolus moves from its original position into more distal branches. This exposes the necrotic tissue to the full force of the arterial blood pressure with resulting haemorrhage from damaged capillaries. Parts of the brain supplied by arteries which are still occluded remain anaemic.

While we agree that this happens in some cases, it is not necessarily the only explanation of the mixture of pale and haemorrhagic infarcts of the grey matter which are often found after sudden obstruction of a large artery. Not all parts of the initially anaemic region are equidistant from the anastomotic vessels. The parts which are very close will receive the greatest quantity of blood after the shortest interval of time and may indeed suffer no permanent damage. Further from the source of returning blood there is a zone where plasma and red blood corpuscles will leak from the damaged capillaries. This region will be haemorrhagic to the naked eye and under the microscope the vessels will be engorged. This histological appearance is not, however, a proof that the blood was circulating. The walls of many capillaries are so damaged and so much plasma has leaked away that the red blood corpuscles within both large and small vessels are stranded, clumped or conglutinated into slowly moving or immovable masses—a state of *pre-stasis* or *stasis*. This pre-stasis or stasis will impede or obstruct the return of blood to distal portions of the capillary bed and to parts which are, in any case, the farthest from the anastomotic vessels. For both these reasons the infarct in the distal portion is likely to remain pale.

While infarction of cortical grey matter, when due to acute arterial obstruction, is often congested or haemorrhagic, the infarction in the underlying white matter is always pale. This appearance is probably due in part to the less dense and therefore less visibly prominent capillary meshwork in the white matter; and in part to the fact that the vessels which supply the white matter have fewer anastomoses and are more in the nature of 'end arteries', so that less blood will return to the white matter when the anastomotic circulation opens up. In the grey matter there are very numerous capillary anastomoses.

It is difficult to be dogmatic upon the role of *spasm* in relation to infarction. From experimental work on animals it is known that the plain muscle in the wall of an artery or arteriole goes into contraction or spasm if it is stretched. This response occurs if the intravascular pressure is raised above the normal, irrespective of whether the pressure is raised from the arterial side (Byrom 1954) or from the venous side (Denny-Brown, Horenstein and Fang 1956). It is also the probable explanation of the spasm which can follow the manipulation of a cerebral artery. It is known that arteriolar spasm can follow the impaction of needle-like emboli made of crushed glass wool in the cerebral arteries of the dog (Villaret and Cachera 1939). It is thus possible that, in man, when an embolus impacts in a cerebral vessel, there is transient overdistension of the vessel wall and transient localized or even propagated spasm.

Arterial embolism

The circulation of the blood through the brain and spinal cord may be impeded by emboli, which may be solitary or multiple. According to their size they become impacted in arteries, arterioles or capillaries. The blood flow is arrested suddenly, so that the ischaemic effects are not mitigated by the previous establishment of a collateral circulation. If emboli reach the brain through the internal carotid artery they usually become impacted in the distribution of the middle cerebral artery. When they come from the heart, they lodge as often in the left cerebral hemisphere as in the right (Jones 1910). The chief types of embolus are blood clot (either bland or infected), fat and gas (air or nitrogen), and atheromatous debris.

Blood clot (bland)
These emboli usually originate from thrombi in the auricular appendages of the heart in patients with auricular fibrillation, from thrombi overlying myocardial infarcts, from thrombosed internal carotid or vertebral or basilar arteries. Cortical infarcts produced by these emboli are usually haemorrhagic; the question of fragmentation of the embolus has already been discussed (p. 105). Infarcts in the basal ganglia are usually pale, but sometimes they are very haemorrhagic (Fig. 3.6) and when this occurs there is usually reason to believe that the embolus has first occluded the striate arteries and then moved on down the middle cerebral artery.

Blood clot (infected)
These emboli usually originate in pulmonary suppuration or bacterial endocarditis or pyaemia. According to their size and virulence they may give rise to brain purpura, suppurative encephalitis or myelitis, abscess or mycotic aneurysm.

Fat embolism
Following fractures (especially of long bones) or trauma to subcutaneous tissues or to fatty viscera, innumerable small globules of fat may appear in

the blood stream. These fatty emboli are held up at capillary level, particularly in the lungs, kidneys and central nervous system. The symptoms of cerebral fat embolism do not immediately follow the trauma: there is usually an interval of time (average 3 to 6 days). Widespread involvement is shown by headache, fatigue and sleepiness progressing to stupor, coma and death. Hemiplegia and ocular palsy can occur. Strauss (1933) found that the prognosis was bad. In his series of 89 cases, 70 died: 12 on the 1st day, 17 on the 2nd day, 19 on the 3rd day, 13 on the 4th day and 9 between the 6th and 11th day. In patients with multiple injuries, including damage to the brain, the possibility of associated fat embolism should always be considered.

In a series of patients who underwent open heart surgery we have observed widespread cerebral fat embolism, the fat being derived from subcutaneous tissues of the thoracic wound; it had been recirculated via the aorta together with escaped blood at the operative site. Air, thrombi, calcified tissue debris and antifoaming agent have all caused cerebral damage in such cases.

In patients who die within the first 3 or 4 days, the white matter of the brain is diffusely studded with petechial haemorrhages, one type of cerebral purpura. Microscopically these are pericapillary, ring, and ball haemorrhages. Numerous fat globules are visible in these capillaries. Sometimes the capillary walls show focal necrosis. Around some capillaries there are zones of myelin pallor; around others the parenchyma is necrotic and infiltrated by numerous polymorphonuclear leucocytes. In the grey matter fat globules are equally numerous, but haemorrhages and tissue damage are not visible. The fact that the haemorrhages are confined to the white matter is probably dependent upon the capillary network. In the grey matter the capillaries are individually short, anastomoses are frequent. Should one segment of capillary be blocked, enough oxygen can usually diffuse out from the closely adjacent capillaries to keep alive the obstructed capillaries and the surrounding tissue. In the white matter the capillaries are long, anastomoses are few and the wall of the blocked capillary is rendered anoxic; the endothelial cells become less firmly bound together, or die, and red blood corpuscles and plasma leak out.

In patients who survive for several days changes may be found in the grey matter. In a case surviving 6½ days (Neubürger 1925) there were miliary foci of necrosis. These were chiefly in the deeper layers of the cortex. Nerve cells had disappeared but glial cells were numerous. Glial shrubs were present in the molecular layer of the cerebellum from which Purkinje cells had disappeared. Fat globules were present in the capillaries both in the lesions and also in vessels in normal regions.

In a case surviving 12 days Winkelman (1942) found small softenings of various ages in the deeper layers of the cortex, in the white matter especially of the frontal lobes, and in the brainstem especially in the pons. The oldest lesions were full of compound granular cells and the capillaries were prominent.

Air embolism

Air may enter the circulation during abortion, following trauma or operation on the lungs, during artificial pneumothorax, from suicidal or surgical damage to the veins of the neck, and during neurosurgical operations on the cervical region with the patient in the sitting position. If the volume of air is small there may be little change in the condition of the patient. If the quantity of air is large, it will rapidly be mixed with the blood in the heart to produce a frothy fluid, which will then be pumped into the coronary arteries and systemic circulation. The patient will immediately become pale, then cyanotic; coma, convulsions, hemiplegia and blindness may develop with great rapidity. Death occurs in 15 to 50% of cases (Hamilton and Rothstein 1935), probably from ventricular fibrillation due to obstruction of the coronary arteries by air bubbles. The prognosis in air embolism is, however, much better than in fat embolism. If the patient can survive the first 10 to 15 minutes the danger has largely passed (Hiller 1936). Severe paralysis and blindness may completely disappear within hours or days, although mental disturbance may persist.

Post-mortem examination of patients with suspected air embolism must be carried out with care. Taylor (1952) recommends X-raying the intact body, when large collections of air will easily be seen. Before the rest of the body is disturbed the pericardial sac should be filled with water and the right ventricle should be incised under water. Air will then bubble out. If there is any possibility of gas having been formed by anaerobic bacilli such as B. welchii, the blood should be cultured. If the amount of air has been large, frothy blood will be present in the right side of the heart and air will be visible in the veins. More gas bubbles than usual will be seen in the cerebral veins.

In patients who die within a few minutes the only abnormality is the excess of air in the veins. There are no haemorrhages and no microscopical abnormalities in the brain.

In Neubürger's patient (1925), who survived for 55 hours, there were small, perivascular, cortical foci of ischaemic neuronal damage. The nerve cells had pale eosinophilic cytoplasm and disintegrating nuclei (the appearances are similar to those seen after temporary recovery from cardiac arrest). In addition to the perivascular distribution of the lesions there was also a laminar pattern of neuronal damage. Lhermitte and Barrelet (1934) found marked changes in the cortex but none in the white matter in a patient who died of pneumonia some weeks after air embolism. There was spongy transformation of the molecular and external granular layers of the cerebral cortex and scattered, small, irregularly shaped foci from which all the nerve cells and glial cells had disappeared; some of these foci contained the remains of a blood vessel, in others there was a vessel filled with blood but with a necrotic wall. Chromatolysis was present in some of the cortical layers, especially the 6th. In one part of the parietal cortex, the nerve cells of the 2nd and 3rd layers had completely disappeared, with replacement by glial cells including rod cells.

Nitrogen embolism (*Decompression sickness*)
When a person has been living for some time in air which is at a pressure greater than the normal atmosphere and then the pressure is rapidly diminished, he often suffers from sensory and motor disturbances of a transient or permanent nature. Sometimes he dies within an hour or two. At necropsy, in patients who have survived for only a short time, the central nervous system is intensely congested and there may be haemorrhages. In patients who have survived for a longer period, there may be regions of softening. These lesions are commoner in the thoracic portion of the spinal cord than elsewhere. Haymaker (1957), whose article should be consulted by all those more deeply interested in the subject, considers that the involvement of the spinal cord is due to embolism by bubbles of nitrogen which appear in the blood stream after the reduction in atmospheric pressure, together with embarrassment of the spino-vertebral venous circulation by

gas bubbles arising in the epidural and/or retroperitoneal fat. Decompression sickness was first noticed in underwater divers and workers in caissons (Caisson disease). It has now to be taken into consideration in high-altitude flyers who may suddenly find themselves in a subnormal atmospheric pressure.

Atheromatous embolism
Disruption of the intima covering an atheromatous patch will often allow excavation of the lesion by the blood stream and the lodgement distally of fatty and crystalline debris. Temporary obstruction by such debris of small vessels in the retina has been observed clinically and blamed for many transient amblyopic or other neurological attacks. The more permanent occlusion of small cerebral arteries (Fig. 3.29) with minor infarcts is a commonplace of routine neuropathological examination (McDonald 1967).

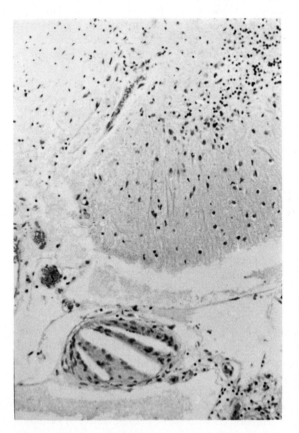

Fig. 3.29 Embolism of small cerebellar artery by three crystals of atheromatous debris. Small old infarct of nearby cortex.

Atherosclerosis

This is a disease process which most commonly affects the largest arteries of the brain. The main stems and branches of the anterior, middle and posterior cerebral arteries are often affected, less commonly the cerebellar arteries and the small arteries of the cerebral hemispheres including the perforating arteries to the basal ganglia. The spinal arteries are very seldom affected.

The changes seen in the cerebral arteries in atherosclerosis are similar to those seen in the rest of the body. To the naked eye there are initially eccentric patches of yellowish opacity of the vessel wall and the calibre of the vessel may be increased. Especially is this noticeable in the basilar artery which becomes dilated, elongated and tortuous.

The earliest lesions in atheroma and the true aetiology are still matters of debate. It is a condition which is more frequently seen with advancing years, although it can occur in the young. It tends to start around the origin of branches of arteries, indicative of a mechanical factor. Duguid (1948) considers that the initial lesion is a deposit of fibrin on the internal surface of the artery, that the endothelium grows over the surface of the fibrinous deposit, which becomes organized, and that red blood corpuscles, entangled in the fibrinous deposit, break down and liberate fatty material.

The other school of thought favours the concept that fatty material from the blood is deposited in the wall of the vessel, a concept which appeared to receive support from the atheroma-like lesions which can occur in rabbits fed on a rich cholesterol diet, and from the finding of a higher incidence of atheroma in people living on a diet rich in fat compared to people living on a low fat diet. Fullerton (1955) has shown that a high fat intake, which produces lipaemia, also produces a marked shortening of the clotting time of the blood. This must, at least, predispose to local intravascular clotting. The 'thrombotic' theory and the 'dietetic' theory may not therefore be as widely separated as was originally supposed. Whatever the initial lesion the subsequent progress of the disease appears to be largely one of repeated

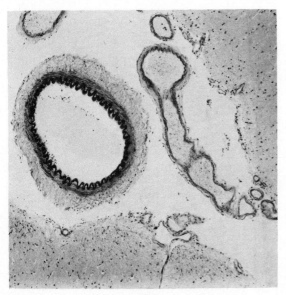

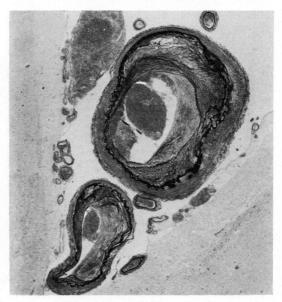

3.30   3.31

Fig. 3.30 Normal arteries and arterioles lying in a sulcus of the brain. Note the internal elastic lamina, the dark staining muscularis, no external elastic lamina, small amount of adventitia. Celloidin; Weigert's elastic van Gieson. × 64.

Fig. 3.31 Atherosclerosis. Cortical arteries and arterioles from a patient with marked atherosclerosis but without hypertension. Note that the abnormalities are in the arteries, which are eccentrically narrowed. The elastica is duplicated. In places the media is thin. Celloidin; Weigert's elastic van Gieson. × 24. (Reproduced by courtesy of Dr W. G. P. Mair.)

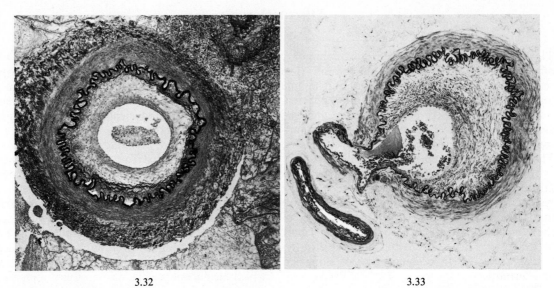

3.32   3.33

Fig. 3.32 Endarteritis obliterans.   Artery at the base of the brain, pneumococcal leptomeningitis, treated sulpha drugs, one month's duration.   Fibrinous exudate is present round the vessel which shows a thickened adventitia, an intact internal elastic membrane and concentric intimal thickening.   Fine elastic fibres are visible in the depths of the intimal thickening.   An adjacent artery, in the upper right-hand side of the picture, shows necrosis and cellular infiltration of its wall.   Paraffin; Weigert's elastic van Gieson.   × 57.

Fig. 3.33 Thrombo-angiitis obliterans.   Branch of the anterior cerebral artery.   The lumen is narrowed by loosely packed cellular fibrous tissue.   The internal elastic lamina and media are intact.   There are no changes in the adventitia or leptomeninges.   A healthy portion of artery lies close to the diseased one.   Paraffin; Weigert's elastic van Giesen.   × 77. (Reproduced by courtesy of Prof. D. S. Russell.)

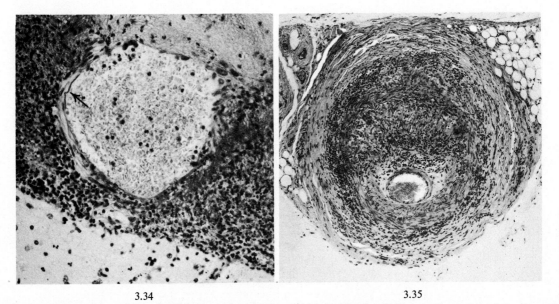

3.34   3.35

Fig. 3.34 Polyarteritis nodosa.   Small leptomeningeal artery which is dilated.   Only a small portion of the internal elastic lamina is visible (arrow) and most of the muscularis is destroyed.   Polymorphonuclear leucocytes infiltrate the outer coats of the artery and the adjacent leptomeninges.   Colloidin; haematoxylin van Gieson.   × 75.

Fig. 3.35 Giant-celled arteritis.   Ciliary artery of eye, showing intimal proliferation and cellular infiltration, including multinucleated giant cells close to the irregularly damaged internal elastic lamina.   There is mononuclear infiltration of the media and, to a lesser extent, of the adventitia.   Celloidin; haematoxylin van Gieson.   × 64.

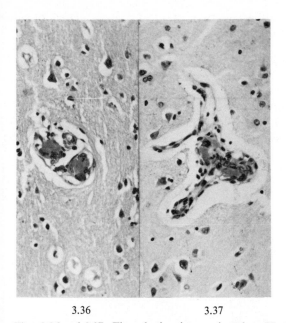 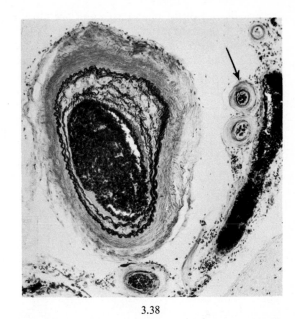

3.36	3.37	3.38

Figs. 3.36 and **3.37** Thrombotic micro-angiopathy. Hyaline eosinophilic thrombus obstructs the dilated lumen at the arteriolocapillary junction zone. There is endothelial hyperplasia. The adjacent grey matter of the brain does not show any noticeable abnormality (apart from artefact due to shrinkage). Paraffin; haematoxylin and eosin. × 200. (Reproduced by courtesy of Prof. W. Symmers.)

Fig. 3.38 Hypertensive vascular disease. Arteries and arterioles in a cerebral sulcus (patient aged 51, blood pressure 190/125, heart weight 470 g, same case as Figs. 3.64 to 3.68). The artery shows hypertrophy of the media, adventitial fibrosis and eccentric splitting and duplication of the elastic lamina. The arterioles (arrow) show an increase in the thickness of the media and adventitia. Celloidin; Weigert's elastic. × 100.

thrombosis upon the surface of the initial plaque. The deposited thrombus becomes organized, elastic tissue is formed within it and endothelium spreads from the edges over its free surface (Fig. 3.31). Regions of fresh or old haemorrhage may be found in the depths of an old plaque. Crystalline esters of cholesterol may also be present and sometimes these excite a foreign body giant cell reaction. Deep to the plaque the media degenerates and undergoes fatty change. The muscularis and internal elastic membrane are weakened and the vessel wall itself dilates, although the lumen may be narrowed by the plaque.

The process of thrombosis upon the surface of the plaque may reduce the blood flow through the artery to such an extent that some or all of the tissues within its bed of supply can no longer live and there is a region of ischaemic necrosis. It is often difficult to differentiate, histologically, between atherosclerosis, organized local thrombosis and a healed embolism. For example a solitary patch of atheroma at the first main point of branching of a middle cerebral artery should always suggest the possibility of carotid artery

thrombosis on the same side with previous embolism and subsequent organization.

Effects of atherosclerosis on the brain

If atherosclerosis is widespread, and almost certainly if the process is of many years' duration, the brain will be atrophic. The ventricles will be dilated and the sulci widened. Foci of softening may be present in the cortex. These may be large or small and are usually of various ages. It is now felt that the general dementia which in the past has been attributed to small artery sclerosis and a presumed reduction of blood flow is caused by a multiplicity of small infarcts probably embolically derived. Around each damaged area will be a zone of failure of blood flow auto-regulation such that cerebral function is disturbed in extensive territories (Hachinski, Lassen and Marshall, 1974). Small, irregularly shaped softenings up to 1·5 cm in diameter are frequently present in the anterior part of the pons, less frequently in the centrum semi-ovale and in the basal grey nuclei. Microscopically these lesions are usually full of fat phagocytes and are always close to a diseased artery or arteriole. These small cystic spaces are quite different from 'état criblé' or 'état lacunaire' which are also found in senile arteriosclerotic brains (Bertrand 1923). Some are clearly the result of obstruction of a

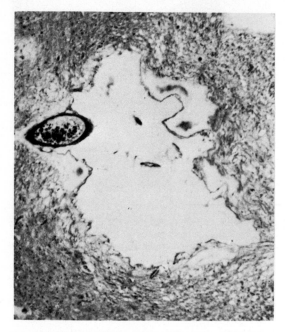

Fig. 3.39 État lacunaire. Small artery lying at one side of the tunnel that its spiralled course now occupies.

small central artery (Fisher 1969); others may show haemosiderin pigment and be associated with more recent small haemorrhages indicating that hypertension and arterial rupture are the cause (Cole and Yates 1967). The term *état lacunaire* (of Pierre Marie) is usually applied to multiple, clearly visible, cavities with irregular contours in the basal grey nuclei; while the term *état criblé* (of Vogt) is applied to similar cavities in the centrum semi-ovale and in other richly myelinated regions. Within each cavity there is an artery or an arteriole (Fig. 3.39). Microscopical examination reveals that the cavity is a greatly dilated perivascular space and that the dilatation is secondary to irregular rarefaction and disintegration of the nervous parenchyma which surrounded the vessel. The artery or arteriole always looks healthy and the cavity contains very few cells. This condition therefore differs from a small softening in respect of its

sites of election, state of the associated blood vessel and cell content within the cavity.

A lesser degree of this condition is sometimes present. The perivascular spaces are not dilated but, in the parenchyma which surrounds the vessel, the myelin sheaths are thin, pale and sinuous. When this change is widespread throughout the basal grey nuclei it is called 'état pre-criblé'. It may be seen less frequently

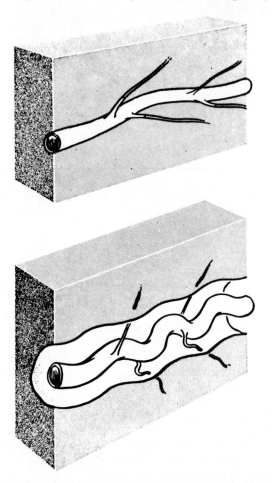

Fig. 3.40 Diagram illustrating the changes in intracerebral arteries that bring about the condition of 'état lacunaire'— elongation, dilatation and spiralling of the artery with distortion of branches and separation from brain tissue.

in the centrum semi-ovale and the deep white matter of the gyri. It thus appears that the initial process is one of slow disintegration of the cerebral parenchyma around blood vessels. We have found that this perivascular atrophy is most common (38%) in hypertensives of all ages and is the result of spiralled elongation of small intracerebral arteries under the effects of raised blood pressure (Fig. 3.40). This process necessitates a dissociation between the artery and adjacent tissue which may be worsened by pulsatile unfolding of the vessel.

Endarteritis obliterans

In meningovascular syphilis, in tuberculous leptomeningitis and in subacute or chronic pyogenic leptomeningitis, when the arteries lie for a long time in tuberculous or purulent exudate, it is not uncommon to find thickening of the arterial wall (Fig. 3.32). The lumen of the artery is reduced in size because the intact endothelium is raised up, in a concentric or eccentric fashion, from the internal elastic lamina by a cellular infiltrate. This may at first be composed of mononuclear cells. In syphilis plasma cells are usually present and eosinophil leucocytes are common. At a later stage, or from the beginning, this cellular infiltrate may be replaced by fibroblasts and collagen with fine elastic fibrils lying internal to the internal elastic lamina, which itself remains intact. The media either appears intact or shows slight inflammatory cell infiltration or slight fibrosis. The adventitia is thickened, either by inflammatory cells or by fibrous tissue.

This condition is called endarteritis obliterans. It shows a stage, or stages, in the reaction of the arteries to infection of the body by more than one type of bacteria. Of itself it is neither diagnostic of any one of the infections named nor is it the only change produced in arteries by these organisms. It is therefore not a specific disease entity and the term should always be qualified by an adjective indicating its cause, if known.

In our opinion the most probable cause of most of the lesions described above is an irritant acting on the arteries from without. A process which is almost certainly due to an externally acting irritant is the paraplegia which may occur as a delayed sequel of *spinal anaesthesia*. In addition to fibrous thickening, and obliteration of the fluid spaces, of the pia arachnoid, extending as far cranially as the base of the brain, these cases often show marked changes in the arteries and less severe changes in the veins.

In Brain and Russell's (1937) patient paralysis came on a month after the anaesthetic, and death occurred $3\frac{1}{2}$ months later. At necropsy there was an endophlebitis and a necrotizing panarteritis of the pial arteries and perforating arterioles of the lumbar region with extensive softening of the grey and white matter of the spinal cord.

In the cases of Greenfield, Rickards and Manning (1955) paralysis came on about 7, 8 and 24 weeks after the anaesthetic and death occurred about 5, 1 and 1 week later. At necropsy the vascular changes were strictly limited to the lower thoracic and lumbosacral segments of the cord, and were confined to the leptomeningeal vessels. The usual change in the arteries consisted of adventitial fibrosis, collagenous replacement of the muscle of the media, stretching and breakage or thickening or reduplication of the elastica, and fibrous thickening (usually concentric) of the intima. One small artery showed coagulative necrosis; evidence of thrombosis was present in only one small artery. The walls of the veins were partially or wholly replaced by fibrous tissue. Haematogenous cellular infiltration was noticeably absent. It was considered that these changes were caused either by the anaesthetic material or by some contaminant introduced along with it. Whether the toxic action was direct or hyperallergic in nature remained undecided.

In order to test the possibility of the condition being due to a contaminant, Hurst (1955) injected a number of detergents and antiseptics in considerable dilution intracisternally into monkeys. He found that many of these substances, although of quite dissimilar chemical type, damaged superficial nervous structures, produced cellular proliferation and fibrosis in the pia arachnoid, and caused necrosis of the media and often of the adventitia of the leptomeningeal arteries with subsequent intimal thickening. The end result was therefore similar to that described in man by Greenfield *et al*. Hurst considered that the experimental lesions were due to the direct irritative action of the chemicals tested; he did not find any evidence of a hyperallergic reaction. He was careful, however, to point out that his experiments did not prove that a contaminant was the cause of the post-anaesthetic changes in man.

Thrombo-angiitis obliterans
(*Winiwarter-Buerger's disease*)

This is a disease of the arteries and veins, of unknown aetiology, characteristically affecting the limbs of young males who are heavy smokers. In the limb vessels the histological changes are different from those in any other disease process. In the early stages there is acute inflammation of the wall and perivascular tissues of both artery and vein, with polymorphonuclear leucocytic infiltration. Thrombosis is present within the vessel and is subsequently organized and re-canalized. At the edge of the thrombus Buerger saw miliary foci not unlike tubercles. In the subacute and chronic stages there is medial and adventitial fibrosis involving and binding together both the artery and its accompanying vein. The internal elastic lamina is not particularly damaged. The lumen of both artery and vein contains organizing thrombus which may be extensively recanalized. The vasa vasorum are prominent and may afford a local collateral pathway.

The disease process can affect vessels other than the limb vessels. When the cerebral vessels are affected the process is confined to the arteries and very rarely involves the veins. This feature may be due to the anatomical fact that the cerebral arteries and veins do not lie as close to each other as do the vessels of the limbs. Involvement of the spinal arteries is extremely rare (Eicke 1957).

In the brain there are two types of distribution: (1) widespread, focal, cortical lesions and (2) in both cerebral hemispheres symmetrically, in the peripheral part of the cortical distribution of the anterior, middle and posterior cerebral arteries, and sometimes in the retinal arteries (Lindenberg and Spatz 1939). The smaller arteries in the sub-arachnoid space are those particularly affected. The process involves considerable lengths of artery at a time and, in the chronic stage, they are shrunken, white and worm-like. Healthy arteries are found close to those which are diseased. The underlying cortex shows many small zones of ischaemic necrosis giving a macroscopical appearance of granular atrophy.

Microscopically, in the central nervous system, the changes are confined to the lumen and to the endothelial and subendothelial layers of the intima; the internal elastic lamina and media are intact. Within the lumen there may or may not be a thrombus, varying in age from recent to old

and recanalized. The endothelium is always affected. In the absence of thrombosis, in the early stages the endothelial cells are swollen and proliferated. In the later stages there is concentric or eccentric narrowing of the lumen by a ring of loosely packed, cellular, fibrous tissue, covered by endothelium (Fig. 3.33). When thrombosis is also present, the thrombotic and intimal proliferative processes are intermingled. Lymphocytic infiltration of the intimal tissues may be visible; occasionally polymorphonuclear leucocytes are present. The lesions vary in apparent age from place to place.

Histologically, the intact media and internal elastic lamina are sufficient to distinguish the condition from polyarteritis nodosa and giant-celled arteritis. Atherosclerosis, even if associated with hypertension, can be distinguished because atherosclerosis almost always affects the large vessels at the base of the brain, which are not involved in thrombo-angiitis obliterans; also when atheroma affects the cortical arteries it does so over short segments, not long distances; and in atherosclerosis the elastica and sometimes the media are damaged. Heubner's arteritis (end-arteritis obliterans), whether due to syphilis or postmeningitic, can usually be diagnosed on the basis of the clinical history, serological changes, widespread cerebral distribution and the histological changes in the media, adventitia and the leptomeninges. The principal difficulty is to distinguish a case of thrombo-angiitis obliterans from a case in which there have been multiple cerebral emboli. Spatz (1935), writing of his own cases, said that, on a purely histological basis, it would be very difficult to distinguish between what he saw and an embolic process (based for example on an endocarditis affecting the aortic valves). When only the brain is available for study the bilateral symmetrical distribution may be suggestive but cannot exclude embolism or local thrombosis. Such a source of emboli or cause of possible local thrombosis may be present in thrombosed carotid arteries, a condition which is usually due to atherosclerosis. It seems doubtful whether the diagnosis of thrombo-angiitis obliterans can properly be made without a full post-mortem examination, including examination of the vessels of the limbs (Fisher 1957).

In view of the doubtful nature of many of the reported cases, we would agree with Adams and Michelson (1952) that a diagnosis of thrombo-angiitis obliterans should not be made, except in the event of (1) an acute inflammatory reaction in cerebral arteries, particularly an obliterating endarteritis with epithelioid and giant cells in the thrombus or intima and with relative sparing of the media (thereby distinguishing it from giant celled arteritis), or (2) obliteration of long stretches of brain arteries in non-atherosclerotic, non-syphilitic patients, with cortical necrosis at the periphery of the field of distribution of the middle cerebral artery, or (3) occlusion of cerebral arteries due to a non-specific endarteritis obliterans in cases with the characteristic findings of thrombo-angiitis obliterans in the limbs.

Polyarteritis nodosa

This is an acute and subacute disease of medium and small sized arteries, especially those of the kidney, liver and splanchnic region. Clinical involvement of voluntary muscle and peripheral nerve is quite frequent (Miller and Daley 1946). Clinical involvement of the central nervous system is considered to be less common, although it was found to be as high as 20% by Foster and Malamud (1941) in their review of 300 cases. In their own case, which came to post-mortem examination, the arteries of the brain were extensively involved histologically, but this in our experience is rare. When present it is usually widespread but focal, so that a muscle biopsy in a suspected case should be cut at several levels. Recent, healing and healed lesions can often be found fairly close together. Hypertension and secondary left sided cardiac hypertrophy are common. Clinical recovery occurs in at least 50% of cases (Miller and Daley 1946) and this has been confirmed histologically.

The primary pathological lesion appears to be subendothelial oedema followed by fibrinoid or hyaline necrosis of the media, destruction of the internal elastic lamina and infiltration of all coats by inflammatory cells. These changes may involve only part of the arterial wall, as seen on cross-section. The cellular infiltration is most abundant in the adventitia (Fig. 3.34). It is composed of neutrophil polymorphonuclear leucocytes, lymphocytes, large mononuclear cells, and a variable number of eosinophil leucocytes which are often present in large numbers. Failure to demonstrate eosinophil leucocytes does not exclude a diagnosis of polyarteritis nodosa. The damage to the vessel coats may include the lining endothelium and secondary thrombus may occlude the vessel. Sometimes the damage to the vessel is so severe that nodular dilatation, aneurysm formation (rare) or rupture may occur. The walls of the arteries of the central nervous system are so thin that, in the few cases in which they are affected, rupture and haemorrhage are common.

In the healing or healed stage the arteries show a concentric or eccentric subendothelial fibrous deposit. The internal elastic lamina is partially or wholly fragmented, or destroyed. Part or all of the media is replaced by fibrous tissue and there is slight fibrous thickening of the adventitia.

Pathogenesis. Polyarteritis nodosa may follow organismal infection (especially streptococcal infection treated with sulphonomides), other drug intoxications and serum sickness. In such cases there is clinical evidence that it is a hypersensitive reaction. This view was supported experimentally by Rich and Gregory (1943), who found the lesions of polyarteritis nodosa in rabbits in which they had established a condition analogous to serum sickness in man. In the human cases it appears that the antigen may vary from case to case but the antigen–antibody reaction remains histologically similar.

Giant-celled arteritis

This subacute inflammatory disease of arteries usually occurs in people over the age of 55 years. It often involves the superficial temporal arteries, which become swollen, tender, tortuous and nodular; pulsation is usually diminished or lost and the artery becomes reduced in size and hard.

The disease is not limited to the temporal arteries. Nearly all the larger arteries in the body, from the aorta downwards, have been found to be involved in an irregular and focal manner. Of the medium and smaller sized arteries which may be affected, those of particular importance are the coronary arteries and the ophthalmic artery and its branches, including the ciliary arteries and the central artery of the retina (Crompton 1959). About 25% of patients become blind in one or both eyes. The arteries of the brain are less often, and those of the spinal cord very rarely, involved. Two cases with involvement of the small meningeal and intracerebral vessels were published by McCormick and Neubürger (1958).

The affected arteries are not diseased throughout their length but in segments. The vessel wall is thickened and the lumen is eccentrically reduced in calibre. It may be blocked by recent thrombus, but this is an uncommon feature and a point of distinction from Buerger's disease.

Histologically, between the endothelium and the internal elastic lamina, there is a zone of intimal proliferation which can often, in the active stage of the disease, be divided into two zones, (1) a thicker inner zone composed of loosely packed, cellular, fibrous tissue with a mucoid intercellular substance, and (2) a thinner outer zone of vascular granulomatous tissue infiltrated by a variable, but usually small, number of large and small mononuclear cells, plasma cells, and a few neutrophil polymorphonuclear leucocytes. Eosinophil leucocytes are very rare, a point of distinction from polyarteritis nodosa.

The internal elastic lamina and the media are always severely damaged, but in an irregular fashion. The internal elastic lamina stains poorly for elastic tissue and is fragmented. The media is infiltrated by small and large mononuclear cells, some of 'epithelioid' type. Giant cells of foreign body type (10 to 100 μm diameter) are almost invariably present, either in the media close to the damaged internal elastic lamina, or in the external portion of the intimal proliferation (Fig. 3.35). Sometimes the histological relationship of a fragment of elastica and a giant cell supports the view that the elastica is undergoing phagocytosis. A lesser degree of inflammatory cell infiltration is often present in the adventitia and giant cells may be found here (Harrison 1948; Heptinstall, Porter and Barkley 1954).

Pathogenesis. This is at present unknown.

Thrombotic micro-angiopathy

Thrombocytic acro-angiothrombosis

This is a rare disease, first described by Moschowitz (1925), with the clinical features of fever, purpura, haemolytic anaemia and thrombocytopenia, together with various neurological disorders such as hemiplegia, convulsions and coma. It runs a rapid course and death occurs within a few days or weeks. It is rather more common in adolescents and young adults than in older persons.

At necropsy there are no specific changes visible to the naked eye, but microscopically, widespread in many organs including the brain, there is thrombosis of the smaller blood vessels. The region affected is the arteriolo-capillary junction zone, where there is an increased cellularity of the vessel wall and obstruction of the lumen by granular or hyaline, eosinophilic, thrombus (Figs. 3.36 and 3.37), which may be undergoing organization. The exact nature of the thrombus is not certain. It has been generally considered that the staining qualities were those of platelets but Stuart and MacGregor-Robertson (1956) have put forward evidence that the thrombi stain more like fibrin. Because of the doubtful nature of the thrombi, Symmers (1952) has proposed that the disease should be called thrombotic micro-angiopathy rather than by any title which implies platelet thrombi.

In the brain the lesions are almost confined to the grey matter (Adams, Cammermeyer and Fitzgerald 1948) and consist of (1) Hyperplasia of endothelial, and probably of adventitial, cells of terminal arterioles and capillaries, with increase in the total diameter of the vessels. Sometimes the vessel wall is necrotic. (2) Occlusion of these vessels by acidophilic thrombi. (3) Foci of nerve cell damage and, in some regions, proliferation of glia. There is, however, a striking disparity between the marked involvement of the vessels and the slight change in the surrounding brain. (4) Occasional petechial haemorrhages.

The aetiology is unknown. The possibility that hypersensitivity can sometimes play a part is suggested by Symmers' (1956) case of thrombotic micro-angiopathy associated with acute haemorrhagic leucoencephalitis and sensitivity to oxophenarsine.

A paper by Timperley, Preston and Ward (1974) describes a similar and apparently much more common intravascular coagulative state in diabetic ketoacidosis. Excessive platelet stickiness would appear to be involved in this condition and treatment with heparin is very effective.

Takayasu's arteritis

Often referred to as Japanese pulseless disease, it has now been reported from other parts of the world. It is a disease of young women affecting mainly but not exclusively the aortic arch and its branches (Fig. 3.41) (Riehl 1963).

All arterial coats are involved by a granulomatous destructive reaction with subsequent fibrosis, cellular intimal thickening, thrombosis and embolic complications (Nasu 1963). The pathological picture is not unlike that found in tertiary syphilis and indeed a false-positive serological test may be found.

The young age of the patients allows a fairly rapid hypertrophy of collateral channels which may by-pass major occluded cerebral arteries; subclavian and other steal syndromes are common. Eventually total obliteration of all vessels arising from the aortic arch may be found. The intracranial cerebral arteries are not directly involved in the process but usually show residual evidence of embolization.

The occurrence of fever, a raised ESR and

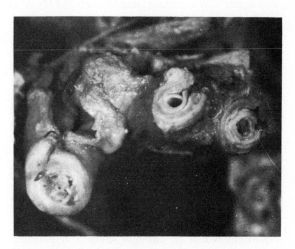

Fig. 3.41 Takayasu's arteritis. Vessels arising from the arch of the aorta showing great thickening of arterial walls and occlusion of lumina. Innominate on the left.

alteration of serum proteins all suggest a response to an infective agent although none has yet been reported.

Other forms of arteritis

A granulomatous angiitis has been described which involves cerebral arteries of all sizes and sometimes veins (Hughes and Brownell 1966; Nurick, Blackwood and Mair 1972). It occurs at all adult ages and runs a course often lasting only weeks or months. The pathological picture resembles that of Takayasu's disease or giant-cell arteritis with lymphocytic and plasma cell infiltration, multinucleated giant-cell systems in the vessel wall and occasional focal destruction of the internal elastic membrane. Less than half the reported cases have shown a generalized system disease involving vessels outside the nervous system.

More specific arterial inflammatory changes follow septic embolization of cerebral vessels and destruction of their walls by bacteria or fungal infiltration; mucor, aspergillus and candida infections are not uncommon complications of modern therapy for Hodgkin's disease, leukaemia and other general neoplasia.

The central nervous system in rheumatic fever

Costero (1949) found that patients who died in the acute stage of rheumatic fever always had swollen oedematous brains in which, microscopically, the perivascular spaces were dilated, the capillaries showed fibrous sclerosis, there were recent and old diapedetic haemorrhages, regions of cellular devastation and foci of softening. Widespread reactive change was present in the microglia. Winkelman and Eckel (1932) had previously reported swelling and proliferation of the endothelial cells of cortical arterioles and capillaries, with thickening and hyalinization of their walls. While none of these changes is specific for rheumatic fever, Costero considered them to be more important than heart failure as a cause of death. One of Winkelman's cases had vegetative endocarditis and a large temporal softening.

Specific lesions, such as the acute necrotic arteritis described in other bodily organs by von Glahn and Pappenheimer (1926), or Aschoff bodies, have not been reported; although Costero, in 6 children out of his 107 cases, found occasional nodules of branched microglia in the brainstem which he thought were a hyperergic response comparable to the Aschoff body; and von Santha (1932) saw fibrinous infiltration of the vessel wall.

Following rheumatic fever, or in patients with recurrent attacks, psychiatric or neurological symptoms may arise. In such cases post-mortem examination may show (Bruetsch 1942, 1949) either:

(1) Widespread obliterative arteritis of the small meningeal and cortical vessels, with proliferation of the endothelial cells, subendothelial fibrosis, and sometimes fibrous thickening of the media; numerous small secondary softenings are present in the brain. A similar change may occur in larger arteries with large secondary softenings. Kernohan (1942) considered that these arterial changes resembled local proliferation, *in situ*, of the endothelial cells rather than those secondary to emboli from the diseased heart. Taken by themselves, the histological appearances in the brain may bear a close resemblance to syphilitic arteritis, or to thrombo-angiitis obliterans, from which they should be separated by an examination of the rest of the body; or

(2) Cerebral embolism, which occurs most often in patients with mitral stenosis in whom auricular thrombi are disturbed by auricular fibrillation; or

(3) Uncommonly, rheumatic meningo-encephalitis, with perivascular and diffuse round cell infiltration through the grey and white matter of the brain.

These changes are also non-specific and by themselves they are not diagnostic of rheumatic infection. Aschoff bodies and acute necrotic arteritis have not been reported.

With the exception of Costero's microglial nodules, most of the lesions in the central nervous system, in both the acute and chronic phases of rheumatic infection, are either directly due to the associated disease of the heart, or are non-specific changes which are found in other toxi-infective conditions. Some of the lesions are undoubtedly due to embolism, some may be due to local thrombosis or anoxia, all of which can be attributed to disease of the heart, especially to endocarditis or to auricular fibrillation or to cardiac insufficiency. Other findings, such as the vascular endothelial proliferation, are also seen in typhoid, toxaemia of pregnancy, erysipelas, Hodgkin's disease and chronic tuberculosis (Winkelman and Eckel 1929) but here also cardiac insufficiency cannot be entirely excluded.

Thrombosis of the veins and dural sinuses of the brain

Thrombosis of a dural venous sinus may occur alone or may be associated with thrombosis of the veins which drain into it or the veins alone may be involved. The thrombus may be (1) *Primary*, local and not infected and probably due to a defect in the circulating blood; or (2) *Secondary* to pyogenic infection, either local or remote, in which case the thrombus may or may not be purulent.

Primary thrombosis

This may complicate malnutrition, dehydration, infectious fevers, tuberculosis, heart disease, usually with right heart failure (Barnett and Hyland 1953), the post-operative state (excluding intracranial operations), head injury, cerebral arterial occlusion, intracerebral haemorrhage, leukaemia, polycythaemia rubra vera and may occur in puerperal women and following abortion. The superior longitudinal sinus is the most commonly involved sinus, with possible extension of the clot into the lateral sinus.

The causes of primary thrombosis are not certain. In some of the associated conditions there is an alteration in the physical state of the blood: it may be more viscous and the circulation may be slow. In the superior longitudinal sinus there may be some significance in the fact that the venous blood enters against the blood stream. In the puerperal period there is an increase in plasma fibrinogen (Plass and Matthew 1926) and both then and following surgical operations there is an increase both in the number and the adhesiveness of the platelets (Wright 1942), which commences on the 4th day and is maximal on the 10th day.

A direct relationship between a changing hormonal state and venous thrombosis is implied in a report that about half of such complications of pregnancy occur in the first 3 months (Carroll, Leak and Lee 1966). Furthermore, the well-reported association between the hormonal contraceptive pill and thrombosis supports such a hypothesis (Atkinson, Fairburn and Heathfield 1970).

The possibility of retrograde venous embolism must be considered. There is known to be anatomical continuity, in the human, between the utero-vaginal veins, the vertebral veins, the intracranial veins and the dural venous sinuses (Batson 1940). It is possible that, during periods of high intra-abdominal pressure, a small embolus might pass from the pelvic veins into the intracranial veins and dural venous sinuses by this route and there form a nidus for a larger thrombus (Martin 1941). Such an embolus could easily originate in one of the thrombosed vessels which are normally to be found in the pelvis following parturition or abortion.

Bland thrombosis confined to a portion of a venous sinus does not necessarily cause much obstruction to the venous drainage of the brain, because, especially over the cortex, there is an abundant anastomotic arrangement of the veins which lead into the sinus. Thus the blood can often find a new pathway and avoid the obstructed segment of the sinus. Extensive thrombosis of a sinus is, however, a danger to life. Thrombosis of the superior sagittal sinus, together with short portions of the lateral sinus, can produce coma and death. We have seen two such cases, in children, who died 9 to 10 days after the onset of the clinical signs, which were principally those of raised intracranial pressure. At necropsy the surface veins were engorged, the brains were swollen and showed gyral flattening. Neither haemorrhage nor infarction was visible externally or on section. Microscopically there was extensive ischaemic damage to the cerebral cortex. The nerve cells were either shrunken, with pale staining cytoplasm and triangular dark staining nuclei, or had disappeared. There was vacuolar swelling of the cytoplasm of the oligodendroglia, and the capillary endothelial cells were swollen.

When both the sinus and considerable lengths of associated veins are obstructed by thrombus, there is serious interference with venous drainage. The affected portion of cortex and underlying white matter becomes congested, swollen, oedematous, and the site of numerous haemorrhages (Figs. 3.42 and 3.43). In venous infarction there are petechial or larger haemorrhages in the white matter and a relatively large amount of blood soon finds its way into the overlying subarachnoid space: two features which distinguish an infarct due to venous obstruction from one due to arterial obstruction. To the naked eye recently thrombosed sinuses and veins are distended by hard clot, mostly bluish in colour but with some flecks of pale material. The necrotic cortex and white matter disintegrate rapidly and are absorbed by the body in the usual fashion so that later the lesion is shrunken, cystic and brownish-yellow in colour (Bailey and Hass 1937). Thrombus in sinuses and veins is rapidly organized and recanalized and it may indeed be difficult to see with the naked eye or even to prove histologically that it was ever there.

Secondary thrombosis

This is most often found as a complication of pyogenic infection, either local or remote. Of local infections the commoner are those of the frontal air sinuses (superior longitudinal sinus), and of the mastoid air spaces or the middle ear (lateral sinus). Secondary thrombosis may also

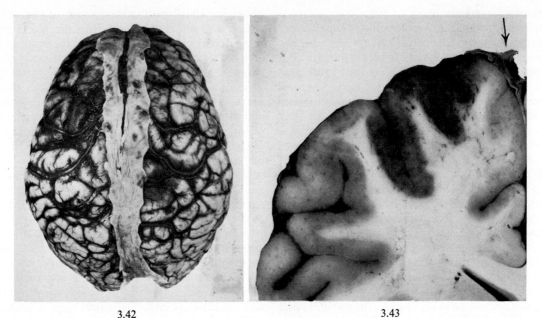

3.42   3.43

Fig. 3.42 Thrombosis of the superior sagittal sinus, and thrombophlebitis of the cortical veins which are distended by partly pale, partly dark thrombus. Note the marked perivenular subarachnoid haemorrhage. Clinically three days' duration. Puerperal woman with breast abscess.
Fig. 3.43 Same case as Fig. 3.42. Coronal section of brain showing thrombus in the superior sagittal sinus (arrow), with swelling and gross haemorrhagic streaking of the cortex and the underlying white matter.

be a sequel to subdural abscess, or to pyogenic infection of the face, especially in the region of the eyes, nose, cheeks and the upper jaw, or to pyogenic infection of ethmoidal or sphenoidal air sinuses (cavernous sinus). The thrombus may spread to the sinus along the veins which drain into it, or sinus thrombosis may arise secondary to inflammation of the wall of the sinus when closely adjacent to a purulent process. The thrombus may not, apparently, be infected: or it may be septic, in which case it is liable to fragment and be carried away in the blood stream to the heart and lungs, giving rise to pyaemia and abscesses.

Superior longitudinal sinus thrombosis
This is usually not septic, except when associated with subdural abscess. This is the sinus usually found thrombosed in primary thrombosis and in puerperal women. The thrombus often extends into the lateral sinus.

Lateral sinus thrombosis
This commonly occurs secondary to otitis media and mastoiditis. It may or may not be septic. If there is no communication between the right and left lateral sinuses at the torcular, thrombosis of the left lateral sinus may obstruct the venous return from the basal ganglia via the great vein of Galen and straight sinus, with resulting infarction of the basal ganglia.

Otitic hydrocephalus
Rarely, patients with otitis media develop weakness of the lateral rectus muscle of one or both eyes and intermittent headache, from which they usually recover. There is papilloedema and the pressure of the lumbar cerebrospinal fluid is raised, but there is no appreciable increase of cells or protein. The ventricles of the brain are not increased in size: indeed, in early cases, they may be smaller than normal. Thrombosis of a lateral sinus has always been demonstrated in the few cases which have been examined *post mortem*. Foley (1955) considered that the obstructed sinus should be the major lateral sinus, or that the thrombus should extend to involve the torcular, thereby severely impeding the venous return from the brain. Symonds (1956), in a critical examination of the cases which have been examined *post mortem*, found that in three cases a lateral sinus, the torcular and the posterior part of the superior

sagittal sinus were all obstructed; and that in two other cases the reports mentioned obstruction of one lateral sinus but gave no details of the findings in the torcular region; in particular it was not possible to judge whether the obstructed sinus was the major lateral sinus. He concluded that the venous obstruction caused cerebral oedema and swelling of the brain, which would account for the intracranial hypertension without ventricular dilatation. He considered that the 6th cranial nerves were damaged by the presence of blood clot in the inferior petrosal sinuses. Further careful post-mortem studies are necessary in this condition, particular attention being paid to the extent of the thrombus, the pattern of anastomosis at the torcular and the condition of the inferior petrosal sinus.

Cavernous sinus thrombosis

Cavernous sinus thrombosis, commonly accompanied by thrombosis of associated veins and venous sinuses, is usually secondary to pyogenic infection of the central half of the face or of the underlying bones and soft tissues. The thrombus usually becomes infected and, in untreated cases, purulent leptomeningitis is generally present at the time of death. The facial and ophthalmic veins are often obstructed and there is oedema of the soft tissues of the orbit, with proptosis. Haemorrhages are found in the retina. It has been suggested that the paralysis, of the 6th or less commonly the 3rd and 4th cranial nerves which may occur, is due to thrombosis of vasa nervorum. Secondary infarction of the pituitary has been reported in a purulent case (Weisman 1944).

Thrombosis of internal cerebral veins

This, in the child, may be primary in the veins, or secondary to thrombosis of the dural sinuses (see lateral sinus thrombosis, above). It may arise with or without pyogenic infection. The usual result is a haemorrhagic infarct in part or the whole of the field of distribution of the veins, which includes the septum pellucidum, the corpus striatum, the thalamus, the ventral portion of the corpus callosum, the medial aspect of the occipital lobe and the superomedial surface of the cerebellum on each side (Ehlers and Courville 1936).

Vascular lesions associated with supratentorial space-occupying lesions

Patients with a rapidly expanding, unilateral or predominantly unilateral, space-occupying lesion, such as intracranial haemorrhage, neoplasm, abscess or cerebral oedema associated with other pathological process, often show clinical evidence of derangement of function at the upper level of the brainstem. If the pressure is not relieved the patient will die and *post mortem* one or more of the following may be found.

(1) *Injury to 3rd cranial nerves.* The 3rd cranial nerve, particularly on the side of the space-occupying lesion, as it passes between the posterior cerebral and superior cerebellar arteries, is flattened and may show haemorrhage within its substance (Fig. 3.44). The appearances suggest that the nerve has been held tightly against one of the arteries or the petroclinoid ligament.

(2) *Temporal or incisural herniation.* A portion of the uncus or hippocampal gyrus will have herniated through the incisura tentorii (Fig. 3.44). This incisural herniation is much more important than any tonsillar herniation which may also be present (Jefferson 1938). Among other effects the herniation compresses the aqueduct and causes supratentorial obstructive hydrocephalus (Smyth and Henderson 1938). When the space-occupying lesion is large and situated in the temporal region it is not uncommon to find that a wedge of uncus has intruded itself between the midbrain and the posterior cerebral artery (Fig. 3.45) (Allison and Morison 1941).

(3) *Anteroposterior elongation of the midbrain.* As a result of the temporal herniation, the incisura tentorii contains both a portion of the hippocampus and the upper part of the brainstem, which is secondarily deformed and elongated anteroposteriorly (Johnson and Yates 1956) (Fig. 3.44).

(4) *Damage to the contralateral cerebral peduncle.* Also as a result of the temporal herniation the cerebral peduncle, on the side opposite to the space-occupying lesion, is pressed against, indented by, and damaged by the free edge of the tentorium cerebelli (Kernohan and Woltman 1929) (Fig. 3.45).

(5) *Vascular lesions in the rostral portion of the*

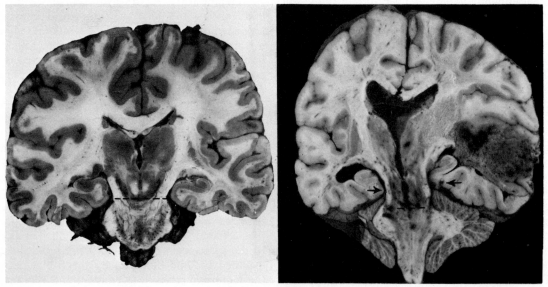

Fig. 3.44 Base of brain from below, right temporal glioblastoma. The third nerves, as they lie caudal to the posterior cerebral arteries, are flattened and haemorrhage has occurred into them; this is more apparent on the right side of the picture (arrow). Temporal herniation is visible on the left side of the picture; arrows indicate the groove formed by the free edge of the tentorium cerebelli. On the right side of the picture there are petechial haemorrhages in the cerebral peduncle which was so soft that it was lacerated *post mortem*. Florid paramedian haemorrhages are visible in the mid-brain. Note the paramedian arteries running posteriorly from the cranial end of the basilar artery and the distortion of the aqueduct (the side of the tumour is on the left of the picture).

Fig. 3.45 Base of brain from below, left temporal glioblastoma. Arrows indicate the line of the free edge of the tentorium cerebelli. A wedge of uncus (U) has intruded itself between the midbrain and the posterior cerebral artery. Note the concavity of the cerebral peduncle on the side of the tumour, the displacement of midline midbrain structures away from the side of the tumour, the narrowing and anteroposterior elongation of the aqueduct, and the bruising of the cerebral peduncle on the side opposite to the tumour.

Fig. 3.46 Edge of ischaemic lesion in rostral pons, case of bilateral frontal glioblastoma. Ischaemic necrosis affects the tissue on the top right of the picture. At the junction of this and the healthier tissue is a swollen axon within a ballooned myelin sheath (circle). Compare with Fig. 3.27. Celloidin; haematoxylin van Gieson. × 100.

Fig. 3.47 Brainstem haemorrhage into the parenchyma and the sheath of an arteriole (A), which is recognised by its internal elastic lamina. A dilated venule (V) is also visible. Paraffin, haematoxylin eosin. × 64.

Fig. 3.48 Normal brain, fixed *in situ*. The dotted line indicates the level of the free edge of the tentorium cerebelli. Note that this line passes through the lowest part of the substantia nigra.

Fig. 3.49 Temporal glioblastoma. Coronal section similar to Fig. 3.48. Arrows indicate the level of the free edge of the tentorium cerebelli. A dotted line indicates the level of the lowest part of the substantia nigra. This is seen to be a considerable distance caudal to the level of the tentorial aperture.

brainstem. In the midbrain and rostral portion of the pons, especially in the paracentral and lateral tegmental regions, there may be florid haemorrhages (Figs. 3.44 and 3.49). In addition, or in less severe cases as the only lesions, there may be sharply delimited foci of ischaemic necrosis. Patients with these vascular lesions usually die within 12 to 72 hours, so that the haemorrhagic lesions are easily seen, but the ischaemic lesions will not be visible to the naked eye. Microscopically, however, in the ischaemic lesions, the myelin sheaths stain poorly with haematoxylin and, at the periphery of the lesion, the myelin sheaths are ballooned and the axons often swollen (Fig. 3.46). Such appearances are similar to those found shortly after thrombosis of the basilar artery. When the patient is saved from rapid death by surgical relief of the supratentorial pressure, and death occurs later, small old regions of necrosis may be found in the brainstem (Wolman 1953).

There are two schools of thought with regard to the nature of the haemorrhages. Scheinker (1945), concentrating attention on the haemorrhage in the tegmental region, considered it venous in origin. While not denying that some of the haemorrhages in this region may be venous, we would agree with Moore and Stern (1938) that the majority, and especially the paracentral haemorrhages, are related to capillaries and arterioles, and occur both into the sheaths of the arterioles and into the surrounding parenchyma (Fig. 3.47). This view is supported by the post-mortem injection experiments of Johnson and Yates (1956).

(6) *Vascular lesions in the occipital and temporal lobes.* A region of haemorrhagic infarction of the cortex and a thin belt of ischaemic necrosis in the underlying white matter are often seen on the medial and inferior aspects of the ipsilateral temporal and occipital lobes. Rarely the condition is bilateral. The lesion is often confined to the distribution of the calcarine branches of the posterior cerebral artery. It commences anteriorly at the margin of the indentation made in the temporal cortex by the free edge of the tentorium cerebelli, and it fans out posteriorly. All authors agree that it is due to obstruction of the posterior cerebral artery or its branches. Examination of the same region, in less florid cases where little or no change is to be seen with the naked eye, will often show, in frozen or celloidin sections, the changes of shrinkage and 'incrusta-

tion of the Golgi network' in the nerve cells. Such changes are known to occur as a result of anoxia.

(7) *Vascular lesions in the thalamus.* Small capillary and arteriolar haemorrhages, usually ipsilateral, are occasionally found in the posterior part of the thalamus, in regions in the distribution of the posterior cerebral artery.

Pathogenesis. The problem is one of explaining the occurrence of ischaemic and haemorrhagic lesions in the rostral portion of the brainstem (within the distribution of the paramedian and short circumferential branches of the basilar, superior cerebellar and posterior cerebral arteries), in the occipital and temporal lobes and the thalamus (within the distribution of the cortical and perforating branches of the posterior cerebral artery), and in the 3rd cranial nerves. Blackwood and Dott (1952, unpublished) consider that all these lesions can usually be explained by a study of the displacements of nervous tissue and arteries which occur in the region of the incisura tentorii.

As a supratentorial space-occupying lesion increases in bulk the volume of the supratentorial contents of the skull increases. In the adult the skull cannot expand to accommodate it, and the dura of the tentorium cerebelli is so well supported by the falx cerebri and by its peripheral attachments that it can only be pushed caudally to a very limited extent. The only aperture of any size in this bony and membranous box is the incisura tentorii and through this aperture the soft brain gradually herniates. The first structure to pass caudally is the midbrain (Figs. 3.48 and 3.49). Post-mortem fixation of brains *in situ* has revealed that the *caudal displacement* may be so marked that the whole midbrain passes below the level of the incisura tentorii. The mobility of the arteries of the circle of Willis and their branches is such that they can follow the displaced brain for a short distance. The circle of Willis is, however, anchored anteriorly to the skull by the internal carotid arteries (Fig. 3.50) and a point will be reached when the posterior communicating arteries and the supporting arachnoid will stretch no further. The caudal movement of the rostral portion of the basilar artery will then be arrested and, as the brainstem continues to be displaced, its paramedian and short circumferential branches will come under tension.

The posterior cerebral arteries also act as anchors for the basilar artery. Both temporal lobes are pressed firmly down on, and are often grooved by, the free edges of the tentorium cerebelli. The laterally placed branches of the posterior cerebral arteries become hooked over these edges and fixed. This prevents any further movement of the posterior cerebral arteries and, through them, limits the caudal movement of the rostral end of the basilar artery. In addition

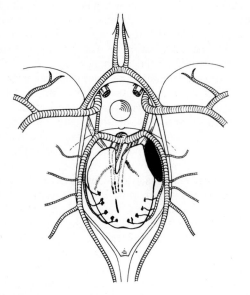

Fig. 3.50 Diagram to illustrate the mechanism of vascular lesions of the rostral brainstem in cases with an intruded wedge of uncus. Compare with Fig. 3.45. Note the antero-posterior elongation of the midbrain and its lateral displacement relative to the basilar artery, which is relatively fixed in relation to the skull and the free edge of the tentorium cerebelli. The midbrain is also displaced caudally (not shown). Abnormal tension develops in the para-median and short circumferential arteries, with ischaemic or haemorrhagic lesions. The posterior cerebral artery, or its branches, may be compressed between the temporal lobe above it and the free edge of the tentorium cerebelli below it.

to being under tension, some of the branches of the posterior cerebral arteries are markedly kinked by the free edges of the tentorium cerebelli and the blood flow through these vessels is impeded, with consequent ischaemic or haemorrhagic

necrosis in their distribution. The calcarine branches are most commonly affected.

Many supratentorial space-occupying lesions are predominantly or wholly unilateral, so that there is a greater degree of temporal herniation on one side than on the other and there is *lateral displacement of the caudal portion of the brainstem*. Such lateral displacement of the midbrain and pons is not only relative to the skull and incisura tentorii, but also relative to the branches of the circle of Willis and of the rostral end of the basilar artery. This factor increases the likelihood of tension in these branches. If in addition a wedge of uncus is intruded between the posterior cerebral artery and the brainstem, the distortion of cerebral tissue relative to the blood vessels is increased.

With temporal herniation, either bilaterally symmetrical or asymmetrical, the upper part of the brainstem is elongated anteroposteriorly (Johnson and Yates 1956) and there is relative displacement of nervous tissue and the blood vessels within its substance.

Thus there are several factors which cause abnormal tension in the arteries and arterioles in question. Such tension on elastic tubes will cause reduction in calibre of the lumen and this, together with any local vasospasm which may occur, will reduce the blood flow to the capillaries and produce ischaemic necrosis. Variations in the degree of tension, the factor of venous obstruction, and in some cases actual tearing or avulsion of arterioles, may be the basis of the haemorrhagic nature of some of the lesions.

Like the circle of Willis the 3rd cranial nerve is anchored anteriorly where it pierces the dura to reach the region of the cavernous sinus. The anterior part of the extramedullary portion of the nerve is pushed down on to the clivus by the herniated hippocampus and it may be flattened or bruised in this region. Nearer the midbrain, the caudally displaced posterior cerebral artery presses down upon the upper surface of the nerve. After leaving the midbrain the nerve has to pass round the postero-inferior and inferior aspect of the artery which flattens it and interferes with its local blood supply.

Oedema in the central nervous system

Organismal infection, recent ischaemic necrosis, traumatic lacerations, and other inflammatory conditions (in the broad sense of the words) of the brain or spinal cord, are often accompanied by localized oedema. More extensive oedema is commonly found in the white matter around abscesses, recent massive haemorrhage, and tumours (Fig. 3.51) especially the metastases of carcinoma, some gliomata and around meningiomata (Greenfield 1939).

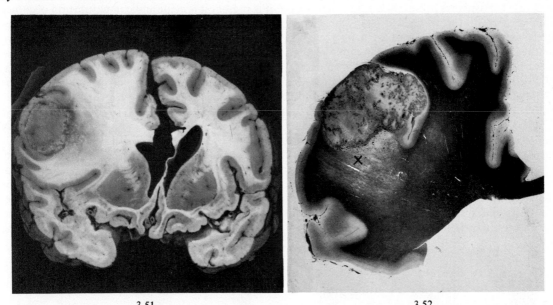

3.51   3.52

Fig. 3.51 Oedema associated with a frontal meningioma. Note the swelling of the white matter, but not the grey matter, adjacent to the tumour. The ventricles are displaced, and subfalcine herniation is visible on the side of the tumour.

Fig. 3.52 Oedema associated with a metastatic bronchial carcinoma, situated in a position similar to that of the tumour in Fig. 3.51. Myelin preparation. Note the pallor of the white matter adjacent to the tumour. This pallor is most marked close to the tumour, tends not to affect the U-fibres on the medial aspect of the tumour, has an indefinite edge, and extends further within the lateral white matter of the hemisphere than it does towards the corpus callosum.

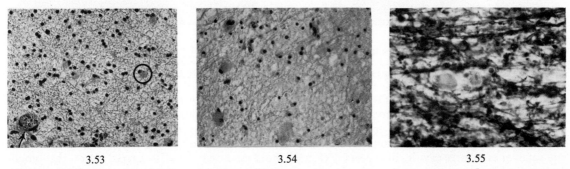

3.53   3.54   3.55

Fig. 3.53 Oedematous white matter from the region of the X in Fig. 3.52. Note the separation of the myelinated nerve fibres, the increase in cytoplasm of the astrocytes (circle), the large number of oligodendroglial nuclei, and the absence of any visible abnormality of the small blood vessels (arrow). Celloidin; haematoxylin van Gieson. × 145.

Fig. 3.54 Oedematous white matter close to a metastatic carcinoma. Note the swelling of the cytoplasm of the astrocytes which are sometimes binucleated, the separation of the myelinated nerve fibres and the numerous oligodendroglial nuclei. Celloidin; haematoxylin van Gieson. × 145

Fig. 3.55 Oedematous white matter close to a secondary carcinoma, myelin preparation. The fibres are separated and often beaded. Two astrocytes with swollen cytoplasm are present near the centre of the picture. Celloidin; Loyez. × 300.

This extensive oedema does not affect grey matter and it noticeably spares the long fibre tracts such as the internal capsules, the corpus callosum and the optic radiations. While confined to the white matter it usually spares the subcortical arcuate fibres. It is most noticeable when it affects the centrum semi-ovale of the cerebral hemispheres (Fig. 3.52) or the deep white matter of the cerebellar hemispheres. It rarely spreads from one cerebral hemisphere to another. The margin of the oedematous change is not clear cut, either macroscopically or microscopically, and in this it differs from, and may be distinguished from, ischaemic necrosis of white matter, which has a sharply defined edge.

In the early stages of oedema the affected white matter is swollen, soft and has a damp appearance on cut section. It may be yellowish in colour. Since it occupies more volume than healthy white matter it acts as a space-occupying lesion causing flattening of the overlying gyri and distortion of the ventricular system. Within oedematous brain there is gradual destruction of axons and myelin

swellings. They may show end bulbs, a sign of loss of continuity. In general they are less severely affected than the myelin sheaths. This damage to myelin and axons, which may be quite severe, is accompanied by a noticeably slight reaction on the part of the microglia and fat phagocytes. Seldom can any interstitial fluid be demonstrated. When it is present it is acidophilic in nature and occupies ovoid spaces. In acute severe cases the astrocytes show swelling of their cytoplasm and degenerative changes: in cases of longer duration and less severity the astrocytes are increased in number, have swollen cytoplasm and lay down astrocytic fibres. Oligodendroglial nuclei are not noticeably affected and blood vessels appear healthy. Changes in the grey matter are very slight but may include swelling of nerve cells.

By chemical examination of oedematous brain, Stewart-Wallace (1939) found that there was an increased fluid content, restricted to the portions of the brain which were microscopically oedematous. There was an increase of water, and also of sodium, chloride and potassium, in the

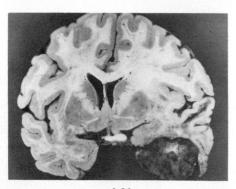
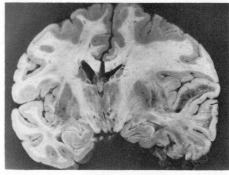

3.56   3.57

Figs. 3.56 and **3.57** Patient with slow growing right meningioma, no surgical treatment. Note the extensive cystic replacement of the white matter of the temporal lobe and insular region. Note the sparing of the grey matter, except immediately overlying the tumour. The most likely cause of these changes is considered to be oedema of long duration.

sheaths, with a moderate amount of astrocytic gliosis. Oedema may be present for many months or years around a very slowly growing meningioma, in which case the destruction predominates and small or even large cavities may develop (Figs. 3.56 and 3.57).

In oedema of short duration (Figs. 3.53–3.55) and varying in severity from case to case, the myelinated fibres are less closely packed than normal and show degenerative changes. Some myelin sheaths are irregularly swollen, beaded, or have broken down into globules or granules. The axons are also widely separated and show irregular

same relative proportions as would be the case if the added fluid was a serum filtrate. This suggests that in cerebral oedema, as in oedema elsewhere, there is an increase in the interstitial fluid and that this is derived from the blood. Cumings (1961), examining water soluble proteins and enzymes extracted from oedematous white matter, found that there was an increase of albumin but no gross alteration of the enzyme content—evidence in favour of the fluid being interstitial (extracellular) and not the result of breakdown of cells.

In *oedema of long standing* the degenerative

process affects most of the tissue. Smaller or larger spaces are found, filled with clear fluid and separated by delicate astrocytic and vascular tissue. Few phagocytes are present (Figs. 3.56 and 3.57).

Pathogenesis. In addition to the interstitial fluid described above, there is also destruction of white matter. The interstitial fluid must come from vessels in some region of the oedematous white matter. Since, however, the oedema is most severe close to the causative lesion, it is reasonable to suppose that most of the fluid comes from vessels which are either close to or even within the causative lesion. Such leakage from damaged vessels may be due to one or more causes. It may be secondary to venous compression (as by a meningioma), to thrombosis (as in a malignant glioma), to damage by toxic metabolites (as in an abscess), or to anoxia (infarct or massive haemorrhage).

Once the fluid has left the vessels it will tend to diffuse. There is experimental evidence in the cat and rabbit (Bertrand 1952) that injected fluid will diffuse rapidly, in a widespread fashion, in the cerebral white matter but not in grey matter. In the experimental animal it tends to pass towards the walls of the lateral ventricle and towards the internal cerebral vein and its branches, where it is absorbed. It is noticeable in his diagrams that the fluid did not diffuse across the corpus callosum. He found also that diffusion ceased at the periphery of the white matter and in grey matter, because here also the fluid was absorbed. The distribution of injected fluid and of cerebral oedema are thus very similar. There is therefore support for the concept that, in cerebral oedema, excessive fluid leaks from the capillaries close to the causative lesion and diffuses widely towards the absorbing

veins and venules, which are found in the walls of the ventricles, at the periphery of the white matter and in the grey matter itself. An excessive macro-pinocytotic vesicular activity in the capillary endothelial cells has been shown by Hills (1964) in experimentally produced lesions. However, no increase of endothelial gaps or stomas has been seen. It may also be postulated that the excess of interstitial fluid interferes with the normal passage of oxygen from the capillaries to the nerve fibres, which will therefore gradually degenerate.

An alternative view, that the swelling in cerebral oedema is the result of an excess of intracellular fluid, is also worthy of consideration. In 1957 Magee, Stoner and Barnes produced experimental cerebral 'oedema' with triethyl tin compounds; in 1958 Klatzo, Piraux and Laskowski produced it by the application of cold to the exposed pia; in 1959 and 1960 Torack, Terry and Zimmerman, using similar techniques, examined brains with the electron microscope and suggested that the initial process, in experimental 'oedema' of the white matter, was an accumulation of fluid, not in the perivascular and intercellular spaces, which they considered to be almost non-existent, but in the swollen perivascular processes of glial cells with clear cytoplasm. Whether these were oligodendroglia or astrocytes is still a matter of debate.

Portions of human cerebral tissue, obtained during neurosurgical procedures from regions close to intracranial tumours have been examined with the electron microscope by Torack *et al.* (1960) and changes were found similar to those seen in experimental triethyl tin 'oedema'. In some regions the cell membranes of the clear glial cells had ruptured but there was no accumulation of extracellular fluid.

Intracranial haemorrhage

There are many causes of intracranial haemorrhage, and the relative frequency of those, which are either the main cause of the symptoms and signs or the cause of death, will vary from hospital to hospital and from time to time, especially with regard to the frequency of those due to mechanical trauma.

In 1954 Russell published her findings of the

causes of spontaneous intracranial haemorrhage from the post-mortem records of the London Hospital (1912-52). She excluded all varieties in which trauma played a part and all neonatal haemorrhages. She recorded only cases in which there were significantly large haemorrhages (in the brainstem of 1·5 cm diameter or more, in the cerebrum 3 cm or more).

Hypertensive		232
Basal ganglia	151	
Cerebral white matter	21	
Subcortical (cerebrum)	4	
Meninges	6	
Pons and midbrain	32	
Cerebellum	18	
Congenital medial defects of cerebral arteries		96
(92 cases with aneurysm)		
Blood diseases		36
Acute leukaemia	15	
Thrombocytopenia	13	
Aplastic anaemia	3	
Other anaemias	3	
Erythrocythaemia	1	
Haemophilia	1	
Mycotic aneurysm		28
Vascular hamartoma		21
Telangiectasis	0	
Multiple cavernous angioma	1	
Arteriovenous angioma	20	
Arteritis (no aneurysm)		13
Pyaemia	10	
Associated purulent leptomeningitis	3	
Neoplasm		9
Arterial degeneration (no cardiovascular hypertrophy)		7
Various		3
Cause not found		16

Comparable figures from the post-mortem records of the National Hospital, Queen Square (1909-69) are:

Hypertensive		143
Cerebrum	113	
Pons	12	
Cerebellum	13	
Pons and cerebellum	5	
Congenital saccular aneurysms		246
Patients with a single aneurysm	200	
Patients with multiple aneurysms	46	

In the 246 patients there were 302 aneurysms distributed as follows:

Internal carotid in cavernous sinus	4	
Junction of terminal portion of internal carotid and its branches	106	
Junction of anterior cerebral and anterior communicating	82	
Middle cerebral at first major branching	73	
Basilar artery and its branches	17	
Vertebral	8	
Anterior cerebral at distal points of branching	5	
Junction of internal carotid and ophthalmic artery	6	
Trigeminal artery (basilar/internal carotid)	1	
Blood diseases		2
Mycotic aneurysm		1
Vascular hamartoma		25
Telangiectasis (cerebellar)	2	

Arteriovenous angioma 23
(cerebral 19, cerebellar 4)
Four of these arteriovenous angiomata also had saccular aneurysms,
1, 2, 3 and 4 in number respectively. In one case an aneurysmal rupture
was the cause of death. These are not included among the congenital
saccular aneurysms.
Arteritis (no aneurysm) 0
Haemorrhage into a neoplasm 14
Arterial degeneration (no cardiovascular hypertrophy) 0
Cause not found 18

The London Hospital is a general hospital and the National Hospital, Queen Square, is a neurological hospital, and this probably accounts for the greater frequency of hypertensive cases, blood diseases and mycotic aneurysms in the London Hospital figures.

In the two series, in 3·5% and 4% of the cases the cause of the haemorrhage was not found. Some of these were probably due to a congenital saccular aneurysm or a small, cryptic, venous or arteriovenous malformation, such as those described by Crawford and Russell (1956), which was destroyed by the haemorrhage.

The central nervous system in hypertensive vascular disease

The arteries of the brain respond to a persistent rise in luminal blood pressure by an appropriate hypertrophy of the muscular medial coat (Fig. 3.59). This physiological reaction is sometimes locally masked by the degenerative changes of atheroma and focal senile arteriosclerosis which appear to be exacerbated by the hypertension (Fig. 3.60). Nevertheless it is always possible to find lengths of artery of all calibres in which the media is hypertrophic. Cook and Yates (1972) measured the medial thickness in cerebral and renal arteries fixed when distended to their normal diameter *in vivo*. They found that a medial/luminal ratio could thus be defined for a vessel of given luminal size, this ratio being much lower for cerebral than for renal arteries presumably because of the additional support provided for the former by the closed intracranial situation and the hydraulic damping that this gives. The ratio was the same for men and women and did not change with age alone. In hypertensive people the ratio increased in both sets of arteries *pari passu* and all arterial sizes were involved (Fig. 3.58).

Arteries within cerebral tissue are almost all relatively thin-walled, of small calibre and generally follow a smooth course; after a short distance from the pial surface they are closely embraced by astrocytic glial cells. Not only do these arteries respond to hypertension by medial hyper-

trophy but there is also elongation which produces a sinusoidal or spiralled course (Fig. 3.69). This phenomenon is most obvious in hypertensives over the age of 30.

Several problems arise for the cerebral circula-

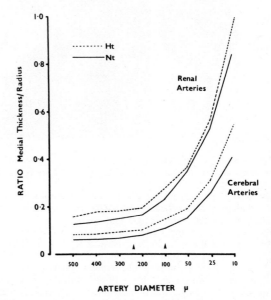

Fig. 3.58 Comparison of the relative medial thickness of cerebral and renal arteries of various diameters in normotensive and hypertensive people. The two arrows indicate the size of intracerebral artery on which microaneurysms are produced.

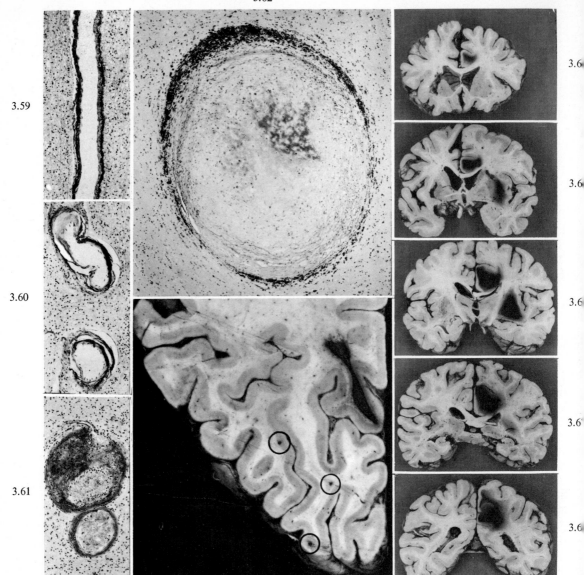

3.62

3.59

3.60

3.61

3.63

3.6

3.6

3.6

3.6

3.6

Figs. 3.59–3.68 Hypertensive vascular disease. These pictures illustrate the progressively more serious lesions which may be found in this condition. Figs. 3.59–3.62 are from one brain, Fig. 3.63 from a different case, Figs. 3.64–3.68 from a third case.

Fig. 3.59 Small artery in the superficial cerebral white matter showing muscular hypertrophy, from a man aged 59, blood pressure 240/60, heart weight 550 g, who died from uraemia. Small frontal and occipital haemorrhages were present. Celloidin; haematoxylin van Gieson. × 40.

Fig. 3.60 Another small artery in the superficial white matter showing fibrous degeneration of the wall. × 40.

Fig. 3.61 Small arteries in the superficial white matter showing degeneration of the wall and aneurysmal dilatation. In the lower vessel the wall is necrotic but the lumen contains fluid blood. In the upper wall the vessel is necrotic and dilated but otherwise intact. The lumen is partly occupied by thrombus. A patient capillary is visible in the upper part of the picture. Its lumen is in continuity with the residual lumen of the artery. × 40.

Fig. 3.62 Microscopic appearance of haemorrhagic lesion in cortex, similar to those in Fig. 3.60. The wall of the original artery is degenerate and there has been haemorrhage into the surrounding tissue. The lumen is completely filled with old thrombus. Around the false aneurysm are phagocytes containing haemosiderin, which appear dark in colour. × 50.

Fig. 3.63 Horizontal section, occipital region, male aged 53, blood pressure 250/150, left ventricular hypertrophy. Note the miliary aneurysms (circles) in the cortex and white matter. In the upper right-hand side of the picture there is a lit haemorrhage, which probably arose from a lesion similar to that which produces a miliary aneurysm.

Figs. 3.64–3.68 Same case as Fig. 3.38. Recent haemorrhages (clinically 10 days' duration) are present in the white matter of the cingulate gyrus and the putamen. The cingulate haemorrhage was 9 cm anteroposteriorly. An old haemorrhagic softening is present in the left corpus striatum.

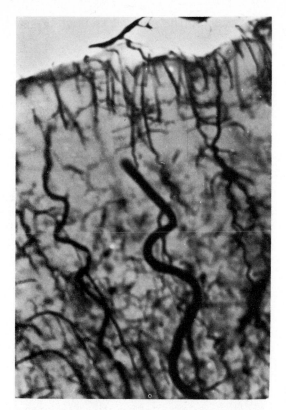

Fig. 3.69 Cleared thick section of cerebral cortex showing arterial spiralling that occurs especially in young hypertensive people. Infected specimen. × 10.

tion. The origins of side branches from such a spiralled artery are shifted and flow into them may be less efficient. The artery becomes separated from adjacent brain tissue by a fluid-filled channel which may be large enough in some areas to be apparent to the naked eye as the condition of 'état criblé' or 'état lacunaire' (Fig. 3.40). This has been reported as recurring in 38% of all hypertensives and only 9% of normotensives (all nine having diastolic pressures over 100 mm Hg) (Cole and Yates 1967a). One consequence of this might be a loss of sensitivity of the artery to changes in nearby O_2 and CO_2 tensions and an inappropriate or inadequate vasodilation.

Elongation and distortion of major cerebral arteries under the combined effect of hypertension and senile atrophy of the medial and elastic coats and its relevance to transient neurological attacks is referred to later.

Hypertensive encephalopathy

The changes described above are those which occur in a gradually developing increase of the blood pressure over a long period of time. Where the time is short as in the acute episodes occurring in cases with a phaeochromocytoma or when severe levels of hypertension are reached rapidly in a period of weeks in primary malignant hypertension or the malignant phases of benign hypertension, changes of a different kind are found. The clinical picture of severe headache, impairment of consciousness, convulsions and sometimes focal neurological signs such as hemiplegia, aphasia and blindness associated with such a sudden rise of blood pressure was given the name 'hypertensive encephalopathy' by Oppenheimer and Fishberg (1928). Adams and Vander Eecken (1953) found a general but patchy oedema with exudates and petechial haemorrhages in addition to many other features of hypertension. The pathological picture is often confused in the

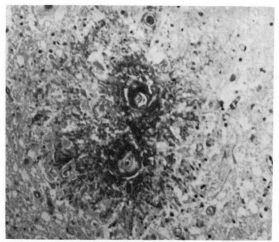

Fig. 3.70 Malignant hypertension. Two branches of a small intracerebral artery showing necrosis of their walls and fibrinous exudate. Surrounding brain shows early oedema and dissolution.

elderly by the presence of multiple infarcts (Rosenberg 1940) and evidence of atherosclerotic disease but in the young hypertensive we have found that patchy necrosis of the walls of quite small arteries allowing escape of blood and oedema fluid seems to be the predominant factor (Fig. 3.70).

Byrom (1954) has pointed out that, in the human, hypertension is not usually associated with a more rapid flow of blood through the brain, so that some degree of arterial or arteriolar constriction must occur. This constriction is due to the fact that arteries have intrinsic local tone, largely dependent on intra-arterial pressure. Byrom made rats hypertensive by means of a renal clamp, and they showed clinical evidence of hypertensive encephalopathy. He observed the cerebral vessels through transparent windows in their skulls and saw arteriolar spasm taking place. By means of *intra vitam* injection of trypan blue he showed that some capillaries were abnormally permeable. Histologically he saw (1) focal cerebral oedema without vascular necrosis, (2) vascular necrosis, (3) haemorrhage.

He considers that hypertensive disease may be divided into two main grades of severity. In the first the underlying peripheral vasoconstriction is diffuse and so controlled that the distribution of the blood to the tissues remains substantially normal, except where it is locally impeded by secondary degenerative changes in the arterial wall, such as atherosclerosis. In the second, more severe, grade there is, superimposed upon physiological vasoconstriction, a state of focal but widespread pathological spasm. This spasm is a direct local response to the physical strain of excessive intra-arterial tension; a morbid response which can be traced to a simple physiological property of arterial muscle, i.e. its faculty of contracting against a filling tension. It is possible that the arteries are also abnormally sensitive.

The effects of the spasm depend upon its intensity, duration, location and extent. They comprise, in increasing order of severity (1) transient disturbance of function, (2) increased capillary permeability with attendant focal oedema and (3) local necrosis of the arterial wall and/or the tissue supplied. An alternative explanation of arterial necrosis is that blood trapped between two zones of constriction may be squeezed into the vessel wall. Byron found that the arterial spasm which underlay these various changes could be abolished in the rat by removing its cause, i.e. by lowering the blood pressure.

However, there is increasing evidence to suggest that Byrom's experimental observations of widespread vasospasm may not apply in man. Lassen and Agnoli (1972) studying regional cerebral blood flow in man found that the autoregulatory mechanisms may break down when an acute rise of blood pressure occurs. They found a general increase in cerebral blood flow which appeared to be inappropriate in terms of the local metabolism.

Disruptive effects of hypertension

(1) *Small haemorrhages up to 1 cm in diameter found in basal ganglia, cerebral cortex and gyral white matter and in pons and cerebellum.* These lesions are sometimes fresh but more usually at necropsy one finds groups of haemosiderin-laden macrophages close to a small vessel or a small gliotic cyst with a pigmented wall (Fig. 3.71).

(2) *Slit haemorrhages.* These are quite often present in the brains of hypertensive patients, in the superficial part of the white matter of the

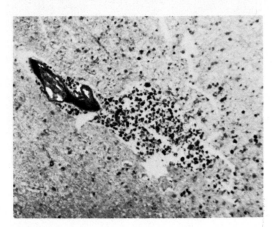

Fig. 3.71 Hypertension. A collection of pigment-laden macrophages lying at the site of a small haemorrhage.

cerebral hemispheres. The blood clot is not rounded but fills a slit-like cavity which runs roughly parallel to the overlying cortex (Fig. 3.63). Their appearance suggests that the blood, after leaving the vessel, found that the path of least resistance was between the fibres of the white matter in a plane parallel to the cortex. The blood clot in these lesions varies from recent to very old; and the lesions vary in size from very small to those extending for about half the anteroposterior length of the brain (Figs. 3.64–3.68). A somewhat similar type of localized haemorrhage may be found involving the region of the putamen (Figs. 3.65 and 3.66), which is partially or completely replaced by blood clot. In this case the haemorrhage is confined to the lentiform nucleus by the more resistant surrounding bundles of white fibres.

(3) *Massive haemorrhage.* The common sites

for massive cerebral haemorrhage of hypertensive origin are (1) the region of the lentiform nucleus, (2) the deep white matter of the cerebellar hemispheres, (3) the pons and midbrain. Courville (1950) gives the relative incidence in his 40,000 autopsies as 938, 124 and 73 respectively.

It is not uncommon, in cases of massive cerebral haemorrhage, to find one or more separate haemorrhages in the midbrain and pons. The brainstem lesion is then secondary to the displacement caused by the cerebral haemorrhage, and is similar to that commonly seen as a terminal event in patients with other kinds of supratentorial space-occupying lesions, e.g. a glioma, abscess, oedema, extradural or acute subdural haemorrhage (see p. 121).

Haemorrhage in the region of the lentiform nucleus has been divided by Courville and Friedman (1942) into a medial ganglionic type, which is usually fatal, and a lateral ganglionic type, which the patient may survive. The medial ganglionic type arises medial to the putamen and usually destroys the hypothalamus and ruptures into the ventricle. Haemorrhages of lateral ganglionic type arise in the putamen, external capsule or claustrum. In some cases the haemorrhage remains relatively localized to the putamen; in other cases it extends posteriorly into the white matter of the occipital lobe.

Massive hypertensive haemorrhage into the cerebellum, or into the pons and midbrain, is almost invariably and rapidly fatal.

Examination of the brain, soon after a massive haemorrhage, reveals clot which is soft and like redcurrant jelly. When such a clot is removed, the walls of the cavity are ragged. Small vessels can often be found projecting into the cavity and, in these vessels, necrosis of the wall and thrombosis of the lumen are often present. Around the main haemorrhage, numerous petechial haemorrhages are visible in the adjacent grey matter, and in the white matter which is soft, swollen and oedematous. On microscopical examination there is ischaemic necrosis of variable extent in the nervous tissue which forms the wall of the cavity; many of the small vessels which are present have necrotic walls; and the petechial haemorrhages, which are principally of ring and ball type, are around capillaries. These changes at the periphery of a recent haemorrhage appear to have occurred at, or about, the time of the massive haemorrhage. If the patient does not die as a result of the haemorrhage, the blood

clot becomes inspissated and turns reddish-brown in colour. Reactionary changes occur in the surrounding tissue, with phagocytosis of haemosiderin and of necrotic cerebral tissue. Astrocytes become swollen, increase in numbers and lay down astrocytic fibres. The amount of nervous tissue which is destroyed is not as much as one might perhaps expect. Massive cerebral haemorrhage has a tendency to track along tissue planes, separating rather than destroying the nervous substance. In this way it differs from a haemorrhagic infarct, due to obstruction of an artery, in which nearly all the tissue within the distribution of the artery undergoes necrosis. This anatomical difference is helpful in deciding whether a lesion, especially an old lesion, was a haemorrhage or a haemorrhagic infarct.

Pathogenesis of hypertensive cerebral haemorrhage

Prehaemorrhagic infarction

The almost inevitable finding of fairly severe atherosclerosis in the vessels of hypertensive patients has suggested to many that large intracerebral haemorrhages may be no more than a very extensive haemorrhagic infarct or at any rate haemorrhage from poorly 'supported' arteries traversing ischaemically softened areas (Globus 1938). Such infarction, it was thought, might be due to thrombosis of central arteries in cases of massive haemorrhage (though such has rarely been demonstrated) or to severe vasospasm of highly irritable vessels (Schwartz 1961).

In the neighbourhood of a large haematoma it is indeed common to find distorted and necrotic vessels and tissues but there is not usually any evidence to suggest that these changes preceded the haemorrhage.

Microaneurysms

The hypothesis that cerebral haemorrhage was due to rupture of intracerebral arterial aneurysms was put forward in 1868 by Charcot and Bouchard, but subsequent authors (Ellis 1909; Russell 1954) doubted that the lesions described by the rather primitive technique of maceration were truly aneurysms. We have repeated the original methods and it became clear that while a few of Charcot and Bouchard's aneurysms were probably real most were forms of blood clot (Cole and Yates 1967b).

However, Green (1930) found three unmistakable aneurysms in a tedious histological search of ten brains of hypertensives. Clarification of the real situation awaited the new technique of post-mortem X-ray angiography used by Ross Russell (1963) to discover very many more aneurysms particularly in elderly patients. A subsequent survey by similar methods (Cole and Yates 1967c) revealed their presence in 46 of 100 hypertensives (but only 2 out of 21 patients under the age of 50 years) and in 7 of 100 normotensives, all 7 having diastolic pressures over 100 mm Hg and being over 66 years of age (Fig. 3.72).

Of 21 patients who had had a massive intra-cerebral haemorrhage 18 showed microaneurysms,

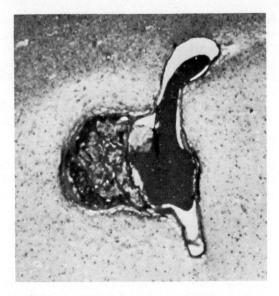

Fig. 3.73 Small intracerebral artery with aneurysm sac on its left side partially occluded by organizing thrombus. (Lumen of vessel contains shrunken gelatin cast.)

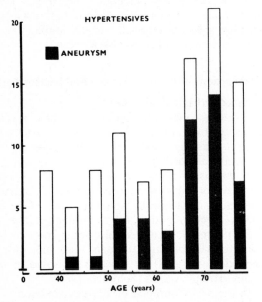

Fig. 3.72 Occurrence of microaneurysms at different ages in the brains of 100 hypertensive people.

one was young and had malignant hypertension and one had an angioma. All the cases in which small and slit haemorrhages were found had microaneurysms (Cole and Yates 1967a). The aneurysms were common in brains where they were found at all—least number 9, largest 80—the usual number being about 20. They were found in basal ganglia, subcortical gyral white matter, pons and cerebellum in that order of frequency. Their diameter was usually about 500 μm and only rarely did they reach 2 mm. Sometimes thrombus could be seen lining the aneurysmal sac but the vessel itself was not occluded (Fig. 3.73).

The significance of these lesions may be two-fold; by a whirlpool effect they may alter the

flow of blood along the vessel; by rupture they undoubtedly cause small haemorrhages, although there is less certain evidence of their role in initiating massive haemorrhage.

The presence of microaneurysms and the occurrence of large cerebral haemorrhages are both uncommon in young hypertensives; it appears that some ageing factor such as a change in the resilience of the arterial elastic lamina is also important. The histological appearance of these microaneurysms is very similar to that of so-called congenital aneurysms of the circle of Willis and it may be that similar degenerative changes allow both types to become apparent in middle age (Fig. 3.74).

Hypertension and number of 'strokes'

It is a well-established clinical observation that hypertensive patients have many more 'strokes' than normotensives, and this applies equally to 'small strokes' as to large ones. Some accentuation of atheromatous arterial disease is thought to be caused by raised blood pressure but little evidence exists to quantify this factor. An attempt to assess these effects was made by Cole and Yates (1968) who examined the brains from 100 hypertensives and from 100 age and sex matched normotensives not selected for any

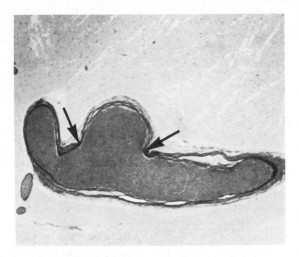

Fig. 3.74 Small artery and aneurysm filled by gelatin cast. Arrows indicate the points where the medial coat and internal elastic membrane stop at the base of the sac which is formed of collagen only.

reason as to cause of death. They found that a quarter of the normotensives had suffered old or recent cerebral infarcts, large or small or cystic scars. About half the hypertensives showed cerebrovascular damage, but as in the normotensive group those with infarction formed about a quarter of the total; the additional quarter had old or recent haemorrhagic lesions or pigmented cysts. There remained only three hypertensive patients who had had both infarction and haemorrhage.

An interesting finding was the number of small lesions of a size likely to have caused a 'small stroke'. In the 100 normotensives there were 19 small infarcts and 59 cystic scars, a total of 78 small lesions occurring in 17 people. The 100 hypertensive brains showed many more lesions per case; 33 small infarcts and 60 cystic scars in 18 people; 69 small haemorrhages (over 1 cm) and 60 pigmented cysts in 23 people.

Apart from the considerable excess of large and small 'stroke' lesions suffered by the group of hypertensive patients the interesting point was made that only three patients had both infarcts and haemorrhages. It seemed that a persistently raised blood pressure either exacerbated a thromboatheromatous tendency or produced arterial microaneurysms and haemorrhage but rarely both in the same patient. Identification of these two groups of people is obviously of

great importance when preventive anticoagulant therapy is contemplated.

Chronic progressive subcortical encephalitis of Binswanger

Described by Binswanger in 1894, this is a very rare type of involvement of the brain in hypertensive vascular disease. Very few cases have been published, the most recent being those of Farnell and Globus (1932) and Davison (1942).

It is found from the age of 50 onwards and affects the cerebrum. The cortex and the subcortical arcuate fibres are intact, or almost intact, but the deep white matter is reduced in amount.

According to Binswanger the disease process is most severe in the occipital and temporal lobes. The condition may be confined to the white matter of one convolution or may affect several convolutions (Fig. 3.75). In severe cases the white matter of whole lobes of the cerebrum is almost completely atrophied, so that there is, in places, very little white matter left. In such cases the temporal and occipital horns of the lateral ventricles will be enormously dilated. In his cases the white matter of the frontal lobes was not significantly affected.

Some of the regions of myelin destruction are

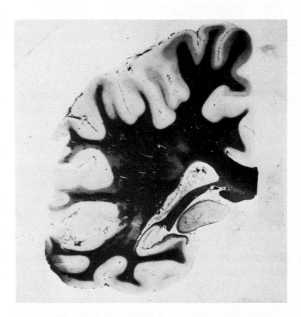

Fig. 3.75 Multiple, often clearly demarcated, foci of myelin destruction in the white matter of a hypertensive patient, of the type seen in Binswanger's subcortical encephalopathy. Celloidin; Loyez.

sharply delimited, like plaques or disseminated sclerosis; some are less well defined. Where myelin is no longer present there are fat granule cells and proliferated astrocytes and their fibres.

The arterioles of the white matter are the site of narrowing, fibrous thickening, and hyaline change, such as is found in hypertension. The arteries of the circle of Willis show atherosclerosis.

Aneurysm

The word aneurysm means a dilatation of an artery. In relation to the central nervous system we are concerned with:

(1) Congenital saccular aneurysms.
(2) Mycotic aneurysms.
(3) Atherosclerotic fusiform aneurysms.
(4) Spontaneous and post-traumatic arterio-venous aneurysms between the internal carotid artery and the cavernous sinus.
(5) Dissecting aneurysms.
(6) Intracerebral micro-aneurysms (see p. 133).

Congenital saccular aneurysms

Frequency. In the large presurgical series, discussed by Fearnsides (1916) and corrected by Turnbull (1918), the incidence of congenital intracranial aneurysm was 0·64% (29 persons with 33 aneurysms in 4547 post-mortem examinations of the head at the London Hospital 1908-13). The extra number of aneurysms is accounted for by 3 persons having 2, 2 and 3 aneurysms respectively, giving an incidence of multiple aneurysms of 11%. Bigelow (1955) found multiple saccular aneurysms in 16% of his cases. Multiple saccular aneurysms of congenital type are also found on the cerebral arteries in association with arteriovenous angiomata. In one such case death was due to rupture of an aneurysm (Brihaye and Blackwood 1957).

Age. Although aneurysms have been recorded at the extremes of life less than 1% present under the age of 20 years (Crompton 1964); they most commonly cause death during the 5th decade (Carmichael 1950). Of those which give rise to clinical symptoms about half are found after the age of 40 (Meadows 1951). They are not markedly more frequent in either sex (Dandy 1944).

Site. Almost all saccular aneurysms arise at, or very close to, the points of division of arteries (Carmichael 1950). The commonest site is on the middle cerebral artery at its first or second point of branching in the Sylvian fissure (about 30%): the next most common is at the junction of an anterior cerebral and an anterior communicating artery (about 25%): next the junction of the terminal portion of the internal carotid artery and its branches (the middle and anterior cerebral and the posterior communicating) is involved in about 20% of cases. The basilar artery and its branches account for about 12 to 15% and other arteries (vertebral, posterior cerebral, posterior communicating) for about 12%. Aneurysms are not appreciably more common either on the left or the right side (Dandy 1944).

Naked eye findings. Saccular aneurysms may vary in size from smaller than a pin's head to 30 mm in diameter, but, as Fearnsides (1916) records, the commonest size is that of a pea.

At necropsy it is occasionally difficult to find the aneurysm, either because of its small size or because, in rupturing, it has disintegrated.*

Initially the sac lies in the subarachnoid space, but with enlargement and possible leakages the major portion of the sac may be buried in the substance of the brain, or a portion of the sac may protrude through the arachnoid into the subdural space. The blood vessels of the circle of Willis may be generally atheromatous, but sometimes almost the only yellowish thickening of the vessels is to be seen close to the neck of the aneurysm. The wall of the aneurysm is usually thin and is composed of fibrous tissue. In larger aneurysms the sac is often partly filled with laminated, organized and organizing blood clot. Embolism of the arteries distal to the aneurysm, by fragments of the clot which form in it, is very rare or perhaps unknown. Calcification may be present. Brownish pigmentation, fibrous thickening and adhesions to surrounding tissues are signs of old leakage. Occasionally at

---

* We recommend an initial careful dissection of the common sites in the unfixed specimen, because after fixation it is more difficult to push away any blood clot which may be present. If this fails to reveal the aneurysm then examine the less common sites; or fix the brain, dissect out the basal vessels and examine all junctional points.

necropsy one finds a small aneurysm filled with old pale fibrous tissue: it appears to be healed.

Aneurysms often rupture, usually near the fundus of the sac.

The blood from a ruptured saccular aneurysm may pass:

(1) Into the subarachnoid space (Fig. 3.76).
(2) Into the overlying brain, sometimes forming a false aneurysm, but more often ploughing through the substance of the brain to enter and fill the ventricular system (Figs. 3.77, 3.78 and 3.79). Richardson and Hyland (1941) emphasized the frequency of intracerebral haemorrhage (19 out of their 27 cases of ruptured aneurysm). They noted the two common sites, frontal and temporal, from aneurysms in the region of the anterior communicating artery, or at the carotid bifurcation, or on the middle cerebral artery in the Sylvian fissure.
(3) Much less commonly, into the subdural space.

Distortion, compression and destruction of neighbouring cranial nerves and brain substance may be produced by the sac and by haemorrhage which is not sufficient to cause death. Rupture of an aneurysm is not invariably fatal.

Cerebral infarction has been reported in about 70% of those who die after a ruptured aneurysm (Crompton 1964). Most often it lies within the territory of the artery bearing the aneurysm but occasionally other parts of either hemisphere are involved. The appropriate vessels are only rarely occluded by thrombus so that vasospasm, which is often seen angiographically in life (Schneck and Kricheff 1964), and general hypotension are thought to be the important causes.

The mortality and morbidity of cases of ruptured congenital saccular aneurysms, which have not been treated surgically, have been investigated by Hyland (1950) and by Walton (1956). After considering the literature and his own cases of subarachnoid haemorrhage (80% of which he considers to be from aneurysms), Walton's conclusions may be summarized as follows. Of 100 persons who come into hospital with ruptured intracranial aneurysms, 45 will die during the next 8 weeks, 55 will survive this period. Of the 45 who die, 28 will die from the initial haemorrhage (12 within 24 hours, 16 between the 3rd and 14th days); 17 will die from a recurrence of the haemorrhage. Of the 55 who survive the

first 8 weeks, 5 will die of a recurrent haemorrhage within the next 6 months, 7 will die for the same reason at a later date (in several cases the follow up was as long as 12 years). Of the remaining 43, one-third will be more or less disabled by residual paralysis, epilepsy, headache or mental symptoms; one-third will suffer from relatively trivial symptoms, and one-third will recover completely.

Microscopical findings. At the neck of the sac the muscle of the media of the artery comes to an abrupt end. At about the same point the internal elastic membrane shows degenerative changes, which appear to be due to the implication of the elastica in an ordinary atheromatous process. The degenerate elastic membrane usually passes only a short distance into the sac, the wall of which is formed of fibrous tissue continuous with the intima and adventitia of the artery. Part of the fibrous wall may be degenerate. In cases where there has been previous leakage, phagocytes filled with haemosiderin, small round-celled infiltration and fibrous thickening are present around the sac.

Pathogenesis. There is general agreement that the chief aetiological factor in the development of these aneurysms is aplasia or hypoplasia of the muscle coat at the point of branching or junction of the arteries. Such developmental defects are not confined to cerebral arteries but are also present in coronary, mesenteric and pulmonary arteries (Forbus 1930). In the circle of Willis, Glynn (1940) found such defects at 80% of bifurcations, both in cases with cerebral aneurysms and in normal controls. The probable reason for the defect is the way in which the medial coat of an artery and its branches develops. It does not grow in continuity, like the bark of a tree, but develops from separate islands of mesenchyme, which subsequently fuse at the points of junction or branching of permanent vessels or of temporary embryonic vessels which are subsequently absorbed (Padget 1944). If fusion is imperfect then, at these points, the arterial wall is composed only of endothelium, the internal elastic lamina, and a small amount of fibrous tissue: for cerebral arteries have no external elastic lamina and only a rudimentary adventitia.

In the majority of people this thin portion of wall is adequate. In a few people, however, there is evidence that this region is further weakened by degeneration of the elastica. This degeneration is almost invariably associated with appearances indistinguishable from atheroma.

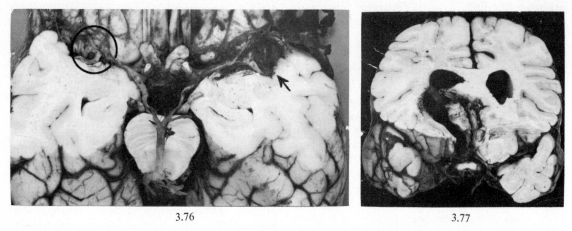

3.76   3.77

Fig. 3.76 Ruptured congenital saccular aneurysm of the left middle cerebral artery (arrow). The blood had passed into the subarachnoid space of the insula and of the basal cisterns (from which it was partly removed to display the aneurysm). The aneurysm arose from the point of branching of the artery in the Sylvian fissure. The corresponding point of branching on the right middle cerebral artery is ringed.

Fig. 3.77 Ruptured congenital saccular aneurysm of the right anterior cerebral/anterior communicating artery. The blood has ploughed through the substance of the frontal lobe into the lateral ventricle.

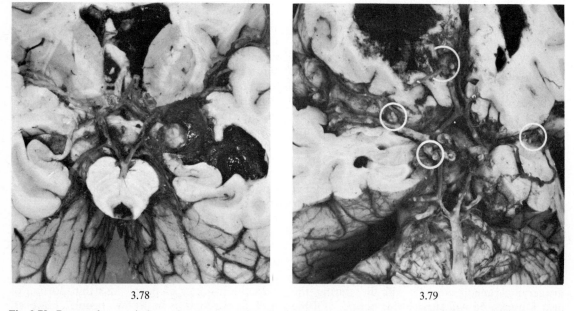

3.78   3.79

Fig. 3.78 Ruptured congenital saccular aneurysm of the left internal carotid/posterior communicating artery. The blood has passed laterally through the choroidal fissure into the left lateral ventricle. A lesser amount of blood was present in the right lateral ventricle. The 3rd ventricle, the aqueduct and the 4th ventricle were full of blood.

Fig. 3.79 Base of the brain in a patient with multiple congenital saccular aneurysms (ringed). An aneurysm on the right anterior cerebral artery has bled into the substance of the right frontal lobe and into the lateral ventricle.

Without the support of the elastica, the endothelium and the fibrous tissue yield before the pressure of the blood and an aneurysm is formed (Carmichael 1950).

Hypertension is present in more than half the cases and must be considered to play an important secondary role in the pathogenesis of these aneurysms and their rupture.

Mycotic aneurysm

A mycotic aneurysm forms when the wall of an artery is weakened from within by pyogenic bacteria. The bacteria usually reach the affected portion of the wall in an infected embolus. The commonest source of such emboli are the aortic heart valves in endocarditis, particularly of subacute bacterial type. Less commonly pulmonary suppuration or pyaemia may be the origin. The organisms are usually of low or attenuated virulence; those of high virulence cause leptomeningitis or cerebral abscess. The aneurysms are usually found on the branches of the middle cerebral artery, especially in the lateral fissure (Stengel and Wolferth 1923). Sometimes they are peripherally situated in the distribution of this artery and are multiple.

The embolus becomes adherent to the wall, which shows the usual histological changes of an acute inflammatory process. When the elastica and the media are sufficiently damaged, the wall of the artery shows a localized dilatation, which may progress to rupture and haemorrhage into the subarachnoid space or into the nervous tissue. Mycotic aneurysms are usually small because the process is a relatively rapid one. Since the aneurysm usually arises from the lodgement of an embolus there will be a varying amount of ischaemic necrosis of nervous tissue in the field of distribution of the artery.

Atherosclerotic fusiform aneurysms of the basilar artery and aneurysms of the intracavernous portion of the internal carotid artery

Fusiform dilatation of the basilar or internal carotid artery is a not uncommon finding in patients with severe atherosclerosis. The elastica and muscularis of the vessel are damaged by the atherosclerotic process and the vessel dilates. The *basilar artery* is often elongated as well as dilated and has a sinuous course and similar changes are seen in the middle cerebral arteries (Fig. 3.80).

These aneurysms may be quite large compressing and distorting cerebral tissue and nerve roots producing for example trigeminal neuralgia. The origins of many of the small branches of the basilar and of the middle cerebral are considerably displaced by the sinuous course of the parent

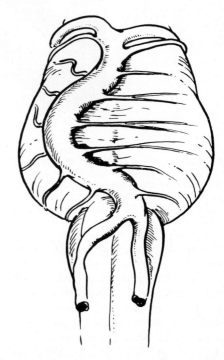

Fig. 3.80 Diagram of fusiform aneurysm of basilar artery showing distortion of its course from the midline and consequent effects on paramedian branches which might be one cause of transient neurological attacks.

vessels. Alterations of the blood pressure will further fold or unfold these vessels (Hughes 1965) perhaps causing temporary cessation of flow into some of the small kinked branches. Such a mechanism has been suggested as a cause of minor transient neurological attacks of the kind that recur frequently and identically in some patients (Yates 1973).

The dilatation of the *internal carotid artery*, which usually affects both arteries, may have serious effects especially in its intracavernous portion where it is closely related to important structures. Aneurysms in this situation may be either fusiform shape and associated with atheroma, or of saccular shape (Fig. 3.81), associated with atheroma but presumably developing upon the basis of a congenital saccular aneurysm (Barr, Blackwood and Meadows 1971). Since the ill

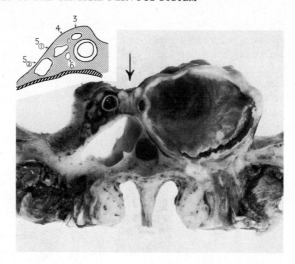

Fig. 3.81 Coronal section of the skull of a patient with an intracavernous saccular aneurysm of the right internal carotid artery. The section passes through the pituitary gland (arrow). On the left of the pituitary can be seen the normal internal carotid artery, the cavernous sinus, and the 3rd, 4th, two divisions of the 5th, and the 6th cranial nerves (see diagram). On the right of the pituitary is the large, partly thrombosed, sac of the aneurysm. The wall of the internal carotid artery is complete at this level, the neck of sac lay further forward. Blood, which had leaked from the aneurysm into the right sphenoidal air sinus, is visible below and medial to the sac of the aneurysm.

effects of both types are essentially similar they are considered together. As the aneurysm enlarges it may damage adjacent 3rd, 4th, 5th and 6th cranial nerves, elevate the dura on the lateral aspect of the cavernous sinus, enlarge the sphenoidal fissure and erode the anterior clinoid process and the lateral portions of the sella turcica (Jefferson 1937, 1938; Rischbeith and Bull 1957). It may enter the sphenoidal air sinus and bleed into it, producing epistaxis. Thrombosis and calcification occur in these aneurysms: rupture is rare.

Carotid-cavernous sinus aneurysm

As it lies within the cavernous sinus the internal carotid artery is surrounded by venous blood. Any breach in the continuity of the artery will result in an arteriovenous aneurysm. This is usually secondary to mechanical trauma, but less commonly it develops spontaneously, with an unexplained predilection for middle-aged women. Some of these spontaneous cases are secondary to rupture of a congenital saccular aneurysm of the internal carotid artery (Dandy and Follis 1941). Some are secondary to atherosclerotic degeneration of the artery. The consequence of such an arteriovenous communication, here as elsewhere, is a rise in the blood pressure in the venous tributaries of the sinus, with dilatation and tortuosity of the veins and the development of a pulsating exophthalmos. The alteration of the flow of the blood produces a murmur. Secondary enlargement of the heart was not present in Dandy's (1937) 8 cases. Histological descriptions are few, but thrombosis within the aneurysm may occur and is the probable cause of the spontaneous cure which occasionally happens.

Dissecting aneurysms

Wolman in 1959 found 14 cases in the literature and added 3 of his own. Subsequently cases have been described by Scott, Neubürger and Denst (1960), Spudis, Schary, Alexander and Martin (1962), Perier, Cauchie and Demanet (1964), Maltais and Giroux (1964) and Hayman and Anderson (1966). Females were involved only slightly more than males, ages ranged from birth to 47 years (more frequent in the 2nd and 3rd decades). Involvement of the middle cerebral artery was twice as often reported as that of the basilar artery. The plane of dissection has been subintimal, splitting the internal elastic lamina and separating it from the media. The cause of the dissection has been ascribed to trauma, syphilitic arteritis and to a congenital defect in the media.

References

Abbie, A. A.   (1933) Clinical significance of the anterior choroidal artery.   *Brain*, **56**, 233-246.

Abbie, A. A.   (1934) The morphology of the forebrain arteries, with special reference to the evolution of the basal ganglia.   *Journal of Anatomy*, **68**, 433-470.

Adams, R. D.   (1943) Occlusion of anterior inferior cerebellar artery.   *Archives of Neurology and Psychiatry (Chicago)*, **49**, 765-770.

Adams, R. D., Cammermeyer, J. & FitzGerald, P. J.   (1948) Neuropathological aspects of thrombocytic acroangiothrombosis; clinico-anatomical study of generalized platelet thrombosis.   *Journal of Neurology, Neurosurgery and Psychiatry*, **11**, 27-43.

Adams, R. D. & Michelson, J. J.   (1952) Inflammatory lesions of the blood vessels of the brain.   *Proceedings of the 1st International Congress of Neuropathology, Rome*, pp. 347-371, Rosenberg & Sellier, Torino.

Adams, R. D. & Vander Eecken, H. M.   (1953) Vascular diseases of the brain.   *Annual Review of Medicine*, **4**, 213-252.

Allison, R. S. & Morison, J. E.   (1941) Cerebral vascular lesions and tentorial pressure cone.   *Journal of Neurology and Psychiatry*, **4**, 1-10.

Anderson, T. W. & Mackay, J. S.   (1968) A critical reappraisal of the epidemiology of cerebrovascular disease.   *Lancet*, **1**, 1137-1141.

Atkinson, W. J.   (1949) Anterior inferior cerebellar artery, its variations, pontine distribution, and significance in surgery of cerebello-pontine angle tumours.   *Journal of Neurology, Neurosurgery and Psychiatry*, **12**, 137-151.

Atkinson, E. A., Fairburn, B. & Heathfield, K. W.   (1970) Intracranial venous thrombosis as complication of oral contraception.   *Lancet*, **1**, 914-918.

Bailey, O. T. & Hass, G. M.   (1937) Dural sinus thrombosis in early life; recovery from acute thrombosis of the superior longitudinal sinus and its relation to certain acquired cerebral lesions in childhood.   *Brain*, **60**, 293-314.

Barnett, H. J. M. & Hyland, H. H.   (1953) Non-infective intracranial venous thrombosis.   *Brain*, **76**, 36-49.

Barr, H. W. K., Blackwood, W. & Meadows, S. P.   (1971) Intracavernous carotid aneurysms: A clinical-pathological report.   *Brain*, **94**, 607-622.

Batson, O. V.   (1940) Function of vertebral veins and their role in spread of metastases.   *Annals of Surgery*, **112**, 138-149.

Batson, O. V.   (1957) The vertebral vein system.   *American Journal of Roentgenology*, **78**, 195-212.

Beevor, C. E.   (1908) On the distribution of the different arteries supplying the human brain.   *Philosophical Transactions of the Royal Society, Series B*, **200**, 1-55.

Bertrand, I.   (1923) *Les Processes de Désintégration Nerveuse*, Masson, Paris.

Bertrand, C.   (1952) Diffusion and absorption within brain; experimental study with prussian blue and india ink in rabbits and cats.   *Journal of Neuropathology and Experimental Neurology*, **11**, 53-61.

Biemond, A.   (1951) Thrombosis of the basilar artery and the vascularization of the brain stem.   *Brain*, **74**, 300-317.

Bigelow, N. H.   (1955) Multiple intracranial arterial aneurysms.   *Archives of Neurology and Psychiatry (Chicago)*, **73**, 76-99.

Binswanger, O.   (1894) Die Abgrenzung der allgemeinen progressiven Paralyse.   *Klinische Wochenschrift (Berlin)*, **31**, 1180-1186.

Blackwood, W. & Dott, N. M.   (1952) Personal communication to Society of British Neurological Surgeons and the Association of British Neurologists.

Bodenheimer, T. S. & Brightman, M. W.   (1968) A blood-brain barrier to peroxidase in capillaries surrounded by perivascular spaces.   *American Journal of Anatomy*, **122**, 249-267.

Brain, W. R. & Russell, D. S.   (1937) Myelomalacia following spinal anaesthesia.   *Proceedings of the Royal Society of Medicine*, **30**, 1024-1030.

Brihaye, J. & Blackwood, W.   (1957) Arteriovenous aneurysms of the cerebral hemispheres.   *Journal of Pathology and Bacteriology*, **73**, 25-31.

Bruetsch, W. L.   (1942) Rheumatic endarteritis of cerebral vessels; sequel of rheumatic fever.   *Transactions of the American Neurological Association*, **68**, 17-20.

Bruetsch, W. L.   (1949) Late nervous system sequelae of rheumatic fever in *Proceedings of the 4th International Congress on Neurology*, Paris, Vol. 3, pp. 297-301, Masson, Paris.

Byrom, F. B.   (1954) Pathogenesis of hypertensive encephalopathy and its relation to malignant phase of hypertension; experimental evidence from hypertensive rat.   *Lancet*, **2**, 201-211.

Carmichael, E. A., Dix, M. R. & Hallpike, C. S. (1956) Pathology, symptomatology and diagnosis of organic affections of eighth nerve system. *British Medical Bulletin*, **12**, 146-152.

Carmichael, R. (1950). The pathogenesis of non-inflammatory cerebral aneurysms. *Journal of Pathology and Bacteriology*, **62**, 1-19.

Carroll, J. D., Leak, D. & Lee, H. A. (1966) Cerebral thrombophlebitis in pregnancy and the puerperium. *Quarterly Journal of Medicine*, **35**, 347-368.

Charcot, J.-M. & Bouchard, C. (1868) Nouvelles recherches sur la pathogénie de l'hémorrhagie cérébrale. *Archives de Physiologie Normale et de Pathologie*, **1**, 110-127, 643-665.

Chiari, H. (1905) Ueber das Verhalten des Teilungswinkels der Carotis communis bei der Endarteriitis chronica deformans. *Verhandlungen der Deutschen Gesellschaft für Pathologie*, **9**, 326-330.

Cole, F. M. (1967) A variation in the course and distribution of the 'lateral striate artery'. *Journal of Anatomy (London)*, **102**, 125-128.

Cole, F. M. & Yates, P. O. (1967a) Intracerebral microaneurysms and small cerebrovascular lesions. *Brain*, **90**, 759-768.

Cole, F. M. & Yates, P. O. (1967b) Pseudo-aneurysms in relationship to massive cerebral haemorrhage. *Journal of Neurology Neurosurgery and Psychiatry*, **30**, 61-66.

Cole, F. M. & Yates, P. O. (1967c) The occurrence and significance of intracerebral microaneurysms. *Journal of Pathology and Bacteriology*, **93**, 393-411.

Cole, F. M. & Yates, P. O. (1968) Comparative incidence of cerebrovascular lesions in normotensive and hypertensive patients. *Neurology (Minneapolis)*, **18**, 255-259.

Cone, W. & Barrera, S. E. (1931) Brain and cerebrospinal fluid in acute aseptic cerebral embolism: experimental and pathologic study. *Archives of Neurology and Psychiatry (Chicago)*, **25**, 523-547.

Cook, T. A. & Yates, P. O. (1972) A histometric study of cerebral and renal arteries in normotensives and chronic hypertensives. *Journal of Pathology*, **108**, 129-135.

Corday, E., Rothenberg, S. F. & Putman, T. J. (1953) Cerebral vascular insufficiency; explanation of some types of localized cerebral encephalopathy. *Archives of Neurology and Psychiatry (Chicago)*, **69**, 551-570.

Costero, I. (1949) Cerebral lesions responsible for death of patients with active rheumatic fever. *Archives of Neurology and Psychiatry (Chicago)*, **62**, 48-72.

Courville, C. B. (1950) *Pathology of the Central Nervous System*, 3rd edition, Pacific Press Publishing Association, Mountain View, California.

Courville, C. B. & Friedman, A. P. (1942) Hemorrhages into the lateral basal ganglionic region. *Bulletin of the Los Angeles Neurological Society*, **7**, 137-149.

Crawford, J. V. & Russell, D. S. (1956) Cryptic arteriovenous and venous hamartomas of brain. *Journal of Neurology, Neurosurgery and Psychiatry*, **19**, 1-11.

Critchley, M. (1930) The anterior cerebral artery and its syndromes. *Brain*, **53**, 120-165.

Critchley, M. & Schuster, P. (1933) Beiträge zur Anatomie und Pathologie der Arteria cerebelli superior. *Zeitschrift für die gesamte Neurologie und Psychiatrie*, **144**, 681-741.

Crompton, M. R. (1959) The visual changes in temporal (giant-cell) arteritis. *Brain*, **82**, 377-390.

Crompton, M. R. (1964) Cerebral infarction following the rupture of cerebral berry aneurysms. *Brain*, **87**, 491-510.

Cumings, J. N. (1961) Water soluble proteins and enzymes in normal and oedematous brain tissue in *Proceedings of the IVth International Congress of Neuropathology, Munich*, Vol. 1, pp. 157-161, Thieme, Stuttgart.

Dandy, W. E. (1937) Carotid-cavernous aneurysms (pulsating exophthalmos). *Zentralblatt für Neurochirurgie*, **2**, 77.

Dandy, W. E. (1944) *Intracranial Arterial Aneurysms*, Comstock Publishing Co., Ithaca.

Dandy, W. E. & Follis, R. H. (1941) On the pathology of carotid-cavernous aneurysms (pulsating exophthalmos). *American Journal of Ophthalmology*, **24**, 365-385.

Davison, C. (1942) Progressive subcortical encephalopathy (Binswanger's disease). *Journal of Neuropathology and Experimental Neurology*, **1**, 42-48.

Davison, C., Goodhart, S. P. & Savitsky, N. (1935) Syndrome of superior cerebellar artery and its branches. *Archives of Neurology and Psychiatry (Chicago)*, **33**, 1143-1174.

Denny-Brown, D. (1960) Recurrent cerebrovascular episodes. *Archives of Neurology (Chicago)*, **2**, 194-210.

Denny-Brown, D., Horenstein, S. & Fang, H. C. H. (1956) Cerebral infarction produced by venous distention. *Journal of Neuropathology and Experimental Neurology*, **15**, 146-180.

Duguid, J. B. (1948) Thrombosis as a factor in the pathogenesis of aortic atherosclerosis. *Journal of Pathology and Bacteriology*, **60**, 57-61.

Earle, K. M., Baldwin, M. & Penfield, W. (1953) Incisural sclerosis and temporal lobe seizures produced by hippocampal herniation at birth. *Archives of Neurology and Psychiatry (Chicago)*, **69**, 27-42.

Ehlers, H. & Courville, C. B.   (1936) Thrombosis of internal cerebral veins in infancy and childhood: review of literature and report of 5 cases.   *Journal of Pediatrics*, **8**, 600-623.

Eicke, W. J.   (1957) Die Endangitis obliterans der Hirngefässe in *Handbuch der speziellen pathologischen Anatomie und Histologie* (Eds. Lubarsch, O., Henke, F. & Rössle, R.), Vol. 13, part 1, B, pp. 1536-1562, Springer Verlag, Berlin.

Ellis, A. G.   (1909) The pathogenesis of spontaneous cerebral haemorrhage.   *Proceedings of the Pathological Society of Philadelphia*, n.s. **12**, 197-235.

Farnell, F. J. & Globus, J. H.   (1932) Chronic progressive vascular subcortical encephalopathy; chronic progressive subcortical encephalitis of Binswanger.   *Archives of Neurology and Psychiatry (Chicago)*, **27**, 593-604.

Fearnsides, E. G.   (1916) Intracranial aneurysms.   *Brain*, **39**, 224-296.

Fisher, C. M.   (1957) Cerebral thromboangiitis obliterans.   *Medicine*, **36**, 169-209.

Fisher, C. H.   (1959) Observations of the fundus oculi in transient monocular blindness.   *Neurology (Minneapolis)*, **9**, 333-347.

Fisher, C. M.   (1969) The arterial lesions underlying lacunes.   *Acta neuropathologica (Berlin)*, **12**, 1-15.

Fisher, C. M., Karnes, W. E. & Kubik, C. S.   (1961) Lateral medullary infarction—the pattern of vascular occlusion.   *Journal of Neuropathology and Experimental Neurology*, **20**, 323-379.

Fisher, M.   (1951) Occlusion of internal carotid artery.   *Archives of Neurology and Psychiatry (Chicago)*, **65**, 346-377.

Fisher, M. & Adams, R. D.   (1951) Observations on brain embolism with special reference to the mechanism of hemorrhagic infarction.   *Journal of Neuropathology and Experimental Neurology*, **10**, 92-94.

Foix, C. & Hillemand, P.   (1926) Contribution à l'étude des ramolissements protubérantiels.   *Revue de Médecine*, **43**, 287-305.

Foix, C., Hillemand, P. & Schalit, I.   (1925) Sur le syndrome latéral du bulbe et l'irrigation du bulbe supérieur.   *Revue Neurologique*, **1**, 160-179.

Foix, C. & Levy, M.   (1927) Les ramolissements sylviens.   Syndromes des lésions en foyer du territoire de l'artère sylvienne et de ses branches.   *Revue Neurologique*, **2**, 1-51.

Foix, C. & Masson, A.   (1923) Le syndrome de l'artère cérébrale postérieure.   *Presse Médicale*, **31**, 361-365.

Foley, J.   (1955) Benign forms of intracranial hypertension—'toxic' and 'otitic' hydrocephalus.   *Brain*, **78**, 1-41.

Forbus, W. D.   (1930) On the origin of miliary aneurysms of the superficial cerebral arteries.   *Bulletin of the Johns Hopkins Hospital*, **47**, 239-284.

Foster, D. B. & Malamud, N.   (1941) Periarteritis nodosa; clinico-pathologic report with special reference to central nervous system; preliminary report.   *University Hospital Bulletin, Ann Arbor*, **7**, 102-104.

Freeman, W. & Jaffe, D.   (1941) Occlusion of superior cerebellar artery; report on case with necropsy.   *Archives of Neurology and Psychiatry (Chicago)*, **46**, 115-126.

Frøvig, A. G.   (1946) Bilateral obliteration of the common carotid artery.   *Acta Psychiatrica et Neurologica, Copenhagen, Suppl.* 39.

Fullerton, H. W.   (1955) The role of diet in the pathogenesis of coronary artery disease.   *Proceedings of the Royal Society of Medicine*, **48**, 664-667.

Gillilan, Lois A.   (1969) The arterial blood supply of the human spinal cord.   *Journal of Neuropathology and Experimental Neurology*, **28**, 295-307.

von Glahn, W. C. & Pappenheimer, A. M.   (1926) Specific lesions of peripheral blood vessels in rheumatism.   *American Journal of Pathology*, **2**, 235-249.

Globus, J. H.   (1938) Massive cerebral haemorrhage in *The Circulation of the Brain and Spinal Cord. Research Publications, Association for Research in Nervous and Mental Diseases*, **18**, 438-470.

Glynn, L. E.   (1940) Medial defects in the circle of Willis and their relation to aneurysm formation.   *Journal of Pathology and Bacteriology*, **51**, 213-222.

Goodhart, S. P. & Davison, C.   (1936) Syndrome of posterior inferior and anterior inferior cerebellar arteries and their branches.   *Archives of Neurology and Psychiatry (Chicago)*, **35**, 501-524.

Gowers, W. R.   (1893) *Diseases of the Nervous System*, 2nd edition, Vol. 2, pp. 436-449, Churchill, London.

Green, F. H. K.   (1930) Miliary aneurysms in the brain.   *Journal of Pathology and Bacteriology*, **33**, 71-77.

Greenfield, J. G.   (1939) Histology of cerebral oedema associated with intracranial tumours (with special reference to changes in nerve fibres of centrum ovale).   *Brain*, **62**, 129-152.

Greenfield, J. G., Rickards, A. G. & Manning, G. B.   (1955) Pathology of paraplegia occurring as delayed sequela of spinal anaesthesia, with special reference to vascular changes.   *Journal of Pathology and Bacteriology*, **69**, 97-107.

Guillain, G., Bertrand, I. & Peron, N.   (1928) Le syndrome de l'artère cérébelleuse supérieure.   *Revue Neuro-logique*, **2**, 835-843.

Hachinsky, V. C., Lassen, N. A. & Marshall, J.   (1974) Multi-infarct dementia.   *Lancet*, **2**, 207-210.

Hamilton, C. E. & Rothstein, E.   (1935) Air embolism.   *Journal of the American Medical Association*, **104**, 2226-2230.

Harrison, C. V.   (1948) Giant-cell or temporal arteritis: a review.   *Journal of Clinical Pathology*, **1**, 197-211.

Hayman, J. A. & Anderson, R. M.   (1966) Dissecting aneurysm of the basilar artery.   *Medical Journal of Australia*, **2**, 360-361.

Haymaker, W.   (1957) Decompression sickness in *Handbuch der speziellen pathologischen Anatomie und Histologie* (Eds. Lubarsch, O., Henke, F. & Rössle, R.), Vol. 13, part 1, B, pp. 1600-1672, Springer Verlag, Berlin.

Heptinstall, R. H., Porter, K. A. & Barkley, H.   (1954) Giant-cell (temporal) arteritis.   *Journal of Pathology and Bacteriology*, **67**, 507-519.

Hiller, F.   (1936) Die Luft- und Fettembolie in Bumke und Foerster *Handbuch der Neurologie*, Vol. 11, pp. 328-331, Springer Verlag, Berlin.

Hills, C. P.   (1964) Ultrastructural changes in the capillary bed of the rat cerebral cortex in anoxic-ischemic brain lesions.   *American Journal of Pathology*, **44**, 531-551.

Holmes, G.   (1934) Representation of the mesial sectors of retinae in calcarine cortex.   *Jahrbuch für Psychiatrie und Neurologie*, **51**, 39-48.

Hughes, W.   (1965) Origin of lacunes.   *Lancet*, **2**, 19-21.

Hughes, J. T. & Brownell, Betty.   (1966) Granulomatous giant cells angiitis of the central nervous system.   *Neurology*, **16**, 293-298.

Hughes, J. T. & Brownell, B.   (1968) Traumatic thrombosis of the internal carotid artery in the neck.   *Journal of Neurology, Neurosurgery and Psychiatry*, **31**, 307-314.

Hultquist, G. T.   (1942) *Über Thrombose und Embolie der Arteria Carotidis und hierbei vorkommende Gehirn-veränderungen*, Fischer, Jena, Stockholm.

Hunt, J. R.   (1914) The role of the carotid arteries, in the causation of the vascular lesions of the brain, with remarks on certain special features of the symptomatology.   *American Journal of Medical Science*, **147**, 704-713.

Hurst, E. W.   (1955) Adhesive arachnoiditis and vascular blockage caused by detergents and other chemical irritants: experimental study.   *Journal of Pathology and Bacteriology*, **70**, 167-178.

Hutchinson, E. C. & Yates, P. O.   (1956) The cervical portion of the vertebral artery: a clinico-pathological study.   *Brain*, **79**, 319-331.

Hutchinson, E. C. & Yates, P. O.   (1957) Carotico-vertebral stenosis.   *Lancet*, **1**, 2-8.

Hutchinson, E. C. & Yates, P. O.   (1961) Cerebral infarction: the role of stenosis of the extracranial cerebral arteries.   *Special Report Series of the Medical Research Council*, London, No. **300**, H.M.S.O., London.

Hyland, H. H.   (1950) Prognosis in spontaneous subarachnoid hemorrhage.   *Archives of Neurology and Psychiatry (Chicago)*, **63**, 61-78.

Jefferson, G.   (1937) Compression of the chiasma, optic nerves, and optic tracts by intracranial aneurysms.   *Brain*, **60**, 444-497.

Jefferson, G.   (1938) On the saccular aneurysms of the internal carotid artery in the cavernous sinus.   *British Journal of Surgery*, **26**, 267-302.

Johnson, R. T. & Yates, P. O.   (1956) Brain stem haemorrhages in expanding supratentorial conditions.   *Acta radiologica (Stockholm)*, **46**, 250-256.

Jones, E.   (1910) The question of the side affected in hemiplegia and in arterial lesions of the brain.   *Quarterly Journal of Medicine*, **3**, 233-250.

Kernohan, J. W.   (1942) Discussion on rheumatic endarteritis of cerebral vessels: sequel of rheumatic fever (paper by W. L. Bruetsch).   *Transactions of the American Neurological Association*, **68**, 18.

Kernohan, J. W. & Woltman, H. W.   (1929) Incisura of the crus due to contralateral brain tumour.   *Archives of Neurology and Psychiatry (Chicago)*, **21**, 274-287.

Kiloh, L. G.   (1953) Syndromes of arteries of brain and spinal cord.   *Postgraduate Medical Journal*, **29**, 65-74 and 119-128.

Klatzo, I., Piraux, A. & Laskowski, E. J.   (1958) The relationships between edema, blood-brain barrier and tissue elements in a local brain injury.   *Journal of Neuropathology and Experimental Neurology*, **17**, 548-564.

Kubik, C. S. & Adams, R. D.   (1946) Occlusion of the basilar artery—a clinical and pathological study.   *Brain*, **69**, 73-121.

Kurtzke, J. F.   (1969) *Epidemiology of Cerebrovascular Disease*, Springer Verlag, Berlin.

Lassen, N. A. (1966) The luxury perfusion syndrome and its possible relation to acute metabolic acidosis localised within the brain. *Lancet*, **2**, 1113-1115.

Lassen, N. A. & Agnoli, A. (1972) The upper limit of autoregulation of cerebral blood flow—on the pathogenesis of hypertensive encephalopathy. *Scandinavian Journal of Clinical and Laboratory Investigation*, **30**, 113-115.

Levine, B., Cheskin, L. J. & Applebaum, I. L. (1949) Clinical syndrome of occlusion of posterior inferior cerebellar artery; report of 3 cases. *Archives of Internal Medicine*, **84**, 431-439.

Lhermitte, J. & Barrelet. (1934) Embolie gazeuse cérébrale d'origine périphérique. Étude anatomique. *Revue Neurologique*, **2**, 851-857.

Lindenberg, R. & Spatz, H. (1939) Über die Thromboendarteriitis obliterans der Hirngefässe (cerebrale Form der v. Winiwarter-Buergerschen Krankheit). *Virchows Archiv für pathologische Anatomie und Physiologie*, **305**, 531-557.

Lowe, R. D. (1962) Adaptation of the circle of Willis to occlusion of the carotid or vertebral artery: its implication in caroticovertebral stenosis. *Lancet*, **1**, 395-398.

McBrien, D. J., Bradley, R. D. & Ashton, N. (1963) The nature of retinal emboli in stenosis of the internal carotid artery. *Lancet*, **1**, 697-699.

McCormick, H. M. & Neubürger, K. T. (1958) Giant-cell arteritis involving small meningeal and intracerebral vessels. *Journal of Neuropathology and Experimental Neurology*, **17**, 471-478.

McDonald, W. Ian. (1967) Recurrent cholestrol embolism as a cause of fluctuating cerebral symptoms. *Journal of Neurology, Neurosurgery and Psychiatry*, **30**, 489-496.

Magee, P. M., Stoner, H. B. & Barnes, J. M. (1957) The experimental production of oedema in the central nervous system of the rat by triethyltin compounds. *Journal of Pathology and Bacteriology*, **73**, 107-124.

Maltais, R. F. & Giroux, J. C. (1964) Dissecting aneurysm of middle cerebral artery. *Journal of Neurosurgery*, **21**, 413-415.

Martin, J. P. (1941) Thrombosis in superior longitudinal sinus following childbirth. *British Medical Journal*, **2**, 537-540.

Meadows, S. P. (1951) In *Modern Trends in Neurology* (Ed. Feiling, A.), pp. 391-465, Butterworth, London.

Merritt, H. & Finland, M. (1930) Vascular lesions of hindbrain (lateral medullary syndrome). *Brain*, **53**, 290-305.

Meyer, J. S., Fang, H. C. & Denny-Brown, D. (1954) Polarographic study of cerebral collateral circulation. *Archives of Neurology and Psychiatry (Chicago)*, **72**, 296-312.

Miller, H. G. & Daley, R. (1946). Clinical aspects of polyarteritis nodosa. *Quarterly Journal of Medicine*, **15**, 255-283.

Moore, M. T. & Stern, K. (1938) Vascular lesions in the brainstem and occipital lobe occurring in association with brain tumours. *Brain*, **61**, 70-98.

Moschowitz, E. (1925) An acute febrile pleiochromic anemia with hyaline thrombosis of the terminal arterioles and capillaries. *Archives of Internal Medicine*, **36**, 89-93.

Nasu, T. (1963) Pathology of pulseless disease. *Angiology*, **14**, 225-242.

Neubürger, K. T. (1925) Ueber cerebrale Fett und Luftembolie. *Zeitschrift für die gesamte Neurologie und Psychiatrie*, **95**, 278-318.

Nurick, S., Blackwood, W. & Mair, W. G. P. (1972) Giant celled granulomatous angiitis of the central nervous system. *Brain*, **95**, 133-142.

Oppenheimer, B. S. & Fishberg, A. M. (1928) Hypertensive encephalopathy. *Archives of Internal Medicine*, **41**, 264-278.

Padget, D. H. (1944) The circle of Willis, its embryology and anatomy in *Intracranial Arterial Aneurysms* (Ed. Dandy, W. E.), pp. 67-90, Comstock Publishing Co., Ithaca, New York.

Pentschew, A. (1933) Die granuläre Atrophie der Grosshirnrinde. *Archiv für Psychiatrie*, **101**, 80-136.

Perier, O., Cauchie, Ch. & Demanet, J. C. (1964) Haematome intramural par dissection pariétale (anéurysme disséquant) du tronc basilaire. *Acta neurologica Belgica*, **64**, 1064-1074.

Plass, E. D. & Matthew, C. W. (1926) Plasma protein fractions in normal pregnancy, labor, and puerperium. *American Journal of Obstetrics and Gynecology*, **12**, 346-358.

Pratt-Thomas, H. R. & Berger, K. E. (1947) Cerebellar and spinal injuries after chiropractic manipulation. *Journal of the American Medical Association*, **133**, 600-603.

Reese, T. S. & Karnovsky, M. J. (1967) Fine structural localization of a blood-brain barrier to exogenous peroxidase. *Journal of Cell Biology*, **34**, 207-217.

Reivich, M., Holling, H. E., Roberts, B. & Toole, J. F. (1961) Reversal of blood flow through the vertebral artery and its effect on cerebral circulation. *New England Journal of Medicine*, **265**, 878-885.

Rich, A. R. & Gregory, J. E.   (1943) Experimental demonstration that periarteritis nodosa is manifestation of hypersensitivity. *Bulletin of the Johns Hopkins Hospital*, **72**, 65-88.

Richardson, J. C. & Hyland, H. H.   (1941) Intracranial aneurysms. *Medicine*, **20**, 1-83.

Riehl, J. L.   (1963) The idiopathic arteritis of Takayasu. *Neurology*, **13**, 873-884.

Riggs, H. E. & Rupp, C.   (1963) Variation in the form of circle of Willis. *Archives of Neurology* (*Chicago*), **8**, 8-14.

Rischbieth, R. H. & Bull, J. W.   (1958) The significance of enlargement of the superior orbital (sphenoidal) fissure. *British Journal of Radiology*, **31**, 125-135.

Rosenberg, E. F.   (1940) Brain in malignant hypertension; clinicopathologic study. *Archives of Internal Medicine*, **65**, 545-586.

Russell, C. K.   (1931) Syndrome of brachium conjunctivum and tractus spinothalamicus. *Archives of Neurology and Psychiatry* (*Chicago*), **25**, 1003-1010.

Russell, D. S.   (1954) In discussion: The pathology of spontaneous intracranial haemorrhage. *Proceedings of the Royal Society of Medicine*, **47**, 689-704.

Russell, W. R.   (1961) Observations on the retinal blood vessels in monocular blindness. *Lancet*, **2**, 1422-1428.

Russell, W. R.   (1963) Observations on intracerebral aneurysms. *Brain*, **86**, 425-442.

von Santha, K.   (1932) Gefässveränderungen im Zentralnervensystem bei Chorea rheumatica. *Virchows Archiv für pathologische Anatomie und Physiologie*, **287**, 405-420.

Scheinker, I. M.   (1945) Transtentorial herniation of the brain stem. *Archives of Neurology and Psychiatry* (*Chicago*), **53**, 289-298.

Schneck, S. A. & Kricheff, I. I.   (1964) Intracranial aneurysm rupture, vasospasm, and infarction. *Archives of Neurology*, **11**, 668-680.

Schwartz, P.   (1961) *Cerebral Apoplexy: Types, Causes and Pathogenesis*, Charles C. Thomas, Springfield, Ill.

Scott, G. E., Neubürger, K. T. & Denst, J.   (1960) Dissecting aneurysms of intracranial arteries. *Neurology*, **10**, 22-27.

Smyth, G. E.   (1939) Systemization and central connections of spinal tract and nucleus of trigeminal nerve; clinical and pathological study. *Brain*, **62**, 41-87.

Smyth, G. E. & Henderson, W. R.   (1938) Observations on cerebrospinal fluid pressure on simultaneous ventricular and lumbar punctures. *Journal of Neurology, Neurosurgery and Psychiatry*, **1**, 226-238.

Spatz, H.   (1935) Über die Beteiligung des Gehirns bei der v. Winiwarter-Buergerschen Krankheit. *Deutsche Zeitschrift für Nervenheilkunde*, **136**, 86-132.

Spillane, J. D.   (1937) Posterior inferior cerebellar artery thrombosis. *Bulletin of the Neurological Institute, New York*, **6**, 529-539.

Spudis, E. V., Schary, J. M., Alexander, E. & Martin, J.   (1962) Dissecting aneurysms in the neck and head. *Neurology*, **12**, 867-875.

Stengel, A. & Wolferth, C. C.   (1923) Mycotic (bacterial) aneurysms of intravascular origin. *Archives of Internal Medicine*, **31**, 527-554.

Stewart-Wallace, A. M.   (1939) Biochemical study of cerebral tissue, and of changes in cerebral oedema. *Brain*, **62**, 426-438.

Stopford, J. S. B.   (1915) The arteries of the pons and medulla oblongata. *Journal of Anatomy and Physiology*, **50**, 131-164 and 255-280.

Stopford, J. S. B.   (1917) The arteries of the pons and medulla oblongata. Part III, Clinical applications of Part I & II. *Journal of Anatomy and Physiology*, **51**, 250-277.

Strauss, H.   (1933) Zur Symptomatologie der Ventrikelblutungen. *Monatschrift für Psychiatrie und Neurologie*, **85**, 1-19.

Stuart, A. E. & MacGregor-Robertson, G.   (1956) Thrombotic thrombocytopenic purpura; hyperergic micro-angiopathy. *Lancet*, **1**, 475-479.

Suh, T. H. & Alexander, L.   (1939) Vascular system of human spinal cord. *Archives of Neurology and Psychiatry* (*Chicago*), **41**, 659-677.

Symmers, W. St. C.   (1952) Thrombotic microangiopathic haemolytic anaemia (thrombotic microangiopathy). *British Medical Journal*, **2**, 897-903.

Symmers, W. St. C.   (1956) Thrombotic microangiopathy (thrombotic thrombocytopenic purpura) associated with acute haemorrhagic leucoencephalitis and sensitivity to oxophenarsine. *Brain*, **79**, 511-521.

Symonds, C.   (1955) Circle of Willis (Harveian oration). *British Medical Journal*, **1**, 119-124.

Symonds, C.   (1956) Otitic hydrocephalus. *Neurology*, **6**, 681-685.

Taylor, J. E. D.   (1952) Post-mortem diagnosis of air embolism by radiography. *British Medical Journal*, **1**, 890-893.

Tichy, F.   (1949) Syndromes of cerebral arteries. *Archives of Pathology*, **48**, 475-488.

Timperley, W. R., Preston, F. E. & Ward, J. D.   (1974) Cerebral intravascular coagulation in diabetic keto-acidosis. *Lancet*, **1**, 952-956.

Torack, R. M., Terry, R. D. & Zimmerman, H. M.   (1959) The fine structure of cerebral fluid accumulation. I. Swelling secondary to cold injury. *American Journal of Pathology*, **35**, 1135-1147.

Torack, R. M., Terry, R. D. & Zimmerman, H. M.   (1960) The fine structure of cerebral fluid accumulation. II. Swelling produced by triethyl tin poisoning and its comparison with that in the human brain. *American Journal of Pathology*, **36**, 273-287.

Torvik, A. & Jörgensen, L.   (1964) Thrombotic and embolic occlusions of the carotid arteries in an autopsy material, Part I (prevalence, location and associated diseases). *Journal of the Neurological Sciences*, **1**, 24-39.

Turnbull, H. M.   (1918) Intracranial aneurysms. *Brain*, **41**, 50-56.

Vander Eecken, H. M. & Adams, R. D.   (1953) The anatomy and functional significance of the meningeal arterial anastomoses of the human brain. *Journal of Neuropathology and Experimental Neurology*, **12**, 132-157.

Villaret, M. & Cachera, R.   (1939) *Les embolies cérébrales*, Masson, Paris.

Walton, J. N.   (1956) *Subarachnoid Hemorrhage*, Livingstone, Edinburgh.

Weisman, A. D.   (1944) Cavernous-sinus thrombophlebitis. *New England Journal of Medicine*, **231**, 118-122.

Williams, D. J.   (1936) The origin of the posterior cerebral artery. *Brain*, **59**, 175-180.

Winkelman, N. W.   (1942) Cerebral fat embolism; clinico-pathologic study of 2 cases. *Archives of Neurology and Psychiatry (Chicago)*, **47**, 57-76.

Winkelman, N. W. & Eckel, J. L.   (1929) Endarteritis of small cortical vessels in severe infections and toxemias. *Archives of Neurology and Psychiatry (Chicago)*, **21**, 863-875.

Winkelman, N. W. & Eckel, J. L.   (1932) The brain in acute rheumatic fever. *Archives of Neurology and Psychiatry (Chicago)*, **28**, 844-870.

Wolman, L.   (1953) Ischaemic lesions in the brainstem associated with raised supratentorial pressure. *Brain*, **76**, 364-377.

Wolman, L.   (1959) Cerebral dissecting aneurysms. *Brain*, **82**, 276-291.

Wright, H. P.   (1942) Changes in adhesiveness of blood platelets following parturition and surgical operations. *Journal of Pathology and Bacteriology*, **54**, 461-468.

Yates, P. O.   (1959) Birth trauma in the vertebral arteries. *Archives of Disease in Childhood*, **34**, 436-441.

Yates, P. O.   (1964) A change in the pattern of cerebrovascular disease. *Lancet*, **1**, 65-69.

Yates, P. O.   (1966) The changing pattern of cerebrovascular disease in the United Kingdom in *Cerebral Vascular Diseases* (Eds. Millikan, C. H., Siekert, R. G. & Whisnant, J. P.), pp. 67-73, Grune & Stratton, New York.

Yates, P. O.   (1973) Effects of vascular pathology on the cerebral circulation. *Verhandlung der Deutschen, Gesellschaft für Kreislaufforschung*, **39**, 29-35.

4

Intoxications, Poisons and Related Metabolic Disorders

Revised by W. Thomas Smith

Drugs of addiction

Ethyl alcohol

Acute alcoholic intoxication seldom leads to death and necropsy reports are rare. Cerebral congestion, oedema and diffuse petechial haemorrhages have been described (Courville and Myers 1954) and when cardiovascular degeneration is present, in particular cerebral arteriosclerosis with hypertension, a toxic dose of alcohol may lead to massive haemorrhage or infarction (Meyer 1963).

According to McIlwain (1966), severe intoxication is accompanied by decreased cerebral blood flow and decreased respiration. The oxidation of ethanol proceeds through acetaldehyde, the blood level of which is normally low but is elevated following ingestion of alcohol. If acetaldehyde is infused and maintained at a certain level, a nausea akin to alcoholic hangover is experienced, which passes off as acetaldehyde is further oxidized. The depressant action of alcohol is, however, due not to these oxidation products but to the presence of the actual compound in cerebral tissue, as also occurs with drugs such as anaesthetics and hypnotics. Acetaldehyde, like other toxic substances such as the heavy metals (see p. 151), probably combines with lipoic acid which is then no longer available for the oxidation of pyruvates, and this, according to Sinclair (1956), may constitute a pathogenic mechanism in some cases of alcoholic polyneuritis.

Chronic alcoholic intoxication. It is said that repetition of acute intoxication can, over many years, lead to irreversible cerebral changes such as thickening of the meninges and a moderate degree of atrophy, which may be general or most marked in the frontal, central and parietal cortex and white matter, and may be accompanied by moderate enlargement of the ventricles. In such cases the cerebral cortex shows a variety of neuronal changes (in particular, pigmentary degeneration), and diffuse loss of the supraradiary and tangential myelinated fibres, with or without increase of fibrous glia. These findings, described by earlier workers (Mott 1910 and others), have been largely confirmed and critically discussed by Courville (1955) and by Lynch (1960). Astrocytic proliferation with some neuronal degeneration, most marked in the third layer of the frontal cortex, was described by Morel (1939) in patients who suffered repeated attacks of delirium tremens followed by memory disturbances, tremor and impairment of speech. A mental syndrome reminiscent of general paresis (alcoholic pseudoparesis) has been described and delusions, particularly of the auditory type, can accompany the general deterioration shown by many chronic alcoholics.

Degeneration may be more marked in the cerebellum than in the cerebrum, as Jakob (1912) first noted. Stender and Lüthy (1931) described a late form of atrophy of the cerebellar cortex in chronic alcoholism. Lhermitte (1935) also emphasized the importance of chronic alcoholism as a cause of cortical cerebellar degeneration and with de Ajuriaguerra and Garnier (1938) experimented on rabbits, giving them continuous toxic doses of absinthe; chromatolysis of posterior root ganglia neurons, Purkinje cells and cortical neurons occurred, but only in animals in which an additional nutritional deficiency was present. Neubürger (1957) found that degeneration of the cerebellar granular layer was a relatively common lesion in his investigation of 42 cases of alcoholism.

The whole question of alcoholic cerebellar degeneration was fully reviewed by Victor, Adams and Mancall (1959) and Allsop and Turner (1966). Lesions are predominant in the anterior–superior vermis and to a lesser degree in the anterior lobe of the cerebellar hemispheres; the earliest change probably affects the granular layer and is followed by the Purkinje-cell degeneration and astrocytic proliferation; the lesions are essentially focal but can coalesce. Degeneration of the inferior olives appears to be secondary. Alcoholic cerebellar degeneration is now accepted as a distinct entity and not as late cortical atrophy occurring by chance in alcoholics. There is no family history of cerebellar disease. Abstention from alcohol can lead to clinical improvement.

It is often difficult to exclude the effects of complicating factors in chronic alcoholism; cerebral arteriosclerosis or senile cerebral degeneration seem to play a part in some cases and associated cirrhosis of the liver with hepatic failure may be a factor in others. The effect of nutritional deficiencies that result from inadequate or unbalanced diet or from chronic gastritis or other gastrointestinal disturbances are relevant and therefore the pathology of chronic alcoholism is related to that of deficiency states (see Chapter 5). The changes of pellagra may predominate, particularly central chromatolysis of neurons and, more rarely, degeneration of posterior and lateral columns of the spinal cord. In other cases the Wernicke syndrome may be more in evidence (Victor and Adams 1961), presenting clinically with ophthalmoplegia, nystagmus, ataxia and Korsakoff's psychosis. Peripheral neuropathies can accompany either of these syndromes or occur alone; degeneration of the optic nerves has been reported (Victor, Mancall and Dreyfus 1960) and in chronic malnourished alcoholics, deficiency of vitamin B_{12} and subacute combined degeneration of the cord has been described. The essential lesion in alcoholic peripheral neuropathy is axonal (Wallerian) degeneration in acute cases; regeneration occurs in chronic cases given a good diet (Walsh and McCleod 1970).

Marchiafava-Bignami disease
Considerable interest was aroused by the description of degeneration of the corpus callosum by Marchiafava and Bignami (1903). Since then eighty-eight cases have been reported according to the detailed review by Ironside, Bosanquet and McMenemey (1961). The earlier cases were almost all Italian by birth; more recently cases have been reported from the Americas, and from other parts of Europe including France, Switzerland and Spain. The racial and national distribution has been instructively outlined by Ironside et al. Although there is no racial preclusion, the high incidence in Latins, and especially Italians, is striking; the disease is rare in North America and also in Britain, where only two cases seem to have been described, one by McLardy (1951) and the other by Ironside et al.; both were Englishmen without traceable Latin or other foreign ancestry. There has been no report of cases from Sweden or Japan.

Almost all reported patients were chronic alcoholics, many of whom were addicted to Italian crude wine and suffered from malnutrition. There are, however, notable exceptions: McLardy's patient had no taste for Italian wine and had not suffered from nutritional deficiency; Ironside's patient, though showing signs of malnutrition, was a heavy drinker of beer and stout. Earlier reports suggested that the disease was confined to males, but subsequently the disease has occurred in females.

The main change is a degeneration of the central fibres of the corpus callosum. In the cases of King and Meehan (1936) and Ironside et al., the well-defined lesion had a closer resemblance to ischaemic softening than to any other pathological process. In many though not all cases, the callosal degeneration is accompanied by degeneration of other symmetrical pathways such as the anterior commissure and the middle cerebellar peduncles (Figs. 4.1 and 4.2); the centrum ovale, the optic chiasma and the frontal and parietal gyri may also be involved (Victor and Adams 1961). Within the lesions demyelination is a consistent feature; the axis cylinders are affected in some cases but are preserved in others. Glial proliferation is not usually marked and myelin breakdown products are often inconspicuous. A striking feature is proliferation and fibrous sclerosis of blood vessels within the lesions.

Jéquier and Wildi (1955) described two cases showing a combination of Marchiafava–Bignami-like changes with the so-called cortical laminar astrocytosis of Morel; among less consistent findings they also noted glial proliferation in the mamillary bodies of one case and slight degeneration of the optic tracts. In the case of Ironside et al., loss of cortical neurons with glial reaction

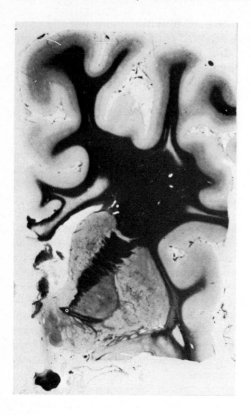

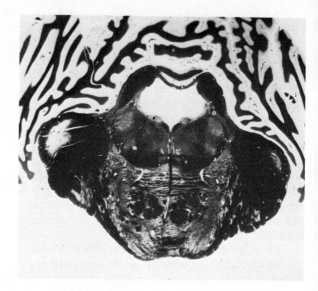

Fig. 4.1 (*left*) Marchiafava–Bignami disease (McLardy's case); degeneration of the central fibres in corpus callosum and anterior commissure, and digital white matter. Heidenhain. × 1·5

Fig. 4.2 (*above*)   McLardy's case; degeneration of middle cerebellar peduncle. Heidenhain. × 2·5

was also recorded and McLardy noted demyelination in the most posterior portion of the optic chiasma. Cirrhosis of the liver is not a constant feature.

The pathogenesis is not known. In many cases there is a history of addiction to Italian crude red wine, associated with malnutrition, which suggests a nutritional deficiency, but, as has been indicated, such a situation does not always apply. Nor is there evidence for vitamin B_1 deficiency, as suggested by Lolli (1941) and Bohrod (1942). Intoxication by a substance so far not identified, which may be present only in Italian red wine, has also been suggested, and it may be relevant that lesions of the white matter, including the corpus callosum and anterior commissure, have been repeatedly described following cyanide intoxication, and less often in carbon monoxide poisoning (p. 68), particularly in lower mammals. Jéquier and Wildi suggested that the development of the lesions may be related to oedema.

Central pontine myelinolysis was described by Adams, Victor and Mancall (1959) in four patients, three of whom were chronic alcoholics

and all had serious malnutrition. The lesion was situated in the centre of the base of the pons and was characterized by demyelination with relative preservation of axons. Oligodendrocytes were grossly reduced in number. Wernicke's syndrome was present in one case. There was no evidence of disseminated sclerosis. Adams *et al.* were cautious regarding the aetiology of the syndrome, but noted the histological resemblance to Marchiafava-Bignami disease. Paguirigan and Lepken (1969) found 69 previous cases and added one more. Conger, McIntyre and Jacoby (1969) noted 'less than' 80 cases in the literature and that alcoholism or malnutrition were not present in all; dehydration, electrolyte disturbances, uraemia and thrombosis of the vein of Galen were possible contributory factors and in their own case there was profound hyponatraemia and inappropriate secretion of antidiuretic hormone. Shurtliff, Ajax, Englert and D'Agostino (1966) described four cases in alcoholics, in all of which hepatic necrosis may have been a contributory factor. Schneck (1966) noted the association of pontine myelinolysis with pontine neuroaxonal dystrophy in three patients with renal transplants:

the significance of terminal infection, malnutrition and uraemia and also of immunosuppression therapy were considered.

Methyl alcohol (methanol)

Methyl alcohol is the most important of the remaining alcohols and its consumption has given rise to serious sociomedical problems in periods of prohibition or war and in poverty-stricken communities. One of the earlier clinical reports added almost 200 personal cases studied in the USA to the 54 fatal or amaurotic cases which had previously been described in the literature (Wood and Buller 1904). Similar descriptions based on smaller numbers also appeared at about the same time in Russia, Hungary and Germany.

The clinical picture of acute methanol poisoning has been detailed by Bennett, Cary, Mitchell and Cooper (1953), who investigated an 'epidemic' of intoxication in 323 patients. After a latent period, lasting on an average 24 hours, patients complained of varying combinations of symptoms that included headache, dizziness, anorexia, nausea, weakness and amblyopia progressing to total blindness. The pupils were dilated and reacted sluggishly; sometimes there was hyperaemia of the optic disc with retinal oedema. In severe cases acidosis was invariably present. The marked variation in the length of the latent period is probably due to the simultaneous or subsequent ingestion of ethyl alcohol, which usually occurs (Røe 1946); this prevents or delays the oxidation of the methanol to formaldehyde and formic acid, which cause both the acidosis and the other toxic effects of this compound. These acidic metabolites inhibit cellular oxidative processes, probably by combining with iron in cytochrome oxydases. In fatal cases there is usually coma and respiratory paralysis.

In most acute cases necropsy reveals severe congestion and oedema of all organs, including the brain, which also shows widespread petechial haemorrhages; these are particularly numerous in the neighbourhood of the 3rd ventricle, the aqueduct and beneath the floor of the 4th ventricle (Meyer 1963). Ischaemic necrosis of all three layers of the cerebellar cortex has been reported and bilateral necrosis of the putamen has been regarded as a selective toxic effect of methyl alcohol.

Degeneration of the ganglion cells in the retina and of optic nerve fibres are frequent and characteristic findings in human cases and in experimental animals (Meyer 1963). Histologically the ganglion cells show central chromatolysis and the degeneration extends into the inner and outer granular layers. The axis cylinders in the optic nerve and its papilla are separated by exudate and show irregular swellings. The changes in the retinal cells and in the optic nerve fibres are probably related.

Morphine and related drugs

In large doses, *morphine* has a depressant action upon respiratory centres in the medulla; acute intoxication may thus lead to respiratory failure, with resultant anoxic and cardiovascular neurological complications.

In chronic poisoning the lesions in the central nervous system are more difficult to interpret. At concentrations comparable to those causing therapeutic analgesia, McIlwain considered morphine to have no adverse effect on the metabolism of cerebral tissue; in such doses it is, however, a powerful inhibitor of cholinesterase and this may explain at least part of its side-effects. There is no doubt that morphine addiction involves complex pharmacological and endocrinological mechanisms which are not yet fully understood.

There have been few histological studies on human cases of addiction or on experimental animals. Acute swelling of oligodendrocytes, fatty degeneration of neurons in the cerebral cortex and Ammon's horn and changes attributable to circulatory disturbances have been noted. Nutritional deficiency, cachexia and the effect of convulsions may sometimes be contributory factors. Experimental studies have not shown specific changes (see Meyer 1963).

Even less is known about the histological effects of *cocaine* intoxication. Like morphine, cocaine depresses the respiratory and circulatory centres in the medulla. In acute poisoning, cerebral congestion and oedema have been described. After chronic intoxication, fatty degeneration and vacuolar shrinkage of neurons have been found in the brains of man and experimental animals.

The changes in chronic *barbiturate* addiction are described on pp. 168 and 222.

Intoxication by heavy metals and related substances

Metals as a class have, according to Jetter (1966), a diffuse systemic toxicity and are referred to as protoplasmic poisons. Their toxic effects are often most severe at sites of entry and elimination, particularly skin, lung, gastrointestinal tract and kidney; the central and peripheral nervous systems are also particularly vulnerable. Many metals act as enzyme inhibitors, and block metabolic processes by combining with sulphydryl groups of enzyme proteins. This effect seems to be confirmed by the therapeutic effect of 2,3-dimercapto-propanol (BAL, British Antilewisite). Peters (1948) and Thompson (1948) have suggested that metals mainly inhibit the pyruvate–oxydase system, the biochemical lesion thus resembling that which occurs in vitamin B_1 deficiency, although the coenzyme cocarboxylase seems not to be involved directly. These complex biochemical relations will be discussed in greater detail in Chapter 5.

From the neuropathological point of view, arsenic, lead, mercury, manganese, thallium, phosphorus and related compounds are the most important toxic substances in this category that need consideration.

Arsenic

Arsenic is widely used in industry. It is a constituent of many weed and vermin killers, and it was formerly used in paints and, as liquor arsenicalis, in the treatment of many diseases. Organic arsenicals (arsphenamines) used to treat syphilis can lead to neurological complications and though there have been many reports of such cases, organo-arsenical neurotoxicity has become uncommon since the introduction of penicillin.

During the second World War arsenical compounds were prepared as war gases. Chloro-phenyldichlorarsine is the so-called lewisite.

There seem to be no qualitative differences between poisoning by inorganic and organic arsenical preparations. In *acute* intoxications, abdominal discomfort and often intense pain, vomiting, diarrhoea and terminal circulatory collapse dominate the picture. Involvement of the brain is indicated by headache, confusion or coma, epileptic convulsions and evidence of raised intracranial pressure. Specific features of chronic poisoning are cutaneous pigmentation, hyperkeratosis, gastrointestinal ulceration and peripheral neuropathies. Chronic gastrointestinal lesions may result in nutritional deficiency and so lead to difficulties in diagnosis, resembling pure vitamin B deficiency. Hepatic necrosis and portal-type cirrhosis have been reported in long-standing poisoning.

The lesions in the central and peripheral nervous systems, which follow arsphenamine intoxication in particular, have been described in a large number of publications (see Meyer 1963 for references). Petechial haemorrhages in the corpus callosum, in the deep cerebral white matter near the inferior and posterior horns of the lateral ventricle, in the internal capsule, in the cerebral peduncles, and in the peripheral parts of pons and medulla are the main feature in the central nervous system. Foci of perivascular demyelination and necrosis in cerebral cortex and white matter may be due to immune sensitization (Russell 1937); they resemble the lesions in postvaccinal encephalomyelitis and that also complicate antirabic treatment.

The amount of arsenic that accumulates in the brain is unusually high. Arsenic and its compounds are also stored in mesenchymal cells, in the Kupffer cells of the liver, in endothelial cells of the sinuses of the spleen and in the capillary endothelium and microglial cells of the central nervous system.

Arsenical polyneuritis has now become very rare. Clinically it presents with pain and paraesthesias, followed by extensor palsy and wasting of forearms or legs, the small muscles of hand and foot being involved first. Histological studies on the cord and peripheral nerves are few. Myelin and axons are involved and the distal ends of the axons degenerate first. Sensory fibres seem to be more affected than motor fibres, and both clinically and histologically there is a resemblance to alcoholic peripheral neuropathy (Greenfield 1958). Chhuttani, Chawla and Sharma (1967) described acute cases that resembled the Landry–Guillain–Barré syndrome. Segmental demyelination may occur but raised CSF protein and hyperpathic foot pains have suggested more proximal involvement in some cases, perhaps of the posterior root ganglia (Jenkins 1966). Anterior horn neuron changes have been noted (Grzycki and Kobusówna 1951).

Harding, Lewis and Done (1968) studied arsanilic acid poisoning in pigs fed doses considerably higher than is given to promote growth or treat dysentery in such animals. Degeneration of the visual pathways and peripheral nerves was identified. As little information is available on experimental arsenical poisoning further studies of the effect of arsanilic acid on a wider range of animals, using different techniques, could be rewarding.

Arsenic probably acts on the tricarboxylic acid cycle at the level of pyruvate metabolism, by inactivating the SH-containing cofactor thioic acid; blood pyruvate levels are high and there is reduced pyruvate tolerance (Cavanagh 1973). A minor site of arsenic binding may be to reactive SH-groups in the enzyme succinate dehydrogenase, as succinate is sometimes excreted in the urine. Folic acid deficiency has been demonstrated in chronic arsenical poisoning, though not in association with neuropathy (van Tongeren, Kunst, Majoor and Schillings 1965).

Lead

Inhalation of inorganic lead was, in the past, a common cause of industrial poisoning, for example in tin plumbers during refining and smelting processes, in the manufacture of many lead-containing articles, and very frequently in painters responsible for stripping old paint. Industrial poisoning has since been effectively checked by appropriate legislation, and lead poisoning is now mainly a non-industrial problem, usually due to accidental ingestion. Interesting clinical examples of domestic occurrences have been published by Gordon and Whitehead (1949), Burrows, Rendle-Short and Hanna (1951), Millichap, Llewellin and Roxburgh (1952), Gibb and MacMahon (1955), Marsden and Wilson (1955) and Turner (1955). Millichap *et al.* listed the sources of plumbism in childhood in order of frequency as painted woodwork, nipple shields, toy soldiers, fumes from burning battery casings, drinking water and toilet powder. The importance of chronic lead poisoning resulting from pica in retarded children, so predisposing to further mental deterioration (Moncrieff, Koumides, Clayton, Patrick, Renwick and Roberts 1964) has not been fully established. Such poisoning needs consideration in children presenting with manifestations of schizophrenia, behaviour disorders or degenerative encephalopathy (White and Fowler 1960).

There is an association between lead intoxication and abnormal porphyrin metabolism, and there are two reports of acute intermittent porphyria occurring with lead poisoning (Galambos and Dowda 1959). Coproporphyrinuria is a recognized feature of lead poisoning though the association is not understood. Porphyria is inherited as a Mendelian dominant and it is possible that extrinsic factors can precipitate the syndrome when the innate trait is present.

Lead is a frequent cause of poisoning in farm animals and usually causes changes in the central nervous system (Howell 1970).

In *acute lead poisoning* there are usually convulsions, delirium and coma, often with papilloedema and meningeal irritation; there are also abnormalities in the CSF, mainly an increase of globulin, cells and sugar.

The well-documented signs of *chronic lead poisoning* are epileptiform convulsions associated with varying degrees of dementia, peripheral neuropathy (particularly in motor nerves and muscles), abdominal colic, a 'lead line' of the gums, and basophilic stippling of the red blood cells. To these may be added evidence of impaired cardiovascular and renal functions.

Pathological changes. Chronic intoxication with lead occasionally leads to lesions of the liver and kidney. In the liver, acid-fast nuclear inclusions, which fill the greater part of the nuclei and stain orange with Masson's trichrome stain, have been found by Wachstein (1949), and also occur in the convoluted and looped tubules of the kidney. Radiological evidence of skeletal deposits is manifest 3 to 6 months after the onset of poisoning. The gastrointestinal tract shows no gross changes. The 'lead line' of the gums is caused by perivascular deposits of lead sulphide in the submucosal papillae, and basophilic stippling of the red blood cells follows the formation of lead phosphate on their surface membranes.

In the *central nervous system*, oedema is a prominent feature in acute fulminating cases, particularly so in the infantile form (Blackman 1937; Akelaitis 1941; Marsden and Wilson 1955). The cerebral and cerebellar white matter may show necrosis, and the histological picture simulate that of Schilder's disease (Verhaart 1941). Severe oedema in the central white matter has been produced experimentally in guinea-pigs (Weller and Christensen 1925). Involvement of the spinal cord can mimic motor neuron disease (Simpson, Seaton and Adams 1964; Livesley and Sissons 1968).

The mechanism of toxicity in subacute and chronic human and experimental lead poisoning has led to much discussion. Direct action on the neuron, resulting in so-called 'severe cell change' has been accepted by many workers from Nissl onwards. Spielmeyer (1922) demonstrated Nissl's severe cell change in a cat poisoned by lead, and, on a different page in the same book, he illustrated

pronounced focal capillary and endothelial proliferation in the deeper layers of the cerebral
cortex, which others have also emphasized. It is
doubtful whether such vascular changes in man
can be distinguished from similar changes caused
by the renal disease and associated hypertension
which so often occur in chronic poisoning (Meyer
1963). Henderson (1954), in a follow-up study
of lead-intoxicated children, found that among
165 who had died, renal or vascular disease was
given as the cause of death in 108. More recently
attention has been focused on proliferation of the
glia (van Bogaert 1956; Pentschew 1958). In van
Bogaert's case, nodular and diffuse proliferation
of glia (mainly astrocytes) was combined with
focal necrosis in the pons and laminar necrosis
in the cerebral cortex; the clinical picture of
Parkinsonism was related to marked gliosis in
the substantia nigra, though this was not accompanied by loss of neurons. It is interesting that
Mott (1909), using Cajal's impregnation techniques, found diffuse astrocytic proliferation
throughout cerebral grey and white matter, in a
lead-poisoned coach painter; this gliosis was most
marked in the outer layers of the cortex, and
disproportionate to the atrophy of neurons.
Unfortunately, Mott's case was complicated by
chronic alcoholism, and perhaps by pellagra, to
which the associated chromatolysis of anterior
horn neurons, Betz cells, and neurons in the
motor nuclei of the brainstem could also be
attributed.

De Villaverde (1927) noted a definite prevalence
of cerebellar lesions following lead intoxication.
In several infants thought to be suffering from
lead poisoning, Verhaart (1941) found necrosis of
the cerebellar white matter through the cerebrum
was unaffected. Pentschew (1958) described an
acute case with severe oedema of the cerebral
cortex and with necrosis of the cerebellar granular
layer and a case of Biemond and van Creveld
(1939) showed definite clinical signs of a cerebellar
syndrome.

Raimondi, Beckman and Evans (1968) studied
brain biopsy specimens from six children with lead
encephalopathy. Electron-microscopy showed
changes in the ergastoplasm of neurons, the basement membranes and pericytes of cortical capillaries and the extracellular space and myelin
sheaths of the white matter.

In the past, experimental investigation of lead
encephalopathy has been hampered by difficulties
in inducing consistent and unequivocal lesions in
the animals used. More recently Pentschew and
Garro (1966) found that lesions were easily
induced in suckling rats, by feeding 4% lead
carbonate to the mothers, who were not affected.
The lesions included glial proliferation, fluid
transudation and microcavitation, which mainly
involved the cerebellum, striatum and central and
callosal white matter. A considerable degree of
resolution and repair occurred on weaning. Brun
and Brunk (1967) found that the activity of acid
phosphatase in the neurons of lead-poisoned
rats was increased, possibly due to lysosomal
rupture with escape of the enzyme into the cytoplasm.

The *peripheral neuropathy* caused by lead
poisoning has been reviewed by Greenfield (1958),
whose account will be closely followed here.
Although wrist drop, which used to occur commonly in painters and other workers with lead
or lead salts, is often said to be due to the direct
action of lead on muscle fibres (Reznikoff and
Aub 1927), lead can also cause a peripheral
neuropathy in which motor nerve fibres are
specially affected.

The work of Gombault (1880-81) is of special
importance and led to the first description of the
nerve fibre lesion which he called periaxial segmental neuritis ('segmental demyelinative neuropathy', Fisher and Adams 1956). He poisoned
guinea-pigs with small doses of lead carbonate
over a period of several months. Although the
animals were not paralysed, their peripheral
nerves, after fixation in osmium tetroxide and
staining with picrocarmine, showed myelin degeneration in a larger or smaller proportion of
fibres. Degeneration was usually limited to a
single internodal segment, with normal myelin
above and below (Fig. 4.3). Gombault did not
study the axons but concluded that in the absence
of Wallerian degeneration they were not seriously
damaged. Axonal changes were studied by de
Villaverde (1926) in guinea-pigs given subcutaneous injections of lead acetate; the distal
parts of the nerves showed severe lesions, but
minor degrees of damage were seen at all levels.
In the most affected nerves the axons had disappeared and only oval or irregular argyrophilic
debris was seen. In less affected nerves the axons
showed irregular swellings or their neurofibrils
were separated by apparently empty spaces. These
changes were more common in the large diameter
axons and could be traced to the motor endplates,
many of which showed complete destruction. The

reaction of the sheath of Schwann was greater than that seen in Wallerian degeneration.

Fullerton (1966) studied lead acetate-poisoned guinea-pigs and noted convulsions and hindlimb

fied. Segmental demyelination was associated with markedly reduced conduction velocities.

Lampert and Schochet (1968b), in an electron-microscope study of chronic poisoning in rats,

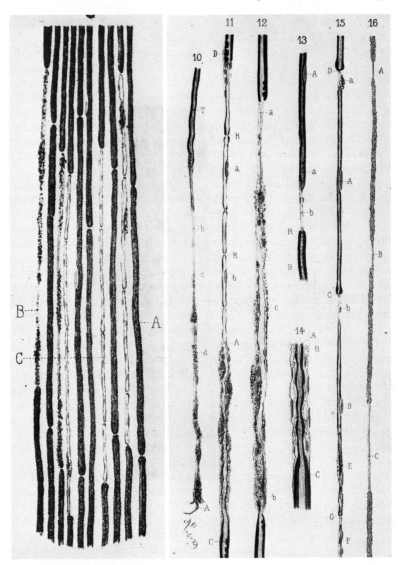

Fig. 4.3 Lead neuropathy; segmental demyelination. Illustrations from Gombault's article on experimental lead neuropathy. Osmic acid and picrocarmine.

paralysis in some animals. She examined the peripheral nerves in 52 animals: 31 were abnormal, 18 showed both segmental demyelination and axonal degeneration, 8 showed only segmental demyelination and 5 only axonal degeneration. Newly formed myelin segments and short intercalated new segments were very frequently identi-

found degeneration and proliferation of Schwann cells, degeneration of related myelin segments beginning at nodes of Ranvier or Schmitt–Lantermann clefts, and separation, disintegration and phagocytosis of myelin lamellas. New lamellas formed later from Schwann cell processes, but some degenerated again. Such repetition of degeneration and regeneration could explain the 'onion bulb' concentric formations sometimes found in chronic neuropathy. Schlaepfer (1968) also carried out a similar EM study, demonstrated more segmental demyelination than axonal degeneration, and concluded that sheath cells and satellite cells in the root ganglia were primarily affected.

Organic lead compounds

The most important of these is tetraethyl lead or lead benzine and inhalation of its vapours has caused fatal poisoning. Tetraethyl lead has its main effect on the central nervous system and causes delirium, convulsive seizures and coma. Bini and Bollea (1947) investigated two cases dying after exposure to lead benzine and found severe neuronal degeneration particularly in the cerebral and cerebellar cortices. Astrocytes and oligodendrocytes showed regressive and progressive changes, and endothelial cells contained excess of fat. Focal lesions, most obvious in the first case, in the mamillary body and the grey matter beneath the floor of the 4th ventricle were reminiscent of the gliomesodermal proliferation that occurs in the Wernicke syndrome. The presence of lead was not proved histochemically and it was concluded that the changes were due to the tetraethyl radical, the toxic action of which appeared to resemble that of acute alcohol or acute ethylbromide intoxications.

Lead encephalopathy has followed repeated self-intoxication by the inhalation of leaded gasoline vapour (Law and Nelson 1968).

Copper

The metabolic defect leading to copper accumulation in the liver and basal ganglia in hepatolenticular degeneration is discussed on p. 172. Otherwise, copper is not important as a neurotoxic substance.

Manganese

Poisoning occurs almost exclusively in workers employed in mining and separating manganese ore and the clinical picture has some resemblance to hepatolenticular degeneration. Couper (1837) gave the first account of its occurrence, but the report aroused little interest until the beginning of the twentieth century, when clinical and clinicopathological observations began to be published (for references see Meyer, 1963).

The neurological picture has been described as a progressive Parkinsonian-like syndrome with a coarse tremor, often of intention type, associated with attacks of uncontrollable laughter; the findings are said to bear a closer resemblance to Wilson's disease than to paralysis agitans. In a case described by Meyer (1930) an extrapyramidal syndrome of rigidity and coarse tremor was accompanied by severe memory and intellectual defect. Mena, Marin, Fuenzalida and Cotziaz (1967) studied manganese miners in Chile and showed that there were severe but apparently temporary psychiatric manifestations followed by a permanently crippling neurological disorder, dominated by extrapyramidal signs. 'Healthy' miners also showed a significant incidence of cogwheel rigidity.

Cotziaz, Horiuchi, Fuenzalida and Mena (1968) measured the rate of disappearance of ^{54}Mn from the blood and serum, from the whole body, from an area representing the liver, from the head area and from the midthigh in normal Chileans, in working manganese miners and in ex-miners with chronic poisoning. The bulk of the tracer was cleared from the blood stream, with a mean halflife ranging between 1·3 and 2·2 minutes, being slower in healthy miners. In contrast, the healthy miners showed faster losses of the isotope from the other areas studied than did the other two groups. These findings indicate that the elevated tissue concentration is not necessary for the continuance of the neurological manifestations; chelation therapy would probably not be effective in reversing the neurological manifestations.

There are few reports of the *pathological changes* in man. Cirrhosis of the liver and chronic interstitial nephritis are described. Focal softenings or gliosis in the cerebral cortex, striatum or cerebellum in association with cardiac or renal disease have been reported and it is then difficult to exclude the effects of the complicating disease. Thus, the available reports are inconclusive. It has been suggested that human intoxication results from inhalation of manganese.

Experimental results are also conflicting. Large doses of manganese chloride have caused necrosis of the liver and smaller doses have induced cirrhosis. Animals have occasionally shown functional signs of a basal ganglia disturbance, though the brain lesions have been slight or absent on histological study. Cerebellar lesions have been found in a monkey poisoned by inhalation of finely sprayed metallic manganese; the liver and kidneys were not involved. Damage to the liver and kidneys in experimental animals may be caused by oral, parenteral or intraperitoneal administration. There is, therefore, suggestive evidence that the distribution and varying combinations of lesions in experimental poisoning is in some way related to the route of injection and the dose administered. Meyer (1963) considered the pathological changes at greater length.

Mercury

Neal (1938) and Brown (1954) gave a detailed account of the history and the sources of mercurial poisoning. Mercurialism, according to Brown, was one of the first recognized industrial diseases. It was known in India in 500 BC and was common among gilders of gold, silver and copper in the sixteenth and seventeenth centuries. Prior to this, most cases occurred in miners of mercury. With the introduction of mercury nitrate in the manufacture of fur felt in France in the seventeenth century, mercurialism became an occupational hazard of the hatting industry; hence the expression 'mad as a hatter'. Mercury and its compounds have many uses today in the electrical, plastics and chemical industries as catalysts in many processes, in dentistry, in laboratories, in agriculture, in photography, in the production of thermometers and barometers and in the criminal investigations of fingerprints.

Mercuric salts, especially the bichloride, are corrosive poisons which exert a local effect upon the gastrointestinal tract and a specific toxic action during excretion on the epithelium of the proximal convoluted tubules of the kidneys.

It has long been known that exposure to metallic mercury or to organic mercury compounds causes a neurological syndrome consisting predominantly of erethysm and tremor ('hatter's shakes'). Erethysm is the term used to describe a florid organic personality change, characterized by fatigue, irritability and emotional instability with variable depressive features; such changes to some extent resemble the frontal lobe syndrome. The tremor, considerably coarser than that occurring in thyrotoxicosis, affects the hands, tongue and legs and may have an intention component. Other systemic signs of mercurialism, such as gingivitis (dark-blue line along the gum margins), stomatitis or phthyalism, are usually associated with the neurological features. The combination of tremor and mental symptoms may give rise to diagnostic difficulties. Brown described amyotrophic lateral sclerosis with chronic mercurialism.

Pathological changes. Before c 1940, knowledge of the toxic effects of mercurial poisoning on the central nervous system was incomplete. Peters (1951) mentioned non-specific neuronal degeneration, softenings, small haemorrhages and perivascular gliosis after chronic intoxication, and degeneration of anterior horn neurons in experimental animals. According to Peters direct toxic effect on the neurons and indirect vascular damage both have to be considered.

Contemporary clinicopathological and experimental investigations with organic mercury compounds, particularly with methylmercury phosphates and nitrates, have clarified the effects of mercurial poisoning (Hunter, Bomford and Russell 1940; Hunter and Russell 1954). Exposure to methylmercury salts by inhalation affects the central nervous system predominantly and gives rise to disturbances that include ataxia, dysarthria and visual disturbances. Rats exposed to methylmercury compounds showed widespread degeneration of the peripheral nerves, posterior columns and the granular layer of the cerebellar cortex, which in one animal contained calcospherites (Hunter *et al.*); a monkey examined by the same workers showed diffuse cerebral cortical change with sparing of the cerebellar cortex.

Hunter *et al.* also studied four patients suffering from neurological disturbances resulting from industrial exposure to methylmercury. The predominant clinical features were gross ataxia combined with severe concentric constriction of the visual fields. In one case (Hunter and Russell 1954), necropsy revealed gross atrophy of the cortex and subcortical white matter of the area striata in the occipital lobe. Foci of similar but more limited cortical atrophy were found in the left precentral, the right postcentral and the left superior temporal gyri; these foci affected the depths of the sulci rather than the summits and are illustrated in Fig. 4.4. The surface of the cerebellum was normal apart from a slight loss of granule cells. The main change, both in the human case and in experimental animals, was a selective atrophy of the granular layer with relative preservation of the Purkinje cells, though the dendrites of the latter often displayed stellate bodies after silver impregnation (Fig. 4.5); this selective lesion of the granular layer appears to be the first example of human granular layer

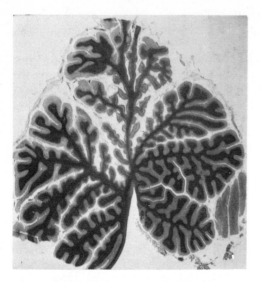 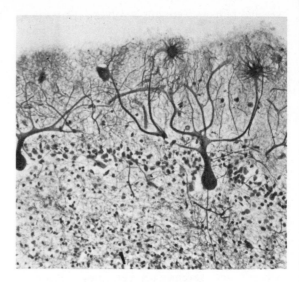

Fig. 4.4 (*left*) Section of vermis showing lobular atrophy in declive extending to adjacent lobules. Loyez' haematoxylation. × 2 approx.
Fig. 4.5 (*right*) Purkinje cell with stellate bodies. Absence of basket fibres around cell body. Hortega's double impregnation. × 180.
(Figs. 4.4 and 4.5 are reproduced by the kindness of Professor Russell.)

degeneration which can be attributed to an exogenous toxin.

Basal ganglia, hypothalamus, brainstem, spinal cord, nerve roots, posterior spinal ganglia and portions of sciatic and ulnar nerve were normal. The focal cerebral cortical lesions and their tendency to occur in the depths of sulci suggest a vascular (ischaemic) factor (Meyer 1963).

Minimata disease (see Shiraki and Takeuchi (1971) for a definitive account). In 1953 fishermen and their families living around the bay of Minimata in Japan first showed evidence of this disease. Clinical features and the pathological lesions suggested mercurial poisoning as a possible cause (McAlpine and Araki 1958). As a result of intensive research at Kumamoto University, toxic organic alkylmercury compounds in the effluent from a fertilizer and plastics factory were isolated from shellfish (Uchida, Hirakawa and Inoue 1961; Miyakawa and Deshimaru 1969). The findings of granular layer atrophy of the cerebellum and of spongiose softenings in the visual cortex and other cortical regions closely resemble those in Hunter and Russell's case (Takeuchi, Morikawa, Matsumato and Shiraishi 1962). Miyakawa (1960) noted that polyneuritis can complicate Minimata disease and most patients with organic mercury poisoning have early sensory disturbances.

Miyakawa, Deshimaru, Sumiyoshi, Teraoka, Udo, Haltori and Tatetsu (1970), in an experimental study of the peripheral nerves in organic mercury poisoning, found widespread degeneration of Schwann cells, myelin and axons in sensory nerves; the changes first affected the nodes of Ranvier. Matsumoto, Koya and Takeuchi (1965) described two infants affected by a congenital form of cerebral palsy who were born in the Minimata bay area; their brains showed lesions very similar to those in florid adult cases of Minimata disease. As the infants had never eaten either fish or shellfish, it was concluded that the changes resulted from mercury intoxication acquired *in utero* from their mothers who did not show evidence of the disease. Miyakawa and Deshimaru (1969) found electron-microscope evidence of ribosomal and nuclear damage in the cerebellar granule cells of rats poisoned with organic mercury; the lesions were consistent with disturbed synthesis of neuronal protein.

In 1971 it was shown that canned tuna fish on sale in Great Britain contained about 0·5 ppm of methylmercury, an amount that was considered to be safe. The level of methylmercury in fish taken from fresh or sea water not known to be contaminated ranges from 0·01 to 0·2 ppm and may rise to 5·0 ppm in fish from contaminated lakes (British Medical Journal 1971). Not all organic mercurial contaminants result from industrial effluents. Natural waters contain many metals, including inorganic mercury, which may act as a receptor for methyl groups from such compounds as cobalamin (vitamin B_{12}) synthesized by microorganisms. The methylated compounds so formed can therefore ascend the food chain and eventually reach fish. Work in Sweden has revealed that certain fish in freshwater lakes contained 10 times more methylmercury than canned tuna, though people consuming it showed no signs of disease. It seems that there is no real prospect of ridding fresh waters or oceans of methylmercury. In future special care must be taken to prevent contamination of water sources by all effluents containing mercury, particularly in areas where fish is the prime source of first-class protein.

Outbreaks of organic mercury poisoning resembling Minimata disease have also occurred in Pakistan, Guatemala and Iraq. In the latter, in 1972, 6000 cases were admitted to hospital and at least 500 died; the cause of the outbreak was the consumption of grain pretreated with an alkylmercury compound (Bakir and colleagues 1973).

Mercury poisoning was also shown to be a major aetiological factor in *erythroedema polyneuritica* (*pink disease, acrodynia*), a disease that is rarely seen today. This condition affected infants and was characterized by insidious onset, occasionally with raised temperature, and by anorexia, insomnia, loss of weight and profuse perspiration, particularly of the extremities. Its popular name 'pink disease' was derived from the red rash (of raw beef colour), and. the swelling, coldness and irritation of the hands, feet, cheeks and nose, which was followed by some desquamation. Mental irritability, photophobia and signs of involvement of the peripheral nerves (such as hypotonia, anaesthesia and loss of tendon reflexes) were consistent features. The prognosis was usually good, with complete recovery; occasional fatal cases reported in the literature usually followed complications such as bronchopneumonia or tuberculosis.

Paterson and Greenfield (1923-4) examined two cases *post mortem* and described polyneuritis affecting the distal part of the peripheral nerve branches; there was considerable degeneration of myelin in the finer nerve bundles. Central chromatolysis of anterior horn neurons was widespread and interpreted as a retrograde reaction to the degeneration of motor nerves. There was some glial proliferation in the spinal grey matter and proliferation of Schwann cells in the ventral roots. Wyllie and Stern (1931) confirmed these findings, and also found central chromatolysis of spinal ganglia and degeneration in the vagal nerve. Kernohan and Kennedy (1928) described central chromatolysis in the Gasserian ganglia and doubtful changes in several nuclei of the brainstem in another case. All investigators found the spinal tracts and the cerebral and cerebellar cortices to be normal. The findings strongly suggest a 'dying-back' process in the peripheral nerves.

With regard to aetiology, Paterson and Greenfield favoured infection and excluded both dietary deficiency and intoxication by lead, arsenic or other chemical substances. Later observations, however, shifted emphasis towards intoxication by mercury sublimate, a constituent of popular 'teething' or 'cooling' powders (*Lancet* 1953). Confirming earlier observations by American and Swiss workers, Holzel and James (1952) found a higher incidence of mercury excretion in active cases of pink disease, in striking contrast to the low rate among healthy infants in the same region of North England. Although mercury was omitted from most teething powders by 1953, sporadic instances of the disease due to mercurialism from other sources have occasionally occurred (Speirs 1959; Forsyth and Savage 1968). It has never been directly established that mercury was the cause of the widespread disease that formerly existed, though the indirect evidence is now seldom questioned.

Phenylmercury. These compounds are also used as fungicides but are less toxic to rats than alkylmercury compounds (Swensson 1952). They more closely resemble inorganic mercury and affect the kidney. A dubious case of motor neuron disease said to result from phenylmercury poisoning has been recorded (Brown 1954) and the problem of motor neuron disease and metallic toxins was discussed by Currier and Haerer (1968).

Mechanism of toxicity of mercuric compounds
The differences between inorganic and organic mercury in relation to their clinicopathological

effects cannot yet be fully explained, though experimental studies have been helpful in clarifying the problem to some extent.

Inorganic mercury mainly affects the proximal convoluted tubule of the kidney (Gritzka and Trump 1968) and also mainly accumulates in the kidney, as compared with liver and brain. Nevertheless, inorganic mercury is much more firmly bound in brain than kidney, so that there seems to be a tendency to selective cerebral accumulation (Cavanagh 1973). Cerebral accumulation of organic methylmercury is also cumulative (Magos and Butler 1972); its distribution elsewhere in the nervous system correlates with the areas subject to histological damage. Electronmicroscopy shows severe alteration of endoplasmic reticulum and mitochondria in anterior horn and posterior root ganglia neurons (Cavanagh). Qualitatively similar EM changes occur in kidney after administration of both inorganic and organic methylmercury, and it is probable that kidney damage due to the latter results from release of inorganic mercury.

In the rat, methylmercury accumulates most in dorsal root ganglia, less in the cerebellum and least in the cerebrum, which accords with the degree of cellular damage; it is likely, as in the kidney, that the release of inorganic mercury is the responsible cytotoxic factor to the nervous system (Cavanagh).

The reason for the differential accumulation cannot be explained, though differences in vascular permeability, metabolic turnover or even neuronal volume may be relevant. Variations in the clinical effects between inhaled organic and ingested inorganic mercury are also puzzling.

The metabolic disorder in affected cells also needs mention. Ultrastructural changes in organelles show some correlation with biochemical evidence that indicates a failure to incorporate and convert available amino acids into protein. This anabolic block may affect liver, kidney and brain similarly, but observed clinical differences, especially in relation to recovery, may be due to incapacity of neurons to regenerate adequately, which does not usually apply to liver or kidney.

Thallium

The neurotoxic effects of thallium salts have been recognized for more than a century, ever since they were first prescribed for 'night sweats' in tuberculosis (Lamy 1863). Since then, their use

as depilating agents in the treatment of ringworm and as rodent or ant killers has led to numerous reports of fatal accidental, suicidal or homicidal poisoning. The continuing availability of thallium salts on an open market should be a matter of public concern.

Large doses (> 1 g) cause death in 1 to 3 days, preceded by acute gastroenteritis, dehydration and shock. Intermediate doses (0.5 to 1.0 g) usually cause death within 4 weeks, preceded by progressive polyneuritis, which develops after about 1 week of less severe gastroenteritis. Therapeutic doses of 8 mg/kg used to be recommended for the depilation of children, who were said to be less susceptible to toxic effects than adults; total or subtotal depilation followed in 2 to 3 weeks, preceded by mild gastroenteritis and 'limb pains'.

In fatal cases the polyneuritis gives rise to severe pain in the feet and back, which is followed by numbness and sensory loss in the lower limbs and, less often, the arms. Paralysis or paresis soon affects the feet, legs and usually arms, trunk and cranial nerves. These features characterize a distal, so-called 'ascending' type of neuropathy. Death follows respiratory failure and/or intercurrent infection, often preceded by bizarre mental changes, including psychotic states. Less severe cases can recover completely.

The neuropathological changes described prior to 1963 included: degeneration of myelin and axons and Schwann cell proliferation in peripheral nerves; degeneration of spinal posterior columns and anterior horn neurons; optic atrophy; neuronal degeneration in vagal, olivary and dentate nuclei; and neuronal chromatolysis and atrophy in cortical or hypothalamic nuclei, associated with variable gliosis (Meyer 1963; Reed, Crawley, Faro, Pieper and Kurlund 1963).

The pathological problem has recently been reassessed in detail by Cavanagh (1973) and Cavanagh, Fuller, Johnson and Rudge (1974) who established that the basic lesion is a 'dying-back' process in peripheral nerves, affecting long axons (e.g. in legs) before short axons (e.g. in cranial nerves), probably affecting large diameter sensory fibres preferentially, and extensively implicating all motor nerves, especially the cranial nerves. There are no significant changes in cerebral or cerebellar cortex or subcortex.

Cavanagh discussed the biochemical background to thallium poisoning. A direct effect of thallium on potassium exchange in cells is an important factor, as thallium ions are in some respects similar to potassium ions, form complex salts with each other and interchange in biological systems. Thallium may also have anticholinesterase activity, but this is probably of less importance than its effect on potassium ion exchange.

The actual mode of damage to cells has still to be worked out, though the entrance of thallium into cells may disturb protein synthesis by damaging organelles. This would impair the efficiency of the perikaryon to maintain a long axon and explain why the longest and to some extent largest diameter axons are affected earlier and more severely.

Tellurium

The neuropathological effects of human poisoning are not known (Osetowska 1971). Experimental evidence suggests that tellurium accumulates in neurons without giving rise to toxic disturbance (Pentschew 1958). In the cat, only the large cells of the red nucleus show structural damage; on macroscopic inspection the grey matter is conspicuous by its blue-grey discoloration, but neurological signs only appear after direct injection of a solution of telluric acid into the cerebrospinal fluid. The storage of tellurium in nerve cells occurs more consistently than with other heavy metals.

Monkeys given intramuscular or intravenous injections of metallic tellurium showed ataxia, tremor and paresis of the tail and hind limbs after 2 to 5 weeks. Axonal dystrophy was present in the nucleus gracilis, along with degeneration in the fasciculus gracilis, Clarke's columns, the spinocerebellar tract and the lateral columns; many neurons showed pigment atrophy and vacuolar degeneration (Pentschew, Ebner and Kovatch 1962). The lesions resembled those described in vitamin E deficient rats, though a satisfactory explanation of the similarities could not be given.

Gold

Roberts (1939) described the deposition of gold in the central nervous system, following the injection of gold salts into animals; the metal was found in neurons and glial cells, particularly in the nuclei of the cranial nerves, the infundibular nuclei, Purkinje cells and anterior horn neurons. Courville and Myers (1957) described focal subcortical degeneration, which they tentatively

suggested was caused by vasospasm, following therapeutic injection of radioactive gold into a pulmonary carcinoma a few weeks earlier.

Walsh (1970) discussed polyneuropathy complicating gold therapy. Gold is often used for the treatment of rheumatoid arthritis, and as this disease is sometimes complicated by 'rheumatoid' neuropathy, diagnosis may be difficult. In the case described by Walsh, electrophysiological studies indicated mainly sensory involvement. Sural nerve biopsy showed a marked reduction in the total fibre count with reduction of both large and small myelinated fibres. Teased fibre preparations confirmed Wallerian-type degeneration with remyelination. Roberts referred to other published cases with polyneuritis, fits, psychiatric disorders, transverse myelitis, Guillain-Barré-like syndromes and/or cranial nerve palsies and suggested that hypersensitivity may be involved in some cases.

Phosphorus

Poisoning with inorganic phosphorus is not frequent but may occur from sources such as rat poisons, phosphorescent paints and the fumes of phosphorous oxide.

Acute poisoning leads rapidly to death, with signs of neurological involvement, especially convulsions, confusional states, coma and respiratory failure. Hepatic failure predominates in subacute or chronic poisoning.

Pathological changes. Even in rapidly fatal cases extensive fatty degeneration occurs in all viscera (including the brain) and is particularly marked in the liver, heart and kidneys. In the liver the degeneration begins in the periphery of the lobules. Lipid accumulation in all neurons was the outstanding feature in a case of suicide described by Wertham (1932), though death occurred only 6 hours after ingestion. In experimental investigations, comparable lipid infiltration of neurons did not occur; there were diffuse degenerative changes in cortical neurons, with little glial reaction, eventually leading to focal areas of cell loss (Meyer 1963). Small perivascular areas of neuronal loss or of softening, endothelial swelling, haemorrhages and hypertrophy of astrocytes have also been found in experimental animals. Swelling of the oligodendrocytes and of the microglia was a prominent feature.

Phosphorus is a potent protoplasmic poison

that damages organelles and impairs cellular oxidative processes; the sequence of biochemical events is, however, still not established.

Organophosphorus compounds

Tri-orthocresyl phosphate (TOCP; an aryl phosphate) intoxication came to be known mainly during the years of prohibition of alcohol in the United States, when the substance was consumed as a substitute for strong liquor. Adulteration of Jamaica ginger with TOCP was the cause of nearly 4000 cases of paralysis in the USA during the year 1930, before the nature of the poison was discovered by Smith, Elvore, Valaer, Frazier and Malory (1930). About the same time cases were seen in Holland (Ter Braak 1931), as well as in other countries on the continent of Europe and in England, where TOCP was sometimes found as an adulterant of 'apiol' or oils used for cooking. Outbreaks of poisoning due to contamination by engine oils in Germany in the second World War (Creutzfeldt and Orzechowski 1941-43), in Switzerland (Moeschlin 1952) and in Morocco (Smith and Spalding 1959) are also well-documented. TOCP was used for its softening, solvent and extracting properties, and at one time preparations containing cresyl phosphate were prescribed in the treatment of pulmonary tuberculosis.

TOCP poisoning has been extensively reviewed by Cavanagh (1964, 1973). In the American cases foot drop, followed by more general weakness of the legs and sometimes also of the extensors of the fingers and wrists, came on progressively over a period of about 2 months. Lesions in the spinal cord sometimes became obvious as the signs of peripheral neuropathy receded, and late cases often resembled amyotrophic lateral sclerosis, with spasticity and peripheral weakness in the legs, deformity of the feet of Friedreich type and wasting of the small muscles of the hands.

According to Meyer (1963), who reviewed the American literature of the 1930s, early human cases were said to show myelin degeneration with slighter changes in the axons in the peripheral nerves and no inflammatory exudate. In the chronic stages constant degeneration of the pyramidal tracts, greater in the lumbar cord than at higher levels and not evident above the cervical segments was noted. The fasciculus gracilis was also degenerated in some cases and here also the degeneration was greater towards the termination of the tract in the cervical segments. The

neurons of the anterior horns were reduced in number and many of those remaining were pyknotic. Similar but less pronounced changes were seen in the nuclei of the lower cranial motor nerves. In the peripheral nerves there was loss of axons and irregularities on many of those remaining. Demyelination was patchy and associated with considerable endoneurial fibrosis which might have hindered regeneration.

Cavanagh (1954) experimented on hens and confirmed that the degeneration of myelin in peripheral nerves was not segmental, as had been suggested by earlier workers, but was continuous along the affected fibres in the part examined and consistent with Wallerian (primary axonal) degeneration. It chiefly affected fibres of large calibre and the peripheral parts of nerves contained more degenerating fibres than proximal parts. In the spinal cord, degeneration was present in the anterior tracts, in the spinocerebellar tracts and less intensely in the fasciculus gracilis; it was greatest towards the termination of the tracts so that ascending tracts degenerated rostrally and descending tracts caudally. Degeneration of individual fibres was seen also in some tracts in the brainstem. In the spinal cord, as in the peripheral nerves, changes in the axons always accompanied degeneration of myelin. Very little chromatolysis was found in the anterior horn neurons.

Histological changes similar to those induced by TOCP have been described as sequelae of poisoning with other organophosphates, including the alkyl compound di-iso-propyl-phosphorofluoridate (or dyflos) and tri-para-ethylphenyl phosphate, an aryl phosphate (Fenton 1955; Cavanagh and Holland 1961). It is of interest that the last mentioned compound, in contrast to the others, has no inhibitory action on cholinesterases. Earl and Thompson (1952) suggested that the paralysis of TOCP poisoning may be caused by the inhibitory effect of pseudo-cholinesterase on myelin, as the enzyme is present in Schwann cells and neuroglia. The hypothesis was unsatisfactory, however, because it did not explain the axonal degeneration, and also because other organophosphorus compounds, though capable of the same inhibitory action, did not cause paralysis. From a histochemical survey of true and pseudo-cholinesterases in the spinal cord and brainstem, Cavanagh, Davies, Holland and Lancaster (1961) concluded that there is no simple relation between the distribution of lesions in organophosphorus poisoning and the localization of these enzymes; nor did they find differences in enzyme distribution between species susceptible and resistant to organophosphorus poisoning.

Ultrastructural studies have indicated that the axonal degeneration precedes chromatolysis in neurons; also that there are accumulations of smooth membranes and other organelles within axons and terminals, which correspond to eosinophilic swellings seen in relation to degenerating axons in the spinal cord (Illis, Patangia and Cavanagh 1966; Prineas 1969; Blakemore and Cavanagh 1969; Bischoff 1970).

The chemical structure, mechanism of action and functional and structural effects of both alkyl and aryl phosphates in different species have been considered by Cavanagh (1964, 1969, 1973). There is a latent period of about 8 to 12 days after the administration of a single dose before neural lesions are manifest and a fundamental question is the nature of the disturbance initiated during this period; unequivocal evidence of a presumed metabolic lesion has not yet been produced. The structural alterations indicate a 'dying-back' of the affected neurons from the periphery centralwards, resembling certain systematized degenerations that afflict man, such as motor neuron disease and Friedreich's ataxia. Although the compounds probably affect all neurons to some degree, the cellular derangement only leads to axonal degeneration in neurons particularly dependent on the metabolic pathways that are deranged by the toxic process. Distal degeneration of the longest and largest diameter fibres suggests that the maintenance of such fibres requires a greater 'work-factor' within the perikaryon and that the capacity to carry this extra metabolic load is impaired. This could involve a defect in synthesis, transport or utilization within perikaryon and axon.

Other compounds inducing organophosphorus (OP) patterns of degeneration

It has recently been shown that the 'dying-back' type of axonal degeneration is not specific for the alkyl and aryl organophosphates but can occur with other compounds that are dissimilar in structure. This may indicate that the different compounds act at similar metabolic loci and so result in similar effects (Cavanagh 1969).

p-*Bromophenylacetyl urea.* The lesions closely resemble those of OP poisoning. However, the rat, though insensitive to OP compounds is very

sensitive, and the hen, sensitive to OP compounds, is insensitive to repeated oral dosage (Cavanagh, Chen, Kyu and Ridley 1968). Another difference is the apparent lack of anticholinesterase activity with p-bromophenylacetyl urea (Cavanagh 1969).

p-*Bromophenylacetylurea (BPAU).* This compound induces paralysis and structural lesions in the rat resembling those that occur in other species poisoned with TOCP and similar organophosphorus compounds. BPAU does not appear to affect species other than the rat (Cavanagh 1973).

p-*Bromophenylisothiocyanate.* Cavanagh (1969) commented on the possibility that the lesions in young lambs fed this compound resemble those of p-bromophenylacetylurea. Rats, hens, rabbits, guinea-pigs and lambs more than 12 weeks old do not appear to be susceptible. As the rumen is not fully functional before 12 weeks, it is possible either that the immature rumen can convert the compound to a toxic form or that the mature rumen can detoxify a compound to which lambs are particularly sensitive.

Acrylamide. There appears to be no essential difference between the effects of this compound and the organophosphorus group. There is less damage to central than to peripheral fibre systems, though this point needs further clarification. The subject is fully reviewed by Cavanagh (1969, 1973).

Sodium diethyldithiocarbamate (NDDC). In experiments designed to influence the levels of tissue copper, this chelating agent was injected repeatedly for many weeks into rabbits and hens (Howell and Edington 1968; Edington and Howell 1969). The hens became ataxic after 7 to 17 weeks and the rabbits after $7\frac{1}{2}$ months. Distal spinal cord degeneration was seen in the ascending posterior and lateral tracts and the descending anterior tracts. Degeneration was present in the peripheral nerves and though the lesions were not analysed quantitatively, from comparison with his own findings in hens poisoned with organophosphorus compounds Cavanagh (1969) tentatively suggested that NDDC intoxication induced a similar degeneration pattern. Rasul and Howell (1973) found that there was a quantitative loss of large diameter peripheral nerve fibres in rabbits subjected to chronic NDDC poisoning, though significant, active Wallerian degeneration was not identified.

Carbon disulphide (CS₂). Workers in the rubber or rayon industries may be subjected to exposure (Davidson and Feinleib 1972) and the sequelae include an increased susceptibility to coronary artery disease and neurological complications. Chronic intoxication affects the peripheral and central nervous systems, leading to a distal sensorimotor neuropathy, mental changes and extrapyramidal features (Cavanagh 1973).

Tetraethylthiuram disulphide (Antabuse; TETD). It seems probable that the appearance of distal neuropathy with Parkinsonian features and mental changes in alcoholic patients treated with this drug are related more to the toxicity of the drug than to that of alcohol; optic atrophy also occurs (Gardner-Thorpe and Benjamin 1971). The clinical picture resembles that of chronic CS_2 intoxication and the causal mechanism may be similar, as there is evidence that CS_2 is released from TETD during its katabolism (Kane 1970; Cavanagh 1973). The analogue tetramethylthiuram disulphide (TMTD) is used as a vulcanizing agent in the rubber industry and also as an antibacterial and antifungicidal agent. TMTD is probably similar to TETD in its toxic propensities (Cavanagh 1973).

Nitrofurans. This group of drugs, which includes nitrofurantoin, nitrofurazone and furaltadone, was introduced as a bacteriostatic but has since been used for the treatment of trypanosomiasis and testicular carcinoma. The toxic effects include cardiac disturbances (not unlike those of beriberi) and a sensorimotor, distal neuropathy (Collings 1960; Ellis 1962) of 'dying-back' type, which has been reproduced experimentally in rats (Behar, Rachmilewitz, Rahamimoff and Deman 1965).

Conclusions. The evidence suggests that the above substances, though not closely resembling organophosphorus compounds either chemically or in their acute toxic effects, seem to affect neurons in a comparable way, but at a slower tempo, after repeated exposure. This problem can only be clarified by further studies using a wider range of techniques, including quantitative methods.

There is a noteworthy resemblance to the peripheral neuropathies of thiamine deficiency and arsenical poisoning and there may be similar

pathogenic mechanisms operating at the metabolic level; abnormalities in pyruvate metabolism have been recorded in poisoning with arsenicals (Joiner, McArdle and Thompson 1950) and with nitrofurans (Robertson and Knight 1964).

Cavanagh (1973) noted that CS_2 readily reacts with pyridoxamine and might lead to a chronic depletion of pyridoxal phosphate and indirectly to a deficiency of available vitamin B_6. The compounds TETD, TMTD and NDDC all probably release CS_2 during their metabolic breakdown and so may lead to similar depletion of pyridoxal phosphate.

The reactivity of CS_2 to amine, sulphydryl or hydroxyl groups is said to result in the formation of various compounds capable of chelating activity. This reaction is of particular interest, because it was the chelating action of dithiocarbamates that first led to experimental investigations into their effects on copper metabolism. Accordingly, it has been postulated that a disturbed balance of polyvalent metal ions (copper, zinc) in the tissues is responsible for the neurotoxicity of CS_2, TETD and dithiocarbamates.

Intoxication by other chemical substances

Isoniazid (isonicotinic acid hydrazide; INAH)

In man INAH appears to result in a predominantly sensory neuropathy (Jones and Jones 1953). In rats, Cavanagh (1967) found that both motor and, to a lesser degree, sensory fibres were affected, medium sized fibres were particularly damaged, large diameter sensory fibres were usually spared and long fibres affected more than short fibres. In severe cases the gracile tracts in the spinal cord were involved, probably indicating distal degeneration of the central axons of sensory posterior root ganglia neurons, the peripheral axons of which were also affected. The pattern of degeneration resembled that found in acute human porphyria but differed from that of organophosphorus poisoning (Cavanagh 1969). Noel, Worden and Palmer (1967) induced oedema and demyelination of the central white matter of dogs, and Kreutzberg and Carlton (1967) and Lampert and Schochet (1968a) found comparable lesions in ducklings fed INAH. The mechanism determining such species differences is obscure. Related hydrazide drugs (thiosemicarbazide, iproniazid, carbohydrazide) induce convulsions and not usually peripheral neuropathy.

Ochoa (1970) studied the sural nerves from 10

patients with isoniazid neuropathy, both qualitatively and quantitatively, by light and electron-microscopy. Myelinated and unmyelinated fibres were damaged in all cases. Fibres showing active degeneration were relatively numerous and the total fibre counts were reduced, with one exception. The most frequent changes were denervation and regeneration of fibres and also degeneration of previously regenerated fibres. Differences between the pattern of true unmyelinated fibres and unmyelinated sprouts from myelinated fibres were noted.

Deficiency of vitamin B_6 (pyridoxine) complicating the clinical use of INAH is noted on p. 205. The INAH inhibits pyridoxal phosphate kinase, the enzyme that phosphorylates pyridoxine to form the active cofactor pyridoxal phosphate; the drug will also chelate with the cofactor to form a hydrazone base, which has an even more inhibitory effect on the enzyme than INAH alone. Thus, the end-result will be a deficiency of cofactor pyridoxal phosphate, necessary for a wide range of decarboxylating and transaminating reactions which occur extensively in nerve and brain tissues. Many metabolic pathways involving amino acids require this cofactor and its deficiency may ultimately disturb the synthesis of fibrous neuroprotein on which the maintenance of axons depends.

Carbon tetrachloride (CCl_4) and related compounds

Carbon tetrachloride is used as an industrial solvent. Its toxic effect on the liver and kidneys has long been known, and has been the subject of many clinicopathological studies. Stevens and Forster (1953) and Cohen (1957) have drawn attention to the early neurological signs of intoxication such as headache, vertigo, ataxia, blurred vision, lethargy and coma, which may appear prior to clinical evidence of either hepatic or renal damage. Stevens and Forster reviewed earlier pathological and experimental investigations, and described foci of perivenous necrosis in the cerebral white matter of one case, not unlike those occurring in perivenous encephalomyelitis. In another case the Purkinje cells were found to be shrunken, pyknotic and reduced in number, without associated glial reaction. Cohen also found similar lesions in his two cases. Luse and Wood (1967) described haemorrhages, apparent demyelination and necrosis in the pons, cerebellum and cerebral white matter, along with non-necrotic spongy foci in the transverse pontine

tracts. But electron-microscopy failed to confirm the demyelination, the light-microscope appearances being due to oedema (extracellular and within myelin sheaths) that separated myelinated axons from each other and from vessel walls. The pathogenesis of the lesions is obscure, though previous investigators have postulated that vascular damage, a direct toxic effect on neuronal metabolism and the indirect influences of hepatic and renal dysfunction are possible factors.

Poisoning by *trichlorethylene* (C_2HCl_3; TCE) a chemically related substance, also used as an industrial solvent, seems also to result in a clinical syndrome of optic atrophy, ataxia, spasticity and confusional states (Baker 1958). In experiments on dogs, the cerebral cortex showed mild diffuse neuronal degeneration; in the cerebellar cortex many Purkinje cells had disappeared, and those remaining showed pyknosis, vacuolation and impaired staining. The problems relating to pathogenesis are similar to those with other solvent poisons, since kidneys and liver are also damaged. Buxton and Hayward (1967) described an industrial accident resulting in exposure to TCE; two of four men developed severe cranial nerve palsies, and necropsy on the one fatal case showed degeneration and loss of neurons in the brainstem nuclei and degeneration of axons and myelin in the stem tracts and emergent nerve roots (especially V, VI and VII). The toxic effect appeared to be on neurons rather than Schwann cells or axons. Smith (1966) gave a detailed review of TCE toxicity.

Baker noted a predilection for Purkinje cell changes in *benzene* and *ethyl acetate* poisoning. *Carbon disulphide* poisoning is described on p. 164.

Aminoquinolines and related substances

The 8-aminoquinoline derivatives including plasmocid (methoxy-diethylamino-propylamino-quinoline), pentaquine, isopentaquine, primaquine and pamaquine (all antimalarial drugs) have been studied by Schmidt and Schmidt (1948, 1951), Richter (1949) and Löken and Haymaker (1949). These investigations all described experiments on monkeys, except for one fatal human case (Löken and Haymaker) following pamaquine poisoning. In general, it was found that variations of the side-chain radical altered the toxic effects: some compounds acted on the heart, others on the haemopoietic system, others on the central nervous system.

In their first report Schmidt and Schmidt described changes in the spinal cord, the nuclei of the brainstem, the diencephalon and the extrapyramidal system following acute, subacute and chronic intoxication. With large doses the histological effects were more widespread than with small doses; at half the maximum tolerated dose, plasmocid caused degeneration that was confined to the brainstem nuclei especially the oculomotor, vestibular and some associated nuclei. In the earlier stages, neuronal degeneration predominated; later, astrocytic and sometimes also microglial proliferation ensued. In their second study, the Schmidts investigated the effects of pentaquine, isopentaquine, primaquine and pamaquine and the main lesions were found in the dorsal motor nucleus of the vagus, supra-optic and paraventricular nuclei and the nucleus of Meynert's commissure; occasionally there was severe injury to the hypoglossal nucleus and mild degeneration of oculomotor nuclei. The Schmidts attributed the functional disturbances of the circulatory system to the lesions of the dorsal vagal nucleus. Using macaques, Richter identified focal lesions in the thalamus, hypothalamus, red nucleus, substantia nigra, oculomotor and trochlear nuclei, nuclei of the abducens, vestibular and cochlear nerves, in the cuneate nucleus and in the reticular system of the pons and medulla. The lesions consisted of foci of incomplete necrosis, with almost complete loss of neurons and microglial proliferation; there was also a remarkable proliferation of capillaries and precapillaries, which had a resemblance to the lesions of Wernicke's encephalopathy and, consequently, raised the possibility of an antithiamine action.

In Löken and Haymaker's fatal human case there was an area of ischaemic necrosis in the pons, less severe necrosis in the globus pallidus, and considerable loss of neurons with gliosis in the abducens, trochlear and lateral oculomotor nuclei. The authors suggested that the lesions were caused indirectly, as a consequence of anaemia associated with methaemoglobin formation; they do not describe lesions in the dorsal vagal nucleus, but Schmidt and Schmidt (1951), who reviewed the findings, suspected the presence of such changes, since the clinical appearances were similar to those shown by their macaques.

Chronic administration of chloroquine (a 4-aminoquinoline derivative) may cause visual loss due to irreversible retinopathy, which may continue to worsen after stopping the drug. Wetter-holm and Winter (1964) found loss of rods and cones similar to that in retinitis pigmentosa, though the pattern of pigment dispersal differed in the latter condition, pigment laden cells accumulating in the outer nuclear and plexiform layers. The drug is apparently bound to the melanin pigment of the eye so that the pigment epithelium is the primary site of damage (Lawwill, Appleton and Altstatt 1968). Bernstein and Ginsberg (1964) confirmed the loss of rods and cones and noted migration of pigment clumps from the pigment epithelium to the inner nuclear layer. The presence of some foveal cones was usual and correlated with the frequent findings of good visual acuity, despite extensive retinal damage. Meier-Ruge (1965) administered subtoxic doses of chloroquine for 4 to 7 weeks to cats and found that there was enlargement of the pigment epithelium followed by decrease in enzyme activity; atrophy of rods and cones finally ensued. Gregory, Rutty and Wood (1970) showed that chloroquine administered to rats rapidly produced abnormal membranous bodies in the cytoplasm of retinal ganglion cells.

A vacuolar myopathy due to chloroquine has been described in man by Eady and Ferrier (1966) and has been reproduced in rabbits by Smith and O'Grady (1966) and in rats by McDonald and Engel (1970). In the human cases evidence of ocular toxicity or lower motor neuron involvement may also be present. An investigation of the short-term effects of chloroquine on rabbit skeletal muscle (Aguayo and Hudgson 1970) showed that serum enzymes (CK and LDH) were usually raised; there was no evidence of vacuolar myopathy but all animals showed many abnormal mitochondria in cardiac and skeletal muscle.

Optic atrophy has followed long-term medication with halogen substituted 8-hydroxyquinolines such as iodochlorhydroxyquinoline (clioquinol) or diiodohydroxyquinoline (Berggren and Hansson 1966; Etheridge and Stewart 1966), sometimes with signs suggestive of a demyelinating process. It has been suggested that these compounds should not be used as a preventative against 'travellers' diarrhoea' (*Lancet* 1968). Although effective in intestinal amoebiasis certain of these preparations are now sold to the public as a broad spectrum prophylactic, even though there is no good evidence for their efficiency in diarrhoea of bacterial, viral or dietetic origin. Tsubaki, Honma and Hoshi (1971), writing from Japan, noted a strong association between clioquinol administration and severe neurological disturbances that have been termed *subacute myelo-optico-neuropathy* (*SMON*). This syndrome first appeared about 15 years previously, had increased markedly in recent years and there were by 1971 more than ten thousand cases in Japan. The patients show a peripheral sensory type neuropathy with ataxia and visual disturbances. Histological studies revealed demyelination and axonal damage in the optic and main peripheral nerves and the lateral and posterior columns of the spinal cord. Of 110 patients given clioquinol for more than 14 days, 40 (35·4%) developed neurological signs. The reason why the syndrome is so common in Japan, if indeed it is due to clioquinol, is far from clear; racial or genetic factors have been suggested. Since banning the sale of clioquinol in Japan in 1970, there has been a marked reduction in the number of new cases. Jones, Searle and Smith (1973*a*) found that rats fed clioquinol and a maize diet developed much more severe neuropathy than rats fed only a maize diet, which seemed to indicate that clioquinol may accentuate other causes of neuropathy. This lends some support to the idea that clustering of cases of SMON in Japan may be due to the combined effects of clioquinol and another factor peculiar to that country (*Lancet* 1971).

Neuropathy has been induced in the mouse by large doses of the antimicrobial agent nitroxline, which is derived from 8-hydroxyquinoline (O'Grady and Smith 1966).

Agenized flour and wheat gluten

Nitrogen trichloride (NCl$_3$; agene) is used in most wheat consuming countries to bleach and soften wheat flour. Mellanby (1946) began a systematic investigation of the possible connection between agene-treated flour and 'canine hysteria', a disease of dogs which manifests itself by 'running fits'. The problem was investigated in several laboratories, particularly in the United States (Silver 1949; Lewey 1950 and others). Lewey reviewed these researches. The NCl$_3$ was found to be toxic to dogs, ferrets and rabbits,- but not to guinea-pigs, cats, monkey or man. Seizures could be produced in susceptible animals by feeding or injecting one of the proteins of flour such as gliadin, glutamine, casein or peptide, after treatment with NCl$_3$.

The toxic agent has now been identified as methionine sulphoximine (Bentley, McDermott and Whitehead 1950), which is an antagonist to glutamine as well as to methionine from which it is derived. The changes in the central nervous system of dogs fed on a diet rich in NCl$_3$-treated flour, consist of necrosis affecting the deep layers of the cerebral cortex and the subcortical arcuate fibres; the hippocampus also shows necrosis, which is identical to that which occurs in anoxia. The Purkinje cells of the cerebellum and the basket cells and their fibres also show severe degeneration, but the nerve cells of the dentate nucleus and the roof nuclei are only mildly affected. The nature and localization of the changes were thought to indicate that a vascular disturbance, anoxia or the inhibition of respiratory enzymes were likely causative factors (Lewey). Similar mechanisms were assumed by Hicks and Coy (1958), who on administration of methionine sulfoximine to rats and mice, induced necrosis that was severe in the cerebral cortex (especially the cingulate gyrus), the corpus striatum and Ammon's horn and less severe in the hypothalamic, subthalamic and thalamic nuclei.

Shatin (1964) noted that the incidence of multiple sclerosis could be correlated with the geography of cereal cultivation and suggested that gluten intolerance interfered with protein biosynthesis and the maintenance of myelin.

Organic tin compounds

Although metallic tin is not a toxic hazard, poisoning from its organic compounds, particularly those with an alkyl radical, has been known since the end of the nineteenth century. Interest has been renewed because of its importance as a source of poisoning from imperfectly canned foodstuffs. Oral diethyl-tin-diiodide has been widely used in France in the treatment of boils and the effects of di- and triethyl tin compounds on rats was investigated by Stoner, Barnes and Duff (1955). Triethyl tin was the more active compound and on injection caused muscular weakness, tremor and convulsions, signs that clearly pointed to involvement of the central nervous system. Naked-eye inspection of the viscera revealed little abnormality and tin was not found in the brain or elsewhere. Magee, Stoner and Barnes (1955, 1957) studied the nervous system of rats and rabbits poisoned with triethyl compounds; histological examination of the cerebral and spinal white matter and the optic nerves showed a remarkable 'interstitial' oedema which, at low magnification, resulted in a reticular appearance, but left myelin and axons intact. When poisoning was discontinued, the animals returned to normal and at necropsy no changes were detected. The cause of these lesions was obscure: there was no evidence of disturbance of the blood–brain barrier. Gruner (1958) studied four human cases (and experimented on monkeys and mice) and Cossa and colleagues (1959) also studied four human cases: the findings of Magee and co-workers were confirmed, but in addition there was more marked ballooning and degeneration of myelin sheaths and axis cylinders, and slight oedema of the cortical grey matter.

Aleu, Katzman and Terry (1963) in an electron-microscope study of rabbit brain, found that the oedema mainly involved the white matter and the fluid was almost wholly in large clefts within the myelin sheaths. 'Clear' glial cells showed mild focal swelling; oligodendrocytes, neurons and vessel walls looked normal and the intercellular space was not increased. Torack, Terry and Zimmerman (1960) showed that in mouse brain, tin oedema was different, the fluid being mainly in 'clear' glial cells. Hirano, Zimmerman and Levine (1968), using rats, found electronlucent myelin clefts after intraperitoneal injection. After implanting pellets of tin compound into rat brain, there was electron-dense inflammatory oedema in the widened extracellular space; myelin clefts did not occur for 4 days and then remained confined to the region of the implant. Simultaneous intraperitoneal injection and intracerebral implantation of the tin compound had an additive effect, causing clefts and oedema. The quantitative effects of triethyl tin acetate and sulphate were similar though qualitatively the clefts were more prominent with the sulphate. Tin compounds seem to act directly on neural tissue and not by an indirect metabolic derangement.

Drugs used in psychiatric and neurological treatment

Some *tranquillizers* of the phenothiazine group are known to induce toxic side-effects, especially extrapyramidal disturbances that may be irreversible (Ayd 1961; Hunter, Earl and Janz 1964; Hunter, Blackwood, Smith and Cummings 1968); these drugs have been said to act on the hypothalamus and on autonomic centres in the lower brainstem. In a survey of 3775 patients receiving phenothiazines, Ayd found that 15% developed Parkinsonism. Pathological investigations on human and experimental cases were reviewed by Roizin, True and Knight (1959): the human cases (consisting of three cases from the literature and six personal cases) died in various ways, including jaundice, agranulocytosis, postelectroconvulsive collapse, etc.; in the central nervous system, diffuse changes such as chromatolysis, increased satellitosis, occasional neuronophagia, and increased lipid in neurons were found, and these findings were more marked in the basal ganglia, the hypothalamus and the mesencephalon than elsewhere. In acute experiments on 62 rats, Roizin and colleagues produced increased sudanophilia of liver cells and widespread chromatolysis and increased satellitosis of cerebral neurons, again with some emphasis on the basal region. A monkey killed after 25 months on the drugs showed a microglial reaction in the outer cortical layers, and astrocytic proliferation in the cerebral white matter. Hunter *et al.* (1968) studied three cases known to have been treated with phenothiazines and found mild chronic degeneration of myelin in the basal ganglia of questionable significance. Christensen, Møller and Fayrbye (1970) studied 28 brains from patients suffering from drug-induced dyskinesias; they found neuronal degeneration in the substantia nigra and gliosis in the midbrain and brainstem. It has been suggested that an association between sudden deaths in psychiatric hospitals and phenothiazine administration is due to myocardial vascular degeneration and mucopolysaccharide infiltration and not to cerebral lesions (*Lancet* 1966).

A retinopathy due to phenothiazines has been described by Mathalone (1966) and Kjaer (1968); this has been confirmed by experiments on cats (Cerletti and Meier-Ruge 1968; Gregory, Rutty and Wood 1970). Other drugs such as haloperidol and tetrabenazine can induce Parkinsonism and a few cases have been attributed to alpha methyldopa (Groden 1963; Peaston 1964).

Davis, Bartlett and Termini (1968) reviewed at length the clinical effects of overdosage of psychotropic drugs, including meprobamate, phenothiazines, chlordiazepoxide and related agents, phenothiazines, tricyclic (imipramine-type) antidepressants, monoamine oxidase (MAO) inhibitors, barbiturates, amphetamine and lithium. They found that relatively little attention has been paid to the neuropathological lesions in fatal human cases, the main changes being attributable ischaemia/anoxia. Simpson and Angus (1970) also reviewed the clinical aspects of drug-induced extrapyramidal disorders.

Palmer and Noel (1963) studied the effects of chronic administration of eight different hydrazine MAO-inhibitors to dogs: focal and bilateral olivary degeneration, cerebellar gliosis, necrosis of cerebellar roof nuclei, cerebral myelin degeneration and oedema, and neuronal vacuolation were seen but the lesions varied according to the drugs used. Haemolytic anaemia occurred with all eight drugs, usually accompanied by convulsions and ataxia. The role of elevated brain serotonin was discussed and it was concluded that this was unlikely to be the cause of all of the changes found. Palmer and Noel (1965) subsequently found similar myelin degeneration in dogs treated with isonicotinic acid hydrazide (isoniazid) and its methanosulphate derivatives, which are not MAO inhibitors; they inferred that such degeneration may not, therefore, be due to elevated serotonin, the chief substrate for MAO.

de Villiers (1966) discussed 29 cases (16 seen personally) of intracranial haemorrhage that occurred during treatment with MAO inhibitors. Six patients died from intracerebral or subarachnoid bleeding, 9 were left with varying disability and 14 recovered completely. The haemorrhages were probably related to hypertensive crises, sometimes precipitated by sympatheticomimetic or imipramine type drugs, or foods containing tyramine such as cheese.

In recent years there has been a large output of papers dealing with biogenic amines, their localization in the brain and the action of psychotropic drugs: the subject is reviewed by Snyder (1967). Localization of amines by the electron-microscope (Aghajanian and Bloom 1967) and the fluorescent microscope (Andea, Dahlström, Fuxe and Hökfelt 1966) and the effect of drugs on amines have been extensively documented (Radouco-Thomas, Singh, Garcin and Radouco-Thomas 1967; Aprison, Kariya, Hingtgen and Toru 1968; Gey and Pletscher 1968; Robinson, Lowinger and Bettinger 1968).

Garland (1957) drew attention to the occurrence of a cerebellar syndrome (dysarthria, nystagmus and ataxia, with or without disturbance of behaviour) in epileptics treated with some of the *hydantoin drugs* (*sodium phenytoin, dilantin*).

Among 31 patients in whom such toxic complications required admission to hospital, overdosage could be incriminated in only four, and there was obvious individual hypersensitivity in three others. In a fatal case, Hofman (1958) found that the Purkinje cells in the cerebellum had practically disappeared, but there was little damage to the cerebral cortex and hippocampus and there were only mild neuronal changes and chronic inflammatory cuffing in striatum and thalamus. The cause of the lesions in this case was difficult to assess, as there was a history of symptomatic epilepsy and a background of an undiagnosed infection. Hofmann concluded that dilantin poisoning was the causal agent, in view of similar findings produced experimentally in cats by Utterback, Ojeman and Malek (1958). This is another example of the selective vulnerability of the cerebellar cortex to toxic processes. A similar predilection has previously been noted in chronic alcoholism, and in poisoning by heavy metals and by some organic compounds. It may be, therefore, that an important factor is interference with a single metabolic pathway by different aetiological agents.

Reynolds (1968, 1970) discussed the neuropsychiatric implications of the anticonvulsant drugs phenobarbitone, phenytoin and pyrimidone. He described in detail the disturbances in folic acid and vitamin B_{12} metabolism that can occur, particularly in relation to the mental disturbances and to the cerebellar, spinal cord and peripheral nerve lesions that can result from treatment.

Anthony (1970) discussed benign and possibly malignant lymphadenopathy that can follow the long-standing use of hydantoin drugs; this complication should be known to neuropathologists.

Thalidomide (Distaval, γ-phthalimidoglutarimide), better known for its teratogenic effects, also results in a predominantly sensory peripheral neuropathy with much less damage to lower motor neurons (Fullerton and Kremer 1961; Fullerton and O'Sullivan 1968). Recovery is often slow and incomplete when use of the drug is withdrawn. There is some evidence that the upper motor neurons can be affected, as several patients have shown Babinski responses or increased reflexes.

Necropsy studies on two cases and also biopsy reports confirm that the affected peripheral nerves undergo Wallerian-type degeneration and that the large diameter fibres are most affected. The two necropsy reports describe degeneration of posterior root ganglia neurons and degeneration in the posterior columns of the spinal cord, mainly gracile tracts. The available evidence strongly suggests a 'dying-back' process though a suitable animal model has not so far been found to confirm this. Cavanagh (1973) has noted that in some respects the human peripheral neurotoxic effects of thalidomide resemble those of methylmercury poisoning in the rat, especially in the severe damage to peripheral sensory neurons and the minimal effects on lower motor neurons.

Drugs and other agents that induce neurofibrillary alterations

This problem was reviewed at length by Wisniewski, Terry and Hirano (1970). Accumulation of argyrophilic fibrillary material is seen on light microscopy in the neurons of the brainstem, spinal cord and posterior root ganglia of patients treated with the drugs vinblastine and vincristine, which are mitotic spindle inhibitors and used against leukaemia and certain other neoplastic disorders; electron-microscopy reveals large aggregates of 9 to 10 nm filaments. Vincristine and vinblastine are derived from *Vinca rosea*, the Madagascan periwinkle. Similar intraneuronal aggregates can be demonstrated in experimental disorders induced in animals by spindle inhibitors (e.g. colchicine, vinblastine, podophyllotoxin), by lathyrogenic agents such as iminodiproprionitrile (IDPN) and after the injection of aluminium compounds into the brain or subarachnoid space. Wisniewski and colleagues compared the 10 nm filaments induced in the above ways with the 20 nm diameter twisted tubules that are constricted every 80 nm, and constitute the characteristic neuronal changes in Alzheimer's disease, Guam-Parkinsonism-dementia complex, postencephalitic Parkinsonism and Pick's disease; in these and in the induced human and experimental disorders there is loss of normal 24 nm neuronal microtubules. The function of microtubules is uncertain. They appear in most cells and seem to have varying roles. The metaphase spindle is composed of relatively unstable microtubules, to enable rapid mitosis to occur. Other intraneuronal cytoplasmic microtubules appear to be continuous with similar tubules in axons and may be concerned with intracellular transport and axoplasmic flow.

Bradley, Lassman, Pearce and Walton (1970)

described in detail the clinical and pathological findings in 23 adults and 14 children with intracranial gliomas given vincristine injections for up to 20 months. Biopsies of the proximal limb muscles showed focal necrosis and phagocytosis; the distal muscles showed denervation atrophy at necropsy. A sural nerve biopsy showed axonal degeneration and phagocytosis. Light microscopy of the brain, cord and posterior root ganglia of five necropsies was normal. Bradley (1970) studied vincristine neuropathy in the guinea-pig; in contrast to the human lesions, the myopathic exceeded the neurotoxic effects.

N-nitroso compounds and the nervous system

Lijinksky and Epstein (1970) summarized the evidence suggesting that human cancer may be caused by nitrosamines or nitrosamides formed in the body from ingested nitrites and secondary amines. Nitrosocompounds have been found in tobacco smoke, grains and alcoholic beverages in concentrations of less than 5 ppm and in higher concentrations in nitrite-preserved fish meal intended for animal feeds. Cooking could be a source of secondary amines. There is experimental evidence that nitrosocompounds can induce malformations and tumours of the nervous system. Koyama, Handa, Handa and Matsumoto (1970) injected pregnant rats with small doses of methylnitrosourea (MNU) and the offspring showed developmental defects of the brain such as encephalocoele, pallial hypoplasia, hydrocephalus and microcephaly. Schiffer, Fabiani, Grossi-Paoletti and Paoletti (1970), Grossi-Paoletti, Paoletti, Schiffer and Fabiani (1970) and Jones, Searle and Smith (1973b), following on the important studies of Druckrey, Ivankovic and Preussmann (1966) and Wechsler and colleagues (1969) induced a wide range of intracranial and spinal neoplasms by injecting pregnant rats or young rats with MNU or ethylnitrosourea; tumours of the Gasserian ganglion were of particular interest. The subject is fully covered by Kirsch, Grossi-Paoletti and Paoletti (1972).

Methylazoxymethanol (MAN) neurotoxicity

Cycasin (methylazoxymethanol-β-D-glucoside) is a naturally occurring methylating agent, derived from the palm-like cycad and related plants. An acute fatal neurological disease has been said to occur in man and cattle from ingestion of materials derived from either seeds or the leaves of the plants (Jones, Mickelson and Yang 1973). A link between cycasin and the variety of motor neuron disease endemic on Guam, has been postulated but not established. However, the toxin certainly has neurotoxic, teratogenic, carcinogenic and hepatotoxic properties, which are fully reviewed by Jones *et al.*

Cycasin and the related synthetic product MAN affect differentiating cells in the central nervous system, especially the cerebellum. MAN has been compared with nitrosocompounds in its toxic effects and both may give rise to alkylating intermediates and so result in methylation of nucleic acids in dividing cells.

Acquired (non-Wilsonian) chronic hepatocerebral degeneration

The neuropathological changes that can complicate various forms of liver disease have been delineated by Waggoner and Malamud (1942), Adams and Foley (1953), Victor, Adams and Cole (1965) and Shiraki and Oda (1968). Episodes of hepatic coma or other manifestations of liver diseases are sometimes followed or preceded by neurological signs such as tremor of the head, asterixis, grimacing, dysarthria, cerebellar ataxia, choreoathetosis or dementia; the pathological changes associated with this clinical state in certain respects resemble those of Wilson's disease. Repeated or prolonged bouts of hepatic failure increase the risk of permanent neurological changes, and in some cases clinical evidence of cerebral damage only becomes obvious after undergoing some form of surgical portal–systemic anastomosis.

Liver lesions. The clinicopathological syndrome has been associated with various types of liver disease, most commonly postnecrotic cirrhosis (including posthepatitis and toxic cases) but also portal cirrhosis, biliary cirrhosis, hepatoma and chronic hepatitis. One patient, in whom neurological signs followed the creation of an Eck fistula during an excision of a carcinoma of pancreas, showed only fatty degeneration of liver at necropsy.

Macroscopic cerebral lesions. Patchy, diffuse, bilateral, band-like, grey-white discoloration in the deeper cerebral cortex or the junction of cortex and white matter, particularly in the parietal and occipital regions, is the most obvious feature. Mild to moderate cortical atrophy and atrophy or focal softening of the basal ganglia have also been noted.

Microscopic cerebral lesions. Victor *et al.* described three main findings: diffuse increase in the size and number of protoplasmic astrocytes; intranuclear inclusions (mainly glycogen) in astrocytes; and diffuse but patchy degeneration of neurons and myelin, especially in the deeper cortex and subcortex, basal ganglia and cerebellum. The abnormal astrocytes were of the Alzheimer type II variety, with large, pale, occasionally lobulated or irregular nuclei, one or two nucleoli and a distinct nuclear membrane, along the outer surface of which lipofuscin-like pigment granules were often seen. Cell cytoplasm was not visible or very scanty in sections stained by routine methods. These astrocytes were most numerous in the deeper cerebral cortex but were also found in variable numbers throughout the basal ganglia, hypothalamus, brainstem, cerebellum and even spinal grey matter. Giant Alzheimer type I astrocytes were rarely seen. The intranuclear glycogen inclusions were easily demonstrated with the periodic acid-Schiff reaction or with Best's carmine stain. In some cases degeneration and loss of neurons and myelin in the deeper cortex were associated with pronounced microcavitation that had a pseudolaminar or laminar distribution, sometimes extending into the subcortical white matter. In places, loss of neurons involved the whole cortex and then microcavitation was not a feature. A variable degree of neuronal loss was usually present in the basal ganglia, together with microcavitation (mainly in the putamen) when cortical cavitation was present. Victor *et al.* also found many Opalski cells in the cerebral cortex and basal ganglia and noted a transition from obvious neurons to Opalski forms.

Shiraki (1968) found central pontine myelinolysis (see p. 150) in cases of acquired hepatocerebral degeneration and in Wilson's disease, which supports the suggestion of Adams, Victor and Mancall (1959) that the pontine disease may result from liver damage. Shiraki also noted that cerebral damage suggestive of 'circulatory inadequacy' and ischaemia were commonly found in all forms of hepatocerebral disease.

Peripheral nerve lesions. Dayan and Williams (1967) found evidence of segmental demyelination in teased single peripheral nerve fibres from ten patients suffering from hepatic failure due to various causes. Clinical evidence of neuropathy was not always present. Patients with clinical signs (sensory impairment, diminished tendon jerks) included all patients with alcoholic cirrhosis and one with haemochromatosis; in these instances multiple factors had to be considered, though alcohol is an unlikely cause of segmental demyelination. It was concluded that the metabolic effects of hepatic failure, perhaps related to disturbed carbohydrate metabolism, were the most likely basis for the neuropathy.

Knill-Jones, Goodwill, Dayan and Williams (1972) studied 14 similar patients with various forms of chronic liver disease and confirmed the presence of indolent demyelination and remyelination; Wallerian-type degeneration was less frequently seen. The occurrence of the neuropathy could not be correlated with either the duration of liver disease or the results of liver function tests, though affected patients showed high immunoglobulin (IgA and IgM) levels. It was concluded that causal factors other than diabetes or excessive alcohol intake were responsible and that collateral shunting of portal blood was important because of the interference with hepatic detoxification which ensues.

Biochemical findings. Liver function tests are invariably abnormal. The blood ammonia levels usually rise to extreme heights during hepatic coma and between such attacks are usually elevated. Serum copper and caeruloplasmin levels and urinary copper excretion are consistently normal. The copper content of fresh brain tissue has also been normal or nearly so (Victor *et al.*).

Although acquired hepatocerebral degeneration and Wilson's disease have features in common there are differences, particularly in the distribution and prominence of the various features. In Wilson's disease the basal ganglia tend to be more affected than the cerebral cortex, but this is not invariable. Necrosis of the lentiform nucleus seems only to occur with Wilson's disease. The presence of Opalski cells and intranuclear glycogen inclusions in astrocytes is not confined to either disease, though in acquired hepatocerebral degeneration the inclusions are more numerous and Opalski cells are less numerous than in Wilson's

disease. Because of the qualitative similarity of the lesions in the two diseases, Victor *et al.* have questioned the role of copper deposition in the induction of the lesions in Wilson's disease. In some cases the clinical features of both processes tend to merge and then a distinction may depend on the family history, the presence or absence of a Kayser–Fleischer ring and the biochemical findings.

When the blood ammonia levels are raised over a long period of time, the function of the ammonium trapping mechanism through the glutamic acid/glutamine system may be interfered with. Accumulation of glutamine in the brain, indicated by raised CSF levels, has been described in man; also in rat brains after portocaval anastomosis by Cavanagh and Kyu (1971*a*, *b*) who found that type II Alzheimer cells were consistently produced if the plasma ammonia nitrogen levels were elevated for more than 5 weeks. Cavanagh and Kyu also noted that when a brain wound was made in these rats, cells resembling type I astrocytes appeared around the wound in numbers that were directly related to the plasma ammonia nitrogen levels. Furthermore, the DNA content of the type I nuclei appeared to be doubled, suggesting that such nuclei were tetraploid. It seemed that the changes leading to this appearance resembled the state of affairs induced in the mitotic spindle by colchicine; it was suggested that a disturbance of microtubular function, perhaps because of the ammonium ion accumulation or some conversion product of this, may be responsible for these changes. Cavanagh, Blakemore and Kyu (1971) studied the electron-microscope appearances of rat brain after portocaval anastomosis; changes (such as aggregates of 4 to 5 nm fibrils and hexagonal arrays of 20 nm tubular structures) were seen in the inner and outer cytoplasmic tongues of myelin sheaths and in the paranodal cytoplasmic loops which conformed with the latter hypothesis. Degeneration of the cerebellar cortex, resembling that described in human acquired hepatic encephalopathy, was also demonstrated in rats after portocaval anastomosis by Cavanagh, Lewis, Blakemore and Kyu (1972). Cellular abnormalities in the brain in liver disease were reviewed by Cavanagh (1972).

Hepatolenticular degeneration (Wilson's disease)

The term hepatolenticular degeneration was applied by Hall of Copenhagen in 1921 to a familial metabolic disease, due to an autosomal recessive gene, in which cirrhosis of the liver is associated with degeneration of the corpus striatum; in both sites there is a great excess of copper, and brown granules containing the metal are also present in the outer zone of the cornea (Kayser–Fleischer ring) in most cases. The disease usually appears towards the end of the second decade but occasional cases have begun in the first decade and onset in the third and fourth decade is not unusual. In untreated cases the duration of the illness is usually between 3 and 10 years but it may be considerably longer. The onset occasionally follows, at an interval of months or years, an attack of febrile jaundice which may be transient. In many instances the hepatic cirrhosis remains occult throughout the course of the disease but there may be variable ascites, swelling of the ankles and/or spleno-megaly. A heavy urinary excretion of amino acids, including types that are not usually found in hepatic cirrhosis, has been noted in the majority of cases.

Clinically there is progressive rigidity and coarse tremor of the limbs, a spastic condition of the face, mouth and pharynx, causing dysarthria and dysphagia and, in the terminal stages of the disease, some degree of dementia.

Historical. Kinnier Wilson (1912) reported six cases with three necropsies and added eight more from the literature. Two or three members of some families were affected but there was no other evidence of hereditary transmission. Hoesslin and Alzheimer (1912) reported a case with full post-mortem examination and termed the condition *pseudosclerosis*. In addition to cirrhosis of the liver, they found widespread degenerative changes in the brain, especially in the striatum; they emphasized the presence in all the degenerated areas of large astrocytes with swollen, vesicular and sometimes multiple nuclei which are now named after Alzheimer (see below). Fleischer (1909, 1912) found the corneal ring of brown pigmentation, which had first been described by Kayser (1902) and himself (1903), in cases of pseudosclerosis associated with cirrhosis of the liver. These various observations were collated by Hall (1921), who added 53 further cases from the literature and four personal cases. In some of these, the lesions were widespread in the brain, involving the cerebral cortex, the other basal ganglia and brainstem nuclei and

the dentate nucleus and superior cerebellar peduncle; but lesions were always most severe in the striatum. Opalski (1930) subsequently described the large phagocytic cells that bear his name, and Haurowitz (1930) and Lüthy (1931) found an excess of copper in both corpus striatum and liver. By 1948, Denny-Brown had found over 150 case reports in the literature and, with Uzman, described the amino aciduria that so often occurs in the disease (Uzman and Denny-Brown 1948). For further details see Cumings (1959), Walshe (1966), Scheinberg and Sternlieb (1965), Schulman (1968), Bergsma (1968) and Bearn (1972).

Pathological changes. The brain usually shows no external abnormality except some sinking-in of the insular cortex. On section the corpus striatum appears shrunken, especially in its middle third, so that on horizontal section the outline of its external border is sinuous, resembling a Cupid's bow. This is less obvious in coronal sections in which the outline is flatter than normal and at some levels may even be concave. The corpus striatum, and sometimes the subthalamic nucleus, have a brownish or brick-red colour according to the duration of formalin fixation. Cavitation is often found in the putamen. In milder form cavitation is chiefly perivascular, but when severe may involve most of the central and anterior parts of the putamen and spread into the caudate nucleus. Very rarely it has been found in other nuclei such as the thalamus and red nucleus (Howard and Royce 1919). The central white matter of the cerebral and cerebellar hemispheres may also show spongy softening or cavitation and the overlying cortex may then be atrophic (Schulman 1968).

Histology. The putamen shows, in most cases, increased cellularity due chiefly to proliferation of astrocytic nuclei. Many of these are larger and more vesicular than normal with one or more basophilic nucleoli, so that they may resemble the nuclei of small nerve cells. Some are considerably larger than this, up to 15 μm in their maximal diameter, and are surrounded by fine yellow-brown granules which appear to be enclosed in tenuous processes. It is not clear whether the granules correspond to the copper-containing cytoplasmic material demonstrated histochemically by Uzman (1956). These nuclei belong to cells of Alzheimer type II, which do not form neuroglial fibres. Large multinucleated cells of Alzheimer's type I are much rarer and are not present in every case; Lapham (1962) demonstrated that such cells had double the normal amount of nuclear DNA. This was confirmed in rats with portocaval shunts and brain wounds (Cavanagh and Kyu 1971a); the reactive astrocytes of such animals are very similar to human type I astrocytes and their nuclear DNA is near-tetraploid, suggesting a 'colchicine-like' interference with nuclear division in hepatic dysfunction. Scharenberg and Drew (1954) studied Alzheimer-type astrocytes by metallic impregnation methods and showed that their cytoplasm and processes are more prominent than routine stains suggest. Both in the putamen and caudate nucleus there is a general reduction in the number of both the large and the small neurons. In some cases this loss falls most heavily on the large neurons, in others on the small neurons, and it varies greatly in degree. There is also a diffuse reaction in the number of myelinated fibres in the corpus striatum. When cavities are present they have ragged edges which show little evidence of reactive scarring by either neuroglial or collagen fibres. Lipophages and siderophages in variable numbers are seen in relation to cavities; old or recent haemorrhages (occasionally extensive) have been described. Lüthy (1931) and Lichtenstein and Gore (1955) found pericapillary concretions which stained heavily for copper in the putamen.

The globus pallidus consistently shows less change, though there is a reduction in the number of its myelinated fibres, and Alzheimer type II nuclei and Opalski cells are usually seen; cystic transformation is rare. In the subthalamic nucleus also, Alzheimer-type astrocytes and Opalski cells may be present and there is often degeneration and loss of neurons. Focal degeneration of the cerebral cortex is not uncommon, especially in the frontal lobes. There may be areas of hypermyelination, status spongiosus or diffuse loss of nerve cells and fibres, both in the cortex and the white matter of the convolutions (Barnes and Hurst 1926). In the thalamus and the nuclei of the brainstem, Alzheimer and Opalski cells may be found. Phagocytes containing iron pigment are commonly found in the globus pallidus and substantia nigra. In the latter nucleus, Lichtenstein and Gore (1955) found unilateral scarring but this is unusual. Degeneration of the dentate nucleus, often associated with Marchi or sudanophilic degeneration of the superior cerebellar peduncle, has been found in a number of cases (Greenfield, Poynton and Walshe 1924).

Careful examination will usually show a variable degree of involvement of the cerebral and cerebellar cortices and white matter, similar to that in the lentiform nucleus, but usually less severe, cystic change being uncommon. The brainstem and spinal cord are rarely affected and only to a limited extent. Victor, Adams and Cole (1965) showed that lesions identical to those found in Wilson's disease can occur with other varieties of cirrhosis in which copper metabolism is not affected; they therefore question the causative effect of copper accumulation, though Popoff, Budzilovich, Goodgold and Feigin (1965) came to the opposite conclusion.

Opalski cells. Opalski (1930) described an unusual cell-type which he found only in cases of hepatolenticular degeneration. These are large cells the nuclei of which are small when compared to the size of the perikarya (in contrast to Alzheimer's glial cells). Opalski cells are oval or rounded, without processes and have a finely granular or slightly foamy cytoplasm, staining a light-rose colour by Nissl's method. The small nucleus is usually oval and central and more darkly-stained than that of Alzheimer type II cells. Very rarely a larger nucleus is present or the cells are multinucleated. Regressive changes in the nucleus and cytoplasm in which the nucleus lies peripherally and the cytoplasm is vacuolated are frequently seen. These cells are very much less frequent than Alzheimer type II cells and Opalski found them mainly in the thalamus, globus pallidus and zona reticulata of substantia nigra but very rarely in the striatum; their presence in hepatolenticular degeneration has been confirmed by numerous subsequent writers. Such cells measure up to 35 μm and stand out prominently when stained with Van Gieson's counterstain by the bright orange-brown colour and rounded outline of the cell body (Fig. 4.7). In the lentiform nuclei they are usually found in relation to foci of degeneration and in association with Alzheimer glia; they are less common in the cerebral cortex and elsewhere in the basal ganglia, though we have seen them in the subthalamus (Fig. 4.7). Their origin is uncertain and they have been regarded as degenerate neurons (Victor *et al.*) or derivatives of either astrocytes (Opalski) or phagocytes (Greenfield 1963).

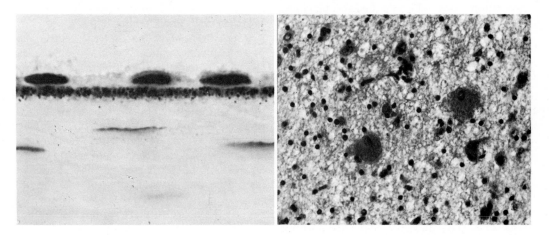

Fig. 4.6 (*left*) Kayser-Fleischer zone of pigment in Descemet's membrane. The pigment lies in the inner layer of the membrane with a few granules more deeply.   × 1200.
Fig. 4.7 (*right*) Opalski cells in subthalamic nucleus. Their cytoplasm is stained a light brown in iron haematoxylin-Van Gieson preparations.   × 250.

Kayser–Fleischer ring. Sections of the cornea show a row of granules of brown pigment in Descemet's membrane near the limbus of the cornea. In some cases the granules appear to lie almost on the inner surface of the membrane but they usually spread into it and never into its endothelial cell covering. They do not give a Prussian blue reaction for iron and do not bleach like melanin granules with oxidizing agents. Brand and Takáts (1951) and Howell (1959) found that the pigment gave the staining reactions of copper with rubeanic acid (black on greenish background) and rhodanin (reddish-brown) and they have been shown to contain copper by spectroscopic analysis (Gerlach and Rohrschneider 1934). In some cases a sunflower cataract, such as is seen when fragments of copper enter the eye, is found in cases of hepatolenticular degeneration (Steger and Steger 1954) (Fig. 4.6). The electron-microscope appearances are described by Uzman and Jakus (1957).

The liver. In the early stages of the disease hepatomegaly may occur, though there is usually atrophy at its termination, when the liver is coarsely cirrhotic with lobules which may vary in size from 1 mm to 2 cm or more. In some cases most are of small size, in others they are coarser than in portal cirrhosis. The colour varies in different cases and the individual lobules may also vary, some being yellow, others brick red, greenish or brown. This appears to be due to differences in the amount of copper storage, fatty degeneration or bile staining. Microscopically the characteristic appearances of multi-lobular cirrhosis are seen, but the fibrous septa are often less heavily collagenous than in most chronic cirrhotic livers, and may contain peri-vascular collections of lymphocytes and numerous small bile-ducts. In some early cases the appearances have been those of subacute hepatitis. Okinawa, Yoshikawa, Toyoda, Mozai, Toyokura and Kamiyama (1954) and Howell (1959) found granules in the liver cells which gave the reactions of copper with rubeanic acid and rhodanin; they varied in number in different lobules. Iron-containing pigment and bile pigment are also often present. Anderson and Popper (1960) studied 19 cases in detail and noted that marked glycogen infiltration of nuclei was an early and typical feature and that the cirrhosis was post-necrotic in type.

Changes in other organs. The spleen is often enlarged, congested and firmer than normal, with fibrosis of the pulp and trabeculae secondary to portal hypertension; in many cases, in which hepatic cirrhosis has been clinically silent, it has shown no abnormality. Böttiger and Möllerberg (1959) described cardiomegaly in this disease; histology showed coarse dark intracellular pigment, which failed to give the staining reactions for iron, around the nuclei of the cardiac muscle cells. Various forms of skeletal disease may occur in association with Wilson's disease including osteoporosis (Rosenoer and Mitchell 1959).

Biochemistry. The chief metabolic abnormality in hepatolenticular degeneration is failure to use the copper absorbed in excess from the intestines to synthesize the serum copper-carrying protein *caeruloplasmin.* Normally copper is taken up from the intestine in loose combination with albumin and after about 24 hours is transferred to globulin, to which it is more firmly bound (Earl, Moulton and Selverstone 1954; Bearn and Kunkel 1954). In the blood serum, copper is attached to the α, β and γ globulins in proportions of about 25%, 50% and 20% and only 2 to 5% remains attached to albumin. In hepatolenticular degeneration, on the other hand, only 40 to 60% of the total serum copper is bound to globulin, chiefly to the β and γ fractions; in four out of five cases Cumings, Goodwin and Earl (1955) found only traces of copper in combination with α-globulin. The remainder is loosely attached to albumin from which it more easily becomes detached and is either taken up by the proteins of the brain and liver or excreted by the kidneys. The urinary excretion therefore rises from the normal 10 to 100 μg Cu/day to amounts of 400 to 600 μg or even higher. Under treatment with BAL or the chelating agent penicillamine these figures may be greatly exceeded. Holmberg and Laurell (1948) isolated from human serum a blue protein substance in which copper was combined with α-globulin. They called this substance caeruloplasmin and found that, using *p*-phenylendiamine as a substrate, it could act as an oxidase. In hepatolenticular degeneration caeruloplasmin is normally absent or present in very small amounts and has no oxidase activity (Scheinberg and Gitlin 1952; Bearn and Kunkel 1954). In 2 out of 40 cases, however, Cumings (1962) found it present in normal quantity and there appears to be poor correlation between caeruloplasmin concentration and the duration and severity of the clinical course of the illness (Cartwright, Markowitz, Shields and Wintrobe 1960). The serum copper level was normal in 4 out of the 40 cases. The amount of serum caeruloplasmin may also be diminished in a patient's siblings who themselves show no sign of the disease (Turpin, Jerome and Schmitt 1953; Bush, Mahoney, Markowitz, Gubler, Cartwright and Wintrobe 1955). The physiology of copper in man and

its relation to Wilson's disease is reviewed by Walshe (1967) and Cumings (1972).

It has been suggested that the caeruloplasmin present in some patients with Wilson's disease is structurally and therefore functionally abnormal. Thus there may be two different alleles mediating the disease, one leading to failure of protein synthesis and one to abnormalities of protein structure: either could result in the same derangement of copper transport (*British Medical Journal* 1967). However, Holtzmann, Naughton, Iber and Gaumnitz (1967) studied the caeruloplasmin from a patient in whom the levels of the protein were near normal and found that the tryptic peptide map, electrophoretic analysis, amino acid and sugar composition, copper content and oxidase activity were all normal and not consistent with the theory that there is a structural abnormality of caeruloplasmin in Wilson's disease; they suggested that there was a reduced rate of caeruloplasmin synthesis in their patient, because treatment with penicillamine caused the protein to disappear from the plasma. Penicillamine lowers body copper stores, and caeruloplasmin synthesis in the normal individual may be stimulated by a fall in body copper. Although caeruloplasmin appears to prevent hepatolenticular degeneration, the precise way it does this remains obscure.

The increase of amino acids in the urine, which may reach 300 to 800 mg of amino acid nitrogen/day (about four to six times normal), affects all those normally present and the abnormal amino acids proline and citralline have also occasionally been found. There is no alteration in the amino acids of the blood serum and it is probable that the increased excretion is related to defective reabsorption in the convoluted tubules of the kidneys. The relation of amino aciduria to the abnormal copper metabolism is not clear. Excess of amino acids appears in the urine in other diseases of the liver, but only when its function is gravely disturbed as in acute yellow atrophy; it is rarely seen in cases of hepatic cirrhosis without jaundice. In hepatolenticular degeneration the amino aciduria is therefore quite out of proportion to the disturbance of liver function, which is usually slight and in many cases is not evident on routine testing. Plasma inorganic phosphate and urate concentrations are reduced and there may be proteinuria, glycosuria, hypercalcuria and hyperphosphaturia (Eastham and Jancar 1968). In untreated cases the blood pyruvate concentrations are increased and pyruvate tolerance is abnormal after glucose ingestion; treatment with penicillamine reverts these features.

Encephalopathy and fatty degeneration of the viscera (Reye's syndrome)

First reported in 1929 by Brain, Hunter and Turnbull, the clinical and pathological features have only recently been defined (Reye, Morgan and Baral 1963; Mowat 1973). The onset is acute, with vomiting, convulsions, disturbance of consciousness and coma. Children of 2 months to 15 years have been affected and about 50% show clinical hepatomegaly. Mortality estimates have varied from 20 to 80% and many survivors show CNS sequelae such as mental impairment, fits or hemiplegia.

The main biochemical findings are high transaminase concentrations, often with hypoglycaemia and prolonged prothrombin time. The CSF is usually normal though the sugar content may be low when hypoglycaemia occurs.

The brain shows severe oedema, usually with anoxic neuronal damage but no inflammatory infiltration or demyelination. The liver is swollen, greasy, shows severe periportal fatty infiltration and in fatal cases (as opposed to biopsy material) is often necrotic. Renal tubules and heart also show fatty infiltration and acute renal failure may occur.

The syndrome is probably commoner than realized and may be misdiagnosed as 'status epilepticus', 'toxic encephalopathy' or 'encephalitis with normal CSF' (*Lancet* 1974).

No infectious, toxic or metabolic agent has been identified. Minor outbreaks occurring over fairly wide areas have been described, suggesting the possibility of an environmental factor. Poisoning by aflatoxin produced by the fungus *Aspergillus flavus* or the viruses of influenza B and varicella have been implicated.

The high concentrations of ammonia in blood and CSF in the acute phase could account for the rapid progression of the encephalopathy. Disturbances of urea cycle pathways have also been proposed, similar to the inherited enzyme deficiency diseases which occur in neonates (*Lancet* 1974) and may be due to deficiency of the mitochondrial enzyme ornithine transcarbamylase, the kinetic properties of which may be altered. Treatment of the hyperammonaemia by liver failure regimens, peritoneal dialysis and exchange transfusion may be indicated if diagnosed early in the disease.

Infantile subacute necrotizing encephalopathy (Leigh's disease)

This disease of infancy, which is sometimes familial, has attracted increasing attention since it was first described by Leigh (1951). The illness is progressive and usually of a few months' duration. When familial, transmission is usually as a Mendelian recessive. A chronic form (Christensen, Melchior and Plum 1963) and adult cases (Harman, Allen, Baughman and Waterman 1968; Feigin and Goebel 1969) have been described.

The chief clinical features in infants are failure to thrive, diarrhoea, immobility, hypotonia or spasticity, absent reflexes, optic atrophy and convulsions (Crome and Stern 1972).

Multiple foci of neuronal degeneration, microglial and astrocytic proliferation, and overgrowth of capillaries are found in the thalamus, subthalamic nuclei and substantia nigra, and in the grey matter of the pons and medulla (Dayan, Ockenden and Crome 1970). There are comparable changes in the posterior columns of the spinal cord. Occasionally, there may be involvement of the corpus striatum, the cerebral cortex, and the white matter of the cerebral and cerebellar hemispheres. The proliferation of capillaries that is so characteristic of the condition suggested the possibility that it might be a chronic form of Wernicke's disease (see p. 196), but the corpora mamillaria have been involved only exceptionally.

Instances of what appears pathologically to be the same disease have recently been reported in siblings (Worsley, Brookfield, Elwood, Noble and Taylor 1965); the clinical manifestations were hyperpnoea, progressive ataxia and convulsions, and these were associated with acidosis (due to excessive glycolytic formation of lactic acid), renal aciduria and hypophosphataemia. The suggestion that an increase in the ratio of phosphorylated hexoses to free glucose in the blood may account in part for the increased rate of glycolysis awaits confirmation.

The disease may not be due to a simple metabolic defect and the biochemical changes so far recorded (lactic acidosis, or elevated plasma alanine, or raised blood acetoacetate and β-hydroxybutyrate) may be the result rather than the cause of the primary disease. For recent reviews see Pincus (1972) and Dunn and Dolman (1972).

The Hallervorden–Spatz syndrome

This disorder was originally described in 1922 by Hallervorden and Spatz. Approximately sixty verified cases have been described to date; it is, however, difficult to give an exact figure, since the position of some cases in the group is still uncertain. In this total are included a few cases described before 1922 and identified retrospectively: a case of Fischer (1911), the macroscopically investigated case of Rothmann (1915) and the case, Oscar M., of the Vogts (1920).

Reviews include those of Kalinowsky (1936), Peters (1951), Eicke (1957), Dreese and Netsky (1968) and Jellinger (1973).

Clinically the condition is characterized by progressive rigidity, first in the lower and later in the upper extremities; an equinovarus deformity of the foot has been recorded as the first presenting sign in several cases. Rigidity is often preceded or accompanied by choreic or athetoid movements, more rarely by torsion dystonia. Both rigidity and involuntary movements may extend to the muscles of the face, tongue and palate, resulting in difficulties in articulation and swallowing. Progressive mental deterioration is a frequent, though not constant manifestation. Epileptic convulsions have been reported only occasionally (Meyer 1963). In most cases the onset was in the first or second decade, and death usually occurred before the thirtieth year of life. Later onset has been recorded by Onari (1925), Hallervorden (1930) and Eicke. Jellinger recognizes three types according to the age of onset: *late infantile* (3 months to 6 years), *classic* (7 to 15 years, duration 6 to 30 years with death at 12 to 39 years) and *adult or late* (22 to 64 years, duration 1 to $7\frac{1}{2}$ years).

In 14 reports the condition was found to be familial (Jellinger) with frequent incidence in other siblings, though infrequent incidence in the ancestors or wider family. Hallervorden and Spatz described a clinically identical condition in five of nine siblings; three more siblings had died early from unknown causes. Onset in the cases they described was between 7 and 9 years, with death occurring at the ages of 16 to 27. Of these one brain was fully investigated, while sections from a second brain revealed identical pathological changes. Familial cases with post-

mortem findings have been reported by Winkelman (1932), Kalinowsky (1927), Urechia *et al.* (1950) and Messing (quoted from Eicke). Eicke also includes the familial cases briefly reported by Fischer (1933), but these were complicated and Fischer himself considered them to be examples of a new syndrome. Other familial cases are listed by Jellinger.

Pathological changes. On macroscopic inspection of the brain a rust-brown discoloration of the globus pallidus and the reticular zone of the substantia nigra is a striking finding in most cases. This discoloration is caused by a great increase of the normal pigment in these areas. In its natural state the pigment has a yellowish-brown colour and, with thionin or cresyl violet, stains in shades of yellow, green and blue. It may be intracellular, in nerve cells, hyperplastic astrocytes, and microglial cells, or may lie free in the tissue, usually as large granules surrounding the blood vessels. Part of it gives a strong iron reaction; it is PAS positive and also often includes sudanophil lipid; reactions for neuraminic acid and acid fastness are negative. This striking picture is in almost all cases enhanced by the presence of strongly siderophilic incrustations of the medium-sized blood vessels and capillaries and of free-lying mulberry concretions (so-called pseudo-calcium).

Apart from the consistent pigmentary increase the other changes within the pallido-reticular zone are more variable. Severe degeneration and loss of nerve cells has been reported in some cases; in others, particularly in familial cases, this may be slight or negligible. Demyelination, particularly of the fine fibres, is usually present, but may be absent in some cases. Proliferation of astrocytes and fibrous gliosis is found in most cases, though to a variable degree.

The finding of large oval or round bodies (spheroids) staining faintly with thionin and lying between the extracellular pigment granules has aroused some discussion: the spheroids are now regarded, as was originally suggested by Hallervorden and Spatz, as being derived from swollen axons. Their occurrence may be widespread beyond the pallido-reticular zone. A histochemical analysis shows them to contain mucoprotein, according to Seitelberger and Gross (1957) and Gross *et al.* (1957), who suggested the term 'neuro-axonal mucoprotoid dystrophy' for the condition. Variable amounts of lipid and carbohydrate have also been identified histochemically and are detailed by Jellinger. Neither the axonal changes nor the pigment deposits alone are regarded by these authors as specific signs; in combination, however, they consider them to have considerable diagnostic value.

Eicke described a remarkable increase of capillaries in the reticular zone in one of his cases: although the resemblance to Wernicke's encephalopathy was striking, the mamillary bodies and other predilective sites of the latter syndrome were not affected.

In many cases histological changes in other parts of the brain and in the spinal cord have been reported, but again they vary greatly in intensity and were slight in some of the familial cases. Hallervorden and Spatz described loss of nerve cells in the cerebral cortex and the Purkinje cell layer of the cerebellum; this finding has been confirmed in other cases. Jervis (1952) found pigment, histochemically indistinguishable from that of the pallido-reticular zone, in the cortex of a case in which the Hallervorden–Spatz syndrome was associated with amaurotic family idiocy. The striatum was found to be involved by Kalinowsky and Onari. The corpus Luysii showed considerable demyelination and gliosis in the cases of the Vogts and that of Meyer and Earl (1936) who also reported gliosis in the dentate nucleus and inferior olives. Retinitis pigmentosa accounted for visual disturbances in the cases of Winkelman (1932), Kalinowsky (1927) and Helfand (1935). Degeneration of the pyramidal tract was seen in five, and of the posterior tracts of the spinal cord in two cases.

Diagnosis and nosology. Although the clinical observation of progressive rigidity with or without involuntary movements and mental deterioration, commencing towards the middle or end of the first decade, may suggest the Hallervorden–Spatz syndrome, a reasonably certain diagnosis can only be made *post mortem*.

Differential diagnosis from the clinically similar progressive juvenile striato-pallidal (Hunt 1917), pallidal and pallido-Luysial (van Bogaert 1946) syndromes is pathologically straightforward. In these conditions the pigment is not appreciably increased, nor is the reticular zone affected.

The separation of the Hallervorden–Spatz syndrome from *état dysmyélinique* of the Vogts presents greater difficulties. In fact, earlier investigators (Hallervorden and Spatz (1922); Hallervorden (1930); Meyer and Earl) more or less identified the two conditions. It is now increasingly realized, however, that *état dysmyélinique* is ill-defined and includes, in addition to possible cases of the Hallervorden–Spatz syndrome, conditions caused by anoxia and injury at birth, by rhesus-factor incompatibility and by other infantile diseases. In such cases the lesions appear soon after birth, are not markedly progressive, and are usually severe and widespread. In contrast, in what is now held to be the Hallervorden–Spatz syndrome, onset is usually towards the second half of the first decade, is preceded by normal development, and progression is marked. The important lesions are more or less confined to the pallidum and the reticular zone; when lesions occur elsewhere they are, on the whole, variable or slight. Within the pallido-reticular zone, emphasis is on the striking increase of pigment rather than on neuronal degeneration. The condition thus approximates to a 'system disease' (though in the form of a localized storage of iron-containing deposits rather than of degeneration), to which Helfand (1935) has given the name of 'status pigmentosus'. Most of the familial cases and some of the sporadic cases (e.g. those of Helfand; Vincent and van Bogaert (1936); and two cases of Eicke) would correspond to this description.

This more restricted definition of the syndrome renders the position of some of the remaining sporadic cases dubious. It is probably no coincidence that in seven of these, almost half of their total, onset was at or soon after birth (Eicke). Their claim to inclusion in the syndrome should therefore be submitted to further scrutiny. Meyer and Earl's case may serve as an example: owing to poor history, no definite statement could be made as to whether the case was sporadic or familial nor whether there had been progression. It is likely, however, that onset had been soon after birth. Selective involvement of globus pallidus and zona reticularis was striking; nerve-cell loss, demyelination and gliosis were severe but pigmentary increase was only moderate. Additional lesions were described in the corpus Luysii, dentate nucleus and inferior olives, a combination which recalled, as the authors noted, the pathology of kernicterus.

Increase of pigment in the globus pallidus and substantia nigra has been reported in other conditions, ranging from central neurofibromatosis (Gamper 1929), myopathies (Hallervorden), dementia praecox (Fünfgeld 1929-30) and epidemic encephalitis (van Bogaert 1939-40) to rheumatic encephalopathy (Benda 1949) and amaurotic family idiocy (Jervis). In each instance the increase was definitely outside the physiological range. In at least one of Benda's cases, and in Jervis's case, the amount of pigment was similar to that described in Hallervorden and Spatz' original publication. Hallervorden suggested that in such circumstances the pigment increase usually is not associated with neuronal or glial changes, but such changes may also be slight in some cases of otherwise indisputable Hallervorden–Spatz syndrome. The question arises, therefore, whether status pigmentosus may be precipitated by other conditions (Benda), or whether there may be a coincidence of two independent conditions, as suggested by Jervis. A relationship to lipid storage diseases seems to have been suggested in some instances and is supported by the histochemical observations of Zeman and Scarpelli (1958), who found widespread ganglioside and sphingomyelin deposits in nerve cells and ependymal cells in two cases of Hallervorden–Spatz disease. The neurons in the corpus striatum, in the fifth and sixth layers of the cerebral cortex and in the reticular substance were ballooned and their nuclei were eccentric.

Relation to infantile neuroaxonal dystrophy and other forms of neuroaxonal dystrophy (NAD)

Jellinger summarized convincing evidence that the spheroids in Hallervorden–Spatz disease are dystrophic axons and identical histologically to those seen in normal ageing human and animal brains; in infantile and late infantile NAD; following human head injury; and in various experimental situations in animals (e.g. vitamin E deficiency; triorthocresyl phosphate or imidodiproprionitrile poisoning). There are, however, minor histochemical differences in this wide range of conditions.

Electron-microscope studies show that the spheroids are granular and surrounded by a single unit membrane. They contain an increased number of cytoplasmic organelles, including normal and enlarged mitochondria, electron-dense patches, vesicles, increased neurofilaments, and accumulations of smooth membranes and tubular and cisternal profiles. Many spheroids show a whorled arrangement of layered smooth membranes and vesiculo-tubular structures, 28 to 40 nm in diameter. The arrangement of the tubulo-membranous systems varies from tightly

packed, whorled lamellae to loose aggregates of hollow cisternae and longitudinal clefts surrounded by neurofilaments (Jellinger). The spheroids probably arise mainly in preterminal axons of ascending fibres, presynaptic areas participating in axodendritic and axoaxonal synaptic complexes, and even in neuromuscular junctions, according to the underlying cause. Tubulomembranous material and abnormal mitochondria may also be found in neuronal perikarya and dendrites.

As random findings in normal ageing human and animal brains, dystrophic axons occur most constantly in Goll's nucleus and in the dorsomedial and dorsomarginal parts of the gracile nucleus; the cuneate, trigeminal and vestibular nuclei, and the grey matter, posterior columns and Clarke's column of the spinal cord are less often affected. In infantile and late infantile NAD the spheroids are generalized throughout the central, peripheral and autonomic nervous systems. In Hallervorden–Spatz disease spheroids are found mainly in the pallidum and reticular part of the substantia nigra and in smaller and variable numbers in the subthalamic nucleus, medullary tegmentum, cerebral cortex, other basal ganglia and spinal cord. The distribution of spheroids in various experimental situations is summarized by Jellinger.

Seitelberger (1971) distinguishes the following types of NAD in man:

(i) infantile NAD (Seitelbergers disease);
(ii) late infantile NAD (also described as late infantile type of Hallervorden–Spatz disease);
(iii) juvenile form of generalized NAD;
(iv) neuroaxonal leucoencephalopathy;
(v) Hallervorden–Spatz disease (juvenile and adult types);
(vi) presenile NAD and Hallervorden–Spatz disease in other disorders.

As pallido-nigral hyperpigmentation associated with NAD have now been described in many different conditions such as chronic CNS disease in childhood (Fadiloglu 1971), Friedreich's ataxia (Netsky, Spiro and Zimmerman 1951), pallido-nigral-subthalamic atrophy (Contamin, Escourolle, Nick and Mignot 1971), Parkinsonism (van Bogaert 1939-40), spongy dystrophy (Jellinger and Seitelberger 1969), etc., the status of Hallervorden–Spatz disease as a clear-cut entity is open to criticism. Typical Hallervorden–

Spatz disease is probably a genetically determined disease; the other listed conditions that show similar structural lesions may be considered as presenile forms of NAD (category (vi) of Seitelberger) due to the effect of exogenous agencies on pallido-nigral axons.

To summarize, NAD seems to represent a nonspecific response of axons to chronic injury, either genetically induced (endogenous) or exogenous. The tubulomembranous structures that accumulate in affected axons closely resemble smooth endoplasmic reticulum. The posterior column nuclei and a few other clearly defined regions are affected 'naturally' as an ageing change (regional predilection). Lesions in other sites occur only in association with various diseases or under experimental conditions: in these circumstances spheroids will be found prematurely and in excess, and the distribution will tend to vary according to the predisposing condition; the sites of regional predilection may also be involved in excess of normal. Classical Hallervorden–Spatz disease is regarded as an example of endogenous NAD occurring prematurely and excessively at the sites of regional predilection.

The distribution and time relationship of dystrophic axons and their association with other lesions are probably determined by the underlying disease or the conditions of the experiment. There is at present no satisfactory general explanation of the basic pathogenetic process that determines the appearance of spheroids and it is not unlikely that several different mechanisms may determine this type of axonal reaction: metabolic or enzymatic axoplasmic deficiencies, axonal injury with redistribution of axoplasm, stasis of axonal flow, altered metabolic activity at axonal terminals with overproduction of smooth endoplasmic reticulum, axoplasmic regeneration, or alterations of synaptic end-complexes have all been proposed as pathogenetic explanations (see Jellinger for details).

West Indian, Indian and African neuromyelopathy

A variety of neuromyelopathy that closely resembles the rare form of neurosyphilis, in which degeneration of the lateral and posterior tracts of the spinal cord is accompanied by variable degrees of periarteritis and arachnoiditis (so-called 'spastic paraplegia of Erb'), has been recognized in the Caribbean region (Montgomery, Cruickshank, Robertson and McMenemey 1964; Robertson and Cruickshank 1972). Its cause is uncertain but a resemblance to neurolathyrism has supported the possibility that ingested toxins may be responsible; other suggested causes include dietary deficiency, an obscure inflammatory process or a multifactorial background. The process may not be a single entity because a comparable syndrome has been recognized in India (Main, Main and Montgomery 1969); in West Africa neuromyelopathy also occurs but sensory neuropathy is commoner than paraplegia (Money 1959; Haddock, Ebrahim and Kapur 1962). Thus, though there are certain resemblances, the view that West Indian, Indian and African neuromyelopathies are variants of the same disorder is not at present fully justified. It has been observed that in parts of Nigeria, a cassava-containing diet is related to the incidence of ataxic sensory neuropathy and because cassava has a relatively high cyanide content it may be that the disorder has some connection with cyanide intoxication (Osuntokun, Monekosso and Wilson 1969; Osuntokun, Langman and Wilson 1970).

The clinical features include weakness and unsteadiness of gait, numbness and burning of the feet and legs and, less commonly, formication or pain in the limbs. Deafness and poor vision are also common. In older patients, spasticity and other upper motor neuron lesions are more common than ataxia and posterior column defects.

Histologically, most cases show inflammatory changes of varying severity, mainly perivascular cuffing with lymphocytes, plasma cells and histiocytes. There is reactive fibroblastic proliferation around blood vessels and in the pia arachnoid. Nerve roots and ganglia and the appropriate cranial nerves usually show inflammatory changes in patients with visual or hearing loss. Loss of myelin is found in the lateral pyramidal tracts, the posterior columns and the spinocerebellar tracts (Robertson and Cruickshank). The spinal grey matter usually shows inflammatory changes and neuronal degeneration. Similar but less severe lesions are often present in the cerebral hemispheres, brainstem and cerebellum. In long-standing cases evidence of active inflammation may be less pronounced, though adventitial and leptomeningeal fibrosis may be prominent and has been attributed to previous burnt-out inflammation. Thickening and opacity of the leptomeninges is often recognizable macro-scopically, particularly in the basal cisterns.

Although the disease often shows a histological resemblance to meningovascular neurosyphilis it is not associated with appropriate CSF and serological changes (Robertson and Cruickshank). Furthermore, Argyll Robertson pupils are not present and there is resistance to penicillin therapy.

The aminoacidurias

Pathological changes affecting the nervous system occur in a number of the aminoacidurias, including phenylketonuria, maple syrup urine disease and a number of other rare metabolic disorders. An excellent account of these is given by Crome and Stern (1972), pp. 352-401, to which the reader is referred.

References

Adams, R. D. & Foley, J. M. (1953) The neurological disorder associated with liver disease. *Research Publications, Association for Research in Nervous and Mental Diseases*, **32**, 198-237.

Adams, R. D., Victor, M. & Mancall, E. L. (1959) Central pontine myelinosis. *Archives of Neurology and Psychiatry*, **81**, 154-172.

Aghajanian, G. K. & Bloom, E. F. (1967) Electronmicroscopic localisation of tritiated norepinephrine in the rat brain: effect of drugs. *Journal of Pharmacology and Experimental Therapeutics*, **156**, 407-416.

Aguayo, A. J. & Hudson, P. (1970) Observations on the short term effects of chloroquine on skeletal muscle. An experimental study in the rabbit. *Journal of the Neurological Sciences*, **11**, 301-325.

Akelaitis, A. J. (1941) Lead encephalopathy in children and adults; clinicopathological study. *Journal of Nervous and Mental Diseases*, **93**, 313-332.

Aleu, F. P., Katzman, R. & Terry, R. D. (1963) Fine structure and electrolyte analysis of cerebral oedema induced by alkyl tin intoxication. *Journal of Neuropathology and Experimental Neurology*, **22**, 403-413.

Allsop, J. & Turner, B. (1966) Cerebellar degeneration associated with chronic alcoholism. *Journal of the Neurological Sciences*, **3**, 238-258.

Andén, N. E., Dahlström, A., Fuxe, K. & Hökfelt, T. (1966) The effect of haloperidol and chlorpromazine and the amine levels of central monoamine neurons. *Acta physiologica scandinavica*, **68**, 419-420.

Anderson, P. J. & Popper, H. (1960) Changes in hepatic structure in Wilson's disease. *American Journal of Pathology*, **36**, 483-497.

Anthony, J. J. (1970) Malignant lymphoma associated with hydantoin drugs. *Archives of Neurology (Chicago)*, **22**, 450-454.

Aprison, M. H., Kariya, T., Hingtgen, N. & Toru, M. (1968) Neurochemical correlates of behavior. Changes in acetylcholine, norepinephrine and 5-hydroxytryptamine. *Journal of Neurochemistry*, **15**, 1131-1139.

Ayd, F. J. (1961) A survey of drug-induced extrapyramidal reactions. *Journal of the American Medical Association*, **175**, 1054-1060.

Baker, A. B. (1958) The nervous system in trichlorethylene intoxication. An experimental study. *Journal of Neuropathology and Experimental Neurology*, **17**, 649-655.

Bakir, F., Damluji, S. F., Amin-zaki, L., Murtadha, M., Khalidi, A. *et al.* (1973) Methylmercury poisoning in Iraq. *Science*, **181**, 230-241.

Barnes, S. & Hurst, E. W. (1926) A further note on hepatolenticular degeneration. *Brain*, **49**, 36-60.

Bearn, A. G. (1972) In *The Metabolic Basis of Inherited Disease* (Ed. Stanbury, J. B., Wyngaarden, J. B. & Fredrickson, D. S.), McGraw-Hill, New York.

Bearn, A. G. & Kunkel, H. G. (1954) Localization of Cu^{64} in serum fractions following oral administration: alteration in Wilson's disease. *Proceedings of the Society for Experimental Biology and Medicine*, **85**, 44-48.

Behar, A., Rachmilewitz, E., Rahamimoff, R. & Deman, M. (1965) Experimental nitrofurantoin neuropathy in rats. *Archives of Neurology*, **13**, 160-163.

Benda, C. E. (1949) Chronic rheumatic encephalitis, torsion dystonia and Hallervorden–Spatz disease. *Archives of Neurology and Psychiatry (Chicago)*, **61**, 137-163.

Bennett, I. L., Cary, F. H., Mitchell, G. L. & Cooper, M. N. (1953) Acute methyl alcohol poisoning. A review based on experiences in an outbreak of 323 cases. *Medicine (Baltimore)*, **32**, 431-463.

Bentley, H. R., McDermott, E. E. & Whitehead, J. K. (1950) Action of nitrogen trichloride on proteins: a synthesis of the toxic factor from methionine. *Nature*, **165**, 735.

Berggren, L. & Hansson, O. (1966) Treating acrodermatitis enteropathica. *Lancet*, **1**, 52.

Bergsma, D. (1968) *Wilson's Disease*, National Foundation for Birth Defects, Vol. 4, No. 2, Williams & Wilkins, Baltimore.

Bernstein, H. N. & Ginsberg, J. (1964) The pathology of chloroquine retinopathy. *Archives of Ophthalmology*, **71**, 238-245.

Biemond, A. & van Creveld, G.   (1939) Cerebellar form of encephalopathy due to lead poisoning.   *Acta paediatrica (Stockholm)*, **27**, 51-62.

Bini, L. & Bollea, G.   (1947) Fatal poisoning by lead benzene.   *Journal of Neuropathology and Experimental Neurology*, **6**, 271-278.

Bischoff, A.   (1970) Ultrastructure of triorthocresyl phosphate poisoning in the chicken.   2. Studies on the spinal cord alterations.   *Acta Neuropathologica (Berlin)*, **15**, 142-155.

Blackman, S. S. Jr.   (1937) The lesions of lead encephalitis in children.   *Bulletin of the Johns Hopkins Hospital*, **61**, 1-61.

Blakemore, W. F. & Cavanagh, J. B.   (1969) 'Neuroaxonal dystrophy' in an experimental 'dying-back' process in the rat.   *Brain*, **92**, 789-804.

Bohrod, M. G.   (1942) Primary degeneration of the corpus callosum (Marchiafava's disease).   *Archives of Neurology and Psychiatry (Chicago)*, **47**, 465-473.

Böttiger, L. E. & Möllerberg, H.   (1959) Increased copper content of hypertrophic myocardium.   *Acta medica scandinavica*, **165**, 413-416.

Bradley, W. G.   (1970) The neuropathy of vincristine in the guinea-pig.   An electrophysiological and pathological study.   *Journal of the Neurological Sciences*, **10**, 133-162.

Bradley, W. G., Lassman, L. P., Pearce, G. W. & Walton, J. M.   (1970) The neuromyopathy of vincristine in man.   Clinical, electrophysiological and pathological studies.   *Journal of the Neurological Sciences*, **10**, 107-131.

Brain, W. R., Hunter, D. & Turnbull, H. M.   (1929) Acute meningo-encephalomyelitis of childhood; report of six cases.   *Lancet*, **1**, 221-227.

Brand, I. & Takáts, I.   (1951) Histochemische untersuchung des Kayser-Fleischerschen Hornhautringes.   *Archiv für Ophthalmologie*, **151**, 391-398.

British Medical Journal   (1967) Leading article.   Blue blood.   **4**, 435-436.

British Medical Journal   (1971) Leading article.   Mercury in edible fish.   **1**, 126.

Brown, I. A.   (1954) Chronic mercurialism.   A cause of the syndrome of amyotrophic lateral sclerosis.   *Archives of Neurology and Psychiatry (Chicago)*, **72**, 674-681.

Brun, A. & Brunk, U.   (1967) Histochemical studies on brain phosphatases in experimental lead poisoning.   *Acta pathologica et microbiologica scandinavica*, **70**, 531-536.

Bush, J. A., Mahoney, J. P., Markowitz, H., Gubler, C. J., Cartwright, G. E. & Wintrobe, M. M.   (1955) Studies on copper metabolism.   XVI. Normal subjects and patients with hepatolenticular degeneration (radioactive copper).   *Journal of Clinical Investigation*, **34**, 1766-1768.

Burrows, N. F. E., Rendle-Short, J. & Hanna, D.   (1951) Lead poisoning in children; report of five cases, with special reference to pica.   *British Medical Journal*, **1**, 329-334.

Buxton, P. H. & Hayward, M.   (1967) Polyneuritis cranialis with industrial triethylene poisoning.   *Journal of Neurology, Neurosurgery and Psychiatry*, **30**, 511-518.

Cartwright, G. E., Markowitz, H., Shields, G. S. & Wintrobe, M. M.   (1960) Studies on copper metabolism.   XXIX. A critical analysis in normal patients and patients with Wilson's disease and their relatives.   *American Journal of Medicine*, **28**, 555-563.

Cavanagh, J. B.   (1954) The toxic effects of triorthocresyl phosphate poisoning on the nervous system.   *Journal of Neurology, Neurosurgery and Psychiatry*, **17**, 163-172.

Cavanagh, J. B.   (1964) The significance of the dying back process in experimental and human neurological disease.   *International Review of Experimental Pathology*, **3**, 219-267.

Cavanagh, J. B.   (1967) On the pattern of change in peripheral nerves produced by isoniazid intoxication in rats.   *Journal of Neurology, Neurosurgery and Psychiatry*, **30**, 26-33.

Cavanagh, J. B.   (1969) Toxic substances and the nervous system.   *British Medical Bulletin*, **25**, 268-273.

Cavanagh, J. B.   (1972) Cellular abnormalities in the brain in chronic liver disease in *The Scientific Basis of Medicine Annual Reviews*, pp. 238-247, Athlone Press, London.

Cavanagh, J. B.   (1973) Peripheral neuropathy caused by chemical agents.   *CRC Critical Reviews in Toxicology*, **2**, 365-417.

Cavanagh, J. B., Davies, D. R., Holland, P. & Lancaster, M.   (1961) Comparison of the functional effects of Dyflos, triorthocresyl phosphate and tri-p-ethyl-phenyl phosphate in chickens.   *British Journal of Pharmacology*, **17**, 21-27.

Cavanagh, J. B. & Holland, P.   (1961) Localisation of cholinesterases in the chicken nervous system and the problem of selective neurotoxicity of organophosphorus compounds.   *British Journal of Pharmacology*, **16**, 218-230.

Cavanagh, J. B., Chen, F. C., Kyu, M. H. & Ridley, A.   (1968) The experimental neuropathy in rats caused by p-bromophenylacetylurea.   *Journal of Neurology, Neurosurgery and Psychiatry*, **31**, 471-478.

Cavanagh, J. B. & Kyu, M. H. (1971a) On the mechanism of Type I Alzheimer abnormality in the nuclei of of rats subjected to porto-caval anastomosis. *Journal of the Neurological Sciences*, **14**, 143-152.

Cavanagh, J. B. & Kyu, M. H. (1971a) On the mechanism of Type I Alzheimer abnormality in the nuclei of astrocytes. *Journal of the Neurological Sciences*, **12**, 241-261.

Cavanagh, J. B. & Kyu, M. H. (1971b) Type II Alzheimer change experimentally produced in astrocytes in the rat. *Journal of the Neurological Sciences*, **12**, 63-75.

Cavanagh, J. B., Lewis, P. D., Blakemore, W. F. & Kyu, M. H. (1972) Changes in the cerebellar cortex in rats after porto-caval anastomosis. *Journal of the Neurological Sciences*, **15**, 13-26.

Cavanagh, J. B., Fuller, N. H., Johnson, H. M. & Rudge, P. (1974) The effects of thallium salts with particular reference to the nervous system changes. *Quarterly Journal of Medicine*, **43**, 293-319.

Cerletti, A. & Meier-Ruge, W. (1968) Toxicological studies on phenothiazine-induced retinopathy. Excerpta Medica International Congress Series No. 145. *Proceedings of the European Society for the Study of Drug Toxicity*, **9**, 170.

Chhuttani, P. N., Chawla, L. S. & Sharma, T. D. (1967) Arsenical neuropathy. *Neurology (Minneapolis)*, **17**, 269-274.

Christensen, E., Melchior, V. C. & Plum, P. (1963) Combined lesions of basal ganglia, medulla oblongata and spinal cord in a 10-year-old boy. *Acta paediatrica (Uppsala)*, **52**, 304-312.

Christensen, E., Møller, J. E. & Fayrbye, A. (1970) Neuropathological investigation of 28 brains from patients with dyskinesia. *Acta psychiatrica scandinavica*, **46**, 14-23.

Cohen, M. (1957) Central nervous system in carbon tetrachloride intoxication. *Neurology (Minneapolis)*, **7**, 238-244.

Collings, H. (1960) Polyneuropathy associated with nitrofuran therapy. *Archives of Neurology*, **3**, 656-660.

Conger, J. D., McIntyre, J. A. & Jacoby, W. I. (1969) Central pontine myelinolysis and inappropriate anti-diuretic hormone secretion. *American Journal of Medicine*, **47**, 813-817.

Contamin, F., Escourolle, R., Nick, J. & Mignot, B. (1971) Atrophie pallido-nigro-luysienne. *Revue Neurologique*, **124**, 107-120.

Cossa, P., Duplay, E. Arfel-Capdeville, Lafon, Passouant, Minvielle & Radermecker, J. (1959) Encephalopathies toxiques au stalinon. *Acta neurologica et psychiatrica belgica*, **59**, 281-303.

Cotziaz, G. C., Horiuchi, K., Fuenzalida, S. & Mena, I. (1968) Chronic manganese poisoning. Clearance of tissue manganese concentrations with persistence of the neurological picture. *Neurology (Minneapolis)*, **18**, 376-382.

Couper, J. (1837) Quoted by Meyer, A. (1963), p. 285.

Courville, C. B. (1955) *Effects of Alcohol on the Nervous System of Man*, Los Angeles.

Courville, C. B. & Myers, R. O. (1954) Effects of extraneous poisons on the nervous system: alcohols. *Bulletin of the Los Angeles Neurological Society*, **19**, 66-95.

Courville, C. B. & Myers, R. O. (1957) Process of demyelination in the nervous system. Focal demyelination and necrosis consequent to injection of radioactive gold (Au[198]). *Neurology (Minneapolis)*, **7**, 323-330.

Creutzfeldt, H. G. & Orzechowski, G. (1941-43) Quoted by Glees, P. & White, W. G. (1961), The absorption of triorthocresyl phosphate through the skin of hens and its neurotoxic effect. *Journal of Neurology, Neurosurgery and Psychiatry*, **24**, 271-274.

Crome, L. & Stern, J. (1972) *The Pathology of Mental Retardation*, 2nd Edn., p. 432, Churchill Livingstone, Edinburgh & London.

Cumings, J. N. (1959) *Heavy Metals and the Brain*, Blackwell Scientific, Oxford.

Cumings, J. N. (1962) The metabolism of copper and Wilson's disease. *Proceedings of the Nutrition Society*, **21**, 29-34.

Cumings, J. N. (1972) Neurochemistry in *Scientific Foundations of Neurology* (Eds. Critchley, M., O'Leary, J. L. & Jennett, B.), p. 433, Heinemann Medical, London.

Cumings, J. N., Goodman, H. J. & Earl, C. J. (1955) Blood copper and its relationship to globulins. *Journal of Clinical Pathology*, **8**, 69-72.

Currier, R. D. & Haerer, A. F. (1968) Amyotrophic lateral sclerosis and metabolic toxins. *Archives of Environmental Health (Chicago)*, **17**, 712-719.

Davidson, M. & Feinlieb, M. (1972) Carbon disulphide poisoning, a review. *American Heart Journal*, **83**, 100-114.

Davis, J. M., Bartlett, E. & Termini, B. A. (1968) Overdosage of psychotropic drugs. *Diseases of the Nervous System*, **29**, 157-164 and 246-256.

Dayan, A. D. & Williams, R. (1967) Demyelinating peripheral neuropathy and liver disease. *Lancet*, **2**, 133-134.

Dayan, A. D., Ockenden, B. G. & Crome, L. (1970) Necrotising encephalomyelopathy of Leigh. Neuropathological findings in 8 cases. *Archives of Disease in Childhood*, **45**, 39-48.

Dreese, M. J. & Netsky, M. G.   (1968) Degenerative disorders of the basal ganglia in *Pathology of the Nervous System* (Ed. Minckler, J.) Vol. 1, pp. 1185-1204, McGraw-Hill, New York.

Druckrey, H., Ivankovic, S. & Preussman, R.   (1966) Teratogenic and carcinogenic effects in the offspring after single injection of ethylnitrosourea to pregnant rats. *Nature*, 210, 1378-1379.

Dunn, H. G. & Dolman, C. L.   (1972) Necrotising encephalomyelopathy. Report of a case with manifestations resembling Behr's syndrome. *European Neurology*, 7, 34-55.

Eady, M. J. & Ferrier, T. M.   (1966) Chloroquine myopathy. *Journal of Neurology, Neurosurgery and Psychiatry*, 29, 331-337.

Earl, C. J. & Thompson, R. H. S.   (1952) Cholinesterase levels in the nervous system in triorthocresyl phosphate poisoning. *British Journal of Pharmacology*, 7, 685-694.

Earl, C. J., Moulton, M. J. & Selverstone, B.   (1954) Metabolism of copper in Wilson's disease and in normal subjects. *American Journal of Medicine*, 17, 205-213.

Eastham, R. D. & Jancar, J.   (1968) *Clinical Pathology in Mental Retardation*, p. 244, Wright, Bristol.

Edington, N. & Howell, J. McC.   (1969) The neurotoxicity of sodium diethyldithiocarbamate, in the rabbit. *Acta Neuropathologica (Berlin)*, 12, 339-347

Eicke, W. J.   (1957) In *Handbuch der speziellen pathologischen Anatomie und Histologie* (Eds. Lubarsch, O., Henke, F. & Rössle, R.), Vol. XIII (i), Springer Verlag, Berlin.

Ellis, F. G.   (1962) Acute polyneuritis after nitrofurantoin therapy. *Lancet*, 2, 1136-1138.

Etheridge, J. E. Jr. & Stewart, G. E.   (1966) Treating acrodermatitis enteropathica. *Lancet*, 1, 261-2.

Fadiloglu, S.   (1971) Sur les formes infantiles précoces de l'atrophie pigmentaire pallido-réticulée. *Acta neurologica belgica*, 71, 392-406.

Feigin, I. & Goebel, H. H.   (1969) Infantile subacute necrotising encephalopathy in the adult. *Neurology (Minneapolis)*, 19, 749-759.

Fenton, J. C. B.   (1955) The nature of the paralysis in chickens following organophosphorus poisoning. *Journal of Pathology and Bacteriology*, 69, 181-189.

Fischer, O.   (1911) Zur Frage der anatomischen Grundlagen der Athetose double und der posthemiplegischen Bewegungstörungen überhaupt. *Zeitschrift für die gesamte Neurologie und Psychiatrie*, 7, 463-486.

Fischer, O.   (1933) Zur Frage der anatomische Grundlagen der Athetose double und der posthemiplegischen Bewegungsstörungen überhaupt. *Münchener medizinische Wochenschrift*, 1, 202.

Fisher, C. M. & Adams, R. D.   (1956) Diphtheritic polyneuritis—a pathological study. *Journal of Neuropathology*, 15, 243-268.

Fleischer, B.   (1903) Quoted by Greenfield, J. G. & McMenemey, W. H. in *Neuropathology* (1963), 2nd edn., p. 580, Arnold, London.

Fleischer, B.   (1909) Die periphere grau-grünliche Hornhautverfärbung als ein Symptom einer eigenartigen Allgemeinerkrankung. *Münchener Medizinische Wochenschrift*, 56, 1120-1123.

Fleischer, B.   (1912) Ueber eine der 'Pseudosklerose' nahestehende bisher unbekannte Krankheit. *Deutsche Zeitschrift für Nervenheilkunde*, 44, 179-201.

Forsyth, Constance C. & Savage, D. C. L.   (1968) Pink disease. *British Medical Journal*, 1, 767.

Fullerton, Pamela M.   (1966) Chronic peripheral neuropathy produced by lead poisoning in guinea pigs. *Journal of Neuropathology and Experimental Neurology*, 25, 214-236.

Fullerton, Pamela M. & Kremer, M.   (1961) Neuropathy after intake of thalidomide (Distaval). *British Medical Journal*, 2, 855-858.

Fullerton, Pamela M. & O'Sullivan, D. J.   (1968) Thalidomide neuropathy: a clinical, electrophysiological and histological follow-up study. *Journal of Neurology, Neurosurgery and Psychiatry*, 31, 543-551.

Fünfgeld, E.   (1929-30) Zur Klinik und Pathologie frühkindlicher, das striäre System bevorzugender Hirnerkrankungen. *Journal für Psychologie und Neurologie (Leipzig)*, 40, 85.

Galambos, J. T. & Dowda, F. W.   (1959) Lead poisoning and porphyria. *American Journal of Medicine*, 27, 803-806.

Gamper, E.   (1929) Zur Kenntnis der zentralen Veränderungen beim Morbus Recklinghausen. *Journal of Psychology and Neurology (Leipzig)*, 39, 39-84.

Gardner-Thorpe, C. & Benjamin, S.   (1971) Peripheral neuropathy after disulfiram administration. *Journal of Neurology, Neurosurgery and Psychiatry*, 34, 253-259.

Garland, H.   (1957) Discussion on the toxic effects of drugs used in neurological and psychiatric practice. *Proceedings of the Royal Society of Medicine*, 50, 611-620.

Gerlach, W. & Rohrschneider, W.   (1934) Besteht das Pigment des Kayser-Fleischerschen Hornhautringes aus Silber? *Klinische Wochenschrift*, 13, 48-49.

Gey, K. F. & Pietscher, A.   (1968) Acceleration of turnover of ^{14}C catecholamines in rat brain by chlorpromazine. *Experientia*, 24, 335-336.

Gibb, J. W. G. & MacMahon, J. F.   (1955) Arrested development induced by lead poisoning.   *British Medical Journal*, **1**, 320-323.

Gombault, A.   (1880-81) Contribution à l'étude anatomique de la névrite parenchymateuse subaigüe ou chronique: névrite segmentaire péri-axile.   *Archives de Neurologie*, **1**, 11-38.

Gordon, I. & Whitehead, T. P.   (1949) Lead poisoning in an infant from lead nipple-shields: association with rickets.   *Lancet*, **2**, 647-650.

Greenfield, J. G.   (1958) In *Neuropathology*, Arnold, London.

Greenfield, J. G.   (1963) In *Neuropathology*, 2nd Edn., Arnold, London.

Greenfield, J. G., Poynton, F. J. & Walshe, F. M. R.   (1924) On progressive lenticular degeneration (hepato-lenticular degeneration).   *Quarterly Journal of Medicine*, **17**, 385-403.

Gregory, M. H., Rutty, P. A. & Wood, R. D.   (1970) Differences in the retinotoxic action of chloroquine and phenothiazine derivatives.   *Journal of Pathology*, **102**, 139-150.

Gritzka, T. L. & Trump, B. F.   (1968) Renal tubular lesions caused by mercuric chloride.   *American Journal of Pathology*, **52**, 1225-1277.

Groden, B. M.   (1963) Parkinsonism occurring with methyldopa treatment.   *British Medical Journal*, **1**, 1001.

Gross, H., Kaltenbäck, E. & Uiberrak, B.   (1957) Über eine spätinfantile Form der Hallervorden-Spatzschen Krankheit. I. Klinisch-anatomische Befunde.   *Deutsche Zeitschrift für Nervenheilkunde*, **176**, 77-103.

Grossi-Paoletti, E., Paoletti, P., Schiffer, D. & Fabiani, A.   (1970) Experimental brain tumours induced by nitrosourea derivatives, Part 2.   *Journal of the Neurological Sciences*, **11**, 573-581.

Gruner, J. E.   (1958) Lésions de nevraxe secondaires à l'ingestion d'éthyl-étain (Stalinon).   *Revue Neurologique*, **98**, 109-116.

Grzycki, S. & Kobusówna, B.   (1951) Histophysiological effects of arsenic and its derivatives on the central nervous system and particularly on the third element of the central nervous system.   *Journal of Neuropathology*, **10**, 325-337.

Haddock, D. R. W., Ebrahim, G. J. & Kapur, B. B.   (1962) Ataxic neurological syndrome found in Tanganyika.   *British Medical Journal*, **2**, 1442-1443.

Hall, H. C.   (1921) *La Dégénérescence Hépato-lenticulaire*, Masson, Paris.

Hallervorden, J.   (1930) Athetose mit eigenartigen pathologisch-anatomischen Befunde.   *Zentralblatt für die gesamte Neurologie*, **56**, 144.

Hallervorden, J. & Spatz, H.   (1922) Eigenartige Erkrankung im extrapyramidalen System mit besonderer Beteiligung des Globus pallidus und der Substantia nigra.   *Zentralblatt für die gesamte Neurologie*, **79**, 254-302.

Harding, J. D. J., Lewis, G. & Done, J. T.   (1968) Experimental arsanilic acid poisoning in pigs.   *Veterinary Record*, **83**, 560-564.

Hardman, J. M., Allen, L. W., Baughman, F. A. & Waterman, D. F.   (1968) Subacute necrotising encephalopathy in late adolescence.   *Archives of Neurology* (*Chicago*), **18**, 478-486.

Haurowitz, F.   (1930) Über eine Anomalie des Kupferstoffwechsels.   *Zeitschrift für physiologische Chemie*, **190**, 72-74.

Helfand, M.   (1935) Status pigmentosus, its pathology and its relation to Hallervorden–Spatz disease.   *Journal of Nervous and Mental Disease*, **81**, 662-675.

Henderson, D. A.   (1954) A follow-up of cases of plumbism in children.   *Australasian Annals of Medicine*, **3**, 219-234.

Hicks, S. P. & Coy, M. A.   (1958) Pathologic effects of antimetabolites. Convulsions and brain lesions caused by sulfoximine and their variation with genotype.   *Archives of Pathology*, **65**, 378-387.

Hirano, A., Zimmerman, H. M. & Levine, S.   (1968) Intramyelinic and extracellular spaces in triethyl tin intoxication.   *Journal of Neuropathology and Experimental Neurology*, **27**, 571-580.

Hoesslin, C. von & Alzheimer, A.   (1912) Ein Beitrag zur Klinik und pathologischen Anatomie der Westphal-Strümpellschen Pseudosklerose.   *Zeitschrift für die gesamte Neurologie und Psychiatrie*, **8**, 183-209.

Hofman, W. W.   (1958) Cerebellar lesions after parenteral dilantin administration.   *Neurology* (*Minneapolis*), **8**, 210-214.

Holmberg, C. G. & Laurell, C. B.   (1948) Investigations in serum copper. II. isolation of the copper-containing protein and a description of some of its properties.   *Acta chemica scandinavica*, **2**, 550-556.

Holzel, A. & James, T.   (1952) Mercury and pink disease.   *Lancet*, **1**, 441-443.

Holtzman, N. A., Naughton, M. A., Iber, F. L. & Gaumnitz, B. M.   (1967) Coeruloplasmin in Wilson's disease.   *Journal of Clinical Investigation*, **46**, 993-1002.

Howard, C. P. & Royce, C. E.   (1919) Progressive lenticular degeneration associated with cirrhosis of the liver (Wilson's disease).   *Archives of Internal Medicine*, **24**, 497-508.

Howell, J. McC.   (1970) Nutrition and the nervous system in farm animals.   *World Review of Nutrition and Diet*, **12**, 377-412.

Howell, J. McC. & Edington, N.   (1968) The neurotoxicity of sodium diethyl-di-thiocarbamate in the hen. *Journal of Neuropathology and Experimental Neurology*, **27**, 464-472.

Howell, J. S.   (1959) Histochemical demonstration of copper in copper fed rats and in hepatolenticular degeneration.   *Journal of Pathology and Bacteriology*, **77**, 473-484.

Hunt, J. R.   (1917) Progressive atrophy of the globus pallidus (primary atrophy of the pallidal system).   A system disease of the paralysis agitans type, characterised by atrophy of the motor cells of the corpus striatum.   *Brain*, **40**, 58-148.

Hunter, D., Bomford, R. R. & Russell, Dorothy S.   (1940) Poisoning by methyl mercury compounds.   *Quarterly Journal of Medicine*, **9**, 193-214.

Hunter, D. & Russell, Dorothy S.   (1954) Focal cerebral and cerebellar atrophy in a human subject due to organic mercury compounds.   *Journal of Neurology and Psychiatry*, **17**, 235-241.

Hunter, R., Earl, C. J. & Janz, D.   (1964) A syndrome of abnormal movements and dementia in leucotomized patients treated with phenothiazines.   *Journal of Neurology, Neurosurgery and Psychiatry*, **27**, 219-223.

Hunter, R., Blackwood, W., Smith, Marion C. & Cumings, J. N.   (1968) Neuropathological findings in three cases of persistent dyskinesia following phenothiazine medication.   *Journal of the Neurological Sciences*, **7**, 263-273.

Illis, L., Patangia, G. N. & Cavanagh, J. B.   (1966) Boutons terminaux and triorthocresylphosphate neurotoxicity.   *Experimental Neurology*, **14**, 160-174.

Ironside, R., Bosanquet, F. Dawn & McMenemey, W. H.   (1961) Central demyelination of the corpus callosum (Marchiafava-Bignami disease).   *Brain*, **84**, 212-230.

Jakob, A.   (1912) Zur Klinik und pathologischen Anatomie des chronischen Alkoholismus, zugleich ein Beitrag zu den Erkrankungen des Kleinhirns.   *Zeitschrift für die gesamte Neurologie und Psychiatrie*, **13**, 132-152.

Jellinger, K.   (1973) Neuronal dystrophy: its natural history and related disorders in *Progress in Neuropathology* (Ed. Zimmerman, H. M.), Vol. 2, p. 129, Grune and Stratton, New York.

Jellinger, K. & Seitelberger, F.   (1969) Juvenile form of spongy degeneration of the CNS.   *Acta Neuropathologica* (*Berlin*), **13**, 276-281.

Jenkins, R. B.   (1966) Inorganic arsenic and the nervous system.   *Brain*, **89**, 479-498.

Jéquier, M. & Wildi, E.   (1955) Deux cas de syndrome de Marchiafava–Bignami et de sclérose laminaire corticale associés; étude anatomo-clinique.   *Schweizerisches Archiv für Neurologie und Psychiatrie*, **75**, 77-88.

Jervis, G. A.   (1952) Hallervorden–Spatz disease associated with atypical amaurotic idiocy.   *Journal of Neuropathology and Experimental Neurology*, **11**, 4-18.

Jetter, W. W.   (1966) In *Pathology* (Ed. Anderson, W. A. D.), 5th Edn., chapter 6, Mosby, St. Louis.

Joiner, C. L., McArdle, B. & Thompson, R. H. S.   (1950) Blood pyruvate estimations in the diagnosis and treatment of polyneuritis.   *Brain*, **73**, 431-452.

Jones, E. L., Searle, C. E. & Smith, W. T.   (1973a) Peripheral neuropathy in ageing rats fed clioquinol and a maize diet.   *Acta Neuropathologica* (*Berlin*), **24**, 256-262.

Jones, E. L., Searle, C. E. & Smith, W. T.   (1973b) Tumours of the nervous system induced in rats by the neonatal administration of N-ethyl N-nitrosourea.   *Journal of Pathology*, **109**, 123-139.

Jones, Margaret, Mickelson, O. & Yang, Modesto   (1973) Methylazoxymethanol toxicity in *Progress in Neuropathology* (Ed. Zimmerman, H. M.), Vol. 2, p. 91, Grune & Stratton, New York.

Jones, W. A. & Jones, G. P.   (1953) Peripheral neuropathy due to isoniazid.   *Lancet*, **1**, 1073-1074.

Kalinowsky, L.   (1927) Familiäre Erkrankung mit besonderer Beteiligung der Stammganglien.   *Monatschrift für Psychiatrie und Neurologie*, **66**, 168-190.

Kalinowsky, L.   (1936) In *Handbuch der Neurologie* (Eds. Bumke, O. & Foerster, O.), Vol. XVI, Springer Verlag, Berlin.

Kane, F. J.   (1970) Carbon disulfide intoxication from overdosage of disulfiram.   *American Journal of Psychiatry*, **127**, 690-694.

Kayser, B.   (1902) quoted by Greenfield, J. G. & McMenemey, W. H. in *Neuropathology*, 2nd Edn., p. 580, Arnold, London.

Kernohan, J. W. & Kennedy, R. L. J.   (1928) Acrodynia (so-called); study of pathology.   *American Journal of Diseases of Children*, **36**, 341-351.

King, L. S. & Meehan, M. C.   (1936) Primary degeneration of the corpus callosum (Marchiafava's disease).   *Archives of Neurology and Psychiatry* (*Chicago*), **36**, 547-568.

Kirsch, W. M., Grossi-Paoletti, E. & Paoletti, P.   (1972) *The Experimental Biology of Brain Tumors*, Charles C. Thomas, Springfield, Ill.

Kjåer, G. C. D. (1968) Retinopathy associated with phenothiazine administration. *Diseases of the Nervous System*, **29**, 316-319.

Knill-Jones, R. P., Goodwill, C. J., Dayan, A. D. & Williams, R. (1972) Peripheral neuropathy in chronic liver disease: clinical electrodiagnostic and nerve biopsy findings. *Journal of Neurology, Neurosurgery and Psychiatry*, **35**, 22-30.

Koyama, T., Handa, J., Handa, H. & Matsumoto, S. (1970) Methylnitrosourea-induced malformations of brain in SD-JCL rats. *Archives of Neurology (Chicago)*, **22**, 342-347.

Kreutzberg, G. W. & Carlton, W. W. (1967) Pathogenetic mechanisms of experimentally induced spongy degeneration. *Acta neuropathologica*, **9**, 175-184.

Lampert, P. W. & Schochet, S. S. (1968*a*) Electromicroscopic observations on experimental spongy degeneration of the cerebellar white matter. *Journal of Neuropathology and Experimental Neurology*, **27**, 210-220.

Lampert, P. W. & Schochet, S. S. (1968*b*) Demyelination and remyelination in lead neuropathy. Electron-microscopic studies. *Journal of Neuropathology and Experimental Neurology*, **27**, 527-545.

Lamy (1863) Sur les effets toxiques duthallium. *Journal de Pharmacie et de Chimie*, **44**, 285-288.

Lancet (1953) Annotation. Teething powders, **2**, 1247 and 1321.

Lancet (1966) Leading article. Sudden death and phenothiazines. **2**, 740.

Lancet (1968) Leading article. Clioquinol and other halogenated hydroxyquinolines. **1**, 679.

Lancet (1971) Leading article. More on S.M.O.N. **2**, 1244.

Lancet (1974) Leading article. Encephalopathy and fatty degeneration of the viscera. **2**, 445.

Lapham, L. W. (1962) Cytologic and cytochemical studies of neuroglia. Part 1: a study of the problem of amitosis in reactive protoplasmic astrocytes. *American Journal of Pathology*, **41**, 1-21.

Law, W. R. & Nelson, E. R. (1968) Gasoline sniffing by an adult. Report of a case with the unusual complication of lead encephalopathy. *Journal of the American Medical Association*, **204**, 1002-1004.

Lawwill, T., Appleton, B. & Altstatt, L. (1968) Chloroquine accumulation in human eyes. *American Journal of Ophthalmology*, **65**, 530-532.

Leigh, D. (1951) Subacute necrotizing encephalomyelopathy in an infant. *Journal of Neurology, Neurosurgery and Psychiatry*, **14**, 216-221.

Lewey, F. H. (1950) Neuropathological changes in nitrogen trichloride intoxication of dogs. *Journal of Neuropathology and Experimental Neurology*, **9**, 396-405.

Lhermitte, J. (1935) Cortical cerebellar degeneration. *Proceedings of the Royal Society of Medicine*, **28**, 379-390.

Lhermitte, J., de Ajuriaguerra, J. & Garnier (1938) Les lésions du système nerveux dans l'intoxication alcoolique expérimentale. *Comptes Rendus des Scéances de la Société de Biologie (Paris)*, **128**, 386-388.

Lichtenstein, B. W. & Gore, I. (1955) Wilson's disease—chronic form. *Archives of Neurology and Psychiatry (Chicago)*, **73**, 13-21.

Lijinsky, W. & Epstein, S. S. (1970) Nitrosamines as environmental carcinogens. *Nature*, **225**, 21-23.

Livesley, B. & Sissons, C. E. (1968) Chronic lead intoxication mimicking motor neuron disease. *British Medical Journal*, **4**, 387-388.

Löken, A. C. & Haymaker, W. (1949) Pamaquine poisoning in man with a clinicopathologic study of one case. *American Journal of Tropical Medicine*, **29**, 341-352.

Lolli, G. (1941) Marchiafava's disease. *Quarterly Journal of Studies in Alcohol*, **2**, 486-495.

Luse, S. A. & Wood, W. G. (1967) The brain in fatal carbon tetrachloride poisoning. *Archives of Neurology (Chicago)*, **17**, 304-312.

Lüthy, F. (1931) Über die hepato-lentikuläre Degeneration (Wilson, Westphal, Strümpell). *Deutsche Zeitschrift für Nervenheilkunde*, **123**, 101-181.

Lynch, M. J. (1960) Brain lesions in chronic alcoholism. *Archives of Pathology*, **69**, 342-353.

McAlpine, D. & Araki, S. (1958) Minamata disease. An unusual neurological disorder caused by contaminated fish. *Lancet*, **2**, 629-631.

McDonald, R. D. & Engel, A. C. (1970) Experimental chloroquine myopatny. *Journal of Neuropathology and Experimental Neurology*, **29**, 479-499.

McIlwain, M. (1966) *Biochemistry and the Central Nervous System*, 3rd Edn., Churchill, London.

McLardy, T. (1951) A case of Marchiafava's disease (primary degeneration of the corpus callosum). *Proceedings of the Royal Society of Medicine*, **44**, 685-686.

Magee, P. N., Stoner, H. B. & Barnes, J. M. (1955) Changes in the central nervous system after poisoning with triethyl tin compounds. *Excerpta Medica, Section 8*, **8**, 859-860.

Magee, P. N., Stoner, H. B. & Barnes, J. M. (1957) Experimental production of oedema of the central nervous system of the rat by triethyl tin compounds. *Journal of Pathology and Bacteriology*, **73**, 107-124.

Magos, L. & Butler, W. H. (1972) Cumulative effects of methylmercury dicyandiamide given orally to rats. *Food and Cosmetics Toxicology*, **10**, 513-517.

Main, K. S., Main, A. J. & Montgomery, R. D.   (1969) A spastic paraplegic syndrome in South India.   *Journal of the Neurological Sciences*, **9**, 179-199.

Marchiafava, E. & Bignami, A.   (1903) Sopra un' alterazione del corpo calloso osservata in sogetti alcoolisti.   *Rivista di Patologia Nervosa e Mentale*, **8**, 544-549.

Marsden, H. B. & Wilson, V. K.   (1955) Lead-poisoning in children; correlation of clinical and pathological findings.   *British Medical Journal*, **1**, 324-326.

Mathalone, M. B.   (1966) Ocular complications of phenothiazines.   *Transactions of the Ophthalmological Society of the United Kingdom*, **86**, 77-88.

Matsumoto, H., Koya, G. & Takeuchi, T.   (1965) Fetal Minamata disease.   A neuropathological study of two cases of intrauterine intoxication by a methyl mercury compound.   *Journal of Neuropathology and Experimental Neurology*, **24**, 563-574.

Meier-Ruge, W.   (1965) Experimental morphogenesis of chloroquine retinopathy.   *Archives of Ophthalmology*, **73**, 540-544.

Mena, I., Marin, O., Fuenzalida, A. & Cotziaz, G. C.   (1967) Chronic manganese poisoning.   Clinical picture and manganese turnover.   *Neurology (Minneapolis)*, **17**, 128-136.

Meyer, A.   (1930) Quoted by Meyer, A. (1963), p. 286.

Meyer, A.   (1963) In *Neuropathology* (Eds. Blackwood, W., McMenemey, W. H., Meyer A., Norman, R. M. & Russell, D. S.), 2nd Edn., p. 261, Arnold, London.

Meyer, A. & Earl, C. J. C.   (1936) Studies on lesions of basal ganglia in defectives; case of état dysmyélinisé (Hallervorden–Spatz disease).   *Journal of Mental Science*, **82**, 798-811.

Mellanby, E.   (1946) Diet and canine hysteria.   *British Medical Journal*, **2**, 885-887.

Millichap, J. G., Llewellin, K. R. & Roxburgh, R. C.   (1952) Lead paint; a hazard to children.   *Lancet*, **2**, 360-362.

Miyakawa, T.   (1960) Experimental study of the pathogenesis of so-called Minimata disease.   *Psychiatria et Neurologia Japonica*, **62**, 1887-1913.

Miyakawa, T. & Deshimaru, M.   (1969) Electromicroscopical study of experimentally induced poisoning due to organic mercurial compound.   Mechanism of development of the morbid change.   *Acta Neuropathologica (Berlin)*, **14**, 126-136.

Miyakawa, T., Deshimaru, M., Sumiyoshi, S., Teraoka, A., Udo, N., Haltori, E. & Tatetsu, S.   (1970) Experimental organic mercury poisoning—pathological changes in peripheral nerves.   *Acta Neuropathologica (Berlin)*, **15**, 45-55.

Moeschlin, S.   (1952) *Klinik und Therapie der Vergiftungen*, Thieme, Stuttgart.

Moncrieff, A. A., Koumides, O. P., Clayton, B. E., Patrick, A. D., Renwick, A. G. C. & Roberts, G. E.   (1964) Lead poisoning in children.   *Archives of Disease in Childhood*, **39**, 1-13.

Money, G. L.   (1959) Clinical aspects of tropical ataxic neuropathies related malnutrition.   *West African Medical Journal*, **8**, 3-17.

Montgomery, R. D., Cruickshank, E. K., Robertson, W. B. & McMenemey, W. H.   (1964) Clinical and pathological observations in Jamaican neuropathy.   A report on 206 cases.   *Brain*, **87**, 425-462.

Morel, F.   (1939) Une forme anatomo-clinique particulaire de l'alcoolisme chronique: sclérose corticale laminaire alcoolique.   *Revue Neurologique*, **71**, 280-288.

Mott, F. W.   (1909) Examination of the nervous system in a case of chronic lead encephalitis.   *Archives of Neurology and Psychiatry (London)*, **4**, 117-130.

Mott, F. W.   (1910) The nervous system in chronic alcoholism.   *British Medical Journal*, **2**, 1403-1408.

Mowat, A. P.   (1973) Encephalopathy and fatty degeneration of the viscera: Reye's syndrome.   *Archives of Disease in Childhood*, **48**, 411-413.

Neal, P. A.   (1938) Mercury poisoning from the public health viewpoint.   *American Journal of Public Health*, **28**, 907-915.

Netsky, M. G., Spiro, D. & Zimmerman, H. M.   (1951) Hallervorden–Spatz disease and dystonia.   *Journal of Neuropathology and Experimental Neurology*, **10**, 125-141.

Neubürger, K. T.   (1957) The changing neuropathologic picture of chronic alcoholism.   *Archives of Pathology*, **63**, 1-6.

Noel, P. R. B., Worden, A. N. & Palmer, A. C.   (1967) Neuropathologic effects and comparative toxicity for dogs of isonicotinic acid hydrazide and its methanosulfonate derivative.   *Toxicology and Applied Pharmacology*, **10**, 183-198.

Ochoa, J.   (1970) Isoniazid neuropathy in man: quantitative EM study.   *Brain*, **93**, 831-850.

O'Grady, F. & Smith, Barbara   (1966) Neuromyopathy in the mouse produced by the antimicrobial agent nitroxoline.   *Journal of Pathology and Bacteriology*, **92**, 43-48.

Okinawa, S., Yoshikawa, M., Toyoda, M., Mozai, T., Toyokura, Y. & Kamiyama, M.   (1954) Pathogenesis of hepatocerebral disease.   *Archives of Neurology and Psychiatry (Chicago)*, **72**, 573-578.

Onari, K.   (1925) Über zwei klinisch und anatomisch kompliziert liegende Fälle von Status marmoratus des Striatum.   *Zeitschrift für die gesamte Neurologie und Psychiatrie*, **98**, 457-486.

Opalski, A.   (1930) Über eine besondere Art von Gliazellen bei der Wilson-Pseudosklerosegruppe.   *Zeitschrift für die gesamte Neurologie und Psychiatrie*, **124**, 420-425.

Osetowska, E.   (1971) Metals in *Pathology of the Nervous System* (Ed. Minckler, J.), Vol. 2, p. 1644, McGraw-Hill, New York.

Osuntokun, B. O., Monekosso, G. L. & Wilson, J.   (1969) Relationship of a degenerative tropical neuropathy to diet.   Report of a field survey.   *British Medical Journal*, **1**, 547-550.

Osuntokun, B. O., Langman, M. J. S., Wilson, J. & Aladetoyinbo, A.   (1970) Controlled trial of hydroxocobalamin and riboflavine in Nigerian ataxic neuropathy.   *Journal of Neurology, Neurosurgery and Psychiatry*, **33**, 663-666.

Paguirigan, A. & Lepken, E. B.   (1969) Central pontine myelinolysis.   *Neurology (Minneapolis)*, **19**,1007-1011.

Palmer, A. C. & Noel, P. R.   (1963) Neuropathological effects of prolonged administration of some hydrazine monoamine oxidase inhibitors in dogs.   *Journal of Pathology and Bacteriology*, **86**, 463-476.

Palmer, A. C. & Noel, P. R.   (1965) Neuropathological effects of dosing dogs with isonicotinic acid hydrazide and with its methanosulphonate derivative.   *Nature*, **205**, 506-507.

Paterson, D. & Greenfield, J. G.   (1923-24) Erythroedema polyneuritis (the so-called pink disease).   *Quarterly Journal of Medicine*, **17**, 6-18.

Peaston, M. J.   (1964) Parkinsonism associated with alpha methyldopa therapy.   *British Medical Journal*, **2**, 168.

Pentschew, A.   (1958) Intoxikationen in *Handbuch der speziellen pathologischen Anatomie und Histologie* (Ed. Scholtz, W.), Vol. 13, 2B, p. 1907, Springer Verlag, Berlin.

Pentschew, A., Ebner, F. & Kovatch, R.   (1962) New aspects of tellurium encephalomyelopathy in *Proceedings of the 4th International Congress of Neuropathology*, Vol. 3, Thieme, Stuttgart.

Pentschew, A. & Garro, F.   (1966) Lead encephalomyelopathy of the suckling rat and its implications on the porphyrinopathic nervous diseases.   *Acta Neuropathologica (Berlin)*, **6**, 266-278.

Peters, G.   (1951) *Spezielle Pathologie der Krankheiten des zentralen und peripheren Nervensystems*, Thieme, Stuttgart.

Peters, R. A.   (1948) Development and theoretical significance of British Anti-Lewisite (BAL).   *British Medical Bulletin*, **5**, 313-318.

Pincus, J. H.   (1972) Subacute necrotising encephalomyelopathy (Leigh's disease): a consideration of clinical features and etiology.   *Developmental Medicine and Child Neurology*, **14**, 87-101.

Popoff, N., Budzilovich, G., Goodgold, A. & Feigin, I.   (1965) Hepatocerebral degeneration.   Its occurrence in the presence and in the absence of abnormal copper metabolism.   *Neurology (Minneapolis)*, **15**, 919-930.

Prineas, J.   (1969) The pathogenesis of dying back neuropathies.   Part 1.   An ultrastructural study of experimental triorthocresyl phosphate intoxication in the cat.   *Journal of Neuropathology and Experimental Neurology*, **28**, 571-597.

Radouco-Thomas, S., Singh, P., Garcin, F. & Radouco-Thomas, C.   (1967) Relation between experimental analgesia and brain monoamines, catecholamines and 5-hydroxytryptamine.   Effects of precursors and monoamine modifying drugs.   *Archives of Biology and Experimental Medicine*, **4**, 42-62.

Raimondi, J. A., Beckman, F. & Evans, J. P.   (1968) Fine structural changes in human lead encephalopathy.   *Journal of Neuropathology and Experimental Neurology*, **27**, 154.

Rasul, A. R. & Howell, J. McC.   (1973) Further observations on the response of the peripheral and central nervous system of the rabbit to sodium diethyldithiocarbamate.   *Acta Neuropathologica (Berlin)*, **24**,161-173.

Reed, D., Crawley, J., Faro, S. N., Pieper, S. J. & Kurlund, L. T.   (1963) Thallotoxicosis; acute manifestations and sequelae.   *Journal of the American Medical Association*, **183**, 516-522.

Reye, R. D. K., Morgan, G. & Baral, J.   (1963) Encephalopathy and fatty degeneration of the viscera.   A disease entity in childhood.   *Lancet*, **2**, 749-752.

Reynolds, E. H.   (1968) Mental effects of anticonvulsants and folic acid metabolism.   *Brain*, **91**, 197-214.

Reynolds, E. H.   (1970) Iatrogenic disorders in epilepsy in *Modern Trends in Neurology* 5 (Ed. Williams, D.), p. 27, Butterworth, London.

Reznikoff, P. & Aub, J. C.   (1927) Lead studies.   *Archives of Neurology and Psychiatry (Chicago)*, **17**, 444-465.

Richter, R.   (1949) The effects of certain quinoline compounds upon the nervous system of monkeys.   *Journal of Neuropathology and Experimental Neurology*, **8**, 155-170.

Roberts, W. J.   (1939) Zum Verhalten des Gehirns nach Injektion von Goldsalzen.   *Archiv für Psychiatrie und Nervenkrankheiten*, **109**, 744-754.

Robertson, D. H. H. & Knight, R. H.   (1964) Observations on the polyneuropathy and disordered pyruvate metabolism induced by nitrofurazone in cases of sleeping sickness due to *T. Rhodesiense*.   *Acta tropica (Basel)*, **21**, 239-263.

Robertson, R. D. & Cruickshank, E. K.   (1972) Jamaican (tropical) myeloneuropathy in *The Pathology of the Nervous System* (Ed. Minckler, J.), Vol. 3, p. 2466, McGraw-Hill, New York.

Robinson, J. D., Lowinger, J. & Bettinger, B.   (1968) Chlorpromazine: differential effects on membrane-bound enzymes from rat brain.   *Biochemical Pharmacology*, **17**, 1113-1116

Røe, O.   (1946) Methanol poisoning: its clinical course, pathogenesis and treatment.   *Acta medica scandinavica, Suppl.* **182**, 1-253.

Roizin, L., True, C. & Knight, M.   (1959) Structural effects of tranquillisers.   *Research Publications, Association for Research in Nervous and Mental Diseases*, **37**, 285-324.

Rosenoer, V. M. & Mitchell, R. C.   (1959) Skeletal changes in Wilson's disease (hepatolenticular degeneration).   *British Journal of Radiology*, **32**, 805-809.

Rothmann, M.   (1915) Demonstration zu den Zwangsbewegungen im Kindesalter.   *Neurologisches Zentralblatt*, **34**, 444-445.

Russell, Dorothy S.   (1937) Changes in the central nervous system following arsphenamine medication.   *Journal of Pathology and Bacteriology*, **45**, 357-366.

Scharenberg, K. & Drew, A. L.   (1954) The histopathology of Wilson's disease.   *Journal of Neuropathology and Experimental Neurology*, **13**, 181-190.

Scheinberg, I. H. & Gitlin, D.   (1952) Deficiency of ceruloplasmin in patients with hepatolenticular degeneration (Wilson's disease).   *Science*, **116**, 484-485.

Scheinberg, I. H. & Sternlieb, I.   (1965) Wilson's disease.   *Annual Review of Medicine*, **16**, 119-134.

Schiffer, D., Fabiani, A., Grossi-Paoletti, E. & Paoletti, P.   (1970) Experimental brain tumours induced by nitrosourea derivatives, Part I.   *Journal of the Neurological Sciences*, **11**, 559-572.

Schlaepfer, W. W.   (1968) Ultrastructural and histochemical studies of a primary sensory neuropathy in rats, produced by chronic lead intoxication.   *Journal of Neuropathology and Experimental Neurology*, **27**, 111-112.

Schmidt, Ida G. & Schmidt, L. H.   (1948) Neurotoxicity of the 8-aminoquinolines I.   *Journal of Neuropathology and Experimental Neurology*, **7**, 368-398.

Schmidt, Ida G. & Schmidt, L. H.   (1951) Neurotoxicity of the 8-aminoquinolines II.   *Journal of Neuropathology and Experimental Neurology*, **10**, 231-256.

Schneck, S. A.   (1966) Neuropathological features of human organ transplantation.   II. Central pontine myelinolysis and neuroaxonal dystrophy.   *Journal of Neuropathology and Experimental Neurology*, **25**, 18-39.

Schulman, S.   (1968) Wilson's disease in *Pathology of the Nervous System* (Ed. Minckler, J.), Vol. 1, p. 1139, McGraw-Hill, New York.

Seitelberger, F.   (1971) Pigmentary disorders in *The Pathology of the Nervous System* (Ed. Minckler, J.), Vol. 2, pp. 1324-1338, McGraw-Hill, New York.

Seitelberger, F. & Gross, H.   (1957) Über eine spätinfantile Form der Hallervorden-Spatzschen Krankheit. II. Histochemische Befunde. Erörterung der Nosologie.   *Deutsche Zeitschrift für Nervenheilkunde*, **176**, 104-125.

Shatin, R.   (1944) Multiple sclerosis and geography.   New interpretation of epidemiological observations.   *Neurology (Minneapolis)*, **14**, 338-344.

Shiraki, H.   (1968) In *The Central Nervous System* (*International Academy of Pathology Monograph*) (Ed. Bailey, O. T. & Smith, D. E.), p. 252, Williams & Wilkins, Baltimore.

Shiraki, H. & Oda, M.   (1968) Neuropathology of hepatocerebral disease with emphasis on comparative studies in *Diseases of the Nervous System* (Ed. Minckler, J.), Vol. 1, p. 1089, McGraw-Hill, New York.

Shiraki, H. & Takeuchi, T.   (1971) Minimata disease in *Pathology of the Nervous System* (Ed. Minckler, J.) Vol. 2, p. 1651, McGraw-Hill, New York.

Shurtliff, L. F., Ajax, E. T., Englert, E. & D'Agostino, A. N.   (1966) Central pontine myelinolysis and cirrhosis of the liver.   *American Journal of Clinical Pathology*, **46**, 239-244.

Silver, M. L.   (1949) Canine epilepsy caused by flour bleached with nitrogen trichloride.   *Journal of Neuropathology and Experimental Neurology*, **8**, 441-445.

Simpson, G. M. & Angus, J. W.   (1970) A rating scale for extrapyramidal side effects.   *Acta psychiatrica scandinavica, Suppl.* **212**, 11-19.

Simpson, J. A., Seaton, D. A. & Adams, J. F.   (1964) Response to treatment with chelating agents of anaemia, chronic encephalopathy and myelopathy due to lead poisoning.   *Journal of Neurology, Neurosurgery and Psychiatry*, **27**, 536-541.

Sinclair, H. M.   (1956) Vitamins and the nervous system.   *British Medical Bulletin*, **12**, 18-23.

Smith, Barbara & O'Grady, F.   (1966) Experimental chloroquine myopathy.   *Journal of Neurology, Neurosurgery and Psychiatry*, **29**, 255-258.

Smith, G. F.   (1966) Trichlorethylene—a review. *British Journal of Industrial Medicine*, **23**, 249-262.

Smith, H. & Spalding, J. M. K.   (1959) Outbreak of paralysis in Morocco due to ortho-cresyl phosphate poisoning. *Lancet*, **2**, 1019-1021.

Smith, M. T., Elvore, E., Valaer, P. J., Frazier, W. H. & Mallory, G. E.   (1930) Pharmaceutical and chemical studies of the causes of the so-called Ginger Jake paralysis. *Public Health Reports*, **45**, 1703-1716.

Snyder, S. H.   (1967) New developments in brain chemistry.   Catechol amine metabolism and the action of psychotropic drugs. *American Journal of Orthopsychiatry*, **37**, 864-879.

Spielmeyer, W.   (1922) *Histopathologie des Nervensystems*, Berlin.

Speirs, A. L.   (1959) Further evidence between the association of mercury and pink disease. *British Medical Journal*, **2**, 142-143.

Steger, J. & Steger, R.   (1954) Die Störungen des Kupfer- und Aminosäuren-Stoffwechsels bei der hepato-cerebralen Degeneration und deren Behandlung mit BAL. *Deutsche Zeitschrift für Nervenheilkunde*, **172**, 321-351.

Stender, A. & Lüthy, F.   (1931) Uber Spätatrophie der Kleinhirnrinde bei chronischem Alkoholismus. *Deutsche Zeitschrift für Nervenheilkunde*, **119**, 604-622.

Stevens, H. & Forster, F. M.   (1953) Effect of carbon tetrachloride on the nervous system. *Archives of Neurology and Psychiatry (Chicago)*, **70**, 635-649.

Stoner, H. B., Barnes, J. M. & Duff, J. I.   (1955) Studies on the toxicity of alkyl tin compounds. *British Journal of Pharmacology and Chemotherapy*, **10**, 16-25.

Swensson, A.   (1952) Investigations on the toxicity of some organic mercury compounds which are used as seed disinfectants. *Acta medica scandinavica*, **143**, 365-384.

Takeuchi, T., Morikawa, N., Matsumoto, H. & Shiraishi, Y.   (1962) A pathological study of Minimata disease in Japan. *Acta Neuropathologica (Berlin)*, **2**, 40-57.

Ter Braak, J. W. G.   (1931) Epidemic of polyneuritis from peculiar cause. *Nederlands Tijdschrift voor Geneeskunde*, **75**, 2329-2339.

Thompson, R. H. S.   (1948) Therapeutic applications of British Anti-Lewisite. *British Medical Bulletin*, **5**, 319-324.

Torack, R. M., Terry, R. D. & Zimmerman, H. M.   (1960) The fine structure of cerebral fluid accumulation. II. Swelling produced by triethyl tin poisoning and its comparison with that in the human brain. *American Journal of Pathology*, **36**, 273-287.

Tsubacki, T., Honma, Y. & Hoshi, M.   (1971) Neurological syndrome associated with clioquinol. *Lancet*, **1**, 696-697.

Turner, J. W. A.   (1955) Metallic poisons and the nervous system. *Lancet*, **1**, 661-663.

Turpin, R., Jerome, H. & Schmidt, H. H.   (1953) Study of the variations of the coeruloplasmin by an easy technique. *Proceedings of the Royal Society of Medicine*, **46**, 1061-1062.

Uchida, M., Hirakawa, K. & Inque, T.   (1961) Quoted in Uchida, M. (1962) Isolation and chemical identification of organic mercury compound in toxic shellfish.   First Asian and Oceanic Congress of Neurology, Tokyo, 1962.

Urechia, C. I., Retezeano, A. & Maller, O.   (1950) La maladie de Hallervorden–Spatz. Deux cas de rigidité progressive familiale avec un examen anatomique. *Encéphale*, **39**, 197-219.

Utterback, R. A., Ojeman, R. & Malek, J.   (1958) Parenchymatous cerebellar degeneration with dilantin intoxication. *Journal of Neuropathology and Experimental Neurology*, **17**, 516-517.

Uzman, L. L.   (1956) Histochemical localization of copper with rubeanic acid. *Laboratory Investigation*, **5**, 299-305.

Uzman, L. L. & Denny-Brown, D.   (1948) Aminoaciduria in hepatolenticular degeneration (Wilson's disease). *American Journal of Medical Science*, **215**, 599-611.

Uzman, L. L. & Jakus, M. A.   (1957) The Kayser Fleischer ring.   A histochemical and electronmicroscope study. *Neurology (Minneapolis)*, **7**, 341-355.

van Bogaert, L.   (1939) Dégénérescence pigmentaire pallido-nigrique (Hallervorden–Spatz) et encéphalite léthargique chronique. *Revue Neurologique*, **72**, 448-456.

van Bogaert, L.   (1946) Aspects cliniques et pathologiques des atrophies pallidales et pallido-luysiennes progressives. *Journal of Neurology and Psychiatry*, **9**, 125-157.

van Bogaert, L.   (1956) Sur le parkinsonisme saturnin avec paralysie des mouvements oculaires associés. *Monatschrift für Psychiatrie und Neurologie*, **131**, 73-88.

van Tongeren, J. H., Kunst, A., Kajoor, C. L. H. & Schillings, P. H. M.   (1965) Folic acid deficiency in chronic arsenical poisoning. *Lancet*, **1**, 784-786.

Verhaart, W. J. C.   (1941) Lead encephalopathy simulating diffuse sclerosis in a Chinese infant. *American Journal of Diseases of Children*, **61**, 1246-1250.

Victor, M. & Adams, R. D.   (1961) On the etiology of the alcoholic neurologic diseases with special reference to the role of nutrition. *American Journal of Clinical Nutrition*, **9**, 379-397.

Victor, M., Adams, R. D. & Mancall, E. L.   (1959) A restricted form of cerebellar cortical degeneration occurring in alcoholic patients. *Archives of Neurology*, **1**, 579-688.

Victor, M., Adams, R. D. & Cole, M.   (1965) The acquired (non-Wilsonian) type of chronic hepatocerebral degeneration. *Medicine*, **44**, 345-396.

Victor, M., Mancall, E. L. & Dreyfus, P. M.   (1960) Deficiency amblyopia in the alcoholic patient. *Archives of Ophthalmology*, **64**, 1-33.

de Villaverde, J. M.   (1926, 1927) Quoted by Meyer, A. (1963), pp. 268-269.

de Villiers, J. C.   (1966) Intracranial haemorrhage in patients treated with monoamine oxidase inhibitors. *British Journal of Psychiatry*, **112**, 109-118.

Vincent, C. & Van Bogaert, L.   (1936) Contribution à l'étude des syndromes du globe pale.   La dégénérescence progressive du globe pâle et de la portion réticulée de la substance noir (maladie de Hallervorden–Spatz). *Revue Neurologique*, **65**, 921-959.

Vogt, C. & Vogt, O.   (1920) Zur Lehre der Erkrankungen des striären Systems. *Journal of Psychology and Neurology (Leipzig)*, **25**, Suppl. 3, 631-896.

Wachstein, M.   (1949) Lead poisoning diagnosed by the presence of nuclear acid-fast inclusion bodies in kidney and liver. *Archives of Pathology*, **48**, 442-446.

Waggoner, R. W. & Malamud, N.   (1942) Wilson's disease in the light of cerebral changes following ordinary acquired liver disorders. *Journal of Nervous and Mental Diseases*, **96**, 410-423.

Walsh, J. C.   (1970) Gold neuropathy. *Neurology (Minneapolis)*, **20**, 455-458.

Walsh, J. C. & McCleod, J. G.   (1970) Alcoholic neuropathy; an electrophysiological and histological study. *Journal of the Neurological Sciences*, **10**, 457-469.

Walshe, J. M.   (1966) In *The Biochemistry of Copper* (Ed. Peisach, J., Aisen, P. & Blumberg, W. E.), p. 475, Academic Press, New York.

Walshe, J. M.   (1967) The physiology of copper in man and its relation to Wilson's disease. *Brain*, **90**, 149-176.

Wechsler, W., Kleihnes, P., Matsumoto, S., Zulch, K. J., Ivankovic, S., Preussman, R. & Druckrey, H.   (1969) Pathology of experimental neurogenic tumors chemically induced in prenatal and postnatal life in Research in the Experimental and Clinical Aspects of Brain Tumors. *Annals of the New York Academy of Sciences*, **159**, 361-408.

Weller, C. V. & Christensen, A. D.   (1925) The cerebrospinal fluid in lead poisoning. *Archives of Neurology and Psychiatry (Chicago)*, **14**, 327-345.

Wertham, F.   (1932) Central nervous system in acute phosphorus poisoning. *Archives of Neurology and Psychiatry (Chicago)*, **28**, 320-330.

Wetterholm, D. H. & Winter, F. C.   (1964) Histopathology of chloroquine retinal toxicity. *Archives of Ophthalmology (Chicago)*, **71**, 82-87.

White, H. H. & Fowler, F. D.   (1960) Chronic lead encephalopathy.   A diagnostic consideration in mental retardation. *Pediatrics*, **25**, 309-315.

Wilson, S. A. K.   (1912) Progressive lenticular degeneration: a familial nervous disease associated with cirrhosis of the liver. *Brain*, **34**, 295-509.

Winkelman, N. W.   (1932) Progressive pallidal degeneration.   A new clinico-pathologic syndrome. *Archives of Neurology and Psychiatry*, **27**, 1-21.

Wisniewski, H., Terry, R. D. & Hirano, A.   (1970) Neurofibrillary pathology. *Journal of Neuropathology and Experimental Neurology*, **29**, 163-176.

Wood, C. A. & Butler, F.   (1904) Poisoning by wood alcohol. *Journal of the American Medical Association*, **43**, 972-977, 1058-1062, 1117-1123, 1213-1221, 1289-1296.

Worsley, H. E., Brookfield, R. W., Elwood, J. S., Noble, R. L. & Taylor, W. H.   (1965) Lactic acidosis with necrotising encephalopathy in two sibs. *Archives of Disease in Childhood*, **40**, 492-501.

Wyllie, W. G. & Stern, R. O.   (1931) Pink disease.   Its morbid anatomy with a note on treatment. *Archives of Disease in Childhood*, **6**, 137-156.

Zeman, W. & Scarpelli, D. G.   (1958) The non-specific lesions of Hallervorden–Spatz disease.   A histochemical study. *Journal of Neuropathology and Experimental Neurology*, **17**, 525-527, 622-630.

5

Nutritional Deficiencies and Disorders

Revised by W. Thomas Smith

Vitamin deficiencies

For a general account the reader is referred to Sebrell and Harris (1967) and György and Pearson (1967). Spillane (1947) and Denny-Brown (1947) have described neurological disorders resulting from nutritional deficiencies that occurred during the second World War and Follis (1948, 1958) has given a comprehensive and critical account of the pathological changes and, in particular, of experimental studies. The effect of vitamins on the nervous system has been reviewed by Sinclair (1956) and McIlwain and Bachelard (1971), with emphasis on experimental and biochemical aspects.

The vitamins were each labelled with a letter as they were discovered, but once a vitamin was identified chemically it was given a specific name, which it is correct to use, but only if it applies to a specific compound. It is sometimes advisable to use the original letters, as certain vitamins (e.g. A, D, E, K, B_{12}) are comprised of several related substances with similar physiological effects. The term 'vitamin B complex' remains useful because the constituent substances, though chemically dissimilar, often occur together in the same food.

From the neurological and psychiatric point of view vitamin B complex is of greater importance than the other vitamins and its main constituents are: thiamine hydrochloride (B_1); nicotinic acid, riboflavin and pantothenic acid (B_2 group); pyridoxine (B_6); and cyanocobalamin and related compounds (vitamin B_{12}). These are the B vitamins principally considered below, since the neuropathological significance of other members of the B complex such as choline, biotin, inositol and para-amino-benzoic acid is at present little understood.

Deficiencies of single vitamins are rare; most deficiencies are multiple or may become so as the result of secondary effects induced by the primary deficiency. Although a particular vitamin is present in the diet, its deficiency can result from lack of absorption, from destruction in the gut, or because *in vivo* synthesis is prevented by an adverse bacterial flora. This bacterial effect has been demonstrated for thiamine by Najjar and Holt (1943), and for nicotinamide by Ellinger, Coulson and Benesch (1944). It has been estimated that more than 80% of the human requirement of nicotinic acid is synthesized in the intestinal tract by the bacterial flora. Variations of storage capacity, rate of excretion and of general requirements may all be increased or reduced in different metabolic conditions and so play an important part in the clinical effects of the deficiency. For example, deficiency of thiamine may result in more severe manifestations if carbohydrates are taken in excess.

Vitamin B complex plays an important role in the metabolism of neurons. Thiamine hydrochloride, in its phosphorylated form, acts as a coenzyme (cocarboxylase) for reactions that involve the carboxylation of pyruvate; pantothenic acid, which is a part of coenzyme A, is also essential for the oxidation of pyruvates. Hyperpyruvaemia is, therefore, a characteristic finding in thiamine and pantothenic acid deficiencies and has been described in beriberi and in the Wernicke syndrome in man (Wortis, Bueding and Jolliffe 1942). According to Sinclair (1961) the oxidation of α-ketoglutaric acid to γ-aminobutyric acid (GABA) is prevented if thiamine is lacking; this may result in depletion of GABA in neurons and so be a factor in the pathogenesis of deficiency neuropathies. Nicotinic acid (niacin), as diphospho- and triphospho-pyridine nucleotide, acts as coenzyme to respiratory enzymes; riboflavin, a dinucleotide, is a component of a number of dehydrogenase enzymes; and pyridoxine is essential for the metabolism of glutamic acid which is present in considerable amounts in the brain.

In most of the above reactions other substances are required. For example, in order to decarboxylate pyruvate, thiamine and pantothenic acid must be supported by lipoic acid (6 : 8-dithio-octanoic acid), which is another coenzyme. Lipoic acid is formed in the liver and its deficiency may be a sequel of liver disease. According to Sinclair (1956) arsenic, mercury, pyruvate, acetaldehyde or acetoacetate readily combine with lipoic acid, which is then no longer available for its reaction with thiamine and pantothenic acid, and thus indirectly prevent the carboxylation of pyruvate. If this is a function of lipoic acid, some of the similarities between the peripheral neuropathies that occur in arsenical and mercurial poisoning, in chronic alcoholism, and in diabetes and that which occurs in vitamin B deficiency might be explained, although, in the strict sense, there is no deficiency of the vitamin in the former conditions. However, this hypothesis has not been confirmed therapeutically (Sinclair 1961), and it is no doubt optimistic to expect that one explanation could account for the mechanism of all these conditions.

Many vitamins are affected by antivitamins (antienzymes). Thiaminase, which destroys thiamine, causes deficiency (Chastek paralysis) in animals fed on raw fish in which this enzyme occurs. Pyrithiamine and oxythiamine are other antagonists of thiamine. Nicotinic acid is 'blocked' by pyridine-3-sulphuric acid (McIlwain 1940) and 3-acetylpyridine (Woolley 1945). Analogues of pyridoxine are deoxypyridoxine and methoxypyridoxine.

In the detailed accounts of deficiency and nutritional disorders that follow, these important metabolic interlinkages will be discussed further but their complexity helps to explain some of the conflicting results described by different workers. Some of the conditions dealt with below (for example, ergotism and lathyrism)

might have found a place in Chapter 4, but they are included here because of their relationship to nutritional problems.

Thiamine deficiency

The syndromes most closely associated with thiamine deficiency are beriberi and the Wernicke syndrome.

Beriberi
Beriberi occurs mainly in the Far East, and in tropical climates, but was prevalent in both World Wars in other localities, particularly during periods of famine that occurred in prisoner-of-war camps and in some occupied countries in Europe. Acute, subacute and chronic forms are described; furthermore, dry and wet beriberi are also recognized, according to whether oedema is present. Peripheral neuropathies more frequently complicate the chronic form, and may be complicated by the characteristic heart condition and oedema. In the infant, beriberi is usually acute and the underlying abnormality is likely to be the sequel of combined protein and thiamine deficiency (Platt 1958a); such cases tend to be very oedematous. Platt and Lu (1935) were probably the first to observe a marked increase of pyruvic acid and of other bisulphite-binding carbonyl compounds in the blood of patients suffering from beriberi.

The heart lesion consists of acute dilatation, particularly on the right side. Symmetrical oedema, starting usually at the ankles, spreads upwards and the scrotum may be involved early. Polyneuritis begins distally in the lower extremities and may become widespread and involve cranial nerves, laryngeal nerves, posterior roots and autonomic nerves.

Retrobulbar neuritis, deafness, the 'burning foot' syndrome, a bulbar myasthenic syndrome and ataxia have all been described in cases of beriberi, but they are now no longer believed to result from thiamine deficiency (Denny-Brown 1947; Follis).

Mental disturbances are said to be rare and Platt and Gin (1934) found such disorders in only 4% of cases; when persistent, it is difficult to exclude the Wernicke syndrome.

The pathology of the peripheral neuropathy was reviewed by Greenfield (1958) and Meyer (1963). In the earlier stages the myelin is mainly affected, but later both myelin and axons are involved. The histological picture is similar to that in Wallerian degeneration, although in the proximal parts of some nerves, Gombault's (1880-1881) segmental demyelination was seen. Degeneration of myelin is associated with greatly increased numbers of nuclei, chiefly belonging to lipophages, but Schwann cell nuclei are also more numerous than normal.

It has been noted that degeneration increases towards the periphery of nerves; it is slight or absent in the large nerve trunks and usually absent in the nerve roots. Greenfield suggested that the primary lesion in this type of neuropathy appears to affect the neuronal perikaryon, and the trophic function of the neuron may be so impaired that it is no longer able to maintain its long axon, which degenerates first in its peripheral part ('dying-back').

Cutaneous and motor nerves are affected and also the terminal branches of the vagus in the pericardium and heart muscle. The vagus might also be severely involved more proximally, for example in its laryngeal branches; in these and the phrenic nerves the changes are usually earlier than in the nerves of the feet and legs.

Robertson, Wasan and Skinner (1968) studied the electron-microscopy of early brainstem lesions in thiamine-deficient rats and noted swelling of myelin sheaths. Tellez and Terry (1968) found early changes in nerve terminals and axons without involvement of neuronal perikarya or vascular lesions. Collins (1967) concluded that the oligodendrocyte may be primarily involved.

With regard to the other pathological manifestations, Buzzard and Greenfield's (1921) description still stands; in the wet form anasarca and hydropericardium are present together with congestion of the spleen and with nutmeg liver. In all fatal cases great dilatation of the right side of the heart has been noted and histologically its muscle shows hydropic swelling of fibres, loss of striations and replacement by granulation and fibrous tissue.

Some of the findings described in the spinal cord are, if not due to other concomitant vitamin deficiency, likely to be secondary to the peripheral neuropathy; for example degeneration of anterior horn neurons, of posterior roots and root ganglia and of posterior spinal tracts.

The brain and its meninges show congestion and oedema. Gross softening within the central nervous system, which was mentioned in earlier reports is likely to have been due to post-mortem artefact.

The Wernicke syndrome

This syndrome was described by Wernicke in 1881 and was named by him *acute superior haemorrhagic polio-encephalitis.* Although in Wernicke's first case the cause of the syndrome was pyloric stenosis complicating sulphuric acid poisoning, the encephalopathy was later attributed exclusively to chronic alcoholism by many workers. Brody and Wilkins (1968) have published a useful transcript of Wernicke's original account. Neubürger (1936) first drew attention to a wider occurrence in 14 non-alcoholic patients, the majority of whom were suffering from carcinoma of the intestinal tract, especially of the stomach. Campbell and Biggart (1939) and Campbell and Russell (1941) stressed that the nutritional aspect was a common aetiological link and even suggested deficiency of vitamin B_1. Since then the syndrome has been shown to complicate many conditions, such as exhausting infectious disease, chronic gastritis, gastric ulcer and gastric carcinoma, persistent vomiting and especially hyperemesis gravidarum, and pernicious anaemia. The condition following breast milk intoxication observed by several Japanese workers seems identical with that of Wernicke (Tanaka 1934).

The Wernicke syndrome may be acute, subacute or chronic. *Clinically*, it is characterized by disturbances of consciousness and in many cases by ataxia and nystagmus; other less consistent signs are disturbances of respiration, of vision and of peripheral nerves. There is considerable clinical variation among different cases, and evidence of Korsakoff's psychosis is extremely common where survival is for longer than a few days.

Pathological descriptions have been given by Wernicke; Spatz (1930); Neubürger (1936); Campbell and Biggart (1939); Victor, Adams and Collins (1971) and many others. The main lesions are found in the regions of the 3rd and 4th ventricles, and of the aqueduct. The mamillary bodies are most consistently involved and often show conspicuous macroscopic petechial haemorrhages. Macroscopic haemorrhages are also occasionally recognizable in the grey matter around the 3rd ventricle and aqueduct (Figs. 5.1 and 5.2), the inferior colliculi, parts of the medial thalamic nuclei and the region of the vestibular and dorsal vagal nuclei. Macroscopic lesions, however, may be absent or scanty.

Histologically, in Nissl preparations the mamillary bodies show increased cellularity (Fig. 5.3) chiefly due to proliferation and dilatation of capillaries, in which the endothelial and adventitial cells are greatly increased. The proliferating capillaries are well demonstrated by reticulin impregnation, haematoxylin–van Gieson staining, and often, as in Fig. 5.4, by Holzer's method for glial fibres. Frequently there is also consider-

when the lesions occur in the other sites mentioned.

Rarely the lesions in the hypothalamus may not be centred on the mamillary body, but on the anterior hypothalamus. The optic chiasma may be involved in such cases and show severe gliosis (Meyer 1944). Involvement of the optic nerves was noted by Campbell and Russell (1941);

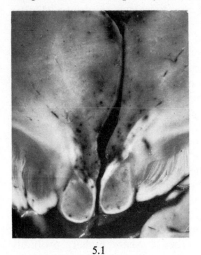

5.1

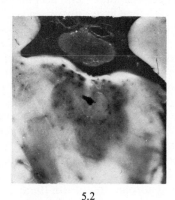

5.2

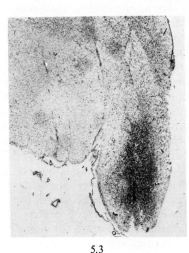

5.3

Figs. 5.1–5.4 Wernicke syndrome.

Figs. 5.1 and 5.2 Macroscopic appearance of haemorrhages around 3rd ventricle and aqueduct. (Reproduced by courtesy of Prof. J. B. Cavanagh.)

Fig. 5.3 Mamillary body. Nissl. × 7.

Fig. 5.4 Mamillary body; capillary proliferation. Holzer. × 60.

5.4

able proliferation of astrocytes and microglia, but transformation of the latter into lipophages is infrequent. The neurons may show degeneration of ischaemic type, but have been found to be relatively spared in a number of cases. Pena (1969) noted marked crowding of neurons in the mamillary bodies associated with changes resembling central chromatolysis. The mamillary bodies are invariably involved when Korsakoff's psychosis has been present.

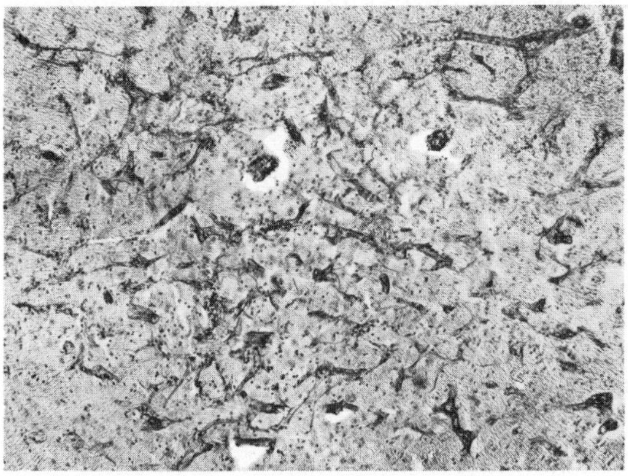

The details of the histological changes is similar

calcification of hypothalamic capillaries was described by Meyer (1944).

The inferior olives are sometimes affected: Riggs and Boles (1944) found this in 11 of 29 cases and Meyer (1963) in 4 out of 5 cases, without appreciable atrophy of the cerebellum. The posteromedial sector of the olive was most affected, showing glial and capillary proliferation and homogenizing degeneration of neurons.

Earlier investigators noted spinal cord involvement. Bonhoeffer (1899), for example, found degeneration in the posterior and lateral tracts, but it is likely that the cause was an associated deficiency of other B complex constituents. Lopez and Collins (1968) described a case associated with central pontine myelinolysis that had complicated haemodialysis for chronic uraemia.

The *pathogenesis* of the lesions remains obscure. Most authors regard the vascular changes as the primary event, followed by secondary degeneration of neurons. Scholz (1949) suggested that increased vascular permeability was the first change, leading to an exudate with a high protein content, which in its turn induced astrocytic, microglial and endothelial proliferation. The circumscribed occurrence of such oedema in selective sites is still, however, unexplained. A toxic effect of pyruvic acid upon the grey matter around the walls and floor of the 3rd and 4th ventricles and the aqueduct or, alternatively, increased requirements of the vitamin by the areas affected have also been suggested, but, so far, there is no proof for either mechanism.

The localization of the Wernicke syndrome in parts of the hypothalamus and in particular in the mamillary bodies has considerable implications in relation to cerebral function. Experimental investigations indicate that the region of the mamillary body and of the posterior nucleus of the hypothalamus is concerned with the maintenance of consciousness and the waking state. Clouding of consciousness, stupor and coma would then be the natural consequence of impairment of these centres. Gamper (1928) first drew attention to the association of mamillary lesion with Korsakoff's psychosis in the chronic forms of the Wernicke syndrome, though it should be remembered that this psychosis may also be caused by lesions different in type and localization.

In five cases of alcoholism with Korsakoff's psychosis, Carmichael and Stern (1931) found widespread neuronal changes in the cerebral cortex (increased lipochrome deposits and central chromatolysis). These changes resembled the lesions of pellagra rather than thiamine deficiency. Although Korsakoff's psychosis is often preceded by delirium tremens, the pathological basis of the latter condition has not been clearly established. Widespread nerve cell degeneration of the type common to toxic conditions, and with no special emphasis on the diencephalon, has been described by many early authors and by Zahnd (1953).

Delirium tremens is often a reversible condition and it may be that during the illness there are temporary biochemical alterations. Such an explanation is consistent with the description of small recent periventricular haemorrhages and perivascular oedema in nine cases of typical alcoholic delirium that were interpreted as an initial stage of the Wernicke syndrome (Huber 1954).

Other clinical features of Wernicke's syndrome are accounted for by the pathological lesions; disturbance of eye muscles by the peri-aqueductal damage, ataxia and nystagmus by changes in the vestibular nuclei, respiratory disturbance by involvement of the dorsal vagal nucleus and occasional impairment of vision by involvement of chiasma and optic nerves or by retinal haemorrhages.

Grunnet (1969) compared Wernicke's disease seen at necropsy in France between 1934-43 and 1965-68 and noted changes: there had been a rise in the number of acute cases in recent years, especially among alcoholics, though the age at death tended to be 10 years higher, probably due to improved nutritional standards. An atypical, more chronic form had appeared since 1965, perhaps due to the ameliorating effects of treatment. Gross evidence of lesions is now less common and the haemorrhagic component may be absent, as noted by Rosenblum and Feigin (1965).

Not all cases of the Wernicke syndrome are fatal. Both Neubürger (1936) and Campbell and Russell (1941) found old cerebral scars in the characteristic sites in several cases of alcoholism or gastric carcinoma dying from intercurrent disease, without clinical evidence of encephalopathy. More recently it has been shown that intensive and early treatment leads to rapid and usually complete recovery, though in some cases the Korsakoff's psychosis may persist for many months or even years (Walton 1969). Ule (1959) described a childhood encephalopathy that he considered to be qualitatively similar to Wernicke's syndrome, although the lesions affected the lower brainstem and not the mamillary bodies. Neither the history nor the clinical symptomatology, however, corresponded to that usually found in cases of the Wernicke syndrome. It is possible that the author was dealing with the infantile subacute necrotizing encephalopathy, first described by Leigh (1951), and which is considered on p. 177.

Alcoholic peripheral neuropathy

The evidence incriminating lack of a vitamin B factor, especially thiamine, in this condition came first from the response of early cases to parenteral treatment with this vitamin and later from the study, in cases of peripheral neuropathy, of the urinary excretion of thiamine or of the blood pyruvate levels, especially after loading doses of glucose (Bueding, Wortis, Fein and Esturonne 1942; Joiner, Thompson and Watson 1950). The clinical and pathological resemblance of alcoholic neuropathy to beriberi has been stressed by Victor and Adams (1953). According to Greenfield (1958), the neuropathy affects motor and sensory neurons in varying proportions; it is most severe in the distal parts of the nerves, so that the extensors of the feet and toes are most commonly affected, and next the extensors of the wrist and fingers. In the ataxic form, position sense may be affected early and severely. This type of sensory loss indicates a greater degeneration of large than of small fibres, and this was confirmed by histograms on myelin-stained sections of the small cutaneous nerve to the toes (Greenfield and Carmichael 1935) (Fig. 5.5). The latter authors and Aring and Spies (1939) found less evidence of axonal lesions. There was prac-tically no regeneration of myelin as long as 11 months after treatment had begun in the cases examined by Aring and Spies. Walsh and McCleod (1970), however, found axonal (Wallerian type) degeneration in acute cases and regeneration in chronic cases given an adequate diet.

In occasional cases the degeneration of the sensory neuron can be traced into the posterior columns of the spinal cord, but these may be intact even in severely paralysed cases (Carmichael and Stern 1931). In severe cases the anterior horn neurons, especially in the lower lumbar and upper sacral segments of the spinal cord, often show a varying degree of chromatolysis.

Apenzeller and Richardson (1966) found abnormal giant neurons showing degeneration, in the sympathetic chain of patients with alcoholic polyneuropathy; there was evidence that such neurons could eventually disappear and that similar changes occurred in diabetic neuropathy, though the clinical significance of such findings was not proven.

Experimental thiamine deficiency

Numerous experimental investigations have been carried out in species ranging from pigeons to

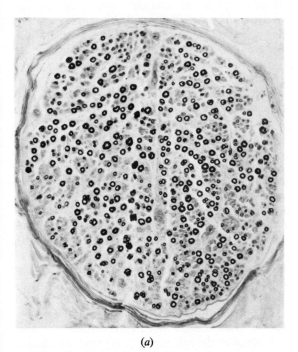
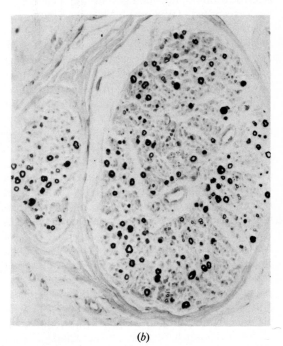

(a)   (b)

Fig. 5.5 Alcoholic neuropathy. Sections of fascicles from terminal cutaneous branch of anterior tibial nerve. (a) Normal nerve; (b) Alcoholic neuropathy. Osmic acid. × 200.

primates and, in a limited way, in man. The pioneer studies by Eijkman (1897) and Fraser and Stanton (1910) showed the nature of the lesions and fundamental investigations in pigeons and rats by Peters and Sinclair (1933), and Peters and Thompson (1934) established the fact that oxidation of pyruvic acid is prevented in the absence of thiamine.

Hyperpyruvaemia has been observed in most species subjected to an appreciable fall of the blood thiamine level. Bradycardia, dilatation of the heart, electrocardiographic changes, atrioventricular block and auricular fibrillation have been demonstrated (Follis, Miller, Wintrobe and Stein 1943) and cardiac abnormalities confirmed at necropsy. Microscopically, the lesions most frequently described have been focal necrosis of heart muscle fibres. Ultrastructural studies in rats have shown mitochondrial abnormalities within individual fibres, culminating in focal areas of cell death (Davies and Jennings 1970). As thiamine deficiency leads to accumulation of lactate and pyruvate in mitochondria and a fall in energy production, it is to be expected that mitochondria would be affected early.

In man, in whom only mild degrees of deficiency have been induced by experiment, clinical and electrocardiographic changes in the heart have been recorded (Williams, Mason, Smith and Wilder 1942).

The significance of polyneuritis has been criticized by Follis (1958) because in the earlier experimental investigations the diets used may have been deficient in factors other than thiamine. In pigeons there have, however, been acceptable descriptions of neuropathy by Bertrand, Liber and Randoin (1934), Swank (1940), Swank and Prados (1942), Zimmerman (1943) and Shaw and Phillips (1945). North and Sinclair (1956) succeeded in inducing degeneration in the distal segments of the sciatic and posterior tibial nerves of rats, but emphasized that the tissue was relatively resistant and yielded lesions only after prolonged deficiency. Even then, only 3 to 5% of the fibres were affected. This may, to some extent, explain the negative results of other experimental investigators. An alternative explanation has been offered by Scriba and Luckner (1949) and Luckner and Scriba (1949), who claimed that a complete experimental equivalent of tropical human beriberi and its triad of heart failure, oedema and peripheral neuropathy could develop in albino rats fed on a diet poor in

protein as well as in thiamine. Their views accord with those of Platt (1958a), though histological detail of the nerve degeneration is not given. North and Sinclair (1957) were unable to induce peripheral nerve degeneration in rats repeatedly subjected to short periods of thiamine (and pantothenic acid) deficiency.

Lesions similar to those seen in the human Wernicke syndrome have been found in many studies on experimental animals with chronic thiamine deficiency: in rats, Prickett (1934) described haemorrhages and unspecified nerve cell changes with a predilection for the vestibular nuclei; in pigeons, Alexander and his collaborators (Alexander, Pijoan, Myerson and Keene 1938; Alexander 1940) induced in the periventricular grey matter haemorrhagic vascular lesions which closely resembled those of the Wernicke syndrome. The latter findings have been confirmed in pigeons and dogs by Zimmerman (1939, 1943); in pigeons by Prados and Swank (1942), in mice by Dunn, Morris and Dubnik (1947), and in rats by Ule and Kammerer (1960). Rinehart (1947) and Rinehart, Friedman and Greenberg (1949) found focal necrosis in the mamillary bodies, corpora quadrigemina, and in the nuclei of the 3rd, 6th, 8th and 10th cranial nerves; they also described similar lesions in unusual sites such as the striatum, globus pallidus and substantia nigra but failed to induce peripheral nerve degeneration. Alexander (1940) considered the vascular changes to be the initial lesion, attributing vasoprotective properties to thiamine. This view was not shared by Prados and Swank, Rinehart and others, who concluded that the vascular proliferation was a reaction to primary neuronal damage, in contrast to the commonly held views on the pathogenesis of the human disease.

Findings resembling those in Wernicke's encephalopathy have also been reported in foxes suffering from Chastek paralysis (Alexander, Green, Evans and Wolf 1941; Evans, Carlson and Green 1942) and in a similar, spontaneous disease of cats (Jubb, Saunders and Coates 1956). In both species, a raw fish diet which contains thiamase, the thiamine-destroying enzyme, was implicated; the benefit from thiamine therapy was demonstrated.

Dreyfus and Victor (1961) reviewed the neuropathological effects of experimental thiamine deficiency in the rat, monkey, pigeon, fox and cat and made a comparison with human Wernicke's disease. They noted striking similarities in all species, the basic lesion being symmetrical focal pan-necrosis of the brainstem nuclei and di-encephalon. Dreyfus (1965) postulated that in progressive thiamine depletion a critical reduction of transketolase activity resulted in defensive oligodendrocyte metabolism which led to irre-versible histological changes. Collins (1967) demonstrated glial alterations but was unable to decide whether the cells affected were oligo-dendrocytes or astrocytes. Warnock and Burk-halter (1968) have found evidence of malfunction of the blood–brain barrier in thiamine-deficient rats with significant impairment of transport systems dependent on this barrier. Such mal-function may allow harmful metabolites to gain access to nerve tissue.

In an electron-microscope study Robertson, Wasan and Skinner (1968) found swelling of glial cytoplasm in the early stages of thiamine deficiency in rats. Later, oedema involved the extracellular spaces and myelin sheaths. They postulated a breakdown of energy-dependent electrolyte transport by perivascular glia, leading to a fluid influx across the blood–brain barrier. This failure of active transport may stem from interference with the production of chemical energy by thiamine-dependent enzymes involved in carbohydrate metabolism. The factors respons-ible for the selective localization of the lesions was undetermined; regional differences in cell meta-bolism were re-emphasized, pointing to systems of separate cell types that react to thiamine deficiency in a specific way.

Most reviewers consider that the experimental evidence strongly supports the view that thiamine deficiency plays a major part or at least is an initiating factor in the aetiology of both beriberi and the Wernicke syndrome.

Vitamins of the B₂ group

Pantothenic acid

Deficiency of pantothenic acid will be considered first, not because it is the most important member of this group, but because it is more closely related to thiamine deficiency than other members. Like thiamine, pantothenic acid is intimately con-cerned with the oxidation of pyruvate, its absence or 'blocking' likewise resulting in hyperpyru-vaemia. As coenzyme A, it is an important catalyser of the acetylation of acetylcholine. For this reason, Follis (1948) thought that many lesions ascribed to thiamine deficiency may be caused by deficiency of pantothenate though this has not been confirmed (North and Sinclair 1957).

Pantothenic acid is indispensable to various animals. Its absence in rats results in alopecia, greying of the hair and generalized dermatitis and may also lead to ulceration of the gastro-intestinal tract, particularly of the colon. Haemor-rhagic necrosis of the adrenal has been reported in rats but not in other animals. An acute syn-drome of sudden prostration, coma, tachycardia and convulsions has been described in dogs de-prived of pantothenic acid (Schaefer, McKibbin and Elvehjem 1942). In monkeys made deficient by McCall, Waisman, Elvehjem and Jones (1946), ataxia was the main clinical sign. Follis and Wintrobe (1945) and Swank and Adams (1948) have observed degeneration of peripheral nerves, the posterior roots and their ganglia and the posterior columns of the spinal cord in pigs; the earliest lesion was central chromatolysis in neurons of the posterior root ganglia, followed by degeneration of myelin and axis cylinders in nerves, spinal roots or spinal cord; central chromatolysis in some anterior horn neurons and occasional degeneration in the pyramidal tracts were also found.

Pantothenic acid deficiency has not been of appreciable significance in man. It has been sug-gested (Gopalan 1946) that the 'burning feet' syndrome may be due, at least in part, to panto-thenic acid deficiency. Human volunteers in whom deficiency was induced by Bean, Hodges and Daum (1955), either by a diet devoid of the vitamin or by administration of its antagonist *co*-methyl pantothenic acid, showed signs of fatigue and paraesthesias of the 'burning feet' type that improved on large doses of the vitamin. Davidson and Passmore (1969), however, con-sider that the syndrome results from prolonged lack of protein and the B group of vitamins.

Nicotinic acid: Pellagra

Pellagra is the complication of most interest in relation to nicotinic acid deficiency. The disease was known in eighteenth-century Spain and re-ceived its present name (*pelle* = skin and *agra* = rough) from peasants in Northern Italy. In-toxication or bacterial infection were originally thought to be the cause, until the clinical studies of Goldberger and Wheeler (1915, 1920) indicated a relation to dietary deficiency, both in human patients and also in dogs with 'black tongue' disease, which has similar clinical features. (A selection of Goldberger's papers written between 1913 and 1928 was edited by Terris in 1963.)

Clinically pellagra is characterized by lesions of the skin and mucous membranes, and by neurological and psychiatric disturbances. The typical skin lesions begin as erythema and are followed by atrophy. Diarrhoea, glossitis, gastric achylia and anaemia are frequent. Changes in the nervous system develop later and polyneuritis, spastic paralysis and ataxia, tremor and rigidity, visual disturbances (particularly retrobulbar neuritis) and deafness have all been described. Mental changes may occur early and are of 'psychoneurotic' type, which later develop into depressive or manic states, followed in severe cases by progressive dementia (Leigh 1952). Epileptic convulsions are not uncommon.

Usually pellagra takes a chronic intermittent course over several years, and morphological lesions of the central nervous system appear only in the later stages.

An acute syndrome has been reported by various authors (Jolliffe, Bowman, Rosenblum and Fein 1940; Sydenstricker and Cleckley 1941; Hardwick 1943; Spillane 1947) and has been termed *nicotinic acid deficiency encephalopathy*. Clinically there is clouding of consciousness, cogwheel rigidity, and grasping and sucking reflexes. The patients are usually elderly, with chronic organic illness and have often been living on an obviously inadequate diet. Signs of other vitamin B complex deficiency states are frequently present. Patients with this encephalopathy may respond dramatically to nicotinic acid therapy.

A syndrome exhibiting pellagra-like symptoms (light-sensitive dermatitis, cerebellar ataxia and psychotic manifestations) has been described by Baron, Dent, Harris, Hart and Jepson (1956). Cases described by Hersov (1955), Rodnight and McIlwain (1955), and Hersov and Rodnight (1960), though originally interpreted differently, have been identified as the same condition, which has been named *Hartnup disease* after one of the affected families. Biochemically, it is characterized by a pronounced and persistent hyperamino aciduria of a special pattern and an abnormally large output of indolic compounds. The basic metabolic defect results from a genetically induced disorder of cell membranes that involves the transport mechanisms of certain neutral amino acids; this defect in the proximal convoluted tubule results in amino aciduria. Malabsorption in the jejunum leads to an intra-luminal increase in tryptophan, which is broken down to indolic compounds by the colonic flora and subsequently excreted in the urine. The abnormal metabolism of tryptophan probably prevents its conversion to nicotinamide, and thus increases the threshold at which the diet becomes inadequate to provide enough nicotinamide for bodily requirements (Milne 1969). Post-mortem investigations have not been traced.

Patients with the carcinoid syndrome due to a malignant argentaffinoma occasionally develop tryptophan deficiency and a pellagra-like state, because of the circulating serotonin.

Pathological studies on pellagra include those made by Wilson (1914), Raubitschek (1915), Pentschew (1928), Greenfield and Holmes (1939), Hsü (1942) and Leigh (1952).

The change most consistently found in the brain is central chromatolysis, first described as 'central neuritis' by Adolf Meyer (1901), though there has been controversy about its distribution. Leigh examined 14 cases and found the highest incidence in Betz cells, followed by pontine nuclei (Fig. 5.7), dorsal vagal nucleus, gracile and cuneate nuclei, nucleus ambiguus, descending trigeminal nucleus, oculomotor nucleus, basal ganglia, vestibular nucleus and reticular and arcuate nuclei in that order. Of the six spinal cords studied, central chromatolysis of anterior horn neurons was seen in four (Fig. 5.6). Hypoglossal and facial nuclei, and the Purkinje cells of the cerebellum, though among the largest neurons, were not affected. Axonal damage is too inconsistent in the central nervous system to account for the chromatolysis, which is more likely to be related to the effect of a metabolic defect on neuronal perikarya.

Proliferation of the neuroglia is not a feature. The fibrosis and hyaline change of the blood vessels emphasized by Hsü was infrequent in Leigh's material; increase of lipofuscin is, according to Hsü, often seen in pellagra, but this also was not a prominent feature in Leigh's material.

In addition to central chromatolysis, degeneration of the posterior and lateral tracts of the cord has received much attention. It was the usual combination of spinal cord lesions in Wilson's cases. In Wilson's and in Greenfield and Holmes' case, the degeneration was most severe in the fasciculus gracilis, with lesions of lesser severity in the spinocerebellar and crossed and uncrossed pyramidal tracts (Fig. 5.8). Most of the 13 Chinese soldiers who died from inanition

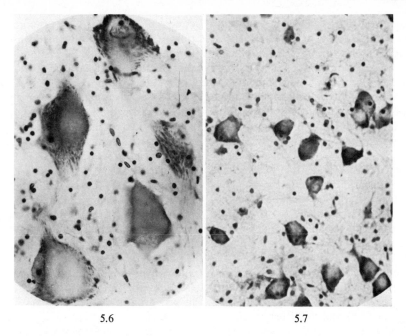

5.6   5.7

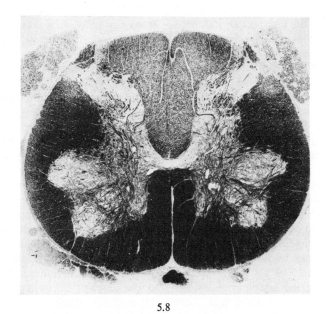

5.8

Figs. 5.6–5.8 Pellagra.

Fig. 5.6 Central chromatolysis in anterior horn cells. Nissl. × 250.
Fig. 5.7 Central chromatolysis in pontine cells. Nissl. × 250. (Reproduced by courtesy of Dr Leigh.)
Fig. 5.8. Lumbar cord in pellagra. Note severe degeneration of the posterior columns and slighter pallor of the pyramidal tracts. Myelin.

and were studied by Hsü, showed degeneration of the posterior columns, Pellagrinous degeneration of posterior and lateral tracts differs histologically from the degeneration of the same fibre systems seen in vitamin B_{12} deficiency. The characteristic honeycombed appearance caused by discontinuous degeneration of myelin sheaths in the latter condition is absent in pellagra, which more closely resembles secondary (Wallerian) degeneration.

Greenfield and Holmes and also Wilson have found that both posterior and anterior roots are affected. Involvement of the peripheral nerves has also been noted by many workers (for example Wilson (1914), Aring, Bean, Roseman, Rosenbaum and Spies (1941), Greenfield and Carmichael (1935)). The latter authors counted the fibres in the cutaneous nerves of the toe and found that in pellagrins the highest count was 5500, whereas in normal nerves the number of fibres was between 6500 and 9000 per mm². In severe cases both myelin and axons showed evidence of degeneration, but in milder cases only the myelin was affected.

Both central and peripheral lesions can occur together, though experience in the second World War has made it clear that certain component syndromes of pellagra can also occur independently. Polyneuritis, for example, is likely to be an admixture rather than an integral part of pellagra and is probably due to deficiency of other vitamins, especially thiamine or other components of the B_2 complex. Combined degeneration of posterior and lateral columns identical to that described in pellagra has been described as an isolated deficiency syndrome, sometimes combined with retrobulbar neuritis and deafness (Spillane).

Biochemical and experimental studies. Since Elvehjem, Madden, Strong and Woolley (1937) showed that nicotinic acid cured black tongue in dogs, it has been accepted that nicotinic acid deficiency is a major aetiological factor in pellagra. Black tongue is not only clinically similar to human pellagra; Denton (1928), who studied Goldberger's dogs, described histological lesions of the skin and mucous membranes that were indistinguishable from those in human pellagra. Histological changes in the central nervous system were not mentioned.

Pentschew (1929) did not find histological abnormalities in the nervous system of a macaque that had developed pellagra-like signs in the course of poisoning with ergotamine. Degeneration of the anterior horn neurons of rats fed on a diet poor in vitamin B_2 was not comparable with the central chromatolysis of human pellagra (Stern and Findlay 1929). Although Scherer (1944) described central chromatolysis in cranial nuclei and in the anterior horns of a chimpanzee showing loss of hair and paralysis, there is no proof that the cause of these signs was nicotinic acid deficiency.

Experiments with antagonistic analogues of nicotinic acid (antinicotinamides) have been equally puzzling. Hicks (1955), using 3-acetyl-pyridine in mice and rats, demonstrated changes such as eosinophilia of cytoplasm and pyknosis of nuclei in neurons of the spinal and sympathetic ganglia, the supraoptic nucleus and the pyramidal layer of Ammon's horn. Changes were less frequent in the medial amygdaloid nucleus and in cell groups of the medulla. The animals had not shown convulsions and the lesions could be prevented by antecedent treatment with nicotinamide. Mice kept on a nicotinamide free diet did not show comparable lesions. Coggleshall and MacLean (1958) also experimenting with 3-acetyl-pyridine in mice and rats, obtained lesions confined almost exclusively to Lorente de No's areas C3 and C4 of Ammon's horn but cell loss in these regions was not accompanied by glial increase; these changes are not comparable to pellagrous lesions. The animals developed weakness, inspiratory rhonchi and urinary incontinence within 6 hours of administration; most of those surviving the acute stage did not show histological changes. Pinsky and Fraser (1960) gave pregnant mice a single dose of another antinicotinamide, 6-amino-nicotinamide, and observed weakness within 6 to 12 hours; their report does not include neurohistological investigations but is interesting because the temporary inactivation of nicotinamide induced congenital malformations in the offspring. Rats, cats and dogs inoculated with 6-amino-nicotinamide showed lesions that differed from those obtained with other antinicotinamides and were confined mainly to the anterior horns and some motor nuclei of the medulla; there were petechial haemorrhages, neuronal chromatolysis (often proceeding to necrosis) and microglial, endothelial and inflammatory reactions (Sternberg and Philips 1958; Wolf, Cowen and Gellar 1959, 1962). Wolf, Cowen and Geller (1962) suggested that the difference in localization and quality of experimental lesions may be due to effects on different nicotinamide radicles.

Dietary deficiency of nicotinic acid is only a partial factor. The greater part of the requirement results from biosynthesis by bacteria in the intestines, and destruction of these bacteria by sulphonamides or antibiotics can result in pellagrous features. The amino acid tryptophan is the source from which nicotinic acid is synthesized (see p. 194) and the absence of tryptophan from maize probably explains why a wholly maize diet often results in pellagra; blood tryptophan levels are relatively low in pellagra (Truswell, Hansen and Wannenburg 1968). Woolley (1946) isolated a pellagra-inducing factor from maize, which may be chemically related to one of the acetyl-pyridin antinicotinamides (see McIlwain 1955).

The complex nature of the deficiency in experimental pellagra was well demonstrated, and to some extent clarified, in experiments under varying conditions by Krehl, Tepley, Sarma and Elvehjem (1945) in dogs and rats and by Wintrobe and his colleagues (1943) in pigs. A diet poor in nicotinamide but adequate in thiamine, riboflavin, pantothenic acid and choline, and with an optimal amount of protein, had few ill effects, but when the protein intake was reduced, signs of deficiency developed. In such animals chromatolysis in the small nerve cells of the posterior root ganglia was reported, but there was no myelin degeneration in peripheral nerves.

Madhaven, Belavady and Gopalan (1968) concluded that pellagra occurring in the Hyderabad region of India is related to consumption of the millet jowar (*Sorglium vulgare*) and that the high leucine content of jowar is a factor. 'Black tongue' was induced in dogs fed diets containing maize, or jowar, or casein-plus-leucine. The animals showed extensive ulceration of the gastrointestinal mucosa. Mild changes were found in the spinal cord, including focal haemorrhages and chromatolysis, satellitosis and neuronal phagocytosis. Excess leucine interferes with tryptophan and nicotinic acid metabolism and so precipitates the pellagra. Gopalan (1969) believes this to be the first evidence that an important deficiency can arise because of particular proportionate amounts of different dietary amino acids.

To conclude, there is reason to believe that pellagra results from a diet that is poor in protein and reduced in nicotinic acid, riboflavin and haemopoetic factors; toxic or antivitamin substances may also be concerned. The neurohistological picture of pure nicotinic acid deficiency is not yet fully known, either in man or in experimental animals. Pellagra is a disease that still needs investigation.

Riboflavin

Riboflavin was the first constituent of an enzyme system to be isolated and synthesized. As riboflavin phosphate it is part of several 'yellow' flavoprotein enzymes and in combination with adenylic acid functions as coenzyme in the dehydrogenase group.

In experimental animals of various species the most prominent changes resulting from deficiency occur in the skin, eyes and nervous system. The skin lesions tend to vary among different species in extent and in quality; usually there is dermatitis followed by atrophy of sebaceous glands and hair follicles. In some species this is most marked in the angle of the mouth and in the nasolabial folds. Bessey and Wolbach (1939) have drawn attention to abnormal capillary growth in the cornea. Cataracts have been noted in rats and pigs.

Myelin degeneration in peripheral nerves and in the fibre tracts of the spinal cord, especially in the posterior columns, has been described in rats (Shaw and Phillips 1941), in dogs (Street, Cowgill and Zimmerman 1941), in mice (Lippincott and Morris 1942) and in young pigs (Wintrobe, Buschke, Follis and Humphreys 1944). All these lesions have been designated 'equivocal' by Follis.

In man the main change, induced experimentally by Sebrell and Butler (1939), is a dermatitis about the mouth resulting in fissure formation (cheilosis) and reddening of the lips. Vascularization of the cornea, occasionally resulting in ulceration, has been reported. It was at one time thought that combined tract degeneration, retrobulbar neuritis and deafness might be due to deficiency of riboflavin, but experimental experience in human volunteers has so far not resulted in any lesion of the peripheral or central nervous system.

Pyridoxine (vitamin B₆)

Goldberger and Lillie (1926) described a pellagra-like condition in rats fed on a maize diet extracted by alcohol. Gyorgy (1934) and his collaborators excluded nicotinic acid and riboflavin as causative agents and showed that another factor, pyridoxine (vitamin B_6) was responsible. Pyridoxine seems to be important in protein metabolism.

Experimental lesions have been described in several species and are most prominent in skin, erythropoietic tissue and the nervous system. The skin lesions consist of pellagra-like symmetrical dermatitis that is not influenced by sunlight. Anaemia (usually normocytic) develops, the liver may show fatty infiltration and there may be extensive deposits of iron pigment in liver, spleen and bone marrow. Rinehart and Greenberg (1956) found intimal proliferation (which closely resembled human atherosclerosis) in many arteries of monkeys completely deprived of pyridoxine for 5 to 6 months. Blood pressure was usually persistently raised and cirrhosis of the liver and dental caries was frequently noted.

Epileptiform fits (grand mal and petit mal) lasting several minutes have been described in deficient rats and pigs (Chick, El Sadr and Worden 1940; Wintrobe *et al*. 1943); the fits responded to replacement therapy. Pyridoxal phosphate is of importance in the conversion of glutamic acid to γ-amino-butyric acid (GABA) which is considered to be an inhibitor of nerve cell function (Roberts 1961; Tower 1961; see also p. 195). Demyelination of peripheral nerves, posterior root fibres and of fibres in the posterior columns has also been described in experiments, but significant chromatolysis in posterior root ganglia were not noted (Follis and Wintrobe 1945; Swank and Adams 1948), even though the neurons later atrophy and may disappear.

Convulsions in human infants may be favourably influenced by pyridoxine (Hunt, Stokes, McCrory and Stroud 1954). Desoxypyridoxine, a synthetic analogue but an antagonist of pyridoxine, has been reported to cause human peripheral neuropathy that is relieved by treatment with this vitamin (Vilter *et al*. 1953). The pathogenesis of the peripheral neuropathy that may complicate the clinical use of the hydrazide, isoniazid, is said to be the combination of isoniazid with pyridoxine to form a stable compound which interferes with the function of pyridoxine (p. 165), but recent studies reveal no evidence of significant vitamin B_6 deficiency during isoniazid therapy (Nutrition Reviews 1968). Pyridoxine deficiency neuropathy has also been noted as a complication of therapy with the antihypertensive drug hydralazine. The hydrazine ($-NHNH_2$) group in the structure of hydralazine relates the drug to the family of compounds, the hydrazines

and hydrazides ($-CONHNH_2$), which have been shown to induce pyridoxine-responsive convulsions in laboratory animals (Raskin and Fishman 1965). Pyridoxal phosphate is also required for the conversion of 5-hydroxytryptophan into 5-hydroxytryptamine (serotonin). Deficiency of pyridoxine may thus reduce the level of serotonin in the brain.

Purpura and Gonzales-Monteagudo (1960) described necrosis in the folium of the hippocampus (areas C2 and C4 of Lorente de No) which developed within 2 hours of a single injection of methoxypyridoxine to cats. In Nissl preparations the nerve cells were shrunken, deeply basophilic and showed complete loss of intracellular architecture. In view of the incidence of convulsions, the authors stress that they failed to produce similar changes within so short a time either by hypoxia or by metrazol and strychnine. The animals had been paralysed with succinylcholine chloride. It is of interest that the lesions occurred in the same localization as those described above, following administration of analogues of nicotinic acid to rodents. Confirmation on a systematic basis seems to be called for.

Vitamin B_{12} neuropathy (subacute combined degeneration of the spinal cord)

Leichtenstern (1884) reported the association of pernicious anaemia with disease of the spinal cord but he considered that the anaemia came on in the course of tabes dorsalis, to which he attributed the spinal lesion. Lichtheim (1887) appears to have been the first to recognize that the spinal lesions of pernicious anaemia differed in several respects from those of tabes. The lesions, which were subacute, as shown both by the short history and by the abundant lipophages in the degenerate tracts of the cord, involved both the dorsal columns and the anterolateral columns; there was no thickening of the leptomeninges and only slight atrophy of the dorsal nerve roots in the lumbar region. Lichtheim's pupil, Minnich (1892), supplemented these observations by examining the spinal cords of five fatal cases of pernicious anaemia with no neurological symptoms or signs, and by finding slight degeneration in the posterior and lateral columns.

The first full clinical and pathological description of the disease was given by Russell, Batten and Collier (1900) who named it *subacute combined degeneration of the spinal cord* (SACD); they were not satisfied with this term but were unable to suggest a better one. Other names that have been suggested such as 'funicular myelopathy' and 'posterolateral sclerosis' have never been generally accepted. The term SACD gives no indication of the association of the spinal lesions with macrocytic anaemia and, in fact, Russell et al. showed that in some cases anaemia cannot be demonstrated. Nor does the term indicate involvement of peripheral nerves or, as occurs in some cases, of the brain. For such reasons, Richmond and Davidson (1958) proposed the term vitamin B_{12} neuropathy and this is now preferred.

Synthesis of crystalline vitamin B_{12} (cyanocobalamin) by Lester-Smith (1948) and Rickes, Brink, Konuisky, Wood and Folkers (1948) marked the culminating point of a great scientific achievement that evolved through the empirical discovery of the value of liver in the treatment of pernicious anaemia by Minot and Murphy (1926), the distinction between intrinsic (gastric) and extrinsic (dietary) factors by Castle (1929) and the identification and eventual synthesis of folic acid in 1946. Vitamin B_{12} has greatly reduced mortality from SACD by prevention, by cure of early cases, and by arrest of the fully developed disease. Folic acid, however, though it has an effect on macrocytic anaemia, is of no value in the treatment or prevention of the neurological complications. Although vitamin B_{12} is now known to be Castle's extrinsic factor, the intrinsic factor is still unidentified. The latter is a glycoprotein, which chelates with and serves as a carrier for vitamin B_{12}, the resultant complex being absorbed in the terminal ileum. In man, intrinsic factor is produced mainly in the fundus of the stomach, but in many animals it is produced near the pylorus or even in the jejunum; this has led to much confusion in experimental research.

The observation by Hurst and Bell (1922) that in cases of SACD achlorhydria was always present led to too rigid an identification with Addisonian pernicious anaemia, in which there is believed to be a genetically determined or autoimmune atrophy of the gastric mucosa. Richmond and Davison demonstrated that Addisonian anaemia is by far the commonest cause of vitamin B_{12} neuropathy, though about one in seven cases had different aetiologies which included other gastric lesions (such as total or subtotal gastrectomy or gastric carcinoma), malabsorption of vitamin B_{12} as a sequel of organic diseases of the intestine (strictures, fistulas, diverticula, tuberculous ulcera-tion, tumour, regional ileitis, idiopathic and tropical sprue), and dietary reduction or absence of the vitamin. Richmond and Davison were able to collect ten cases (not verified histologically) from the literature which came within these non-Addisonian categories and were able to add three new cases that were confirmed by histology. Olivarius and Roos (1968) described SACD following partial gastrectomy and Verjaal and Timmermans-Van Den Bos (1967) following dietary deficiency.

Vegetarian diets are poor in vitamin B_{12}. Wokes, Badenoch and Sinclair (1955) and Wokes (1956) found the serum values of the vitamin significantly low in British vegans, who showed also an excess of p-hydroxylphenylpyruvic acid in the blood serum. These abnormalities were most marked during the first 6 to 10 years of the dietary regime and tended to disappear in later years. Anaemia was slight and no definite signs of neuropathy were recorded. Badenoch (1954) has recorded definite clinical signs of neuropathy in a 15-year-old boy who was a strict vegetarian and who improved dramatically following treatment with vitamin B_{12}. Electroencephalographic abnormalities were noted in vegans (West and Ellis 1966) but unlike those of pernicious anaemia such changes were not corrected by treatment with vitamin B_{12}.

Clinical features. The term *subacute* describes the course of most untreated cases in which functional disturbances increase fairly rapidly and cause severe disability in a few weeks or months. The course may be more rapid so that the patient is unable to stand after 2 to 3 weeks or it may be more gradual and allow the patient to continue at work for a year or more. Russell et al. distinguished three stages in the disease. (1) A stage of spastic paraparesis and slight ataxia, with marked paraesthesias in the lower limbs. The latter symptoms consist of numbness, stiffness or tingling and may precede the onset of motor disability by several months. The upper limbs may be similarly affected at the same time as, or (more often) later than, the lower limbs. Clumsiness in writing is often an early feature. (2) A stage of severe ataxic paraplegia with marked anaesthesia of the legs and trunk, which may come on very rapidly so that a patient who was able to walk on going to bed at night is unable to stand the next morning. This disability is due more to ataxia than to weakness. (3) The final stage, that of complete paraplegia with absolute anaesthesia leading to bedsores and death from infection of the urinary tract, is seldom seen in treated patients. The chief danger to patients is in the first stage, when the anaemia is slight and the significance of the early, largely subjective, symptoms is not recognized. Recovery from the first stage is usually remarkably complete under adequate treatment, but the transition in untreated patients from the first to the second stage may be so rapid that it cannot be arrested before grave and irremediable damage has been done to the spinal cord.

Heaton, McCormick and Freeman (1958) found the serum level of vitamin B_{12} to be lower in 13 patients suffering from tobacco amblyopia than in normal controls. Their patients did not show other neurological abnormalities; amblyopia, however, may be an early indication of B_{12} deficiency. Freeman and Heaton (1961) suggested that the 'optic neuritis' sometimes found in pernicious anaemia was tobacco amblyopia due to cyanide intoxication (see below) from tobacco smoke.

Various mental changes have been observed and range from neurasthenia and depression to confusional states, amnesic syndromes and dementia ('megaloblastic madness'); several workers (Ferraro, Arieti and English 1945; Mayer-Gross, Slater and Roth 1954) stressed the frequency of paranoid psychoses. The overall incidence of mental disorder was estimated by Woltman (1924) to be 4% of nearly 1500 cases of pernicious anaemia seen at the Mayo Clinic, but it is not clear whether this estimate includes minor affective aberrations. Epileptic seizures occasionally occur. Henderson, Strachan and Beck (1966) suggested that a relatively inexpensive and reliable screening procedure for the detection of occult vitamin B_{12} deficiency in psychiatric practice would be primary screening with the immuno-fluorescence antigastric–antibody test, secondary screening with the augmented histamine test meal and final diagnosis by serial serum vitamin B_{12} assays. Shulman (1967), however, concluded from a prospective controlled investigation that routine screening is not indicated.

Pathology. Russell *et al.* noted that the disease mainly involved the midthoracic segments of the cord, where a zone of destruction of white matter might extend all round the cord, affecting not only the long tracts but endogenous and exogenous fibres alike. In severe cases the only intact fibres at this level were those in close relation to the grey horns (Fig. 5.11). On tracing the degeneration upwards it diminished, especially in the antero-lateral columns, until in the upper cervical segments only the posterior columns, especially the funiculus gracilis, and the spinocerebellar tracts were demyelinated. Degeneration in the pyramidal tract began in some cases as high as the medullary pyramids, but these were usually normal. On passing downwards the lesions again became more limited until in the lower lumbar segments only the pyramidal tracts were degenerated.

The early lesions consist of swelling of myelin sheaths with little change in the axons. The lipid in these swollen sheaths at first retains the characters of myelin, staining darkly with Weigert's chrome-haematoxylin and with iron-haematoxylin lakes, and giving the appearance of four bright sectors of a circle under polarized light. At this stage longitudinal sections show a number of fusiform swellings along the course of the myelin sheaths (Fig. 5.12). In some of these, but by no means all, the axons have similar fusiform swellings, but they do not fill the swollen myelin sheaths to the same degree as in traumatic or in early ischaemic lesions. The next stage is the breakdown of the myelin sheath into its constituent lipids and the disappearance of the axons. In this way empty spaces form and these tend to fuse together giving the tissue a loose, vacuolated appearance. The myelin breaks down in the same manner as in Wallerian degeneration; numerous lipophages appear and gradually come to lie within the perivascular spaces of the small vessels. As a result of the damage to the axons at the levels involved in the primary lesion (usually the midthoracic segments) there is secondary Wallerian degeneration in the long tracts, which may be the only lesions in the cervical and lumbar segments.

The distribution of the lesions is remarkably constant. The earliest evidence usually appears in the centres of both posterior columns, as irregular oval areas separated both from the grey horns and from the surface by intact fibres (Michell Clarke 1904) (Fig. 5.9). In the lateral columns lesions may appear, at the same time or slightly later, in areas on the surface of the cord immediately anterior to the posterior horns (Fig. 5.10). Thence they spread inwards and forwards and may in severe cases eventually surround the anterolateral columns. More commonly, small, distinct foci of degeneration appear on the surface

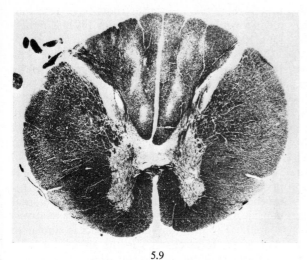
5.9

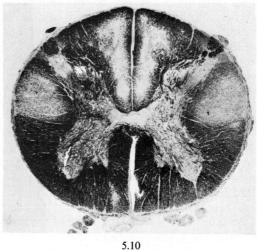
5.10

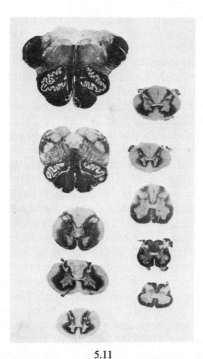
5.11

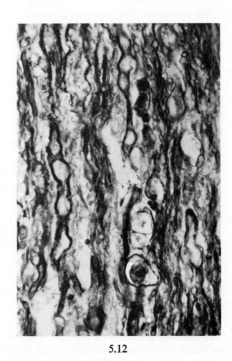
5.12

Figs. 5.9–5.12   Cord in subacute combined degeneration.   Myelin.

Fig. 5.9   Early degeneration limited to the posterior columns.

Fig. 5.10   Fairly early degeneration in posterior and lateral columns and very early degeneration in one anterior column.

Fig. 5.11   Severe case.   Note that there is only Wallerian degeneration in the medulla and the lower lumbar segments.

Fig. 5.12   High power view of longitudinal section of the posterior columns in an early case, showing irregular swellings of the myelin sheaths.

of the cord or in the lips of the anteromedian fissure. Neither in the posterior nor in the anterolateral columns do the early lesions have the distribution of tract degenerations, although they may come to involve much of the posterior columns and of the pyramidal and spinocerebellar tracts.

There has been some discussion about demyelination without damage to the axons in SACD. Although its pathogenesis is probably different from that of demyelinating diseases, there may be, as has been described, early changes in the myelin without evident lesions of the axon; if the disease is arrested at this stage it is probable that some loss of myelin will remain. But lesions in the axons follow soon after those of the myelin and lead to typical Wallerian degeneration. In some very early cases, in which the plantar reflexes were of extensor type, Greenfield and O'Flynn (1933) found very slight and early lesions in the lateral columns and it was suggested that under treatment signs of involvement of the pyramidal tracts might have disappeared. Therefore, the remission and apparently complete cure of early cases by adequate treatment may mean no more than the arrest of the disease at a stage when only a small proportion of the axons in any tract is damaged.

It has also been said that neuroglial scarring only occurs during remissions and especially as a result of treatment. However, Russell et al. observed fibrous gliosis in some of their cases, and it has been seen by others in untreated cases that had progressed steadily but not very rapidly. The astrocytic reaction seems to depend on the tempo of the disease process. In cases with a short history of rapid increase in disability, the astrocytes may appear inactive or undergo regressive changes. In less acute cases the cell bodies of the astrocytes swell slightly and their fibres become thicker and more numerous. In the more slowly progressive cases there is often considerable fibrous gliosis in the areas first affected although none may be seen in areas of recent degeneration.

There are insignificant changes in the meninges, nerve roots or the grey matter of the cord. The anterior horn neurons often contain some excess of lipofuscin but their Nissl granules stain well and there is no displacement of nuclei. In severe cases there may be chromatolysis of the neurons of Clarke's column due to axonal lesions. Similar changes may be seen in the Betz cells of the precentral gyrus. Posterior roots have occasionally shown loss of fibres (Putnam 1891; Zimmerman 1943).

More extensive changes in the brain have been reported in a relatively small number of cases by Barrett (1912-13), Woltman (1918), Adams and Kubik (1944), Ferraro, Arieti and English (1945) and others. The most characteristic lesions are small, ill-defined, often perivascular foci of demyelination within the cerebral white matter. They may be scanty, detectable only on careful search, or they may be disseminated over wide areas of the corona radiata (Fig. 5.13). The large ascending and descending tracts in the internal capsule, cerebral peduncles and pons are relatively spared. The histology of these foci is similar to that of the focal changes in the spinal cord, i.e. fusiform swelling of myelin sheaths and axis cylinders in recent foci, followed by destruction of myelin and axons and proliferation of lipophages in older foci. In some cases there may be perivascular and diffuse fibrous gliosis of greater severity than is usually seen in the spinal cord. Degeneration of the optic nerves (papillomacular bundle) was described by Bickel (1914) and Adams and Kubik (1944).

Apart from these foci of demyelination, fibrosis of capillaries and small arterioles, and haemorrhages may be found. Ferraro et al. described widespread degeneration of cortical neurons.

Pernicious anaemia is one of the conditions associated with the Wernicke syndrome (p. 196).

Peripheral nerves. Clinical observations have indicated that the peripheral nerves can be significantly affected (Ungley 1949) and the finding of decreased nerve conduction velocity in cases of pernicious anaemia (Mayer 1965) accords with this finding. Russell et al. (1900) found the peripheral nerves normal or only slightly degenerated in most of their cases, but in a more chronic case there was considerable degeneration in the larger nerves and in their small intramuscular branches. Van der Scheer and Kock (1938), Foster (1945) and Coërs and Woolf (1959) also found peripheral nerve changes. Greenfield and Carmichael (1935), examined the small peripheral cutaneous branch of the anterior tibial nerve and found a constant reduction in the number of myelin sheaths in four cases of SACD (Fig. 5.14). In these the average count ranged from 3000 to 4400 per mm² whereas in normal subjects of the same age the range was from 5500 to 9600 per mm². In two affected cases the loss was greatest in fibres with diameters of more than 3 μm but in one case it was more evenly spread. (In cases of alcoholic peripheral neuropathy examined at the same time a rather greater loss was found, with average counts of 2000 to 3200 per mm². In these the special incidence of the disease on the large fibres was even more marked.)

Clinical pathology. The cerebrospinal fluid

Pathogenesis. The concentration of vitamin B$_{12}$ in normal human tissues obtained at necropsy has been found to be least in brain (Hsu, Kawin, Minor and Mitchell 1966). Radioactive B$_{12}$ studies suggest that the body contains about 5 mg of the vitamin and loses 1 to 2·6 μg daily. Depletion of vitamin B$_{12}$ in the spinal cord may account for SACD, though it is not known how such depletion might cause the characteristic

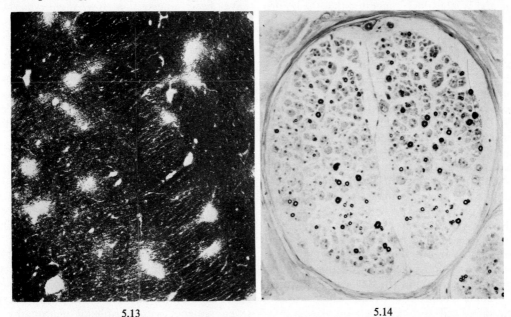

5.13   5.14

Fig. 5.13 Subacute combined degeneration. Ill-defined foci of demyelination in the occipital white matter. Heidenhain's myelin. × 20.

Fig. 5.14 Fascicle of peripheral cutaneous branch of the anterior tibial nerve in subacute combined degeneration. Osmic acid. × 200. Compare with Fig. 5.5*a*.

(CSF) usually shows a slight excess of protein. Vitamin B$_{12}$ levels in the CSF have been studied by various authors (see Girdwood 1968) and though there have been discrepancies, most are agreed that in both normal and affected patients, the CSF levels are considerably less than the serum levels. The blood picture varies greatly and examination of the bone marrow is always indicated in difficult cases. Estimations of the blood serum show reduction, but rarely complete absence, of vitamin B$_{12}$. Biopsy of the gastric mucosa and measurement of the absorption rate of radioactive vitamin B$_{12}$ proved helpful to Badenoch (1954) in separating non-Addisonian cases from those associated with Addison's pernicious anaemia. Only in the latter were the parietal glands in the mucosa atrophied or absent.

changes. SACD has no direct relationship to the degree of anaemia, as is shown by the appearance of disabling neurological lesions in patients with only slight anaemia or in those whose anaemia has responded to treatment with folic acid. Vitamin B$_{12}$ is known to take part in the metabolism of fats, proteins, carbohydrates and nucleic acids. Its absence inhibits the synthesis of RNA and might be expected to have a profound effect on cells such as neurons which have a high RNA content and a rapid protein turnover (Lester-Smith 1956). But an effect on the neuron as a whole or on its axon should produce a predominantly peripheral neuropathy such as is seen with deficiency of vitamin B$_1$ and pantothenic acid. Alexander (1957) observed absence of myelination in the sciatic nerves of 17-day-old B$_{12}$ deficient chicks, and reversible chromatolysis of neurons in the anterior horn and spinal and sympathetic ganglia, together with increase of sudanophilic lipid, in the peripheral nerves of deficient young rats. This points to a role of vitamin B_{12} in the formation and maintenance of myelin and Nissl bodies. Chicks made B_{12} deficient by Ferguson, Rigdon and Couch (1955) showed non-specific lesions (multiple haemorrhages) in the spinal cord and brain.

Cox and White (1962) suggested that the lesions in SACD may result from accumulation of methylmalonic acid and not from the direct effect of deficiency. Methylmalonic acid is excreted in excess in the urine in vitamin B_{12} deficiency, is a metabolite which consistently accumulates in B_{12} deficiency, and according to Vivacqua, Myerson, Prescott and Rabinowitz (1966) can be found in abnormal amounts in peripheral nerves from patients with pernicious anaemia. The long-term effects of methylmalonic acid on neural tissue are unknown.

Wilson and Langman (1966) produced evidence that the metabolism and detoxication of cyanide may be linked to vitamin B_{12}. Wilson and Matthews (1966) proposed that there was a reciprocal relationship between cyanide or thiocyanate and vitamin B_{12} concentrations in plasma. If this is so, it is possible that some neuropathological effects of vitamin B_{12} deficiency may arise from cyanide intoxication. Thiocyanate oxidase, present in red cells, probably acts on plasma thiocyanate (derived from the diet) to form the small normal, metabolically active cyanide pool. Ingested or inhaled cyanide (e.g. from tobacco) is metabolized via the I–C pathway, apparently by conversion of hydroxocobalamin to cyanocobalamin: thus in B_{12} deficiency the plasma cyanide concentration may rise excessively. It is possible that cyanide accumulation depends on thiocyanate oxidase (red cell mass) and thiocyanate concentrations; severe anaemia may therefore protect against the neurotoxic effects of cyanide; and the adverse effects of treating vitamin B_{12} deficiency anaemia with folic acid may follow an increase in thiocyanate oxidase concentrations, consequent on haematological remission increasing the red cell mass. Optic atrophy and retrobulbar neuritis in Addisonian pernicious anaemia occur mainly in smokers and there is a relative excess of male smokers with subacute combined degeneration of the cord, compared with the sex incidence of uncomplicated pernicious anaemia. For the above reasons hydroxocobalamin is to be preferred to cyanocobalamin in the treatment of neurological disease.

A spontaneous disease histologically indistinguishable from SACD has been observed in monkeys during captivity (cage paralysis); cerebral lesions also occur. Hamerton (1938-39, 1942) and Scherer (1944) gave full reports on the disease. The clinical investigations in previous reports have been uneven; a few monkeys showed achlorhydria but macrocytic anaemia was not usually described. However, Oxnard and Smith (1966) showed that vitamin B_{12} deficiency was present in animals with cage paralysis and that a high percentage of non-paralysed, vegetarian-fed, deficient animals showed occult histological lesions. In the peripheral nerves the main lesion was segmental demyelination, though limited Wallerian-type degeneration also occurred (Oxnard, Smith and Torres 1970; Torres, Smith and Oxnard 1971).

Folic acid

Derivatives of folic acid are involved in the formation of methionine from homocysteine and in the construction of purines and pyrimidines and hence of DNA and RNA (Girdwood 1968). There are a few reports suggesting that folic acid depletion can lead to neurological diseases and Grant, Hoffbrand and Wells (1965) described seven patients with peripheral neuropathy and paraplegia and mentioned others in the literature. Anticonvulsant drugs cause folic acid depletion by metabolic competition and may precipitate neurological complications. Psychiatric disorders, particularly in the elderly, have been associated with folate depletion (Girdwood) and in some parts of Britain such depletion is a considerable problem, possibly owing to regional variations in the diet. The folate level of the CSF is two to three times that of the serum, even in folate deficiency. Pathological lesions in human deficiency have not been traced.

The remaining deficiencies

Biotin

Spontaneous deficiency in man appears not to occur, but in experiments on volunteers, itching, scaling of the skin, anorexia, lassitude and sleeplessness were noted. Lesions of the nervous system have not been described in experimental animals, but muscle fibres in rats have shown necrosis and atrophy, and a corresponding proliferation of sub-sarcolemmal nuclei. The changes were similar to those seen in α-tocopherol deficiency (Follis 1948); biotin deficiency may, therefore, not be the only factor.

Choline

Its metabolism is linked with the sulphur-containing amino acid methionine. Deficiency of either substance leads to disturbance of phospholipid metabolism and to delay in the transport of fatty acids to fat deposits. Choline is important also for the synthesis of acetyl-choline. Experimental animals deprived of choline have shown lesions in liver and kidneys. In the liver, there was fatty infiltration and necrosis of the parenchymal cells, associated with a finely granular cirrhosis (Himsworth and Glynn 1944; Himsworth 1946). Pathological changes in the nervous system have not been found, but might nevertheless occur indirectly if hepatic and/or renal failure resulted.

Vitamin A

This substance, a carotene, is the precursor of the light-sensitive pigment rhodopsin, which is present in the rods of the retina. Deficiency of the vitamin leads to nyctalopia and also to keratinizing metaplasia of the conjunctival and corneal epithelium (xerosis). Vitamin A is also necessary in the synthesis of active sulphate (Sundaresen 1966) which is transferred to galacto-ceramide, thus forming sulphatide. Melchior and Clausen (1968) attempted to reduce sulphatide synthesis in human metachromatic leucodystrophy: they fed a diet poor in vitamin A but failed to induce significant clinical improvement.

Experimental deficiency in animals has been associated with degeneration of the cranial and peripheral nerves and grey and white matter of the brain and of the spinal cord (Mellanby 1944; Wolbach and Bessey 1941) but this is the result of selective cessation of growth of bone and subsequent increase of pressure and not to a direct effect of deficiency on the neural tissue. Hayes, Nielsen and Eaton (1968) found that optic nerve lesions in vitamin A deficient calves resulted from raised CSF pressure due to an increased resistance to bulk absorption of the CSF and an abnormal development of the sphenoid bone. Howell and Thompson (1967a, b) found cerebral herniation, thinning of cerebellar flocculi and

ridging of the lumbosacral spine in chicks, cockerels and hens fed vitamin A deficient diets. Fluorescence microscopy detects very little of this vitamin in the normal central nervous system (Popper 1941).

Hydrocephalus in young rabbits whose mothers had suffered from vitamin A deficiency was described by Millen, Woollam and Lamming (1953) and Millen and Woollam (1956); the hydrocephalus was not caused by stenosis of the aqueduct, and its pathogenesis is obscure.

Vitamin D

Deficiency has no known effect on the nervous system.

Ascorbic acid (vitamin C)

This is normally found in appreciable amounts in the cytoplasm of neurons, microglia, oligodendrocytes, and the epithelial cells of the choroid plexus, though these amounts are less than those present in the pituitary gland, adrenal cortex and the interstitial cells of the testes. The close relationship of ascorbic acid (demonstrated by a special silver nitrate impregnation method as silver granules) to the Golgi apparatus and mitochondria is of histochemical interest (Bourne 1951), particularly in view of the *in vitro* increase of oxygen consumption by cerebral tissue containing mitochondria in the presence of ascorbic acid (McIlwain 1955). Despite these indications of its presence in normal brain tissue, the pathological findings in vitamin C deficiency (scurvy) are not particularly striking, consisting only of petechial haemorrhages.

Vitamin K

Similar diapedetic haemorrhages in numerous sites have been reported by Ferraro and Roizin (1943) in the brains of fowls and cats deprived of vitamin K; the haemorrhages are related to the reduction of blood prothrombin levels that follow deficiency of the vitamin. Hypoprothrombinaemia with similar haemorrhagic manifestations is occasionally seen in patients suffering from obstructive jaundice, diarrhoea, sprue, etc., and in such cases therapy with vitamin K has been successful.

α-Tocopherol (vitamin E)

This vitamin was first described by Evans and Bishop (1922) and termed 'the reproduction factor'. Later, Evans and Burr (1928) reported muscular paralysis in young offspring of vitamin E depleted rats.

α-Tocopherol is necessary for the development of the embryo, the maintenance of the germinal epithelium in the male and the metabolism of striated muscle. In the absence of the vitamin, marked retardation and underdevelopment of the embryo ensue. Verma and Wei King (1967) showed that vitamin E deficiency in rats had a deleterious effect on the developing nervous system, and hydrocephalus due to narrowing of the aqueduct of Sylvius was noted. There were gliosis, reduction in the number of neurons and abnormalities of the choroid plexus. Acid phosphatase (lysosomal) activity was increased but cholinesterase activity decreased. Previous workers described chromatolysis and nuclear changes in spermatozoa; also hyaline degeneration and necrosis of striated muscle (including heart muscle), associated with accumulation of acid fast, fluorescent, ceroid pigment. Similar pigment has been found in the brain and cord in neurons, glial cells and blood vessels (Einarson and Ringstead 1938; Einarson 1953; Einarson and Telford 1960). Miyagishi, Takahata and Iizuka (1967) studied the electron-microscope appearances of lipopigments in cerebral neurons of vitamin E deficient rats and concluded that the pigment was similar to that seen in senile rats. Pigment formation began with the deposition of lipid-containing materials in neuronal cytoplasm, and lysosomes participated in the intermediate stages of the process. Einarson and Ringstead described degeneration of the posterior roots and of the posterior spinal tracts; this was confirmed by Luttrell and Mason (1949) and by Malamud, Nelson and Evans (1949).

Thus, there is support for Einarson's hypothesis that the paralysis is not only myogenic

but also neurogenic, but the significance of the widespread pigmentary degeneration of cells in the brain and spinal cord of rats suffering from advanced deficiency of the vitamin requires further clarification. In this respect, it is of interest that free cholesterol is markedly increased in the muscle and brain of deficient rats (Heinrich and Mattil 1943).

Terminal degeneration of mainly afferent axons was the most obvious finding in the grey matter of the spinal cord and the medulla of rats kept on a vitamin E deficient diet for $14\frac{1}{2}$ to 23 months (Pentschew and Schwartz 1962). The nerve cells were not materially affected, but hypertrophic fibrous astrocytes, some of very large size, were demonstrated. By electron-microscopy Lampert, Blumberg and Pentschew (1964) showed severe changes in terminal axons in the sensory nuclei of the spinal cord and medulla; there was an increase in neurofilaments, foci of dense bodies and mitochondria, and collections of vesicular profiles. Lampert *et al.* discussed the resemblance of the axoplasmic alterations to those seen in regenerating axons. The findings suggested a state of increased metabolic activity confined to the terminal sensory axons, and induced in some way by the lack of vitamin E.

There is no evidence that vitamin E deficiency neuropathy occurs in man and there seems to be no connection between such deficiency and human dystrophic and amyotrophic syndromes. A possible exception is in infants suffering from diseases such as cystic fibrosis of the pancreas or biliary atresia, which can lead to malabsorption. In such infants the serum level of α-tocopherol (indicated by degree of haemolysis of erythrocytes in H_2O_2) has been found to be persistently low (Nitowsky, Gordon and Tildon 1956), and Oppenheimer (1956) described muscle necrosis in such a patient aged two years.

Protein and related deficiency disorders

Brain growth takes place mainly in the first months of life and is dependent on protein synthesis. Marasmus in early life results in a small head due to impaired brain growth (Mönckeberg 1969). The central nervous system of malnourished animals shows changes in chemical composition, cellularity and weight (Dobbing

1964; Dobbing and Widdowson 1965; Benton, Dodge and Carr 1966; Dickerson and Walmsley 1967; Chase, Lindsley and O'Brien 1969). In severe human malnutrition there are alterations in learning and behaviour, and it has been suggested that dietary deprivation in early life, especially in underdeveloped countries, affects the expression of genetic potential not only in physical maturation but also in intellectual maturation (Mönckeberg). Myelin deposition can be affected by severe early undernutrition (Platt and Wheeler 1967; Fishman, Prensky and Dodge 1969). Animal experiments suggest that the effect of malnutrition on the nervous system depends on the stage of development reached before the diet is restricted and on the severity and duration of the restriction. If myelination is complete, then the effects of dietary restriction on composition are minimal; when malnutrition begins before the brain has reached mature composition (during myelination) the chemical composition, weight, cellularity, etc., resemble that of younger animals and subsequent rehabilitation may not correct the defect (Dickerson and Walmsley).

Two main conditions need consideration in this section: the so-called hunger oedema and kwashiorkor, which represent, however, only two aspects of a wide range of syndromes.

Hunger oedema

Hunger oedema has been a prominent feature of many famines and occurred as a consequence of impoverished diets in Europe during and immediately after the two World Wars. Reduction in plasma protein has been held to be its main cause, but according to McCance (1951) this may not be as important a factor as the replacement of fat and of tissue volume by fluid; posture, renal function, salt intake and perhaps hormonal imbalance all play their part. The central nervous system is the last region to lose weight and tissue volume and there are no specific neuropathological changes. The central and peripheral neuropathies of vitamin B deficiencies are uncommon.

Kwashiorkor

In contrast, kwashiorkor, of which useful clinicopathological descriptions have been given by Trowell, Davies and Dean (1954), Follis (1958) and Platt (1958b), is caused by a diet deficient mainly in protein, but adequate or even excessive in starchy foodstuffs. The 'starch dystrophy syndrome' and the 'Mehlnährschaden' of German writers are identical conditions. Kwashiorkor has been reported from poverty-stricken areas in Africa, India, Jamaica and elsewhere and usually affects children between the ages of 6 months and 4 years; an adult form has also been recog-

nized. Clinically kwashiorkor is characterized by retardation in growth, muscular wasting, oedema, diarrhoea, a dermatosis resembling pellagra (though not sensitive to sunlight), enlargement of the liver, and a mental apathy and behaviour disturbance which may be profound. If left untreated, the condition is fatal, but severe manifestations of the syndrome may respond favourably to an adequate diet.

Investigation of the nervous system in kwashiorkor has been neglected in the past and it appears that neurological signs are not prominent, although a rhythmic and coarse tremor, hypotonia and areflexia have been described during the recovery period (Kahn 1954; Udani 1960); these signs usually disappeared. The electroencephalogram may show a cerebral dysrhythmia, which occasionally persists after recovery (Udani). Balmer, Howells and Wharton (1968) described acute encephalopathy with drowsiness deepening into coma and asterixis. In fatal cases the brain showed no macroscopic changes. There was circumstantial evidence that hyponatraemia was a factor. Garrow (1967) suggested that mental signs in kwashiorkor may be related to deficiency in brain potassium.

The pathological changes in kwashiorkor are distinct from those of the marasmus of low calorie diet. According to Davies (1954), subcutaneous fat deposits are not exhausted. The liver shows considerable fatty infiltration, the fat being deposited first in the periphery of the lobules, leading to a fine periportal fibrosis, which is usually halted at an early stage. The pancreas shows gross atrophy which may even precede the affection of the liver (Davies); there is atrophy of pancreatic xymogen-secreting cells, and of mucosal glands in the small intestine, and the salivary and lacrimal glands. The brain usually shows oedema and congestion. In one case cysts and sclerosis were present in the occipital cortex (Udani) but were likely to be an unrelated finding. Histological investigation of a case with rhythmic tremor during life showed only minor histological change, which may have been the sequel to terminal acute gastroenteritis (Khan).

Van Bogaert, Radermecker, Janssen and Gatera (1962) investigated the muscles of Congolese infants with kwashiorkor and found changes that they considered to be characteristic; the muscle fibres showed foamy and eosinophilic degeneration, accompanied by an intermysial oedema which was later associated with septal sclerosis. These lesions were not seen in other types of oedema and/or malnutrition.

The salient signs of kwashiorkor have been reproduced in experimental animals, and with particular ease in young pigs, fed on a 'Gambia diet'. Platt and his associates were able to study many of the features of this syndrome in strictly controlled conditions. The central nervous system was only slightly (though consistently) affected (Meyer, Stewart and Platt 1961): there was chromatolysis, especially in the neurons of the anterior horns in the spinal cord, and slight activation of astrocytes and oligodendrocytes. These changes have been interpreted as a reversible adaptation to deficient nutrition, rather than as evidence of progressive degeneration and glial replacement. Similar, though more severe changes were found in the pups of bitches fed on a low protein diet (Meyer, Pampiglione, Platt and Stewart 1961). Stewart and Platt (1968) noted neurological disorders (tremors, abnormal gait, ataxia, convulsions) in protein-calorie deficient pups. Platt and Stewart (1969) subsequently reviewed the whole question of experimental protein–calorie deficiency: as well as the chromatolysis and neuroglial hyperplasia in the cord mentioned above, they noted thinning of myelin sheaths and similar though less pronounced brain involvement; the peripheral nerves showed widening of the nodes of Ranvier. It was suggested that malnutrition during intrauterine or early postnatal life may lead to irreversible neuroglial changes.

Miscellaneous Disorders

Copper Deficiency

Deficiency of copper in sheep has been established by Bennetts and Beck (1942) as the cause of *enzootic ataxia or swayback*—a condition that occurs not only in Australia and England but also in Greece and Iceland (Spais, Palsson and van Bogaert 1961). In Australia the condition occurs in sheep kept on pastures low in copper but in Britain it is found irrespective of the copper content, which may even be high. Hypocupraemia is found, however, in both Australian and English ewes. Some conditioning factor may be involved which in Britain reduces the availability of copper to the animal (see Barlow 1958). The neurological manifestations consist of spastic paralysis, especially of the hindlimbs, severe incoordination and blindness occurring in newborn or very young lambs. In the Australian cases severe anaemia was a predominant sign (Bennetts and Chapman 1937). The pathology has been investigated by Innes (1934, 1936, 1939) and Howell (1968). Demyelination of the white matter is the most consistent feature, varying from circumscribed symmetrical foci of demyelination to complete destruction of myelin. In the severest cases liquefaction takes place and the cerebral cortex and a narrow strip of subcortical white matter may line a cavity which replaces the central white matter. Lipophages are present in small numbers, but are not a conspicuous feature, probably because of the rapid course of the disease. Nerve cells in the cortex and elsewhere are little affected, and the basal ganglia, the brainstem nuclei and the spinal cord are usually spared except for Wallerian degeneration of the descending motor tracts. There is no evidence of dysmyelination, the demyelination representing destruction of myelin already formed. Howell and Davidson (1959) found that cytochrome oxidase was significantly reduced in the CNS of swayback lambs and it has also been noted that cavitation only occurs with severe copper-depletion of the ewe and fetus *in utero*, leading to impaired copper oxidase activity (Howell 1968). This may also account for the chromatolysis and necrosis of large neurons in the brainstem and cord of all affected lambs. There has been some controversy about the demyelination found in the anterior and lateral columns of the spinal cord. This change may be due to impaired lipid synthesis and faulty myelination rather than descending degeneration of motor tracts. It seems, however, that if affected lambs are kept alive from 3 to 8 months, the faulty myelin may undergo degeneration, which is detectable by the Marchi or related techniques.

Cancilla and Barlow (1966*a, b*) in electron-microscope studies on affected lambs showed filamentous hyperplasia of the neurons of the lower brainstem and cord and segmental or diffuse alteration of neuronal and astrocytic processes in the cerebral cortex, with the formation of structural profiles.

Swayback must be distinguished from aplasia of myelin described in lambs by Markson, Terlecki, Shand, Sellers and Woods (1959) as 'hypomyelinogenesis congenita' and from the superficially similar demyelination of the 'Border' disease (Hughes and Kershaw 1959), in which hypocupraemia of the ewes is not a feature.

Roberts, Williams and Harvard (1966) described an acute fatal neurological disease of lambs characterized by hypocuprosis, by brain swelling and neuronal degeneration due to acute 'oedema', and by myelin degeneration in the spinal cord. The brain showed secondary changes attributable to 'pressure/anoxia' but changes in the stem and cord were ascribed to chronic subclinical swayback. It seemed possible that oedematous inhibition followed by spongy transformation and degeneration and subsequent necrosis of the white matter were the predominant change in swayback and that 'oedema' is fundamental to its pathogenesis. Swayback is not really comparable, therefore, with human demyelinating diseases.

Neuropathies associated with diabetes mellitus

Peripheral neuropathies commonly occur, frequency having been estimated by Martin (1953) and Matthews (1955) to be between 30 and 40% of unselected cases of diabetes; Hirson, Feinmann and Wade (1953) and Garland and Tavener (1953) found neurological abnormalities among an even higher percentage (50 to 60%). Cases present predominantly with sensory abnormalities such as pain, paraesthesias, sensory loss and areflexia, which are often bilateral. The ankle jerks are lost in most and the knee jerks in about a third of these cases (Martin). Trophic lesions are not uncommon, and may be the first evidence of sensory loss; ataxia and paralysis (foot or wrist drop) are less common. Pupillary abnormalities, including Argyll-Robertson pupils, were found in 9% of a series of 150 cases with objective evidence of neuropathy (Martin).

Evidence of diabetic neuropathy may occur at any age, but is most frequent in the fifth and sixth decades and in mild chronic cases. About a third of all cases with neuropathy show a diabetic retinopathy (Martin). The rate of fetal death and of congenital malformation in the offspring of diabetic mothers is high and in four surviving infants Dekaban and Magee (1958) found either severe mental deficiency or cerebral diplegia.

Detailed necropsy studies on early cases of diabetic peripheral neuropathy have been few; more has been reported on severe forms of the disease which are usually complicated by other factors such as arterial degeneration. Fraser and Bruce (1895) found degeneration of peripheral nerve myelin extending over many internodes, and associated with varicosity, but with preservation of continuity of the axons. Woltman and Wilder (1929) examined three fatal cases in detail and also the nerves of six limbs amputated for gangrene. Usually the degeneration of peripheral nerves was diffuse, but in two cases it was patchy; there was also consistent thickening of the walls of the small intraneural arteries. Other workers, however, have found no more evidence of arterial degeneration in cases of neuropathy than in other diabetics of the same age. Fagerberg (1960) examined sural nerve biopsies and found that the vasa nervorum showed a specific occlusive angiopathy, demonstrable by the periodic acid-Schiff (PAS) staining method.

Bosanquet and Henson (1957) found degeneration in posterior columns, posterior root ganglia, posterior roots (Fig. 5.15) and peripheral nerves of a 71-year-old woman who had suffered from severe sensory ataxia. It was considered likely that the primary lesion was in the posterior root ganglia. Anterior horn neurons and anterior roots were virtually intact in this case, although degeneration in some muscles suggested associated motor involvement. There was no arterial disease in the affected ganglia, though moderate thickening of arterial walls without atheroma occurred elsewhere. Woolf and Malins (1957), in biopsy material, described swelling and fusion of the terminal expansions of the endplates, with 'soap bubble' formations; they suggested that this change might indicate early 'dying-back' of axons from the periphery.

Greenbaum, Richardson, Salmon and Urich (1964) studied six cases (including five necropsies), and found loss of axons in the peripheral nerves, and changes in the neurons of the anterior horns and posterior root ganglia, without significant occlusive changes in the vasa nervorum. They concluded that the whole neuron and not just the myelin sheath was affected and that ischaemia was not the cause. Thomas and Lascelles (1965, 1966) have since examined teased nerve fibre preparations from one of Greenbaum's patients and cutaneous nerve biopsies from eight others: they demonstrated segmental demyelination and re-myelination, axonal loss and Wallerian-type

firmed that there was focal demyelination of the third nerve, probably due to ischaemia consequent upon severe hyalinization and thickening of arteriolar and capillary walls.

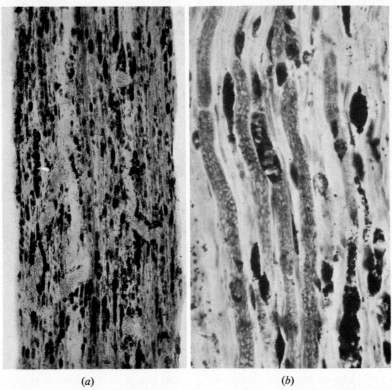

(a)　　　　　　　　　　　　　　　　　　(b)

Fig. 5.15 Diabetic neuritis. (a) Low and (b) high power views of posterior nerve root. The grey cylinders in (b) are intact myelin sheaths. Scharlach R. haematin. (Reproduced by the kindness of Dr Bosanquet.)

degeneration in some cases, and proliferation of Schwann cells on two occasions. Segmental demyelination and less significant axonal loss were confirmed by Chopra, Hurwitz and Montgomery (1969).

Thus, it seems that diabetic neuropathy probably results from primary degeneration of the myelin sheath, which in some cases precedes loss of axons. Demyelination without loss of axons accords with the well-recognized facts that clinical remission can occur and that motor conduction velocities are reduced. In contrast, chronic persistent neuropathy may result from permanent loss of axons. The part played by axonal and muscle fibre regeneration in inducing clinical remission in some patients is at present not understood.

Asbury, Aldredge, Hershberg and Fisher (1970) studied oculomotor palsy in diabetes and con-

Neuropathies associated with carcinoma

The association of neurological lesions with carcinoma has been known for a long time, but only for about 20 years has systematic attention been paid to this concurrence, which is generally held to be more than a coincidence. The problem and the literature have been reviewed by Henson, Russell and Wilkinson (1954), Heathfield and Williams (1954), Brain and Henson (1958), Brain and Norris (1965), Wilkinson, Croft and Urich (1967) and Henson (1970). Brain and Henson emphasized the surprisingly small size of the carcinoma in many cases. Precise classification of the various types of lesion is difficult, since different parts of the nervous system and also the muscles may be affected at the same time. To indicate this problem they used the term *neuromyopathy*. Nevertheless, it is possible to distinguish several main categories. Microscopical metastases, not seen on naked eye inspection, sometimes infiltrate the brain, cord or meninges (carcinomatous meningitis), or microscopic tumour emboli sometimes result in ischaemic lesions of the brain. Such possibilities should be excluded before making a firm diagnosis.

Cortical cerebellar degeneration (Greenfield 1934; Brain, Daniel and Greenfield 1951; Brain and Henson 1958; Brain and Wilkinson 1965)
This may occur as a relatively pure form or it may be associated with other lesions in subcortical centres of the brain (subthalamic nuclei and other brainstem nuclei) and in the spinal cord (degeneration of the spinocerebellar, pyramidal and posterior tracts, and of the motor neurons in the anterior horns). The clinical picture indicates subacute or even acute cerebellar dysfunction and mental changes (initial agitation, confusion, memory defect and eventual dementia) are often prominent. The associated carcinoma has been in various sites, most frequently the bronchus, ovary or breast; the disorder may also occur with Hodgkin's disease (Rewcastle 1963; Brain and Wilkinson 1965). Excess of cells and protein and a paretic Lange curve are frequently found, but the CSF is sterile on culture. On histological examination, degeneration and disappearance of Purkinje cells are found to be widespread, with moderate loss of granular cells, damage to basket cells and tangential fibres, and some glial proliferation (Figs. 5.16 and 5.17). In some cases only the dentate nuclei or the inferior olives are affected. The direct spinocerebellar tracts frequently degenerate in the cord. Meningeal and perivascular lymphocytic infiltration is so frequent that Brain and Henson (1958) refer to an encephalomyelitic form. Henson, Hoffman and Urich (1965) separated such cases into a special category of encephalomyelitis with carcinoma, and also included cases of sensory neuropathy, and limbic and bulbar encephalitis (see below).

Peripheral neuropathy
This can occur with carcinoma in many sites, particularly the bronchus; it has also been described with malignant lymphomas such as Hodgkin's disease and with multiple myelomatosis. In recent years, carcinoma has ranked second, after the Guillain-Barré syndrome, as a cause of peripheral neuropathy; malignant disease

must be sought persistently in obscure cases of neuropathy (Henson 1970). Croft, Urich and Wilkinson (1967) and Henson and Urich (1968) detailed the clinical and pathological features, which are dealt with on p. 718. The peripheral nerves showed loss of axons and, in teased preparations, segmental demyelination. The loss of myelin sheaths usually exceeds axonal loss and is accompanied by Schwann cell proliferation, commensurate fibrosis and sparse lymphocytic infiltration.

Neuropathy associated with 'malignant lymphomas' was recently studied by Walsh (1971); electrophysiological evidence of generalized peripheral neuropathy was found in 22 (35%) of 62 subjects. Nerve biopsy studies on five patients showed axonal degeneration and segmental demyelination of myelinated fibres but no lesions of unmyelinated fibres.

Encephalomyelitis with carcinoma
Sensory neuropathy, involving peripheral sensory nerves, posterior roots, spinal ganglia and the posterior columns of the cord was first delineated by Denny-Brown (1948). Henson et al. (1965) concluded that the frequent association of sensory neuropathy with encephalomyelitis supports the view that the two conditions constitute a single entity showing a common pathogenesis. The lesions were summarized as follows:

 (i) Limbic encephalitis, affecting the hippocampal formation, amygdaloid nucleus and cingulate and orbital cortices (as reviewed by Corsellis, Goldberg and Norton 1968).
 (ii) Bulbar encephalitis affecting mainly the lower brainstem.
(iii) Myelitis affecting the anterior horn neurons at various levels and in some cases other cell groups.
(iv) Ganglioradiculitis destroying the posterior root ganglia sensory neurons and causing Wallerian degeneration in the sensory roots, posterior columns and peripheral nerves.

Lesions may occur in one or more, or even all of the above sites.

Histological changes consist mainly of lymphocytic and microglial infiltration, with loss of neurons and secondary demyelination. As noted, some cases may also show cerebellar cortical degeneration. In a series of 33 cases, 31 had bronchial carcinoma and 24 showed sensory

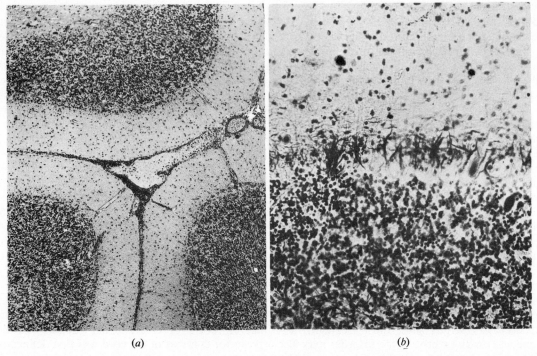

(a)   (b)

Fig. 5.16 Subacute spinocerebellar degeneration; $3\frac{1}{2}$ months' history. (Case 1 of Brain *et al.* 1951.) (a) Cerebellar cortex showing widespread loss of Purkinje cells and lymphocytic exudate in the meninges. (b) Higher power view showing empty baskets of hypertrophied fibres replacing Purkinje cells. Bielschowsky's silver impregnation.

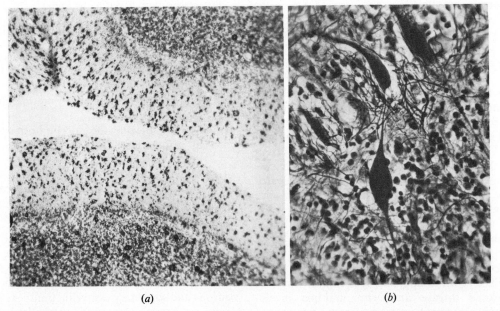

(a)   (b)

Fig. 5.17 Subacute cerebellar degeneration; 6 months' history. (Case 2 of Brain, Daniel and Greenfield 1951.) (a) Cortex of cerebellum showing loss of Purkinje cells and phagocytosis of lipid. Scharlach R. haemalum. (b) Degenerated Purkinje cell with torpedo-like swelling on its axon.

neuropathy (Henson 1970). Predictably, the clinical features tend to be mixed, and include symptoms and signs of limbic lobe, bulbar, cord and posterior root ganglia lesions. The cord signs are usually limited to the motor neurons. The CSF may show mild lymphocytosis; in the CSF and serum, raised protein and brain-specific complement-fixing antibodies have been demonstrated and the latter induce granular fluorescence of the neurons of guinea-pig nervous system with the fluorescent antibody sandwich technique. The cause of the encèphalomyelitis has prompted much speculation and either a viral infection or an autoimmune reaction have been suggested. Nuclear inclusions and viral particles have not so far been identified and virus isolation tests have been negative.

Myelopathy

Brain, Croft and Wilkinson (1965) described an atypical form of motor neuron disease associated with carcinoma. Urich (1967) found that upper and lower motor neurons, pyramidal tracts, posterior root ganglia and posterior columns were involved to various degrees and in various combinations on histological examination. It is by no means firmly established that there is a relationship between carcinoma and classical motor neuron disease (Henson 1970). Hoffman (1955) described the association of cancer and subacute necrotic myelopathy, which must be distinguished from other pathological processes such as post-irradiation necrosis of the cord or metastatic deposits.

Disorders of muscle

A variety of muscular disorders are recognized. In a subgroup termed *polymyositis* by Brain and Adams (1965) the limb girdles show symmetrical weakness and wasting that antedates evidence of carcinoma by months or years. The clinical picture can vary from true polymyositis to florid dermatomyositis. Differentiation from a motor neuropathy can be difficult and in some cases electrodiagnostic evidence of neural involvement is also found (*neuromuscular disorder*). Other cases show a *myasthenia-like syndrome* (Denny-Brown 1948; Henson *et al.* 1954; Heathfield and Williams 1954; Lambert and Rooke 1965) and a potentially hazardous sensitivity to muscle relaxants (Wise and MacDermot 1962). Muscle weakness may also be a feature of the various endocrine and metabolic syndromes that have in recent years been shown to occur with carcinoma. These include the ectopic ACTH syndrome, a hyponatraemic syndrome, hypercalcaemia, the carcinoid syndrome and thyrotoxicosis (Croft 1967; Henson 1970).

Urich (1967) drew attention to the fact that disuse atrophy, wasting due to malnutrition and cachexia, and decubital changes, are to be distinguished from specific lesions. Hildebrand and Coërs (1967), using vital (*in vivo*) stains and qualitative and quantitative methods on muscle biopsies, found increased collateral branching of axons and abnormal volumetric variations of muscle fibres that were subclinical and attributable to malnutrition. Various other changes have been described: single fibre atrophy, degenerative lesions such as vacuolation, hyalinization and necrosis, regeneration, and grades of inflammatory infiltration occur in differing combinations and call for cautious judgement by the pathologist.

Mental disorders

The dementias that accompany cerebellar degenerations have already been mentioned. Mental changes of organic type also occur with other forms of carcinomatous neuropathy or in the absence of neurological signs. Not infrequently, they are early manifestations of carcinoma, particularly of the bronchus. In the clinical and pathological analysis of several cases, Charatan and Brierley (1956) found no clear-cut histological substrate and suggested that the effects of toxic or metabolic abnormalities were responsible.

Miscellaneous disorders

As noted above, neoplasms are sometimes associated with endocrine or metabolic disturbances: these include hyperadrenalism, hypercalcaemia, hyponatraemia, hypoglycaemia and macroglobulinaemia, all of which can result in neurological disorders (Brain and Adams 1965). Some neoplasms, particularly those of the gastrointestinal tract, lead to deficiency states such as Wernicke's encephalopathy. Associated immunological defects occasionally facilitate secondary invasion of the central nervous system by opportunistic bacteria, viruses or fungi. A disseminated thrombotic syndrome can also complicate carcinoma and lead either to occlusion of veins and/or arteries of macro- or microscopical size, or to the deposition on the heart valves of abacterial thrombotic vegetations that are a source of emboli; the brain may be the site of infarcts in such cases (Smith 1961). Primary tumours or metastases can damage organs such as the liver (Bickerstaff and Woolf 1966) or kidneys and result in hepatic or uraemic encephalopathy.

Incidence. Croft *et al.* (1967) found that 6·6% of 1465 cases with carcinoma of different sites had carcinomatous neuromyopathy. Carcinomas of lung, ovary and stomach had the highest incidence and carcinomas of rectum, cervix and uterus the lowest. Males with bronchial carcinoma showed 15% overall incidence (6% excluding ill-defined syndromes). Henson (1970) mentioned an incidence of 5·3% of peripheral neuropathy alone in patients with bronchial cancer, 2·8% with gastric cancer and 1·2% with breast and large bowel cancers; he estimated that the combined incidence of peripheral neuropathy and encephalomyelitis would probably not exceed 1 to 2% in an unselected group of bronchial cancer cases. Currie, Henson, Morgan and Poole (1970) found non-metastatic neurological disorders of obscure origin in 2% of 774 patients with 'reticuloses'.

The *aetiology* of these 'neuromyopathies' is still a matter of speculation. A nutritional or related metabolic disorder caused by the carcinoma has been much discussed. Denny-Brown (1947, 1948) implicated pantothenic acid because of the close similarity of the posterior root and posterior column changes to experimentally induced changes in pigs deprived of the vitamin. He also noted the resemblance of the carcinomatous myopathies to the bulbar myasthenia-like syndrome that can occur in beriberi and pellagra. Other vitamins that have been considered are α-tocopherol, thiamine and nicotinic acid. However, apart from occasional cases with overt Wernicke's syndrome or pellagra, deficiency of these or other vitamins has not so far been proved, and extensive therapy with all known vitamins has had no conclusive effect. There may be an indirect deficiency, in so far as a carcinoma competes with the demands of normal tissues and may divert substances essential for the metabolism of the neuron. Brain and Henson (1958) noted that if a tumour deprived the body of essential nutritional factors or induced other metabolic or 'toxic' changes, one might expect that such effects would be in direct proportion to the size of the tumour, which is clearly not the case. However, Hildebrand and Coërs' (1967)

finding of subclinical neuropathic changes, apparently related to loss of weight and malnutrition, serves to emphasize the need to consider malnutrition as at least a contributory factor.

The inflammatory changes encountered in the neuroencephalomyelitic lesions are so marked that the possibility of a *virus infection* cannot be ruled out. It may occur in combination with an additional constitutional factor to which only a small proportion of the exposed population is susceptible; or with a process of sensitization of particular neuromuscular tissue to some product of the tumour; or as a consequence of immunological depression.

Autoimmune or hypersensitivity mechanism have also been suggested as causes of polymyositis and of some cases of demyelinating peripheral neuropathy. So far, the evidence available is inconclusive but it merits further consideration. Field and Caspary (1971) have recently described sensitization of blood lymphocytes to basic proteins derived from central and peripheral neural tissue in patients with various malignant neoplasms. This sensitization is independent of clinical evidence of non-metastatic neuropathy and can persist for years after successful surgical treatment of the neoplasm.

Acute porphyria

Porphyria, to which Vannotti (1954) has devoted a monograph, may be congenital or manifest itself as an acute form in later life. The congenital variety results in haemolysis, photosensitivity, etc., and neurological complications do not occur. The acute porphyria of later life is inherited as a Mendelian dominant; among exogenous factors, alcoholism, ingestion of certain barbiturates, sulphonamides, hepatic adenoma, intoxication by fungicides and the contraceptive pill have been cited. Macalpine and Hunter (1968) suggested that King George III of England suffered from psychosis due to porphyria and that the disorder afflicted many members of the Royal Houses of Hanover, Prussia and Stuart.

In the acute idiopathic form sleeplessness and acute abdominal pain may be the initial symptoms, followed by polyneuritis or, when severe, by acute ascending paralysis of the Landry type, with confusional states, coma and convulsions (Ridley 1969).

Erbslöh (1903) examined the spinal cord and

peripheral nerves of a case with 10 days' history of weakness. He found no definite changes in the cord or nerve roots, but variable degeneration of myelin and axons in the more peripheral parts of the nerves.

Since then many neuropathological reports have been made, among the most important being those by Baker and Watson (1945), Denny-Brown and Sciarra (1945), Gibson and Goldberg (1956), Hierons (1957), Cavanagh and Mellick (1965) and Cavanagh and Ridley (1967). Some of these authors emphasize irregular, often patchy, degeneration in peripheral nerves, a special effect on myelin sheaths, and irregular swelling or fragmentation of axons in the more chronic or severe lesions. Cavanagh and Mellick (1965) and Cavanagh (1973) drew attention to the Wallerian-type degeneration and resultant denervation that occurs; motor axons are more extensively involved than sensory axons and motor axons may degenerate as far back as the anterior roots. Sensory axons only die back to the spinal roots in exceptionally severe cases. In severe cases, loss of motor nerve fibres may be almost complete in distal muscles. The large diameter fibres from muscle spindles are usually spared, even in muscles showing great loss of motor and other sensory fibres. Long nerve fibres are more affected than short fibres so that in the spinal cord the columns of Goll are more degenerate than those of Burdach which contain the shorter fibres. Central chromatolysis of motor neurons, the extent of which depends on the duration and severity of the lesion in the related peripheral nerves, is found at necropsy. Evidence of axonal regeneration and collateral sprouting may be found in the muscles in chronic cases.

In many cases, especially those with cerebral symptoms and signs, lesions that appear to be ischaemic in character have been found in cerebral and cerebellar cortex, basal ganglia and in the white matter of the hemispheres. Rarely these consist of small areas of infarction (Hierons); more often of focal cell loss, associated with ischaemic type neuronal degeneration in the cortex or of focal pallor of myelin staining in the white matter. Atherosclerosis may be a complicating factor in older patients (Smith and Whittaker 1964).

Involvement of cranial nerve and autonomic neurons may occur and be responsible for certain clinical features such as tachycardia, transient hypertension or even abdominal pain (Cavanagh 1973).

The pathogenesis of porphyric neuropathy is not clear. It has been suggested that the lesions in the brain are anoxic and result from constriction of small arterioles, since Baker and Watson and also Denny-Brown and Sciarra observed localized spasm in the retinal arteries during attacks of porphyria. The latter authors considered the lesions in the peripheral nerves to have a similar pathogenesis, as in some ways they resemble those produced by experimental ischaemia in nerves (Denny-Brown and Brenner 1944). But although in many cases the blood pressure is raised during an attack, in others it remains normal. Other authors have suggested an interference with the Krebs cycle of glucose metabolism and Hierons found abnormal pyruvate metabolism in two cases. The findings of Cavanagh and Mellick are against a primary demyelinating process. The Wallerian-type dying-back process that they describe indicates a lesion in the neuronal perikaryon or axon. The pattern of degeneration closely mimics that of isoniazid toxicity (Cavanagh 1967, 1973) and Cavanagh and Ridley (1967) suggested that, as in the latter case, porphyria may lead to deprivation of the co-factor pyridoxal phosphate. This could result from excessive activity of δ-amino-laevulinic acid synthetase, an enzyme requiring pyridoxal phosphate as a co-factor (Cavanagh 1973). It is interesting that there are similarities between lead poisoning and porphyria (Dagg, Goldberg, Lockhead and Smith 1965) and that in both conditions the urinary excretion of δ-amino-laevulinic acid is considerably increased.

Lesions similar to those described in human porphyria were found in rats in which porphyria was induced by allyl-iso-prophylacetyl carbamide or griseofulvin (Lehoczky, Sos, Selmeci and Halasy 1967).

Steatorrhoea and allied gastrointestinal disorders

Adult coeliac disease

Cooke and Smith (1966) described the clinical and laboratory findings in 16 patients with adult coeliac disease; there was evidence of peripheral neuritis with pain and weakness, sensory loss and ataxia. Three cases showed cerebellar dysfunction and five cases had unexplained attacks of unconsciousness. Necropsies on nine fatal cases showed various lesions, including patchy or more diffuse degeneration of the spinal cord (mainly posterior columns, Fig. 5.18), demyelination of nerve roots, degeneration of the hypothalamus reminiscent of Wernicke-type encephalopathy, neurons; the spongiform degeneration of myelin and the lateral column involvement seen in typical vitamin B_{12} deficiency were not present in this case.

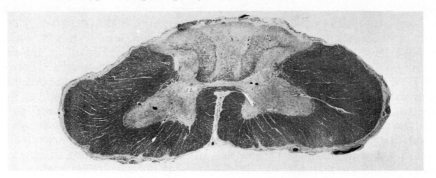

Fig. 5.18 Degeneration of the posterior columns of the cervical cord. The patient had a twelve-year history of adult coeliac disease, neuropathy for two years, and developed intestinal obstruction due to multifocal ileojejunal histiocytic lymphoma (reticulosarcoma) a few weeks before death. The concurrence highlights the similarities between coeliac and carcinomatous neuropathies. Luxol fast blue-cresyl fast violet. $\times 8\frac{1}{2}$. (Reproduced by courtesy of the Editor, *Brain*.)

astrocytic hypertrophy (Alzheimer type II astrocytes) in the basal ganglia, cerebellar cortical atrophy and atrophy and loss of neurons in the cerebral cortex. There were certain clinical and pathological similarities between the above cases and the carcinomatous neuropathy group. Farmer and Richards (1964) and Binder, Solitaire and Spiro 1967) discussed the psychiatric manifestations of adult and childhood coeliac disease, though such features do not usually have a pathological substrate. (An exception was the Wernicke-like lesions present in one of Cooke and Smith's cases). Cooke, Johnson and Woolf (1966) studied muscle biopsies from the patients described by Cooke and Smith and found collateral branching and diffuse swelling of terminal axons, and electron-microscope evidence of severe alteration of the internal fine structure of the terminal axonic expansions.

Postgastrectomy states
Williams, Hall, Thompson and Cooke (1969) reported on 14 patients with neuropathy which appeared many years after gastrectomy. The lower limbs were mainly affected, with weakness, wasting, paraesthesias, difficulty in walking and posterior column deficit. Vitamin B_{12} deficiency occurred in most patients. Little is known of the pathological lesions in such cases. A case which I examined showed demyelination of the posterior columns and posterior roots and atrophy of posterior root ganglia and anterior horn

Whipple's disease
This is a well-known cause of steatorrhoea and can be associated with cerebral involvement leading to psychiatric manifestations resembling Wernicke's encephalopathy (Badenoch, Richards and Oppenheimer 1963; Smith, French, Gottsman, Smith and Wakes-Miller 1965). It is not clear whether the Wernicke-like complications result from infiltration of the brain with PAS-positive material similar to that present in the intestinal tract, or from secondary nutritional deficiency. The intracerebral infiltrate tends to aggregate into granular microfoci that contain Gram-positive particles on light microscopy (Smith *et al.* 1965). The particles resemble bacteria on electron-microscopy (Groodt-Lasseel and Martin 1969) as do the PAS-positive granules in the intestinal macrophages (Roberts, Themann and Knust 1970).

Primary amyloidosis
The clinical and pathological findings are described by French, Hall, Parish and Smith (1965). Infiltration and degeneration of the intestinal autonomic nerves and plexuses can lead to severe diarrhoea and steatorrhoea. The spinal nerve roots and ganglia, peripheral nerves and main autonomic nerves and ganglia can also be infiltrated leading to sensory motor polyneuritis, postural hypotension, anhydrosis, etc. For further details see p. 731.

Lathyrism

This condition has been known from ancient times; since the nineteenth century epidemics have been reported in France, Italy, Algiers and Russia. It is still endemic in India, where it occurs most frequently during famines in the central provinces and in Mysore. A considerable literature has accumulated which has been fully reviewed by Denny-Brown (1947).

Lathyrus sativus, a pea which in times of shortage has been added to bread, has been implicated in most of the outbreaks. However, only a proportion of those who consume bread contaminated by the pea develop signs of disease. Except in times of famine, *L. sativus* seems to have no toxic effect, which suggests that other factors are involved in lathyrism. Shah (1939) described an epidemic of lathyrism in which *L. sativus* was absent from food. Lathyrism occurs also in herbivorous animals (horses, pigs, geese, ducks, etc.) which have fed on *L. sativus* or related peas.

In man, the onset of clinical symptoms has been described by Denny-Brown and others as sudden and characterized by pain and paraesthesias of the lower extremities, progressing to spastic paraplegia. Loss of sphincter control, impotence and muscular atrophy may follow. Filimonoff (1926) described degeneration of the ventral and lateral pyramidal tracts as the main necropsy findings in a patient dying 35 years after the onset of the disease. Buzzard and Greenfield (1921), in addition to degeneration of the anterior and lateral pyramidal tracts, noted involvement of ascending fibres in the direct cerebellar and posterior tracts. They emphasized the resemblance of the lesions to those seen in ergotism, but also observed a honeycombed appearance in marginal parts of the cord.

Experimental investigations (well reviewed by Selye 1957 and German 1960) have become numerous since Geiger, Steenbock and Parsons (1933) observed the retardation of growth and abnormalities of bone, cartilage and other mesodermal tissues in rats fed with sweet pea (*Lathyrus odoratus*). From this paper stems the origin of experimental *osteolathyrism* which was subsequently elaborated by Ponseti and Baird (1952), Ponseti (1954), Menzies and Mills (1957), and many others. According to the last-named authors the fundamental change in this osteolathyrism is the excessive accumulation of inter-cellular ground substance, chondroitin sulphate, which leads to a general breakdown of collagen fibrils. Among the resulting lesions are slipped epiphyses, kyphoscoliosis, degeneration of intervertebral discs, thoracic deformities and a high incidence of dissecting aneurysms of the aorta following the degeneration of elastic fibres. Compression and lesions of the cord by protruding discs or exostoses have been recorded. Osteolathyrism can also be produced experimentally by certain amino-nitriles such as, for example, amino-aceto-nitrile (Selye).

These experimental results were obtained in rats, which are vulnerable to *L. odoratus* but not to *L. sativus*, and so cannot be directly compared with human cases. The clinical symptomatology of sensory and motor disturbances and the postmortem finding of a combination of ascending and descending tract degeneration might be interpreted as the result of local compression of the cord. Alternatively, there has been evidence of a neurotoxic action (Selye's 'neurolathyrism') of *L. odoratus*. Several amino-nitriles, in particular β-amino-proprionitrile, have been suggested as the active neurotropic principle of the sweet pea. β-cyano-ethylamine, an analogue of this nitrile, administered to rats by Hartmann, Lalich and Akert (1958), caused hyperactivity, circling movements and intermittent spasms of neck muscles, which were followed by weakness of the hindlimbs; histologically, there was chromatolysis of anterior horn neurons and degeneration of nerve roots, which were considered to be due to direct neurotoxic action, as vertebral deformities were minimal or absent.

Chou and Hartmann (1964, 1965) showed that imidodiproprionitrile (IDPN) caused ballooning of proximal segments of axons in the brainstem and anterior horns due to accumulation of axoplasmic constituents; the phenomena was termed 'axostasis' and was presumed to result from a disturbance and stasis of axonal flow of protein. Electron-microscopy showed that the axonal balloons contained focal accumulations of neurofibrils, mitochondria and small vesicles; the related cell bodies looked normal. Slagel and Hartmann (1965) also studied the distribution of neuroaxonal lesions in mice given IDPN, particularly in the vestibular system. Slagel, Hartmann and Edström (1966) found that the RNA content and base composition of mesencephalic V cells of mice, which showed axonal lesions after injection with IDPN, and also of anterior horn cells, adjacent glial cells and axonal balloons in rats fed IDPN, were similar to the results in control animals; previous workers had suggested that there was increased synthesis of axonal proteins in such experiments. The axonal balloons in the rat contained RNA that was different in composition from the RNA of anterior horn neurons and adjacent glial cells.

There is hope that such studies will eventually throw light on human axonal disorders such as neuroaxonal dystrophy.

Ergotism

Intoxication by the common 'fungus of rye' has in the past given rise to epidemics, particularly in Europe. The toxic principles seem to be cornutine and sphacelinic acid: cornutine results in convulsions; sphacelinic acid has a constrictor action on muscle fibres, particularly those of the vessel wall, and results in gangrene.

A consistent finding is degeneration of the long spinal tracts, particularly of the posterior columns (Buzzard and Greenfield). The change has been likened to tabetic myelopathy, but the lesions are less selective and are usually more recent; the arteries show thickening of the media, and the smaller arteries are thrombosed.

The causal mechanism is not yet known in detail. The toxic effect may be an interference or blocking of enzyme systems in which vitamins are intimately involved (Denny-Brown 1947). Mellanby (1931) pointed out that the toxic action of ergot is more effective if there is also vitamin A deficiency, and Pentschew (1929) described the clinical features of pellagra in a monkey poisoned by ergot. Jervis and Kindwall (1942) considered that excessive ergotamine administration in migraine may have been a factor in producing Schilder-like demyelination of the cerebral white matter in a case that they studied, though coincidental occurrence could not be excluded.

References

Adams, R. D. & Kubik, C. S. (1944) Subacute degeneration of the brain in pernicious anemia. *New England Journal of Medicine*, **231**, 1-9.

Alexander, L. (1940) Wernicke's disease. Identity of lesions produced experimentally in pigeons with hemorrhagic polioencephalitis occurring in chronic alcoholism in man. *American Journal of Pathology*, **16**, 61-70.

Alexander, L., Green, R. G., Evans, C. A. & Wolf, L. E. (1941) Alcoholic encephalopathy in man and fish-diet disease in foxes and fishes; a study in comparative neuropathology. *Transactions of the American Neurological Association*, **67**, 119-122.

Alexander, L., Pijoan, M., Myerson, A. & Keene, H. N. (1938) Beri-beri and scurvy; experimental study. *Transactions of the American Neurological Association*, **64**, 135-138.

Alexander, W. F. (1957) In *Vitamin B₁₂ and Intrinsic Factor* (Ed. Heinrich, H. C.), p. 372, Thieme, Stuttgart.

Apenzeller, O. & Richardson, E. P. (1966) The sympathetic chain in patients with diabetic and alcoholic polyneuropathy. *Neurology (Minneapolis)*, **16**, 1205-1209.

Aring, C. D., Bean, W. B., Roseman, E., Rosenbaum, M. & Spies, T. D. (1941) Peripheral nerves in cases of nutritional deficiency. *Archives of Neurology and Psychiatry (Chicago)*, **45**, 772-787.

Aring, C. D. & Spies, T. D. (1939) Critical review: vitamin B deficiency and nervous disease. *Journal of Neurology and Psychiatry*, **2**, 335-360.

Asbury, A. K., Aldredge, H., Hershberg, R. & Fisher, C. M. (1970) Oculomotor palsy in diabetes mellitus: a clinicopathological study. *Brain*, **93**, 555-566.

Badenoch, J. (1954) The use of labelled vitamin B₁₂ and gastric biopsy in the investigation of anaemia. *Proceedings of the Royal Society of Medicine*, **47**, 426-427.

Badenoch, J., Richards, W. C. D. & Oppenheimer, D. R. (1963) Encephalopathy in a case of Whipple's disease. *Journal of Neurology, Neurosurgery and Psychiatry*, **26**, 203-210.

Baker, A. B. & Watson, C. J. (1945) The central nervous system in porphyria. *Journal of Neuropathology and Experimental Neurology*, **4**, 68-76.

Balmer, S., Howells, G. & Wharton, B. I. (1968) The acute encephalopathy of kwashiorkor. *Developmental Medicine and Child Neurology*, **10**, 766-771.

Barlow, R. M. (1958) Recent advances in swayback. *Proceedings of the Royal Society of Medicine*, **51**, 748-752.

Baron, D. N., Dent, C. E., Harris, H., Hart, E. W. & Jepson, J. B. (1956) Hereditary pellagra-like skin rash with temporary cerebellar ataxia, constant renal aminoaciduria and other bizarre biochemical features. *Lancet*, **2**, 421-428.

Barrett, A. M. (1912-13) Mental disorders and cerebral lesions associated with pernicious anemia. *American Journal of Insanity*, **69**, 643-651.

Bean, W. B., Hodges, R. E. & Daum, K. (1955) Pantothenic acid deficiency induced in human subjects. *Journal of Clinical Investigation*, **34**, 1073-1084.

Bennetts, H. W. & Beck, A. B. (1942) Enzootic ataxia and copper deficiency of sheep. *Bulletin. Council for Scientific and Industrial Research, Melbourne*, **147**, 1-52.

Bennetts, H. W. & Chapman, F. E. (1937) Copper deficiency in sheep in Western Australia: a preliminary account of the aetiology of enzootic ataxia of lambs and an anaemia of ewes. *Australian Veterinary Journal*, **13**, 138-149.

Benton, J. W., Dodge, P. R. & Carr, S. (1966) Modification of the schedule of myelination in the rat by early nutritional deprivation. *Pediatrics*, **31**, 801-807.

Bertrand, I., Liber, A. F. & Randoin, L. (1934) Altérations anatomiques du système nerveux au cours de l'avitaminose B expérimentale. *Archives d'Anatomie Microscopique et de Morphologie Expérimentale*, **30**, 297-380.

Bessey, O. A. & Wolbach, S. B. (1939) Vascularization of the cornea of the rat in riboflavin deficiency, with a note on corneal vascularization in vitamin A deficiency. *Journal of Experimental Medicine*, **69**, 1-12.

Bickel, H. (1914) Funikuläre Myelitis mit bulbären und polyneuritischen Symptomen. *Archiv für Psychiatrie und Nervenkrankheiten*, **53**, 1106-1117.

Bickerstaff, E. R. & Woolf, A. L. (1966) Severe cerebral degeneration associated with primary hepatic carcinoma. *Journal of Neurology, Neurosurgery and Psychiatry*, **29**, 556-559.

Binder, H. J., Solitaire, G. B. & Spiro, H. M. (1967) Neuromuscular disease in patients with steatorrhoea. *Gut*, **8**, 605-611.

Bonhoeffer, K. (1899) Pathologisch- anatomische Untersuchungen an Alkohol-deliranten. *Monatschrift für Psychiatrie*, **5**, 265-284, 379-387.

Bosanquet, F. D. & Henson, R. A. (1957) Sensory neuropathy in diabetes mellitus. *Folia psychiatrica neurologica et neurochirurgica neerlandica*, **60**, 107-117

Bourne, G. H. (1951) In *Cytology and Cell Physiology*, Clarendon Press, Oxford.

Brain, W. R. & Adams, R. D. (1965) In *The Remote Effects of Cancer on the Nervous System* (Eds. Brain, W. R. & Norris, F. H.), page 216, Grune and Stratton, New York.

Brain, W. R., Croft, P. B. & Wilkinson, M. (1965) Motorneurone disease as a manifestation of neoplasm. *Brain*, **88**, 479-500.

Brain, W. R., Daniel, P. M. & Greenfield, J. G. (1951) Subacute cortical cerebellar degeneration and its relation to carcinoma. *Journal of Neurology, Neurosurgery and Psychiatry*, **14**, 59-75.

Brain, W. R. & Henson, R. A. (1958) Neurological syndromes associated with carcinoma. *Lancet*, **2**, 971-974.

Brain, W. R. & Norris, F. H. (1965) *The Remote Effects of Cancer on the Nervous System*, Grune and Stratton, New York.

Brain, W. R. & Wilkinson, M. (1965) Subacute cerebellar degeneration associated with neoplasms. *Brain*, **88**, 465-478.

Brody, I. A. & Wilkins, C. H. (1968) Wernicke's encephalopathy. *Archives of Neurology (Chicago)*, **19**, 228.

Bueding, E., Wortis, H., Fein, H. D. & Esturonne, D. (1942) Pyruvic acid metabolism in diabetes mellitus. *American Journal of Medical Science*, **204**, 838-845.

Buzzard, E. F. & Greenfield, J. G. (1921) In *Pathology of the Nervous System*, Constable, London.

Campbell, A. C. P. & Biggart, J. H. (1939) Wernicke's encephalopathy (polioencephalitis haemorrhagica superior): its alcoholic and nonalcoholic significance. *Journal of Pathology and Bacteriology*, **48**, 245-262.

Campbell, A. C. P. & Russell, W. R. (1941) Wernicke's encephalopathy: clinical features and their probable relationship to vitamin B deficiency. *Quarterly Journal of Medicine*, **34**, 41-64.

Cancilla, P. A. & Barlow, R. M. (1966a) Structural changes of the central nervous system in swayback (enzootic ataxia) of lambs; electronmicroscopy of the lower motor neuron. *Acta Neuropathologica (Berlin)*, **6**, 251-259.

Cancilla, P. A. & Barlow, R. M. (1966b) Structural changes of the central nervous system in swayback (enzootic ataxia) of lambs: electronmicroscopy of the cerebral lesions. *Acta Neuropathologica (Berlin)*, **6**, 260-265.

Carmichael, E. A. & Stern, O. (1931) Korsakoff's syndrome; its histopathology. *Brain*, **54**, 189-213.

Castle, W. B. (1929) Extrinsic factor in pernicious anaemia. *American Journal of Medical Science*, **178**, ·148.

Cavanagh, J. B. (1967) On the pattern of change in peripheral nerves produced by isoniazid intoxication in rats. *Journal of Neurology, Neurosurgery and Psychiatry*, **30**, 26-33.

Cavanagh, J. B. (1973) Peripheral neuropathy caused by chemical agents. *C.R.C. Critical Reviews in Toxicology*, 365-417.

Cavanagh, J. B. & Mellick, R. S.   (1965) On the nature of the peripheral nerve lesions associated with acute intermittent porphyria. *Journal of Neurology, Neurosurgery and Psychiatry*, **28**, 320-327.

Cavanagh, J. B. & Ridley, A.   (1967) The nature of the neuropathy complicating acute intermittent porphyria. *Lancet*, **2**, 1023-1024.

Charatan, F. B. & Brierley, J. B.   (1956) Mental disorder associated with primary lung carcinoma. *British Medical Journal*, **1**, 765-768.

Chase, H. P., Lindsley, W. F. B. & O'Brien, D.   (1969) Undernutrition and cerebellar development. *Nature*, **221**, 554-555.

Chick, H., El Sadr, M. M. & Worden, A. N.   (1940) Occurrence of fits of an epileptiform nature in rats maintained for a long period on diets deprived of vitamin B_6. *Biochemical Journal*, **34**, 595-600.

Chopra, J. S., Hurwitz, L. J. & Montgomery, D. A. D.   (1969) The pathogenesis of sural nerve changes in diabetes mellitus. *Brain*, **92**, 391-418.

Chou, S. M. & Hartmann, H. A.   (1964) Anoxal lesions and waltzing syndrome after IDPN administration in rats. *Acta Neuropathologica (Berlin)*, **3**, 428-450.

Chou, S. M. & Hartmann, H. A.   (1965) Electronmicroscopy of focal neuroaxonal lesions produced by β-β'-iminodiproprionitrile (IDPN) administration in rats. *Acta Neuropathologica (Berlin)*, **4**, 590-603.

Clarke, J. M.   (1904) On the spinal cord degenerations in anaemia. *Brain*, **27**, 441-459.

Coërs, C. & Woolf, A. L.   (1959) In *The Innervation of Muscle*, p. 91, Blackwell Scientific, Oxford.

Coggeshall, R. E. & MacLean, P. D.   (1958) Hippocampal lesions following administration of 3-acetylpyridine. *Proceedings of the Society of Experimental Biology and Medicine*, **98**, 687-689.

Collins, G. H.   (1967) Glial cell changes in the brainstem of thiamine deficient rats. *American Journal of Pathology*, **50**, 791-814.

Cooke, W. T., Johnson, A. G. & Woolf, A. L.   (1966) Vital staining and electronmicroscopy of the intramuscular nerve endings in the neuropathy of adult coeliac disease. *Brain*, **89**, 663-682.

Cooke, W. T. & Smith, W. T. (1966) Neurological disorders associated with adult coeliac disease. *Brain*, **89**, 683-722.

Corsellis, J. A. N., Goldberg, G. J. & Norton, A. R.   (1968) Limbic encephalitis and its association with carcinoma. *Brain*, **91**, 481-496.

Cox, E. V. & White, A. M.   (1962) Methylmalonic acid excretion: an index of vitamin B_{12} deficiency. *Lancet*, **2**, 853-856.

Croft, P. B.   (1967) The remote effects of cancer on the nervous system. Clinical syndromes. *Proceedings of the Royal Society of Medicine*, **60**, 686.

Croft, P. B., Urich, H. & Wilkinson, M.   (1967) Peripheral neuropathy of sensorimotor type associated with malignant disease. *Brain*, **90**, 31-66.

Currie, S., Henson, R. A., Morgan, H. G. & Poole, A. J.   (1970) The incidence of non-metastatic neurological syndromes of obscure origin in the reticuloses. *Brain*, **93**, 629-640.

Dagg, J. H., Goldberg, A., Lockhead, A. & Smith, J. A.   (1965) The relationship of lead poisoning to acute intermittent porphyria. *Quarterly Journal of Medicine*, **34**, 163-175.

Davidson, L. S. P. & Passmore, R.   (1969) *Human Nutrition and Dietetics*, 4th Edn., Livingstone, Edinburgh and London.

Davies, J. N. P.   (1954) In *Malnutrition in African Mothers, Infants and Young Children* (2nd International African O.C.T.A. Conference), p. 109, London.

Davies, M. J. & Jennings, R. B.   (1970) The ultrastructure of the myocardium in the thiamine-deficient rat. *Journal of Pathology*, **102**, 87-95.

Dekabalan, A. S. & Magee, K. R.   (1958) Occurrence of neurological abnormalities in infants of diabetic mothers. *Neurology (Minneapolis)*, **8**, 193-200.

Denny-Brown, D.   (1947) Neurological conditions resulting from prolonged and severe dietary restriction. (Case reports in prisoners of war and general review.) *Medicine (Baltimore)*, **26**, 41-113.

Denny-Brown, D.   (1948) Primary sensory neuropathy with muscular changes associated with carcinoma. *Journal of Neurology, Neurosurgery and Psychiatry*, **11**, 73-87.

Denny-Brown, D. & Brenner, C.   (1944) Paralysis of nerve induced by direct pressure and by tourniquet. *Archives of Neurology and Psychiatry (Chicago)*, **51**, 1-26.

Denny-Brown, D. & Sciarra, D.   (1945) Changes in the nervous system in acute porphyria. *Brain*, **68**, 1-16.

Denton, J.   (1928) A study of tissue changes in experimental black tongue in dogs compared with similar changes in pellagra. *American Journal of Pathology*, **4**, 341-352.

Dickerson, J. W. & Walmsley, A. L.   (1967) The effect of undernutrition and subsequent rehabilitation on the growth and composition of the central nervous system of the rat. *Brain*, **90**, 897-906.

Dobbing, J.   (1964) The influence of early nutrition on the development and myelination of the brain. *Proceedings of the Royal Society*, Series B, **159**, 503-509.

Dobbing, J. & Widdowson, E. M.   (1965) The effect of undernutrition and subsequent rehabilitation on myelination of rat brain as measured by its composition.   *Brain*, **88**, 357-366.

Dreyfus, P. M.   (1965) The regional distribution of transketolase in normal and the thiamine deficient nervous system.   *Journal of Neuropathology and Experimental Neurology*, **24**, 119-129.

Dreyfus, P. M. & Victor, M.   (1961) Effects of thiamine deficiency on the central nervous system.   *American Journal of Clinical Nutrition*, **9**, 414-425.

Dunn, T. B., Morris, H. P. & Dubnik, C. S.   (1947) Lesions of chronic thiamine deficiency in mice.   *Journal of the National Cancer Institute*, **8**, 139-155.

Eijkman, C.   (1897) Eine Beriberi-ähnliche Krankheit der Hühner.   *Virchows Archiv für pathologische Anatomie*, **148**, 523-532.

Einarson, L.   (1953) Deposits of fluorescent acid-fast products in the nervous system and skeletal muscles of rats with chronic vitamin E deficiency.   *Journal of Neurology, Neurosurgery and Psychiatry*, **16**, 98-109.

Einarson, L. & Ringstead, A.   (1938) *Effect of Chronic Vitamin E Deficiency on the Nervous System and the Skeletal Musculature in Adult Rats*, Copenhagen.

Einarson, L. & Telford, I. R.   (1960) *Structural Changes in the Nervous System of Monkeys deprived of Vitamin E*, Aarhus.

Ellinger, P., Coulson, R. A. & Benesch, R.   (1944) Production and release of nicotinamide by intestinal flora in man.   *Nature*, **154**, 270-271.

Elvehjem, C. A., Madden, R. J., Strong, F. M. & Woolley, D. W.   (1937) Relation of nicotinic acid and nicotinic acid amide to canine black tongue.   *Journal of the American Chemical Society*, **59**, 1767-1768.

Erbslöh, W.   (1903) Zur pathologie und pathologischen Anatomie der toxischen Polyneuritis nach Sulfonalgebrauch.   *Deutsche Zeitschrift für Nervenheilkunde*, **23**, 197-204.

Evans, C. A., Carlson, W. E. & Green, R. G.   (1942) The pathology of Chastek paralysis in foxes.   A counterpart of Wernicke's hemorrhagic polioencephalitis in man.   *American Journal of Pathology*, **18**, 79-91.

Evans, H. M. & Bishop, K. S.   (1922) On the existence of a hitherto unrecognized dietary factor essential for reproduction.   *Science*, **56**, 650.

Evans, H. M. & Burr, G. O.   (1928) Development of paralysis in the suckling of young mothers deprived of vitamin E.   *Journal of Biological Chemistry*, **76**, 273-297.

Fagerberg, S. E.   (1960) Diabetic neuropathy: a clinical and histological study on the significance of vascular alterations.   *Acta medica Scandinavica, Suppl.* **345**, **164**, 1-97.

Farmer, R. G. & Richards, H. G.   (1964) Malabsorption syndrome and peripheral neuropathy: report of two cases.   *Cleveland Clinical Quarterly*, **31**, 163-168.

Ferguson, T. M., Rigdon, R. H. & Couch, J. R.   (1955) Pathologic study of vitamin B_{12} deficient chick embryos.   *Archives of Pathology*, **60**, 393-400.

Ferraro, A., Arieti, S. & English, W. H.   (1945) Cerebral changes in the course of pernicious anaemia and their relationship to psychic symptoms.   *Journal of Neuropathology and Experimental Neurology*, **4**, 217-239.

Ferraro, A. & Roizin, L.   (1943) Histopathology of central nervous tissue in experimental vitamin K deficiency (vitamin K deficiency haemorrhagic diathesis).   *Journal of Neuropathology and Experimental Neurology*, **2**, 392-410.

Field, E. J. & Caspary, E. A.   (1971) Lymphocyte sensitisation: an in vitro test for cancer?   *Lancet*, **1**, 189-190.

Filimonoff, I. N.   (1926) Zur pathologisch-anatomischen Charakteristik des Lathyrismus.   *Zeitschrift für die gesamte Neurologie und Psychiatrie*, **105**, 76.

Fishman, M. A., Prensky, A. L. & Dodge, P. L.   (1969) Low content of cerebral lipids in infants suffering from malnutrition.   *Nature*, **221**, 552-553.

Follis, R. H. Jr.   (1948) *The Pathology of Nutritional Disease*, Thomas, Springfield, Ill.

Follis, R. H. Jr.   (1958) *Deficiency Disease*, Thomas, Springfield, Ill.

Follis, R. H. Jr., Miller, M. H., Wintrobe, M. M. & Stein, H. J.   (1943) Development of myocardial necrosis and absence of nerve degeneration in thiamine deficiency in pigs.   *American Journal of Pathology*, **19**, 341-357.

Follis, R. H. Jr. & Wintrobe, M. M.   (1945) A comparison of the effects of pyridoxine and pantothenic acid deficiencies on the nervous system of swine.   *Journal of Experimental Medicine*, **81**, 539-552.

Foster, D. B.   (1945) Degeneration of peripheral nerves in pernicious anemia.   *Archives of Neurology and Psychiatry*, **54**, 102-109.

Fraser, H. & Stanton, A. T.   (1910) The etiology of beriberi.   *Philippine Journal of Science, Series B*, **5**, 55-61.

Fraser, T. R. & Bruce, A.   (1895) A case of multiple diabetic neuritis.   *British Medical Journal*, **1**, 1149.

Freeman, A. G. & Heaton, J. M.   (1961) The aetiology of retrobulbar neuritis in Addisonian pernicious anaemia.   *Lancet*, **1**, 908-911.

French, J. M., Hall, G. S., Parish, D. J. & Smith, W. T.   (1965) Peripheral and autonomic nerve involvement in primary amyloidosis associated with uncontrollable diarrhoea and steatorrhea. *American Journal of Medicine*, **39**, 277-284.

Gamper, E. (1928) Zur Frage der Polioencephalitis haemorrhagica der chronischen Alkoholiker. *Deutsche Zeitschrift für Nervenheilkunde*, **102**, 122-129.

Garland, H. & Taverner, D. (1953) Diabetic myelopathy. *British Medical Journal*, **1**, 1405-1408.

Garrow, J. S. (1967) Loss of brain potassium in kwashiorkor. *Lancet*, **2**, 643-644.

Geiger, B. J., Steenbock, H. & Parsons, H. T. (1933) Lathyrism in the rat. *Journal of Nutrition*, **6**, 427-442.

German, W. J. (1960) Lathyrism: a review of recent developments. *Journal of Neurosurgery*, **17**, 657-663.

Gibson, J. B. & Goldberg, A. (1956) Neuropathology of acute porphyria. *Journal of Pathology and Bacteriology*, **71**, 495-509.

Girdwood, R. H. (1968) Abnormalities of vitamin B_{12} and folic acid metabolism—their influence on the nervous system. *Proceedings of the Nutrition Society*, **27**, 101-107.

Goldberger, J. & Lillie, R. D. (1926) A note on an experimental pellagra-like condition in the albino rat. *Public Health Reports, Washington, D.C.*, **41**, 1025-1029.

Goldberger, J. & Wheeler, G. A. (1915) Experimental pellagra in the human subject brought about by a restricted diet. *Public Health Reports, Washington, D.C.*, **30**, 3336-3339.

Goldberger, J. & Wheeler, G. A. (1920) Experimental pellagra in white male convicts. *Archives of Internal Medicine*, **25**, 451-471.

Gombault, A. (1880-81) Contribution à l'étude anatomique de la névrite parenchymateuse subaiguë ou chronique: névrite segmentaire péri-axile. *Archives de Neurologie*, **1**, 11, 177-190.

Gopalan, C. (1946) The 'burning feet' syndrome. *Indian Medical Gazette*, **81**, 22-26.

Gopalan, C. (1969) Possible role for dietary leucine in the pathogenesis of pellagra. *Lancet*, **1**, 197-199.

Grant, H. C., Hoffbrand, A. V. & Wells, D. G. (1965) Folate deficiency and neurological disease. *Lancet*, **2**, 763-767.

Greenbaum, D., Richardson, P. C., Salman, M. V. & Urich, H. (1964) Pathological observations on six cases of diabetic neuropathy. *Brain*, **87**, 201-214.

Greenfield, J. C. (1934) Subacute spinocerebellar degeneration occurring in elderly patients. *Brain*, **57**, 161-176.

Greenfield, J. G. (1958) In *Neuropathology*, Arnold, London.

Greenfield, J. G. & Carmichael, E. A. (1935) Peripheral nerves in cases of subacute combined degeneration of the cord. *Brain*, **58**, 483-491.

Greenfield, J. G. & Holmes, J. M. (1939) A case of pellagra. Pathological changes in the spinal cord. *British Medical Journal*, **1**, 815-819.

Greenfield, J. G. & O'Flynn, E. (1933) Subacute combined degeneration and pernicious anaemia. *Lancet*, **2**, 62-63.

Groodt-Lasseel, M. & Martin, J. J. (1969) Étude ultrastructurale des lésions du système nerveux centrale dans la maladie de Whipple. *Pathologie-Biologie (Paris)*, **17**, 121-132.

Grunnet, M. L. (1969) Changing incidence, distribution and histopathology of Wernicke's polioencephalopathy. *Neurology (Minneapolis)*, **19**, 1135-1139.

György, P. (1934) Vitamin B_2 and pellagra-like dermatitis in rats. *Nature*, **133**, 498-499.

György, P. & Pearson, W. N. (1967) *The Vitamins*, Vols 6 and 7, Academic Press, New York.

Hamerton, A. E. (1938-39) Report on the deaths occurring in the Society's Gardens during the year 1937 (Diseases of the nervous system). *Proceedings of the Zoological Society of London, Series B*, **108**, 512-515.

Hamerton, A. E. (1942) Primary degeneration of the spinal cord in monkeys: a study in comparative pathology. *Brain*, **65**, 193-204.

Hardwick, S. W. (1943) Pellagra in psychiatric patients. Twelve recent cases. *Lancet*, **2**, 43-45.

Hartmann, H. A., Lalich, J. J. & Akert, K. (1958) Lesions in the anterior motor horn cells of rats after administration of the bis-β-cyanoethylamine; study of a nitrile closely related to the lathyrus factor. *Journal of Neuropathology and Experimental Neurology*, **17**, 298-304.

Hayes, K. C., Nielsen, S. W. & Eaton, H. D. (1968) Pathogenesis of the optic nerve lesions in vitamin A deficient calves. *Archives of Ophthalmology*, **80**, 777-787.

Heathfield, K. W. G. & Williams, J. R. B. (1954) Peripheral neuropathy and myopathy associated with bronchogenic carcinoma. *Brain*, **77**, 122-137.

Heaton, J. M., McCormick, A. J. A. & Freeman, A. G. (1958) Tobacco amblyopia: a clinical manifestation of vitamin B_{12} deficiency. *Lancet*, **2**, 286-290.

Heinrich, M. R. & Mattil, H. A. (1943) Lipids of muscle and brain in rats deprived of tocopherol. *Proceedings of the Society for Experimental Biology and Medicine*, **52**, 344-346.

Henderson, J. G., Strachan, R. W. & Beck, J. S. (1966) The antigastric-antibody test as a screening procedure for vitamin B_{12} deficiency in psychiatric practice. *Lancet*, **2**, 809-813.

Henson, R. A. (1970) In *Modern Trends in Neurology—5* (Ed. Williams, D.), p. 209, Butterworth, London.

Henson, R. A., Hoffman, H. L. & Urich, H. (1965) Encephalomyelitis with carcinoma. *Brain*, **88**, 449-464.

Henson, R. A., Russell, D. S. & Wilkinson, M. (1954) Carcinomatous neuropathy and myopathy: a clinical and pathological study. *Brain*, **77**, 82-121.

Henson, R. A. & Urich, H. (1968) Peripheral neuropathy and carcinoma. *Proceedings of the Australian Association of Neurologists*, **5**, 399-402.

Hersov, L. A. (1955) A case of childhood pellagra with psychosis. *Journal of Mental Science*, **101**, 878-883.

Hersov, L. A. & Rodnight, R. (1960) Hartnup disease in psychiatric practice: clinical and biochemical features of three cases. *Journal of Neurology, Neurosurgery and Psychiatry*, **23**, 40-45.

Hicks, S. P. (1955) Pathologic effects of antimetabolites; acute lesions in hypothalamus, peripheral ganglia and adrenal medulla caused by 3-acetyl pyridine and prevented by nicotinamide. *American Journal of Pathology*, **31**, 189-197.

Hierons, R. (1957) Changes in the nervous system in acute porphyria. *Brain*, **80**, 176-192.

Hildebrand, J. & Coërs, C. (1967) The neuromuscular function in patients with malignant tumours. *Brain*, **90**, 67-82.

Himsworth, H. P. (1946) Protein metabolism in relation to disease. *Proceedings of the Royal Society of Medicine*, **40**, 27-34.

Himsworth, H. P. & Glynn, L. E. (1944) Toxipathic and tropopathic hepatitis. *Lancet*, **1**, 457-461.

Hirson, C., Feinmann, E. L. & Wade, H. J. (1953) Diabetic neuropathy. *British Medical Journal*, **1**, 1408-1413.

Hoffman, H. L. (1955) Acute necrotic myelopathy. *Brain*, **78**, 377-393.

Howell, J. McC. (1968) Observations on the histology and possible pathogenesis of lesions in the CNS of sheep with swayback. *Proceedings of the Nutrition Society*, **27**, 85-88.

Howell, J. McC. & Davidson, A. W. (1959) The copper content and cytochrome oxidase activity of tissues from normal and swayback lambs. *Biochemical Journal*, **72**, 365-368.

Howell, J. McC. & Thompson, J. N. (1967a) Lesions associated with the development of ataxia in vitamin A deficient chicks. *British Journal of Nutrition*, **21**, 741-750.

Howell, J. McC. & Thompson, J. N. (1967b) Observations on the lesions in vitamin A deficient fowls with particular reference to changes in bone and central nervous system. *British Journal of Experimental Pathology*, **48**, 450-454.

Hsu, J. M., Kawin, B., Minor, P. & Mitchell, J. A. (1966) Vitamin B_{12} concentrations in human tissue. *Nature*, **210**, 1264-1265.

Hsü, Y. K. (1942) Pathologic anatomy of the human nervous system in avitaminosis. *Archives of Neurology and Psychiatry* (*Chicago*), **48**, 271-319.

Huber, G. (1954) Zur pathologischen Anatomie des Delirium tremens. *Archiv für Psychiatrie und Nervenkrankheiten*, **192**, 356-368.

Hughes, L. E. & Kershaw, G. F. (1959) 'B' or border disease: an undescribed disease of sheep. *Veterinary Record*, **71**, 313-317.

Hunt, A. D., Stokes, J., McCrory, W. W. & Stround, H. H. (1954) Pyridoxine dependency: report of a case of intractable convulsions in an infant controlled by pyridoxine. *Pediatrics*, **13**, 140-145.

Hurst, A. F. & Bell, J. R. (1922) The pathogenesis of subacute combined degeneration of the spinal cord. *Brain*, **45**, 266-281.

Innes, J. R. M. (1934) The pathology of swayback: a congenital demyelinating disease of lambs with affinities to Schilder's encephalitis. *Reports of the Institute of Animal Pathology, University of Cambridge*, **4**, 227-250.

Innes, J. R. M. (1936) 'Swayback': congenital demyelinating disease of lambs with affinities to Schilder's encephalitis. *Proceedings of the Royal Society of Medicine*, **29**, 406-409.

Innes, J. R. M. (1939) Swayback: demyelinating disease of lambs with affinities to Schilder's encephalitis and its prevention by copper. *Journal of Neurology and Psychiatry*, **2**, 323-334.

Jervis, G. A. & Kindwall, J. A. (1942) Schilder's disease and ergotamine poisoning. *American Journal of Psychiatry*, **98**, 650-655.

Joiner, C. L., Thompson, R. H. S. & Watson, D. (1950) Pyruvate tolerance in peripheral neuropathy and other conditions. *Guy's Hospital Reports*, **99**, 62-76.

Jolliffe, N., Bowman, K. M., Rosenblum, A. & Fein, H. D. (1940) Nicotinic acid deficiency encephalopathy. *Journal of the American Medical Association*, **114**, 307-312.

Jubb, K. V., Saunders, L. Z. & Coates, H. V. (1956) Thiamine deficiency encephalopathy in cats. *Journal of Comparative Pathology and Therapeutics*, **66**, 217-227.

Kahn, E. (1954) Neurological syndrome in infants recovering from malnutrition. *Archives of Disease in Childhood*, **29**, 256-261.

Krehl, W. A., Tepley, L. J., Sarma, P. S. & Elvehjem, C. A. (1945) Growth retarding effect of corn in nicotinic acid low rations and its counteractions by tryptophane. *Science*, **101**, 489-490.

Lambert, E. H. & Rooke, E. D.   (1965) In *Remote Effects of Cancer on the Nervous System* (Eds. Brain, W. R. & Norris, F. H.), Grune and Stratton, New York.

Lampert, P., Blumberg, J. M. & Pentschew, A.   (1964) An electronmicroscopic study of dystrophic axons in the gracile and cuneate nuclei of vitamin E deficient rats. *Journal of Neuropathology and Experimental Neurology*, **23**, 60-77.

Lehoczky, T., Sos, J., Selmeci, L. & Halasy, M.   (1967) Experimental porphyria and its relationship to human disease. *Brain*, **90**, 795-798.

Leichtenstern, O.   (1884) Über progressive perniciöse Anämie bei Tabeskranken. *Deutsche medizinische Wochenschrift*, **10**, 849.

Leigh, D.   (1951) Subacute necrotizing encephalomyopathy in an infant. *Journal of Neurology, Neurosurgery and Psychiatry*, **14**, 216-221.

Leigh, D.   (1952) Pellagra and the nutritional neuropathies: a neuropathological review. *Journal of Mental Science*, **98**, 130-142.

Lester-Smith, E.   (1948) Purification of antipernicious anaemia factors from liver. *Nature*, **161**, 638-639.

Lester-Smith, E.   (1956) Vitamin B$_{12}$. *British Medical Bulletin*, **12**, 52-56.

Lichtheim, H.   (1887) Zur Kenntnis der perniciösen Anämie. *Verhandlungen der deutschen Gesellschaft für innere Medizin*, p. 84.

Lippincott, S. W. & Morris, H. P.   (1942) Pathologic changes associated with riboflavin deficiency in the mouse. *Journal of the National Cancer Institute*, **2**, 601-610.

Lopez, R. I. & Collins, G. H.   (1968) Wernicke's encephalopathy. A complication of chronic hemodialysis. *Archives of Neurology (Chicago)*, **18**, 248-259.

Luckner, H. & Scriba, K.   (1949) Über die hydropische und cardiovasculäre Form der Beriberi und ihre Entstehung. Tierexperimentelle Untersuchungen zur Ätiologie der Beriberi. *Deutsches Archiv für klinische Medizin*, **194**, 396-433.

Luttrell, C. N. & Mason, K. E.   (1949) Vitamin E deficiency, dietary fat and spinal cord lesions in the rat. *Annals of the New York Academy of Sciences*, **52**, 113-120.

Macalpine, I. & Hunter, R.   (1968) *Porphyria. A Royal Malady*, British Medical Association, London.

McCall, K. B., Waisman, H. A., Elvehjem, C. A. & Jones, E. S.   (1946) Study of pyridoxine and pantothenic acid deficiencies in the monkey (Macaca mulatta). *Journal of Nutrition*, **31**, 685-697.

McCance, R. A.   (1951) The history, significance and aetiology of hunger oedema. *Medical Research Council Special Report Series*, **275**, 21-82.

McIlwain, H.   (1940) Pyridine-3-sulphonic acid and its amide as inhibitors of bacterial growth. *British Journal of Experimental Pathology*, **21**, 136-147.

McIlwain, H.   (1955) *Biochemistry and the Central Nervous System*, Churchill, London.

McIlwain, H. & Bachelard, H. S.   (1971) *Biochemistry and the Central Nervous System*, 4th Edn., Churchill/Livingstone, Edinburgh and London.

Madhaven, T. V., Belavady, B. & Gopalan, C.   (1968) Pathology of canine black tongue. *Journal of Pathology and Bacteriology*, **95**, 259-263.

Malamud, N., Nelson, M. M. & Evans, H. M.   (1949) The effect of chronic vitamin E deficiency on the nervous system in the rat. *Annals of the New York Academy of Sciences*, **52**, 135-138.

Markson, L. M., Terlecki, S., Shand, A., Sellers, K. C. & Woods, A. J.   (1959) Hypomyelinogenesis congenita in sheep. *Veterinary Record*, **71**, 269-271.

Martin, M. M.   (1953) Diabetic neuropathy: clinical study of 150 cases. *Brain*, **76**, 594-624.

Matthews, J. D.   (1955) Neuropathy in diabetes mellitus. *Lancet*, **1**, 474-476.

Mayer, R. F.   (1965) Peripheral nerve function in vitamin B$_{12}$ deficiency. *Archives of Neurology*, **13**, 355-362.

Mayer-Gross, W., Slater, E. & Roth, M.   (1954) *Clinical Psychiatry*, Cassell, London.

Melchior, J. C. & Clausen, J.   (1968) Metachromatic leucodystrophy in early childhood. Treatment with a diet deficient in vitamin A. *Acta paediatrica scandinavica*, **57**, 2-8.

Mellanby, E.   (1931) Experimental production and prevention of degeneration in spinal cord. *Brain*, **54**, 247-290.

Mellanby, E.   (1944) Croonian Lecture: Nutrition in relation to bone growth and nervous system. *Proceedings of the Royal Society, Series B*, **132**, 28-46.

Menzies, D. W. & Mills, K. W.   (1957) Aortic and skeletal lesions of lathyrism in rats on a diet of sweet pea. *Journal of Pathology and Bacteriology*, **73**, 223-237.

Meyer, Adolf   (1901) On parenchymatous systemic degenerations mainly in the central nervous system. *Brain*, **24**, 47.

Meyer,   (1944) The Wernicke syndrome: with special reference to manic syndromes associated with hypothalamic lesions. *Journal of Neurology and Psychiatry*, **7**, 66-75.

Meyer, A., Pampiglione, G., Platt, B. S. & Stewart, R. J. C.   (1961) In *Excerpta Medica International Congress Series*, No. 39, p. 15.

Meyer, A.   (1963) In *Neuropathology* (Eds. Blackwood, W., McMenemey, W. H., Meyer, A., Norman, R. M. & Russell, D. S.), 2nd Edn., Arnold, London.

Meyer, A., Stewart, R. J. C. & Platt, B. S.   (1961) The spinal cord of pigs on low-protein diets. *Proceedings of the Nutrition Society*, **20**, xviii.

Millen, J. W. & Woollam, D. H. M.   (1956) The effect of the duration of vitamin A deficiency in female rabbits upon the incidence of hydrocephalus in their young. *Journal of Neurology, Neurosurgery and Psychiatry*, **19**, 17-20.

Millen, J. W., Woollam, D. H. M. & Lamming, G. E.   (1953) Hydrocephalus associated with deficiency of vitamin A. *Lancet*, **2**, 1234-1236.

Milne, M. D.   (1969) Hartnup disease. *Biochemical Journal*, **111**, 3-4P.

Minnich, W.   (1892) Kenntnis der im Verlaufe der perniciösen Anämie beobachteten Spinalerkrankungen. *Zeitschrift für klinische Medizin*, **21**, 264-314.

Minot, G. R. & Murphy, W. P.   (1926) Treatment of pernicious anaemia by a special diet. *Journal of the American Medical Association*, **87**, 470-476.

Miyagishi, T., Takahata, N. & Iizuka, R.   (1967) Electronmicroscope studies on the lipopigments in the cerebral cortex nerve cells of senile and vitamin E deficient rats. *Acta Neuropathologica (Berlin)*, **9**, 7-17.

Mönckeberg, F. B.   (1969) Malnutrition and mental behaviour. *Nutrition Reviews*, **27**, 191-193.

Najjar, V. A. & Holt, L. E.   (1943) Biosynthesis of thiamine in man and its implications in human nutrition. *Journal of the American Medical Association*, **123**, 683-684.

Neubürger, K.   (1936) Über die nichtalkoholische Wernickesche Krankheit, insbesondere über ihr Vorkommen beim Krebsleiden. *Virchows Archiv für pathologische Anatomie*, **298**, 68-86.

Nitowsky, H. M., Gordon, H. H. & Tildon, J. T.   (1956) Studies of tocopherol deficiency in infants and children; effect of alpha tocopherol on creatinuria in patients with cystic fibrosis of pancreas and biliary atresia. *Bulletin of the Johns Hopkins Hospital*, **98**, 361-371.

North, J. D. & Sinclair, H. M.   (1956) Nutritional neuropathy: chronic thiamine deficiency in the rat. *Archives of Pathology*, **62**, 341-353.

North, J. D. & Sinclair, H. M.   (1957) The effect of combined deficiency of thiamine and pantothenic acid on the nervous system of the rat. *Journal of Nutrition*, **61**, 219-234.

Nutrition Reviews.   (1968) Leading article. Vitamin B_6 deficiency following isoniazid therapy. **26**, 306.

Olivarius, B. de F. & Roos, D.   (1968) Myelopathy following partial gastrectomy. *Acta neurologica Scandinavica*, **44**, 347-362.

Oppenheimer, E. H.   (1956) Focal necrosis of striated muscle in infant with cystic fibrosis of pancreas and evidence of lack of absorption of fat-soluble vitamins. *Bulletin of the Johns Hopkins Hospital*, **98**, 353-359.

Oxnard, C. E. & Smith, W. T.   (1966) Neurological degeneration and reduced serum vitamin B_{12} levels in captive monkeys. *Nature*, **210**, 507-509.

Oxnard, C. E., Smith, W. T. & Torres, I.   (1970) Vitamin B_{12} deficiency in captive monkeys and its effect on the nervous system and blood. *Laboratory Animals*, **4**, 1-12.

Pena, C.   (1969) Wernicke's encephalopathy. Report of 7 cases with severe nerve cell changes in the mamillary bodies. *American Journal of Clinical Pathology*, **51**, 603-609.

Pentschew, A.   (1928) Über die Histopathologie des Zentralnervensystems bei der Psychosis pellagrosa. *Zeitschrift für die gesamte Neurologie und Psychiatrie*, **118**, 17-48.

Pentschew, A.   (1929) Experimentelle Untersuchungen über Pellagra, Ergotismus, und Bleivergiftung. II. Pellagraähnliche Erkrankung eines mit vitaminreicher Nahrung gefütterten Affens. *Krankheitsforschung*, **7**, 415-423.

Pentschew, A. & Schwarz, K.   (1962) Systemic axonal dystrophy in vitamin E deficient adult rats. *Acta Neuropathologica (Berlin)*, **1**, 313-334.

Peters, R. A. & Sinclair, H. M.   (1933) Studies in avian carbohydrate metabolism: further studies upon the action of catatorulin in the brain. *Biochemical Journal*, **27**, 1910-1926.

Peters, R. A. & Thompson, R. H. S.   (1934) Pyruvic acid as an intermediate metabolite in the brain tissue of avitaminous and normal pigeons. *Biochemical Journal*, **28**, 916-925.

Pinsky, L. & Fraser, F. C.   (1960) Congenital malformations after a two-hour inactivation of nicotinamide in pregnant mice. *British Medical Journal*, **2**, 195-197.

Platt, B. S.   (1958*a*) Clinical features of endemic beriberi. *Federation Proceedings*, **17** (*Suppl. 2, part 2*), 8-20.

Platt, B. S.   (1958*b*) Malnutrition and the pathogenesis of disease. *Transactions of the Royal Society of Tropical Medicine and Hygiene*, **52**, 189-216.

Platt, B. S. & Gin, S. Y.   (1934) Some observations on a preliminary study of beriberi in Shanghai.   *Transactions of the Ninth Congress of the Far-East Association of Tropical Medicine*, **2**, 407-413.

Platt, B. S. & Lu, G. D.   (1935) Quoted by Platt, B. S. (1958*a*).

Platt, B. S. & Stewart, R. J. C.   (1969) Effects of protein calorie deficiency on dogs.   2. Morphological changes in the nervous system.   *Developmental Medicine and Child Neurology*, **11**, 174-192.

Platt, B. S. & Wheeler, E. F.   (1967) Protein calorie deficiency and the nervous system.   *Developmental Medicine and Child Neurology*, **9**, 104-105.

Ponseti, I. V. & Baird, W. A.   (1952) Scoliosis and dissecting aneurysm in lathyrus rat.   *American Journal of Pathology*, **28**, 1059-1077.

Ponseti, I. V.   (1954) Lesions of skeleton and other mesodermal tissues in rats fed sweet pea (*Lathyrus odoratus*) seeds.   *Journal of Bone and Joint Surgery*, **36**A, 1031-1058.

Popper, H.   (1941) Histologic distribution of vitamin A in human organs under normal and under pathologic conditions.   *Archives of Pathology*, **31**, 766-802.

Prados, M. & Swank, R. L.   (1942) Vascular and interstitial cell changes in thiamine deficient animals.   *Archives of Neurology and Psychiatry (Chicago)*, **47**, 626-644.

Prickett, C. O.   (1934) The effect of deficiency of vitamin B_1 upon the central and peripheral nervous system of the rat.   *American Journal of Physiology*, **107**, 459-470.

Purpura, D. P. & Gonzalez-Monteagudo, O.   (1960) Acute effects of methoxypyridine on hippocampal end-blade neurons; an experimental study of 'special pathoclisis' in the cerebral cortex.   *Journal of Neuropathology and Experimental Neurology*, **19**, 421-432.

Putnam, J. J.   (1891) A group of cases of system scleroses of the spinal cord associated with diffuse collateral degeneration.   *Journal of Nervous and Mental Disease*, **22**, 51.

Raskin, N. H. & Fishman, R. A.   (1965) Pyridoxine deficiency neuropathy due to hydralazine.   *New England Journal of Medicine*, **273**, 1182-1185.

Raubitschek, H.   (1915) Pathologie, Entstehungsweise und Ursachen der Pellagra.   *Ergebnisse der allgemeinen Pathologie und pathologischen Anatomie*, **18**, 662-786.

Rewcastle, N. B.   (1963) Subacute cerebellar degeneration with Hodgkin's disease.   *Archives of Neurology (Chicago)*, **9**, 407-413.

Richmond, J. & Davidson, S.   (1958) Subacute combined degeneration of the spinal cord in non-Addisonian megaloblastic anaemia.   *Quarterly Journal of Medicine*, **27**, 517-531.

Rickes, E. L., Brink, N. G., Konuisky, F. R., Wood, T. R. & Folkers, K.   (1948) Vitamin B_{12}, a cobalt complex.   *Science*, **108**, 134.

Ridley, A.   (1969) The neuropathy of acute intermittent porphyria.   *Quarterly Journal of Medicine*, **38**, 307-333.

Riggs, H. E. & Boles, R. S.   (1944) Wernicke's disease.   A clinical and pathological study of 42 cases.   *Quarterly Journal of Studies on Alcohol*, **5**, 361-370.

Rinehart, J. F.   (1947) Experimental thiamine deficiency in the rhesus monkey.   *American Journal of Pathology*, **23**, 879-881.

Rinehart, J. F., Friedman, M. & Greenberg, L. D.   (1949) Effects of experimental thiamine deficiency on the nervous system of the rhesus monkey.   *Archives of Pathology*, **48**, 129-139.

Rinehart, J. F. & Greenberg, L. D.   (1956) Arteriosclerotic lesions in pyridoxine deficient monkeys.   *American Journal of Pathology*, **25**, 481-489.

Roberts, D. M., Themann, H. & Knust, F. J.   (1970) An electronmicroscope study of bacteria in two cases of Whipple's disease.   *Journal of Pathology*, **100**, 249-255.

Roberts, E.   (1961) In *Chemical Pathology of the Nervous System* (Ed. Folchi-Pi, J.), Pergamon Press, Oxford.

Roberts, H. E., Williams, B. M. & Harvard, A.   (1966) Cerebral oedema in lambs associated with hypocuprosis and its relationship to swayback: 2, histopathological findings.   *Journal of Comparative Pathology and Therapeutics*, **76**, 285-290.

Robertson, D. M., Wasan, S. M. & Skinner, D. B.   (1968) Ultrastructural features of early brainstem lesions of thiamine deficient rats.   *American Journal of Pathology*, **52**, 1081-1097.

Rodnight, R. & McIlwain, H.   (1955) Indicanuria and psychosis of pellagra.   *Journal of Mental Science*, **101**, 884-889.

Rosenblum, W. I. & Feigin, I.   (1965) The hemorrhagic component of Wernicke's encephalopathy.   *Archives of Neurology*, **13**, 627-632.

Russell, J. S. R., Batten, F. E. & Collier, J.   (1900) Subacute combined degeneration of the spinal cord.   *Brain*, **23**, 39-110.

Schaefer, A. E., McKibbin, J. M. & Elvehjem, C. A.   (1942) Pantothenic acid deficiency in dogs.   *Journal of Biological Chemistry*, **143**, 321-330.

Scherer, H. J.   (1944) *Vergleichende Pathologie des Nervensystems der Säugetiere unter besonderer Berücksichtigung der Primaten*, Thieme, Leipzig.

Scholz, W.   (1949) Histologische und topische Veränderungen und Vulnerabilitätsverhältnisse im menschlichen Gehirn bei Sauerstoffmangel, Ödem und plasmatischen Infiltrationen.   *Archiv für Psychiatrie und Nervenkrankheiten*, **181**, 621-665.

Scriba, K. & Luckner, H.   (1949) Das Beriberiherz im Tierexperiment.   *Deutsches Archiv für klinische Medizin*, **196**, 193-211.

Sebrell, W. H. & Butler, R. E.   (1939) Riboflavin deficiency in man (ariboflavinosis).   *Public Health Reports, Washington D.C.*, **54**, 2121-2131.

Sebrell, W. H. Jr. & Harris, R. S.   (1967) *The Vitamins*, Vols. 1-4, Academic Press, New York.

Selye, H.   (1957) Lathyrism.   *Revue Canadienne de Biologie*, **16**, 1-82.

Shah, S. R. A.   (1939) A note of some cases of lathyrism in a Punjab village.   *Indian Medical Gazette*, **74**, 385-388.

Shaw, J. H. & Phillips, P. H.   (1941) The pathology of riboflavin deficiency in the rat.   *Journal of Nutrition*, **22**, 345-358.

Shaw, J. H. & Phillips, P. H.   (1945) Neuropathologic studies of acute and chronic thiamine deficiencies and of inanition.   *Journal of Nutrition*, **29**, 113-125.

Shulman, R.   (1967) Psychiatric aspects of pernicious anaemia: a prospective controlled investigation.   *British Medical Journal*, **3**, 266-270.

Sinclair, H. M.   (1956) Vitamins and the nervous system.   *British Medical Bulletin*, **12**, 18-23.

Sinclair, H. M.   (1961) In *Chemical Pathology of the Nervous System* (Ed. Folchi-Pi, J.), Pergamon Press, Oxford.

Slagel, D. E. & Hartmann, H. A.   (1965) The distribution of neuroaxonal lesions in mice injected with imidoproprionitrile, with special reference to the vestibular system.   *Journal of Neuropathology and Experimental Neurology*, **24**, 599-620.

Slagel, D. E., Hartmann, H. A. & Edstrom, J. E.   (1966) The effect of imidoproprionitrile on the ribonucleic acid content and composition of mesencephalic V cells, anterior horn cells, glial cells and axonal balloons.   *Journal of Neuropathology and Experimental Neurology*, **25**, 244-253.

Smith, W. T.   (1961) Cerebral lesions due to the thrombotic syndrome associated with carcinoma in *Proceedings of the IVth International Congress of Neuropathology*, Vol. 3, p. 151, Thieme, Stuttgart.

Smith, W. T., French, J. M., Gottsman, M., Smith, A. J. & Wakes-Miller, J. A.   (1965) Cerebral complications of Whipple's disease.   *Brain*, **88**, 137-150.

Smith, W. T. & Whittaker, S. R. F.   (1964) Diffuse degeneration of cerebral white matter resembling so-called Binswanger's disease and symmetrical necrosis of the globus pallidus associated with acute porphyria and cerebral atherosclerosis.   *Journal of Clinical Pathology*, **16**, 419-422.

Spais, A., Palsson, P. A. & van Bogaert, L.   (1961) Pathology of enzootic ataxia of lambs, *Acta Neuropathologica* (*Berlin*), **1**, 56-72.

Spatz, H.   (1930) Encephalitis in *Handbuch der Psychiatrie* (Ed. Bumke, O.), Vol. 2, Springer, Berlin.

Spillane, J. D.   (1947) *Nutritional Disorders of the Nervous System*, Livingstone, Edinburgh.

Stern, R. O. & Findlay, G. M.   (1929) Nervous system in rats fed on diets deficient in vitamins B_1 and B_2.   *Journal of Pathology and Bacteriology*, **32**, 63-69.

Sternberg, S. S. & Phillips, F. S.   (1958) 6-aminonicotinamide and acute degenerative changes in the central nervous system.   *Science*, **127**, 644.

Street, H. R., Cowgill, G. R. & Zimmerman, H. M.   (1941) Further observations on riboflavin deficiency in the dog.   *Journal of Nutrition*, **22**, 7-24.

Stewart, R. J. & Platt, B. S.   (1968) The influence of protein calorie deficiency on the nervous system.   *Proceedings of the Nutrition Society*, **27**, 95-101.

Sundaresen, P. S.   (1966) Vitamin A and sulphate activating enzymes.   *Biochimica et biophysica acta*, **113**, 95-109.

Swank, R. L.   (1940) Avian thiamin deficiency. A correlation of the pathology and clinical behaviour.   *Journal of Experimental Medicine*, **71**, 683-702.

Swank, R. L. & Adams, R. D.   (1948) Pyridoxine and pantothenic acid deficiency in swine.   *Journal of Neuropathology and Experimental Neurology*, **7**, 274-286.

Swank, R. L. & Prados, M.   (1942) Avian thiamine deficiency. II. Pathologic changes in the brain and cranial nerves (especially vestibular) and their relation to clinical behaviour.   *Archives of Neurology and Psychiatry* (*Chicago*), **47**, 97-131.

Sydenstricker, V. P. & Cleckley, H. M.   (1941) The effect of nicotinic acid in stupor, lethargy and various other psychiatric disorders.   *American Journal of Psychiatry*, **98**, 83-92.

Tanaka, T.   (1934) So-called breast milk intoxication.   *American Journal of Diseases of Children*, **47**, 1286-1298.

Tellez, I. & Terry, R. D.   (1968) Fine structure of the early changes in the vestibular nuclei of the thiamine deficient rat.   *American Journal of Pathology*, **52**, 777-794.

Terris, M.   (1963) *Goldberger on Pellagra*, State University Press, Louisiana.

Thomas, P. K. & Lascelles, R. G.   (1965) Schwann cell abnormalities in diabetic neuropathy. *Lancet*, **1**, 1355-1357.

Thomas, P. K. & Lascelles, R. G.   (1966) The pathology of diabetic neuropathy. *Quarterly Journal of Medicine*, **35**, 489-509.

Torres, I., Smith, W. T. & Oxnard, C. E.   (1971) Peripheral neuropathy associated with vitamin B_{12} deficiency in captive monkeys. *Journal of Pathology*, **105**, 125-146.

Tower, D. B.   (1961) In *Chemical Pathology of the Nervous System* (Ed. Folchi-Pi, J.), Pergamon Press, Oxford.

Trowell, H. C., Davies, J. N. P. & Dean, R. F. A.   (1954) In *Kwashiorkor*, Arnold, London.

Truswell, A. S., Hansen, J. D. & Wannenburg, P.   (1968) Plasma tryptophan and other aminoacids in pellagra. *American Journal of Clinical Nutrition*, **21**, 1314-1320.

Udani, P. M.   (1960) Neurological manifestations in kwashiorkor. *Indian Journal of Child Health*, **9**, 103-112.

Ule, G.   (1959) Über eine der Wernickeschen Pseudoencephalitis entsprechende Encephalopathie bei Kindern. *Virchows Archiv für pathologische Anatomie*, **332**, 204-215.

Ule, G. & Kammerer, V.   (1960) Wernicke's encephalopathy in experimental thiamine deficiency in rats. *Virchows Archiv für pathologische Anatomie*, **333**, 190-194.

Ungley, C.   (1949) Subacute combined degeneration of the cord. *Brain*, **72**, 382-427.

Urich, H.   (1967) The remote effects of cancer on the nervous system. Pathology. *Proceedings of the Royal Society of Medicine*, **60**, 690-692.

van Bogaert, L., Radermecker, M. A., Janssen, P. & Gatera, F.   (1962) The muscular lesions of kwashiorkor compared with those of other oedematous conditions and malnutrition in the Congolese infant. *Acta Neuropathologica (Berlin)*, **1**, 363-383.

van der Scheer, W. M. & Kock, H. C.   (1938) Peripheral nerve lesions in cases of pernicious anaemia. *Acta psychiatrica et neurologica*, **13**, 61-92.

Vannotti, A.   (1954) *Porphyrins: Their Biological and Chemical Importance* (Trans. Rimington, C.), Hilger and Watts, London.

Verjaal, A. & Timmermans-Van Den Bos, A. H. C. C.   (1967) Combined degeneration of the spinal cord due to deficiency and alimentary vitamin B_{12}. *Journal of Neurology, Neurosurgery and Psychiatry*, **30**, 464-467.

Verma, K. & Wei King, D.   (1967) Disorders of the developing nervous system of vitamin E deficient rats. *Acta anatomica (Basel)*, **67**, 623-635.

Victor, M. & Adams, R. D.   (1953) The effect of alcohol on the nervous system. *Research Proceedings of the Association for Research in Nervous and Mental Disease*, **32**, 526-573.

Victor, M., Adams, R. D. & Collins, G. H.   (1971) *The Wernicke-Korsakoff Syndrome*, Blackwell Scientific, Oxford.

Vilter, R. W., Mueller, J. F., Glazer, H. S., Jarrold, T., Abraham, J., Thompson, C. & Hawkins, V. R.   (1953) The effect of vitamin B_6 deficiency induced by desoxypyridoxine in human beings. *Journal of Laboratory and Clinical Medicine*, **42**, 335-357.

Vivacqua, R. J., Myerson, R. M., Prescott, D. J. & Rabinowitz, J. L.   (1966) Abnormal proprionic-methyl-malonic-succinic acid metabolism in vitamin B_{12} deficiency and its possible relationship to the neurologic syndrome of pernicious anaemia. *American Journal of Medical Science*, **251**, 507-515.

Walsh, J. C.   (1971) Neuropathy associated with lymphoma. *Journal of Neurology, Neurosurgery and Psychiatry*, **34**, 42-50.

Walsh, J. C. & McLeod, J. G.   (1970) Alcoholic neuropathy; an electrophysiological and histological study. *Journal of the Neurological Sciences*, **10**, 457-469.

Walton, J. W.   (1969) In *Brain's Diseases of the Nervous System*, 7th Edn., p. 729, Oxford University Press, London.

Warnock, L. J. & Burkhalter, V. J.   (1968) Evidence of malfunctioning blood brain barrier in experimental thiamine deficiency in rats. *Journal of Nutrition*, **94**, 256-260.

Wernicke, C.   (1881-83) *Lehrbuch der Gehirnkrankheiten*, Band. 2, Fischer, Kassel and Berlin.

West, E. D. & Ellis, F. R.,   (1966) The electroencephalogram in veganism, vegetarianism, vitamin B_{12} deficiency and in controls. *Journal of Neurology, Neurosurgery and Psychiatry*, **29**, 391-397.

Wilkinson, M., Croft, P. B. & Urich, H.   (1967) The remote effects of cancer on the nervous system. *Proceedings of the Royal Society of Medicine*, **60**, 683-686.

Williams, J. A., Hall, G. S., Thompson, A. G. & Cooke, W. T.   (1969) Neurological disease after partial gastrectomy. *British Medical Journal*, **3**, 210-212.

Williams, R. D., Mason, H. L., Smith, B. F. & Wilder, R. M.   (1942) Induced thiamine (vitamin B_1) deficiency and thiamine requirement of man: further observations. *Archives of Internal Medicine*, **69**, 721-738.

Wilson, J. & Langman, M. J. S.   (1966) Relation of subacute combined degeneration of the cord to vitamin B_{12} deficiency. *Nature*, **212**, 787-789.

Wilson, J. & Matthews, D. M.   (1966) Metabolic inter-relationships between cyanide, thiocyanate and vitamin B_{12} in smokers and non-smokers. *Clinical Science*, **31**, 1-7.

Wilson, S. A. K.   (1914) The pathology of pellagra. *Proceedings of the Royal Society of Medicine*, **7**, 91.

Wintrobe, M. M., Bushke, W., Follis, R. H. Jr. & Humphreys, S.   (1944) Riboflavin deficiency in the swine with special reference to the occurrence of cataracts. *Bulletin of the Johns Hopkins Hospital*, **75**, 102-114.

Wintrobe, M. M., Follis, R. H. Jr., Miller, M. H., Stein, H. J., Alcayaga, R., Humphreys, S., Suksta, A. & Cartwright, G. E.   (1943) Pyridoxine deficiency in swine with particular reference to anaemia, epileptiform convulsions and fatty liver. *Bulletin of the Johns Hopkins Hospital*, **72**, 1-25.

Wise, R. P. & MacDermot, V.   (1962) A myasthenic syndrome associated with bronchial carcinoma. *Journal of Neurology, Neurosurgery and Psychiatry*, **25**, 31-39.

Wokes, F.   (1956) Diet and anaemia: anaemia and vitamin B_{12} dietary deficiency. *Proceedings of the Nutrition Society*, **15**, 134-141.

Wokes, F., Badenoch, J. & Sinclair, H. M.   (1955) Human dietary deficiency of vitamin B_{12}. *American Journal of Clinical Nutrition*, **3**, 375-382.

Wolbach, S. B. & Bessey, O. A.   (1941) Vitamin deficiency and the nervous system. *Archives of Pathology (Chicago)*, **32**, 689-722.

Wolf, A., Cowen, D. & Gellar, L. M.   (1959) The effects of an antimetabolite, 6-aminonicotinamide, on the central nervous system. *Transactions of the American Neurological Association*, **84**, 140-145.

Wolf, A., Cowen, D. & Geller, L. M.   (1962) Structural and functional effects of 6-aminonicotinamide and other antimetabolites on the central nervous system. *Proceedings of the IVth International Congress of Neuropathology*, Vol. 3, p. 477, Thieme, Stuttgart.

Woltman, H. W.   (1918) Brain changes associated with pernicious anemia. *Archives of Internal Medicine*, **21**, 791-843.

Woltman, H. W.   (1924) The mental changes with pernicious anemia. *American Journal of Psychiatry*, **3**, 435.

Woltman, H. W. & Wilder, R. M.   (1929) Diabetes mellitus. Pathologic changes in the spinal cord and peripheral nerves. *Archives of Internal Medicine*, **44**, 576-603.

Woolf, A. L. & Malins, J. M.   (1957) Changes in the intramuscular nerve endings in diabetic neuropathy: a biopsy study. *Journal of Pathology and Bacteriology*, **73**, 316-319.

Woolley, D. W.   (1945) Observations on growth-stimulating action of certain proteins added to protein-free diets compounded with aminoacids. *Journal of Biological Chemistry*, **159**, 753-754.

Woolley, D. W.   (1946) Occurrence of 'pellagragenic' agent in corn. *Journal of Biological Chemistry*, **163**, 773-774.

Wortis, H., Bueding, E. & Jollife, N.   (1942) Pyruvic acid studies in peripheral neuropathy of alcohol addicts. *New England Journal of Medicine*, **226**, 376-379.

Zahnd, G.   (1953) Über die Hirnbefunde beim Delirium tremens. *Monatschrift für Psychiatrie*, **125**, 103-125.

Zimmerman, H. M.   (1939) The pathology of the nervous system in vitamin deficiencies. *Yale Journal of Biology and Medicine*, **12**, 23-28.

Zimmerman, H. M.   (1943) Pathology of vitamin B group deficiencies. *Research Publications of the Association for Research in Nervous and Mental Disease*, **22**, 51-79.

6

Bacterial Infections of the Central Nervous System

Revised by D. G. F. Harriman

The central nervous system offers less resistance to infection than any other tissue of the body. As a consequence microorganisms, such as *Fusobacterium fusiforme*, which are commonly regarded as feebly pathogenic, may, when they obtain access to the brain, cause abscesses or meningitis which are often fatal. Other organisms of comparatively mild pathogenicity, such as *N. meningitidis* (*meningococcus*) and *Brucella abortus*, rarely cause fatal illness unless they invade the nervous system; it is fortunate therefore that the central nervous system is well shielded from infection from without by its bony and dural coverings and that the blood–brain barrier also gives some protection against infection by the blood stream.

In the history of most infectious diseases the search for the causative agent has followed a presumptive diagnosis based largely on the character of the cellular exudate. This remains true for many individual cases in which the clinical diagnosis is uncertain. It is therefore important first to decide, as far as possible, what type or degree of cellular exudate can be accepted as evidence of infection by a living organism. This question has arisen especially in some forms of demyelinating disease and of peripheral neuropathy and in the more acute cases of systemic degeneration, in all of which some degree of cellular infiltration is commonly found, especially round the vessels and in the meninges.

It is now recognized that cellular exudation, especially of lymphocytes, can be excited by many stimuli, one of which may be the rapid breakdown of nervous tissue. The reaction is comparable to those seen in acute degenerations and ischaemic necroses in other organs such as the liver, kidney and heart. In doubtful cases the first question is whether the destruction of nervous tissue precedes the cellular exudate or whether both appear at the same time. When this cannot be ascertained, an assessment of the relative intensities of exudate and destruction of nervous tissue may give valuable evidence. The type of cell forming the exudate is also important. For example, acute demyelinating processes are often associated with quite thick cuffs of lymphocytes round the vessels in the neighbourhood, but polymorphonuclear leucocytes and plasma cells are usually absent or very scarce. On the other hand mild inflammatory reactions in which plasma cells and their derivatives, Russell and mulberry cells, are prominent, as in some forms of subacute encephalitis, are strong evidence of an infectious aetiology.

Reaction either to infectious or other acutely destructive processes is not confined to leucocytes and other wandering cells. The supporting tissues of the central nervous system also react either by regressive changes or by hyperplasia. Some of the reactions of astrocytes and microglia have already been discussed. Reticulin and collagenous tissue are only present in the meninges and the walls of the vessels, and their reactions are less constant and usually slighter than those of astrocytes, but with the more severe infections and other serious lesions of nervous tissue their reaction may be of major importance. The fact that the only available supply of fibroblastic tissue is in the walls of the vessels delays and may prevent the fibrous tissue encapsulation which plays an important part in the healing of acute inflammatory foci here as elsewhere in the body. In many milder infections, and in demyelinating lesions also, there is some thickening of the walls of small vessels and limited outgrowth of collagen from them into the surrounding nervous tissue.

Virchow–Robin space

The perivascular or Virchow–Robin space, which surrounds the arteries and veins within the central nervous system, but not the capillaries, is a structure peculiar to the central nervous system. It may be considered as a continuation of the subarachnoid space along the vessel walls as they leave this space to enter the nervous tissue, and it contains cerebrospinal fluid. Its inner wall is the adventitia of the vessel walls. Externally it is bounded by a thin layer of collagen or reticulin fibres between which cells may be able to enter and leave the space. When it is empty of cells, as it normally is, its thin outer wall is not easily distinguished from the adventitia of the vessel wall, but when it is filled with lymphocytes or lipid phagocytes, these cells are seen to lie between the adventitia and an enclosing connective tissue layer which stains red with van Gieson's picro-fuchsin and is usually also argyrophilic. Fine trabeculae can be seen under these conditions to join the inner and outer walls of the space in a manner similar to the trabeculae of the subarachnoid space.

The Virchow–Robin space normally contains occasional mononuclear cells and numerous mesenchymal or reticulo-endothelial cells lie in its walls. Under many conditions these cells may be seen undergoing mitotic division. It is probable that they also play an active part in the absorption and katabolism of lipids in areas of demyelination or softening. Whether lymphocytes can multiply in the space is less certain.

The manner in which lymphocytes and lipid phagocytes are confined within the space in pathological conditions and the fact that it may be filled by injecting indian ink or colloidal carbon into the subarachnoid space (Millen and Woollam 1954) make it certain that a potential space, in communication with the subarachnoid space, normally exists around the intracerebral and intramedullary arteries and veins. It is thought that the current in this space is normally from within outwards so that lymphocytes or other cells which collect around the smaller vascular branches pass along the larger vessels into the subarachnoid space. The Virchow–Robin space appears to be wider round these larger vessels, and cuffs of lymphocytes two, three or more cells thick may be seen around them in cases where only a single layer of cells surrounds the small venules and arterioles.

The Virchow–Robin spaces may be considered both in constitution and in function as the lymphatic channels of the central nervous system. It seems probable that some protein substances, as well as lymphocytes, plasma cells and lipid phagocytes, may be carried along them to the subarachnoid space since, in its passage over the brain and spinal cord, the cerebrospinal fluid always receives an addition of protein. This is shown very clearly by comparing protein values in cerebrospinal fluid taken from the ventricles and the lumbar subarachnoid space (15 mg/100 ml and 45 mg/100 ml respectively). The γ globulin, which the cerebrospinal fluid often contains in subacute forms of encephalitis, may well be formed within the brain and pass into the cerebrospinal fluid along the Virchow–Robin spaces (Field 1954).

The term Virchow–Robin space is used in preference to perivascular space for the invagination of the arachnoid space around the larger vessels. Perivascular space or space of His is the name sometimes given to the cleavage space between smaller vessels and the nervous parenchyma; this is seen in paraffin, but never in nitrocellulose, sections and is generally considered to be an artefact. Under certain conditions a space may be formed in that situation by haemorrhage or pools of plasma, entailing rupture of the foot-plate processes of perivascular astrocytes, but it is very doubtful whether any true space exists there under normal conditions.

Anatomical considerations

The brain and spinal cord are protected from infections from outside by their membranous coverings. The skull also provides an effective shield although emissary veins may carry infection through it to the brain. The dura mater is a valuable barrier against infection and, especially in the spinal cord, may prevent the spread of infection through it for a considerable time. The external layer of arachnoid, possibly largely owing to the layer of endothelial cells which covers its external surface, provides a check to infection passing either from the subdural to the arachnoid space or vice versa, and the pia mater, in much the same manner, acts as a temporary barrier preventing subarachnoid infections from spreading into the brain. Infections in these four situations, *epidural, subdural, subarachnoid* and *intracerebral* or *intramedullary*, are therefore discussed separately, although in many cases they are combined.

Routes of infection

1. Infections of the central nervous system or meninges may come from the blood stream either directly or via the choroid plexus.
2. Infections may be derived from local sources
(a) by erosion of the thin plate of bone overlying infected middle ear, mastoid, or paranasal air sinuses;
(b) by transmission along anastomotic veins from the face, scalp, or air sinuses;
(c) by fractures which may open channels from the exterior to the meninges;
(d) by transmission along cranial nerves, e.g. the olfactory filaments.

Epidural infections and suppurations

Infections of the intracranial epidural space may produce abscesses which are flattened between the bone and the dura mater and are usually of small size. They most often result from infection of air sinuses, but may be secondary to osteomyelitis of the cranial bones. The frontal and mastoid air sinuses not infrequently give origin to an epidural abscess over their deep walls, but infection of the other air sinuses is more likely to burst through the dura mater into the subdural or subarachnoid space. The reason for this is not clear, but may simply be that the dura is more easily detached from the bone in the frontal and mastoid situations.

Within the spinal canal epidural infections are usually secondary to osteomyelitis of the laminae or bodies of the vertebrae, and are most often caused by *Staphylococcus aureus*. The less acute staphylococcal infections in this situation may be granulomas rather than abscesses, containing at most only small pockets of pus in inflammatory fibroblastic or fibrous tissue. They are most frequently found in the thoracic region and may extend over several segments of the cord. The focus of osteomyelitis which gave rise to the epidural infection may be small and difficult to find. Sometimes the pus tracks downwards in the epidural space so that the largest collection lies within the lumbar theca, whence it may be drained by lumbar puncture. Infection of the vertebrae with *Salmonella typhi* may also produce an epidural abscess or granuloma. The resistance of the dura mater to infection in these cases, as well as in epidural abscesses within the cranium, is demonstrated by the commonly favourable results of surgical procedures which expose the

dura mater. In occasional cases there may be a wide spread of infection within the layers of the dura mater. A case of chronic infection in the sacral region spreading in this way to the posterior cranial fossa, and revealing itself first by signs of damage to the lower cranial nerves, was an unusual instance. In this case the dura mater throughout its intraspinal portion was greatly thickened and inflamed and contained numerous small staphylococcal abscesses.

Infections of the pleural cavities or in the sub-diaphragmatic and perirenal tissues may extend through the intervertebral foramina into the spinal epidural space. Infection in the reverse direction, from the epidural space to the thoracic or abdominal cavities, is rare.

Epidural granulomas due to *tuberculosis* and *syphilis* will be discussed under those headings.

Subdural infections

Infection of the subdural space is commonly widespread (subdural empyema) and usually secondary to infections of the paranasal air sinuses (Fig. 6.1a). Sometimes the infection may reach the subdural space by way of veins, for the anterior end of the sagittal sinus is often thrombosed when the source is the frontal sinus, as are the circular or petrosal sinuses in the case of the sphenoidal air sinus. Subdural abscesses resulting from sphenoidal sinusitis may in this way involve both middle fossae. Infection of the subdural space is also a common result of osteomyelitis of the cranial bones. All subdural infections are liable to spread widely and to cause phlebitis of veins at some distance from the original focus of infection. Pus often collects in unsuspected pockets, or in situations which are difficult to drain, especially alongside the falx or on the upper surface of the tentorium. As the dura is a poorly vascularized structure, antibiotics have little access to the subdural space unless placed directly in it; in consequence, subdural infections continue to have a high mortality (Bhandari and Sarkari 1970). The most common causative organisms here also are *staphylococci* and *streptococci*.

Pathological changes

The absence of any endothelial lining and the vascular character of its innermost layer make the dura mater the protagonist in the reactions to subdural infection. In the less acute infections

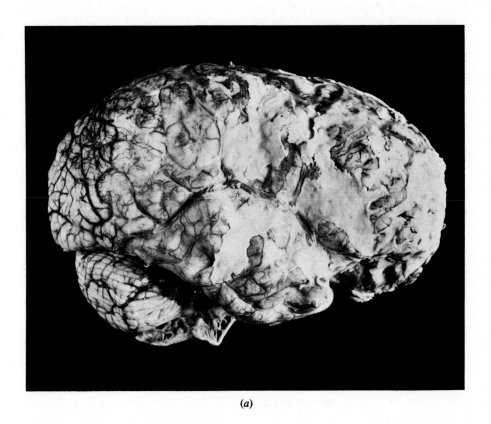

(*a*)

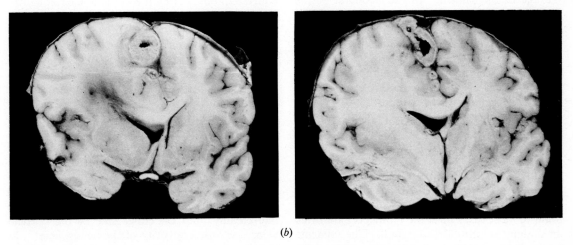

(*b*)

Fig. 6.1 Subdural empyema. (*a*) The pus is clearly on the surface of the arachnoid and not within it. (*b*) Loculated collections of pus in the subdural space have led to the formation of multiple abscesses.

it rapidly forms an inflammatory granulation tissue by which the infection may become loculated. As this tissue becomes adherent to the underlying arachnoid the latter becomes involved in the inflammatory tissue and localized abscesses may thus be formed (Fig. 6.1*b*). More frequently pus extends widely and can usually be wiped off the arachnoid, leaving a smooth glistening surface. In treated cases which recover at this stage the subdural space remains patent, and at necropsy the dura mater shows few residua except fibrous thickening of its inner layer.

Leptomeningitis

The leptomeninges offer comparatively little resistance to infection, although the pia mater contains a vascular bed from which polymorphonuclear leucocytes can migrate freely. In fact, the cerebrospinal fluid provides a good culture medium for many organisms. When virulent microorganisms invade the subarachnoid space they often cause death within a few hours, and many kinds of microorganisms, which have a low pathogenicity for other tissues, may produce serious or even fatal meningitis. Even an organism such as *Brevibacterium fermentans*, generally considered non-pathogenic, may be introduced at operation and be responsible for prolonged postoperative fever (Fleurette, Moulin, Mounet and Lapras 1969).

To some extent the microorganism varies with the age of the patient. In the neonatal period Gram-negative organisms are commonly found (*E. coli*), whereas in children respiratory tract organisms such as *H. influenzae* are predominant (de Kalbermatten and Piolino 1969). In adolescence and adulthood the meningococcus and pneumococcus are more frequently encountered. Meningococcal meningitis is almost always blood-borne, and is still the most frequent form of meningitis, although decreasing (Jensen, Ranek and Rosdahl 1967). It follows a stage of bacteraemia during which, in severe infections, macular rashes may appear, giving rise to the old name *spotted fever*. It seems probable that the choroid plexus is the site of invasion of the brain in most cases since the diplococci are often most abundant in ventricular fluid. The subacute form of the disease, in which meningeal inflammation is almost confined to the neighbourhood of the cisterna magna, is most easily explained on this theory. It may be assumed that in these

cases the meningococcus is of low virulence or the child's resistance high, so that although capable of survival in the ventricles the diplococci are quickly destroyed when they reach the more vascular meninges. The pneumococcus may reach the meninges from an infected middle ear or from a pulmonary infection. Rarer causes of meningitis are *B. anthracis*, *Brucella abortus*, *Salmonellae* (Beine, Hansen and Fulton 1951), and *Listeria monocytogenes* (Gray and Killinger 1966). The last-named causes a meningitis or meningo-encephalitis usually in neonates or in adults over 40, and because of difficulties in its isolation and culture may in fact be responsible for more cases than is at present apparent. The organism may be found in many domestic and wild animals.

Macroscopic appearances

In a typical case of pyogenic meningitis of a few days' duration the appearance of the brain and spinal cord is quite characteristic. The cisterns at the base of the brain are filled with creamy pus which covers the blood vessels and appears to stretch the arachnoid membrane which covers them but there is little if any pus on the surface of this membrane. On the convexity of the hemispheres the pus may be confined to the fissures and their lips, exposing the convolutions. In some cases, however, these also are covered, sometimes more over one hemisphere than the other. Where exposed the cortex may appear congested, but is often less so than in encephalitis. Pus may be found in the ventricles in flakes mixed with cerebrospinal fluid or lying on the ventricular walls. The choroid plexus may be covered by a more firmly attached layer of pus. The spinal cord is similarly covered by subarachnoid pus especially on its dorsal surface. In more acute cases the quantity of pus is less and the congestion of the meninges greater. Purulent infiltration is often most obvious in the cisterna basalis and over the dorsal surface of the spinal cord. In very acute cases purulent infiltration of the meninges may be much less obvious. The pia arachnoid covering the base of the brain appears congested and cloudy and there may be fine creamy lines on either side of the cortical veins, over the convexity of the hemispheres. In some such cases the diagnosis of meningitis can be confirmed only by histological examination. On section the brain appears soft, the cortical congestion may be more obvious and the white matter is often oedematous. Small cortical infarcts may be seen in the cerebrum and cerebellum. In cases of longer standing some dilatation of the ventricles with softening of the subependymal tissues may be present. In many cases of *meningococcal meningitis* petechial haemorrhages in the white or grey matter, focal softenings or even small abscesses caused by septic embolism of the smaller vessels, may be seen. In infections due to *B. anthracis* the haemorrhagic nature of the exudate and the rapidly fatal course may suggest a spontaneous subarachnoid haemorrhage. In *pneumococcal meningitis* cerebral arteritis and phlebitis have been described (Cairns and Russell 1946) and may explain the infarction that occasionally occurs in this and other forms of purulent meningitis. The hypersensitivity reaction responsible has been attributed to the use of antibiotics or sulphonamides, but vasculitis has occurred in untreated patients, and a reaction to the organism or its products is a more likely explanation.

Histological characteristics

These are similar to those of pyogenic inflammation in other body cavities. Large numbers of polymorphonuclear leucocytes, with an admixture of plasma cells, lymphocytes and macrophages, lie between the outer layer of the arachnoid and the pia mater. The causative bacteria may be seen in or among the pus cells. The meningeal vessels are dilated and there is a varying amount of fibrinous exudate. In some cases the inflammation spreads into the walls of the smaller meningeal vessels causing thrombosis, but this is more often seen in tuberculous meningitis. There may be some infiltration along the Virchow–Robin spaces of the cortical veins, and some microglial reaction in the outer cortical layers. Otherwise there is little evidence of inflammatory reaction in the nervous parenchyma. In the walls of the ventricles some stripping of ependymal cells and infiltration of the subependymal veins may be seen. During the later stages mononuclear cells, some of which are phagocytic, appear in greater number. Some of these may be derived from the histiocytes of the meninges, and others from the blood stream.

In more chronic infections, especially in subacute cases of meningococcal meningitis in which diagnosis is retarded or treatment inadequate, there is proliferation of fibroblasts and eventually of collagen fibres in the meninges. This may lead to loculation of cerebrospinal fluid and so produce well-recognized sequelae. (1) When the meningeal thickening takes place round the basal cisterns it may prevent the free flow of cerebrospinal fluid in an upward and downward direction. Hydrocephalus in such cases may result either because the cerebrospinal fluid cannot escape from the cisterna magna, in which case it is *noncommunicating*, or because it is prevented by adhesions and meningeal thickening around the ventral aspect of the pons and midbrain from passing upwards into the middle cranial fossa. This is a common cause of acquired *communicating hydrocephalus* in childhood. (2) Loculation of fluid in pockets of the thickened meninges around the spinal cord may cause paraplegia by pressure. In some epidemics of meningococcal meningitis this sequela has not been uncommon, especially when intrathecal antiserum was the only treatment. In cases treated by antibiotics it is probably rarer, especially when frequent lumbar punctures are performed, but it may still occur. It may also be seen in infections by staphylococci and other pyogenic organisms. Some of the cases of progressive spinal arachnoiditis which occur as sequelae of spinal anaesthesia may be due to infections by microorganisms of low virulence. In other cases, however, the normal condition of the cerebrospinal fluid during the early period after the anaesthetic excludes bacterial infection. Irritation of the meninges by a chemical contaminant is the most probable cause of this condition (see p. 113). The leptomeninges may be very sensitive to chemical irritants and, unless these are quickiy eliminated, progressive thickening and adhesions of the pia arachnoid may cause symptoms of paraplegia or hydrocephalus after an interval of several months.

Encysted loculations of fluid, either in the spinal canal or over the base of the brain, have for long been recognized as a cause of paraplegia, hydrocephalus, vertiginous attacks or symptoms due to pressure on the oculomotor or optic nerves and chiasma. The cause of most cases is unknown. Syphilis used to be blamed for many, but at the present time only a small proportion can be attributed to this cause, and the majority appear to be due to minor meningeal infections. Some seem to be related to trauma. Elkington (1936), in 41 cases of spinal arachnoiditis, obtained a history of spinal injury in 9, of syphilis in 4, of gonorrhoea in 4 and of other systemic infections in 6. In 18 no cause could be ascertained. A rare situation of such encysted collections of cerebrospinal fluid is over the surface of the hemispheres where they cause symptoms of intracranial pressure. In two cases of this kind a rounded depression, filled with clear fluid and 5 to 6 cm in width, was found on the surface of the parietal lobe. This appeared to be the only cause of the symptoms of intracranial pressure which led to death. These examples of cystic arachnoiditis have to be distinguished from true arachnoid cysts, some of which are lined by a simple epithelium and are thought to be derived from ectopic glial tissue nests containing ependymal clefts (Jabukiac, Dunsmore and Beckett 1968).

Other rarer sequelae of meningitis include diffuse necrosis of the subcortical white matter (Buchan and Alvord 1969), resulting from venous sinus occlusion. Meningococcal septicaemia may be associated with intravascular coagulation (McGehee, Rapaport and Hjort 1967), and in fatal meningococcal infection myocarditis, formerly thought to be rare, is now common (Hardman and Earle 1969).

Cerebral abscess

Aetiology and pathogenesis

Pyogenic microorganisms may gain access to the tissues of the brain, as to the meninges, either from the blood stream, from foci of infection in overlying tissues, or from wounds which communicate either directly or indirectly with the outside air. Before antibiotics came into general use the great majority of cerebral abscesses were due to infections of the middle ear and paranasal and aural air sinuses, and these are still common routes of infection. In fact, the advent of the antibiotic era has made little difference to the incidence of brain abscess according to Liske and Weikers (1964), who found it to be the same as prior to antibiotics. The source of the abscess in the series of 47 cases reported by Kerr, King and Meagher (1958) was identified with certainty in 72%, with suspicion in a further 17%. In the remainder nothing could be found to indicate a primary site. The middle ear was responsible for 10; the paranasal sinuses for 10; trauma for 6; blood spread from lungs, 7; teeth, 3; osteomyelitis, 1; septic abortion, 1; ? tonsils, 1; upper respiratory tract, 1. Two patients had meningitis but it was not clear whether this was cause or result. Brain abscess may still carry a high mortality,

depending on the organism. Liske and Weikers mention 13 deaths in 17 brain abscesses caused by beta-haemolytic streptococci, and 50% mortality when staphylococci or 'Gram-negative rods' were found. Infection of the middle ear may spread through the tegmen tympani to cause a temporal abscess, or via the mastoid air sinuses, especially in children in whom the bone is thinner, to produce an abscess in the cerebellar hemisphere. Disease of the frontal, ethmoidal or sphenoidal air sinuses or fractures of the roof of the nasopharynx, especially the cribriform plate of the ethmoid, may cause abscesses in the frontal lobe. As with meningitis, the causative organism varies greatly.

Abscesses arising from blood-borne infection may occur anywhere in the brain but especially at the junction of the grey and white matter. They are commonly but not always multiple. In most cases they are secondary to chronic septic diseases of the respiratory tract such as bronchiectasis, but sometimes the focus of infection is less obvious or more recent (Fig. 6.2). Metastatic staphylococcal cerebral abscesses may occur also after osteomyelitis or other severe staphylococcal infections, or without evidence of previous infection. They are less commonly multiple than those secondary to disease of the respiratory tract.

Solitary abscesses due to various organisms are sometimes found in the parietal lobe. They form an uncommon and mysterious group, for no source, local or metastatic, can usually be found. Predisposition to cerebral abscess occurs in cyanotic congenital heart disease, and here again the source is often unidentified (Newton 1956). Cerebrovascular thrombosis is twice as common as abscess in these patients (Abbott and Stern 1969) but the reason for the increased susceptibility of cyanotic cerebral tissue to abscess formation is not known.

At present *chronic granulomatous disease* is a rare cause of recurrent infections including cerebral abscess in children, mainly males (Blattner 1969). This familial condition predisposes to infection by certain organisms only, including staphylococci, and is due to a deficiency of nicotinamide adenine dinucleotide (NADH) in leucocytes which renders them unable to digest the organisms. There is an associated hypergammaglobulinaemia.

Abscesses form much more commonly in the white than the grey matter of the brain. Even when infection has to pass through the cerebral

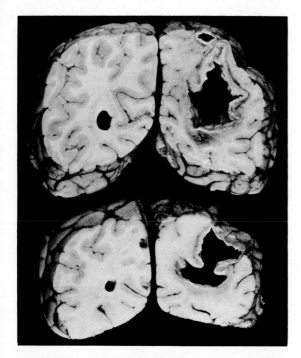

Fig. 6.2 Capsulated abscess in the right parieto-occipital region, secondary to bronchiectasis.

cortex the main bulk of the abscess is deep to this and the channel leading to it through the cortex may be very narrow and difficult to find. The reason for this choice of situation may be that the white matter has a poorer vascular supply than the grey. This not only restricts the migration of phagocytes from the blood stream but also delays the encapsulation of a focus of infection by fibrous tissue, since in the brain fibroblasts can only be formed from the meninges or the walls of the blood vessels. The delay in capsule formation and the softening of brain tissue which occurs round an abscess often allow the infection to spread more deeply into the white matter and to produce secondary abscesses, which are connected to the primary abscess either by a narrow channel or by an area of inflamed and softened brain tissue. Occasionally a chain of such abscesses may be found. This tendency to spread inwards makes rupture into the ventricles one of the chief dangers in cerebral abscesses.-

It is not uncommon to find a firmer capsule around the primary than around the secondary abscesses, or the capsule may be better formed on

the superficial than on the deep side of the abscess. Thorotrast, which was often injected into the abscess cavity to make its position and size visible to X-rays, appeared also to have a value in encouraging encapsulation. The walls of an abscess treated in this manner often show a zone, several millimetres thick, of concentric layers of collagen fibres between which are innumerable phagocytes filled with thorotrast. This substance has now been replaced by an iodinated radio-opaque compound which is also ingested by phagocytes but whose fibrosing effect is not established.

The earliest stage of an abscess is an area of septic encephalitis, that is of softening and congestion of brain tissue, often with numerous petechial haemorrhages. The centre of this area becomes deliquescent and an abscess cavity is thus formed. Its wall is at first poorly defined and may be quite irregular in outline. Gradually a firmer wall appears, sometimes more at one side than the other, and as this grows thicker and more complete the abscess becomes encapsulated. Chronic abscesses, especially those of staphylococcal origin, may be surrounded by a firm concentric capsule of fibrous tissue from 1 to 3 mm or more in thickness. The rate of development of the capsule is variable but as a rough guide it may be taken as 1 mm per month in the earlier stages.

The white matter in the zone surrounding an abscess is usually softened and oedematous so that the capsule may strip from it very easily. Sometimes a firmly encapsulated abscess may appear at necropsy as if lying loose in a cavity in the brain tissue. The oedema around an abscess is often very severe and extensive so that, on section of the brain, the white matter is seen to be swollen and often has a yellow or greenish discoloration.

Microscopically the appearances of the wall of a cerebral abscess vary greatly. In the most acute abscesses there is an inner layer of pus, usually with a narrow irregular layer of inflammatory granulation tissue external to it. But in some abscesses, and around some part of the wall in many, this layer may be scarcely recognizable. The brain tissue is infiltrated with polymorphonuclear leucocytes and plasma cells near the abscess and with lymphocytes in the more peripheral zones, and there is usually heavy lymphocytic cuffing of the veins both in the neighbourhood and extending some distance from the abscess. The oedema of the white matter appears as a loosening of texture with pools of faintly eosinophilic plasma in some places and swelling of the cell bodies of the astrocytes. Those in the zone nearest to the abscess may have undergone clasmatodendrosis. Along with this there is pallor in the staining of myelin around the abscess.

In more chronic abscesses the layer of granulation tissue is more definite and passes gradually into a collagenous capsule which varies considerably in thickness and density over different parts of the abscess. This has a fairly well defined outer border, but fibroblasts and reticulin fibres may be seen intertwined with neuroglial fibres in the zone outside it. In such cases there is often considerable swelling of the cell bodies of astrocytes, which may assume large spider forms and often have more than one nucleus. Perivascular cuffing with lymphocytes may still be seen in the zone around the abscess in spite of good encapsulation.

The chief differences between abscesses in the brain and those in other parts of the body are thus seen to be due (1) to the paucity of fibrous tissue and the consequent tardiness of fibroblastic activity in the encapsulation of the abscess; and (2) to the very vulnerable nature of the nervous parenchyma. The neuroglial reaction is slow and has little value in the encapsulation of the abscess; in fact the astrocytes are easily destroyed by infection and in the early stages show more degenerative than proliferative change.

Septic embolism

In cases of malignant endocarditis multiple septic emboli may lodge in the small cerebral arteries. These may cause mycotic aneurysms (see p. 139) which may enlarge and burst, or multiple small infarcts. It may be difficult to distinguish these from aseptic emboli since neutrophil leucocytes can be seen round both. But septic emboli are more often multiple, they are more heavily infiltrated with neutrophil leucocytes, and streptococci can usually be found in them.

Cerebrospinal fluid

In bacterial infections of the brain or its coverings the constancy and severity of inflammatory changes in the cerebrospinal fluid vary with the site of the infection. When the subarachnoid space is involved evidences of inflammation, in cell count and protein, are always found, as also in many cases of subdural infection. In cases of cerebral or subdural abscess they are more variable and when infection is confined to the cranial epidural space the fluid is usually normal.

Spinal epidural infections, when granulomatous or localized, usually produce the compression syndrome of raised protein with or without xanthochromia (Froin–Nonne syndrome) and some degree of spinal block. More purulent collections may gravitate to the lumbar theca where they may be tapped by lumbar puncture. The pus in such cases is not under pressure and may have to be aspirated; this and its creamy consistency distinguish it from purulent cerebrospinal fluid. Rarely a mixture of epidural pus and normal cerebrospinal fluid is obtained on lumbar puncture. This can be distinguished from the fluid of purulent leptomeningitis by the fact that it contains normal percentages of glucose and chlorides, although pus cells and staphylococci are present in the deposit.

In *purulent meningitis* the most important characteristics of the fluid, apart from the pressure, are (1) its tendency to form a fibrinous or stringy coagulum, (2) the diminution or absence of glucose and (3) the presence of visible bacteria in the deposit. The cell excess may be of any degree and the more purulent fluids contain several thousand cells per mm³. But in late cases and in some subacute cases the cell count may be comparatively low and may contain a varying proportion of lymphocytes and large mononuclear cells, including plasma cells. The protein rises in proportion to the cell count. Glucose always falls rapidly and often disappears from the fluid. The chlorides also often fall to 650 mg per 100 ml or below. The causative organism can usually be seen in films of the centrifuged deposit either extra- or intracellularly and can be grown on culture. In meningococcal meningitis when diplococci are scanty and, as is usual, intracellular, they are best demonstrated by counterstaining after Gram's method with Pappenheim's methyl green pyronin, which stains the cocci a brilliant red against the green (or purple) of the nucleus. The reason for the sharp fall in cerebrospinal fluid glucose in bacterial meningitis is not entirely clear. In their paper on experimental pneumococcal meningitis in dogs Prockup and Fishman (1968) discuss this point in detail, including the effect of infection on the blood–cerebrospinal fluid barrier. The traditional view is that the fall in glucose value is due to glycolysis by polymorphs in the presence of bacteria, but additional factors have been suggested such as an alteration in the membrane transfer of glucose from the blood.

In *cerebral abscess* the changes in the fluid vary with the location of the abscess. In general it is not possible to culture organisms from the cerebrospinal fluid, which shows either: (1) a white cell count of less than 50 per mm³ with 25% or more of neutrophil leucocytes along with a rise in protein to the neighbourhood of 100 mg per 100 ml, absence of a coagulum and normal glucose and chlorides; or (2) a purulent fluid which does not form the stringy coagulum of meningitis, which contains over 30 mg glucose per 100 ml and in which no bacteria can be seen in the deposit. Purulent fluids of this kind are not uncommon when the abscess is near the meningeal or ventricular surface and are sometimes responsible for an erroneous diagnosis of generalized meningitis. But all variations between these types of fluid, or more normal fluids, may be found. Since neutrophil leucocytes may also be found in the fluid from cases of cerebral glioma or embolism, they do not of themselves indicate infection. The formation of a fibrin coagulum is rare, whereas it is the rule in generalized meningitis. The chlorides are usually normal but may fall temporarily when the blood chlorides are lowered by vomiting or other cause. The glucose is little reduced and a fall below 25 mg per 100 ml, or disappearance, is usually evidence of spread of infection to the leptomeninges and generalized meningitis.

Tuberculous infection

The acid-fast *Mycobacterium tuberculosis* of human, bovine or, rarely, avian type may affect the epidural space, leptomeninges or substance of the brain. Nervous system involvement is, however, never primary, and must always follow a lesion formed via the usual portals of entry, the respiratory and alimentary tracts. The primary infection is often unnoticed and secondary spread to the nervous system may occur after many years, with or without involvement of other organs; or the primary infection may be fulminant with rapid spread to the brain. The incidence and severity of all forms of tuberculosis have been reduced by improved standards of living, by vaccination and by modern therapy, although resistant strains are occasionally encountered. In this country not only the incidence but the presenting features of tuberculosis have changed in recent years, partly due to the development of primary lesions in adults, and partly to immigration from countries where the disease often presents in unfamiliar ways (Kocen and Parsons 1970).

Epidural infection

Tuberculous disease of the vertebral bodies or spinal caries (Pott's paraplegia) will be considered later (Chapter 15) as a cause of spinal compression. It is very frequently associated with an epidural tuberculous granuloma. In the majority of cases this does not spread more deeply, but in rare cases it may give rise to tuberculous meningitis. In the cranial cavity epidural tuberculosis is very rare except when related to otitis media.

Subdural tuberculous infection

This occurs during the somewhat rare passage of an infection through the dura mater towards the subarachnoid space. Miliary tubercles are also frequently found on the inside of the dural covering of the floor of the cranium in cases of tuberculous meningitis. They may assist in the macroscopical diagnosis of this form of meningitis. More widespread granulomas attached to the inner surface of the dura mater, usually with some spread to the leptomeninges and sometimes to the cerebral cortex, have been described. Pardee and Knox (1927) in reporting a case of this kind used the term *tuberculoma en plaque*. These granulomas form fairly large flattened, sometimes nodular, masses, adherent to the dura externally and in varying degree to the leptomeninges and the cerebral cortex internally. Their outer margin can often be lifted free from the surface of the brain when their central area is more adherent. In some cases their relation to the cerebral sulci suggests a subarachnoid spread.

Meningeal tuberculoma and tuberculous leptomeningitis

Isolated tuberculomas of varying size are occasionally found in the leptomeninges, and may give rise to generalized meningitis. Single tuberculomas on the surface of the brain may originate either in the leptomeninges or in the cerebral cortex and may form rounded or oval masses up to 7 or 8 cm in diameter. They compress and destroy the underlying brain tissue and, except for their attachment to the leptomeninges, do not differ from tuberculomas found more deeply within the brain. Multiple isolated meningeal tuberculomas, a few millimetres in diameter, are not very rare as necropsy findings in patients who die of tuberculosis without showing clinical evidence of intracranial disease. They may lie in the fissures of the brain or along the line of the larger vessels. In most cases they are associated with tuberculomas of similar size within the brain tissue.

Generalized tuberculous meningitis

This common form of meningitis used almost always to be fatal before antibiotic and chemotherapy was discovered. It occurs in young children, especially between the ages of 6 months and five years, but no age is exempt and in recent years it has become a greater problem in the elderly; it may also occur in patients under treatment by steroids. It is always secondary to disease elsewhere in the body, but in some cases the primary focus may be small and difficult to find, for example a small Ghon's focus in one lung, or infection of a cervical or mediastinal lymph node. In children it is most often part of a generalized miliary tuberculosis; in the large series collected by Blacklock and Griffin (1935) 68% of all cases of meningitis were associated with a miliary spread of disease in the organs of the body and in 81% of all cases of miliary tuberculosis there was also meningitis. In a smaller series with a more varied age incidence, Rich and McCordock (1933) found miliary tuberculosis in 78%. In adults the association with miliary tuberculosis is rather less common. The primary focus is usually in the lung (Blacklock and Griffin, 74%), but cases of abdominal or genito-urinary infection or of tuberculosis apparently limited to lymph nodes or bones and joints may end with meningitis.

The majority of cases of tuberculous meningitis are caused by human *M. tuberculosis*, and although this is usually antibiotic-sensitive a drug-resistant strain has recently been isolated from an affected patient (Bonforte, Karpas and Gribetz 1968). In England a few cases are still caused by the bovine type.

Various theories of *pathogenesis* have been put forward.

(1) A direct spread to the meninges would appear to be the most obvious cause when their infection is part of a generalized miliary tuberculosis. But Rich and McCordock (1929, 1933) showed that in animals the injection of tubercle bacilli directly into the carotid artery does not cause primary tuberculous meningitis, although it produces miliary tubercle nodules in the brain, meninges and elsewhere in the body. On the other hand, an injection of bacilli directly into the subarachnoid space constantly produces generalized meningitis. They therefore postulated that in the majority of cases meningitis was secondary to a small focus in the cortex or leptomeninges, and they found evidence for this theory in 90% of their cases. Others have been unable to find foci of this kind in so large a percentage of cases. Beres and Metzler (1938) in 28 cases of tuberculous meningitis found no intracerebral foci in 14 and none in contact with the surface in 3 others. In cases of tuberculous meningitis which have been treated with streptomycin and relapsed or died of hydrocephalus some months later, caseous tuberculous nodules are commonly found among the exudate either over the base of the brain or in the depths of the sulci on the convexity of the hemispheres, but such tuberculomas have probably developed during the course of the clinical disease.

(2) A primary focus in the choroid plexus with secondary spread to the walls of the ventricles and subarachnoid space has been postulated. In fact, the choroid plexus is frequently involved but usually with miliary tubercles which might be no older than the disease in the subarachnoid space.

The macroscopical appearance of the brain of a case of tuberculous meningitis is usually typical (Fig. 6.3a). There is a diffuse grey-green opacity of the meninges over the convexity of the hemispheres, and a green gelatinous exudate fills the basal cistern and spreads out from this into the neighbouring parts of the subarachnoid space, covering the front of the pons. The membranes over the cisterna magna are also infiltrated and the dorsal surface of the spinal cord is covered by a gelatinous exudate which is often especially thick in the cervical region. In this exudate individual tubercle nodules may not easily be seen. They are most common in the lips of the Sylvian fissures and near the pre- and postcentral veins over the convexity of the hemispheres. They are also common on the inner surface of the dura mater covering the basisphenoid, or other part of the floor of the skull, and these may show the nature of the infection in cases in which the

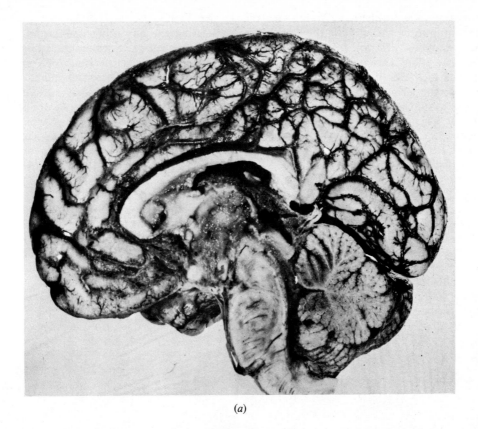

(a)

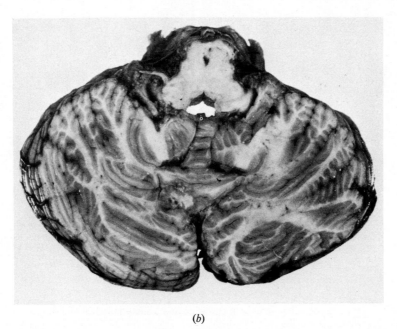

(b)

Fig. 6.3 Tuberculous meningitis. (a) view of the mesial surface of the brain. The cisterna basalis is filled with exudate and glistening tubercles are seen on the walls of the dilated ventricle and septum pellucidum. (b) Rich's focus.

exudate looks more purulent. The amount of meningeal infiltration varies with the length of history of meningitis. In rare early cases it may be limited to a small area of the surface of the brain, sparing the base. In such cases it usually lies in the neighbourhood of a tuberculoma of the brain or meninges. On section of the brain the tissue is usually soft, especially that surrounding the lateral ventricles which are somewhat dilated.

Microscopically in cases which have lasted for a few weeks the meningeal exudate consists of lymphocytes, plasma cells and epithelioid cells lying in a matrix of degenerated and partly caseated fibrin. Giant-celled tuberculous nodules may be seen in this exudate, but are often scanty and may be absent. The degree of cellular exudate and of caseation varies from case to case. It is often concentrated around the meningeal vessels. *M. tuberculosis* may be abundant or scanty. In the latter case they are most often found in the tuberculous nodules.

The meningeal arteries show inflammatory changes in the adventitia and media, and often also in the intima, or subintimal fibrous hyperplasia may occur as in Heubner's arteritis (see p. 258) (Fig. 6.4). These inflammatory changes both in arteries and veins may go on to fibrinoid necrosis or complete caseation. The resulting thrombosis leads to infarctions which may be superficial, but often involve the basal ganglia when the perforating vessels are involved. They are most often seen at the base of the brain and the lips of the Sylvian fissures (Smith and Daniel 1947; Dastur and Udani 1966). Elsewhere the outer layers of the cerebral cortex and some of the superficial folia of the cerebellum show microglial reaction, and there is usually some lymphocytic infiltration of the entering veins. Small tuberculous nodules are not uncommonly seen in relation to these, but widespread involvement of the cortex is rare.

In streptomycin-treated cases, dying more than 10 weeks after the onset of the illness, the exudate

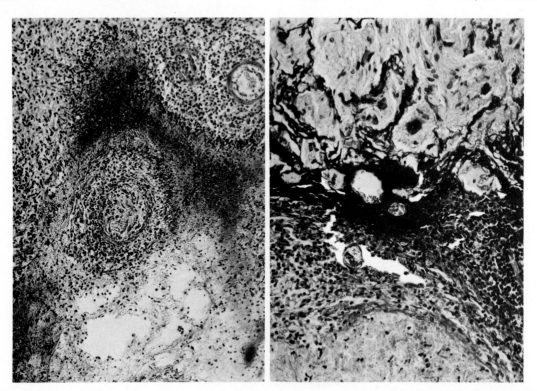

Fig. 6.4 Tuberculous meningitis, showing an area of caseation and a small inflamed and thrombosed meningeal artery. Note the absence of Langhans giant cells.

Fig. 6.5 Margin of a cerebellar tuberculoma. Zones of lymphocytic infiltration, collagenous fibrous tissue and neuroglial reaction with large irregular glial cells are seen round the caseated central mass (bottom of the photograph).

is more fibrous and may be of woody hardness (Daniel 1949). It is especially thick round the base of the brain and the cisterna ambiens, where it obstructs the circulation of cerebrospinal fluid and thus often leads to hydrocephalus. Occasionally tuberculous meningitis predominates around the spinal cord with compression of roots and cord by a thick exudate (Dastur and Wadia 1969).

Cerebrospinal fluid. The importance of early diagnosis of cases of tuberculous meningitis has been greatly increased since the advent of drug therapy. The typical cerebrospinal fluid in tuberculous meningitis is under increased pressure, often over 300 mm. It is clear or very slightly opalescent, and on standing forms a fine cobweb coagulum. The cell count is usually between 50 and 200 cells per mm³ and consists chiefly of lymphocytes with plasma cells and other large mononuclear cells; neutrophil leucocytes may also be present in considerable numbers. The total protein is only moderately increased in the early stages, but as the disease progresses it often exceeds 200 mg per 100 ml. The glucose almost always falls to 20 or 30 mg or lower but is rarely completely absent. The chlorides fall progressively and often very considerably so that levels below 600 mg of NaCl are not uncommon. But in the early stages they may be in the region of 700 mg. They are therefore less reliable than the level of glucose. *M. tuberculosis* may be found either in the spread out coagulum or in slides made by scraping and drawing up the centrifuged deposit with a Pasteur pipette. The percentage of cases in which tubercle bacilli can be found varies with the technique and with care may exceed 90%. Guinea pig injection and culture of the deposit are even more reliable.

The chief diseases which may cause difficulty in differential diagnosis are various forms of meningo-encephalitis due to viruses, including poliomyelitis, cerebral abscess and subacute meningitis due to organisms other than *M. tuberculosis* (e.g. cryptococci). Virus meningitis and cerebral abscess are most easily distinguished by the normal level of glucose and usually of chlorides in these conditions, as also by the absence of the typical cobweb coagulum, although this may form rarely in cases of poliomyelitis and other virus conditions. The nature of the cell count and the presence of organisms are the most valuable criteria in distinguishing tuberculous from other forms of ingravescent meningitis. But

these very seldom come into question on clinical grounds.

Some children who show all the signs of an incipient meningitis, and in whom tuberculous meningitis is suspected, have a normal cerebrospinal fluid apart from a raised cell count up to 300 per mm³. Although tubercle bacilli have never been shown in the cerebrospinal fluid these patients are sometimes later found to have a tuberculoma. The condition has been referred to as *serous tuberculous meningitis*, and carries a good prognosis (Lincoln and Sewell 1963).

Tuberculomas of the brain and spinal cord

Tuberculous granulomas used to be a very common form of intracranial tumour and remain far from rare in areas where tuberculosis is still rife (Dastur and Desai 1965). Cerebellar tuberculomas used to be the most frequent form of intracranial growth in children and the cerebellum is still the commonest site. Supratentorial tuberculomas often cease to enlarge after a time and may become calcified in their outer parts, but cerebellar masses probably less often become quiescent. It is rather more common to find multiple than single intracerebral tuberculomas. They may form rounded or oval masses or may have a more lobular shape from the fusion of several smaller nodules. On section the centre is necrotic but firm and of a creamy colour. The capsule, which may be from 1 to 3 mm in thickness, is grey, gelatinous and rather tough, and a narrow zone of greyish gliotic tissue is present around it; there is much less softening in this zone than in cerebral abscesses. A tuberculoma can often be separated almost cleanly from the brain tissue at operation, but before streptomycin was used this procedure was almost always followed by tuberculous meningitis in cerebellar cases and very frequently also in supratentorial cases.

Microscopically the capsule of an intracerebral tuberculoma contains varying proportions of collagenous tissue and of giant-celled tubercle nodules. The capsule may vary considerably in thickness round different parts of the mass. Its contents have the usual necrotic appearance of caseous material, and external to it there is a zone of gliosis in which large spider-like astrocytes with thick processes are often found (Fig. 6.5). There is a varying amount of lymphocytic infiltration of the vessel walls in the neighbourhood. In old-standing cases the capsule becomes more collagenous and loses more or less completely its giant-celled nodules and other inflammatory infiltrations. At this stage calcospherites may be present in large numbers, especially in the outer parts of the necrotic centre, and bone may be formed in occasional cases.

Tuberculous abscess

True abscesses of the brain as opposed to tuberculomata have been described but are very rare (Rand 1935). The tubercle bacilli proliferate in large numbers and pus is formed; eventually a capsule develops exactly similar to that produced by pyogenic organisms, but without any sign of systematized follicles. A solitary abscess has been described (Bannister 1970), but others have been multiple (Rand). It is doubtful whether the three tuberculous abscesses 'with or without definite tuberculomas' mentioned by Sinh, Pandya and Dastur (1968) belong to the same category, as they may have been examples of liquefaction of caseous tissue. The absence of the usual granulomatous reaction to the tubercle bacilli suggests a failure of an immune mechanism; complete failure of any cellular reaction has also been noted in tuberculous infections not necessarily overwhelming but with abnormal blood pictures (O'Brien 1954).

Sarcoidosis
(*Schaumann's disease*)

Sarcoidosis has been recognized for many years as the most usual cause of the syndrome of uveoparotitis. In these cases the facial nerve is often involved in its course in or near the parotid gland. More recently a considerable number of cases have been reported in which sarcoidosis has affected the meninges, brain or spinal cord. Some of these cases have been associated with the syndrome of uveoparotitis, others with a spread of the disease to lungs, spleen or bones, but in a few there has been no evident disease outside the cranial cavity. The diagnosis rests on clinical evidence, for example diabetes insipidus or papilloedema complicating the uveoparotid syndrome, and on investigations such as the serum calcium level, the Kveim and Mantoux reactions or lymph node biopsy (Silverstein, Feuer and Siltzbach 1965). The disease is frequently self-limited, but autopsy reports are now available (Ross 1955; Herring and Urich 1969). In the majority of these cases the disease has been localized in one of two situations: (1) the leptomeninges, most often round the base of the brain and in the posterior fossa; (2) the infundibulum and the floor and anterior part of the walls of the third ventricle (Fig. 6.6a). The optic nerves and chiasma may also be invaded in these cases. The Virchow–Robin spaces of the vessels in the basal ganglia and pons may be distended with granuloma, with little invasion of the meninges, or there may be a similar perivascular invasion of the cerebral and cerebellar cortex with lesions in the overlying meninges. Aszkanazy (1952)

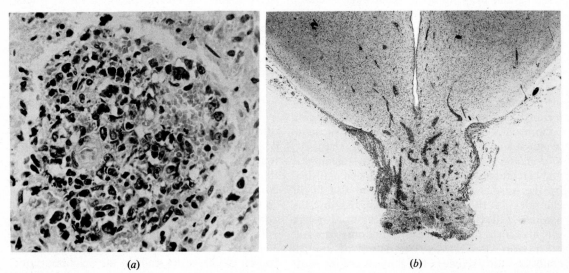

(a)   (b)

Fig. 6.6 Sarcoidosis. (a) Infiltration of the basal meninges and infundibular region. (b) Mainly perivascular infiltration of the hypothalamus.

reported a case in which the spinal cord at the upper thoracic level was infiltrated by granulomatous nodules with slighter meningeal lesions. He noted that giant cells may be small and scarce in the nervous tissue and that reticulin is not so abundant as in sarcoid lesions elsewhere in the body. The lesions are always closely related to blood vessels, and even within the brain may be confined in the Virchow–Robin spaces (Fig. 6.6*b*). Granulomas in the floor of the 3rd ventricle may not be recognized as sarcoid lesions unless more typical lesions are found in other organs.

The course of the intracranial disease is usually slow and there may be clinical remissions or arrest of progress, but some cases are fatal within a few weeks. When the disease is limited to the meninges the symptoms are usually those of hydrocephalus or cranial nerve palsies; Jacksonian epilepsy due to meningeal lesions near the vertex of the brain has been reported by Aszkanazy. When the infundibulum and the floor of the 3rd ventricle are invaded there may be diabetes insipidus or other signs of damage to the hypothalamus. Direct invasion of the optic chiasma or nerves may lead to hemianopia or blindness.

Neurosyphilis

The incidence of the various types of neurosyphilis has changed since the turn of the century, and certain forms such as the cerebral gumma and tabes dorsalis have almost disappeared. This change was brought about by the introduction first of arsenical drugs, and later of penicillin. Neurosyphilis causing psychotic illness is now rare (Dewhurst 1969) and tends to cause depression, dementia and confusional states rather than the grandiose delusions of classical GPI. But neurosyphilis in general has not disappeared. Heathfield (1968) reported seeing 30 cases between 1964 and 1968, of which 10 were tabes dorsalis, 13 meningovascular syphilis, 2 cerebral 'meningosyphilis', 3 GPI, 1 syphilitic paraplegia, and 1 ?syphilitic labyrinthitis. Significantly, half were aged over 60, and six over 70.

Primary and secondary stages
It is generally agreed that the meningeal spaces are invaded by the *Treponema pallidum* during the first two years after infection in a very large percentage of cases. There is much evidence to show that inflammatory changes are present in

the cerebrospinal fluid during this stage of the disease in from 30% to 60% of all infected persons. This percentage varies with the adequacy of early treatment and the stage of infection at which it is begun. In some clinics early lumbar puncture is considered inadvisable owing to the supposed risk of encouraging meningeal invasion, and the statistics in these clinics are limited to cases in which lumbar puncture was performed after thorough early treatment. Under these circumstances the percentage of cases with abnormal fluids may fall to 13·9% (Dattner 1944). These figures are taken from days before large doses of penicillin were given in early treatment, and may well now have been reduced. In the majority of cases the increase of cells and protein, which is found in the fluid at early lumbar puncture, disappears rapidly under treatment and does not reappear after this is terminated. It is probable that neurosyphilis is a rare sequel in such cases.

The invasion of the meninges during the secondary or latent stage is usually clinically silent. But in a small number of cases meningeal symptoms such as headache and drowsiness or amaurosis, often associated with papilloedema, or cranial nerve palsies or hemiplegia may appear abruptly. In such cases the cerebrospinal fluid shows clear evidence of inflammation, usually containing several hundred cells per mm³ and giving strongly positive globulin and Wassermann reactions (Merritt, Adams and Solomon 1946). Moore (1929) in a follow-up study of 28 cases with 'neuro-recurrences' of this kind found that they were especially prone to develop some form of neurosyphilis after a comparatively short interval. Fifty per cent of cases, in which he considered that treatment had been inadequate, had developed tabes or meningovascular syphilis and 30% of well-treated cases had general paralysis, tabes or other form of neurosyphilis. In most of these cases signs of the disease had appeared within five years of the neuro-recurrence.

In a few cases which have come to necropsy during the neuro-recurrence a more or less widespread infiltration of the meninges with lymphocytes and sparse plasma cells has been found. The infiltration, which was chiefly lymphocytic, followed the vessels into the brainstem and spinal cord as thick cuffs, chiefly confined in the Virchow–Robin spaces. In one case the vessels of the corpus striatum and those under the walls of the ventricles were heavily infiltrated. In another there was infiltration and degeneration, going on to necrosis, of the media of some small meningeal vessels along with swelling and concentric proliferation of the intima; numerous treponemas were found in the walls of these vessels (Heubner's arteritis). Swelling of the cell bodies of astrocytes and microglial hyperplasia were seen in the subpial zone of the cerebral cortex, but no deeper lesions. In the spinal cord swollen-bodied astrocytes were more abundant; there were reactionary changes in the nerve cells of the ventral horns and some myelin degeneration around heavily infiltrated vessels in the dorsal and lateral columns. In a case with amaurosis and papilloedema heavy lymphocytic infiltration of the connective tissue septa and meninges of the optic nerve was found. In other cases temporary visual impairment with or without papilloedema may be due to hydrocephalus.

Tertiary neurosyphilis

The later forms of neurosyphilis are usually divided into (1) meningovascular and (2) parenchymatous, which includes general paralysis and tabes dorsalis. All types of neurosyphilis have certain features in common such as thickening of meninges and lymphocytic infiltration of these and of the perivascular spaces of small vessels. But in other ways there is a remarkable histological distinction between the meningovascular and parenchymatous types. Thus gummata and the grosser forms of cerebral vascular disease are very rare in cases of parenchymatous neurosyphilis, whereas the typical parenchymatous lesions of the cerebral cortex or posterior columns of the cord are rarely found in cases in which the lesions are chiefly meningovascular. It has been suggested that these differences depend on a difference in the local or general immunity reactions of the patient to the treponema. The lesions in meningovascular cases are essentially the same as those of tertiary syphilis elsewhere in the body and are often combined with such changes, whereas the diffuse exudative and inflammatory process in the cerebral cortex, and the abundance of viable organisms which can usually be found there in general paralysis, link the disease to the mucocutaneous lesions of the secondary stage. But these analogies with the secondary stage do not explain the concentration of the lesions of general paralysis in parts of the brain, such as the prefrontal cortex and striatum, which are phylogenetically newest. Nor is

syphilitic aortitis less commonly found in parenchymatous than in meningovascular cases. It seems clear, however, that in general paralysis there is less tendency than in other forms of late syphilis for the development of those immune reactions which kill off the majority of organisms and hedge in those that remain with dense connective tissue barriers. Dattner (1944) found that the absence of hypersensitivity in cases of general paralysis was of a more general character, since 80% of cases failed to give a skin reaction to tuberculin which was positive in more than 80% of the general population. Other evidence in the same direction is given by the fairly numerous cases in which miliary or larger gummata or ulcerations have appeared in general paralytics after treatment with malaria, which by destroying the treponema may stimulate immunity reactions.

The classification of tabes dorsalis among the parenchymatous forms of neurosyphilis is justified by the concentration of the lesions on the dorsal roots and columns. But although it shares with general paralysis certain characteristics such as absence of gummatous lesions, there are few other resemblances between the pathology of the two diseases. It is true that tabetic degeneration of the dorsal columns may be found in occasional cases of general paralysis, but in most of the cases in which cerebral symptoms appear during the course of tabes, and which are often diagnosed clinically as taboparesis, the cerebral lesions are those of meningovascular syphilis. It is also recognized that primary optic atrophy is commonly associated with tabes dorsalis and sometimes with meningovascular syphilis, but rarely with otherwise uncomplicated general paralysis. It is, however, impossible to classify tabes dorsalis more exactly until its pathogenesis is better understood.

Meningovascular syphilis. As the name implies, meningovascular syphilis attacks the meninges and vessels primarily. The lesions which occur in the brain and spinal cord are as a rule secondary, but certain changes in the subpial zone of the cord and brainstem and in the floor of the fourth ventricle may be an exception to this. Tertiary syphilitic meningitis takes a great variety of forms which are to some extent separable both clinically and pathologically, although all kinds of grouping of lesions and transition forms between those of different kinds are found. In all forms there is widespread, often diffuse, thickening of the pia arachnoid and infiltration of its meshes with lymphocytes and plasma cells. This is usually concentrated around the meningeal vessels and may follow their branches for a short distance into the brain and spinal cord along the Virchow–Robin spaces. The small meningeal vessels especially show thickening and infiltration of the adventitia and in some there is also intimal proliferation.

In the description which follows the various forms are treated separately, although it is recognized that they are no more than variants in distribution and concentration of the same type of lesion. Clinical symptomatology must also be taken into account in classifying these cases, since they usually come to necropsy owing to a different train of symptoms such as those of intracranial pressure or paraplegia.

Diffuse basal meningitis. The basal meningitis of the secondary stage may be carried over into the tertiary stage with increased fibrosis of the meninges and the formation of small, often miliary, gummata in them. A series of cases of this kind, in which death was due directly or indirectly to hydrocephalus, was reported by Greenfield and Stern (1932). They found the meninges around the fourth ventricle to be so thickened and felted that in most cases the foramina of exit of cerebrospinal fluid from the fourth ventricle were sealed off and the cisterna magna contained little or no fluid. The meningeal thickening was continued over the front of the pons to the cisterna basalis, but was less evident above this level. The basilar artery might be buried in a felt-work of thickened meninges. Firm white or greyish gummatous thickenings in the meninges were also seen, especially in the region of the acoustic nerve and over the front of the pons. On microscopic examination, giant-celled miliary gummata, which were scarcely visible to the naked eye, might be found in the thickened meninges and sometimes also in the superficial parts of the medulla and cerebellum. The floor of the fourth ventricle was covered over, especially towards its lower end, by an outgrowth of neuroglial cells and fibres and often also by a layer of fibroblastic and collagenous tissue, heavily infiltrated with lymphocytes and plasma cells. This formed a diffuse smooth pad which filled the calamus scriptorius, and in some cases covered the greater part of the floor of the ventricle (see Fig. 1.24b). On naked eye examination this appeared at first sight to be not much altered but it had lost its glistening appear-

ance. Small ependymal granulations, like those seen in general paralysis, were also seen in the upper and lateral parts of the floor of the ventricle and perivascular infiltration or miliary gummata might be found under the floor of the ventricle. A very characteristic lesion seen in these cases was an outgrowth of neuroglia into the subarachnoid space over the ventral surface of the medulla through irregular breaks in the thickened pia mater. Collagen strands were often intermingled with neuroglial fibres in these outgrowths (Fig. 6.7).

In cases of basal meningitis the meningeal thickening is often continued over the upper cervical segments but is usually less evident over

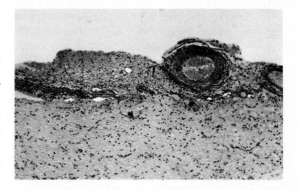

Fig. 6.7 Chronic meningovascular syphilis. Outgrowth of neuroglia through breaks in the pia mater on the ventral surface of the medulla.

the lower part of the spinal cord. The hydrocephalus may be of the communicating type, but in some cases the foramina of Luschka and Magendie seem to be completely covered by fibrous tissue.

In many such cases symptoms of hydrocephalus are associated with loss of vision due to papilloedema and secondary optic atrophy. The blindness in such cases should be distinguished from the so-called primary optic atrophy of syphilis although the two forms may be combined. Basal meningitis also often causes paralysis of cranial nerves especially the oculomotor, abducens and acoustic.

Diffuse syphilitic spinal arachnoiditis usually involves principally the leptomeninges. It may reveal its presence by root symptoms and signs or by pressure effects. The nerve roots may be enclosed in small gummata or strangled by local thickening of the meninges. Pockets of cerebrospinal fluid may form in the subarachnoid space and cause local pressure effects on the spinal cord or occlusion of small vessels may cause local softenings. In more chronic cases diffuse degenerative lesions may be found in the spinal cord, which on macroscopic examination appears shrunken and has lost its firm consistency. In transverse sections of such cords there is general pallor of myelin staining along with a narrow zone of more complete destruction of myelinated fibres under the pia mater. This may be most evident in the ventrolateral columns but often surrounds the cord in what has been called a 'syphilitic halo'. Although it involves the fibres of the spinocerebellar tract it is clearly not a systemic degeneration as it passes around both the ventral and dorsal surfaces of the cord and often also along the lips of the ventromedian fissure. Some overgrowth of neuroglial fibres may be seen in this zone but there is seldom the dense sclerosis which might be expected from the amount of myelin loss. This marginal degeneration may be seen throughout the length of the cord or may be most extensive in the cervical or thoracic segments. In cases associated with muscular atrophy, which is most often seen in the upper limbs, the corresponding ventral roots appear grey and atrophic and the ventral horns in the affected segments are also shrunken and have lost the majority of their motor neurons. Those that remain may be atrophic or show the peripheral type of chromatolysis. These lesions are often associated with hyaline changes in the walls of the intramedullary vessels. In some cases the vascular lesion may be severe enough to cause local ischaemic softenings in the cord, most often at the thoracic level. The classical picture of syphilitic meningomyelitis is a combination of these meningeal and vascular changes in which either may preponderate.

The pathogenesis of the more diffuse lesions is not clear. Merritt, Adams and Solomon (1946), in an early case of spastic paraplegia without amyotrophy, found heavy infiltration not only of the meninges but also along the vessels in the periphery of the cord. They considered that the syphilitic inflammation of the pia mater directly affected the more superficial parts of the cord. This seems more probable than theories which invoke constriction by thickened meninges or purely ischaemic effects since the meninges are not always greatly thickened and the peculiar peripheral distribution of the degeneration is not seen in vascular occlusions. Although atrophy of the ventral horns and roots is often combined with the characteristic subpial degeneration, it cannot be easily explained by the meningitis, which would be expected to damage the dorsal as severely as the ventral roots. In rare cases of *tabetic amyotrophy* the subpial zone of degeneration may be associated with the lesions of tabes dorsalis, but in many cases of syphilitic amyotrophy there is no systemic degeneration of the dorsal roots or columns.

Pachymeningitis cervicalis hypertrophica. This name was given by Charcot and Joffroy (1869) to a fairly well-defined form of syphilitic disease of the spinal cord. It is somewhat confusing, as the inflammatory thickening is not confined to the dura mater and is more evident in the pia arachnoid. In this condition the membranes over the cervical region of the cord form a thick sleeve, in which all three membranes are so united by dense fibrous adhesions that it is impossible to separate them. Its outer layer may be unduly adherent to the posterior common ligament of the vertebrae. Necrotic foci may be found in this gummatous thickening. The cord to which the membranes are firmly adherent is usually reduced in size but may be oedematous. The nerve roots passing through the thickened membranes are atrophied and the walls of the blood vessels share in the fibrous thickening. As a result of vascular stasis and compression the white columns of the spinal cord undergo degeneration, which is usually greatest near the surface, and there is also atrophy of the grey matter and its neurons. This condition is now quite rare but in typical cases as in those of classical literature, it is not clear why the disease was much more evident at the cervical level of the cord than elsewhere. It was usually combined with diffuse leptomeningitis over the lower part of the cord and the base of the brain without involvement of the dura mater at either of these levels.

The symptomatology of pachymeningitis cervicalis hypertrophica was well described by older writers (Gowers 1899). It is closely related to the pathology, in that symptoms of paraplegia are associated with root pains or paraesthesiae in the upper limbs and with progressive amyotrophy in these or in the shoulders and neck. This may or may not be symmetrical. Areas of anaesthesia or analgesia may be found in the same segmental areas as the muscular wasting. As Gowers pointed out, the loss of skin sensibility differs from that of syringomyelia in affecting all modalities and in being less extensive than the muscular wasting.

Large meningeal gummata are now rare. They most often occur either over the convexity of the cerebrum or over the cerebellum, and are usually attached both to the dura mater and to the brain, in which they become embedded. More rarely gummata are confined to the dura mater and skull and produce cerebral symptoms by pressure. Similarly gummata involving the spinal cord usually grow from the leptomeninges and invade the tissue of the cord, but in some cases they are confined to the dura mater or grow from the vertebrae. Gummata of sufficient size to cause pressure symptoms may be associated with other smaller gummatous masses, and a few cases have been described of multiple meningeal gummata of the size of a pea or a bean. Such cases are now very rare, but it is not unusual, in cases of meningeal syphilis, to find small flat gummata resembling dense fibrous thickenings of the lepto-meninges; these may be adherent to the dura mater.

Meningeal gummata are usually less sharply circumscribed than tuberculomata and the sur-rounding meninges are more diffusely thickened. On section they are tough, rubbery and often difficult to cut. The capsule is irregular in thick-ness and is continuous with fibrous trabeculae which run into or through the gumma. Caseous areas may be seen but do not constitute the greater part of the mass, as they do in tuberculo-mata. When gummata are embedded in the brain or cerebellum they are surrounded by a zone of oedematous softening which may extend for a considerable distance into the white matter. This may be to some extent ischaemic in origin, and may be determined by involvement of the meningeal veins and arteries in the syphilitic process. *Microscopically* they contain much more collagen than tuberculomas. There is consider-able infiltration of the outer layers with lympho-cytes and plasma cells; giant cells may also be seen; it is seldom possible to find treponemas. Lymphocytic infiltration of the Virchow–Robin spaces may be found in the surrounding nervous tissue, and there is always a widespread meningeal infiltration which may, however, have a rather focal distribution.

Syphilitic vascular disease

Lesions of the cerebral vessels of varied severity may accompany any form of neurosyphilis, but are most common in meningeal and gummatous forms. In some cases they are the chief cause of cerebral or spinal symptoms. Syphilis was at one time considered to be a common cause of cerebral vascular accidents, since a positive Wassermann reaction was found in a considerable proportion of such cases. Syphilitic vascular

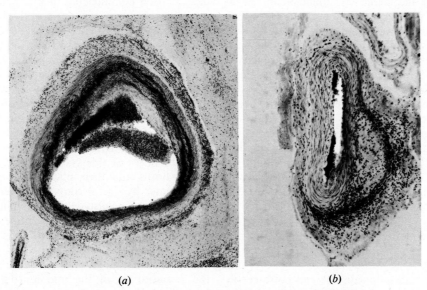

(a) *(b)*

Fig. 6.8 Syphilitic arteritis. (*a*) Heubner's arteritis in a vessel on the surface of the cerebellum. There is infiltration and thickening of the adventitia, thinning of the media, duplication of the elastica and proliferation of the intima. Elastin. (*b*) A small gumma in the wall of the anterior spinal artery. Haematoxylin van Gieson.

disease is not now a common cause of cerebral thrombosis, and is a rare cause of cerebral haemorrhage.

The classical lesion of syphilis in the large- and medium-sized meningeal vessels was described by Heubner in 1874 and is often called *endarteritis obliterans*. It consists of a fibroblastic and eventually collagenous thickening of the intima, which is usually greater on one side of the vessel but may be concentric. This is associated with fibrosis or thinning of the media. The elastica is usually intact. There is an excess of fibrous tissue in the adventitia and lymphocytes and plasma cells infiltrate this coat and often penetrate into the media (Fig. 6.8). In the larger vessels they may be most numerous round the vasa vasorum. Although it is usually called an endarteritis, the lesion is due in most cases to a primary inflammation of the middle and outer coats, to which the intimal thickening is for the most part secondary. The arteritis appears in fact to be due to an extension of the meningeal inflammation to the vessels which lie in the subarachnoid space. It is possible that this inflammation sometimes spreads inwards and directly stimulates the fibroblastic proliferation of the intima and, as in tuberculosis, inflammation of the intima may in some cases be the only early lesion. It follows from this view of the pathogenesis that Heubner's arteritis may result in weakening of the media and aneurysmal dilatation. When such syphilitic aneurysms form they are usually fusiform and are not so liable to rupture and cause haemorrhage as berry aneurysms. More often the encroachment of the thickened intima on the lumen of the vessel leads to ischaemia or thrombosis.

In the late stages the affected vessels appear firm and creamy white in colour. Although usually more widespread than the lesions of atheroma in the cerebral vessels, syphilitic arteritis rarely affects all the vessels in a uniform manner. In some cases the typical change may be seen only in some of the medium-sized vessels. At this stage lymphocytic infiltration may be scanty and the lesions may be most evident in the media and elastica.

Tabes dorsalis

The lesions in tabes dorsalis are concentrated on the dorsal roots and columns, most often at the lumbosacral and lower thoracic levels. In a typical case there is a moderate or slight diffuse meningeal thickening which is greater over the dorsal than the ventral surface of the spinal cord. The dorsal roots of the lumbosacral enlargement are thin and grey and contrast with the normal thick white ventral roots. The spinal cord is flattened from before backwards owing to shrinkage of the dorsal columns, which appear grey throughout their width, especially in the lower part of the cord. At higher levels the funiculus gracilis may be more severely degenerated than the funiculus cuneatus. The dorsal root ganglia of the lumbar segments may be smaller than normal, but usually they show little change.

In early cases, transverse sections of the lumbar segments of the cord, stained for myelin, show a very characteristic pattern of degeneration. Pierret (1871) found the earliest degeneration in a bundle of fibres which passed ventromedially along the inner border of the dorsal horn, and which he called the *ruban externe*. After Flechsig (1876) had described the zones in the dorsal columns in which myelination occurred at different stages of fetal development, it was realized that the *bandelette of Pierret* corresponded to the outer part of *Flechsig's middle root zone*. Flechsig's view, that the fibres from this zone passed to the cells of Clarke's column, has been neither confirmed nor refuted by more recent work. The association, both in tabes dorsalis and Friedreich's ataxia, of predominantly ataxic symptoms with degeneration commencing in this zone, makes it probable that it carries proprioceptive impressions. In the lumbar segments Flechsig's middle root zone forms a wedge-shaped cap of rather large fibres, lying ventral to the superficial, lenticular, posterior root zone and separated both from the dorsal horns and to a less extent from the dorsal median septum by finer fibres probably of intrinsic origin. When degenerated in both dorsal columns it forms an area shaped like a butterfly, or like a broad letter 'W'. On passing up the cord the fibres of this system disappear into the dorsal horns and their place is taken by fibres which enter by dorsal roots at higher levels. In the cervical region also degeneration in this system of fibres is often seen in the central part of the funiculus cuneatus in cases in which the upper limbs are involved in the disease (Fig. 6.9).

In some cases degeneration appears as early in the posterior as in the middle root zone. In later cases the posterior root zone degenerates and in long-standing cases the whole of the dorsal columns except a narrow *cornucommissural* zone, near the bases of the dorsal horns and the grey commissure, may become cleared of myelinated fibres and filled with a dense felt-work of fibrous neuroglia. On passing up the cord the degeneration becomes greatest in the funiculus gracilis and it may be confined to this tract at the cervical level. In early cases, in which the degeneration in the lumbar segments is almost confined to the middle root zone, the degeneration of the funiculus gracilis at the cervical level may be slight or even absent. In cases of *cervical tabes*, degeneration in the middle root zone of the funiculus cuneatus appears at this level and occasionally this funiculus may be severely degenerated.

Lesions in the dorsal root ganglia are less definite. They were denied by many of the early workers and do not appear to be at all commensurate with the degeneration in the dorsal roots and columns. But atrophic cells may be found in the lumbar ganglia in severe cases; it is probable that some also have disappeared, but shrinkage of the ganglia makes it difficult to assess the degree of cell loss.

Lymphocytic and plasma-celled infiltration of the leptomeninges varies greatly in intensity from case to case. Perivascular infiltration within the cord is also common and is not limited to the degenerated tracts. The meningeal vessels in

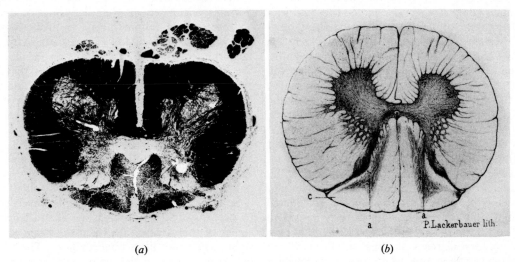

(a)   *(b)*

Fig. 6.9 Tabes dorsalis. (*a*) Drawing from Pierret's (1871) article showing sclerosis in *bandelette externe* in a case of cervical tabes. Probably picro-carmine. (*b*) Section of lumbar cord in early tabes showing degeneration in the middle root zone. Myelin.

Degeneration of dorsal roots is found to correspond closely to that in the dorsal columns but in the early stages it is less obvious. It has been frequently observed, in sections stained for myelin, that the dorsal root fibres become less deeply stained on passing through the pia mater. This has been described as the *zone of paling*. It is, however, difficult to be certain whether there is in early tabes a greater disparity than normal between the staining of myelin sheaths external to and internal to the pia mater, or whether the scarcity of large myelinated fibres in this disease makes a normal difference more evident. In later cases or those with severe and rapid onset of symptoms, there may be degeneration of a large proportion of the fibres in the dorsal roots, especially those of larger calibre.

early cases usually show little change except lymphocytic infiltration and some thickening of the adventitia. In cases of longer standing this adventitial thickening, as well as the fibrous thickening of the pia arachnoid, often become more intense, while the cellular infiltrations may be less, especially in burnt out and well treated cases. In cases of tabes with cranial nerve palsies, these nerves undergo a similar grey atrophy to that seen in the dorsal roots. The pathological basis of the Argyll-Robertson pupil is not clear, but has been attributed to syphilitic ependymitis and subependymal gliosis in the anterior midbrain (Walsh and Hoyt 1969). The pretecto-oculomotor fibres on the dorsal side of the Edinger Westphal nucleus would be involved, abolishing the light reflex, whereas the near vision fibres which approach this nucleus slightly more ventrally would be spared.

Pathogenesis. Various theories of the pathogenesis of tabes dorsalis have been put forward but none has been generally accepted. The earlier writers considered that the disease began in the spinal cord but did not explain why the dorsal roots also underwent atrophy. Obersteiner and Redlich (1894) considered that both the symptomatology and pathology of tabes could be explained by an inflammatory lesion of the dorsal roots. They placed the lesion at the site where the root pierces the pia mater. Emphasizing the *zone of paling*, which has already been discussed, they considered that syphilitic thickening of the pia mater could strangle the nerve fibres and lead to their degeneration. Their theory did not, however, explain the absence of degeneration in the dorsal columns in meningovascular syphilis. Nageotte (1894) held that the main lesion was in what he called the *radicular nerve*, that is in that part of the spinal root which lies between the dorsal root ganglion and the subarachnoid space. In this part of its course the roots are covered by a dural sheath and by an extension into this of mesothelial cells which cover the arachnoid. Nageotte, at this point, found an interstitial radiculitis consisting of an infiltration of lymphocytes and plasma cells and what he considered as embryonic cells, along with fibrosis limited to the posterior root. He considered that the inflammatory changes in this situation varied from time to time and, when severe, damaged a certain number of dorsal root fibres, which were unable to regenerate since most of their course ran in the dorsal columns. If any fibres of the ventral roots were also damaged they were capable of regeneration, as the degenerated segment was in them peripheral. While it is possible to accept a lesion of the radicular nerve as playing some part in the pathogenesis of tabes dorsalis, the limitation of the disease in almost every case to the dorsal component of the nerve and its special emphasis on fibres going to the middle root zone are not easily explained.

Paretic dementia (General paralysis of the insane)
Paretic dementia has been a recognized form of insanity for more than 150 years, but its relation to syphilis was not confirmed until the introduction of the Wassermann reaction. Noguchi and Moore (1913) by finding treponema in the cortex of general paralytics, provided the final proof that the disease was a direct result of syphilitic infection of the brain.

When a patient dies demented after several years of illness the brain presents a very typical appearance. It is shrunken and firmer than normal and is covered with opaque, thickened pia arachnoid (Fig. 6.10). This thickening partly conceals a convolutional atrophy and, like it, is usually most evident in the frontal lobes and temporal poles, diminishing on passing towards the occipital poles. The vessels may be generally thickened, but are not always much altered. There is considerable dilatation of the lateral ventricles, and the ependyma, especially of the frontal horns and the 3rd and 4th ventricles, presents a coarsely granular appearance due to the presence of innumerable fine projections on its surface (see Fig. 1.24a). These are most evident near the foramen of Monro and in the floor of the 4th ventricle. In old descriptions the dura mater was said to be greatly thickened, containing on section several brownish layers of altered blood. This *pachymeningitis haemorrhagica* appears to have been due to repeated head injuries and is an unfortunate name for a subdural haematoma. Abnormal adhesion of the dura mater to the bone has also been described, but this is too common a finding *post mortem* to be significant.

Some cases of general paralysis, however, come to necropsy for various reasons at much earlier stages of the disease. In them the brain at first sight may show little abnormality. There may be slight opacity of the leptomeninges especially over the frontal poles, the base of the brain and the dorsal surface of the spinal cord. On careful examination ependymal granulations will usually be found in the floor of the 4th ventricle and near the foramina of Monro. Otherwise the brain may appear normal. There may be no alteration in the vessels at the base or in the size of the ventricles.

Microscopical examination, at any stage of the disease, shows the lesions to be concentrated on the cerebral cortex, striatum and hypothalamus. In the cerebral cortex the lesions, like the meningeal thickening, are most intense in the prefrontal cortex, and diminish on passing toward the occipital pole, but they often vary greatly in intensity in different areas. All the cellular elements of the cortex, neurons, neuroglia, microglia, blood vessels and meninges, are involved in the process. With low magnifications the most obvious change is loss of the cortical

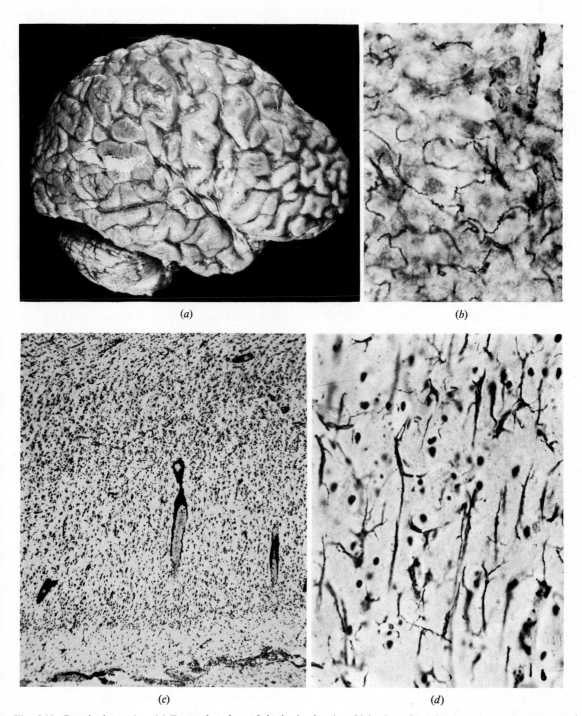

(a)

(b)

(c)

(d)

Fig. 6.10 Paretic dementia. *(a)* External surface of the brain showing thickening of arachnoid and atrophy of frontal convolutions. *(b)* Treponemas in cortex. Jahnel's silver method. *(c)* Low power view of the cortex showing loss of definition of the cell layers and perivascular infiltration. Nissl. × 50. *(d)* Rod cell forms of microglia. Silver carbonate. × 400.

architecture so that the different layers cannot easily be distinguished (Fig. 6.10c). Examination with higher magnifications shows this to be due to loss of many nerve cells, shrinkage and degeneration of others, and increase in the number of the nuclei of astrocytes and microglial cells. There is also thickening of the walls of the small vessels, many of which contain a single ring of plasma cells in their Virchow–Robin spaces. Heavier cuffs of lymphocytes and plasma cells may be seen round many of the larger cortical venules.

With special stains further details of the lesion can be made out. Many of the nerve cells are sclerotic with hyperchromic nuclei and corkscrew-like apical dendrites. The protoplasmic astrocytes of the deeper cortical layers are not only more numerous, but their processes are thickened and Ranvier–Weigert fibres appear in some of the foot-plate processes. There is also thickening of the subpial layer of fibrous neuroglia, and from this layer neuroglial fibres pass inwards in the outer cortical layers for a varying distance.

The changes in the microglia are even more characteristic. These cells are increased both in number and in size. The bipolar forms which normally are orientated perpendicularly to the surface have proliferated and become greatly elongated; their nuclei also have increased to twice or more their normal length, and their cytoplasm is often visible, even with basic aniline dyes, for some distance at either pole of the nucleus (Fig. 6.10d). To this form of hypertrophic microglial cell Nissl gave the name rod cell (Stäbchenzell). Other forms of microglial cell are similarly enlarged and their nuclei tend to assume unusual trilobed or horseshoe forms. This microglial hyperplasia and the infiltration of many of the small cortical vessels with plasma cells and lymphocytes link paretic dementia to other forms of subacute encephalitis such as encephalitis lethargica or sleeping sickness due to Trypanosoma gambiense. Even more characteristic of paretic dementia, but in no sense diagnostic, is the demonstration, by the Prussian blue or Turnbull's blue method, of unmasked or easily unmasked iron as fine granules in the cytoplasm of many of the microglial cells and in larger irregular masses in the walls of many cortical vessels. This iron-containing material does not stain with haematoxylin as does that which is commonly found in dead cortical nerve cells or in the walls of vessels in the globus pallidus. It

may be difficult to demonstrate in the microglia in brains which have remained for some months in formalin, and for this reason Merritt, Adams and Solomon (1946) recommend fixation in alcohol. The vascular deposits are less soluble in watery fixatives, and are usually readily demonstrated even in brains which have remained in formalin for years.

The meningeal lesions in general paralysis differ from those of diffuse meningeal syphilis only in the larger proportion of plasma cells which they contain, but this varies from case to case. In some early cases, especially those dying in convulsive attacks, both meninges and cortical vessels may be very heavily infiltrated with cells, the majority of which are lymphocytes, whereas in more chronic or quiescent cases infiltrations may be very scanty in both situations. Heubner's arteritis is found in about a quarter of the cases.

Lesions which are similar in all respects to those in the frontal cortex, but which may be less severe, are usually present in the striatum. No lesions except perivascular infiltration are usually found in the globus pallidus, and the line of demarcation in this respect between the two nuclei is often quite striking. Neuronal degeneration, microglial hyperplasia and perivascular infiltration are also frequently present in the thalamus and hypothalamus. In some cases the thalamic lesions are confined to the neurons, and these may be secondary to cortical lesions.

The treponema pallidum has been found in the cortex of many cases of paretic dementia (Fig. 6.10b). Although this organism has been identified in most parts of the brain it is usually most abundant in the frontal cortex, and if absent there it is unlikely to be found elsewhere.

Ependymal granulations consist of small hummocks of neuroglial fibres containing a few astrocyte nuclei. They either raise the ependymal cells over them or more often break through their line and lie over those that remain. They are usually about 0·5 to 1 mm at the base and rise 0·3 to 0·5 mm above the level of the ependyma. Except for a small celled infiltration of underlying blood vessels there is no evidence of inflammation either in or around these granulations and the term granular ependymitis which has sometimes been given to the lesion is to that extent a misnomer. In severe cases the median V of the 4th ventricle may be filled with neuroglial overgrowth, but the diffuse neuroglial pad which is common in chronic meningovascular syphilis is rare in paretic dementia. It seems probable that ependymal granulations are formed by the reaction of astrocytes to treponemas which have been deposited on the wall of the ventricle, but Stern (1932) was unable to find any organisms in them in her cases.

The effects of malarial treatment on the lesions of paretic dementia have been studied by a number of workers, all of whom agree that treponemas disappear rapidly after treatment has begun. Stern was able to find a few degenerated forms in the brain of one patient who died 16 days after inoculation with malaria, but none in 22 other cases so treated. They may, however, be present in large numbers in the brains of patients who relapse after a course of malarial therapy. Few observations have been made on the histology of paretic brains after treatment with penicillin, but in some of these little or no evidence of an inflammatory reaction can be found. The changes are confined to foci of neuronal loss, gliosis and persistent rod cell formation.

Norman, Urich and Heaton-Ward (1959) examined a congenital case in whom the treatment appeared to have been sufficient to arrest the paretic process but not to eradicate the infection completely.

Pathogenesis. Paretic dementia has the histological features of a subacute encephalitis due to infection of the cortex and striatum with the *Treponema pallidum.* The meningeal and perivascular infiltrations, microglial and astrocytic hyperplasia and proliferation and the degeneration and disappearance of nerve cells are similar to those found in other forms of subacute or chronic encephalitis such as sleeping sickness due to *Trypanosoma gambiense* and subacute sclerosing panencephalitis. In the former the iron reaction in the cortex also resembles that seen in paretic brains. The concept of paretic dementia as a syphilitic encephalitis, however, leaves many of its special features unexplained. The local emphasis on the frontal lobes and striatum with relative sparing of the occipital lobes and globus pallidus may be compared with that of Alzheimer's and Pick's forms of cortical atrophy, in which the phylogenetically newer areas and those which mature last tend to be specially affected. The damage to nerve cells in the cortex in paretic dementia may be considered as the direct effect of toxins emanating from the spirochaetes or as the result of narrowing of the small cortical vessels by endothelial proliferation. The clearing of the mental confusion which is seen after any treatment which kills the spirochaetes might be explained by either theory. But obvious reduction in the calibre of the cortical vessels is far from being constant and shows little correlation with the mental state.

Another problem concerns the presence of large numbers of spirochaetes in the cerebral cortex at a long interval after the original infection. This may be considered as a prolongation of the secondary stage of the disease in the brain alone. It is possible that any spirochaetes which gain access to the cerebral cortex during the early stages of the disease are protected by the blood–brain barrier from the processes of immunity which normally bring the secondary stage to an end. It has also been suggested (Dattner 1944) that patients with paretic dementia have less tendency to acquire hypersensitivity reactions than the general population. Whatever the explanation, it is evident that in paretic dementia there is either failure to produce neutralizing or destructive antibodies, or, if these are formed, they fail to reach the spirochaetes. In spite of much investigation this problem still remains unsolved.

The change in the clinical pattern of the illness is to some extent found pathologically also, for the severe cerebral atrophy classically described in this condition is now rarely seen even in patients who have survived for many years.

Lissauer's dementia paralytica

Lissauer and Storch (1901) described a rare form of general paralysis characterized clinically by epileptic or apoplectiform attacks followed by focal signs such as hemiplegia or aphasia. Pathologically, in addition to the usual appearances of general paralysis, there was severe atrophy of convolutions in one or both temporal lobes and the neighbouring parts of the parietal lobe. Merritt and Springlova (1932) studied eight cases of this kind, two of which were caused by congenital syphilis. In their cases epilepsy was a constant early symptom and hemiplegia, aphasia, apraxia or hemianopia might follow as immediate sequelae, or come on more gradually. In some cases these focal signs were at first temporary but later became permanent. The course of the disease was more prolonged in their cases (7·9 years) than is usual in paretic dementia.

Post-mortem examination showed atrophy which was always greatest in the temporal lobes, but usually involved also the postcentral, supra-marginal and angular gyri. In six of their eight cases it was unilateral. The frontal lobes were involved in only two cases. The distribution of the atrophy differed from that of Pick's disease in not sparing the first temporal convolution or the cornu Ammonis, in being usually asymmetrical and in rarely involving the medial surface of the frontal pole.

Microscopically there was a pseudolaminar degeneration in the atrophic convolutions affecting chiefly the second and third layers and, where it was most severe, causing a *status spongiosus* of the cortex. Nerve cells with distended cell bodies, in which nucleus and Nissl granules were displaced to the periphery, were found in the fifth and sixth layers. They resembled the cells of Pick's disease but did not contain argyrophilic inclusions. Other nerve cells had undergone sclerotic changes. There was an increase in numbers and size of the protoplasmic astrocytes, and some formation of neuroglial fibres in the spongy areas. Although the usual exudative changes of general paralysis were present in the less damaged areas of cortex they were slight in the atrophic convolutions. Iron was not seen there, either in the microglia or in the walls of the blood vessels, nor could treponemas be found. Degeneration of white matter was present under the areas of cortex showing status spongiosus and in small foci elsewhere. The pathogenesis of this lesion is not clear, but it may be related to the lobar or more local atrophies which sometimes follow repeated convulsive attacks.

Syphilitic optic atrophy

Syphilis may produce optic atrophy in several different ways.

(1) *Syphilitic hydrocephalus* and *cerebral gummas* may cause excess of intracranial pressure which leads to papilloedema and secondary optic atrophy. In some cases of hydrocephalus direct pressure on the chiasma and intracranial portions of the optic nerves may cause primary optic atrophy or there may be considerable loss of vision with slight papilloedema (Fig. 6.11*a*).

(2) The condition known as *optico-chiasmatic arachnoiditis* is occasionally due to syphilis. In it the optic chiasma and the intracranial portion of the optic nerves are surrounded by thickened pia arachnoid. Pockets of fluid, collected in the meshes of this tissue, may compress the nerves

or they may be stretched or pressed on by contraction of the fibrous tissue. In either case loss of vision, which is usually bilateral, comes on fairly rapidly, but in some cases there are periods of remission. Bitemporal hemianopia, horizontal field losses or central scotomata are common. The optic discs most often show a combination of papilloedema and optic atrophy.

(3) The classical *primary optic atrophy* of syphilis is often called *tabetic optic atrophy* as it is more often associated with tabes dorsalis than with other forms of neurosyphilis. It is rare in otherwise uncomplicated cases of general paralysis; it may accompany chronic meningo-vascular syphilis, or may be the sole clinical manifestation of neurosyphilis.

Until the end of the nineteenth century syphilitic optic atrophy was considered by most neurologists to be due to primary atrophy of the ganglion cells in the retina, with secondary degeneration of their fibres in the optic nerves. The work of Leri (1904) and Stargardt (1913), however, showed that the primary lesion was a chronic inflammation of the pia mater in the intracranial part of the nerve and the chiasma. They found lymphocytic and plasma-celled exudate concentrated around the vessels in this situation, with fibrous thickening of the meninges and intraneural septa. Leri laid great emphasis on the accompanying endo- and peri-arteritis and considered that the degeneration of the nerve was due to ischaemia. Stargardt found that inflammatory exudate into and around the nerve always preceded degeneration, but he thought that neither was secondary to the other; both, in his view, were directly caused by the treponema. At that time the organism had not been found in or around the nerve, but later Igersheimer (1921) demonstrated treponemas in the sheaths of the optic nerves in a large proportion of cases. Stargardt rarely found evidence of inflammation extending forwards from the optic foramen into the orbit or backwards to the optic tracts and external geniculate bodies.

This work has been fully confirmed by later workers. In long-standing cases there may be considerable fibrous thickening of the pia arachnoid covering the intra-orbital part of the nerve, with adhesion of these membranes to the dural sheath. But the intraneural septa show little thickening and lymphocytic exudate is slight and usually confined to the neighbourhood of the optic foramen. The exudate is much more evident in the intracranial part of the nerve and

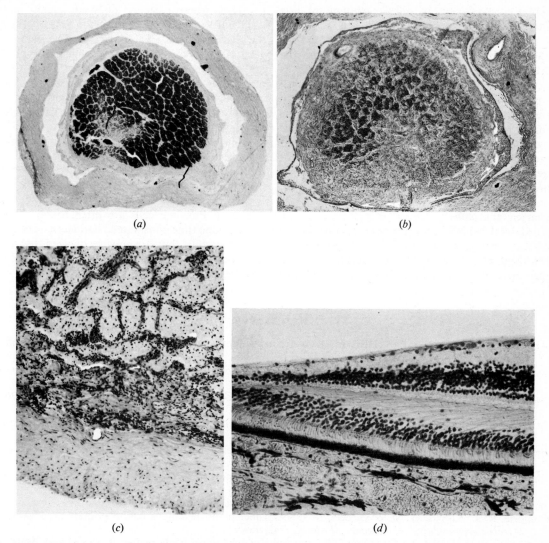

Fig. 6.11 Optic atrophy in syphilis. (*a*) Central atrophy of the optic nerve secondary to syphilitic hydrocephalus. The arachnoid is thickened but not adherent to the dural sheath. Myelin. (*b*, *c* and *d*) Syphilitic optic atrophy. (*b*) Section of the optic nerve showing relative sparing of the more central fibres. W.P. carmine. (*c*) Higher power view of the optic nerve showing fusion of dura and arachnoid membranes and lymphocytic infiltration of these and the connective tissue septa. Haematoxylin van Gieson. (*d*) Section of retina at the macula in chronic case with almost complete disappearance of nerve cells in the ganglion cell layer, but no other obvious change. Haematoxylin van Gieson.

may extend into it along the septa or the vessels (Fig. 6.11*c*). Degeneration of nerve fibres, in which the myelin sheaths are usually more severely damaged than the axons, is commonly greatest in the peripheral zone of the nerves, but is often eccentric or irregular; and the whole cross-section of the nerve usually stains poorly for myelin (Fig. 6.11*b*). The degeneration becomes less severe on passing towards the nerve head. It is associated with heavy fibrous gliosis. In the retina there is

simple atrophy of many nerve cells, and others show chromatolysis, but even when the degeneration of the nerve appears complete near the chiasma many nerve cells may still be present in the retina (Leri) (Fig. 6.11*d*). There is little gliosis of the layers of nerve cells and fibres, and the outer retinal layers show no changes. In some cases a subpial zone of degeneration extends along the optic tracts. The resemblance of this subpial zone of degeneration to that seen in the spinal cord in cases of diffuse meningomyelitis suggests a similar pathogenesis.

Syphilitic optic atrophy often begins in one eye and may be far advanced in this eye before the other is affected. In most cases the progress is slow and vision may not be completely lost for some years. There is evidence that modern treatment may arrest the disease, at least in the earlier stages. The visual fields commonly show peripheral restriction which may be concentric or greater in the temporal fields. Quadratic loss or hemianopia is less common and central scotomas are seldom if ever found.

Congenital syphilis

Congenital syphilis may produce lesions in the central nervous system similar to those seen in the acquired disease. Hydrocephalus due to basal meningitis may occur in early infancy. General paralysis, when it occurs, does not usually show itself until towards the end of the first or during the second decade. Tabes is rare. The lesions of general paralysis, when due to congenital syphilis, are often very severe. They differ from those due to the acquired form in being more diffuse and in attacking the cerebellar cortex, often severely. There is considerable loss of Purkinje and granule cells and gross, often irregular, shrinkage of the cortex. A rather dense neuroglial overgrowth is seen throughout the cortex. In the molecular layer it is usually quite irregular, with little of the parallel orientation of fibres which is seen in the cortical glioses of adult life. Binucleated Purkinje cells are often found. They were at one time considered characteristic of congenital syphilis, but it is now recognized that they may occur when the cerebellum is involved at any age or at any stage of the disease.

References

Abbot, M. & Stern, W. E. (1969) Hemorrhage associated with brain abscess. *Journal of the American Medical Association*, **207**, 1111-1114.

Aszkanazy, C. L. (1952) Sarcoidosis of the central nervous system. *Journal of Neuropathology and Experimental Neurology*, **11**, 392-400.

Bannister, C. M. (1970) A tuberculous abscess of the brain. Case report. *Journal of Neurosurgery*, **33**, 203-206.

Beine, M. L., Hansen, A. E. & Fulton, MacD. (1951) Salmonella meningitis. *American Journal of Diseases of Children*, **82**, 567-573.

Beres, D. & Metzler, T. (1938) Tuberculous meningitis and its relation to tuberculous foci in the brain. *American Journal of Pathology*, **14**, 59-70.

Blacklock, J. W. S. & Griffin, M. A. (1935) Tuberculous meningitis in children. *Journal of Pathology and Bacteriology*, **40**, 489-502.

Blattner, R. J. (1969) Chronic granulomatous disease. *Journal of Pediatrics*, **74**, 315-318.

Bonforte, R. J., Karpas, G. M. & Gribetz, I. (1968) Tuberculous meningitis due to primary drug-resistant *Mycobacterium tuberculosis hominis*. *Pediatrics*, **42**, 969-975.

Buchan, G. C. & Alvord, E. C. (1969) Diffuse necrosis of subcortical white matter associated with bacterial meningitis. *Neurology (Minneapolis)*, **19**, 1-9.

Cairns, H. & Russell, D. S. (1946) Cerebral arteritis and phlebitis in pneumococcal meningitis. *Journal of Pathology and Bacteriology*, **58**, 649-665.

Charcot, J. M. & Joffroy, A. (1869) Deux cas d'atrophie musculaire progressive avec lésions de la substance grise et des faisceaux anterolateraux de la moelle epinière. *Archives de Physiologie*, **2**, 354-367, 629-649, 744-760.

Daniel, P. M. (1949) Gross morbid anatomy of the central nervous system of cases of tuberculous meningitis treated with streptomycin. *Proceedings of the Royal Society of Medicine*, **42**, 169-174.

Dastur, D. K. & Udani, P. M. (1966) The pathology and pathogenesis of tuberculous encephalopathy. *Acta Neuropathologica (Berlin)*, **6**, 311-326.

Dastur, D. K. & Wadia, N. H. (1969) Spinal meningitides with radiculo-myelopathy. Part 2: Pathology and pathogenesis. *Journal of the Neurological Sciences*, **8**, 261-297.

Dastur, H. M. & Desai, A. D. (1965) A comparative study of brain tuberculomas and gliomas based on 107 case records of each. *Brain*, **88**, 375-396.

Dattner, B. (1944) *The Management of Neurosyphilis*, Grune and Stratton, New York.

Dewhurst, K. (1969) The neurosyphilitic psychoses today: a survey of 91 cases. *British Journal of Psychiatry*, **115**, 31-38.

Elkington, J. St. C.   (1936) Meningitis serosa circumscripta spinalis (spinal arachnoiditis).   *Brain*, **59**,181-203.

Field, E. O.   (1954) The production of gamma-globulin in the central nervous system.   *Journal of Neurology, Neurosurgery and Psychiatry*, **17**, 228-232.

Flechsig, P.   (1876) *Die Leitungsbahnen im Gehirn and Rückenmark des Menschen*, Leipzig.

Fleurette, J., Moulin, A., Mounet, P. & Lapras, C.   (1969) Meningite postoperatoire et fièvre prolongée. Isolement répété de *Brevibacterium fermentens*.   Hypothèse pathogénique.   *Annales de l'Institut Pasteur*, **116**, 327-330.

Gowers, W. R.   (1899) *A Manual of Diseases of the Nervous System*, 1, 3rd edition, Churchill, London.

Gray, M. L. & Killinger, A. H.   (1966) *Listeria monocytogenes* and listeric infections.   *Bacteriological Reviews*, **30**, 309-382.

Greenfield, J. G. & Stern, R. O.   (1932) Syphilitic hydrocephalus in the adult.   *Brain*, **55**, 367-390.

Hardman, J. M. & Earle, K. M.   (1969) Myocarditis in 200 fatal meningococcal infections.   *Archives of Pathology*, **37**, 318-325.

Heathfield, K. W. G.   (1968) Changing clinical picture of neurosyphilis.   *British Medical Journal*, **1**, 765-766.

Herring, A. B. & Urich, H.   (1969) Sarcoidosis of the central nervous system.   *Journal of the Neurological Sciences*, **9**, 405-422.

Heubner, O.   (1874) *Die Luetische Erkrankung der Hirnarterien*, Vogel, Leipzig.

Igersheimer, J.   (1921) Spirochätenbefunde an der Sehbahn bei Paralyse.   *Deutsche Medizinische Wochenschrift*, **47**, 738.

Jabukiac, P., Dunsmore, R. H. & Beckett, R. S.   (1968) Supratentorial brain cysts.   *Journal of Neurosurgery*, **28**, 129-136.

Jensen, K., Ranek, L. & Rosdahl, N.   (1967) Bacterial meningitis.   A study of 356 cases seen at Blegdams Hospitalet between 1960-1965.   *Nordisk Medicin*, **77**, 693-699.

de Kalbermatten, J. P. & Piolino, M.   (1969) Considérations sur la meningite purulente de l'adulte.   *Schweizerische Medizinische Wochenschrift*, **99**, 101-110.

Kerr, F. W. L., King, R. B. & Meagher, J. N.   (1958) Brain abscess: a study of 47 consecutive cases.   *Journal of the American Medical Association*, **168**, 868-872.

Kocen, R. S. & Parsons, M.   (1970) Neurological complications of tuberculosis: some unusual manifestations.   *Quarterly Journal of Medicine*, **39**, 17-30.

Leri, A.   (1904) Etude de la retine dans l'amaurose tabétique.   *Nouvelle Iconographie de la Salpetrière*, **17**, 304-310.

Lincoln, E. M. & Sewell, E. M.   (1963) *Tuberculosis in Children*, Blakiston/McGraw-Hill, New York.

Liske, E. & Weikers, N. J.   (1964) Changing aspects of brain abscesses.   Review of cases in Wisconsin 1940 through 1962.   *Neurology (Minneapolis)*, **14**, 294-300.

Lissauer, H. & Storch, E.   (1901) Ueber einige Fälle atypischer progressiver Paralyse.   *Monatschrift für Psychiatrie und Neurologie (Berlin)*, **9**, 401-434.

McGehee, W. G., Rapaport, S. I. & Hjort, P. F.   (1967) Intravascular coagulation in fulminant meningococcaemia.   *Annals of Internal Medicine*, **67**, 250-260.

Merritt, H. H. & Springlova, M.   (1932) Lissauer's dementia paralytica.   *Archives of Neurology and Psychiatry (Chicago)*, **21**, 117-136.

Merritt, H. H., Adams, R. D. & Solomon, H. C.   (1946) *Neurosyphilis*, Oxford University Press, London.

Millen, J. W. & Woollam, D. H. M.   (1954) The reticular perivascular tissue of the central nervous system.   *Journal of Neurology, Neurosurgery and Psychiatry*, **17**, 286-294.

Moore, J. E.   (1929) The relation of neurorecurrences to late syphilis—a clinical study of eighty-one cases.   *Archives of Neurology and Psychiatry (Chicago)*, **21**, 117-136.

Nageotte, J.   (1894) La lésion primitive du tabes.   *Bulletin de la Société d'Anatomie de Paris*, **69**, 808-820.

Newton, E. J.   (1956) Haematogenous brain abscess in cyanotic congenital heart disease.   *Quarterly Journal of Medicine*, **25**, 201-220.

Noguchi, H. & Moore, J. W.   (1913) A demonstration of treponema pallidum in the brain in cases of general paralysis.   *Journal of Experimental Medicine*, **17**, 232-238.

Norman, R. M., Urich, H. & Heaton-Ward, W. A.   (1959) Neuropathological findings in a case of juvenile general paresis treated with penicillin.   *British Journal of Venereal Diseases*, **35**, 231-237.

Obersteiner, H. & Redlich, E.   (1894) Ueber Wesen und pathogenese der tabischen Hinterstrangsdegeneration.   *Arbeiten aus dem Institut für Anatomie und Physiologie des Zentralnervensystems an der Wiener Universität*, **2**, 158-172.

O'Brien, J. R.   (1954) Non-reactive tuberculosis.   *Journal of Clinical Pathology*, **7**, 216-225.

Pardee, I. & Knox, L. C.   (1927) Tuberculoma en plaque.   *Archives of Neurology and Psychiatry (Chicago)*, **17**, 231-238.

Peirret, M.   (1871) Note sur la sclerose des cordons posterieurs dans l'ataxie locomotrice progressive.   *Archives de Physiologie*, **4**, 364-379.

Prockup, L. D. & Fishman, R. A.   (1968) Experimental pneumococcal meningitis.   Permeability changes influencing the concentration of sugars and macromolecules in cerebrospinal fluid.   *Archives of Neurology (Chicago)*, **19**, 449-463.

Rand, C. W.   (1935) Tuberculous abscesses of the brain secondary to tuberculosis of the caecum.   *Surgery, Gynecology and Obstetrics*, **60**, 229-235.

Rich, A. R. & McCordock, H. A.   (1929) An enquiry concerning the role of allergy, immunity and other factors of importance in the pathogenesis of human tuberculosis.   *Bulletin of the Johns Hopkins Hospital*, **44**, 273-424.

Rich, A. R. & McCordock, H. A.   (1933) Pathogenesis of tuberculous meningitis.   *Bulletin of the Johns Hopkins Hospital*, **52**, 5-37.

Ross, J. A.   (1955) Uveoparotid sarcoidosis with cerebral involvement.   *British Medical Journal*, **2**, 593-596.

Silverstein, A., Feuer. M. M. & Siltzbach, L. E.   (1965) Neurologic sarcoidosis: study of 18 cases.   *Archives of Neurology (Chicago)*, **12**, 1-11.

Sinh, G., Pandya, S. K. & Dastur, D. K.   (1968) Pathogenesis of unusual intracranial tuberculomas and tuberculous space-occupying lesions.   *Journal of Neurosurgery*, **29**, 149-159.

Smith, H. V. & Daniel, P. M.   (1947) Some clinical and pathological aspects of tuberculosis of the central nervous system.   *Tubercle*, **28**, 64-80.

Stargardt, K.   (1913) Ueber die Ursachen des Sehnervenschwundes bei der Tabes und der progressiven Paralyse.   *Archiv für Psychiatrie und Nervenheilkunde*, **51**, 711-976.

Stern, R. O.   (1932) Certain pathological aspects of neurosyphilis.   *Brain*, **55**, 145-180.

Walsh, F. B. & Hoyt, W. F.   (1969) *Clinical Neuro-Ophthalmology*, 3rd Edn., Vol. I, p. 511, Williams and Wilkins Co., Baltimore.

7

Parasitic and Fungal Infections of the Nervous System

Revised by J. Hume Adams

Protozoal infections

Toxoplasmosis

Wolf and Cowen (1937) described a case of granulomatous encephalitis in a 1-month-old baby in which minute nucleated crescentic bodies resembling *Toxoplasma gondii* were found in the lesions. On re-examining a similar case in a 7-week-old infant, which had been reported in 1936 by Richter, parasites of the same kind were found. Since then many cases in newborn infants have been reported from North and South America, Great Britain and the continent of Europe, and from some of these cases the disease has been transmitted to laboratory animals. Toxoplasmosis may be due to congenital or to acquired infection. Acute acquired toxoplasmosis may present in three main ways: lymphadeno-pathy, lymphadenopathy with involvement of another organ, and generalized toxoplasmosis (Beverley 1973). Lymph node involvement is the most common (Siim 1951, 1955; Gard and Magnusson 1951) but the parasite may also cause acute encephalitis in older children (Sabin 1941) or pulmonary infection in adults (Pinkerton and Henderson 1941). For congenital toxo-plasmosis to occur, a woman must have a primary infection in pregnancy. The outcome of infection depends on the virulence of the infecting strain and the age of the fetus at the time of infection (Beverley 1973). Infection in early pregnancy may lead to abortion, later to a miscarriage, a little later to a stillborn child, and still later to a live born child with clinical manifestations. If infection occurs near the end of pregnancy, an apparently healthy child may be born which then develops disease in the early weeks of life. In babies who survive congenital or neonatal infec-tion there may be radiological evidence of the disease in the form of small, diffusely scattered or periventricular, calcifications within the brain. These are often associated with epilepsy and mental retardation. They may be accompanied by choroidoretinitis with some degree of optic atrophy, or this may be the only clinical evidence of the disease.

Aetiology. *Toxoplasma gondii* (Gr. *toxon* = a bow) is a coccidian parasite (Hutchison, Dunachie, Siim and Work 1970). It is a cres-centic, oval or elongated protozoon consisting of an acidophilic cell body and a polar mass of chromatin. With Wright's or Leishman's stain the cell body stains blue and the polar chromatin red. In some parasites a smaller red staining granule can be seen at the pole opposite to the nucleus. The absence of a kinetoplast distin-guishes the parasites from the leishmania stage of trypanosomes. With methylene blue-eosin the cell body stains pink and the chromatin blue. The parasites divide by longitudinal fission which begins in the nucleus. In sections they measure 2 to 3 μm in length by 1·5 to 2 μm in width. Wolf and Cowen give the measurement of the smallest as 0·9 μm × 0·7 μm and of the largest 3·5 μm × 1·8 μm. In smears of tissue or of the deposit from the cerebrospinal fluid they appear rather larger. In the tissues they occur either in endothelial cells or free in the tissues. In either situation they may be isolated or in small groups. More rarely pseudocysts containing closely packed parasites or rosettes of parasites, which may arise from the disappearance of the cell membrane enclosing the pseudocyst, are seen. The pseudocysts vary in size from 6 μm × 7 μm to 15 μm × 17 μm. The encysted parasites are rather smaller than those that lie free (Fig. 7.1).

The name *Toxoplasma gondii* is taken from the first mammalian species in which the parasite was found. At first toxoplasmas from different animal species received the name of the species in which they occurred, but according to modern views there is no difference between these various strains.

Toxoplasma gondii is widely spread in nature among both mammals and birds. It has been found in the urine and faeces of domestic animals and in the milk of laboratory animals. Every mammalian species which has been tested is susceptible but primates appear to be less so than lower animals, and rodents, especially mice, guinea pigs and rabbits are particularly susceptible. Under natural conditions infection is widespread among rabbits with the result that dogs and cats which feed on rabbits may become infected. Until recently, little was known of how infection was transmitted from one host to another. Transplacental transfer from mother to fetus and accidental laboratory infections were recognized, as was infection by eating uncooked or undercooked meat. How infection was transmitted to herbivores and vegetarians was not known since both trophozoites and zoites in cysts are very susceptible to drying, heat, and changes in tonicity (Beverley 1973). Then Hutchison *et al.* (1970) reported a life cycle of the parasite in cats leading to the excretion of highly resistant oocysts. It seems probable that these cysts are an important source of human infections. In all species the young are more easily infected and more liable to develop cerebral lesions than older animals; for example vaginal infection of pregnant mice may cause a predominantly cerebral infection in their offspring. The same rule applies in human cases. Mothers with only glandular or subclinical infection may give birth to babies with cerebral lesions but all fetuses are not equally susceptible, and one twin may be severely affected when the other shows little evidence of disease.

Pathology. In babies with congenital or neonatal involvement of the central nervous system, naked eye examination of the brain may show yellowish, depressed and softened cortical areas which vary in size from a few millimetres to 3 cm in diameter. The pia-arachnoid over these areas is thickened and discoloured. On section

of the brain areas of granulomatous inflammation may be seen in all parts of the brain, brainstem and spinal cord. They are often most numerous in the cerebral cortex and basal ganglia and may be confined to these situations. Some are well defined and may have a caseous or cystic centre. Others are more diffuse. A zone of inflammation and necrosis of tissue round the lateral ventricles is not uncommon. These lesions often feel gritty to the knife when sectioned.

Histological examination may show lesions of three kinds. (1) Large granulomatous areas with a necrotic centre. (2) More diffuse inflammation of the tissues. (3) Miliary granulomas. The last are the most widespread and characteristic. They are often present in the more superficial layers of the cortex where they blend with the thickened and inflamed pia-arachnoid but may be abundant also in the white matter and may be found in the basal ganglia, brainstem, and spinal cord. They are usually about 100 μm in diameter. They consist chiefly of large endothelial or epithelioid cells of irregular, oblong or oval shape, along with an admixture of lymphocytes and occasional plasma and other mononuclear cells. Eosinophil leucocytes may also be seen in them. They do not contain giant cells. The large endothelial cells appear to arise from the capillaries and the adventitia of the arterioles which show swelling of their endothelium. The larger granulomas are made up of inflammatory cells of all kinds including neutrophil leucocytes near necrotic areas. The outer zones are invaded by fibroblasts and show capillary dilatation and sprouting. They are surrounded by a zone of oedematous brain tissue in which miliary granulomas may be present. The meninges are diffusely infiltrated and, where they overlie granulomatous areas of cortex, share in this type of inflammation. Parasites may be found in all areas of inflammation. They are chiefly extracellular but many are seen in large endothelial cells (Fig. 7.1). In the larger lesions amorphous deposits of calcium salts are often present, both in necrotic areas and more diffusely; they are rare in the meninges. Many of the nerve cells in the neighbourhood of granulomas are encrusted with calcium or iron salts.

In the *eye* toxoplasmosis may attack the choroid, ciliary body or retina producing small foci of granulomatous inflammation followed by scarring.

Clinical pathology. In infants with severe congenital encephalomyelitis the cerebrospinal fluid is usually xanthochromic and contains a great excess of protein and some increase in cells. In children who survive intra-uterine infection, or who acquire the disease later, the diagnosis may be established by complement fixation tests which should be positive in a dilution of 1 in 8 or more.

Amoebiasis

Primary amoebic meningo-encephalitis

This is a relatively recently discovered disease of man caused by free-living amoebae traditionally typed have been *N. fowleri*. It is generally accepted that meningo-encephalitis in man results from spread of amoebae by the olfactory route from the nasal sinuses, and that amoebae reach the nasal sinuses as a result of exposure to contaminated water. Once the infection is acquired, the progress of the disease tends to be rapid, the great majority of patients dying within about a week. Recovery is rare (Apley *et al.* 1970), perhaps partly because diagnosis early in the course of the disease has not often been achieved. Diagnosis is based on the identification of amoebae in cerebrospinal fluid.

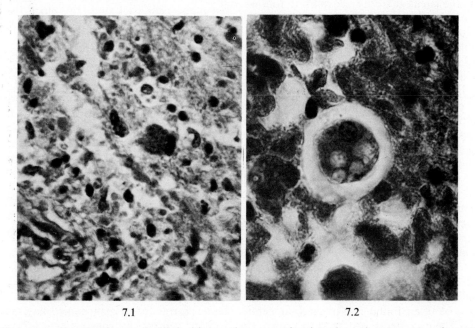

7.1   7.2

Fig. 7.1 Toxoplasmosis. Two large cells filled with toxoplasma parasites (pseudocysts) are seen near the centre of the photograph.
Fig. 7.2 Amoeba histolytica in cerebral abscess.

regarded as being non-pathogenic in man (Carter 1972). Before the first human cases were reported (Fowler and Carter 1965), however, it had been demonstrated by Culbertson and his group (Culbertson, Smith, Cohen and Minner 1959; Culbertson 1961) that such free-living amoebae could produce a fatal meningo-encephalitis in experimental animals if instilled intranasally. Numerous cases have now been described from many parts of the world (see Carter 1972) including the United Kingdom (Apley *et al.* 1970). The amoebae isolated from human cases usually belong to the Naegleri group, and Carter has argued that the great majority of those accurately

Post mortem the brain may be swollen and the meninges diffusely hyperaemic. There is a variable amount of purulent exudate that is often inconspicuous except within sulci and in the basal cisterns. The olfactory bulbs and tracts may be haemorrhagic. Microscopical examination shows a fibrinopurulent exudate in which mononuclear cells are often as numerous as polymorphs. The inflammatory exudate may extend for a short distance along perivascular spaces in the cerebral cortex where there may also be some necrotizing vasculitis and necrosis. Amoebae are often found in large numbers, particularly around blood vessels in necrotic foci. They tend to be very similar in appearance to lipid phagocytes (Butt 1966). Pathological findings are restricted to the central nervous system, there being no convincing evidence of systemic infection by the amoebae.

Primary encephalitis (Robert and Rorke 1973) and brain abscess (Jager and Stamm 1972) due to free-living amoebae have also been reported.

Amoebic abscess of the brain

Infection of the brain by *Entamoeba histolytica* causes a rapidly growing abscess and is the most frequently fatal complication of amoebic dysentery. In the great majority of cases it follows abscess of the liver, but sometimes infection spreads to the brain from the lungs. Of the 61 cases collected from the literature by Halpert and Ashley (1944) an abscess was found in the liver in all except five. When these figures are compared with the prevalence of amoebic dysentery it is clear that abscess in the brain is a very rare complication, but certainly many cases have gone unrecorded. A brain abscess may make its appearance many years after the first attack of amoebic dysentery, in fact it is much more often a late than an early complication of the disease. In many cases the patient does not know that he is a chronic carrier of amoebae, or fails to let his physician know this, so that the cause of the abscess is not recognized until it is too late. This is one of several factors which make amoebic abscess of the brain so often a fatal disease. Amoebic abscesses, in the brain as in the liver, are usually single. They may occur anywhere but are most often found in the cerebral hemispheres. Their contents are reddish-brown or pinkish, creamy fluid, often paler than the characteristic 'strawberry ice cream' contents of liver abscesses. No coagulum forms when this fluid is allowed to stand. It consists of necrotic cells, which are chiefly mononuclear, and unrecognizable débris. Amoebae are not easily recognizable in smears of this material but may be found in wet films. The abscess cavity has ragged and inflamed walls and is surrounded by a wide zone of oedema.

Microscopically the wall of the cavity is ill-defined and irregular and shows little or no evidence of encapsulation by fibrous tissue. There is an inner zone of necrotic tissue with little nuclear staining and a broad outer zone of vascular congestion, degeneration and necrosis of the nervous tissue and diffuse infiltration by lymphocytes, plasma cells and other mononuclear cells. Neutrophil leucocytes are usually scanty. The astrocytes in the surrounding white matter show the swelling of the cell body characteristic of cerebral oedema. Amoebae can be recognized by their large size and relatively small, usually eccentric, palely stained nucleus (Fig. 7.2). They are found both in the necrotic tissue and among the infiltrating cells of the abscess wall.

Malaria

Cerebral malaria is almost always due to infection by *Plasmodium falciparum*. The heavily infected red blood cells pack and may block the cerebral capillaries and, in typical cases, this may give the brain tissue, especially the cortex, a greyish colour to the naked eye. In most cases there are also numerous petechial haemorrhages both in the meninges and on the cut surfaces of the brain.

Microscopically granules of brightly anisotropic, dark malarial pigment (related to haematin) lie in lines along every capillary. In addition to ring and ball haemorrhages, small necrotic foci ringed with microglial cells are seen around the blocked capillaries. These resemble the perivascular areas of necrosis seen in fat embolism. In cases that recover from the acute attack they become invaded by microglial cells and form small glial nodules. Small foci of demyelination and rarefaction of the white matter are also commonly found.

Trypanosomiasis

Three forms of trypanosome may attack the human central nervous system, *Trypanosoma gambiense*, *T. rhodesiense* and *T. cruzi* (*Chagas*). The method and results of the attack differ to some extent in the three forms. The African forms produce an initial meningitis which, in the Gambian form, gradually goes on to meningo-encephalitis, the well-known *sleeping sickness* of Zaire and Uganda. Infection by *T. rhodesiense* is more acute and when untreated usually ends fatally from involvement of the heart before any nervous symptoms appear. When inadequately treated the disease is more subacute and signs of nervous disease may appear for a short time before death.

T. cruzi appears to reach the brain by the blood stream and produces multiple inflammatory foci in its substance. The heart muscle is also involved in most cases.

Trypanosoma gambiense and *rhodesiense*

These forms of trypanosome seem not to have a leishmania stage in their life cycle but in the insect vector develop a crythidial stage in which they multiply. The tsetse fly which is the usual vector of *T. gambiense* is *Glossina palpalis* and that carrying *T. rhodesiense* is *Glossina morsitans*. Both infections are usually transmitted from man to man, but there may be a reservoir in antelopes and domestic animals. Koppisch (1953) divides cases into three clinical types: (1) Those with a chronic course of several years and with changes in the cerebrospinal fluid, but no serious symptoms. (2) Those with severe early symptoms and a course of more than a year, later passing into the stage of *sleeping sickness*. These two forms are commonly caused by *T. gambiense*. (3) Those with an acute or subacute course, fatal in a few months from involvement of the heart and other viscera. Most cases of this kind are caused by *T. rhodesiense*. Changes in the cerebrospinal fluid may be the only evidence during life of infection of the nervous system in these cases, even in those which on necropsy show intra-cerebral as well as meningeal lesions. In some cases of infection by *T. rhodesiense*, especially those which have received insufficient early treatment, there is a terminal stage of dementia passing into coma (Calwell 1937).

Pathology of African sleeping sickness (T. gambiense). On naked eye examination of the brain there is no wasting or convolutional atrophy. In some cases oedema has been observed. The pia-arachnoid is diffusely thickened, or more opaque than normal. Ependymal granulations are not seen. On section of the brain some of the vessels in both the white and grey matter may appear to be surrounded by a grey sleeve, owing to intense infiltration of Virchow–Robin spaces. Haemorrhages or softenings are not usually present.

On *histological examination* the most striking abnormality is the perivascular infiltration which is very widespread throughout the central nervous system, but more intense in some areas than in others. In some cases it is greatest in the white matter and it may also be especially severe in the basal ganglia. In some cases there are selectively severe inflammatory changes in the spinal cord. Around the smaller vessels the infiltration consists almost entirely of plasma cells, but in the thick cuffs around larger vessels lymphocytes are also found. Large histiocytic phagocytes engulfing plasma cells may be seen in these heavier infiltrations (Bertrand, Bablet and Sicé 1935). Where perivascular infiltration is intense, plasma cells are also found free in the tissues.

Morular cells, which were first described in this disease by Mott (1906), are present in considerable numbers both within and outside the Virchow–Robin spaces in the nervous tissue and in the subarachnoid space. They are more numerous in this disease than in any other condition. They are large spherical or ovoid cells measuring from 12 to 20 μm. The hyperchromic nucleus lies under the cell membrane and the cytoplasm is filled with numerous small globules which measure from 1·5 to 3 μm in diameter, and give the cell the appearance of a mulberry, whence the name. In some all the globules are of the same size; in others they vary considerably. They may appear encapsulated so that the cell has a smooth contour or may, as in a mulberry, form rounded projections on the surface (Fig. 7.3). The globules are acidophilic, staining strongly with acid fuchsin, eosin and phloxin, and also with all stains for neuroglial fibres such as phosphotungstic acid haematoxylin and Holzer's stain. They remain uncoloured by silver impregnations and by fat stains, and are pale blue or unstained in Nissl sections. These cells, which are probably derived from plasma cells, appear to be either the same as Russell bodies or a stage in their formation.

Some hypertrophied microglial cells and rod cells are present in the cortex. The astrocytes also are hypertrophied and may be binucleated. There is little loss of cortical neurons; the changes which have been described in nerve cells appear to be chiefly of a terminal character such as Nissl's acute swelling, but a few cells show chronic changes. Some loss of tangential fibres and hyperplasia of neuroglial fibres in the molecular layer of the cortex have also been described but are of minor degree.

Jansen, van Bogaert and Haymaker (1956) found lesions of parenchymatous as well as interstitial character in the cranial and spinal nerve roots and dorsal root ganglia. The interstitial changes consisted of inflammatory exudate and fibrous tissue thickening similar to that found elsewhere in the meninges. In addition there was degeneration of nerve fibres, isolated or in groups and varying in degree from the segmental peri-axial demyelination of Gombault to Wallerian degeneration. This seemed to be primary and independent of the interstitial changes. Both were probably caused by neuro-toxins produced by the disintegration of trypano-somes. The changes in the nerve cells of the ganglia of the dorsal roots and cranial nerves appeared to be secondary to lesions of their axons. In one case a peripheral nerve showed a degree of degeneration of nerve fibres which was quite out of proportion to the degree of inflammatory exudate in and around it.

per mm³. Hawking and Greenfield (1941) found that trypanosomes did not survive *in vitro* at 37° in cerebrospinal fluid with a protein level of 100 to 150 mg per 100 ml for more than 2 to 4 hours, but remained active for more than 24 hours when the protein level was raised by the addition of serum to 3500 mg per 100 ml. The critical percentage of protein appeared to be about 400 mg per 100 ml. Even in cerebrospinal fluid which naturally contained trypanosomes

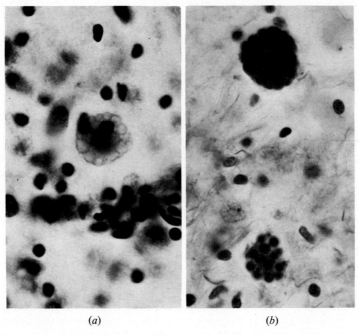

(a)   (b)

Fig. 7.3 Morular cells in subacute encephalitis. (*a*) Thionin. (*b*) Phosphotungstic acid haematoxylin.

Clinical pathology. The diagnosis of Gambian trypanosomiasis is best established by finding parasites in the centrifuged deposit of blood serum or in the juice of enlarged glands. Parasites may be found in the cerebrospinal fluid during the later stages of the disease. Neujean (1950) rarely found trypanosomes in the fluid when the cell count was below 30 per mm³ and only in about 10% of cases in which it was between 30 and 100 per mm³. With higher cell counts the percentage of positive findings rose sharply and when more than 1000 cells per mm³ were present trypanosomes could always be found. The total protein in the cerebrospinal fluid in trypanosomiasis rises with the cell count and the colloidal benzoin reaction also is usually positive when the cell count has risen above 20

they died in 1 to 2 hours at 37°. From this it would appear that their normal habitat in the subarachnoid space during the early stages of invasion is intracellular rather than free in the fluid.

T. rhodesiense

In two untreated cases of infection by this parasite, in which trypanosomes abounded in the cerebro-spinal fluid shortly before death, Hawking and Greenfield (1941) found pericardial and pleural effusions with very little fibrin or adhesions, and severe myocardial infiltration and degeneration. The central nervous system was normal except for mild diffuse meningeal infiltration in both cases and petechial haemorrhages in the occipital lobe in one. There was also slight infiltration of the choroid plexus. The meningeal infiltration consisted chiefly of large histiocytic cells, varying from the size of the large mononuclears of the blood to cells 30 to 40 μm in diameter which were often binucleated or multinucleated. Lymphocytes and plasma cells were relatively scanty. Some of the latter had a vacuolated cytoplasm and resembled morular cells.

Calwell (1937) examined the brains of 17 cases in most of which inadequate treatment had been given in the early stages of the disease. In these the meningeal exudate was usually greatest towards the vertex of the brain. In only one case was it basal. The chief intracerebral lesion was perivascular infiltration which might be found in any part of the central nervous system including the spinal cord. It was common in the medulla and cerebellum, and morular cells were most often seen in those sites, but might also be found in the cortex, meninges, corpus callosum and basal ganglia in descending order of frequency. The choroid plexus was usually infiltrated with plasma cells and fibrinous exudate was sometimes found in it. Calwell found narrow, irregular zones of demyelination around small vessels, most often in medulla, pons, or cortex in 11 of his cases. Trypanosomes were never found in the brain, although they were commonly present in the cerebrospinal fluid during life. In his cases the cell count in the cerebrospinal fluid never exceeded 500 per mm³. He noted that with inadequate treatment the Rhodesian type of disease tended to approach the typical picture of *sleeping sickness.*

Manuelidis *et al.* (1965) have described six cases. They found that lymphocytes and plasma cells were conspicuous in the subarachnoid space and cerebral cortex early in the disease. Inflammatory changes were more prominent in the white matter and tended to increase with the duration of the disease. Gliosis was also severe in the white matter although myelin was well preserved. Perivascular cuffing was intense in the basal ganglia—in the striatum, the thalamus and the globus pallidus in decreasing order of severity. There was also conspicuous microglial hyperplasia in the basal ganglia. Manuelidis *et al.* (1965) also comment on the absence of neuronophagia and gliomesenchymal cellular nodules.

Chagas' disease

T. cruzi, the cause of South American trypanosomiasis or Chagas' disease, is conveyed by house bugs (usually *Triatoma megista*) which excrete it in their faeces. Mammals, especially the armadillo, are much more commonly infected than man and provide the reservoir of the disease. The human disease, which is relatively rare, usually begins with conjunctivitis and goes on to lymphadenopathy and oedema of the face and limbs. It may undergo spontaneous cure or relapse. When it becomes chronic the heart and nervous system are commonly affected.

The parasite may appear in the blood as a trypanosome, often curved like a letter C, or in cells in leishmania form. The latter form is that usually seen in sections of tissues. Cases in which there is involvement of the nervous system usually end fatally. Post-mortem examination shows congestion and oedema of the brain. Numerous small inflammatory foci, consisting of collections of mononuclear cells of various kinds, are found scattered through the substance of the brain, more in the white matter than the grey. They are commonly seen in the cerebellum, brainstem and spinal cord. They do not appear to be related to vessels. Leishmania may be found in swollen neuroglial cells and large mononuclear cells in these foci. In chronic cases Chagas found old scarred foci as well as recent foci containing leishmania. The *heart* usually shows intense myocarditis, with necrosis and phagocytosis of muscle fibres in some areas. Leishmania may be found in the muscle cells. The skin, spleen, lymph nodes, endocrine glands and voluntary muscle may also contain parasites in leishmania form.

Metazoal infections

Cestodes

Taenia solium (*Cysticercosis*)

The encysted larval stage of the common human tapeworm, *Taenia solium*, is usually passed in the pig; but if ova are ingested by man their shells are dissolved in the stomach and the embryos penetrate the wall of the intestine and are carried to all the organs of the body, including the brain and muscles. In most cases the resulting cysts remain small and in time the larvae die and become calcified. In the brain the cysts may grow for some time but here also they usually remain small, and soon die. In such cases the only symptoms are epileptic attacks, and when these begin in middle life in patients who have lived in India or Central or South America, the possibility of cysticercosis should be considered. Less often cysticerci develop as thin-walled, usually sterile, racemose cysts in the basal cisterns, causing hydrocephalus or cranial nerve palsies. In children, and more rarely in adults, they may develop into larger cysts in the brain, which can act as expanding lesions and lead to a fatal termination within a few months of the first appearance of symptoms. These three forms or any two of them may be combined.

In the case described by Bickerstaff, Cloake, Hughes and Smith (1952) in which hydrocephalic symptoms were present for 7 years before death, racemose cysts were removed from the cisterna magna at operation, and necropsy revealed numerous small calcified nodules in the brain and a cyst, containing a larva, in the head of the caudate nucleus.

The incidence of human cysticercosis varies greatly in different parts of the world. MacArthur (1933) observed numerous cases of subacute or chronic type in soldiers infected in India. Obrador (1948) in Mexico found that 25% of cases submitted to operation for symptoms of raised intracranial pressure proved to have cerebral cysticercosis, and large series of surgical cases have also been reported from Chile by Arana and Asenjo (1945) and from Poland by Stepien and Chorobski (1949).*

Clinical pathology. Although in chronic cases the cerebrospinal fluid is usually normal, in acute and subacute cases the cell count is raised to between 15 and 100 cells per mm³ and the total protein is also moderately increased. The glucose is often slightly, and may be considerably reduced. Examination of the deposit often reveals the presence of eosinophil leucocytes, which occasionally form a third of the cells present. The fluid may give colloidal gold curves of meningitic or even paretic type. The complement fixation test is more specific and constant. Obrador (1948), using alcoholic extract of pig cysticerci

as antigen, obtained positive results in all his cases, in more than half with a 1 : 5 dilution of cerebrospinal fluid. Eosinophilia in the blood is less constant and when present is usually low (2 to 5%, Stepien and Chorobski 1949).

In chronic cases diagnosis often rests on the presence of cysts in the muscles which may be palpable or appear radiographically as small oval, elongated or carrot-shaped opacities. Calcified intracerebral nodules are less easily shown up owing to the density of the skull shadow.

Pathology. External examination of the brain shows in some cases small colourless cysts in the subarachnoid space. When closely grouped they are attached to a central pedicle and resemble a bunch of grapes. They are most often seen in the cisterna magna but may be present in the pontine or basal cisterns or in the Sylvian fissure. The leptomeninges are thickened in their neighbourhood. In other cases small cysts project from the cortex. These may be greyish and glistening with a white mural nodule, or more opaque. On section of the brain numerous cysts measuring about 1 cm in diameter or smaller spherical nodules may be found. They are most common in the cerebral cortex but a few may be seen in the basal ganglia or white matter and they sometimes project into the cavities of the ventricles. They are rare in the cerebellum. Occasionally cysts lie free in the fourth ventricle and still more rarely in the lateral or third ventricles. The smaller nodules measure 2 to 4 mm in diameter and most have a thin greyish corrugated capsule surrounding a paler centre. Some may show no capsule. In chronic cases many of these nodules are calcified and gritty on section. Larger cysts have a tense grey capsule on which, unless they are sterile, there is a mural nodule in which the embryo lies. They contain a little clear fluid.

Microscopically the meningeal racemose cysts and the larger intracerebral cysts have a cyst wall composed of a very thin outer cuticular layer, averaging 3 μm in thickness, lined by a wider parenchymatous layer consisting of a meshwork of fine fibrils. This is heavily nucleated immediately under the cuticular layer and more sparsely throughout. The larva in the mural nodule shows a double perioral row of hooklets. Most of the subarachnoid racemose cysts, however, are sterile. Around the intracerebral cysts there is a collagenous capsule derived from the host's tissues. So long as the larva is alive there is little inflam-

---

* These authors recall that Paracelsus in 1650 had noted epilepsy as a symptom of cysticercosis.

matory reaction and, apart from some gliosis, the neighbouring tissue shows little abnormality. If the parasite has recently died the cyst is surrounded by an inner zone of dead leucocytes, large mononuclear cells and foreign body giant cells, and an outer more vascular zone of granulation tissue forming collagenous fibres. Eosinophil leucocytes may be present in this zone but are rarely numerous (Menon and Veliath 1940). In the smaller nodules a fibrous tissue capsule is separated by a space containing foreign body giant cells from an inner mass of necrotic débris, cholesterol clefts and granules of calcium salts surrounding the remains of the parasite. There is no evidence of the cyst wall. The capsule is infiltrated by plasma cells and scanty lymphocytes and large mononuclear cells. Some old nodules consist only of a fibrous tissue scar which in the cortex may be continuous with the fibrous tissue of the meninges. Although calcification usually begins in the remains of the larva, it may start in the capsule. According to MacArthur it is not seen during the first two or three years after infection.

Cysticercus endarteritis is a characteristic reaction seen in the small intracerebral arteries close to cysts, as well as in the meningeal arteries in the neighbourhood of racemose cysts. The affected vessels show concentric or eccentric fibroblastic or collagenous thickening of the intima or local excrescences sometimes forming bridges across the lumen. The elastica is not duplicated as in Heubner's arteritis but may be discontinuous in places. There is usually little fibrosis of the media. The adventitia is infiltrated with plasma cells. This form of arteritis differs from that of syphilis in the greater severity of the intimal changes and the slighter lesions in the media. This may be associated to some extent with its greater chronicity.

Echinococcus granularis

Hydatid disease is not uncommon in sheep-rearing countries and numerous reports have come from Australia, New Zealand, Uruguay and the Argentine (Arana-Iniguez and San Julian 1955). In the British Isles, Wales and Shetland provide the majority of cases. The mature worm lives in the intestine of the dog and ova passed in the dog's faeces infect herbage eaten by sheep in whose liver, lungs or abdominal organs the ova develop into encysted embryos. If dogs are allowed to eat the offal of infected sheep the parasite matures in the dog's intestine and its life cycle is repeated. Human infection arises from the contamination of food by dust containing viable ova or by licking the hands after fondling dogs. The latter method of infection probably accounts for the fact that in the great majority of cases infection is acquired in childhood.

Cases of *primary hydatid cyst of the brain* form about 5% of all cases showing evidence of infestation during childhood, but are much rarer in adults (0·7%, Dew 1934). Of 29 such cases collected by Phillips (1948) from those reported in Australia and New Zealand, only two were in adults. This may be explained by the more rapid growth of hydatid cysts in the brain than in the body organs or bones. In many cases a cerebral hydatid cyst is associated with a cyst in the liver. The cerebral cysts are usually single, spherical and unilocular, and may be of considerable size. They rarely cause serious symptoms until they reach the size of a hen's egg and they are often very much larger. In Phillips' series two had a diameter of 10 cm, two contained 600 ml of fluid and two were described as being the size of an orange. Half of these large cysts were successfully removed by operation. Langmaid and Rogers (1940) found two cysts side by side, one 8 cm and the other 6 cm in diameter. Even larger cysts almost filling a cerebral hemisphere have been described. They are almost always found in the cerebral hemispheres, where they favour the region supplied by the middle cerebral artery, especially the parietal lobe. Owing to their large size they usually lie only a few millimetres below the cortex which is flattened over them and appears bluish. Their outer surface has a characteristic greyish wash-leather appearance. The contents of most cysts are a clear colourless fluid which usually contains small daughter cysts and a granular deposit of scolices. A few cysts are sterile, and some contain turbid or, more rarely, yellowish fluid. If the cyst contents are allowed to infect the brain tissue at operation new cysts are likely to form and may grow rather rapidly. In a case of this kind which came to autopsy 8 months after operation, Phillips found numerous new cysts, some of which were 2·5 cm in diameter. This gives some indication of the possible rate of growth of hydatid cysts in the brain.

When the scolex is examined under the microscope the head of the embryo, which is usually invaginated, is seen to have a double perioral row of hooklets (Fig. 7.4). The wall of the cyst is 2 to 3 mm thick and is readily detached from the surrounding brain tissue: in fact when the cyst is emptied it may free itself spontaneously. It is made up of three layers: (1) The germinal layer which usually has brood capsules attached to its inner surface. (2) A chitinous or cuticular, laminated layer. (3) An adventitial layer of fibrous tissue derived from the tissues of the host. In the brain this layer is usually very thin. The surrounding brain tissue shows little evidence of

or, by growing into the spinal canal, may compress the spinal cord. Most of them appear to start in childhood but they grow very slowly and rarely cause symptoms before adult life is reached.

Clinical pathology. In cases of hydatid cysts of the brain without disease elsewhere in the body, the Casoni reaction and complement fixation reactions are usually negative and there is no eosinophilia in the blood. The cerebrospinal fluid also is normal and, except for its increased pressure, gives little help in the diagnosis.

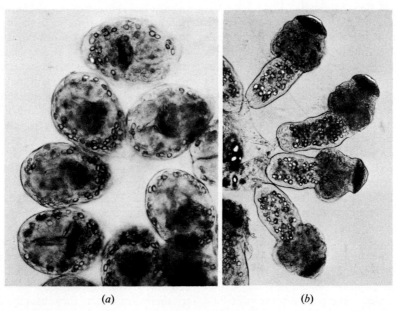

(a)   (b)

Fig. 7.4 Echinococcus granularis. (a) Scolices from the deposit of the fluid from a cerebral hydatid cyst. (b) The same after protrusion of the heads.

reaction to the presence of the cyst except fibrous gliosis and lymphocytic infiltration of occasional vessels in the neighbourhood.

Secondary hydatid cysts of the brain, which are usually multiple, result from rupture of a hydatid cyst in the heart wall into the cavity of the left ventricle. They are usually seen in adults and are much rarer than primary cerebral cysts.

Hydatid cysts of the vertebrae occur in from 0·3 to 1% of all cases (Woodland 1949). They most often grow in the spongy tissue of the vertebrae in the thoracic or lumbar region and may lead to fracture or subluxation of the spine

Multiceps multiceps (*Coenurus cerebralis*)

In some sheep-rearing countries, especially South Africa, *Multiceps multiceps* is the common tapeworm of dogs. Its life history is similar to that of *Echinococcus granularis* and it may have an intermediate host in sheep, goats, cattle, horses, gazelles, antelopes and monkeys. In these animals, cysts form in the cerebral ventricles or subarachnoid spaces (*Coenurus cerebralis*). Occasional human cases of this kind have been reported (Becker and Jacobson 1951; Kuper, Mendelow and Proctor 1958).

The cysts, which are unilocular, may be single or multiple, and may vary in size from a few millimetres to 2 or more centimetres. They are most often found in the 4th ventricle or the sub-arachnoid space of the posterior cranial fossa, but may lie in the cisterna basalis where they may compress the optic chiasma. The arachnoid surrounding them is thickened and may form a grape-like collection of vesicles which closely resembles the racemose type of cysticercus. It can, however, be distinguished by the fact that coenurus cysts are always unilocular and often contain several scolices, whereas cysticercus cysts only contain a single embryo.

Microscopical examination of the pedicle will therefore show it to be composed only of con-nective tissue derived from the arachnoid. The cyst wall is similar to that of a cysticercus, being composed of a thin outer cuticular layer and an inner germinal layer, rich in nuclei. From this scolices project into the lumen of the cyst. The head of these carries a rostellum armed with a double row of hooklets. The cysts may, however, be sterile. In infestations of this type the cerebro-spinal fluid is often normal or shows only a slight increase of cells. The complement fixation reaction on the serum with hydatid antigen is usually positive.

Trematodes

Paragonimus westermanii

Owing to its common situation in the lung the ova of this fluke worm are commonly deposited in the brain or meninges, where they become encysted in a fibrous tissue capsule. This later becomes calcified and may thus be visible by X-rays. Kim (1955) in reporting four cases with multiple cysts of this kind states that Japanese literature contains reports of about 150 similar cases.

Schistosomiasis

The central nervous system is one of the rarer sites of schistosomal infection but Herskowitz (1972) traced 104 cases in the literature. Granu-lomas are most often found in the brain and are usually caused by S. japonicum but recently Ghaly and El-Banhawy (1973) have reported seven veri-fied cases of schistosomiasis of the spinal cord. Cord lesions are usually caused by S. haematobium and S. mansoni. The adult worm has not been found in the central nervous system in human infestations. Involvement of the brain in Japanese schistosomiasis was recognized as a cause of focal

epilepsy by Yamagiwa in 1890, but very few cases were confirmed either by operation or post-mortem examination before 1944. In that year the campaign on Leyte Island in the Philippines resulted in about 1200 cases of schistosomiasis among American soldiers, among which were 27 cases (2·3%) with cerebral involvement. Kane and Most (1948) studied 17 cerebral cases at a hospital where 800 cases of schistosomiasis had been treated (2%). Some who have observed small groups of cases have found cerebral involve-ment to be more common. Chu (1931) found 2 cases in 39, Egan (1936) 2 cases in 12 and Thomas and Gage (1945) 2 cases in 41. In a disease with which, in some parts of China, a large number of the population are infected (Houghton 1910), even such small proportions of cerebral cases as 2 to 5% would be impressive, but Houghton did not find many such cases in native Chinese.

In some patients signs of brain involvement occur, along with the typical gastrointestinal symptoms, from 1 to 2 months after infestation with S. japonicum. In such cases ova are usually abundant in the faeces and the diagnosis is easily made. But when nervous symptoms appear at a longer interval, up to 2 or 4 years after infesta-tion, there may be no evidence of disease else-where in the body and ova may be difficult to find in the faeces. The cerebrospinal fluid usually shows an excess of protein with a slight to moderate rise in lymphocyte count. Neither eosinophil leucocytes nor ova have been found in the cerebrospinal fluid.

Kane and Most describe an unusual ophthalmo-scopic appearance which may have been evidence of invasion of the choroid or retina by ova. It appeared as 'a billowy white mass which measured 1 by 1½ disc diameters, was triangular and lay in the fork made by branches of the inferior temporal vein, with oedema of the surrounding retina'.

Invasion of the brain by the ova of S. japonicum may be diffuse or focal. When diffuse, miliary granulomas may be found in all parts of the cerebrum. They are most common in the grey matter of the cortex and basal ganglia, but may occur also in the white matter. Bassett and Lowenberg (1949) describe the appearances at operation as 'innumerable, shotty, yellow-orange, glistening, discrete nodules ranging in size from 1 to 2 mm to a half centimetre in diameter' scattered over the exposed cortical surface which included parietal, temporal and occipital lobes. In other cases a localized, fairly large mass of granuloma, at first sight resembling a glioblastoma multiforme, has been found at operation, or an agglomeration of smaller nodules up to 3 cm in diameter has been seen on the surface of the brain. Occasionally the dura mater is invaded by granulomas.

On naked-eye examination multiple white nodules of pinpoint or pinhead size, or cream-coloured areas resembling minute abscesses, may be seen on the surface of the brain or on section

enclosed in a multinucleated foreign body giant cell. When several lie together there is a central zone of pyknotic and necrotic nuclei and around this a zone of fibroblastic and endothelial cells. A few foreign body giant cells may be present in this zone. External to this there is a wall of varying thickness consisting of collagen fibres infiltrated with inflammatory cells. These vary greatly from case to case. In early lesions the cellular exudate, which consists predominantly of eosinophil leucocytes, is very abundant and there is relatively little collagen. In more chronic

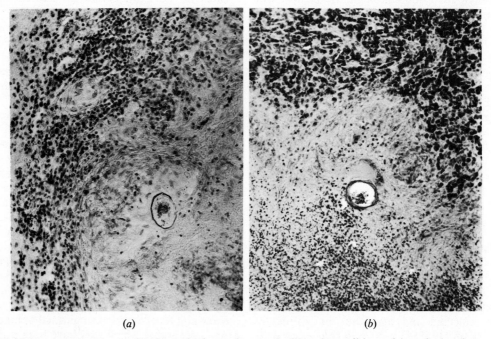

(a)   (b)

Fig. 7.5 *Schistosoma japonicum.* Ova in cerebral granulomas. In (b) a giant cell is partly enveloping the ovum. (a) Haematoxylin van Gieson. (b) Nissl. (Case of Greenfield and Pritchard, 1937.)

of the excised tissue. This is usually firm and rubbery and when cut may feel gritty from the deposition of calcium salts.

Histological sections show a number of small granulomas containing a smaller or larger number of ova. These are oval measuring 60 to 90 μm in length by 40 to 60 μm in width. Many have a blunt spine midway between the centre and the anterior pole. Paired salivary glands may be seen near the anterior end and a number of germ cell nuclei in the centre and towards the posterior end of the ovum (Fig. 7.5). When they lie singly they may be surrounded by a zone of radially arranged fibroblasts or may be partly

lesions the amount of collagen increases and the exudate consists chiefly of lymphocytes and plasma cells with a small number of neutrophil and eosinophil leucocytes. This zone may be very wide, forming the greater part of the granuloma, and giving the mass a firm rubbery texture. It passes externally into a zone of more normal brain tissue in which degenerated or chromatolytic neurons and swollen-bodied astrocytes are seen near the granuloma.

It is clear that the granuloma is formed by the reaction of the tissues to an irritant or toxic substance in the ova. This appears to be present only when they are alive, as, under treatment with antimony, neurological symptoms usually clear up rapidly even when no decompressive craniotomy is performed. The method by which ova reach the brain presents some difficulty. It is unlikely that they come from adult worms lying in their usual situation in superior mesenteric veins, but embolism of ova to the brain might occur if adult worms lay in the pulmonary venules. In this case diffuse dissemination of small lesions would be expected. The larger more focal lesions have usually been found in the occipital, temporal or posterior parietal lobes, and more often on the left side than the right. The condensation of very numerous ova in a localized area of the brain in these cases suggests deposition *in situ* by the female worm lying in a cerebral venous sinus, or large superficial cerebral vein (Greenfield and Pritchard 1937). The usual arrangement at the torcular by which the larger volume of blood passes into the right lateral sinus may account for the preference for the left side.

Symptomatic involvement of the central nervous system is less common in infestations with either *S. haematobium* or *S. mansoni* but diffuse deposition of ova may occur without any clinical manifestations. Gelfand (1950) in Rhodesia, by digesting tissue from various parts of the brain and brainstem, found ova in 28 out of 50 brains from cases with bilharzial infection. One of these cases died in coma but most were asymptomatic and in none were granulomas macroscopically visible. He also reported a case of myelitis with invasion of the dorsolumbar cord by ova of *S. haematobium*. A few other cases of paraplegia have been reported in which granulomas surrounding ova of *S. haematobium* or *S. mansoni* have been found. Martinez-Niochet and Potenza (1956) collected from the literature six such cases which had occurred in Brazil and Venezuela while Ghaly and El-Banhawy (1973) have reported six cases of spinal compression from Egypt. The granulomas are usually intramedullary and appear to be relatively common in the conus medullaris. Ghaly and El-Banhawy believe that the ova reach the spinal cord by way of venous anastomoses between the vesical and pericolic veins and the vertebral and intraspinal plexuses.

Nematodes

Invasion of the brain by larval forms of round worms is rare compared with the frequency of infestation of other organs, but scattered case reports include instances of cerebral invasion by a great variety of nematodes. In many cases they have been chance findings and there has been little evidence that they have contributed in any way to the fatal disease. In other cases symptoms of cerebral disease have been present before or during the final illness or the patient has died in coma. There have also been a number of clinical reports of organic neurological disease which has been attributed, with some evidence, to this cause. In these cases the predominant nervous symptoms may be those of hemiplegia, encephalitis, meningitis or acute psychosis. These symptoms may be transient or there may be recurrent attacks. In some cases with symptoms of encephalitis or meningitis larvae have been found in the cerebrospinal fluid. These cases as well as those of fatal cerebral disease have been most often caused either by larvae of *trichinella* or by one of the forms of *microfilaria*, usually *Loa-loa* or *Wuchereria bancrofti*.

Trichinella spiralis

The rather rare cases of cerebral disease due to invasion by larvae of trichinella have been reviewed by Most and Abeles (1937) who reported a fatal case. They found granulomatous nodules scattered through the brain especially in the white matter and the deeper layers of the cortex. These were of two kinds. Some were composed entirely of microglia and contained no larvae. Others consisted of a more solid collection of mononuclear cells including lymphocytes, histiocytes and plasma cells and often contained larvae. Perivascular lymphocytic infiltrations, which might be quite heavy, were found in the brain and meninges. In addition, round and oval cavities filled with amorphous mucinoid material were diffusely distributed in the subcortical white matter and the midbrain. Similar cavities were found by Hassin and Diamond (1926) in the frontal lobes and pons. These authors also noted various degenerative changes in the nerve cells near granulomas. They found numerous trichinella larvae free in the tissues without any cellular reaction round them.

Filariasis

Microfilariae, circulating in the blood, must pass through the cerebral vessels, but they only cause cerebral lesions if they are so numerous as to plug capillaries or if they die and disintegrate in the brain. The latter effect may be produced by therapeutic drugs when the infestation is heavy as in a case reported by van Bogaert *et al.* (1955) from the Congo, in which the cerebral lesions were severe and widespread. They consisted of small granulomatous nodules not visible to the naked eye, in most of which one or more microfilariae could be found. In addition there were more diffuse inflammatory and vascular lesions. The granulomas were usually perivascular and were made up of microglial cells and lymphocytes with occasional leucocytes. In some there was a tendency to necrosis of the walls of the central vessel and, when microfilariae were numerous, giant cells, probably of histiocytic origin, were formed in them. They were scattered throughout the cerebral and cerebellar hemispheres, including the basal ganglia, but were less abundant in the brainstem. Some folia of the cerebellum showed ischaemic atrophy, and many of the Purkinje cells in the neighbourhood of granulomatous nodules either had disappeared or showed homogenizing change. In the cerebral cortex there was a diffuse microgliosis with the formation of rod cells and a more focal increase in astrocyte nuclei. Perivenous lymphocytic infiltrations were found both in the meninges and the brain tissue. In the white matter honeycomb or spongy areas, in which the myelin had undergone lysis, were seen round many blood vessels. Of the lesions in other organs the most characteristic were in the liver where multiple small necrotic areas surrounded by lymphocytes and containing degenerated microfilariae were found in the portal spaces.

Infections by fungi

Some fungi may produce disease in man in the absence of any apparent predisposing factors other than increased exposure to a particular fungus due either to occupation or domicile. However, fungi which are not normally pathogenic for man may become so if the natural defences of the body are lowered. This may occur as a result of chronic debilitating diseases such as diabetes mellitus, leukaemia, the lymphomas or other disseminated malignant processes, or by the prolonged use of antibiotics, corticosteroids, cytotoxic drugs or immunosuppressive agents. Infections of this type are referred to as *opportunistic* and, in such infections, the nervous system is frequently affected. Greater attention has been paid to these infections since fungicidal agents have become increasingly available.

Fungal infections of the nervous system are invariably secondary to infection elsewhere in the body but lesions at the portal of entry may be small and readily overlooked during life or at autopsy. The brain, therefore, may appear to be the only organ involved. In other cases infection of the nervous system may simply be one manifestation of a systematized infectious process especially when the latter is opportunistic. It is generally accepted that fungi usually reach the nervous system by the blood stream, and that the primary focus is most often in the lung. Occasionally invasion is direct from a primary focus in the paranasal sinuses or the orbit, or when the spinal cord is involved from osteitis in the vertebral column. An excellent survey of fungal infections of the nervous system is that by Fetter, Klintworth and Hendry (1967). In the account which follows, fungus infections which tend to occur in the absence of any known predisposing factors will be described before the opportunistic infections.

Cryptococcus neoformans
Cryptococcosis is probably the commonest fungal infection of the nervous system. It has a worldwide distribution but most reported cases have occurred in the more southern parts of the United States and in Australia (Cox and Tolhurst 1946; Mosberg and Arnold 1950). According to Fetter *et al.* (1967) over 500 cases have been documented. *Cryptococcus neoformans*—known in the past as *Torula histolytica* or Torulosis—is a pathogenic yeast that was first isolated in fermenting fruit juices. It has also been recovered from milk, pigeon manure and mucous membranes in man. Pigeon manure may be an important reservoir of infection, but although *Cryptococcus neoformans* may cause disease in various domestic and wild animals, it has not

been shown to produce a naturally occurring disease in birds.

Cryptococcus neoformans is a round or oval body usually varying in diameter from about 2 to 15 μm and surrounded by a thick polysaccharide capsule. In culture, occasional organisms develop short abortive germ tubes which mimic pseudohyphae (Moss and McQuown 1953). It increases by budding which may be clearly seen in histological sections, and does not form spores. It usually gains access to the body through the respiratory tract but pulmonary cryptococcosis is less commonly encountered clinically than infection of the nervous system. The commonest clinical presentation in man is as a subacute meningitis. In a few cases the disease appears to have been limited to the spinal cord (Ley, Jacas and Oliveras 1951; Carton and Mount 1951). Primary infections of the skin and mucous membranes occur, and invasion may take place through the skin (Greenfield, Martin and Moore 1938).

The cerebrospinal fluid varies greatly from case to case. In some there is a clear fluid with only a small excess of lymphocytes and protein, whereas in others the fluid is turbid and contains large numbers of lymphocytes. There may also be some polymorphonuclear leucocytes. Cryptococci may be seen in the counting chamber or in the centrifuged deposit, and may be cultured from the fluid even when the cell count is low. In dried films the cryptococci may be mistaken for lymphocytes unless their capsules are sought by the appropriate techniques. The protein also varies greatly (from normal to more than 500 mg per 100 ml) and the glucose tends to be reduced or even absent (Rose, Grant and Jeanes 1958).

Pathological findings
On macroscopic examination there is usually diffuse or more localized opacity of the leptomeninges, and flattening of the convolutions and other evidence of raised intracranial pressure. The cerebrospinal fluid is turbid, sometimes yellowish and often glairy, with the result that the surface of the brain is slippery to the touch. Small tubercle-like granules or nodules 2 to 3 mm in diameter may be seen particularly in the interpeduncular fossa and within sulci. On section the typical abnormality is the presence of numerous cystic spaces measuring up to 2 to 3 mm in diameter. They tend to be particularly numerous in the superficial layers of the cortex where they

appear as distensions of perivascular spaces with mucoid material. Deeply placed cysts of similar appearance also occur. In the basal ganglia and sometimes in the white matter the lesions may follow vessels for some distance as sleeves of mucoid material with localized cyst formation in places (Fig. 7.6*a*). Stevenson, Vogel and Williams (1950) described small single subcortical cysts measuring 1 cm or less in diameter as a chance post-mortem finding in three cases, and larger apparently single cysts in the cerebellum or spinal cord have been found at operation.

On histological examination encapsulated cryptococci (Fig. 7.6*c* and *d*) are scattered throughout the meninges either as isolated units or as small collections. The flask-shaped cysts in the superficial layers of the cortex and some of the more deeply placed cysts may contain little except masses of encapsulated cryptococci which appear to push the surrounding tissues aside rather than destroy them. There is often no significant reactive gliosis around these cysts. Reactive inflammatory changes are also often only minimal but in other cases, probably due to the length of the illness, there may be an irregular granulomatous reaction in the subarachnoid space and around some of the perivascular intracerebral lesions. Multinucleate giant cells occur in addition to lymphocytes and occasional plasma cells (Fig. 7.6*b*). The nuclei of the multinucleate cells are sometimes more centrally placed than in typical Langhans-type cells, while cryptococci often without capsules can frequently be seen within them. The cryptococci in the subarachnoid space and in cysts stain well with basic blue dyes and, when lightly stained, may show small dark granules near their surface. When more deeply stained, the capsules owing to shrinkage artefact may appear as radial spicules which stain metachromatically (Fig. 7.6*d*). Cryptococci also stain with the periodic-acid Schiff (PAS) method.

Coccidioides immitis
This is a natural inhabitant of the soil in the semi-arid regions of some parts of the South-Western United States, Mexico and South America. The disease coccidioidal mycosis is endemic in the San Joaquin Valley of California, parts of Arizona, New Mexico and West Texas and in parts of the Argentine and Paraguay. The fungus exists as spherules containing endospores, and hyphae with arthrospores. The latter may

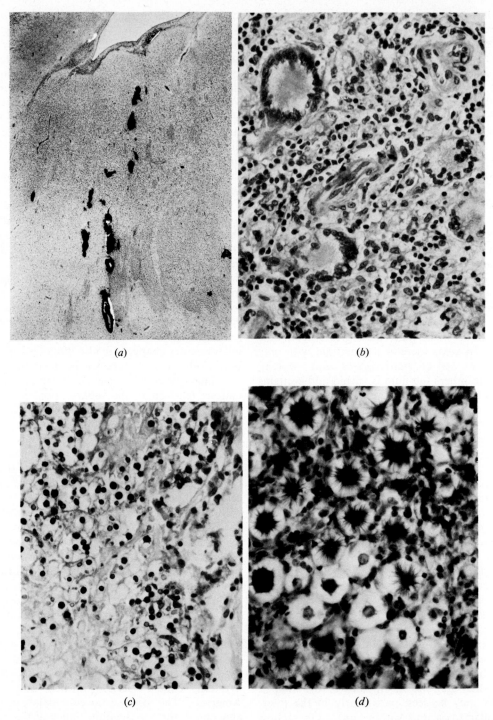

Fig. 7.6 Infection of the brain with *Cryptococcus neoformans*. (*a*) Low power view to show granulomatous infiltration around subventricular veins. Cresyl violet. (*b*) Granulomatous reaction with multinucleate giant cells in the subarachnoid space. H and E. ×250. (*c*) Masses of encapsulated cryptococci in the subarachnoid space. H and E. ×250. (*d*) Higher magnification of cryptococci to show metachromatic spicules of mucopolysaccharide in capsule. Toluidin blue. ×400.

be carried for a considerable distance by the wind and thus give rise to a dust-borne disease. The arthrospores have a high degree of infectivity and are capable of provoking disease in the absence of any underlying predisposing factors. Although coccidioides usually cause only a mild transient febrile illness, this is followed in a significant number of cases by a more chronic form of disease with granulomatous lesions in the lungs. The fungus may then be carried to the brain by the blood stream. The spinal cord may be involved either by haematogenous dissemination or by extradural granulomas arising from the vertebrae (Rand 1930).

Within the cranial cavity coccidioides usually causes a granulomatous meningitis, but more solid granulomas may also occur within the substance of the brain. Histologically the lesions closely resemble those of tuberculosis but many of the giant cells contain the organisms which appear as spherules about 10 to 60 μm in diameter filled with endospores. Organisms may be observed in the cerebrospinal fluid or cultured from it but the diagnosis is more easily made by skin tests or complement fixation tests with the antigen coccidioidin.

Blastomyces dermatidis

This is the causative agent of North American blastomycosis which is restricted to the United States, Canada and Mexico. The regions of high endemicity lie east of the Mississippi. The fungus exists as a filamentous growth and as a yeast but in human infections appears almost invariably as the latter. The round or oval yeast-like bodies are about 10 to 25 μm in diameter and are surrounded by a refractile capsule. Budding is frequently seen.

Blastomyces dermatidis generally gains access to the body via the respiratory tract, where it may produce a primary pulmonary granulomatous disease. Blastomycosis also occurs as a rather rare cause of skin lesions. Involvement of the brain and spinal cord may be due either to haematogenous dissemination or to direct spread of the infection from osteitis in the overlying bone. When paraplegia occurs it is usually due to compression of the spinal cord by an extradural granuloma arising in the vertebrae. A dumb-bell shaped granuloma partly in the spinal canal and partly in the thoracic cavity was described by Craig, Dockerty and Harrington (1940).

Pathological findings

The lesions have a considerable resemblance to those of tuberculosis both macroscopically and microscopically. When the nervous system is involved, meningitis is common but there may also be granulomas or suppurative lesions within the substance of the brain. Microscopic examination shows a combination of granulomatous and suppurative reactions. The centres of more recent nodules in the brain contain neutrophil and eosinophil leucocytes or pus cells, and groups of fungi are usually seen among these. Around the suppurative or caseous cores of nodules there is a zone of macrophages, fibroblasts and giant cells of Langhans type. If the lesions have been present for some time, a denser capsule of hyalinized connective tissue infiltrated with plasma cells forms round the nodule. The yeasts occur free or within giant cells or mononuclear cells. They vary greatly in size, and many may have the single bud which is distinctive for this yeast.

Histoplasma capsulatum

Systemic infections by this fungus are common in the Southern and Middle Western States of America, and a number of cases have also been reported from Brazil, the Argentine, Panama, Southern Rhodesia and Australia. It has appeared in small epidemics in the Middle West States by infection from underground mines, cellars or towers, some of which were full of pigeon droppings (Schwartz and Spitz 1952). Infection probably usually takes place by inhalation. Despite the frequency of this fungus infection in the heavy endemic zones in the United States, involvement of the central nervous system is uncommon. It may take the form of isolated granulomata in the brain or of a more diffuse meningitis. In 23 fatal cases of histoplasmosis occurring in Tennessee, Sprofkin, Shapiro and Lux (1955) found invasion of the brain or the leptomeninges in six. When meningitis is well established, there is a thick yellow exudate over the base of the brain with occasional discrete greyish white opacities resembling tubercles along the lines of vessels particularly in the Sylvian fissures. Microscopically there are large mononuclear phagocytes, lymphocytes and a few polymorphonuclear leucocytes and plasma cells. There may also be small granulomas around vessels in the leptomeninges, and spread along the vessel walls for a short distance into the brain. In chronic cases there may be marked

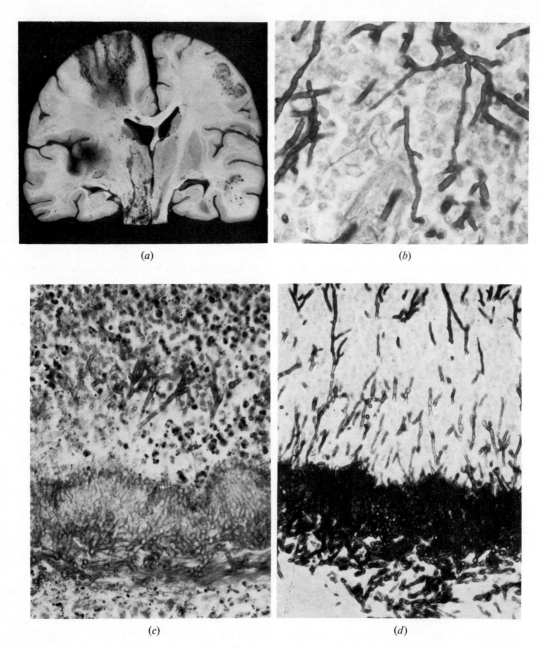

Fig. 7.7 Candidiasis. (a) Note numerous focally haemorrhagic regions in brain. (b) Pseudohyphae in necrotic areas seen in (a). Methenamine silver. × 400. (c) and (d) Meningeal vessel. The vessel wall (bottom) is necrotic and almost totally replaced by fungus. (c) H and E. (d) Methenamine silver. × 250.

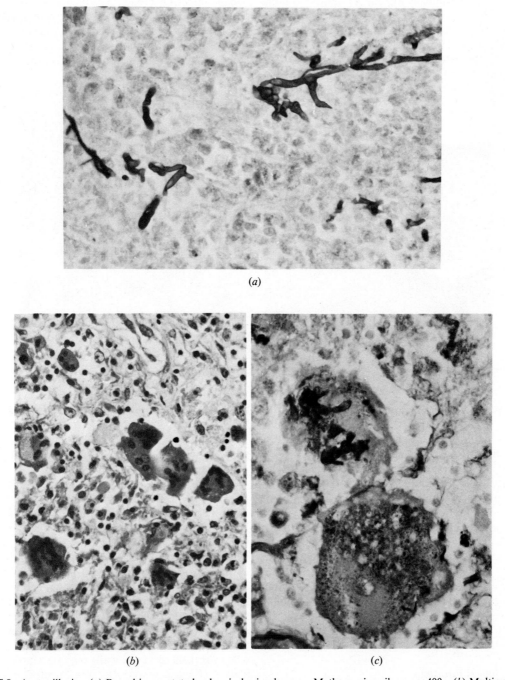

(a)

(b)

(c)

Fig. 7.8 Aspergillosis. (*a*) Branching septate hyphae in brain abscess. Methenamine silver. × 400. (*b*) Multinucleate giant cells at edge of abscess. H and E. × 250. (*c*) Remnants of fungus within giant cells. Methenamine silver. × 400.

meningeal fibrosis. Granulomas within the brain may be single or multiple. Suppuration does not occur. The organisms appear as lightly staining basophilic structures measuring 2 to 5 μm in diameter, ovoid, pyriform or crescentic, and surrounded by a clear halo. They are most often found in the cytoplasm of macrophages.

of any predisposing factors. Infection of the brain may simply be one feature of a systematized fungal infection (Black 1970), or it may appear to be the only manifestation (Mukoyama, Gimple and Poser 1969). In the latter circumstances, the 'primary' lesion, e.g. in the lung, may be small and inconspicuous. Infection of the

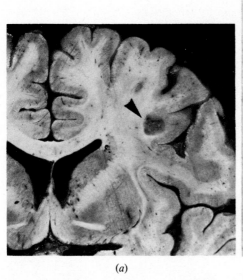

(a)

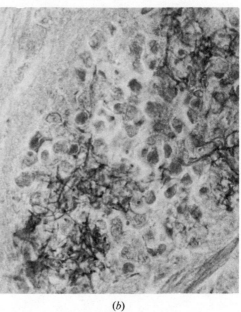

(b)

Fig. 7.9 Nocardiosis. (a) Small abscess in brain (arrow). (b) Delicate branching hyphae in the abscess. Methenamine silver. ×540.

Actinomycosis

This is a chronic suppurative disease which occurs principally in cervicofacial or alimentary forms and only rarely spreads to the nervous system, either directly from cervicofacial lesions or by the blood stream from infection of the alimentary tract. The pathology of cerebral abscess or meningitis is similar to that elsewhere in the body. Abscesses are often multilocular, and the pus contains colonies of actinomyces (sulphur granules) which consists of delicate branching hyphae. Around the 'sulphur granules' the hyphae are radially disposed and often have club-shaped outlines.

Other fungal infections

These are mainly *opportunistic infections*, the commonest being caused by *Candida albicans*, *Aspergillus fumigatus* and *Nocardia asteroides* although nocardia may infect man in the absence

nervous system is usually attributed to haematogenous spread from a primary lesion.

These three fungi generally produce abscesses of varying size, often multiple, in the brain. Early in the disease process, the lesions resemble haemorrhagic infarcts (Fig. 7.7a). Later they usually become well-defined abscesses (Fig. 7.9a). Microscopical examination shows varying degrees of infarction, including necrosis of vessel walls, and a dense infiltrate of polymorphonuclear leucocytes. Aspergillus may provoke a granulomatous reaction characterized by the presence of multinucleate giant cells (Figs. 7.8b and c). Candida may also produce a florid meningitis when necrosis of vessel walls may be a prominent feature (Figs. 7.7c and d). The purulent exudate usually contains easily identifiable mycelia. The larger of these fungi, candida and aspergillus, may be seen in sections stained by haematoxylin and eosin, but they are most easily seen in sections stained by Grocott's methenamine silver technique (Figs. 7.7b and 7.8a). Candida appears in tissue as yeast forms with pseudohyphae which may virtually replace necrotic vessel walls, aspergillus as branching septate hyphae without yeast forms, and nocardia as rather delicate branching hyphae that readily fragment into coccal and bacillary forms (Fig. 7.9b).

Accurate identification of the fungus can only be based on its characteristics in culture.

A further rarer opportunistic infection of the nervous system is *mucormycosis* (phycomycosis). It has a particular propensity to infect uncontrolled diabetic patients but is not confined to them (Gregory, Golden and Haymaker 1943; Vorreith 1968). It may cause a more or less localized meningitis by spread from an infected paranasal air sinus (Wolf and Cowen 1949), but then extends into the inferior parts of the frontal lobes where it produces extensive necrosis of brain tissue. When the fungus reaches the brain by the blood stream, it characteristically produces extensive haemorrhagic infarction. Microscopical examination shows necrosis of tissue and vessel walls, often only mild inflammatory changes, and large branching non-septate hyphae.

References

Apley, J., Clarke, S. K. R., Roome, A. P. C. H., Sandry, S. A., Saygi, G., Silk, B. & Warhurst, D. C. (1970) Primary amoebic meningoencephalitis in Britain. *British Medical Journal*, **1**, 596-599.

Arana, R. & Asenjo, A. (1945) Ventriculographic diagnosis of cysticercosis of the posterior fossa. *Journal of Neurosurgery*, **2**, 181-190.

Arana-Iniguez, R. & San Julian, J. (1955) Hydatid cysts of the brain. *Journal of Neurosurgery*, **12**, 323-335.

Bassett, R. C. & Lowenberg, K. (1949) Cerebral schistosomiasis. *Journal of Neuropathology and Experimental Neurology*, **8**, 220-225.

Becker, B. J. B. & Jacobson, S. (1951) Infestation of the human brain with *Coenurus cerebralis*. *Lancet*, **2**, 1202-1204.

Bertrand, I., Bablet, J. & Sicé, A. (1935) Lésions histologiques des centres nerveux dans la trypanosomiase humaine. *Annales de l'Institut Pasteur*, **54**, 91-144.

Beverley, J. K. A. (1973) Toxoplasmosis. *British Medical Journal*, **2**, 475-478.

Bickerstaff, E. R., Cloake, P. C. P., Hughes, B. & Smith, W. T. (1952) The racemose form of cerebral cysticercosis. *Brain*, **75**, 1-18.

Black, J. T. (1970) Cerebral candidiasis: case report and review of literature. *Journal of Neurology, Neurosurgery and Psychiatry*, **33**, 864-870.

Bogaert, L. van, Dubois, A., Janssens, P. G., Radermecker, J., Tverdy, G. & Wanson, M. (1955) Encephalitis in loaloa filariasis. *Journal of Neurology, Neurosurgery and Psychiatry*, **18**, 103-119.

Butt, C. G. (1966) Primary amebic meningoencephalitis. *New England Journal of Medicine*, **274**, 1473-1476.

Calwell, H. G. (1937) The pathology of the brain in Rhodesian trypanosomiasis. *Transactions of the Royal Society of Tropical Medicine and Hygiene*, **30**, 611-624.

Carter, R. F. (1972) Primary amoebic meningo-encephalitis: an appraisal of present knowledge. *Transactions of the Royal Society of Tropical Medicine and Hygiene*, **66**, 193-208.

Carton, C. A. & Mount, L. A. (1951) Neurosurgical aspects of cryptococcosis. *Journal of Neurosurgery*, **8**, 143-156.

Chu, C. F. (1931) Schistosomiasis japonica in Nanking. *Chinese Medical Journal*, **52**, 651-664.

Cox, L. B. & Tolhurst, J. C. (1946) In *Human Torulosis*, Oxford University Press, London.

Craig, W. McK., Dockerty, M. B. & Harrington, S. W. (1940) Intravertebral and intrathoracic blastomycoma simulating dumb-bell tumour. *Southern Surgeon*, **9**, 759-766.

Culbertson, C. G. (1961) Pathogenic *Acanthamoeba* (*Hartmanella*). *American Journal of Clinical Pathology*, **35**, 185-197.

Culbertson, C. G., Smith, J. W., Cohen, H. K. & Minner, J. R. (1959) Experimental infection of mice and monkeys by *Acanthamoeba*. *American Journal of Pathology*, **35**, 185-197.

Dew, H. R. (1934) Hydatid disease of brain. *Surgery, Gynecology and Obstetrics*, **59**, 321-329.

Egan, C. H. (1936) An outbreak of *Schistosomiasis japonicum*. *Journal of the Royal Naval Medical Service*, **22**, 6-18.

Fetter, B. F., Klintworth, G. K. & Hendry, W. S. (1967) *Mycoses of the Central Nervous System*, Williams and Wilkins, Baltimore.

Fowler, M. & Carter, R. F. (1965) Acute pyogenic meningitis probably due to *Acanthamoeba* sp.: a preliminary report. *British Medical Journal*, **2**, 740-742.

Gard, S. & Magnusson, J. H.   (1951) A glandular form of toxoplasmosis in connection with pregnancy.   *Acta medica Scandinavica*, **141**, 59-64.

Gelfand, M.   (1950) *Schistosomiasis in S. Central Africa*, Juta, Cape Town.

Ghaly, A. F. & El-Banhawy, A.   (1973) Schistosomiasis of the spinal cord.   *Journal of Pathology*, **111**, 57-60.

Greenfield, J. G. & Pritchard, E. A. B.   (1937) Cerebral infection with *Schistosoma japonicum*.   *Brain*, **60**, 361-372.

Greenfield, J. G., Martin, J. P. & Moore, M. T.   (1938) Meningo-encephalitis due to cryptococcus meningitidis (torula histolytica) with a report of a case.   *Lancet*, **2**, 1154-1157.

Gregory, J. E., Golden, A. & Haymaker, W.   (1943) Mucormycosis of the central nervous system: report of three cases.   *Bulletin of the Johns Hopkins Hospital*, **73**, 405-419.

Halpert, B. & Ashley, J. D.   (1944) Amebic colitis complicated with abscess of the brain.   *Archives of Pathology*, **38**, 112-114.

Hassin, G. B. & Diamond, I. B.   (1926) Trichinosis encephalitis: a pathological study.   *Archives of Neurology and Psychiatry (Chicago)*, **15**, 34-47.

Hawking, F. & Greenfield, J. G.   (1941) Two autopsies on Rhodesiense sleeping sickness; visceral lesions and significance of changes in cerebrospinal fluid.   *Transactions of the Royal Society of Tropical Medicine and Hygiene*, **35**, 155-164.

Herskowitz, A.   (1972) Spinal cord involvement with *Schistosoma mansoni*.   *Journal of Neurosurgery*, **36**, 494-498.

Houghton, H. S.   (1910) Notes on infections with Schistosomum japonicum.   *Journal of Tropical Medicine and Hygiene*, **13**, 185-187.

Hutchison, W. M., Dunachie, J. F., Siim, J. C. & Work, K.   (1970) Coccidian-like nature of *Toxoplasma gondii*.   *British Medical Journal*, **1**, 142-144.

Jager, B. V. & Stamm, W. B.   (1972) Brain abscess caused by free-living amoeba probably of the genus *Hartmannella* in a patient with Hodgkin's disease.   *Lancet*, **2**, 1342-1345.

Jansen, P., Bogaert, L. van & Haymaker, W.   (1956) Pathology of peripheral nervous system in African trypanosomiasis; study of 7 cases.   *Journal of Neuropathology and Experimental Neurology*, **15**, 269-287.

Kane, C. A. & Most, H.   (1948) Schistosomiasis of the central nervous system.   *Archives of Neurology and Psychiatry (Chicago)*, **59**, 141-184.

Kim, S. K.   (1955) Cerebral paragonimiasis.   *Journal of Neurosurgery*, **12**, 89-94.

Koppisch, E.   (1953) Protozoal and helminthic infections in *Pathology* (Ed. Anderson, W. A. D.), Kimpton, London.

Kuper, S., Mendelow, H. & Proctor, N. S. F.   (1958) Internal hydrocephalus caused by parasitic cysts.   *Brain*, **81**, 235-242.

Langmaid, C. & Rogers, L.   (1940) Intracranial hydatids.   *Brain*, **63**, 184-190.

Ley, A., Jacas, R. & Oliveras, C.   (1951) Torula granuloma of the cervical spinal cord.   *Journal of Neurosurgery*, **8**, 327-335.

MacArthur, W. P.   (1933) Cysticercosis as seen in the British Army with special reference to the production of epilepsy.   *Transactions of the Royal Society of Tropical Medicine and Hygiene*, **27**, 343-363.

Manuelidis, E. E., Robertson, D. H. H., Amberson, J. M., Polak, M. & Haymaker, W.   (1965) *Trypanosoma rhodesiense* encephalitis.   *Acta Neuropathologica (Berlin)*, **5**, 176-204.

Martinez-Niochet, A. & Potenza, L.   (1956) Bilharziasis mansoni de la médula espinal simulando tumour.   *Acta Neurológica Latinoamericana*, **2**, 72-76.

Menon, T. B. & Veliath, G. D.   (1940) Tissue reactions to Cysticercus cellulosae in man.   *Transactions of the Royal Society of Tropical Medicine and Hygiene*, **33**, 537-544.

Mosberg, W. H. & Arnold, J. G.   (1950) Torulosis of the central nervous system: review of literature and report of five cases.   *Annals of Internal Medicine*, **32**, 1153-1183.

Moss, E. S. & McQuown, A. L.   (1953) In *Atlas of Medical Mycology*, Williams and Wilkins, Baltimore.

Most, H. & Abeles, M. M.   (1937) Trichiniasis involving nervous system: clinical and neuropathologic review, with report of 2 cases.   *Archives of Neurology and Psychiatry (Chicago)*, **37**, 589-616.

Mott, F. W.   (1906) Reports of Sleeping Sickness Commission, No. 7.   Bale and Danielsson, London.

Mukoyama, M., Gimple, K & Poser, C. M.   (1969) Aspergillosis of the central nervous system: report of a brain abscess due to A. fumigatus and review of literature.   *Neurology (Minneapolis)*, **19**, 967-974.

Neujean, G.   (1950) Contribution à l'étude des liquides rachidiennes cephaliques dans la maladie du sommeil à 'trypanosoma gambiense'.   *Annales de la Société belge de médicine tropicale*, **30**, 1125-1387.

Obrador S.   (1948) Clinical aspects of cerebral cysticercosis.   *Archives of Neurology and Psychiatry (Chicago)*, **59**, 457-468.

Phillips, G.   (1948) Primary cerebral hydatid cysts.   *Journal of Neurology and Psychiatry*, **11**, 44-52.

Pinkerton, H. & Henderson, R. G.   (1941) Adult toxoplasmosis: a previously unrecognised disease entity simulating the typhus spotted fever group.   *Journal of the American Medical Association*, **116**, 807-814.

Rand, C. W. (1930) Coccidioidal granuloma: two cases simulating tumour of spinal cord. *Archives of Neurology and Psychiatry (Chicago)*, **23**, 502-511.

Robert, V. B. & Rorke, L. B.   (1973) Primary amebic encephalitis, probably from *Acanthamoeba*.   *Annals of Internal Medicine*, **79**, 174-179.

Rose, F. C., Grant, H. C. & Jeanes, A. L.   (1958) Torulosis of the central nervous system in Britain.   *Brain*, **81**, 542-555.

Sabin, A. B.   (1941) Toxoplasmic encephalitis in children.   *Journal of the American Medical Association*, **116**, 801-807.

Schwartz, B. & Spitz, L. J.   (1952) Histoplasmosis in epidemic form.   *Archives of Internal Medicine*, **89**, 541-546.

Siim, J. C.   (1951) Acquired toxoplasmosis: report of seven cases with strongly positive serological reactions. *Journal of the American Medical Association*, **147**, 1641-1645.

Siim, J. C.   (1955) Discussion on toxoplasmosis.   *Proceedings of the Royal Society of Medicine*, **48**, 1067-1071.

Sprofkin, B. E., Shapiro, J. L. & Lux, J. J.   (1955) Histoplasmosis of the central nervous system: case report of Histoplasma meningitis.   *Journal of Neuropathology and Experimental Neurology*, **14**, 288-296.

Stepien, L. & Chorobski, J.   (1949) Cysticercosis cerebri and its operative treatment.   *Archives of Neurology and Psychiatry (Chicago)*, **61**, 499-527.

Stevenson, L. D., Vogel, F. S. & Williams, V.   (1950) Cryptococcosis of the central nervous system and incidental cryptococcic granuloma.   *Archives of Pathology*, **49**, 321-332.

Thomas, H. M. & Gage, D. P.   (1945) Symptomatology of early *Schistosomiasis Japonica*.   *Bulletin of the U.S. Army Medical Department*, **4**, 197-202.

Vorreith, M.   (1968) Mycotic encephalitis.   *Acta Neuropathologica (Berlin)*, **11**, 55-68.

Wolf, A. & Cowen, D.   (1937) Granulomatous encephalomyelitis due to Encephalitozoon; new protozoan disease of man.   *Bulletin of the New York Neurological Institute*, **6**, 306-371.

Wolf, A. & Cowen, D.   (1949) Mucormycosis of the central nervous system.   *Journal of Neuropathology and Experimental Neurology*, **8**, 107-110.

Woodland, L. J.   (1949) Hydatid disease of vertebrae.   *Medical Journal of Australia*, **2**, 904-910.

8

Virus Diseases of the Nervous System

Revised by J. Hume Adams

Encephalitis, or brain fever, has been a common clinical diagnosis for several centuries, but knowledge of the aetiology of most forms has only been acquired during the last fifty years. Epidemics of encephalitis may have occurred on the continent of Europe in 1580 and in London in the 1670s. In the eighteenth and nineteenth centuries there were clinical descriptions of epidemics of sleeping sickness and of encephalitis which appeared to be specially related to an influenzal type of illness. The first viral encephalitis to be recognized clinically appears to have been rabies. It was also the first viral encephalitis confirmed by inoculation and transfer. However, until the advent of encephalitis lethargica, pathological descriptions of encephalitis were rare and, by modern criteria, unsatisfactory. A major advance was made by Landsteiner and Popper (1908, 1909) and by Flexner and Amos (1914) when they demonstrated that poliomyelitis was due to a virus. Clinicians and laboratory workers were thus prepared to recognize the viral origin of encephalitis lethargica in the pandemic between 1917 and 1926, but despite the intensive virological studies that were undertaken during this period, no virus was consistently isolated from patients with this disease.

It is now known that many viruses may be pathogenic for the central nervous system in man. The reservoir of some of these viruses is man himself when their distribution is worldwide: common examples are herpes simplex virus and poliovirus. Other viruses have an animal reservoir. Some of these are arthropod-borne and are known as arboviruses: they are restricted to those parts of the world in which the arthropod concerned is endemic. A further group of viruses, such as rabies or B virus, may be transmitted by animal secretions. This group may also have a worldwide distribution since the animal which harbours the virus, e.g. the monkey in the case of B virus, may be transported by man far beyond its natural habitat. In the first half of the twentieth century viruses were generally classified as pantropic, viscerotropic or neurotropic, but increasing knowledge of the way in which viruses proliferate in the body has shown that these clearly defined subdivisions are no longer tenable. The term neurotropic has, however, tended to be retained for viruses which produce significant and consistent lesions in the nervous system.

Viruses affecting the nervous system produce a meningo-encephalitis but the majority of patients with acute virus infections of the nervous system present as cases of aseptic meningitis *or* of encephalitis. In some types of encephalitis due, for example, to the polioviruses or other enteroviruses, the most severe lesions occur in the spinal cord when the term 'paralytic disease' is often appropriate clinically. Although *aseptic meningitis* is the commonest clinical illness, due for example to mumps virus or the enteroviruses, relatively little is known about the neuropathology of these diseases since they are rarely fatal unless there has been some complicating episode such as status epilepticus; in such circumstances hypoxic damage will probably be more conspicuous than inflammation on microscopical examination of the brain. The various types of virus *encephalitis* (including paralytic disease) present essentially similar microscopical abnormalities but the distribution of the more severe lesions in the central nervous system is different. Indeed, it is mainly on the basis of the distribution of lesions in the nervous system that the neuropathologist can hazard a guess as to the type of viral encephalitis he has encountered, but he cannot often diagnose a specific type of encephalitis: thus, while he may be able to conclude on the basis of the clinical, radiological, neuropathological and ultrastructural findings that a patient has almost certainly died of herpes simplex encephalitis, he will be unable to distinguish a case of paralytic disease caused by poliovirus from one due to one of the other enteroviruses. Fortunately the need for such a decision is rare now that isolation of virus and serological tests are pursued much more actively than in the past.

As chemotherapy can now control most bacterial infections of the nervous system, greater attention is being paid to virus diseases, and much new information has been gained by the combined efforts of clinicians, virologists, biochemists, cell biologists, immunologists and neuropathologists. Furthermore, since potential antiviral agents have become available such as idoxuridine and cytosine arabinoside in the treatment of herpes simplex encephalitis (Rappel 1973), the retrospective and, in a way, academic diagnosis of particular virus diseases of the nervous system may have to be replaced by a more active approach aimed at making an early positive diagnosis. In the hope that more effective antiviral agents will become available in the future, early diagnosis must be the aim of the clinician, the virologist and the neuropathologist, and this often requires brain biopsy through a burr hole (Adams 1972; Adams and Miller 1973; Ross 1973). Early diagnosis, however, can only be achieved on the basis of a clearer understanding of the clinical and neuropathological features of acute virus infections of the nervous system.

Aseptic meningitis and encephalitis have been recognized for many years, but only relatively recently have *persistent virus infections* of the nervous system such as subacute sclerosing panencephalitis, and *slow virus infections* such as kuru, been widely recognized as important in diseases of the nervous system in man. This section will deal with the commoner acute viral infections, persistent virus infections and slow virus infections of the nervous system.

Pathogenesis

Many aspects of the pathogenesis of some acute virus diseases of the nervous system such as the source of infection, the sites of implantation and of primary and secondary viral multiplication, the route of spread of virus to the nervous system, and its distribution in the brain, spinal cord and meninges are not yet fully understood. One reason is that the clinical features indicative of involvement of the nervous system are often observed late in the course of the infection. Indeed, the fact that clinical symptoms tend not to occur until viraemia is subsiding, and antibody has started to circulate, has led to the concept that inflammation and oedema resulting from the reaction of virus antigen and antibody in the walls of small vessels are important factors contributing to brain damage (Webb 1969). A second reason is that only a proportion of individuals infected by a potentially neurotropic virus develop clinical evidence of disease of the nervous system.

Viruses which cause encephalitis may gain access to the body by various routes, e.g. infection of the surface of the skin or of a mucosa (herpes simplex virus or enteroviruses), infection through injured skin (B virus or rabies), or introduction through the skin by the bite of an arthropod (arboviruses). A few viruses travel along peripheral nerves to the nervous system, e.g. rabies virus, but it is generally accepted that most viruses reach the nervous system by way of the blood stream, often after primary viral multiplication in lymphoid tissue. In the experimental situation some viruses, e.g. polioviruses, may readily spread along nerve trunks (Howe and Bodian 1942) but it does not necessarily follow that this is the natural route of infection in man (Wright 1959).

The general pathological features of virus infections of the central nervous system

The reactions of the brain and spinal cord to inflammation are somewhat stereotyped and tend to be similar in all forms of virus encephalitis. However, they vary both in the emphasis on one or other type of reaction, and in their distribution throughout the cerebrospinal axis.

In a patient who has died as a result of an acute virus infection of the nervous system, the brain may appear macroscopically normal, particularly if death occurs within a few days of the onset of the disease. In other cases there may be diffuse or localized swelling and slight softening of brain tissue, and sometimes frank necrosis (Fig. 8.2a). The latter, however, may be difficult to recognize if it is not haemorrhagic, particularly if the brain is not properly fixed. There are, however, several characteristic histological abnormalities, the intensity of reactive changes and the types of cell present depending largely on the duration of the illness.

Infiltration by inflammatory cells

This is usually the most conspicuous histological abnormality and, even in those types of encephalitis in which some parts of the brain are selectively and severely involved, cellular infiltration is usually seen diffusely throughout the brain and spinal cord. In the earliest stages of one of the more acute forms of encephalitis, the cellular infiltrate may consist largely of neutrophil leucocytes some of which lie free in the tissues. At a slightly later stage in acute forms, and in less acute forms, the exudate consists almost entirely of mononuclear cells—lymphocytes, plasma cells and large mononuclear phagocytes. A single layer of mononuclear cells in the Virchow–Robin space of small venules, and thicker cuffs of mononuclear cells around the larger vessels (Fig. 8.1*a*) are particularly characteristic features, this infiltration being referred to as *perivascular cuffing*. After the first week or so plasma cells, which may be mature or immature, become more numerous around the vessels. In the absence of tissue necrosis, inflammatory cells tend to be restricted to perivascular spaces but, when necrosis is present, lymphocytes and plasma cells stream out into the abnormal brain tissue. Another typical histological feature of encephalitis is diffuse infiltration of the leptomeninges by inflammatory cells: mononuclear cells again predominate but polymorphonuclear leucocytes may be numerous in the early stage of acute infections.

Hyperplasia and proliferation of microglia

This is frequently seen throughout the cortex, and often also in the basal ganglia and brainstem, in patients who have survived for more than a few days after the onset of encephalitis. The microglia become hypertrophied to form rod cells and cells with long, curved and slightly convoluted nuclei. Microglial activity is particularly intense in and around regions of tissue destruction where many lipid phagocytes will be seen if the patient survives long enough. Other characteristic features brought about by reactive changes in the microglia are neuronophagia and the formation of small microglial stars. *Neuronophagia* is the term used to describe a dense mass of hyper-

trophied microglial cells around and obscuring a dead nerve cell (Fig. 8.1*b*). In particularly acute infections, e.g. a rapidly fatal case of poliomyelitis, polymorphonuclear leucocytes contribute to the mass of cells. *Microglial stars* are collections of hypertrophied microglial cells not specifically related to a nerve cell and occurring mainly in the white matter (Fig. 8.1*c*). Neuronophagia and microglial stars, however, are not restricted to virus encephalitis as both may occur in hypoxic brain damage, while microglial stars occur in the white matter in large numbers in patients with diffuse white matter damage as a result of a head injury (Mitchell and Adams 1973). In some types of encephalitis, e.g. St Louis and equine encephalomyelitis, there may be larger accumulations of microglia, lymphocytes and other mononuclear cells: these may be referred to as *glio-mesenchymal nodules*.

Alterations in astrocytes

In acute encephalitis, reactive changes in astrocytes are usually restricted to regions of tissue destruction. In subacute encephalitis, e.g. subacute sclerosing panencephalitis, there may be considerable and diffuse hypertrophy of astrocytes, and a fibrous gliosis (Fig. 8.9*b*).

Changes in neurons

These are of frequent occurrence but are by no means characteristic unless there is actual necrosis of nerve cells and neuronophagia. Various nonspecific changes such as some loss of Nissl granules, swelling of the perikaryon, and eosinophilia of the cytoplasm have been described, but these should be interpreted with caution because of the possibility that they are not related directly to the virus infection but to terminal disturbances of the cerebral circulation. Autolysis may also play a part, particularly in the present era of intensive nursing care and assisted ventilation.

Inclusion bodies

Various forms of inclusion body may be found in neurons, astrocytes and oligodendroglia in virus encephalitis. The great majority are intranuclear but probably the only inclusion body that is pathognomonic of a specific infection is the intracytoplasmic Negri body of rabies. Intranuclear inclusions are conventionally divided into type A and type B (Cowdry 1934). While the majority of intranuclear inclusion bodies are eosinophilic, some appear as almost unstained but clearly defined homogeneous masses within the nucleus.

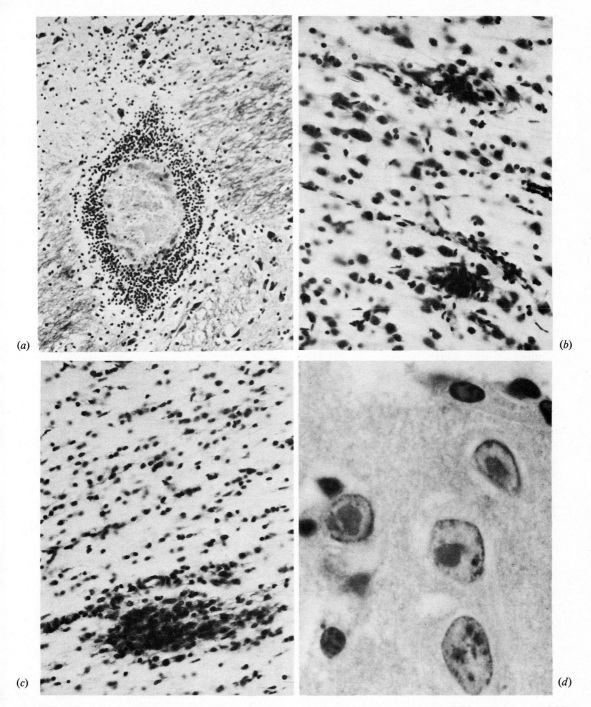

Fig. 8.1 (*a*) Perivascular cuffing in a case of acute necrotizing encephalitis. Note the mononuclear cells around a fairly large vessel in the pons (from Adams 1973). H and E. ×150. (*b*) Neuronophagia in a case of subacute sclerosing panencephalitis. Two neurons in the cerebral cortex are obscured by microglia (from Adams 1973). Cresyl violet. ×250. (*c*) Microglial star in a case of acute necrotizing encephalitis. Note the large aggregate of microglial cells in the white matter in the brain stem. There is also diffuse hypertrophy of microglia (from Adams 1973). Cresyl violet. ×250. (*d*) Type A intranuclear inclusion bodies in a case of acute necrotizing encephalitis. Three neuronal nuclei contain inclusion bodies. H and E. ×1200.

Type A inclusions may be amorphous or finely granular; they are usually spherical or oval, have a clearly defined edge, and are sometimes surrounded by a clear halo (Fig. 8.1*d*). The nuclear chromatin is collected in granules under the nuclear membrane. When fully developed the inclusion may occupy the greater part of the nucleus leaving a clear zone between it and the nuclear membrane, or it may entirely fill the nucleus except for a ring of fine chromatin granules. Type A inclusions strongly suggest a virus infection and are seen in several types of encephalitis including those due to herpes simplex virus, B virus, and cytomegalovirus, and in subacute sclerosing panencephalitis.

Type B intranuclear inclusions are small and spherical, and may be multiple. They do not cause displacement of nuclear chromatin or of the nucleolus. They may become as large as, or slightly larger than, the nucleolus of the large motor neurons in which they are most often found, e.g. in poliomyelitis.

It is still uncertain whether inclusion bodies are a product of viral metabolism or whether they consist of virus particles suspended within a matrix.

Necrosis
This is frequently seen in the brain in several types of acute viral encephalitis, and may range from selective neuronal necrosis to frank infarction of grey and white matter with varying degrees of necrosis of vessel walls. Necrosis may have a characteristic distribution as in herpes simplex encephalitis, or it may conform to no particular pattern as in equine encephalomyelitis. Terminal rarefaction necrosis or selective neuronal necrosis in susceptible parts of the brain such as the Sommer sector of the hippocampus, the Purkinje cells of the cerebellum, or the thalamus are more likely to be a manifestation of an inadequate supply of oxygen to the brain as a result of other factors such as circulatory disturbances and raised intracranial pressure than to the virus infection *per se*. In cases in which tissue necrosis is an integral part of the encephalitis, the histological features are those of infarction combined with those of inflammation as shown by the presence of cells of inflammatory type and sheets of lipid phagocytes: reactive changes tend to be most intense at three sites—at the edge of the necrotic zone, immediately deep to the pia, and around vessels within the affected tissue (Fig. 8.3*c*). If the patient survives the acute stage, the dead tissue progressively disintegrates and becomes replaced by shrunken, rarefied partly cystic tissue (Fig. 8.2*d*).

Aseptic meningitis
Aseptic meningitis is rarely fatal unless there is some complication such as status epilepticus. There are no specific macroscopic abnormalities. Histological abnormalities are virtually restricted to infiltration of the leptomeninges by mononuclear inflammatory cells, and perivascular cuffing spreading into the superficial layers of the cortex (Fig. 8.3*d*). There may also be aggregates of polymorphonuclear leucocytes in the molecular layer. Neuronophagia, necrosis or inflammatory changes in the deeper structures in the brain are not features of aseptic meningitis.

Cerebrospinal fluid
Alterations in the cerebrospinal fluid are also rather stereotyped in acute viral infections of the central nervous system. The *pressure* may be normal or it may be slightly raised. The fluid is clear and colourless in the majority of cases but in some types of encephalitis, e.g. herpes simplex encephalitis in the acute phase, it may be slightly blood-stained (Adams and Jennett 1967). A coagulum rarely forms. The *cell count* is increased in varying degrees but rarely to more than 200 to 250 per mm^3. In the very early stages, polymorphonuclear leucocytes may sometimes form a proportion of the cells, rarely more than 40 to 50%, but they soon disappear. The cells then consist of lymphocytes, large mononuclear cells and a varying proportion of plasma cells. Mononuclear cells with a remarkably primitive appearance, based on the morphology of the nucleus and a high nucleocytoplasmic ratio, are sometimes seen in acute encephalitis, as are occasional binucleate cells and mitotic figures (Adams and Jennett 1967). The *protein* is slightly raised. *Glucose* and *chlorides* are characteristically normal unless the blood levels of glucose and chlorides are abnormal. The colloidal gold curve may be of mid-zone type or, rarely, paretic.

In subacute encephalitis, e.g. subacute sclerosing panencephalitis, the protein and cell count may be only very slightly increased, but in this disease the colloidal gold curve is often paretic in type. In slow virus infections such as kuru, the cerebrospinal fluid is normal.

Infection of the nervous system by viruses of the herpes group

The central nervous system may be affected by at least four viruses in the herpes group—herpes simplex, varicella–zoster, B virus of monkeys, and cytomegalovirus. All are DNA viruses of similar morphology, that is icosahedrons with axial symmetry. The complete virion has a diameter of 130 to 180 nm. Herpes simplex virus and varicella–zoster commonly affect the central nervous system and have several features in common. There are two antigenically distinguishable subtypes of herpes simplex: type 1 is usually associated with primary oropharyngeal and cutaneous lesions and with acute encephalitis in children and in adults; type 2 is usually associated with genital and perineal lesions and with disseminated neonatal infections (Juel-Jensen and MacCallum 1972). Varicella–zoster produces varicella as a primary infection. The natural host of herpes simplex virus and of varicella–zoster is man, and most individuals acquire their primary infection in childhood. With either virus, the primary infection may be associated with transient systemic symptoms: dissemination of infection via the blood stream is rare but herpes simplex virus may produce acute encephalitis at this time, and varicella–zoster sometimes causes meningo-encephalitis. After the primary infection, circulating antibodies to the viruses remain. Herpes simplex virus remains latent to give rise to sporadic or recurrent labial herpes. Varicella–zoster appears to behave in a similar fashion, zoster being a reactivation of latent virus in a partially immune individual (Hope-Simpson 1965). It has, however, not yet been fully established if sporadic cases of acute herpes simplex encephalitis in adults are due to reactivation of latent virus or to a late primary infection; both probably occur.

B virus is a natural parasite of monkeys and, in them, behaves in a manner very similar to herpes simplex virus in man. When man is infected with B virus, it produces a rapidly progressive myelitis and encephalitis. Cytomegalovirus also causes persistent latent infections (Stern 1972), but significant brain damage probably occurs only as a result of intra-uterine and neonatal infections.

Infection of the central nervous system with herpes simplex virus

Herpes simplex virus affects the central nervous system in one of three ways. The commonest manifestation is a fulminating encephalitis that may occur in any age group with the exception of infants and very young children; this type of encephalitis is often known as *acute necrotizing encephalitis*. There has been considerable discussion about the relationship between acute herpes simplex virus encephalitis and the descriptive term acute necrotizing encephalitis, but this has been based mainly on earlier reports in which detailed virological studies had not been carried out. In a personal experience of some 25 cases with the typical neuropathological features of acute necrotizing encephalitis over the past 10 years (Adams and Miller 1973; Ross 1973), herpes simplex virus has been implicated in every case either as a result of virus isolation from brain biopsy, or a significant increase of complement-fixing antibodies to herpes simplex virus, or the identification of herpes virus particles in brain tissue by electron-microscopy. This is not to say, however, that herpes simplex virus always produces this type of encephalitis in man, as the neuropathological pattern can only be defined in fatal cases.

The second type of involvement of the central nervous system by herpes simplex virus is an encephalitis associated with disseminated infection by the virus in infants. The third is aseptic meningitis which is the least important of the three since it is uncommon and appears to be a benign and self-limiting infection (Juel-Jensen and MacCallum 1972). The precise neuropathology of the condition remains unknown.

Acute necrotizing encephalitis

This appears to be the commonest type of acute encephalitis in Western Europe at the present time and probably also in other temperate latitudes. It mainly affects adolescents and adults of all ages. The typical clinical picture (Adams and Miller 1973) is the sudden onset of an acute febrile encephalitic illness, the most conspicuous early features of which are confusion, headache and meningeal irritation. About half the cases have a history of a preceding mild febrile illness. The patient's conscious level deteriorates rapidly, and focal motor neurological signs and focal epilepsy are common. The distribution of necrosis and swelling in the brain is such that patients fre-

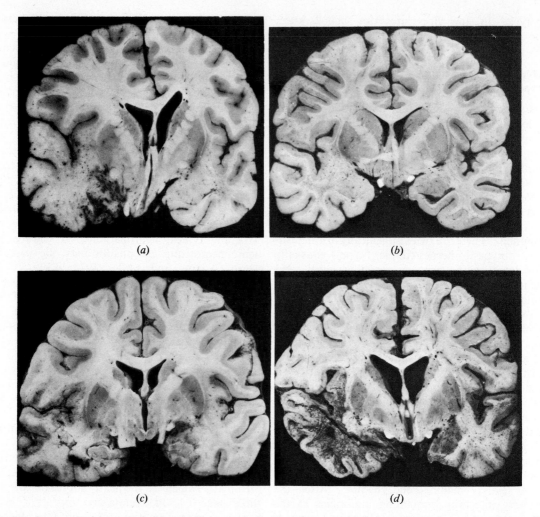

Fig. 8.2 Acute necrotizing encephalitis. (*a*) Short survival. The left temporal lobe is swollen and necrotic and its medial part is focally haemorrhagic. The midline structures are shifted to the right and there are tentorial and supracallosal (subfalcine) herniae (from Adams 1973). (*b*) Short survival. In this case there is no focal haemorrhage or midline shift. Necrosis was more severe in the left hemisphere. Note the loss of definition between cortex and white matter in the medial part of the left temporal lobe compared with the right temporal lobe (from Adams and Miller 1973). (*c*) A few weeks' survival. The abnormal tissue in the more severely affected left hemisphere (temporal lobe, insula and cingulate gyrus) is beginning to disintegrate. Similar but much less severe abnormalities are seen in the right parahippocampal gyrus and in the insula. (*d*) Several weeks' survival. The abnormal regions are now cystic. Note the extensive cavitation in the left temporal lobe and insula compared with the much smaller lesions in the right hemisphere. Necrosis is also clearly seen in the cingulate gyri (from Adams 1973).

quently display many of the clinical and radiological features of an expanding lesion in one temporal lobe (Bennett, ZuRhein and Roberts 1962; Carmon, Behar and Beller 1965; Adams and Jennett 1967). The mortality rate in acute cases is high, while many of the survivors have severe and permanent intellectual and neurological disability (Oxbury and MacCallum 1973).

Pathological findings

These are highly characteristic, the distinctive feature being widespread and asymmetrical necrosis, particularly in the temporal lobes (Haymaker, Smith, van Bogaert and de Chenar 1958; Adams 1969). The distribution of the necrosis is most easily seen in large celloidin sections of brain (Figs. 8.3*a* and *b*). In the more

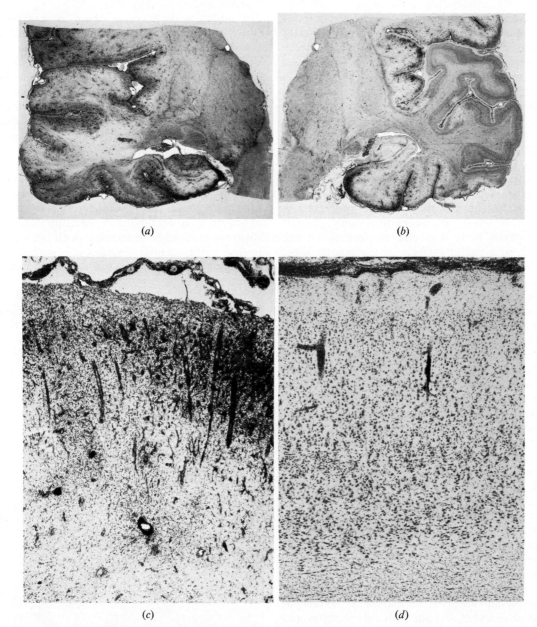

Fig. 8.3 (a) Acute necrotizing encephalitis (a few weeks' survival). Photomicrograph of left temporal lobe to show total necrosis of the cortex of the left temporal lobe, the insula, and the adjacent part of the inferior frontal gyrus (from Adams 1973). Cresyl violet. (b) Same case as (a). In the right temporal lobe, necrosis is much less extensive than on the left, being restricted principally to the parahippocampal, fusiform and inferior temporal gyri and to the insula (from Adams 1973). Cresyl violet. (c) Acute necrotizing encephalitis. Reactive changes—perivascular cuffing and microglial proliferation—are most conspicuous immediately deep to the pia and around vessels (from Adams 1973) Cresyl violet. × 25. (d) Aseptic meningitis. Infiltration by mononuclear cells is restricted to the leptomeninges and to the perivascular spaces in the outer layers of the cortex (from Adams 1973). Cresyl violet. × 40.

severely affected hemisphere, necrosis charac-teristically affects the anterior parts of the parahippocampal, the fusiform and the inferior and middle temporal gyri and the posterior orbital cortex; it may also extend through the superior temporal gyrus to become continuous with necrosis in the insula. The necrosis is not restricted to the neocortex but involves the digitate white matter, the hippocampus, the amygdaloid nucleus and the inferior pole of the putamen. In the less severely affected hemisphere, necrosis in the temporal lobe tends to be restricted to the parahippocampal and fusiform gyri and to the adjacent part of the inferior temporal gyrus. Other areas fairly consistently affected by necrosis are the insulae and the cingulate gyri: this is usually bilateral. In the more severely affected hemisphere, there may also be necrosis on the medial and lateral surfaces of the frontal lobe. Necrosis in other regions is uncommon unless it is secondary to raised intracranial pressure.

In a patient dying in the acute stage the more severely affected temporal lobe is soft and swollen, and there are frequently many of the macroscopic abnormalities conventionally associated with an acute expanding lesion, e.g. a tentorial hernia and a shift of the midline structures. The medial part of the other temporal lobe is soft. The necrotic tissue is sometimes focally haemorrhagic but on other occasions it is pale and therefore not very apparent macroscopically, particularly if the brain is not adequately fixed (Figs. 8.2a and b). The microscopical features in the early stages are essentially those of rarefaction necrosis associated with a conventional diffuse meningo-encephalitis, the inflammatory reaction being characteristically intensified in and adjacent to the necrotic tissue. If the patient survives for a week or two, the dead tissue becomes softer and starts to disinte-grate (Fig. 8.2c). Microscopical examination now shows intense reactive changes in and around the necrotic tissue in the form of microglial hyperplasia, with the formation of sheets of lipid phagocytes, and abundant lymphocytes and plasma cells in the meninges and around vessels. Numerous plasma cells stream out into the affected tissue. Reactive changes are particularly intense immediately deep to the pia (Fig. 8.3c). Even at this stage, however, there may still be regions of what appears to be recent rarefaction necrosis which suggests that the virus may spread pro-gressively or in episodes to susceptible parts of the brain. If the patient survives for several

weeks or more, the affected tissue becomes shrunken and cystic (Fig. 8.2d).

In addition to necrosis, there is a typical diffuse meningo-encephalitis as shown by infiltra-tion of the leptomeninges by lymphocytes, plasma cells and large mononuclear cells, perivascular cuffing, neuronophagia, and diffuse microglial hyperplasia. Intranuclear inclusion bodies occur but in a personal experience of some 25 cases, they have been seen only in the minority of cases. When present, they occur as type A inclusions, mainly within the nuclei of neurons, and are most numerous immediately adjacent to regions of tissue necrosis (Fig. 8.1d). Inclusion bodies also occur in astrocytes and in oligodendrocytes. Other pathological abnormalities often found in the brains of patients dying in the acute stage are those conventionally associated with an acute increase in intracranial pressure, e.g. necrosis of the medial occipital cortex and infarction in the brainstem.

Virus is rarely isolated from CSF but can be isolated in most cases from brain tissue removed at biopsy (Ross 1973), even from brain tissue that

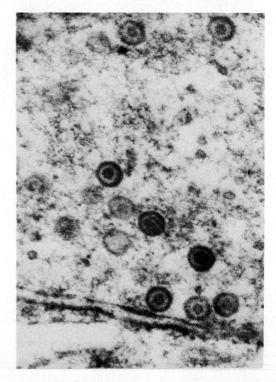

Fig. 8.4 Electronmicrograph to show herpes virus particles within the nucleus of a neuron in a case of acute necrotizing encephalitis. × 80,000.

is histologically normal. Provided an exhaustive search is carried out, herpes virus particles (Fig. 8.4) can usually be found in brain tissue removed at biopsy or *post mortem* for electron-microscopy (Harland, Adams and McSeveney 1967).

Disseminated infection with herpes simplex virus

This follows a primary infection and is commonest in neonates. Type 2 virus is usually implicated. The characteristic pathological features are necrotic lesions disseminated throughout the body, the liver and the adrenal glands often being particularly severely affected. The brain is not always involved but in some cases there may be widespread necrosis throughout the central nervous system (Haymaker *et al.* 1958). Disseminated herpes simplex virus infection can also occur occasionally in older babies and in adolescents and adults (Juel-Jensen and Mac-Callum 1972), but although a proportion of those affected may show the clinical features of meningo-encephalitis, a definite link between acute necrotizing encephalitis and disseminated infection by herpes simplex virus appears not to have been established.

Herpes zoster

This common condition consists of a vesicular skin rash in the distribution of one dermatome and accompanied, or preceded, by pain in a similar distribution. It was shown by Von Baerensprung (1863) to be associated with a lesion of the posterior root ganglion corresponding to the level of the skin eruption. This was confirmed by Head and Campbell (1900) in their detailed pathological study.

Virus was first isolated from a case of zoster by Weller and Stoddard (1952), and in 1954 Weller and Coons concluded that viruses isolated from cases of zoster and of varicella were indistinguishable. It is now generally accepted that zoster is due to the same virus as causes varicella —hence the name varicella–zoster virus. The disease has its highest incidence between the sixth and eighth decades; it occurs in about 50% of individuals who have previously had varicella, and second attacks are quite common (McCarthy 1972). It is believed that all patients with zoster have had varicella in the past (Hope-Simpson 1965). As a history of contact with chickenpox in patients with zoster is uncommon (Juel-Jensen and MacCallum 1972), it is generally accepted that the disease is a recrudescence of an earlier

varicella infection, and that the virus has remained latent in the body during the intervening years. McCarthy (1972) believes that the virus persists after an attack of varicella in a form which preserves the genome of the virus unaltered, and that zoster arises when the restriction on virus replication is removed. He also suggests that the path taken by virus to and from sensory ganglia is probably the Schwann cells surrounding sensory nerves, and that the more likely site of long-term persistence is in the nerve cell body. When the virus is reactivated it produces an acute necrotizing inflammatory response in the posterior root ganglion and travels antidromically down the sensory nerve causing neuritis and, when it reaches the skin, the characteristic vesicular rash (Hope-Simpson 1965). Esiri and Tomlinson (1972), using electron-microscopic and direct fluorescent antibody techniques, found virus in the nerve and ganglion of a patient 4 days after the onset of unilateral ophthalmic zoster. What produces reactivation of the virus is not clear although in 65 of the 100 cases reported by Juel-Jensen (1970) there was some precipitating factor in the 2 weeks preceding the onset of the clinical disease. Physical trauma to the affected part was particularly common (in 38% of patients), but malignancy was not: a high incidence of zoster has, however, been reported in association with malignant lymphoma (Williams, Diamond and Craver 1958). Immunological imbalance may therefore be a factor leading to the onset of zoster, and in some patients with malignant lymphoma, particularly those treated with cyto-toxic drugs and corticosteroids, the lesions may become disseminated and lead to a fatal generalized varicelliform rash (Merselis, Kaye and Hook 1964).

Pathological findings

The pathological changes in zoster are usually limited to one dorsal root ganglion or to the sensory ganglion of a cranial nerve, to the nerve and the nerve root close to it, and to the skin. Head and Campbell (1900) noted that certain of the spinal root ganglia were more often attacked than others. These were the 2nd, 3rd and 4th cervical, the thoracic from the 2nd downwards, and the 1st lumbar. As a rule only one ganglion is markedly involved but less severe lesions may occur in the immediately adjacent ganglia. Of the cranial ganglia, the Gasserian is most commonly affected, usually in its internal part which is related to the ophthalmic division. Otic and geniculate zoster also occur.

In the acute stage the affected ganglion is swollen and congested and may be haemorrhagic. Microscopically there is intense inflammation with lymphocytic infiltration both within and around the ganglion. This may be associated with necrosis which, in severe cases, may be massive and involve the entire ganglion, the appearances resembling those of an infarct. There may also be a few plasma cells and polymorphonuclear leucocytes. Adjacent to areas of necrosis, the nerve cells show various forms of degeneration of which loss of Nissl granules with eosinophilia of the cytoplasm, and neuronophagia are the most common. Type A intranuclear inclusion bodies are sometimes found in neurons and in their satellite cells in the dorsal root ganglia (Dayan, Morgan, Hope-Stone and Boucher 1964). Inflammation may extend for a short distance into the posterior nerve root and into the spinal nerve as well as into surrounding tissues. After the acute stage, minor lesions heal completely. If, however, there has been severe inflammation and necrosis there is loss of neurons and fibrosis. This is often associated with persistent post-herpetic neuralgia.

In most patients who die during or soon after the acute stage of the disease, abnormalities are commonly seen within the spinal cord at the level of the affected ganglion. The abnormalities consist of perivascular cuffing by lymphocytes, neuronophagia in the dorsal horn and occasionally in the ventral horn, central chromatolysis in ventral horn neurons, and an excess of microglial cells especially in the dorsal horns and around Clarke's column. The brainstem may be similarly involved in cases of trigeminal zoster. Occasionally widespread involvement of the central nervous system occurs. This takes the form of a multifocal often necrotizing encephalomyelitis in which inclusion bodies can be seen in glial nuclei, and virus particles can be demonstrated microscopically (Perier, Vanderhaeghen, Franken and Parmentier 1966; McCormick, Rodnitzky, Schochet and McKee 1969). A further abnormality that may be found in the spinal cord is ascending Wallerian-type degeneration in the posterior columns corresponding to the dorsal root involvement.

Involvement of motor nerves occurred in about 5% of Thomas and Howard's (1972) series of over 1200 patients with zoster. The patients developed segmental muscle weakness usually within 2 weeks of the onset of the rash. Facial palsy was particularly common. In the remaining cases the upper and lower limbs were affected equally, and proximal myotomes were affected as often as distal myotomes. The reason for muscle weakness is not fully established. Denny-Brown, Adams and Fitzgerald (1944) found focal infiltration by lymphocytes along the course of the facial nerve in a case in which paralysis of the facial and hypoglossal nerve on the side of the lesion occurred 11 days after zoster in the upper cervical dermatomes. In cases of thoracic herpes they found infiltration and degeneration of the motor nerve in the neighbourhood of the affected ganglion. However, the diseased dermatome and myotome may be widely separated, and this suggests that the virus may be able to attack motor neurons directly.

The skin lesions in chickenpox and zoster are identical and are similar to those caused by herpes simplex virus. The epithelial cells in and near the Malpighian layer swell and become ballooned or disintegrate. The fluid, which contains virus, collects between the epithelial cells to form a multiloculated vesicle, and there is invasion of the epithelium and dermis by neutrophil leucocytes. Some of the ballooned cells at the base of the vesicle and occasional connective tissue cells may contain the type A intranuclear inclusions described by Lipschutz (1925) but these are not always present. Electron-microscopy has shown that the virus replicates in the cells of the striatum germinativum and the stratum spinosum. Degeneration of small cutaneous nerve bundles may be another cause of post-herpetic pain (Juel-Jensen and MacCallum 1972).

B virus encephalomyelitis

B virus (herpes virus simiae) was first isolated by Sabin and Wright (1934) from the central nervous system of a laboratory worker who died after a bite from an apparently healthy rhesus monkey. With the increasing use of monkeys for various purposes a number of similar cases, nearly all fatal, have since been reported in animal handlers and laboratory workers. B virus is a natural parasite of monkeys and, in them, behaves very similarly to herpes simplex virus in man causing stomatitis and viraemia with latent infection induction in various organs. Transmission to man is by a monkey bite or by contamination of a skin wound by saliva or tissues from an infected monkey.

In man the clinical signs take the form of an encephalitis or an encephalomyelitis which usually progress very rapidly to paralysis of cranial nerves and respiratory muscles, coma and death within a few days to 3 weeks (Hartley 1966; Juel-Jensen and MacCallum 1972).

The essential pathological feature in man is a multifocal necrotizing encephalitis affecting grey and white matter, sometimes with a particular predilection for the spinal cord.

Cytomegalovirus

Cytomegalovirus is a common infection in both children and adults. Infection is predominantly subclinical and it is another virus that causes persistent latent infections (Stern 1972). Involvement of the central nervous system is mainly restricted to newborn infants, but polyneuritis in adults associated with cytomegalovirus infections has been reported by Leonard and Tobin (1971). Neonatal cytomegalic inclusion disease sometimes runs a rapid and very severe course, and in the majority of cases the infection is probably congenital in origin (Dudgeon 1971). If the infant dies in the neonatal period, there is often a severe disseminated necrotizing encephalitis with selective involvement of periventricular tissue. Calcification which is also predominantly periventricular can clearly occur early, as it may be observed in radiographs of the skull even in the neonatal period. Other microscopical features are perivascular infiltration with lymphocytes and plasma cells, the occurrence of microscopic granulomas, and the appearance of cytomegalic inclusions in various cell types (Haymaker et al. 1958). Survivors are often mentally retarded (Crome and Stern 1972): in such cases the principal abnormalities in the brain are periventricular calcification and hydrocephalus. In utero infection early in pregnancy may lead to developmental malformations such as microgyria and porencephaly (Crome 1961; Stern, Booth, Elek and Fleck 1969).

Infection of the nervous system by arboviruses

Some 200 arboviruses (arthropod-borne) are recognized. Their only shared attributes are that they are transmitted from host to host by blood-sucking insects, and that they are all probably RNA viruses (Cruickshank 1972). They replicate in the cytoplasm and give rise to a wide variety of diseases including several named types of encephalitis. Arboviruses multiply in both vertebrate and invertebrate hosts. An arthropod vector is infected by ingesting blood from the vertebrate reservoir and, after an incubation period, the virus reaches the salivary glands of the arthropod. The virus is then inoculated into a new host and, after an interval during which viral proliferation occurs, there is a period of viraemia during which a further arthropod may become infected. So the cycle is continued. Man is not the natural host for any arbovirus infection but, during periods of epizootic spread among the natural hosts, he may become infected. Arbovirus infections tend to have a seasonal occurrence, as climatic factors exert a strong influence in maintaining the cycle by directly affecting both vectors and hosts. As with other forms of virus encephalitis, only a proportion of individuals infected develop clinical evidence of encephalitis.

Mosquito-borne arbovirus encephalitis
St. Louis encephalitis

A severe epidemic of encephalitis involving over 1000 cases occurred in St. Louis and the surrounding country during the late summer of 1933. A smaller epidemic which was shown to be due to the same virus occurred in Paris, Illinois, in 1932. Since that time there have been numerous sporadic cases and small epidemics in the Central and Western United States. The mortality rate in recent epidemics has been low. The epidemic that occurred in Texas in 1966 has been fully reported (Southern, Smith, Luby, Barnett and Sanford 1969). The primary reservoirs of the virus have not yet been fully elucidated but are probably wild birds and possibly some mammals, and the principal vectors are C. tarsalis and C. pipiens (Nieberg and Blumberg 1972). The encephalitis mainly affects adults, and the chief clinical features are headache, fever, neck rigidity, confusion and tremor. There is a pleocytosis in the cerebrospinal fluid, the cell type changing from polymorphonuclear leucocytes to mononuclear cells as the disease progresses.

Pathological findings

The brain may appear normal to the naked eye. The histological features are those of a meningo-encephalitis with no particular identifying features. The meninges and the perivascular spaces are infiltrated with lymphocytes and plasma cells (there may be some polymorphs in the early stages), and there are numerous cellular nodules composed essentially of microglia throughout the grey and white matter. The most severe lesions are usually found in the thalamus, the striatum and the midbrain, but damage to neurons is not severe and neuronophagia is rare. Necrosis of brain tissue is uncommon. The precise diagnosis can only be made as a result of virological studies.

Equine encephalomyelitis

Man may be affected by three types of equine encephalomyelitis: Eastern equine encephalomyelitis which occurs mainly on the eastern seaboard of North America and in parts of South America; Western equine encephalomyelitis which occurs over most of the United States to the west of the Appalachian mountains and in Southern Canada; and Venezuelan equine encephalomyelitis which occurs in the northern part of South America. The principal natural reservoirs for the viruses of the Eastern and Western types appear to be wild birds and small mammals but the reservoir of the Venezuelan type has not been definitely established. The horse seems not to be a reservoir for any type of equine encephalomyelitis, and it is now usually considered as no more than a highly susceptible host. The disease may be spread by several types of mosquito. The viruses are antigenically distinct and were each identified between 1933 and 1938. Eastern equine encephalomyelitis is the most fulminating type, having a mortality rate in man as high as 74%. In Western equine encephalomyelitis the mortality is about 10% although it has risen to 40% in some epidemics. The mortality of Venezuelan encephalomyelitis rarely exceeds 3%. The diagnosis of each type of equine encephalomyelitis depends on virological investigations.

Pathological findings
Eastern type
Macroscopically the brain is congested and swollen. Microscopically there is a severe meningo-encephalitis, polymorphonuclear leucocytes being prominent in the acute stage. There is also an acute vasculitis with necrosis of, and fibrin deposition in, vessel walls. In addition there are many discrete or confluent areas of necrosis infiltrated with polymorphonuclear leucocytes and microglia. Selective neuronal necrosis and neuronophagia are common. All parts of the brain are involved: in some cases abnormalities are greatest in the brainstem and basal

ganglia, but in others the cerebral cortex may be the most severely involved region.

At a later stage the perivascular and meningeal infiltrations are mononuclear in type. There may also be scattered regions of infarction within which there are many mononuclear cells and lipid phagocytes.

Western type
Abnormalities are similar in character and distribution to the Eastern type but they are usually less acute. The inflammatory reaction is less intense and is composed essentially of mononuclear cells. The greatest damage is usually seen in the basal ganglia and in the white matter of the cerebral hemispheres where there may be numerous small regions of demyelination or, less commonly, of frank necrosis of tissue; these are usually perivascular and may form small cysts at a later stage (Weil and Breslich 1942; Noran and Baker 1945). More extensive cystic degeneration of the white matter has been described in patients who are afflicted with the disease during the first year of life.

Venezuelan type
Relatively little is known about the pathological abnormalities in man; there is simply a mild encephalomyelitis with mononuclear cells and microglial hyperplasia. Inflammation is most prominent in the putamen and in the cerebral white matter (Haymaker 1961).

Japanese B encephalitis
Severe epidemics of encephalitis have occurred in Japan during the late summer since 1871. The name Japanese B encephalitis was established by Kaneko and Aoki (1928) when they recognized it as different from encephalitis lethargica which had spread to Japan during the pandemic, and which they called encephalitis A. The letter B is often omitted to minimize any possible confusion between Japanese encephalitis and B virus encephalitis. The disease is very similar to Australian X disease (which is the same as Murray Valley encephalitis), the virus of which is antigenically related to but distinct from Japanese encephalitis. The virus is probably maintained by a wild bird–mosquito cycle, outbreaks of encephalitis sometimes being attributable to the migration of birds (Rivers and Horsfall 1959).

Japanese encephalitis and Murray Valley encephalitis have very similar clinical features and, in acute cases, the mortality is between about 30% and 40%. The virus of Japanese encephalitis occurs widely in the Far East including Continental and Sub-Asia and the off-shore Pacific islands extending from Southern Siberia as far south as the Philippine islands and westward to India. A distressing feature of Japanese encephalitis is the frequency of neuropsychiatric sequelae, particularly when the encephalitis affects children under the age of 10 (Shiraki, Goto and Narabayashi 1963).

Pathological findings
Macroscopic examination of the brains and spinal cords of acutely fatal cases may show nothing apart from congestion, but in patients who have survived for more than a few weeks there are often numerous small pale granular or gritty areas throughout the cortex and basal ganglia. Quite large areas of softening have also been described (Uchiyama 1925). In long-surviving cases the lesions may become so heavily calcified that it is impossible to cut the brain with a knife (Zimmerman 1946, 1948). This has also been noted in cases of Murray Valley encephalitis.

Microscopically there is usually a moderate leptomeningeal mononuclear infiltrate concentrated in sulci. Perivascular infiltration is widespread in the grey matter but mostly restricted to the subcortical zone in the white matter. Early in the disease there may be some polymorphonuclear leucocytes. There are also nodular collections of cells scattered throughout the cortex, the basal ganglia, the brainstem and the spinal cord: they consist of varying numbers of macrophages and mononuclear inflammatory cells. In addition to these nodules, there is a more diffuse increase of cells, particularly microglia, in the basal ganglia and in some nuclei of the brainstem; the most severely affected regions are the thalamus, the globus pallidus, the substantia nigra and the nuclei pontis. There may also be some loss of cells in these nuclei. In the cerebellum nodules of microglia and mononuclear cells of inflammatory type tend to be confined to the molecular layer, and may be accompanied by some loss of Purkinje cells. In the spinal cord neuronophagia is common especially in the ventral horns.

The calcification described by Zimmerman (1948) occurred either as clumps or as long wide bands along the cortical laminae. Foreign body giant cells might be seen among these deposits. In these cases he also found extensive loss of Purkinje cells. Uchiyama (1925) described sclerosis and calcification of the walls of small blood vessels and deposition of iron-containing material in many vessels in the white matter of the cerebral and cerebellar hemispheres.

Encephalitis due to tick-borne viruses
Tick-borne viruses are responsible for Russian (Far Eastern) Spring–Summer encephalitis, Central European tick-borne encephalitis and louping-ill encephalitis. The natural virus cycle is maintained between ticks and various warm blooded mammals. Most clinical cases occur in people exposed to infection in forests or in the laboratory (Webb, Connolly, Kane, O'Reilly and Simpson 1968). The viruses are closely related antigenically. The clinical features of the various types of encephalitis are very similar ranging from aseptic meningitis to a frank encephalitis with paralysis. The disease may be clinically indistinguishable from poliomyelitis.

Pathological findings
On macroscopic examination of the nervous system there may be congestion and petechial haemorrhages in the medulla and in the spinal cord. Microscopically abnormalities tend to be confined to the grey matter of the precentral cortex, the basal ganglia, the brainstem, the cerebellum and the spinal cord. All stages of neuronal necrosis are seen along with neuronophagia, perivascular cuffing with mononuclear cells, foci of microglial hyperplasia and occasionally necrotizing vasculitis. In the spinal cord inflammation is usually greatest in the cervical and the lower lumbar segments.

Infection of the central nervous system by enteroviruses

The most important enteroviruses are the polioviruses (Types 1, 2 and 3), the Coxsackie viruses and the Echo viruses. They are small RNA viruses measuring some 22 to 27 nm in diameter, and they replicate in the cytoplasm. They are a frequent cause of acute disease of the central nervous system in man, the commonest clinical illness being a mild aseptic meningitis. They may also cause severe clinical illness, paralytic poliomyelitis being classically associated with the polioviruses. According to Flewett (1972), however, no overt clinical illness occurs in about

95% of individuals infected with polioviruses. Virus, however, may continue to be excreted in the faeces for several weeks, serum antibodies appear, and the patient becomes immune to subsequent infection. He also estimates that about 5% experience a brief febrile illness with or without aseptic meningitis, and that overt paralysis occurs in no more than about 1% of infected individuals. Classical paralytic poliomyelitis may also be produced occasionally by some of the other enteroviruses, particularly Coxsackie A7 virus. Indeed, in countries where an intensive vaccination programme against poliovirus has been pursued, Coxsackie virus may now be a commoner cause of paralytic disease than the polioviruses.

Enterovirus infections are usually contracted by ingesting the virus which multiplies in the pharynx and in the cells lining the gastrointestinal tract, particularly in the ileum. Within a few days virus is present in pharyngeal and cervical lymph nodes, in the Peyer's patches and in mesenteric lymph nodes. Whether or not there is always a transient viraemia is not fully established but there is little doubt that enteroviruses reach their target organs, e.g. the central nervous system or the myocardium, by the blood stream and not by travelling along nerves.

Poliomyelitis

Poliomyelitis is a relatively common form of encephalomyelitis which has an almost worldwide distribution and which, in its classical overt clinical form, is associated with paralysis. It was described in England by Badham as long ago as 1836 and then more completely by Heine in 1840 and 1860. Epidemics were reported in 1891 and in 1905 in Sweden, and in 1907 Wickman gave a classical description of the pathological changes. Since that time there have been many local epidemics in Europe. Severe epidemics have also occurred in the United States, Canada, Australia, New Zealand and South Africa. During the second World War there was a high incidence of poliomyelitis among British, Dominion and American troops in the Near East, while a severe epidemic in South Africa in 1944-45 was attributed to the return of service personnel from the Near East. Great Britain had its first severe epidemic in 1947 and further epidemics in 1950 and 1955. Epidemics no longer occur in countries where an active vaccination programme has been pursued.

Pathogenesis

Poliomyelitis was first shown to be a virus disease by Landsteiner and Popper (1908, 1909), and it is now known that paralytic poliomyelitis may be caused by the three types of poliovirus (1, 2 and 3) and by other members of the enterovirus group. No intermediate host or significant reservoir of poliovirus has been identified, it being generally accepted that virus is spread directly or indirectly from individual to individual. Spread of the virus is greatly facilitated by the fact that it may be excreted in the faeces for 2 or 3 months by individuals who do not have any apparent clinical illness.

The seasonal incidence of poliomyelitis during the late summer months has led to the suggestion that flies as faecal feeders and contaminators of food may be an important factor in spreading the infection. A few small outbreaks have been traced to water supplies contaminated by sewage, while bathing in polluted streams or in swimming baths has also been blamed for individual cases but without conclusive evidence. Although poliomyelitis has an almost worldwide distribution, most epidemics have occurred in temperate climates. Present evidence suggests that in more primitive communities infection takes place during infancy, chiefly in a sub-clinical form. The absence of epidemics in these communities may therefore be due to general immunity of the population. In these communities the disease is endemic and occurs most often in children under the age of 5 years. On the other hand, where sanitary and hygienic controls are stricter there is less immunity; there is therefore a greater tendency to epidemic spread and a higher age incidence. Several factors appear to contribute to the distribution and severity of paralysis: infants are less liable to develop severe paralysis than older patients; males are more susceptible to paralysis than females in the ratio of 3 to 1; poliomyelitis occurring in the third trimester of pregnancy is associated with severe paralysis; and trauma, including tonsillectomy and injections, and excessive exertion, especially swimming, also appear to be associated with severe paralytic disease (Flewett 1972). It has been suggested that these latter factors produce reflex vasodilatation in the corresponding motor and sensory nuclei of the cord and brainstem thus reducing the efficiency of the blood–brain barrier in preventing spread of virus from the blood stream to the nervous system.

Poliomyelitis has probably been studied in greater detail experimentally than any other virus encephalitis of man. This has been greatly aided by the fact that the responses of the chimpanzee seem to be virtually identical to those in man (Bodian 1955, 1956, 1972). When chimpanzees are fed with virulent poliovirus, virus multiplies primarily in the mucosa of the throat and the ileum, and can be isolated from faeces and throat secretions within a few days, i.e. 1 to 2 weeks before the onset of paralysis. Virus then spreads to regional lymph nodes and, after a further few days there is a period of viraemia during which the virus is disseminated throughout the body, particularly to systemic lymph nodes, brown fat and the nervous system. Although poliovirus can, in the experimental situation, travel along a nerve, it is generally accepted that the principal if not the only route by which virus reaches the nervous system after it has been ingested, as in a natural infection, is by the blood stream. Virus then multiplies in the nervous system, there being a sharp rise in viral concentration therein on the day prior to the appearance of paralysis. Related to this increase in viral concentration, histological changes in nerve cells and paralysis precede the appearance of an inflammatory response. Damage to neurons, however, must attain a certain severity before paralysis is observed, since it is known that neuronal damage and inflammatory changes may occur in its absence (Bodian 1972).

Pathological findings
There may be no macroscopic abnormalities in the central nervous system of a patient dying in the acute stage of the disease, but not infrequently there are congestion and small haemorrhages in the ventral grey horns of the spinal cord and sometimes also in the medulla. In cases which come to autopsy months or even years after paralytic poliomyelitis, the striking macroscopic abnormalities are grey, shrunken ventral nerve roots emerging from the affected segments of the spinal cord and a reduction in size of the associated ventral grey horns.

Microscopically there is a typical encephalomyelitis. In the first few days there is diffuse infiltration of the ventral horns and the base of the dorsal horns of the spinal cord with lymphocytes and hypertrophied microglial cells and, if survival has been very short, numerous polymorphonuclear leucocytes (Fig. 8.5a). Polymorphs are often a very conspicuous element in

the numerous neuronophagic nodules that are seen early in the disease. The cellular infiltration may be so dense that many nerve cells are obscured, but some may appear to be little damaged. There are varying degrees of infiltration of the leptomeninges by inflammatory cells.

At a later stage, when death occurs after several days of paralysis, the cellular infiltration may be slightly less intense and neuronophagia more evident (Fig. 8.5b). Changes in other nerve cells range from a moderate degree of central chromatolysis to complete loss of Nissl granules along with degenerative changes in the nucleus. Nevertheless other nerve cells in the same ventral horn may appear normal. Some nerve cells may contain type B intranuclear eosinophilic inclusion bodies. At a rather later stage (21 days) their presence in otherwise normal neurons has been taken as evidence that these cells were attacked by the virus but have recovered (Bodian 1952). Perivascular infiltration with lymphocytes and a few plasma cells, and the inflammatory cell infiltrate in the leptomeninges may persist for weeks or even months.

In cases which come to autopsy long after the onset of paralysis the most obvious change is loss of neurons in the ventral horns. There may be small cysts in the ventral horns some of which may be surrounded by haemosiderin. There is also loss of myelinated fibres in the ventral horns. The axons of neurons which have been destroyed undergo Wallerian degeneration, and the affected muscles show the typical features of denervation atrophy.

Distribution of lesions
The most severe lesions are usually found in the anterior two-thirds of the grey matter of the spinal cord. They vary from one level to another and are often conspicuously asymmetrical in the same section of spinal cord. The lower sacral segments are usually relatively or completely spared. In early fatal cases, intense inflammation is also seen in the formatio reticularis, especially in the medulla but to a lesser degree also in the pons and sometimes in the midbrain, in the tectal nuclei and sometimes in the dentate nucleus of the cerebellum, in the hypothalamus, in the thalamus and in the globus pallidus. Inflammatory changes are almost constant in the precentral gyrus where some Betz cells may undergo neuronophagia. Abnormalities are rarely seen elsewhere in the cerebral cortex. In cases of

bulbar poliomyelitis, dense cellular infiltrations are seen in relation to most of the nuclei of the motor cranial nerves. In some cases the sensory nuclei are also infiltrated but, whereas there is usually degeneration or neuronophagia of many neurons in the motor nuclei, the nerve cells of the sensory nuclei appear unaffected.

In convalescent cases the loss of nerve cells in the spinal cord often has a rather characteristic distribution. Although in the most severely

Western Europe—they are practically unknown in the British Isles—and in the United States, but in Central and Eastern Europe, Siberia and India and in some parts of North and South America rabies is still a problem. The great majority of human cases can be traced to the bites of dogs, the virus being transmitted in the saliva. But although the dog is the prime source of human infections, the major reservoir of infection is often other types of wildlife, particularly

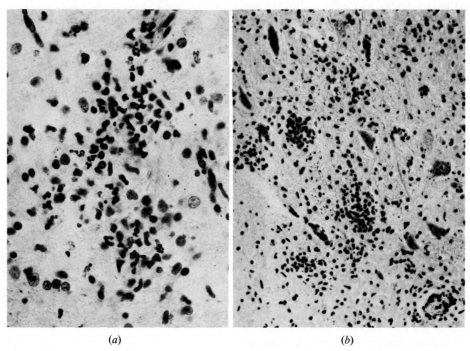

(a)   (b)

Fig. 8.5 Poliomyelitis. Ventral horns of spinal cord in acute stages. (a) Very early neuronophagia with many poly-morphonuclear leucocytes. (b) Slightly later stage of established neuronophagia without leucocytes. Note the normal appearance of some neurons.

damaged segments of the cervical and lumbo-sacral enlargements every motor neuron may have disappeared, there is in general a tendency for the greatest cell loss to be found in the more medially placed cell groups (Peers 1943; Elliott 1947). This may be due to selectively severe hypoxia of the more medially placed neurons, since the blood flow from arterioles to venules through the ventral horns is from their lateral to their medial parts.

Rabies

Of all the zoonoses, rabies has for centuries been the most feared. Human cases are now rare in

the fox in Europe and the Eastern seaboard of the United States, the skunk in the Midwest, the Southwest and the far West of the United States, and the jackal in India. In Central and South America, however, the most important reservoir is the dog. Vampire bats seem to be important in maintaining the circulation of the virus in some regions: rabies is usually transmitted to cattle by vampires, but some human cases have been directly attributed to contact with bats (Blattner 1961). In the informative report on 49 cases of human rabies encephalitis published by Dupont and Earle (1965), however, there was no history of animal exposure in 19 patients (38·8%). Dogs transmitted the disease in 50% of their cases but the disease was also transmitted by cats, skunks and bats.

The incubation period of the disease varies greatly. It is rarely as short as 2 weeks, more commonly 1 to 3 months, and sometimes more than a year. The widely accepted belief that the length of the incubation period is related to the site of the bite, i.e. the nearer the focus of infection is to the central nervous system the shorter the incubation period, was not supported by the series reported by Dupont and Earle. The average incubation period in their series was 57·3 days. The disease may assume a restless type corresponding to the furious rabies of dogs, or a paralytic type. As the old name hydrophobia implies, spasm of the muscles of deglutition on attempting to drink water may be the first or at least a prominent and early symptom.

Rabies is one of the larger viruses, measuring between 100 nm and 150 nm. It is generally accepted that the virus reaches the central nervous system by travelling along peripheral nerves. The evidence for this derives from the original observations of Pasteur, Chamberland and Roux (1884) who found virus in the nerves after subcutaneous inoculation. This work was extended by Nicolau, Nicolau and Galloway (1929) who found the peripheral nerves to be infected after intracerebral inoculation of virus.

Pathological findings
The brain may appear normal macroscopically or may be congested. Microscopically rabies encephalitis is predominantly a polioencephalomyelitis (Dupont and Earle 1965) since inflammatory changes consisting of perivascular cuffing by lymphocytes and plasma cells, and microglial hyperplasia occur predominantly in the grey matter. Neuronophagia is common as are the so-called Babe's nodules which are no longer considered to be lesions specific to rabies but merely accumulations of microglial cells of the type seen in most forms of virus encephalitis. Meningitis is uncommon. The pathognomonic histological feature of rabies, however, is the Negri body (Fig. 8.6).

Negri bodies are seen only after infection by 'street virus' and do not occur after the virus has become 'fixed' by laboratory passage. As they are not found in every case—they were present in 70·9% of Dupont and Earle's cases—the diagnosis of rabies sometimes has to be based on

virological studies. In both the dog and man Negri bodies are usually most numerous in the pyramidal layer of the hippocampus but they are also common in the cerebral cortex and in Purkinje cells. In contrast they tend to be scarce in the parts of the central nervous system which bear the chief brunt of the inflammatory disease. They are more abundant and larger in cases surviving for more than 4 or 5 days, and may be difficult to find in patients who succumb during the first 48 hours. Negri bodies alone, without any evidence of inflammation, occur in some cases of human rabies (Dupont and Earle 1965).

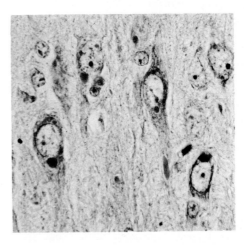

Fig. 8.6 Rabies. Negri and Lyssa bodies within neurons in the Ammon's horn of a guinea pig.

Negri bodies are sharply defined, rounded or oval acidophilic cytoplasmic inclusions varying in size from 1 nm to 20 nm but usually between 5 and 10 nm. They may lie anywhere in the cytoplasm of the cell body or its dendrites and two or more may be seen in one cell. The largest bodies are seen in the pyramidal cells of the hippocampus, in the adjacent temporal cortex and in the Purkinje cells. When present in motor neurons of the spinal cord they may also be very large. Their form is adapted to their surroundings, e.g. they may be oval in dendritic processes. The cells in which they lie may show little other abnormality or only minor degrees of chromatolysis.

The nature of the Negri body is still not fully understood. Negri (1903) originally considered that they represented a stage in the life cycle of a protozoal parasite. Both RNA and DNA have been demonstrated in Negri bodies, and rabies virus antigen has been identified in them by the fluorescent antibody technique which is the most useful technique for the rapid diagnosis of rabies (Goldwasser, Kissling, Carski and Hosty 1959). Morecki and Zimmerman (1969) could not find virus particles in Negri bodies examined with the electron microscope. Conversely, sites of viral synthesis were easily identified with the electron microscope but could not be visualized optically. They concluded that Negri bodies contained nucleoproteins, probably ribonucleoproteins, and suggested that these structures might represent sites where nucleoproteins are stored and modified until a proper template for virus assembly is formed.

The name Lyssa bodies has been given to simple acidophil cytoplasmic inclusions with no internal structure. They may be the only recognizable type of inclusion in some cases of rabies but they are not so characteristic as Negri bodies, since similar acidophilic droplets may be seen in nerve cells in a variety of degenerative conditions which are not related to virus infections. According to Dupont and Earle (1965), Lyssa bodies are more numerous than Negri bodies, and both types are usually observed in the same material.

The distribution of the lesions differs to some extent in the two chief clinical types of the disease. In the classical type with restlessness and dysphagia the principal inflammatory lesions are found in the jugular, Gasserian and dorsal root ganglia, in the lower two-thirds of the medulla and in the pons, and in the hypothalamic and tuberal nuclei usually in that order of severity. Inflammatory cells may also be seen in the peripheral nerves, the spinal cord and the cerebral and cerebellar hemispheres. In all the affected areas the nerve cells show varying degrees of degeneration and destruction. There may also be degeneration of neurons in dorsal root ganglia with or without multiplication of capsule cells. Neuronophagia is common in the jugular ganglion and may also be seen in other dorsal root ganglia as well as in the spinal cord and the medulla. In the central nervous system inflammatory lesions are particularly severe in relation to the sensory and motor nuclei of the 9th, 10th and 12th cranial nerves.

The pathology of the paralytic form of rabies was described by Hurst and Pawan (1932) *Post mortem* the spinal cord was congested and its lower half extremely softened. Microscopically there were perivascular accumulations of lymphocytes and microglial proliferation in the grey and white matter of the spinal cord. Many nerve cells were swollen and showed severe central chromatolysis, the neurons of the dorsal horns being as severely affected as the motor neurons. In the caudal part of the medulla lesions were almost as severe as in the spinal cord. There was also considerable inflammatory change in the tegmentum of the pons and the midbrain, but in the basis and in the cerebral peduncles only small glial stars were seen. Many of the neurons in the lower brainstem had undergone degeneration of varying degrees but neuronophagia was not seen. The cerebellum was normal. In the cerebral cortex abnormalities were restricted to perivascular infiltration with lymphocytes, and chromatolysis of the larger pyramidal cells. Negri bodies were not found but the hippocampus was not available for examination. The sciatic nerves from the limb which had been bitten showed lymphocytic infiltration.

Encephalitis lethargica

It has never been established that a virus was the cause of encephalitis lethargica but it is generally assumed that the disease was a virus encephalitis.

A small epidemic of encephalitis with a mortality of 50% occurred in Vienna in the winter of 1916-17 and was studied by von Economo (1931) and von Wiesner (1917). The disease then spread to Western Europe and to Great Britain, where 126 cases (20% of which were fatal) occurred during the first six months of 1918. The pathology of these cases was described by Marinesco and McIntosh (1918) and by Buzzard and Greenfield (1919). Towards the end of 1918 the disease spread to North America. The epidemic reached its peak in Britain in 1924 during which 541 cases were notified in London, 398 in Glasgow, and 301 in Sheffield. Thereafter it became less common and very few cases have been known to occur in the British Isles since 1926. Most cases occurred during the winter and early spring months. The disease was protean in its clinical manifestations but in many cases was characterized by a peculiar somnolent state from which the patient could be wakened easily and completely so as to answer questions rationally but then would quickly relapse into sleep. In mild cases this condition soon passed off, but in other patients it persisted for many days, and sometimes for weeks or months. In severe cases sleep might deepen to coma leading to death. The lethargic state from which the disease received its name was often associated with other symptoms and signs, especially oculomotor palsies and myoclonus either of the limb or trunk muscles. A mask-like facies was observed in some early cases and this often passed into a more widespread Parkinsonism rigidity, or Parkinsonism might appear after an interval of apparently complete recovery lasting for weeks or months. Another characteristic sequela was an 'oculogyric crisis' or forced adversive movements of the eyes.

In sections, congestion was evident not only in the grey matter of the cortex and basal ganglia but also in the brainstem especially adjacent to the aqueduct and in the floor of the fourth ventricle. Minute haemorrhages around congested vessels were not uncommon.

Microscopically the most conspicuous abnormality was perivascular infiltration, mainly by lymphocytes but also by plasma cells (Fig. 8.7a). There was also increased cellularity of the brain parenchyma around vessels due to the presence of lymphocytes, plasma cells and probably also microglia but this cell was not generally recog-

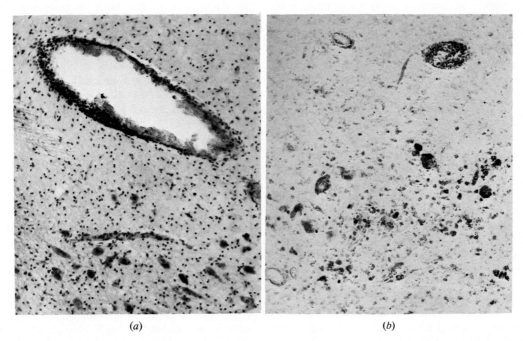

(a)

(b)

Fig. 8.7 Encephalitis lethargica. Substantia nigra. (a) Perivascular cuffing but little loss of neurons. (b) Severe destruction of pigmented neurons with extraneuronal pigment in a subacute case.

Mental retardation often with a marked psychopathic component was displayed by many children who contracted the disease.

Von Wiesner (1917) and McIntosh and Turnbull (1920) claimed to have infected monkeys by intracerebral inoculation but did not pass the disease to other animals. Later workers either failed to infect animals or produced an encephalitis from which herpes simplex virus was passaged.

Pathological findings
In cases dying during the first two weeks, the cerebral cortex appeared to be intensely congested and was sometimes described as plum-coloured.

nized during the years when the epidemic was at its height. Infiltration of the meninges by inflammatory cells was always patchy and rarely intense. In cases dying in the course of the first three or four days, perivascular haemorrhages were often more in evidence than cellular infiltrations (von Economo 1931). Inflammatory changes were usually greatest in the midbrain both in the tegmentum and in the substantia nigra but they were also seen in the cerebral cortex, in the basal ganglia and the lower brainstem, and in many cases in the cervical segments of the spinal cord.

Lesions of neurons were less obvious; they

were present in most cases but extensive selective neuronal necrosis or tissue necrosis was not a feature of this type of encephalitis. Von Economo used the term neurophthoria to describe a degeneration of neurons which often progressed to their disappearance but was rarely associated with neuronophagia. Marinesco found a diminution in the number of neurons in many nuclei in the brainstem, especially in the locus ceruleus where phagocytic cells filled with melanin granules were evidence of cell destruction. He was also one of the first to note the special incidence of cellular infiltration and neuronal degeneration in the substantia nigra (Fig. 8.7*b*) and in the oculomotor nuclei. In a case fatal on the 23rd day, Greenfield found that most of the cells of the substantia nigra had disappeared and that melanin pigment lay free in the tissues or was in the process of being absorbed by phagocytic cells. Cortical lesions were less constant but Buzzard and Greenfield (1919) found areas of astrocytic hyperplasia and intense perivascular infiltration in a patient who survived for 6 weeks. In one which survived for 4 months they found thrombosis and calcification of many small cortical vessels: similar but more severe changes were seen in the lentiform nucleus. Many of the calcified vessels were also ringed by lymphocytes. Durck (1921) reported calcification most often in the corpus striatum but also in the dentate nucleus, the hippocampus and the thalamus. It was also shown that these encrustations contained iron, but Hurst (1926) questioned their relationship to encephalitis.

In post-encephalitic Parkinsonism there is a severe diffuse loss of nerve cells from the substantia nigra. In asymmetrical cases this loss may be greater on the side opposite to the greater clinical disability. Some loss of nerve cells and gliosis in the lenticular nucleus and hypothalamus may also be found and neurofibrillary changes resembling those of Alzheimer's disease can usually be seen in some of the pigmented cells of the brainstem (Greenfield and Bosanquet 1953). Post-encephalitis Parkinsonism is described in greater detail on p. 614.

Subacute sclerosing panencephalitis

In 1933 and 1934 Dawson reported two subacute progressive cases of encephalitis in children in Tennessee. They were characterized clinically by involuntary jerking movements of the limbs and mental regression, and pathologically by an encephalitis with type A intranuclear inclusion bodies in many cortical neurons. This disease was referred to as subacute inclusion body encephalitis. In 1945 van Bogaert, under the title 'subacute sclerosing leucoencephalitis', reported three cases with similar clinical histories. It is now generally accepted that these are variants of the same disease and that the most appropriate name is subacute sclerosing panencephalitis. In the Dawson type cortical damage with inclusion bodies predominate while in the van Bogaert type inflammation in and gliosis of the white matter are more conspicuous than cortical damage.

Clinical features

Subacute sclerosing panencephalitis is a rare disease but it has several unusual clinical features which may make the diagnosis evident during life. The great majority of cases so far reported have been children or young people between the ages of 4 and 20 years. The first stage of the disease is characterized by personality changes and intellectual deterioration. The second stage is characterized by periodic involuntary movements: these may consist of jerking of the face, fingers or limbs, or rapid torsion spasms of the trunk, or of loss of tone causing the patient to stumble or fall. They tend to occur at regular intervals, often once every 5 to 10 seconds, and the interval may remain the same for many days at a time. A characteristic EEG has been found during the middle stages of the disease in a large proportion of cases, its special feature being the periodic succession of high voltage complexes which are usually synchronous in all leads with the involuntary movements. Like the latter they retain a definite interval which is usually between 5 and 10 seconds. A colloidal gold curve of paretic type is often found in the cerebrospinal fluid. The cell count, however, is usually low and the total protein content is often normal or only slightly raised. In most cases the disease progresses steadily to a fatal termination in from 6 weeks to 6 months, the third and final stage being characterized by profound dementia and decerebrate rigidity.

Aetiology

The presence of type A intranuclear inclusions naturally led to the idea originally that subacute sclerosing panencephalitis might be due to herpes simplex virus, but this idea soon had to be abandoned. It is now clear that subacute sclerosing panencephalitis is caused in some way by a paramyxovirus closely similar to or identical with measles virus. Bouteille, Fontaine, Vedrenne and Delarue (1965) observed myxovirus-like particles in affected brain tissue, but the first definite evidence linking measles virus with subacute sclerosing panencephalitis came from the observations of Connolly, Allen, Hurwitz and Millar (1967, 1968), who found measles antigen in the brains of three patients with subacute sclerosing panencephalitis, and high levels of measles antibody in their sera and cerebrospinal fluid. They found measles antigen in neurons and glial cells by the direct fluorescent antibody test. These observations have been confirmed and expanded in several laboratories (Zeman and Kolar 1968; Herndon and Rubinstein 1968). Measles virus antigen has also been found by fluorescent antibody techniques in cells in the cerebrospinal fluid in patients with subacute sclerosing panencephalitis. The final link in the chain was the isolation of complete measles virus from brain biopsy tissue from cases of subacute sclerosing panencephalitis (Horta-Barbosa, Fuccillo, Sever and Zeman 1969).

Although there is now a firmly established link between measles virus and subacute sclerosing panencephalitis, the mechanism and sequence of events whereby a patient develops the disease some years after clinical measles have not yet been clarified. The levels of serum antibody to measles virus in patients with subacute sclerosing panencephalitis have usually been considerably higher than is usually seen after primary measles infection. Furthermore, increases in the level of serum antibody have been found in the course of the disease, and there are high levels of antibody to measles virus in the cerebrospinal fluid. Measles IgM and IgG are both abnormally high in serum and cerebrospinal fluid (Connolly, Haire and Hadden 1971). These findings suggest that there is a continuous or repeated antigenic stimulus over a period of time and that there is synthesis of immunoglobulins in the central nervous system (Dick 1969). Connolly (1972), in a recent review of the experimental work on subacute sclerosing panencephalitis, considers that the disease results from a persistent measles virus infection associated with an abnormal immunological response by the patient. Brody and Detels (1970) found that measles had occurred at an unusually early age in their series of patients with subacute sclerosing panencephalitis, and that in 15% of the cases there was no history of clinical measles. They suggest that this excess of inapparent or early onset measles may reflect an initial exposure to measles before complete loss of passive immunity of maternal origin. The existence therefore of some degree of passive immunity inhibits the development of full active immunity. The resulting partial immunity is apparently sufficient to protect the individual from a second attack of clinical measles, but not sufficient to prevent the persistence of measles virus genomic material in certain cells. They have also suggested (Detels, Brody, McNew and Edgar 1973) that some as yet undetermined factor which most frequently affects rural males may precipitate the clinical expression of subacute sclerosing panencephalitis.

Pathological findings

On macroscopic examination the brain may appear normal but often it feels unusually firm in its fresh state. Some convolutions may be shrunken and discoloured while more rarely there is local necrosis of the cortex. In many cases no abnormalities may be seen in slices of the brain but the white matter may sometimes be granular, particularly in the occipital lobes, or firmer than normal and slightly translucent. The more severely damaged areas of white matter may be covered by shrunken sclerotic cortex.

Microscopical examination shows the features of a subacute encephalitis. Perivascular spaces in grey and white matter are infiltrated, often heavily, with lymphocytes and plasma cells, and there is usually a slight degree of infiltration of the meninges by mononuclear cells. In the more severely affected parts of the cortex there may be considerable loss of neurons, and astrocytic and microglial hyperplasia. Neuronophagia is common. Neurofibrillary degeneration of Alzheimer type in many nerve cells, not only in the cerebral cortex but also in the thalamus and brainstem, has been reported by Malamud, Haymaker and Pinkerton (1950) and by Corsellis (1951). Type A intranuclear inclusion bodies (Figs 8.8a and b) are most frequently seen in neurons but they occur also in oligodendroglia. They are most numerous in cases which pursue a rapidly fatal course. In the most severely damaged cells the nucleus is filled with the acidophilic inclusion which compresses the chromatin against the nuclear membrane. In less severely affected areas of the cortex, the most obvious changes are a focal increase in microglial nuclei, neuronophagia and perivascular cuffing. Even in such slightly damaged areas, however, a few nerve cells may contain intranuclear inclusions.

A wide range of abnormalities may be found in the white matter: thus there may be no more than mild perivascular cuffing with lymphocytes and plasma cells, or there may be a prominent inflammatory infiltrate associated with numerous hypertrophied astrocytes (Fig. 8.9c), with or without a diffuse isomorphic gliosis, i.e. sclerosing leucoencephalitis. Gliosis tends to be much

The ventral half of the brainstem is more involved than the dorsal. In most cases microglial proliferation is conspicuous among the nuclei pontis and, but less constantly, in the substantia nigra, and in the dentate and inferior olivary nuclei. Inclusion bodies have been found in the nerve cells of many nuclei in the brainstem, particularly in the nuclei pontis. The spinal cord is not severely affected but Brain, Greenfield and Russell (1948) and van Buren (1954) described inclusions in the nerve cells of the ventral and dorsal horns of the cervical enlargement. Degeneration and loss of ventral horn cells, and glial stars in the white matter have been described,

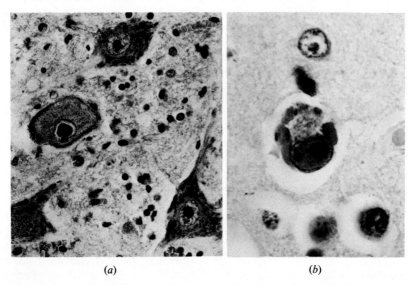

(a)   (b)

Fig. 8.8 Subacute sclerosing panencephalitis. (a) Inclusion body and central chromatolysis in a ventral horn neuron from the 8th cervical segment. (b) Intranuclear and intracytoplasmic inclusion bodies in a cortical neuron.

more conspicuous than myelin destruction, this often being particularly apparent when sections from the same case are stained for myelin and for glial fibrils (Figs. 8.9a and b). The white matter may be deep blue in Holzer preparations yet myelination may appear almost normal to the naked eye. Nevertheless, there are usually scattered microglial cells containing sudanophilic lipid, while areas of more complete demyelination occur occasionally (Foley and Williams 1953; Allen 1969).

In addition to abnormalities in the neocortex and in the white matter, the hippocampus and the medial thalamus may be quite severely involved. Lesions are usually slight in the corpus striatum and in the globus pallidus.

while Radermecker (1949) found lesions in dorsal root ganglia, in spinal nerve roots and in peripheral nerves.

Progressive multifocal leucoencephalopathy

Progressive multifocal leucoencephalopathy was not established as a clearly defined entity until Astrom, Mancall and Richardson described three cases in 1958. Since that time a great many cases have been reported from almost all parts of the world. The condition has been reviewed in detail by Richardson (1970) and by ZuRhein (1969, 1972). It is a relentlessly and usually rapid progressive condition characterized by multiple foci of degeneration in the brain, particularly in

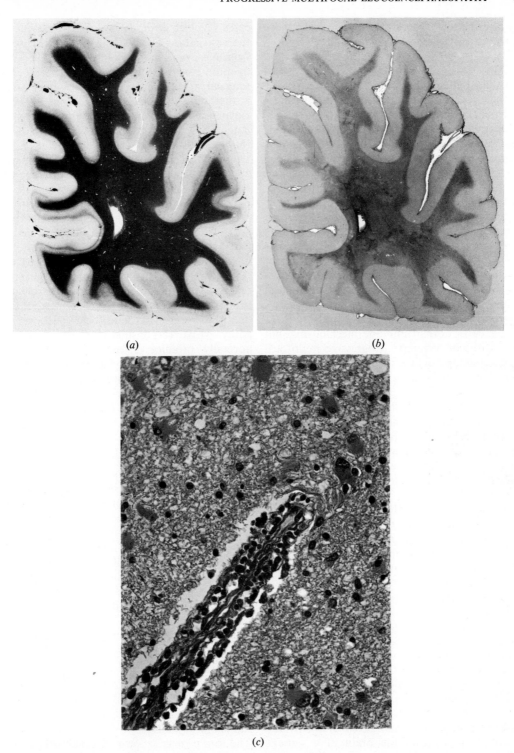

Fig. 8.9 Subacute sclerosing panencephalitis. (*a*) Occipital lobe. Note preservation of myelin staining. Heidenhain. (*b*) Same section as (*a*). Note diffuse gliosis in white matter. Holzer. (*c*) Note hypertrophied astrocytes and perivascular cuffing in the white matter.

the white matter. There are also several highly characteristic cytological changes.

Aetiology

More than half of the patients with progressive multifocal leucoencephalopathy have been suffering from a pre-existing malignant lymphoproliferative disease such as lymphosarcoma, Hodgkin's disease or lymphatic leukaemia. Others have had allied diseases such as myeloid leukaemia, multiple myelomatosis, polycythaemia vera or primary hypersplenism. Progressive multifocal leucoencephalopathy has also been associated with other diseases which involve the reticuloendothelial system such as miliary tuberculosis or widespread sarcoidosis, carcinomatosis and Whipple's disease. The frequent co-existence of diffuse diseases of the lymphoreticular system led Cavanagh, Greenbaum, Marshall and Rubinstein (1959) to conjecture that the disease was in some way related to a disturbance in normal immune mechanisms, but several cases of 'primary' progressive multifocal leucoencephalopathy, i.e. cases apparently arising de novo have now been described (Faris and Martinez 1972). Cavanagh et al. also suggested that viral parasitism might be a factor because of the occurrence of inclusion bodies within oligodendroglial nuclei but at that time they agreed that the evidence was tenuous. However, there is now a wealth of evidence supporting the idea that a virus plays an important part in the causation of the disease.

ZuRhein and Chou (1965) were the first to find virus particles in formalin-fixed brain tissue by electron microscopy. At about the same time Silverman and Rubinstein (1965) independently found similar virions in autopsy tissue processed immediately for electron-microscopy. These results were rapidly confirmed by others. The virions all had similar morphological appearances and were thought to be papovaviruses. Further investigations suggested that the virions belonged to the polyomavirus subgroup of papovaviruses, and ZuRhein (1969) suggested that the progressive multifocal leucoencephalopathy virus might therefore be a new papovavirus specific to man. In 1971 Padgett et al. reported the isolation of a polyoma-like virus which they labelled JC virus from the brain of a patient with progressive multifocal leucoencephalopathy. Virus almost identical to polyoma SV40 virus was then isolated from the brains of two further

cases (Weiner et al. 1972). Further evidence of the association of viruses with the disease came from Narayan et al. (1973) who identified mainly by fluorescent antibody and electron microscopical agglutination techniques papovaviruses in the brains of 13 cases. Field et al. (1974) have isolated a further strain of polyoma virus, designated COL and antigenically similar to JC from the brain of a case, while Marriott et al. (1975) have isolated JC virus. There is thus a remarkably consistent association of polyoma-type viruses with progressive multifocal leucoencephalopathy.

The precise relationship between this virus and progressive multifocal leucoencephalopathy has not yet been established. ZuRhein maintains that papova virions have been found in all cases in which ultrastructural studies have been undertaken, and that such virions have never been reported in any other brain disease or in any systemic disease in man. She suggests therefore that the progressive multifocal leucoencephalopathy virus responsible for the disease may normally produce a latent infection in man, and when some other factor is superimposed such as an immunological deficiency, cytotoxic drug therapy or immunosuppressive treatment, the virus may attack the brain.

Clinical features

The typical clinical picture is the appearance of a progressive diffuse disease of the central nervous system of insidious onset usually in a patient already known to be suffering from some other diffuse disease of the reticuloendothelial system. The symptoms include deterioration in mental functions such as confusion, amnesia and dementia, abnormalities of speech, visual disturbances that may lead to blindness, and involvement of the pyramidal tracts. There may often be evidence of cerebellar dysfunction. The usual duration of the disease is from 3 to 6 months. It has, however, been suggested that the disease may occasionally have an intermittently progressive course or that there may actually be remission (Hedley-White, Smith, Tyler and Peterson 1966).

Pathological findings

The brain may appear normal externally but there may be some cortical atrophy. In sections the most characteristic macroscopic feature is the presence of multiple small grey foci often occurring in groups (Fig. 8.10). These are distributed widely but asymmetrically in the white matter of the cerebrum and to a lesser extent in the cerebellum and brainstem. They also occur in grey matter, but here they are less conspicuous to the naked eye. These small foci may coalesce to form large rather soft grey areas which can, on occasion, progress to become frankly cystic (Adams and Short 1965).

Microscopical examination shows multiple, in places confluent, foci of demyelination (Fig. 8.11a). The most striking cytological feature in small lesions is the presence of abnormal oligodendrocytes. Their nuclei are larger than normal, they are hyperchromatic and devoid of a normal chromatin pattern, and some contain ill-defined

cortex, there is no sparing of the arcuate fibres. Neurons in general are well preserved, and changes of inflammatory type, e.g. perivascular cuffing by mononuclear cells are usually minimal or absent.

The smallest discernible lesions appear to be composed of a small group of abnormal oligodendrocytes and hypertrophied microglia. Their relation to vessels varies but the great majority are not perivascular.

Kuru

The discovery and investigation of kuru can be claimed with considerable justification to be the most dramatic occurrence in the entire field of

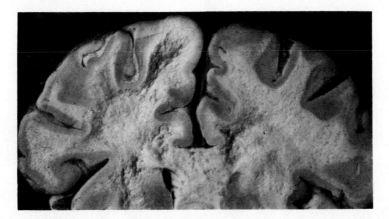

Fig. 8.10 Progressive multifocal leucoencephalopathy. Section of brain to show many small abnormal foci in the white matter. Some are coalescing to form larger confluent partly cystic lesions (Adams and Short 1965).

intranuclear inclusions of varying density and colour (Fig. 8.11c). They may be basophilic eosinophilic or amphophilic. Such oligodendrocytes are not seen within large confluent lesions but they are numerous at their periphery and in the immediately adjacent brain. The predominant cell types within large lesions are large reactive astrocytes and macrophages laden with neutral fat. The most striking cytological feature here is bizarre enlargement of astrocytes (Fig. 8.11d): they are often multinucleate and they may also show mitotic figures. Within the zones of demyelination there is relative sparing of axons but some of the residual axons may be coarsely beaded. Retraction balls are also seen. Lesions in grey matter are much more easily seen in microscopical preparations (Fig. 8.11b) and, where foci of demyelination extend into the

diseases of the nervous system in the course of the last two decades. The condition is restricted to the Fore tribe and their tribal neighbours in the eastern highlands of New Guinea and, although known to the native population for several decades (Alpers 1969), was reported for the first time by Gajdusek and Zigas in 1957. Its peculiar importance is that it was the first progressive degenerative disease of the central nervous system in man to be transmitted to another animal, first to the chimpanzee but later from passaged material and human material to several species of New World monkey and to the rhesus monkey (Gibbs and Gajdusek 1972). The agent which is filterable and capable of replicating has not been identified, but kuru is now generally accepted as being a slow virus infection; the epidemiology suggests that there

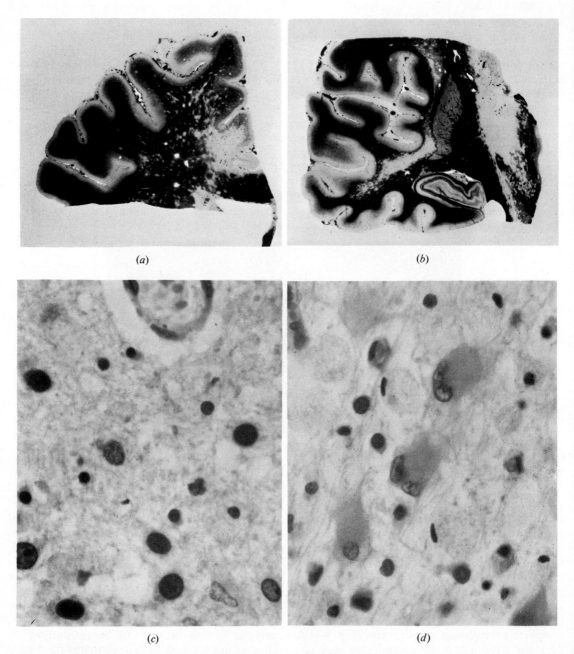

Fig. 8.11 Progressive multifocal leucoencephalopathy. (*a*) Posterior part of left frontal lobe. There are many small foci of demyelination in the white matter, and confluent demyelination in the cingulate gyrus. Heidenhain. (*b*) Left temporal lobe. Note the confluent demyelination in the thalamus. Heidenhain. (*c*) Edge of demyelinated area to show atypical oligodendroglia with large dense hyperchromatic nuclei and ill-defined intranuclear inclusion bodies. H and E. × 525. (*d*) Large binucleated astrocytes and lipid phagocytes within a focus of demyelination. H and E. × 525. (All from Adams and Short 1965.)

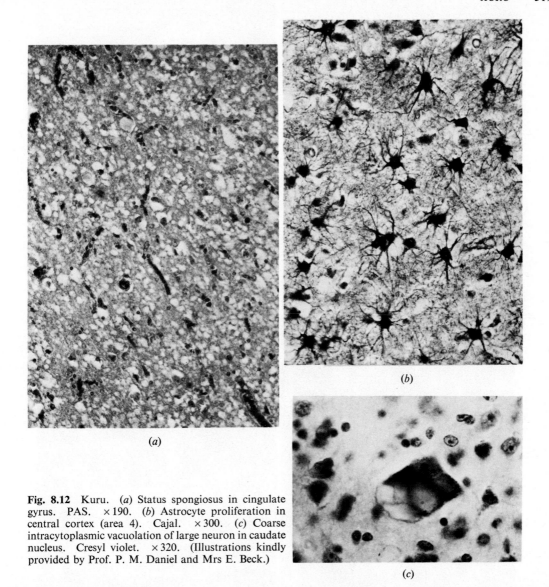

Fig. 8.12 Kuru. (*a*) Status spongiosus in cingulate gyrus. PAS. ×190. (*b*) Astrocyte proliferation in central cortex (area 4). Cajal. ×300. (*c*) Coarse intracytoplasmic vacuolation of large neuron in caudate nucleus. Cresyl violet. ×320. (Illustrations kindly provided by Prof. P. M. Daniel and Mrs E. Beck.)

is also a genetic component in its determination (Gajdusek 1972).

It is now generally accepted that cannibalism was the primary mode of transmission of the agent, and the incidence of the disease has considerably subsided since this practice ceased. When kuru was rife it is said to have been responsible for approximately 1% of deaths in the entire Fore population and probably for as many as 50% in some regions. The disease affects mainly adult women and children and adolescents of both sexes. This is attributed to the fact that adult males tended not to cannibalize their dead relatives and, if they did, only to eat muscle.

In contrast the women and young children ate all parts of the body, including brain and viscera often inadequately cooked (Alpers 1969). It may be that the agent was not ingested but entered the body through abrasions on the skin during the ritual. Cases encountered recently, since the abolition of cannibalism, are presumably due to exposure to the agent many years previously, since clinical disease can probably develop between 4 and 20 years after ingestion of the agent (Matthews, Glasse and Lindenbaum 1968).

The disease—kuru in the Fore language means trembling with cold or fear—takes the form of a

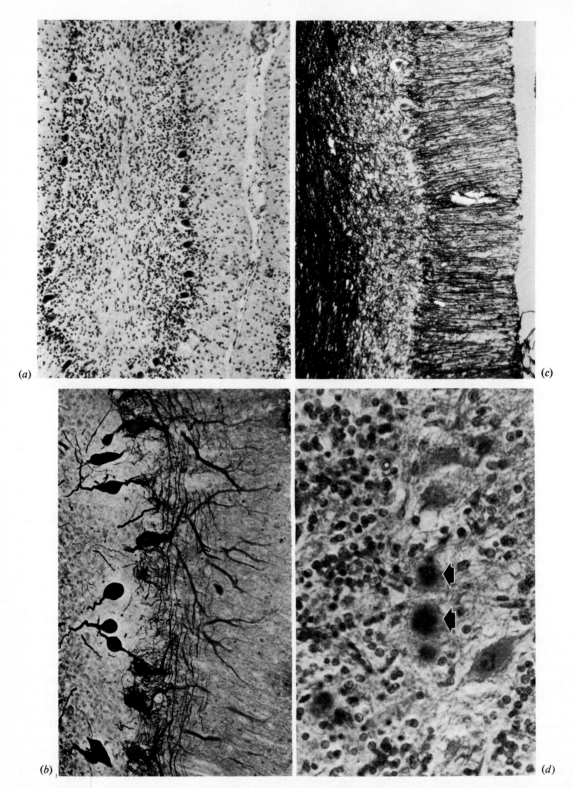

Fig. 8.13 Kuru. (*a*) Loss of granule cells and Purkinje cells in the cerebellar vermis. Cresyl violet. × 120. (*b*) Swellings on axons of Purkinje cells, and thickened dendrites. Gros Bielschowsky. × 190. (*c*) Dense fibrillary gliosis in cerebellar vermis. Holzer. × 120. (*d*) Plaques in cerebellum (arrowed). PAS. × 300. (Illustrations kindly provided by Prof. P. M. Daniel and Mrs E. Beck.)

subacute progressive cerebellar degeneration. It is uniformly fatal, and has an average duration of 1 year. The clinical stages have been fully described by Alpers (1969). After a prodromal period characterized by headache, malaise and vague limb pains, the patient develops postural instability, ataxia of gait and tremor. As the disease progresses walking and standing become impossible, and the patient ultimately becomes unable even to sit without support or to speak intelligibly. Terminally there may be dysphagia and urinary and faecal incontinence.

Pathological findings
Pathological studies have established that the disease is restricted to the nervous system and that it is a subacute degenerative condition (Klatzo, Gajdusek and Zigas 1959; Fowler and Robertson 1959; Beck and Daniel 1965; Beck, Daniel, Alpers, Gajdusek and Gibbs 1969). Macroscopically the brain may appear normal apart from some atrophy of the cerebellum, particularly in the phylogenetically old vermis and flocculonodular lobe. Histologically the disease process involves grey matter in general but, because it has a selectively severe effect on the cerebellar system, it has been suggested that kuru might be classified as a 'system degeneration' (Beck and Daniel 1965; Beck, Daniel and Gajdusek 1965). The widespread generalized changes in the cerebral hemispheres are characterized by a mild status spongiosus (Fig. 8.12a), particularly in the limbic and paralimbic cortex and in the thalamus. The status spongiosus is associated with loss of neurons, a great excess of hypertrophied astrocytes (Fig. 8.12b), and the presence of rod-shaped microglial cells many of which contain lipid. In all of the cases examined by Beck, Daniel, Gajdusek and Gibbs (1970) there were, however, large areas of cortex where status spongiosus was not obvious and where the cyto-architecture was well preserved. There is often coarse vacuolation of the large neurons in the caudate nucleus and putamen (Fig. 8.12c). Neuronal loss is often severe in the heads of the caudate nuclei and in the anterior and medial nuclei of the thalamus. As evidence of an abnormality in the hypothalamo–hypophyseal tract there is an excess of neuro-secretory material in the median eminence but the supraoptic and paraventricular nuclei remain of normal appearance (Beck and Daniel 1965). Plaques of the type described below in the cerebellum may also be found in the cerebral hemispheres.

The most dramatic histological abnormalities occur in the cerebellum, particularly in the palaeocerebellum. Loss of granule cells is more conspicuous than loss of Purkinje cells although many of the latter which survive appear abnormal and have torpedo-like swellings on their axons and antler-like thickenings of their dendrites (Fig. 8.13a and b). A particularly characteristic feature of kuru is the presence of plaques: these are most numerous in the granule cell layer but they also occur in the molecular and Purkinje cell layers and in the subcortical white matter (Fig. 8.13d). Each plaque consists of a solid rather homogeneous core surrounded by a halo of delicate radially arranged fibrils: they are readily apparent in sections stained with haematoxylin and eosin, are strongly PAS positive even after pretreatment with diastase, moderately argentophilic, and birefringent. They also stain selectively with congo red when they fluoresce with a pale orange colour. There is fibrous gliosis in the cortex and in the subcortical white matter and a little myelin breakdown in the white matter (Fig. 8.13c). Sections stained for myelin, however, appear normal on macroscopic examination. In the brainstem there is degeneration of all of the nuclei with cerebellar connections, particularly the pontine and the inferior olivary nuclei. In some cases there is degeneration of the corticospinal tracts.

Kuru has been classified as one of the spongiform virus encephalopathies in a recent review by Gajdusek (1972) in which he draws attention to similarities between kuru, Creutzfeldt-Jakob disease, scrapie and mink encephalopathy. All appear to be due to slow viruses, have an exceptionally long incubation period, and have a characteristic unremitting and always fatal progressive course. Kuru and Creutzfeldt-Jakob disease are the only two human diseases of this type that have been regularly transmitted to other species. Furthermore naturally occurring and experimental kuru, Creutzfeldt-Jakob disease and scrapie are characterized by a primary degeneration of grey matter associated with a florid astrocytosis but without any conventional inflammatory response in the brain (Beck, Daniel, Gajdusek and Gibbs 1970; Adams, Beck and Shenkin 1974). The agents have so far not been shown to be antigenic in that antibody has not yet been demonstrated.

References

Adams, J. H.   (1969) Acute necrotising encephalitis.   *British Journal of Psychiatry*, special publication no. 4, 35-39.

Adams, J. H.   (1972) Brain biopsy in *Scientific Foundations of Neurology* (Eds. Critchley, M., O'Leary, J. L. & Jennett, B.), pp. 427-433, Heinemann Medical, London.

Adams, J. H.   (1973) The neuropathology of viral infections of the nervous system.   *British Journal of Hospital Medicine*, **10**, 392-401.

Adams, J. H., Beck, E. & Shenkin, A. M.   (1974) Creutzfeldt-Jakob disease.   Further similarities with kuru. *Journal of Neurology, Neurosurgery and Psychiatry*, **37**, 195-200.

Adams, J. H. & Jennett, W. B.   (1967) Acute necrotising encephalitis: a problem in diagnosis.   *Journal of Neurology, Neurosurgery and Psychiatry*, **30**, 248-260.

Adams, J. H. & Miller, D.   (1973) Herpes simplex encephalitis: a clinical and pathological analysis of twenty-two cases.   *Postgraduate Medical Journal*, **49**, 393-397.

Adams, J. H. & Short, I. A.   (1965) Progressive multifocal leucoencephalopathy.   *Scottish Medical Journal*, **10**, 195-202.

Allen, I. V.   (1969) Pathological findings in subacute sclerosing panencephalitis in *Virus Diseases and the Nervous System* (Eds. Whitty, C. W. M., Hughes, J. T. & MacCallum, F. O.), pp. 157-162, Blackwell Scientific, Oxford.

Alpers, M.   (1969) Kuru: clinical and aetiological aspects in *Virus Diseases and the Nervous System* (Eds. Whitty, C. W. M., Hughes, J. T. & MacCallum, F. O.), pp. 83-97, Blackwell Scientific, Oxford.

Astrom, K. E., Mancall, E. L. & Richardson, E. P.   (1958) Progressive multifocal leuko-encephalopathy. *Brain*, **81**, 93-111.

Badham, J.   (1836) Paralysis in childhood.   Four remarkable cases of suddenly induced paralysis in the extremities occurring in children without any apparent cerebral or cerebro-spinal lesion.   *London Medical Gazette*, **17**, 215-218.

Baerensprung, von   (1863) Beiträge zur Kenntniss der Zoster (Dritte Folge) *Charité-Annales*, **11**, 96-116.

Beck, E. & Daniel, P. M.   (1965) Kuru and scrapie compared: are they examples of system degeneration? in *Slow, Latent and Temperate Virus Infections*, NINDB monograph no. 2 (Eds. Gajdusek, D. C., Gibbs, C. J. Jr. & Alpers, M.), pp. 85-93.

Beck, E., Daniel, P. M., Alpers, M. P., Gajdusek, D. C. & Gibbs, C. J. Jr.   (1969) Neuropathological comparisons of experimental kuru in chimpanzees with human kuru in *Pathogenesis and Etiology of Demyelinating Diseases*: addendum to International Archives of Allergy, **36**, 553-562, Karger, Basel/New York.

Beck, E., Daniel, P. M. & Gajdusek, D. C.   (1965) A comparison between the neuropathological changes in kuru and in scrapie, a system degeneration.   *Proceedings of the Vth International Congress of Neuropathology*, pp. 213-218, Excerpta Medica, Amsterdam.

Beck, E., Daniel, P. M., Gajdusek, D. C. & Gibbs, C. J. Jr.   (1970) Subacute degenerations of the brain transmissible to experimental animals: a neuropathological evaluation.   *Proceedings of the VIth International Congress of Neuropathology*, pp. 858-873, Masson, Paris.

Bennett, D. R., ZuRhein, G. M. & Roberts, T. S.   (1962) Acute necrotising encephalitis.   *Archives of Neurology (Chicago)*, **6**, 22-39.

Blattner, R. J.   (1961) Rabies infection transmitted by insectivorous bats.   *Journal of Pediatrics*, **58**, 433-437.

Bodian, D.   (1952) Virus and host factors determining the nature and severity of lesions and of clinical manifestations.   Poliomyelitis.   *Proceedings of the 2nd International Poliomyelitis Conference*, pp. 61-87, Lippincott, Philadelphia.

Bodian, D.   (1955) Emerging concept of poliomyelitis infection.   *Science*, **122**, 105-108.

Bodian, D.   (1956) Poliovirus in chimpanzee tissues after virus feeding.   *American Journal of Hygiene*, **64**, 181-197.

Bodian, D.   (1972) Poliomyelitis in *Pathology of the Nervous System* (Ed. Minckler, J.), vol. 3, chap. 170, McGraw-Hill, New York.

Bogaert, L. van   (1945) Une leuco-encéphalite sclérosante subaigüe.   *Journal of Neurology, Neurosurgery and Psychiatry*, **8**, 101-120.

Bouteille, M., Fontaine, C., Vedrenne, C. & Delarue, J.   (1965) Sur un cas d'encéphalite subaigüe à inclusions: étude anatomo-clinique et ultrastructurale.   *Revue Neurologique*, **113**, 454-458.

Brain, W. R., Greenfield, J. G. & Russell, D. S.   (1948) Subacute inclusion encephalitis (Dawson type).   *Brain*, **71**, 365-385.

Brody, J. A. & Detels, R.   (1970) Subacute sclerosing panencephalitis: a zoonosis following aberrant measles. *Lancet*, **2**, 500-501.

Buren, J. M. van   (1954) Case of subacute inclusion encephalitis studied by metallic methods. *Journal of Neuropathology and Experimental Neurology*, **13**, 230-247.

Buzzard, E. F. & Greenfield, J. G.   (1919) Lethargic encephalitis: its sequelae and morbid anatomy. *Brain*, **13**, 305-338.

Carmon, A., Behar, A. & Beller, A. J.   (1965) Acute necrotizing haemorrhagic encephalitis presenting clinically as a space-occupying lesion. *Journal of the Neurological Sciences*, **2**, 328-343.

Cavanagh, J. B., Greenbaum, D., Marshall, A. H. E. & Rubinstein, L. J.   (1959) Cerebral demyelination associated with disorders of the reticuloendothelial system. *Lancet*, **2**, 524-529.

Connolly, J. H.   (1972) Subacute sclerosing panencephalitis. *Journal of Clinical Pathology*, **25** Suppl. (Roy. Coll. Path.) **6**, 73-77.

Connolly, J. H., Allen, I. V., Hurwitz, L. J. & Millar, J. H. D.   (1967) Measles virus antibody and antigen in sub-acute sclerosing panencephalitis. *Lancet*, **1**, 542-544.

Connolly, J. H., Allen, I. V., Hurwitz, L. J. & Millar, J. H. D.   (1968) Subacute sclerosing panencephalitis: clinical, pathological, epidemiological and virological findings in three patients. *Quarterly Journal of Medicine*, **37**, 625-644.

Connolly, J. H., Haire, M. & Hadden, D. S. M.   (1971) Measles immunoglobulins in subacute sclerosing panencephalitis. *British Medical Journal*, **1**, 23-25.

Corsellis, J. A. N.   (1951) Subacute sclerosing leucoencephalitis: clinical and pathological report of 2 cases. *Journal of Mental Science*, **97**, 570-583.

Cowdry, E. V.   (1934) The problem of intranuclear inclusions in virus diseases. *Archives of Pathology*, **18**, 527-542.

Crome, L.   (1961) Cytomegalic inclusion body disease. *World Neurology*, **2**, 447-458.

Crome, L. & Stern, J.   (1972) Disorders of gestation in *Pathology of Mental Retardation*, 2nd Edition, chap. 2, Churchill Livingstone, Edinburgh and London.

Cruickshank, J. G.   (1972) The nature of viruses in *The Pathological Basis of Medicine* (Eds. Curran, R. C. & Harnden, D. G.), chap. 35, Heinemann Medical, London.

Dawson, J. R.   (1933) Cellular inclusions in cerebral lesions of lethargic encephalitis. *American Journal of Pathology*, **9**, 7-15.

Dawson, J. R.   (1934) Cellular inclusions in cerebral lesions of epidemic encephalitis. *Archives of Neurology and Psychiatry* (*Chicago*), **31**, 685-700.

Dayan, A. D., Morgan, H. G., Hope-Stone, H. F. & Boucher, B. J.   (1964) Disseminated herpes zoster in the reticuloses. *American Journal of Roentgenology*, **92**, 116-123.

Denny-Brown, D., Adams, R. D. & Fitzgerald, P. J.   (1944) Pathological features of herpes zoster: a note on 'geniculate herpes'. *Archives of Neurology and Psychiatry* (*Chicago*), **51**, 216-231.

Detels, R., Brody, J. A., McNew, J. & Edgar, A. H.   (1973) Further epidemiological studies of subacute sclerosing panencephalitis. *Lancet*, **2**, 11-14.

Dick, G.   (1969) Subacute sclerosing panencephalitis in *Virus Diseases and the Nervous System* (Eds. Whitty, C. W. M., Hughes, J. T. & MacCallum, F. O.), pp. 149-155, Blackwell Scientific, Oxford.

Dudgeon, J. A.   (1971) Cytomegalovirus infection. *Archives of Disease in Childhood*, **46**, 581-583.

Dupont, J. R. & Earle, K. M.   (1965) Human rabies encephalitis: a study of forty-nine fatal cases with a review of the literature. *Neurology* (*Minneapolis*), **15**, 1023-1034.

Durck, H.   (1921) Ueber die Verkalkung von Hirngefässen bei der akuten Encephalitis Lethargica. *Zeitschrift für die gesamte Neurologie und Psychiatrie*, **72**, 175-192.

Economo, C. von   (1931) *Encephalitis Lethargica.   Its Sequelae and Treatment*, Oxford University Press, London.

Elliot, H. C.   (1947) Studies on the motor cells of the spinal cord V: poliomyelitic lesions in the spinal motor nuclei in acute cases. *American Journal of Pathology*, **23**, 313-325.

Esiri, M. M. & Tomlinson, A. H.   (1972) Herpes zoster: demonstration of virus in trigeminal nerve and ganglion by immunofluorescence and electron microscopy. *Journal of the Neurological Sciences*, **15**, 35-48.

Faris, A. A. & Martinez, A. J.   (1972) Primary progressive multifocal leukoencephalopathy. *Archives of Neurology* (*Chicago*), **27**, 357-360.

Field, A. M., Gardner, S. D., Goodbody, R. A. & Woodhouse, M. A.   (1974) Identity of a newly isolated human polyomavirus from a patient with progressive multifocal leucoencephalopathy. *Journal of Clinical Pathology*, **27**, 341-347.

Flewett, T. H.   (1972) Cell and tissue reactions to viruses in *The Pathological Basis of Medicine* (Eds. Curran, R. C. & Harnden, D. G.), chap, 36, Heinemann Medical, London.

Flexner, S. & Amos, H. L.   (1914) Localisation of the virus and pathogenesis of epidemic poliomyelitis. *Journal of Experimental Medicine*, **20**, 249-268.

Foley, J. & Williams, D.   (1953) Inclusion encephalitis and its relation to subacute sclerosing leucoencephalitis. *Quarterly Journal of Medicine*, **22**, 157-194.

Fowler, M. & Robertson, E. G.   (1959) Observations on kuru III.   Pathological features in five cases.   *Australasian Annals of Medicine*, **8**, 16-26.

Gajdusek, D. C.   (1972) Spongiform virus encephalopathies.   *Journal of Clinical Pathology*, **25**, Suppl. (Roy. Coll. Path.), **6**, 78-83.

Gajdusek, D. C. & Zigas, V.   (1957) Degenerative disease of the central nervous system in New Guinea: the endemic occurrence of kuru in the native population.   *New England Journal of Medicine*, **257**, 974-978.

Gibbs, C. J. Jr. & Gajdusek, D. C.   (1972) Isolation and characterisation of the subacute spongiform virus encephalopathies of man: kuru and Creutzfeldt-Jakob disease.   *Journal of Clinical Pathology*, **25**, Suppl. (Roy. Coll. Path.), **6**, 84-96.

Goldwasser, R. A., Kissling, R. E., Carski, T. R. & Hosty, T. S.   (1959) Fluorescent antibody staining of rabies virus antigens.   *Proceedings of the Society of Experimental Biology and Medicine*, **98**, 219-223.

Greenfield, J. G. & Bosanquet, F. D.   (1953) The brain-stem lesions in Parkinsonism.   *Journal of Neurology, Neurosurgery and Psychiatry*, **16**, 213-226.

Harland, W. A., Adams, J. H. & McSeveney, D.   (1967) Herpes simplex particles in acute necrotising encephalitis.   *Lancet*, **2**, 581-582.

Hartley, E. G.   (1966) 'B' virus: herpes virus hominis.   *Lancet*, **1**, 87.

Haymaker, W.   (1961) Mosquito-borne encephalitides in *Encephalitides* (Eds. van Bogaert, L., Radermecker, J., Hozay, J. & Lowenthal, A.), pp. 38-56, Elsevier, Amsterdam.

Haymaker, W., Smith, M. G., Bogaert, L. van & de Chenar, C.   (1958) Pathology of viral disease in man characterised by nuclear inclusions in *Viral Encephalitis* (Eds. Fields, W. S. & Blattner, R. L.), pp. 95-201, Thomas, Springfield, Illinois.

Head, H. & Campbell, A. W.   (1900) The pathology of herpes zoster and its bearing on sensory localisation.   *Brain*, **23**, 353-523.

Hedley-White, E. T., Smith, B. P., Tyler, H. R. & Peterson, W. P.   (1966) Multifocal leukoencephalopathy with remission and five year survival.   *Journal of Neuropathology and Experimental Neurology*, **25**, 107-116.

Heine, J. von   (1840) *Beobachtungen ueber Lähmungszustande der untern Extremitaeten und deren Behandlung*, Kohler, Stuttgart.

Heine, J. von   (1860) *Spinal Kinderlähmung*, Cotta, Stuttgart.

Herndon, R. M. & Rubinstein, L. J.   (1968) Light and electron microscopy observations on the development of viral particles in the inclusions of Dawson's encephalitis (subacute sclerosing panencephalitis).   *Neurology* (*Minneapolis*), **18**, 8-18.

Hope-Simpson, R. E.   (1965) The nature of herpes zoster: a long term study and a new hypothesis.   *Proceedings of the Royal Society of Medicine*, **58**, 9-12.

Horta-Barbosa, L., Fuccillo, D. A., Sever, J. L. & Zeman, W.   (1969) Subacute sclerosing panencephalitis: isolation of measles virus from a brain biopsy.   *Nature* (*London*), **221**, 974.

Howe, H. A. & Bodian, D.   (1942) *Neural Mechanisms in Poliomyelitis*, Oxford University Press, London.

Hurst, W.   (1926) On the so-called calcification in the basal ganglia of the brain.   *Journal of Pathology and Bacteriology*, **29**, 65-85.

Hurst, E. W. & Pawan, J. L.   (1932) A further account of the Trinidad outbreak of acute rabic myelitis: histology of the experimental disease.   *Journal of Pathology and Bacteriology*, **35**, 301-321.

Juel-Jensen, B. E.   (1970) The natural history of shingles: events associated with reactivation of varicella-zoster virus.   *Journal of the Royal College of General Practitioners*, **20**, 323-327.

Juel-Jensen, B. E. & MacCallum, F. O.   (1972) *Herpes Simplex Varicella and Zoster*, Heinemann Medical, London.

Kaneko, R. & Aoki, Y.   (1928) Über die Encephalitis epidemica in Japan.   *Ergebnisse der inneren Medizin und Kinderheilkunde*, **34**, 342-456.

Klatzo, I., Gajdusek, D. C. & Zigas, V.   (1959) Pathology of kuru.   *Laboratory Investigation*, **8**, 799-847.

Landsteiner, K. & Popper, E.   (1908) Mikroscopische Praeparäte von einem menschlichen und zwei Affenrückenmarken.   *Wiener Klinische Wochenschrift*, **21**, 1830.

Landsteiner, K. & Popper, E.   (1909) Uebertragung der Poliomyelitis acuta auf Affen.   *Zeitschrift für Immunforschung*, **2**, 377-390.

Leonard, J. C. & Tobin, T. O'H.   (1971) Polyneuritis associated with cytomegalovirus infections.   *Quarterly Journal of Medicine*, **40**, 435-442.

Lipschutz, B.   (1925) Weitere Untersuchungen ueber die Aetiologie des Zoster.   Ueber die Mikroskopie der Impfreaktien und des generalisierten Bläschenexanthem nach Impfung mit Zoster.   *Archiv für Dermatologie und Syphilis, Wien*, **149**, 196-206.

McCarthy, K.   (1972) Varicella-zoster and related viruses.   *Journal of Clinical Pathology*, **25**, Suppl. (Roy. Coll. Path.), **6**, 46-50.

McCormick, W. F., Rodnitzky, R. L., Schochet, S. S. & McKee, A. P.   (1969) Varicella-zoster encephalomyelitis: a morphologic and virologic study.   *Archives of Neurology (Chicago)*, **21**, 559-570.

McIntosh, J. & Turnbull, H. M.   (1920) The experimental transmission of encephalitis lethargica to a monkey.   *British Journal of Experimental Pathology*, **1**, 89-102.

Malamud, N., Haymaker, W. & Pinkerton, H.   (1950) Inclusion encephalitis with a clinicopathologic report of three cases.   *American Journal of Pathology*, **26**, 133-153.

Marinesco, G. & McIntosh, J.   (1918) *Report of an enquiry into an obscure disease Encephalitis Lethargica*. Report to the Local Government Board.   New Series, 121, 74 pp., HMSO, London.

Marriot, P. J., O'Brien, M. D., Mackenzie, I. C. K. & Janota, I.   (1975) Progressive multifocal leucoencephalopathy: remission with cytarabine.   *Journal of Neurology, Neurosurgery and Psychiatry*, **38**, 205-209.

Matthews, J. D., Glasse, R. & Lindenbaum, S.   (1968) Kuru and cannibalism.   *Lancet*, **2**, 449-452.

Merselis, J. G., Kaye, D. & Hook, E. W.   (1964) Disseminated herpes zoster: a report of 17 cases.   *Archives of Internal Medicine*, **113**, 679-686.

Mitchell, D. E. & Adams, J. H.   (1973) Primary focal impact damage to the brainstem in blunt head injuries: does it exist?   *Lancet*, **2**, 215-218.

Morecki, R. & Zimmerman, H. M.   (1969) Human rabies encephalitis: fine structure study of cytoplasmic inclusions.   *Archives of Neurology (Chicago)*, **20**, 599-604.

Narayan, O., Penney, J. B., Johnson, R. T., Herndon, R. M. & Weiner, L. P.   (1973) Etiology of progressive multifocal leukoencephalopathy: identification of papovavirus.   *New England Journal of Medicine*, **289**, 1278-1282.

Negri, A.   (1903) Beitrag zum Studium der Aetiologie der Tollwuth.   *Zeitschrift für Hygiene und Infektionskrankheiten*, **43**, 507-528.

Nicolau, S., Nicolau, O. & Galloway, I. A.   (1929) Etude sur les septinévrites à ultravirus neurotrope.   *Annales de l'Institut Pasteur*, **43**, 1-88.

Nieberg, K. C. & Blumberg, J. M.   (1972) Viral encephalitides in *Pathology of the Nervous System* (Ed. Minckler, J.), Vol. 3, chap. 169, McGraw-Hill, New York.

Noran, H. H. & Baker, A. B.   (1945) Western equine encephalomyelitis: the pathogenesis of the pathological lesions.   *Journal of Neuropathology and Experimental Neurology*, **4**, 269-276.

Oxbury, J. M. & MacCallum, F. O.   (1973) Herpes simplex virus encephalitis: clinical features and residual damage.   *Postgraduate Medical Journal*, **49**, 387-389.

Padgett, B. L., Walker, D. L., ZuRhein, G. M., Eckroade, R. J. & Dessel, B. H.   (1971) Cultivation of papova-like virus from human brain with progressive multifocal leucoencephalopathy.   *Lancet*, **1**, 1257-1260.

Pasteur, L., Chamberland & Roux, E.   (1884) Nouvelle communication sur la rage.   *Comptes rendues hebdomadaires des séances de l'Académie des sciences*, Ser. D., **98**, 457-463.

Peers, J. H.   (1943) The pathology of convalescent poliomyelitis in man.   *American Journal of Pathology*, **19**, 673-695.

Perier, O., Vanderhaeghen, J. J., Franken, L. & Parmentier, N.   (1966) Etude clinique et anatomique de deux cas d'encéphalite zosterienne.   *Acta neurologica et psychiatrica Belgica*, **66**, 53-75.

Radermecker, J.   (1949) Leucoencéphalite subaigue sclérosant avec lesions des ganglions rachidiens et des nerfs.   *Revue Neurologique*, **81**, 1009-1017.

Rappel, M.   (1973) The management of acute necrotizing encephalitis: a review of 369 cases.   *Postgraduate Medical Journal*, **49**, 419-427.

Richardson, E. P.   (1970) Progressive multifocal leukoencephalopathy in *Handbook of Clinical Neurology* (Eds. Vinken, P. J. & Bruyn, G. W.), Vol. 9, chap. 18, North-Holland Publishing Company, Amsterdam.

Rivers, T. M. & Horsfall, F. L.   (1959) in *Viral and Rickettsial Infections of Man*, 3rd ed., Lippincott, Philadelphia.

Ross, C. A. C.   (1973) Virological diagnosis of herpes simplex encephalitis in Glasgow (1962-71).   *Postgraduate Medical Journal*, **49**, 401-402.

Sabin, A. B. & Wright, A. M.   (1934) Acute ascending myelitis following a monkey bite, with the isolation of a virus capable of reproducing the disease.   *Journal of Experimental Medicine*, **59**, 115-136.

Shiraki, H., Goto, A. & Narabayashi, H.   (1963) Etat passé et présent de l'encéphalite au Japon.   *Revue Neurologique*, **180**, 633-696.

Silverman, L. & Rubinstein, L. J.   (1965) Electron microscopic observations on a case of progressive multifocal leukoencephalopathy.   *Acta neuropathologica (Berlin)*, **5**, 215-224.

Southern, P. M., Smith, J. W., Luby, J. P., Barnett, J. A. & Sanford, J. P.   (1969) Clinical and laboratory features of epidemic St. Louis encephalitis   *Annals of Internal Medicine*, **71**, 681-689.

Stern, H.   (1972) Cytomegalovirus: a cause of persistent latent infection.   *Journal of Clinical Pathology*, **25**, Suppl (Roy. Coll. Path.), **6**, 34-38.

Stern, H., Booth, J. C., Elek, S. D. & Fleck, D. G.   (1969) Microbial causes of mental retardation.   *Lancet*, **2**, 443-448.

Thomas, J. E. & Howard, F. M.   (1972) Segmental zoster paresis—a disease profile.   *Neurology (Minneapolis)*, **22**, 459-466.

Uchiyama, T.   (1925) Pathological studies of encephalitis epidemica of 1924 in Japan.   *Japan Medical World*, **5**, 345-348.

Webb, H. E.   (1969) The pathogenesis of the viral encephalitides in *Virus Diseases and the Nervous System* (Eds. Whitty, C. W. M., Hughes, J. T. & MacCallum, F. O.), pp. 169-177, Blackwell Scientific, Oxford.

Webb, H. E., Connolly, J. H., Kane, F. F., O'Reilly, K. J. & Simpson, D. I. H.   (1968) Laboratory infections with louping-ill with associated encephalitis.   *Lancet*, **2**, 255-258.

Weil, A. & Breslich, P. J.   (1942) Histopathology of the central nervous system in the North Dakota epidemic encephalitis.   *Journal of Neuropathology and Experimental Neurology*, **1**, 49-58.

Weiner, L. P., Herndon, R. M., Narayan, O., Johnson, R. T., Shah, K., Rubinstein, L. J., Preziosi, T. J. & Conley, F. K.   (1972) Isolation of virus related to SV40 from patients with progressive multifocal leuco-encephalopathy.   *New England Journal of Medicine*, **286**, 385-390.

Weller, T. H. & Coons, A. H.   (1954) Fluorescent antibody studies with agents of varicella and herpes zoster propagated in vitro.   *Proceedings of the Society for Experimental Biology and Medicine*, **86**, 789-794.

Weller, T. H. & Stoddard, M. B.   (1952) Intranuclear inclusion bodies in cultures of human tissue inoculated with varicella vesicle fluid.   *Journal of Immunology*, **68**, 311-319.

Wickman, I.   (1907) Beiträge zur Kenntniss der Heine.   *Medizinische Krankheit*, Karger, Berlin.

Wiesner, R. R. von   (1917) Die Aetiologie der Encephalitis Lethargica.   *Wiener Klinische Wochenschrift*, **30**, 933-935.

Williams, H. M., Diamond, H. D. & Craver, L. F.   (1958) Pathogenesis and management of neurological complications in patients with malignant lymphomas and leukaemia.   *Cancer*, **11**, 76-82.

Wright, G. P.   (1959) Movements of neurotoxins and neuroviruses in the nervous system in *Modern Trends in Pathology* (Ed. Collins, D. H.), chap. 11, Butterworth, London.

Zeman, W. & Kolar, O.   (1968) Reflections on the etiology and pathogenesis of subacute sclerosing panencephalitis.   *Neurology (Minneapolis)*, **18**, 1-7.

Zimmerman, H. M.   (1946) The pathology of Japanese B encephalitis.   *American Journal of Pathology*, **22**, 965-991.

Zimmerman, H. M.   (1948) Japanese B encephalitis.   *Journal of Neuropathology and Experimental Neurology*, **7**, 106.

ZuRhein, G. M.   (1969) Association of papova-virions with a human demyelinating disease (progressive multifocal leukoencephalopathy) in *Progress in Medical Virology* (Ed. Melnick, J. L.), chap. 11, Karger, Basel.

ZuRhein, G. M.   (1972) Virions in progressive multifocal leukoencephalopathy in *Pathology of the Nervous System* (Ed. Minckler, J.), vol. 3, chap. 207, McGraw-Hill, New York.

ZuRhein, G. M. & Chou, S.-M.   (1965) Particles resembling papova viruses in human cerebral demyelinating disease.   *Science*, **148**, 1477-1479.

9

Cerebral Trauma

S. J. Strich

The pathological findings following head injury may be classified in various ways. Firstly there are those lesions which are due to direct *mechanical damage* inflicted at the time of the injury. These include fractures of the skull, contusions, tearing of blood vessels leading to haemorrhage, and tearing of nerve fibres. Then there are lesions consequent upon the development of intracranial *space occupying haematomas*. These have their own particular complications such as distortion and sometimes swelling of the brain, downward displacement of the parahippocampal gyrus with compression of the brainstem and secondary brainstem haemorrhages, or herniation of the cerebellar tonsils through the foramen magnum. Further, one must remember that head injuries seldom occur in isolation but may be accompanied by injuries elsewhere. These affect the patient's general condition which in turn affects the brain. Thus the patient may suffer from episodes of *hypotension* due to blood loss, from *respiratory difficulties* due to an obstructed airway or due to chest injuries, or there may be systemic *fat embolism*. In many accidents a combination of physical damage and secondary factors operate and it is often difficult to sort out the pathogenesis of every lesion seen in the brain of a case of head injury.

Damage caused by physical forces

The first event in a head injury, whatever may happen later, is that physical forces act on the skull and its contents and may damage either in various ways. Few physicists have concerned themselves with the problem. The set-up is complex: the head is hinged on the neck; the rigid, irregularly shaped and buttressed skull is divided into communicating compartments by dural folds; the brain, jelly-like but not uniformly structured, is tethered to the skull here and there and filled and surrounded by cerebrospinal fluid of almost the same density as brain substance. The physical properties of the object with which the head collides are also important. There is no agreement as to which of the possible physical forces are injurious to brain tissue and how exactly any damage is produced. A measure of the perplexity felt by physicians, experimentalists and engineers can be gained by reading the discussion on the mechanical aspects of head injury in any symposium (Caveness and Walker 1966). An extensive review of the early literature will be found in Jakob's (1913) paper and an excellent summary of the theories concerning concussion in the paper by Pudenz and Shelden (1946).

The problem was clearly set out by the physicist Holbourn (1943, 1945), who came to the conclusion that significant damage to the brain is likely to be due to (1) *local deformation* of the skull at the site or sites of impact, and fractures producing local damage; (2) *shear stresses* mainly due to rotation of the brain, producing damage at distant sites and throughout the brain; (3) *decrease in intracranial pressure*, but only if great enough to cause cavitation, by the liberation of bubbles of vapour or dissolved gas. Holbourn estimated that this last was unlikely to occur in the ordinary run of head injuries and considered that distortion and movement of the brain caused the most damage. Brain substance is a fluid and as such is very incompressible, and it needs enormous forces to reduce the brain in volume. Therefore the brain cannot rattle about inside the skull, nor can it pull away from the skull during linear acceleration of the head. The brain has, however, little rigidity and is easily changed in shape or distorted. This results in shear strains which are highly injurious. Shear stresses and strains are produced particularly during rotational movement of the head when the brain lags behind the skull and 'makes the only lagging movement open to an incompressible substance in an enclosed space, viz. a whirling movement' (Holbourn 1945). Some rotation of the head occurs in most head injuries and in many accidents the magnitude of the shear stresses are sufficient to tear blood vessels, nerve fibres and synapses.

Holbourn's theoretical considerations have been tested on animals. If the head is free to move after an impact a remarkable degree of swirling and gliding of the cerebral convolutions takes place. This was demonstrated cinematographically by Pudenz and Shelden (1946) and by Ommaya and co-workers (Ommaya 1966) in rhesus monkeys whose skull caps had been replaced by translucent material. Signs of concussion, and contusions and haemorrhages have been produced in animals subjected to rotational acceleration without impact to the head (Ommaya, Faas and Yarnell 1968; Unterharnscheidt and Higgins 1969). Ommaya further showed that concussion did not occur if the head was prevented by a plaster collar from rotating during acceleration. There is much clinical evidence (summarized by Strich 1956, 1961) that movement of the head is an important factor in producing concussion and presumably also more severe brain damage. Crush injuries (Russell and Schiller 1949) and penetrating injuries may lead to skull fractures and to much loss of brain substance without loss of consciousness.

Most workers have accepted parts of Holbourn's theories, but some have placed more emphasis on changes in intracranial pressure immediately after impact, which Holbourn regarded as relatively harmless to brain tissue. It must be emphasized that the supporters of 'pressure gradient theories' are not concerned with generalized brain damage but confine themselves almost entirely to explaining the distribution of surface damage (contusions) to the cerebral hemispheres, especially those at sites distant to the impact. The practical importance of such theories is limited since these contusions are not the cause of concussion, nor usually of serious neurological deficits.

It seems generally agreed that it is the development of *negative* pressure inside the head that will damage the brain tissue. Sjövall (1943) and Sellier and Unterharnscheidt (1963) for example, point out that because of its inertia the brain tends to lag behind when the skull is set in motion and negative pressure develops at the leading end during acceleration and at the trailing end during deceleration, only linear motions being considered. The cavitation theory (Gross 1958) proposes that negative pressure at the point opposite the impact produces temporary cavities which, on collapse, would release large amounts of energy which damages the tissue. An extension of the cavitation theory, by which 'resonance cavitation' due to gas bubbles is set up, would provide a mechanism for diffuse brain damage, but apparently this only works if there is no fracture of the skull. Sellier and Unterharnscheidt have attempted to explain some internal brain damage (haemorrhages near the ventricles) by the 'pressure gradient' theory.

Negative pressure certainly develops in the skull after a blow although not only opposite the site of impact (Lissner and Evans 1960), but there seems to be doubt whether cavitation ever occurs in the brain (Caveness and Walker 1966) unless the head is subjected to extraordinary forces, as for example in some aircraft accidents. The negative pressure theories do not in fact provide a satisfactory explanation for the localization of contusions as found in the human brain after head injury.

The time course of pressure changes and the transmission of pressure waves in a simple model (rigid, fluid-filled sphere) subjected to a blow have been analysed mathematically (Anzelius 1943; Güttinger 1950), and there has been some experimentation both on simple models and on cadaver heads (Holbourn 1943; Gross 1958; Lissner and Evans 1960; Sellier and Unterharnscheidt 1963; Goldsmith 1966).

Fractures of the skull

Although the importance of fractures of the skull has been exaggerated in the past, cases of head injury with such fractures tend to have more complications and end fatally more often than those without. The presence of skull fractures is evidence that the impact to the head had considerable force. It is common to find areas of bruising (contusions) under fractures (Lindenberg and Freytag 1960) even when they are no more than linear fissures (Fig. 9.1). Depressed fractures raise the incidence of many complications of

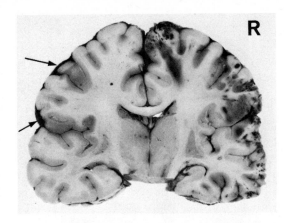

R

Fig. 9.1 Assault with blunt object causing extensive fractures of the right side of the skull; very short survival. There are numerous cortical haemorrhages (contusions) on the right and a little subarachnoid haemorrhage (arrows) on the left. The ventricles are small and both hemispheres are swollen.

head injury such as intracranial haematoma (due to laceration of meningeal arteries), infection, laceration of dural sinuses, and traumatic epilepsy (Miller and Jennett 1968). Fractures of the base have a special significance; not only are they evidence of a severe impact, but as they often pass through the sphenoidal air sinus or the middle ear they may open up channels for infection, and damage cranial nerves at the base of the brain. Fracture of the ethmoid bone or the thin inner walls of the frontal air sinuses, which may be caused by a comparatively mild blow, similarly may allow infection to spread to the meninges and an initial rhinorrhoea is a danger signal in such cases. The defect of bone may become closed by granulation tissue which allows infection to pass into the cranial cavity even months after the injury.

The patterns of skull fracturing have been worked out both for blunt and for penetrating injuries on embalmed cadaver heads and skulls (Gurdjian and Webster 1958).

Growing skull fracture of infancy

In infants and young children the dura is firmly attached to the skull and is readily torn when the skull breaks. If dura and arachnoid get caught in the fracture an arachnoid cyst can form. This prevents the fracture from healing and indeed enlarges it. The patient then presents with a pulsating swelling at the site of the fracture some months after the injury. Brain tissue may be

found herniated into such a swelling (Goldstein, Rosenthal, Garancis, Larson and Brackett 1970).

Contusions

These are areas of superficial damage to the brain found at the crests of cerebral cortical convolutions and occasionally on the surface of the cerebellum. They consist of streaks of haemorrhage at right angles to the cortical surface or of groups of punctate haemorrhage (Figs. 9.2-9.4), often sparing the superficial layers, and are accompanied by variable amounts of tissue necrosis. Like other destructive lesions, contusions are surrounded by a zone of oedema and this may become an important aspect of the injury if the contusions are numerous and widespread. Contusions heal in a few weeks; once they are healed their age cannot be determined. In the course of healing blood vessels proliferate, blood and necrotic tissue are removed by macrophages (Fig. 9.7) and the floor of the defect is covered by a glial and occasionally by a thin collagenous scar. The result is the characteristic shallow, often slightly yellow, defect running along the crests of gyri (Figs. 9.5, 9.6). In this contusions differ from areas of necrosis due to small vascular lesions which are found at the bottom of sulci (Spatz 1932). At the edge of old contusions the cortex is often gliosed, and calcified neurons or binucleated nerve cells (Gaupp 1933) may be present.

Incidence and distribution of contusions

Contusions of the brain are extremely common in fatal head injuries but also occur frequently in non-fatal injuries. Healed contusions were reported as an incidental finding in 2·5% of 2000 consecutive necropsies in a general hospital (Welte 1948). There appears to be little relation between cortical contusions and clinical signs in head injury, and the lesions usually leave no significant neurological deficit (other than anosmia which is frequent after orbital contusion), but they are sometimes the only naked-eye evidence of brain injury and their distribution has fascinated pathologists for centuries (Louis 1788). This distribution has been described by various workers (Welte 1948; Krauland 1950; Gurdjian, Webster and Lissner 1955; Lindenberg and Freytag 1960; Sellier and Unterharnscheidt 1963). Contusions are found near fracture lines and under the area of impact (Fig. 9.1). In addition, they are commonly seen at sites other than that

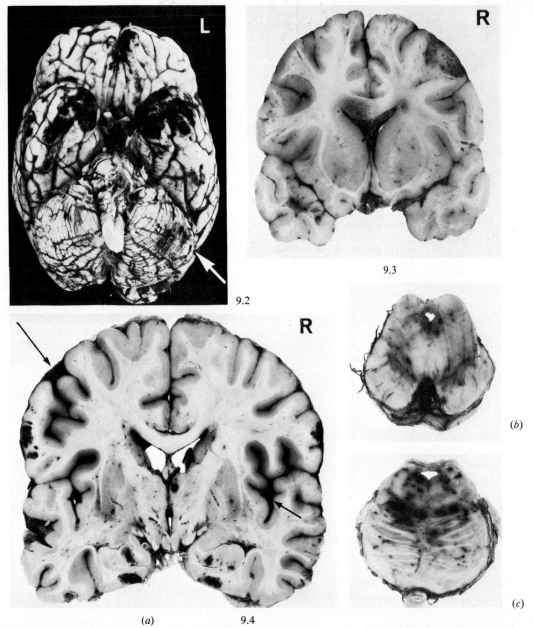

(a)   9.4

Fig. 9.2 Acute head injury, base of brain. Contusions are seen on the anterior parts of both temporal lobes, on the under-surface of the frontal lobes (involving the olfactory bulbs), on the left cerebellar hemisphere (arrow). The impact had been to the left parieto-occipital region and there was a fracture of the left occipital bone extending into the posterior fossa. (Reproduced by courtesy of Dr J. A. N. Corsellis.)

Fig. 9.3 Girl aged 14. Traffic accident, unconscious until death at 8 days. Note wedge-shaped area of necrosis on the right (underlying a fracture). There is a traumatic tear in the left half of the corpus callosum.

Fig. 9.4 Male aged 47. Multiple fractures of both sides of the skull. (*a*) Coronal section of the brain. Notice contusions in right and left parietal regions and in the parahippocampal gyri (related to the edge of the tentorium cerebelli). Haemor-rhages are present in the hippocampi and in the right thalamus. Subarachnoid blood (arrows) and a little intraventricular blood are also seen. (*b*) Midbrain. There are several haemorrhages. (*c*) Pons. Numerous haemorrhages in the floor of the 4th ventricle and in the tegmental region.

of impact. These are the so-called contre-coup lesions which tend to occur in certain regions of the brain no matter where the blow. These regions are the undersurface of the frontal lobes, the tip of the temporal poles, the lips of the Sylvian fissures (Fig. 9.2), the unci and the under-edge of the falx. In the absence of fractures, contusions are rarely seen over the vertex, the occipital lobes, or the cerebellum. Well-marked contusions under the site of impact are more commonly found when the head is hit by a small object such as a hammer (Fig. 9.1) or a cricket

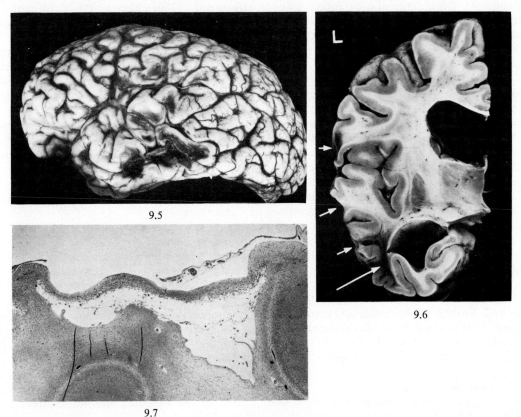

9.5

9.6

9.7

Fig. 9.5 Male aged 70. Head injury, with 3 days unconsciousness, 20 years ago. No obvious sequelae. Lateral surface of the left hemisphere with old contusions showing as shallow cortical defects, and a healed laceration at the border of the temporal lobe leaving a deeper defect. (Reproduced by courtesy of Dr J. A. N. Corsellis.)

Fig. 9.6 Coronal section of the same hemisphere as Fig. 9.5 showing cortical defects involving the crests of gyri (short arrows) and the deeper cavity seen on the surface (long arrow) going down as far as the ependyma. The body and inferior horn of the lateral ventricle are enlarged and the corpus callosum is thin. (Reproduced by courtesy of Dr. J. A. N. Corsellis.)

Fig. 9.7 Male aged 65. Head injury 5 years before death. Old contusion. The cortical ribbon shows a wedge shaped defect which is bridged by a layer of glial tissue and normal looking meninges. There is no excess reticulin. (cf. Fig. 9.32). Reticulin stain. × 23.

surface and lateral surface of the temporal lobes (Fig. 9.5). The lesions are usually found on both hemispheres but may be more pronounced on the side contralateral to the one which received the blow. Contusions or haemorrhages are also characteristically found on the undersurface of the temporal lobe related to the edge of the tent (Fig. 9.4a), and in the cingulate gyri, below the ball than when it hits a large object such as a brick wall. In the latter case distant and contra-lateral contusions predominate.

One of the explanations for the distribution of the contre-coup contusions is that they are due to negative pressure, possibly causing cavitation (see above) which develops in the area directly opposite the site of the impact. This theory is difficult to test in practice because the direction of the blow and thus the true location of the 'area opposite the site of impact' is rarely known in human accidents, and it seems that the lines customarily drawn from the site of the blow to the contusion as found on the brain are based on prejudice. The absence of occipital contusions after frontal blows, and the relatively constant localization of contusions in spite of the variety of blows, argue against any negative pressure theory.

A more satisfactory theory to explain the distribution of contusions, other than those due to distortion of the skull, is that they are rotational injuries. Contusions are unlikely to occur where the brain slides over a smooth surface, but where the skull is moulded to the convolutions as in the anterior and middle fossae and where the sphenoidal ridge sticks into the brain, shear strains will be produced in the brain substance during rotational acceleration or deceleration. Analysis of the distribution of surface lesions on the brain after frontal or occipital blows to the monkey head supports these ideas (Ommaya, Grubb and Naumann 1971). Experimental work with a gelatin model of the brain in a plaster skull (Holbourn 1943) and with monkeys (Ommaya, Faas and Yarnell 1968; Unterharnscheidt and Higgins 1969) has confirmed that contusions can be produced by rotation of the skull without impact to the head (whiplash injuries).

Subarachnoid haemorrhage
This is very common in head injuries and is due to tearing of leptomeningeal blood vessels (Figs. 9.1 and 9.4a). It is usually most marked over the vertex of the brain in the parasagittal regions where there is most movement. The organization of subarachnoid haemorrhage with the formation of fibrous adhesions may lead to frank obstruction of the cerebrospinal fluid pathways or to more subtle disturbances of circulation and reabsorption of cerebrospinal fluid as seen in the '*normal pressure hydrocephalus*' syndrome. Patients with this syndrome frequently have a history of head injury (Ojemann, Fisher, Adams, Sweet and New 1969).

Intracerebral haemorrhages
These are common in head injuries. They may be so small that they can only be seen with the microscope, or so large that they constitute serious space-occupying lesions, particularly if they are multiple or surrounded by zones of oedema. They may occur anywhere in the brain but are uncommon below the middle pons. These haemorrhages are thought to be of primary traumatic origin and torn blood vessels have in fact been seen microscopically in serial sections (Krauland 1950; Mayer 1967; Minauf and Schacht 1966). When there are macroscopic haemorrhages a search with the microscope will frequently reveal widespread tearing of nerve fibres in the cerebral hemispheres and brainstem. Statements about brain damage due to head injuries based on naked-eye appearances alone are very misleading.

The clinical importance of traumatic haemorrhages depends on their location in the brain and not only on their size. Very small haemorrhages in the hypothalamus (Crompton 1971) in the optic nerves (Crompton 1970) or in the pituitary (see p. 599) may produce obvious clinical signs.

Brainstem haemorrhages
Primary traumatic haemorrhages visible with the naked eye are common in the pons, midbrain and hypothalamus in fatal head injuries. Their incidence reaches almost 100% in series in which these areas have been examined histologically (Tomlinson 1970). Such haemorrhages tend to lie in the lateral parts of the tegmental region of the brainstem, frequently involving one or both cerebellar peduncles. Haemorrhages, usually small ones, are also common in the subependymal region of the aqueduct and 4th ventricle (Figs. 9.4b and c).

Cases in which there are primary brainstem haemorrhages often also show evidence of torn nerve fibres not directly associated with the haemorrhage (Tomlinson 1970).

Brainstem lesions *secondary* to supratentorial space-occupying haematomas can usually be distinguished from primary lesions. In acute cases there is compression of the midbrain from the side by parahippocampal gyri which have herniated through the tentorial opening. The haemorrhages tend to occur near the midline or to spread out from there (Figs. 9.22, 9.25), and they are often associated with multiple irregular areas of necrosis.

It is sometimes stated that brainstem lesions are responsible for prolonged or permanent disturbances of consciousness after head injury. There are, however, no cases of prolonged post-traumatic coma on record in which the only pathological lesions were in the brainstem and in which the hemispheres were shown to be normal histologically as well as macroscopically.

Corpus callosum haemorrhages
Haemorrhages are seen in the corpus callosum in about 18% of fatal head injuries (Lindenberg, Fisher, Durlacher, Lovitt and Freytag 1955; Schacht and Minauf 1965). They usually lie to one or other side of the midline (Fig. 9.3) and on the undersurface of the corpus callosum and may involve a part or its whole length. In the splenium, where haemorrhages are usually centrally situated and where the falx comes close to the corpus callosum, they may be due to direct damage by the edge of the falx.

Other sites. Haemorrhages may lie in the territory of the perforating vessels at the base of the brain and are also not uncommonly seen in the hippocampus (Fig. 9.4a). Occasionally they are present in the subependymal tissue of the ventricular system.

Haemorrhages have been described in the dorsal root ganglia (Spicer and Strich 1967), but it is not known whether these were traumatic or secondary to raised intracranial pressure.

Tearing of nerve fibres
There is good evidence that the violent movement of the brain which occurs in many head injuries can result in tearing of nerve fibres and their subsequent degeneration.

Widespread degeneration in white matter was first reported in patients who had had apparently uncomplicated head injuries and yet had remained in a state of extreme dementia ('akinetic mutism', 'coma vigil', 'apallic syndrome') with gross neurological abnormalities until they died some months later (Rosenblath 1899; Strich 1956; Ule, Döhner and Bues 1961; Girard, Tommasi and Trillet 1963; Jellinger 1965; Jellinger and Seitelberger 1970). Evidence of damaged nerve fibres has now been seen in patients with short survival times (Strich 1961; Tomlinson 1964; Nevin 1967; Peerless and Rewcastle 1967), and also after mild head injuries, including patients who were concussed but who recovered consciousness and died of other causes later. It may be that microscopic damage to white matter is present in as many as two-thirds of cases of head injury (Nevin 1967; Oppenheimer 1968).

There may be little to see in the brain macroscopically, though lesions in the corpus callosum are very common in this type of case and there may be small haemorrhages elsewhere in the hemispheres or in the brainstem. In patients with longer survival the ventricles are dilated and the degenerated tracts in brainstem and spinal cord look chalky white macroscopically.

The histological changes are those of Wallerian degeneration. In the early stages, that is from 18 hours to 3 or 4 weeks after injury, the most obvious histological feature is the presence of eosinophilic and argyrophilic swellings on nerve fibres (Figs. 9.8, 9.9) which probably represent the extrusion of axoplasm occurring at the proximal and distal ends of severed nerve fibres. The natural history of these structures was described by Ramon y Cajal (1928) who named them 'retraction balls or bulbs'. Retraction balls do not invariably form, they are often absent at the edge of haemorrhages or infarcts and are unusual underneath contusions. From 18 hours after injury onwards clusters of microglial cells (Fig. 9.10) will be seen in suitably impregnated silver preparations (Oppenheimer 1968) and these are thought to be the reaction to minute tissue tears. For the first five to six weeks Wallerian degeneration in the central nervous system is difficult to recognize histologically because the cellular reaction is inconspicuous and because the myelin sheaths retain their usual staining characteristics. Severed axons become fragmented and myelin sheaths break up into sausage-shaped masses, hollow spheres and solid balls (Fig. 9.13). The nuclei of the astrocytes enlarge and their cytoplasm swells. Clusters of glial cells (Figs. 9.11, 9.12) are seen at this stage even without using special stains. As in Wallerian degeneration due to other causes neutral fat does not appear for six to eight weeks (Daniel and Strich 1969). After this time the site of the degenerated myelinated nerve fibres is marked by macrophages (Figs. 9.15, 9.16) containing myelin breakdown products (cholesterol esters) which may remain in the tissues for at least two years. After two to three months Wallerian degeneration becomes easy to detect in myelin stained preparations (Fig. 9.14), but its pattern stands out particularly clearly (Figs. 9.17, 9.18) with the Marchi method (Strich 1968).

The distribution of the white matter degeneration is not random and its pattern is remarkably similar in most of the reported cases. Apart

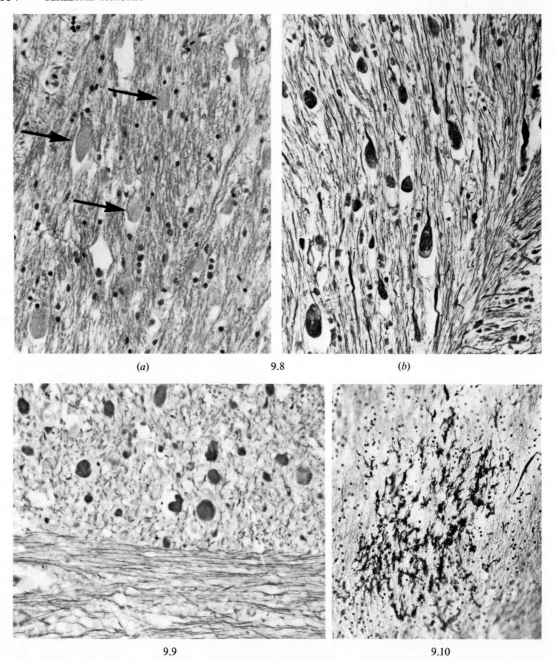

(a)   9.8   (b)

9.9   9.10

Fig. 9.8 Woman aged 35 who died 11 days after head injury without having recovered consciousness. Section through internal capsule. (*a*) Haematoxylin and eosin. Large eosinophilic blobs, so-called retraction balls (arrows), can be seen. They are more conspicuous in sections impregnated with silver as in (*b*). (*b*) Silver impregnation. There are many argyrophilic swellings (retraction balls), some clearly at the ends of nerve fibres. × 225. (Reproduced by courtesy of the Editor, *Journal of Clinical Pathology*.)

Fig. 9.9 Head injury, survival 20 days. Horizontal section through the pons. Retraction balls are seen in the transversely cut (descending) tract whereas neighbouring longitudinally cut fibres are normal. Silver impregnation. × 200. (Reproduced by kind permission from Walker, *Late Effects of Head Injury*, Charles C Thomas.)

Fig. 9.10 Male aged 66. Mild head injury, post-traumatic amnesia 20 minutes, conscious until death from bronchopneumonia three days later. Section through corpus callosum. A cluster of microglial cells is seen. Such clusters were also present in the brainstem. Silver impregnation. × 190.

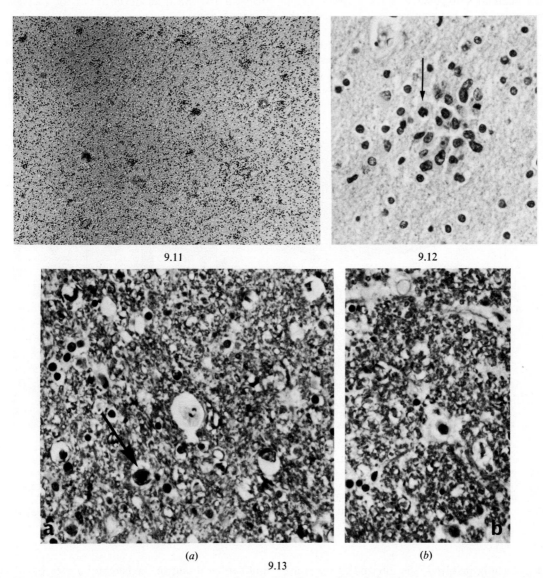

9.11

9.12

(a)

9.13

(b)

Fig. 9.11 Road accident, patient survived in coma for 6 weeks. Section through the centrum semiovale shows numerous 'glial stars' or 'clusters', evidence of degeneration in the white matter. There are generally more glial nuclei than normal. No stainable fat is seen at this stage and myelin stains show no pallor. Nissl. × 85.

Fig. 9.12 Male aged 25, survived in coma following a head injury, for 5 weeks. Section of the hemisphere white matter. There is a cluster of glial cells, one of which is in mitosis (arrow). Haematoxylin and eosin. × 320. (Reproduced by courtesy of the Editor, *Journal of Clinical Pathology*.)

Fig. 9.13 Head injury 5 weeks before death. (a) Transverse section through pyramidal tract undergoing Wallerian degeneration. Myelin sheaths show varying and irregular outlines. There are many spaces some of which contain debris. The tract is more cellular than normal. Some sheaths have collapsed to form solid masses (arrow). (b) Normal pyramidal tract. Luxol Fast Blue. × 360.

from bilateral involvement of the cerebral hemispheres which is not uniform but may spare the whole or parts of some convolutions, any of the long tracts may be involved on one or both sides. The corpus callosum always shows extensive degeneration even in areas remote from focal lesions; the anterior commissure, the fornices, the internal and external sagittal strata in the occipital lobes

account for the tract degeneration or the hemisphere lesions.

The body of a nerve cell whose axon has been interrupted undergoes 'chromatolysis'. The nucleus becomes eccentric in position and the Nissl bodies disappear or break up, the fragments accumulating near the cell membrane. These changes are more readily seen in large nerve cells

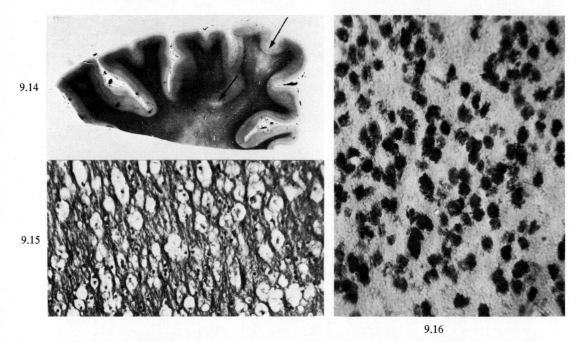

9.14

9.15

9.16

Fig. 9.14 Male aged 27, head injury; quadriplegic and mute until death 15 months later. Parietal region to show severe patchy loss of myelin. Small cortical lesions (arrows) are present at the bottom of two sulci. Myelin stain. × 12.
Fig. 9.15 Portion of degenerated white matter from the same brain as Fig. 9.14. Numerous lipid containing macrophages are still present (see Fig. 9.16). PTAH. × 190.
Fig. 9.16 Frozen section from the same region as Fig. 9.15 showing that the macrophages are full of myelin breakdown products (cholesterol esters). Marchi. × 190.

are frequently involved; the internal capsules are affected (Fig. 9.18), bundles of normal nerve fibres are here seen side by side with degenerated ones. Degeneration of tracts in the lower brainstem is often strikingly *asymmetrical*, one pyramidal tract and the corresponding medial lemniscus (an ascending tract) showing more degeneration than the other (Figs. 9.17*b*, *c*). The superior cerebellar peduncles are usually affected but unequally so; other tracts such as the central tegmental tract and the medial longitudinal bundles may show degeneration. Haemorrhages and small softenings may be seen here and there but are not present in every case. They are never enough to

and can be found in the cerebral cortex or in the brainstem during the first month or so after a head injury. In some anatomical sites, notably the thalamus, nerve cells which have had their axons interrupted actually die and disappear, so-called retrograde degeneration.

The evidence available at present suggests that the degeneration found in the white matter after head injury is secondary to stretching or tearing of nerve fibres at the time of the accident (Strich 1956, 1963, 1969). Since the damage will depend on the direction of shear strains in relation to fibre direction certain patterns of injury may arise (Fig. 9.9) and bundles of nerve fibres could be

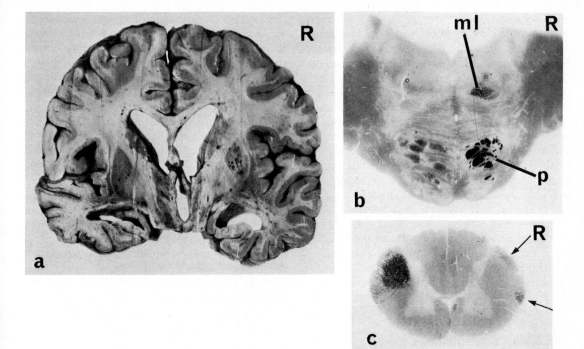

Fig. 9.17 Man aged 18. Motor cycle accident; impact to right side of head, no fractures. Unconscious, generalised epileptic fits becoming localized to the right side. Left spastic hemiplegia. Akinetic mutism until death 13 months later. (*a*) Coronal section through brain showing dilatation of both lateral ventricles and the 3rd ventricle. The cortical ribbon of the left temporal lobe is very thin and the underlying white matter looks granular (long-standing infarction). (*b*) Pons of the same case stained for myelin breakdown products. There is asymmetrical degeneration of the long tracts, the right pyramidal tract (p) and medial lemniscus (ml) being more affected than the left. Marchi. × 1·3. (*c*) Spinal cord of the same case. Note severe degeneration of the left pyramidal tract. There is a little degeneration in the right spinocerebellar tracts (arrows) indicating that the spinal cord itself had been damaged. Marchi. × 1·3. (Part (*b*) reproduced by courtesy of the Editor, *Journal of Clinical Pathology*.)

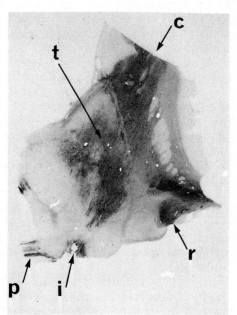

Fig. 9.18 Male aged 16. Decerebrate and mute from time of head injury until death 15 months later. Coronal section through right posterior basal ganglia to show degenerating myelinated nerve fibres in the thalamus (t), the posterior limb (c) and retrolenticular parts of the internal capsule, the optic radiation (r) and the posterior commissure (p). There is a small infarct (i) in the subthalamic region. Marchi. × 1·3.

selectively involved in one or other half of the brain. No other physical theories to account for internal brain damage have been proposed. Some authors feel that cerebral oedema and circulatory disturbances play a major part in the pathogenesis of this white matter lesion (Ule, Döhner and Bues 1961; Jellinger 1965). There is, however, no clinical or pathological evidence for this, once patients with massive intracranial haematomas are excluded. In such patients cerebral oedema and subsequent white matter degeneration do occur but the histology (see below) is unlike that seen in Wallerian degeneration.

Occasionally patients who have had an obviously severe head injury with weeks in coma make a good recovery. The pathological findings in such cases have not been reported and it is not known whether the lesions in patients who recover differ in distribution or only in quantity from those seen by the pathologist in the patients who die in consequence of the injury.

In infants under 5 months old who have had blunt head injuries actual tears may be seen in the white matter extending into the cortex. The healed lesions present as smooth-walled cavities or clefts (Lindenberg and Freytag 1969).

Concussion

The structural or the exact physiological lesions which accompany concussion are still not known. Some signs of concussion (Denny-Brown 1945), such as irregularity or momentary cessation of breathing, changes in blood pressure, slowing of the heart, show that the lower brainstem is implicated. Stimulation of a system of neurons in the reticular formation of pons, midbrain and thalamus arouses a sleeping animal (Lindsley 1960) and conversely lesions anywhere in the brainstem, including the thalamus, may produce coma along with other neurological signs (Cairns 1952; French 1952). Whether the temporary loss of consciousness characteristically associated with concussion is entirely or only due to disturbances in the brainstem is not clear, however. Other important concomitants of concussion such as retrograde and post-traumatic amnesia certainly suggest a more widespread cerebral dysfunction.

Symonds (1962) thought it doubtful on clinical grounds, that the brain in concussion ever escaped some physical damage. Since concussion is by definition a reversible affair very few accounts of its pathology are available in the human. Clusters of microglial cells (Fig. 9.10), probably marking the site of tiny tears, and retraction balls, that is evidence of torn nerve fibres, have in fact been seen in the brainstem and hemispheres of patients who were briefly concussed and died of other causes some days later (Oppenheimer 1968). Such lesions are permanent but they may not leave any detectable neurological sequelae. The lesions are not themselves the cause of concussion, they merely provide obvious evidence of physical damage to the brain. It is possible that there are more widespread reversible lesions which interfere with the function of the nervous system. Thus concussion might be due to physical derangement of cell organelles and synapses or to stretching, rather than tearing, of nerve fibres, changes which can only be elucidated by use of the electron microscope.

The pathology of the *post-concussion syndrome* (Taylor 1967) is unknown.

Concussion in animals

It has proved difficult to produce severe concussion in animals, the margin between a stunning blow and fatal injury being very small. This difficulty was foreseen by Holbourn (1956), who maintained that shear strains due to rotational acceleration are the most likely causes of diffuse brain damage. Such stresses are inversely proportional to the mass$^{\frac{2}{3}}$ of the brain, that is the smaller the brain the less vulnerable it is to rotational forces (Ommaya 1966), and the larger the forces necessary to concuss its owner. Difficulties also arose because, until the work of Denny-Brown and Russell (1941), the importance of movement of the head in head injury was not appreciated. These workers showed, among other things, that it requires less force to concuss an animal if the head is free to move when struck than when it is fixed. Even when applying blows to the mobile head the duration of reversible cerebral dysfunction of the nervous system in all published experiments is a matter of seconds or at most a few minutes, stronger blows causing death. Long periods of coma after a single head injury have not been produced in animals.

Histological changes have been seen in the brains of concussed animals, particularly the lower brainstem on which most authors have focused their attention. Clumping of Nissl bodies was demonstrated in nerve cells in the brainstem of guinea pigs perfused with fixative immediately after a concussive blow (Windle, Groat and Fox 1944). Twenty-four hours after single or multiple blows there was a chromatolysis in certain brainstem nuclei, apparently different from that seen after interruption of the axon. Changes were always found in the lateral vestibular nuclei and in the large cells of the reticular formation of midbrain, pons and medulla. Large pyramidal cells of the cerebral cortex also showed cytological changes. Eventually there was loss of nerve cells, confirmed by cell counts (Windle and Groat 1945; Groat and Simmons 1950). Similar changes were observed in the brainstem and cortex of monkeys that had been concussed once (Groat, Windle and Magoun 1945) and in the spinal cord of cats after a blow to the back (Groat, Rambach and Windle 1945). Windle (1948) also described nerve fibre degeneration in many long tracts of the brain. All these changes were attributed to direct injury. Chromatolysis of large nerve cells and accumulation of glycogen in dendrite and axon terminals has also been seen in electronmicrographs in concussed guinea pigs (Brown, Yoshida, Canty and Verity 1972). Friede (1960, 1961) also found chromatolysis of nerve cells in the brainstem in cats subjected to head injury. He interpreted these changes as true axonal reaction since he found evidence of damage to nerve fibres in the cervical region. He argued that bending and stretching of the neck with damage to the upper spinal cord is the basic mechanism for concussion, at least in cats, in which the cranio-cervical anatomy is, however, different from that of primates.

Because of the difficulties in producing experimental concussion and brain damage with single blows, several workers have administered repeated blows, either on the same or on successive days. Jakob (1913), in a classical study, allowed known weights to fall on to the heads of rabbits or monkeys daily until permanent neurological signs appeared. He found widespread degeneration of nerve fibres which he thought was secondary to physical damage. More recently Unterharnscheidt (1963) subjected cats to a large number of concussive blows over many days. At necropsy there were focal ischaemic lesions in the cerebellum and cerebral cortex. These experiments seem of limited relevance to the problem of human head injuries.

In some of their experiments Windle and associates (and others, for example Chason, Haddad, Webster and Gurdjian 1957) produced the physical signs of 'concussion' by a blow directly on to the exposed dura through a burr hole. This produces a sudden rise in intracranial pressure and distortion of the brain. Chromatolysis was again found in nerve cells in the brainstem. The relevance of such experiments to the effects of blows to the intact head is doubtful.

Damage to the pituitary gland

In fatal head injuries haemorrhages are frequently found in the posterior lobe of the pituitary. Infarction of the anterior lobe is occasionally observed and may be due to actual rupture of the pituitary stalk or to impairment of the blood supply during periods of hypotension etc (see p. 599).

Intracranial haematoma

Extradural (epidural) haematoma

This is a collection of blood between the skull and the dura mater. It is caused by tearing of a blood vessel, usually an artery but sometimes a vein, and this is almost invariably associated with a fracture of the overlying skull bone which may involve the inner table only. Extradural haematoma occurs in 1 to 3% of all head injuries and was found in 15% of 1367 fatal head injuries by Freytag (1963a). Classically these haemorrhages are due to tearing of the middle meningeal artery in the temporal region where the bone is thin and easily fractured. It is important to realize, however, that in 20 to 30% of cases the haemorrhage is not situated in the temporal region (Lewin 1949; McKissock, Taylor, Bloom and Till 1960). Because the dura strips off the skull with difficulty, extradural haematomas remain circumscribed bun-shaped masses (Fig. 9.19). Since the blood accumulates rapidly the effects of raised intracranial pressure and of brain displacement quickly become serious, and the patient will die unless the haematoma is found and removed promptly. The mortality of patients with extradural haematoma varies in different series, but is around 15 to 30% (McKissock et al.). Mortality is high in patients with a short interval between injury and onset of symptoms due to the expanding mass, and it is higher in adults than in children. The prognosis is also worse if there is additional traumatic brain damage but an extra-dural haematoma may develop after a mild head injury and often no brain damage other than that attributable to the effects of a space-occupying lesion is found at necropsy (cf. subdural haema-toma).

cases have fractures of the skull (Freytag 1963*a*). The source of bleeding is often from torn blood vessels in lacerations or contusions of the brain which are frequently present in this type of case. Another cause of bleeding is tearing of bridging veins between cortex and venous sinuses due to

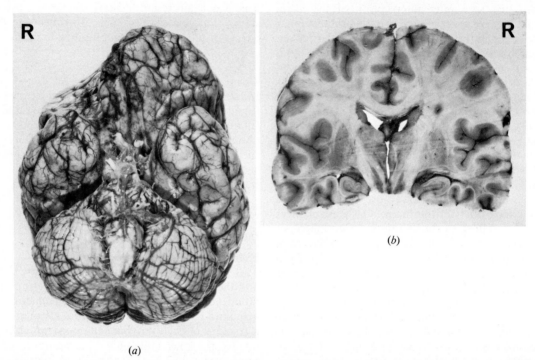

(a)

(b)

Fig. 9.19 Man aged 18. Head-on collision on football field. Dazed, unconscious within a few hours. Clinical diagnosis: cerebral swelling. Died 3 days later. At necropsy a large right subfrontal extradural haematoma and a fracture of the right orbital plate were discovered. (*a*) Base of brain. Note the marked indentation and distortion of the right frontal lobe produced by the haematoma. Small contusions are seen on the gyri recti. (*b*) Coronal section of the same brain at a level posterior to the extradural haematoma. The right hemisphere is swollen, the right lateral ventricle is smaller than the left and the 3rd ventricle is shifted to the left. The boundary between cortex and white matter is indistinct in places.

Subdural haematoma
This is a blood clot lying between the dura and the arachnoid mater, a space normally occupied by a film of fluid. This space is easily opened up, in contrast to the extradural space, and several hundred millilitres of blood may collect in it. A subdural haematoma can consist of a film of blood or a thick mass, but it is usually extensive and may cover a whole cerebral (or cerebellar) hemisphere.

Acute subdural haematoma
This is usually preceded by an obvious head injury and symptoms of a space-occupying lesion appear within hours or days. About half the

movement of the brain at the time of the accident. Subdural haematoma has been reported following whiplash, a violent movement of the head without impact (Ommaya and Yarnell 1969). The lesion has also been described in 'battered babies' who have been shaken violently, rather than hit (Guthkelch 1971).

Recent mortality figures are not available but personal enquiry suggests that the mortality is still between 50 and 80%—a very high figure for a potentially treatable lesion (Loew and Wüstner 1960; McLaurin and Tutor 1961).

Because subdural haematomas tend to be voluminous and extensive, they displace and distort the underlying brain, possibly to a greater extent than do extradural clots. However, both types of haematoma are liable to produce all the complications of rapidly expanding space-occupying lesions which may lead to death. One basis pedunculi may be pressed against the rim of the tentorial opening (Fig. 9.20) giving rise to one of the classical false localizing signs—hemiparesis on the same side as the space-occupying lesion. In fatal cases there is nearly always herniation of the parahippocampal gyrus through the tentorial opening (Fig. 9.20) with compression of the midbrain which may occlude the cerebral

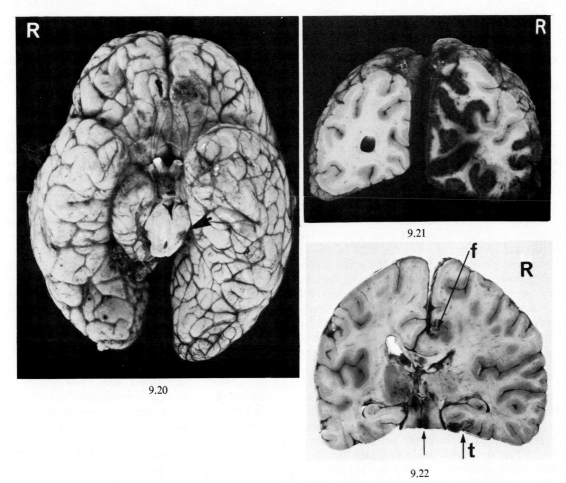

Fig. 9.20 Two-year-old child. Fell off swing, unsteady and drowsy at first, later deeply unconscious. Partial evacuation of right subdural haematoma. Died 5 days after admission. Large right subdural haematoma at necropsy. Base of brain showing pale, widened convolutions on the right (oedema). Note severe right hippocampal herniation with distortion and compression of the midbrain. There is a haemorrhagic lesion (arrow) on the *left* side of the midbrain, caused by pressure against the tentorium cerebelli (Kernohan's notch). Contusions are seen on the undersurface of both frontal lobes. (Reproduced by courtesy of Dr J. A. N. Corsellis.)

Fig. 9.21 A case of acute right sided subdural haematoma. Coronal section through occipital lobes. There is extensive haemorrhagic infarction of the medial and undersurfaces of the right occipital lobe. (Reproduced by courtesy of Dr J. A. N. Corsellis.)

Fig. 9.22 Male aged 74. Head injury, no loss of consciousness. Lapsed into coma 1 hour later. Right subdural haematoma evacuated, brain not swollen then. Died 12 hours later without regaining consciousness. At necropsy only a thin film of subarachnoid blood was found. Coronal section through the brain shows marked swelling of the right hemisphere, its ventricles are almost obliterated. Tentorial herniation has produced haemorrhage and necrosis (t) in the right parahippocampal and fusiform gyri related to the edge of the tent. The right cingulate gyrus has been pushed to the left and there is an area of necrosis (f) above it, related to the edge of the falx. Midline haemorrhages (arrow) have damaged part of the midbrain. Note haemorrhage in corpus callosum.

aqueduct leading to a further rise in supra-tentorial pressure. Midbrain and pontine haemorrhages (rarely found below the middle of the pons) are seen. There may be distortion and downwards shift of the hypothalamus which may contain small haemorrhages (Fig. 9.22). Haemorrhagic cortical infarction of the medial and under surface of the occipital lobes (Fig. 9.21) is a frequent finding. Infarcts in the pituitary gland due to distortion of the stalk have also been described (Wolman 1956).

Oedema surrounding lacerated brain tissue which is so often present contributes to the poor prognosis of these patients. A serious and ill-understood complication is the development of generalized cerebral oedema (Figs. 9.19, 9.22) often *after* the successful evacuation of an extra-dural or subdural clot (Putnam and Cushing 1925; Browder and Rabiner 1951; McLaurin and Tutor 1961). This widespread oedema responds poorly to treatment with steroids, hyperventilation or dehydrating agents, and contributes to the high mortality and morbidity. It may also produce permanent histological changes, that is loss of myelin and gliosis (Fig. 9.24) in the white matter.

Patients can survive all these complications but may be left with varying degrees of disability including states of 'akinetic mutism' or 'apallic syndrome' (Courville and Amyes 1952; Jellinger 1965; see Strich, 1969 for references to further case reports). The pathologist, of course, only sees the brains of patients who have sustained very severe damage and eventually die of this weeks or months after evacuation of an extra-dural or subdural haematoma. In such cases large irregular healed areas of necrosis or haemorrhage are found in the upper pons and midbrain (Fig. 9.25), frequently extending into the hypothalamus or thalamus. Healed cortical infarction is frequently found on the medial surface of one or both occipital lobes and there are often multiple areas of cortical necrosis, sometimes in both hemispheres; healed contusions (Fig. 9.23) may of course also be present. A further source of damage to the brain is the necrosis, probably due to venous obstruction, in tissue which had herniated through a craniotomy which is sometimes made in this group of patients (Fig. 9.23). In addition, there is gross demyelination, probably the consequence of cerebral oedema (Fig. 9.24) most marked in the brain under the evacuated space-occupying lesion, but by no means always confined to this site.

Chronic subdural haematoma

If the accumulation of blood is slow or small, and particularly if there is a large subarachnoid space as in the elderly, the haematoma does not produce immediate symptoms but becomes organized. In such cases there is often a history of only a trivial or even no injury and there may be no obvious damage to the brain (Fig. 9.26). At times the trauma is not to the head, but there may have been a sudden jar as in a fall on the buttocks. Patients on anticoagulants or with blood-clotting disorders are also liable to develop haematomas after very slight blows to the head (Wiener and Nathanson 1962).

Chronic subdural haematomas may be very large (Fig. 9.26) and are often bilateral. The clot becomes surrounded by endothelial cells and granulation tissue begins to grow in, almost entirely from the dural aspect (Putnam and Cushing 1925). The haematoma, which may liquefy, becomes enclosed by a highly vascular membrane containing much iron pigment, the membrane on the dural (outer) aspect of the clot is thicker and more vascular than the inner membrane (Fig. 9.27). Once the membranes have formed (2 to 3 weeks) it is not possible to determine their age. Fresh blood is often seen in these membranes (Fig. 9.27) and continuing bleeding or transudation of plasma (Putnam and Cushing 1925) may be the reason why a chronic subdural haematoma may present as a slowly expanding space occupying lesion.

A subdural haematoma may re-absorb completely without surgical intervention, and all that is left eventually is a thin yellow membrane. At times the final stage is a thick walled sac containing clear fluid and calcified or ossified haematomas have also been reported (Chusid and de Gutiérrez-Mahoney 1953).

Chronic subdural haematoma in infancy

There is usually a history of a traumatic delivery or of a fall on the head. An important physical sign is enlargement of the head due to the accumulation of blood which is frequently bilateral. Brain damage and mental retardation is sometimes seen in children who have had a haematoma in infancy (Ingraham and Matson 1944; Phillips 1955), particularly when the lesion developed in the first month or two of life. In such cases there is no good evidence that the haematoma was itself harmful to the brain;

rather it is thought that it accompanies brain damage due to other causes, e.g. birth trauma or neonatal asphyxia (Christensen and Husby 1963; Mealey 1968).

Experimental acute extradural or subdural space-occupying lesions

These have been produced by introducing inflatable balloons into the skull (Ishii, Hayner, Kelly

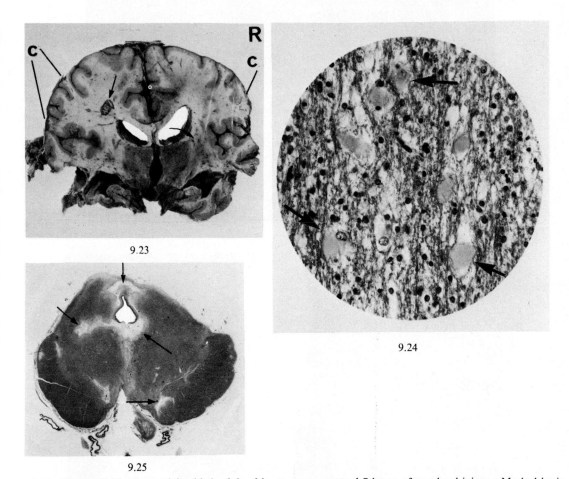

9.23

9.24

9.25

Fig. 9.23 Man aged 55. Large right-sided subdural haematoma removed 7 hours after a head injury. Marked brain swelling postoperatively, bilateral temporal decompression. Survived 3 months in a state of 'akinetic mutism'. Coronal section through the brain shows much loss of tissue of both temporal lobes, partly due to lacerations, partly due to necrosis secondary to herniation through the surgical decompression. Notice cyst in white matter (arrow) and healed contusions (c) on apices of gyri. The ventricles are dilated.

Fig. 9.24 White matter from the brain seen in Fig. 9.23. There is loss of myelinated fibres. Numerous swollen astrocytes (arrows to some) are present but there are no lipid-laden macrophages. These appearances are probably the consequence of severe cerebral oedema. PTAH. × 250.

Fig. 9.25 Man aged 24, fell off a lorry, unconscious soon afterwards. Extradural and subdural haematoma removed 12 hours later. Raised intracranial pressure for many days. Died without recovering consciousness 84 days after the accident. The brain showed severe loss of white matter with gliosis and many areas of cortical infarction. Midbrain shows several healed areas of haemorrhage and necrosis (arrows to some). PTAH. × 1·3.

Subdural hygroma. This consists of a pool of cerebrospinal fluid which has collected in the subdural space from which it cannot be absorbed. It is thought to be due to a tear in the arachnoid.

and Evans 1959; Langfitt, Shawaluk, Mahoney, Stein and Hedges 1964; Klintworth 1965). Herniation of the hippocampal gyrus, brainstem haemorrhages, and papilloedema have been pro-

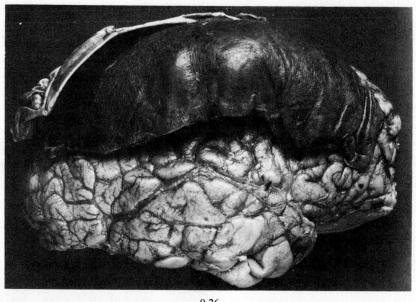

9.26

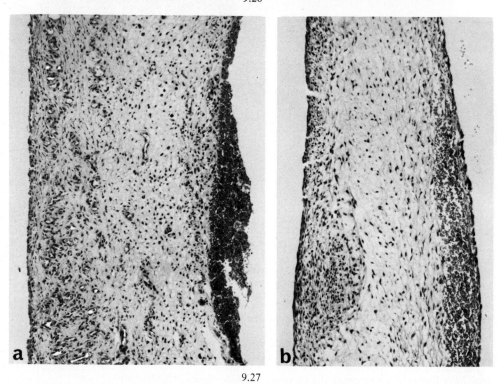

9.27

Fig. 9.26 Chronic subdural haematoma. There was no history of injury, but progressive symptoms went back for nearly a year. Note the complete encapsulation, freedom from the arachnoid and clean separation from the dura mater.
Fig. 9.27 Subdural haematoma, mild head injury 4 weeks before operation. (*a*) Outer membrane consists of well vascularized granulation tissue and collagen. Well preserved blood clot is seen on the inner (right) surface. (*b*) Inner membrane is thinner and consists of loose connective tissue with few blood vessels. Fresh haemorrhage into the membrane is seen at the right. Haematoxylin and eosin. × 105.

duced in this way. As in the human, severe uni-lateral cerebral oedema occurs, usually after the removal of the balloon, and this in the absence of brain lacerations. It has been confirmed with the electron microscope that the brain swelling is due to an accumulation of fluid both within cells and in the extracellular space (Tani and Evans 1965).

Cerebral oedema after head injury
Regional oedema
Regional oedema occurs in the white matter sur-rounding lacerations and contusions, and under-neath intracerebral and extracerebral haematomas

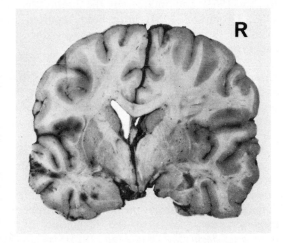

Fig. 9.28 Man aged 20, motorcycle accident; multiple skull fractures; survived 10 hours. The brain was swollen, there were severe lacerations in left occipital and frontal lobes. Coronal section shows contusions and haemor-rhages in the left temporal lobe. The right hemisphere is swollen although there was little macroscopic damage to that side of the brain. Midline structures are shifted to the left, the right cingular gyrus is herniated to the left.

(Figs. 9.19, 9.22, 9.28) (see above). In acute cases the white matter is increased in bulk and looks wet and often slightly yellow. Microscopically the myelin sheaths are irregular and are spaced far apart. The astrocytes have enlarged nuclei and swollen cytoplasm (Fig. 9.24). Astrocytes react quickly (Klatzo, Piraux and Laskowski 1958) and this is useful in the histological diag-nosis of cerebral oedema. After some weeks there is atrophy of the white matter with rarefac-tion of myelin and even cyst formation (Fig. 9.23). The astrocytes remain enlarged and there is well-marked fibrous gliosis. Very little neutral fat

(myelin breakdown products) is seen at any stage and this is in marked contrast to the large amounts of neutral fat seen in traumatic white matter degeneration due to tearing of nerve fibres. The mechanism by which myelin disappears in cerebral oedema is not known.

The course of events in oedema due to traumatic lesions has been investigated experimentally (Klatzo 1967). Oedema fluid leaks out of the damaged blood vessels in the actually injured tissue. From there it apparently seeps far into the surrounding white matter the vascular per-meability of which is not abnormal. A rise in systemic blood pressure which may accompany the rise in intracranial pressure increases the out-pouring of fluid and makes the oedema worse (Schutta, Kassell and Langfitt 1968).

Generalized cerebral oedema
After uncomplicated head injury this is probably rare in adults (Greenfield 1938) though it is diffi-cult to ascertain how common it is. Cerebral oedema is a dangerous complication which is difficult to treat and which produces its harmful effects partly by causing distortion, displacement and herniation of brain substance. In addition, raised intracranial pressure, which can now be monitored continuously in patients (Lundberg, Troupp and Lorin 1965), may compromise the cerebral circulation. This is because the effective cerebral perfusion pressure is the difference between the intracranial pressure and the arterial blood pressure. It has been shown that the rise in blood pressure which usually occurs when the intracranial pressure rises (the Cushing response) does not take place in some cases of severe head injury (Johnston, Johnston and Jennett 1970) so that the blood flow through the brain becomes inadequate. The evidence that oedema occurs in experimental concussion (always a slight affair compared with most human cases) is contradic-tory. The subject has recently been reviewed and re-investigated by Faas and Ommaya (1968) who found no change in brain water or electrolyte content after concussion in monkeys. Langfitt, Tannanbaum and Kassell (1966) have produced evidence that raised intracranial pressure seen in experimental head injury may be 'vasogenic', that is, due to an increased intracranial blood volume. This cerebral vascular engorgement may be due to vasodilatation caused by vasoparalysis or CO_2 retention caused by impaired respiration. Con-

gestion can certainly contribute to raised intra-cranial pressure seen in some human patients and is important because it is amenable to treatment. Evans and Scheinker (1945) have reported cases of disability after head injury associated with cystic white matter. They regarded venous stasis as an important factor in the production of demyelination.

Patients with head injury may pass through hypoxic episodes due to injuries of the chest, or to obstructed airway due to inhaled vomit, faulty positioning of the head while unconscious, etc. Such hypoxic brain damage may also lead to cerebral oedema (see Chapter 2).

Marked generalized brain swelling occasionally occurs in *children* (Pickles 1950; Mealey 1968) after a head injury which may have been quite trivial. If the patients die, the brain is large and pale and shows marked flattening of con-volutions and small symmetrical ventricles, but usually no obvious signs of injury. Parahippo-campal and tonsillar herniation are not usually seen.

Vascular lesions

Areas of necrosis are often seen in the brains of patients who have died from head injuries. Lesions may be small and involve only the cortex at the bottom of a few sulci or part or the whole territory of a major cerebral artery (Fig. 9.17) may be affected (Lewin 1968). Sometimes the infarcts are situated at the boundary zones (Fig. 9.29) between the territories of adjacent cerebral arteries (Graham and Adams 1971). Large irregular areas of necrosis may be seen near lacerations. Rarely multiple small ischaemic lesions develop in grey matter after a trivial head injury. These lesions may be severe enough to cause death or to produce post-traumatic dementia (Denst, Richey and Neubuerger 1958; Nyström 1960). We have seen two patients who suddenly lapsed into coma minutes after a trivial head injury; the brain in each case showed innumerable areas of necrosis (Fig. 9.30) strictly confined to grey matter.

The pathogenesis of vascular lesions in head injuries is still debated and no doubt combinations of different factors are at work in different cases. Causes which have to be considered include spasm of blood vessels, systemic hypotension (q.v.), pre-existing atheroma, thrombosis, em-bolism, and a drop in perfusion pressure due to a combination of raised intracranial and low or normal blood pressure (Johnston *et al.* 1970). Vascular spasm can never be demonstrated *post mortem*, but it is well known that it can be induced by kinking or stretching a vessel as may happen during movement of the brain at the time of the accident, or for example by direct damage of the vessel wall by bone frag-ments. Evidence that mechanical strains occur around vessels in cerebral trauma is provided by the finding of torn nerve fibres (retraction balls) and clusters of microglial cells in tissue immedi-ately adjacent to blood vessels. Massive subarach-noid haemorrhage may also be important in this connection since vasospasm during life (du Boulay 1963) and infarcts in the brain (Smith 1963; Crompton 1964) have been reported in cases of subarachnoid haemorrhage due to aneurysm.

Thrombosis of a carotid artery (Yamada, Kindt and Youmans 1967) or a vertebral artery in the neck is seen occasionally, especially in injuries involving hyperextension of the neck or in penetrating injury of that region.

The internal carotid artery may be torn where it lies in the cavernous sinus by a fracture passing through the base of the skull, giving rise to an *arteriovenous aneurysm* (Krauland 1955). Rarely damage to the tunica media of a peripheral cerebral artery leads to the formation of a *traumatic aneurysm* (Krauland 1955) within a week or two. This has also been reported follow-ing surgical trauma (Burton, Velasco and Dorman 1968.)

Delayed cerebral haemorrhage (Spät-Apoplexie), that is a stroke some days or weeks after a head injury, is a rare but well-documented event (Morin and Pitts 1970). The patients are usually children or young people and the injuries to the head tend to have been slight. The pathogenesis is not clear.

Cysts. A cyst may form in the white matter under a traumatic or surgical bony defect when-ever some degree of cerebral herniation has taken place. Such cysts were observed in otherwise normal rabbits when a craniotomy with opening of the dura mater had been followed by transitory herniation (Falconer and Russell 1944). In some examples the cysts communicated with the lateral ventricle. Their formation was explained by

Holbourn (1944) as the result of stresses set up in the hernia which would tend to cause splitting at the junction of cortex and white matter: the site, in fact, where the cysts were observed to originate. If there is raised intracranial pressure as well as a bony defect the venous return of the herniated tissue is obstructed leading to its infarction (Fig. 9.23). A cystic cavity communicating

Post-traumatic epilepsy

There are many reviews of the incidence and clinical aspects of post-traumatic epilepsy (Phillips 1954; Caveness, Walker and Ascroft 1962; Jennett 1962) but the underlying pathology and electrophysiology of fits occurring within hours of an injury, or of those following years later, are not well understood. In uncomplicated head

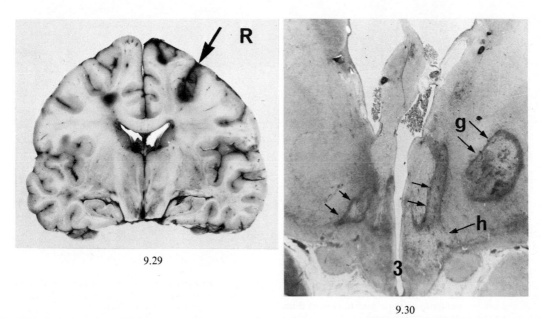

9.29

9.30

Fig. 9.29 Girl aged 15. Head injury. Unconscious. Evacuation of small subdural haematoma on 4th day. Died 8 days after the accident. The brain was swollen. Coronal section shows that the convolutions are flattened. There are a few haemorrhages and an area of cortical necrosis (arrow) at the boundary zone between the territories of the right anterior and middle cerebral arteries.

Fig. 9.30 Boy aged 18. Trivial head injury on football field, lapsed into coma a few minutes later. Decerebrate and unconscious until death 10 days later. There were innumerable small areas of necrosis in the grey matter of cerebral hemispheres and brain stem. This section is through the hypothalamus. Areas of necrosis (arrows) surrounded by a rim of granulation tissue are seen, some in the hypothalamus (h) and globus pallidus (g). 3 = 3rd ventricle. Nissl. × 3.

with the subarachnoid or subdural space will then be left.

Brain tissue which has been destroyed, for example by indriven pieces of bone, is removed by macrophages and eventually a cyst is formed. If this cyst is in continuity with the ventricle a diverticulum (Fig. 9.31) develops which is lined with glial fibrils, not with ependyma. Such a cyst may be in direct communication with one of the air sinuses (aerocele) and a spontaneous air ventriculogram may be discovered on a skull X-ray. Infection may obviously also reach the ventricles in this way.

injuries the incidence of epilepsy is low. Intracranial haematoma, depressed fracture (Miller and Jennett 1968) and particularly penetration of the dura and infection of the wound greatly increase the incidence of both early and late epilepsy. These conditions are likely to produce fibrous tissue scars in the cerebral cortex (simple contusions usually leave a thin glial scar (Fig. 9.7) over the cortical defect) or between cortex and meninges (Fig. 9.32) and these are liable to distort and pull on the brain (Penfield 1927; Foerster and Penfield 1930). Excision of the scar will often relieve the epilepsy. Occasionally

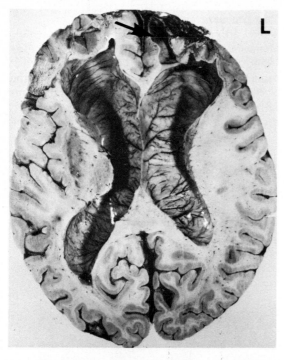

Fig. 9.31 Male aged 65. Head injury. Comminuted fractures of left orbital plate and frontal bone. Bilateral subdural haematomas. Remained decerebrate and almost mute and died 10 weeks after the accident. Horizontal section through the brain shows dilated ventricles, old necrosis and contusions of the left frontal lobe. There is a diverticulum from the left anterior horn (arrow). It is closed off by granulation tissue and thickened dura which lay on the shattered frontal bones.

a trivial head injury will precipitate a series of fits and this (like status epilepticus from other causes) may produce widespread damage in the nervous system especially in children (Small and Woolf 1957, personal observations).

Cerebral fat embolism

This serious complication, which may affect the brain as well as other organs, occurs when there have been bone fractures or when marrow-containing bone has been operated upon as in splitting of the sternum during cardiac surgery. If the patients survive, they usually recover completely and only few cases with residual neurological signs have been reported (Harnett, Paterson, Lowe, Stewart and Uytman 1959; McTaggart and Neubuerger 1970). The patho-genesis of lesions seen in cerebral fat embolism has not been satisfactorily explained. Histologically, fat emboli are found in profusion in

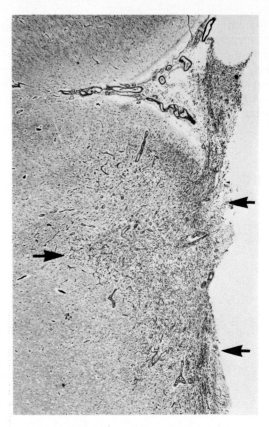

Fig. 9.32 An early meningo-cerebral cicatrix (1 month). There is a wedge-shaped area of destruction of the cerebral cortex (outlined by arrows) which is being organized by ingrowth of fibrous tissue and blood vessels from the arachnoid which is itself thickened. Compare with Fig. 9.7 which shows a cortical contusion without meningeal involvement. Reticulin. × 23.

the grey matter (Fig. 9.34a) and the posterior lobe of the pituitary, structures in which but a few areas of necrosis are seen (Neubuerger 1925; Winkelman, Henn and Spann 1965). On the other hand few emboli are found in the white matter which is the seat of numerous perivascular areas of necrosis which may be confluent and in which the walls of the blood vessels often appear to be necrotic (Figs. 9.34-9.36). In addition there may be a few or very many ball and ring haemorrhages (Fig. 9.33). The necrotic foci heal with the formation of a collagenous scar in which fat containing macrophages are enmeshed. The haemorrhages leave minute clusters or scattered macrophages containing haemosiderin. It seems that it is the areas of necrosis rather than the petechiae which cause the brain damage seen in survivors (McTaggart and Neubuerger 1970,

7-year survival). Fat can be seen in capillaries for at least 2 weeks after the onset of clinical signs.

Cerebral embolism to lung
Brain tissue is found in the lungs of about 2% of patients who have died after severe head injuries. Laceration of dural sinuses as well as lacerated brain is usually found (McMillan 1956). The emboli may be large enough to be seen with the naked eye (Wacks and Bird 1970) and to cause pulmonary infarcts. Emboli may also appear after neurosurgical operations.

Progressive neurological disease after head injury
There are a number of instances where a single injury is said to have been followed by a progressive neurological disorder. The reader will find many of the case reports unconvincing, however, either because the injury was too trivial (or not even to the head), or because the time interval between trauma and onset of the disease was too long. Diseases for which an association with head injury has been claimed include Alzheimer's disease (Corsellis and Brierley 1959; Hollander and Strich 1970), Pick's disease (McMenemy, Grant and Behrman 1965), Parkinson's disease (Grimberg 1934), motor neuron disease and Creutzfeldt-Jakob disease (Behrman, Mandybur and McMenemy 1962). In these cases the pathology is that of the particular disease rather than that of trauma though it has been suggested that haemorrhage in the substantia nigra and the globus pallidus might be the cause of post-traumatic Parkinsonism (Lindenberg 1964; Jellinger 1966).

It is well established that persons subjected to repeated concussive or sub-concussive blows such as boxers and footballers may develop neurological signs and progressive dementia, the 'punch-drunk' syndrome (Mawdsley and Ferguson 1963; Roberts 1969). This dementia tends to become apparent in the early years of retirement from boxing, and affects amateur as well as professional boxers, especially those with long careers. Most of the brains examined have shown some cortical atrophy and there is a remarkably high incidence of a cavum in the septum pellucidum (Fig. 9.37) which is often torn (Spillane 1962; Mawdsley and Ferguson 1963).

Many of the brains that have been examined histologically show that a large number of neurons contain neurofibrillary tangles especially in the temporal lobes (Fig. 9.38). Senile plaques, like those seen in Alzheimer's disease, however, are commonly absent in these cases—a finding worthy of comment (Brandenburg and Hallervorden 1954; Grahmann and Ule 1957; Constantinides and Tissot 1967; Corsellis, Bruton and Freeman-Browne 1973).

The pathogenesis of neurofibrillary thickening in this, as in other conditions, is quite obscure. Hallervorden and Quadbeck (1957) proposed a theory involving thixotropy by which repeated disturbance of the gel–sol equilibrium leads to irreversible changes in nerve cell colloid, but this was before anything was known about cell organelles and the theory may now be of no more than historical interest. Another change which has frequently been reported in the brains of 'punch-drunk' boxers is degeneration of the substantia nigra. Atypical Pick's disease has been suggested in one case (Neuberger, Sinton and Denst 1959), and small cortical infarcts of doubtful significance have been described in some brains (Payne 1968).

Trauma and intracranial neoplasms
Microscopic nodules of meningeal cells, sometimes with psammoma bodies, readily develop at the site of any injury. From time to time trauma is invoked as a cause for large meningiomas and gliomas. The published case reports have been reviewed by Zülch (1970) and by Russell and Rubinstein (1971) who state that 'it must be concluded that these few cases are more curious than significant'.

Penetrating wounds
Damage caused by bullets, or by fragments of shells or bomb casing varies chiefly according to size, and the velocity of the missile as it strikes the head. Small flying objects which have a high kinetic energy but impart little momentum will produce much local damage but little rotational (distant) damage since there will be little movement of the head. The extreme example of this is the high-velocity bullet which may traverse the head without knocking the victim down or causing impairment of consciousness. A large cavity momentarily forms in the bullet's wake due to radial acceleration of the traversed tissue. This and heat generated produce a wide sleeve of necrotic and haemorrhagic tissue (Fig. 9.39)

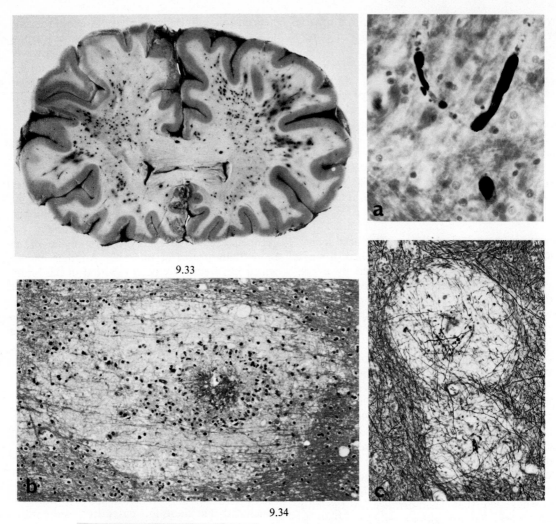

9.33

9.34

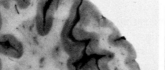

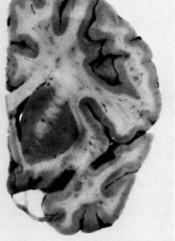

9.35

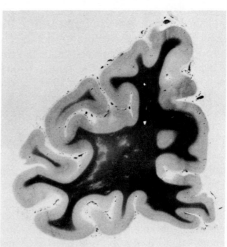

9.36

Fig. 9.33 Male aged 55. Fat embolism, 4 days' survival. Coronal section of the brain shows numerous small haemorrhages confined to white matter. A few haemorrhages were seen in cerebellum and brainstem.

Fig. 9.34 Woman aged 28. Fat embolism. Fall from a great height. Multiple fractures of long bones, not unconscious. Became comatose after 3 days and died 7 days after the injuries. (*a*) Section through *pons* stained for fat to show the fat emboli. Oil-red-0. × 176. (*b*) White matter showing an apparently necrotic blood vessel surrounded by a sharply demarcated zone of demyelination. A few intact myelin sheaths are running through the abnormal zone. Myelin stain. × 100. (*c*) White matter with two punched-out lesions showing severe but not complete loss of nerve fibres. There was very little fat in the white matter. Palmgren. × 100.

Fig. 9.35 Man aged 74. Fat embolism. Fractured femur, became unconscious that evening and remained so until death 14 days later. Coronal section through right frontal lobe. There were numerous small grey areas in the white matter. No haemorrhages were seen. Areas of perivascular demyelination were seen microscopically and numerous fat emboli could be demonstrated.

Fig. 9.36 Male aged 34. Multiple fractures. Concussed. Fat embolism. Became unconscious and remained so for 3 weeks. Gradual, almost complete recovery. Died of pulmonary embolus 5 months after the accident. Section through frontal lobe shows multiple confluent areas of demyelination and diffuse loss of myelin in the lateral part of the lobe. Myelin stain. × 1·5.

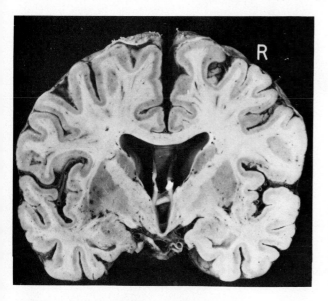

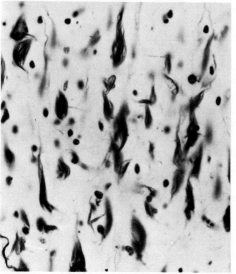

Fig. 9.37 Well-known boxer, died aged 83. Dysarthria, ataxia, aggressive outbursts, and poor memory developed towards end of boxing career. Coronal section through the brain shows cortical atrophy, moderately dilated ventricles, and a wide cavum, with torn walls, in the septum pellucidum (under the corpus callosum).

Fig. 9.38 Professional boxer and world champion, died aged 63. Vagrant since end of boxing career, demented. Section of the cortex of the temporal lobe. Almost every neuron contains thick tangles of neurofibrils. There are no sensile plaques. Bielschowsky. × 325.

around the track. The enormous rise in intra-cranial pressure (40 atmospheres or more) which accompanies the passage of a high-velocity missile may cause fractures of the orbital roofs uncon-nected with those made by the missile. Contusions are sometimes seen in distant parts of the brain, mainly on its undersurface and on the cerebellar tonsils (Freytag 1963*b*). A bullet fired at long range, smaller calibre bullets or pellets from shot-guns as used in hunting leave only a narrow track (if they penetrate the skull at all). The

it becomes clear that there has been very little new since 1900. Many of the important experi-ments on concussion were done by Polis (1894) and by Witkowski (1877). Witkowski observed the pial arteries through a trephine hole during concussion and also produced permanent neuro-logical signs—tremulousness and loss of will-power—in frogs by subjecting them to repeated head injuries. Scagliosi (1898) described clumping of Nissl substance in nerve cells within an hour of experimental concussion, followed later by

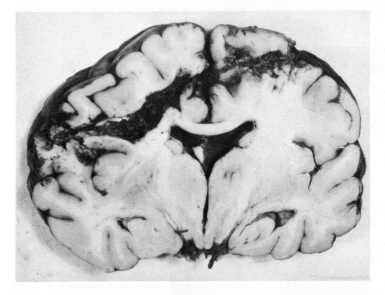

Fig. 9.39 Track of bullet wound through frontal lobes, from right to left.

entrance hole is conical and fractures of the inner table of the skull may be many times larger than the hole in the outer table. Injuries from low-velocity missiles tend to be complicated by frag-ments of bone (and scalp and clothing) driven into the brain (Sights 1969). The result is severe laceration of the brain with damage to blood vessels causing haemorrhage and necrosis. Low-velocity missiles often have not enough energy to leave the skull, and the bullet may ricochet from the skull and traverse the brain several times. Haemorrhage in the track and infection of the brain (Cairns, Calvert, Daniel and Northcroft 1947) are serious complications of any kind of penetrating wound and make early surgical débridement essential.

Historical perspective
On looking through the literature on head injuries

chromatolysis. Retraction balls on severed nerve fibres were described by Schmaus in 1890 in experimental spinal concussion and by Hauser in 1900 in a human case of head injury. Bikeles (1895) reported that lesions in the cervical spinal cord and brainstem were consistently seen after concussion in guinea pigs. Cerebral oedema and brain swelling due to vascular engorgement in head injuries were discussed fully by Courtney (1899). The first case report in which there were infarcts in the brain underlying a subdural haematoma was made by Köppen in 1900, and the first case of traumatic white matter degenera-tion was described by Rosenblath in 1899. His patient survived in a 'sleep-like' state for 8 months. During this time he had to be fed by stomach tube, one of the items fed being soup made of dried meat extract.

    The pre-nineteenth century literature on head

injuries and on concussion, post-concussion syndrome and post-traumatic brain damage has been collected by Courville (1953).

to the nervous system for neoplasms, has led to necrosis of nervous tissue (Pennybacker and Russell 1948; Crompton and Layton 1961; Afra,

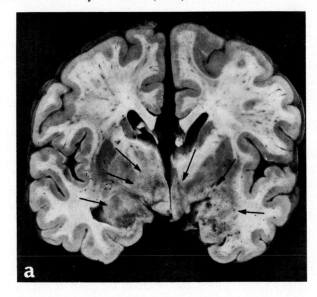

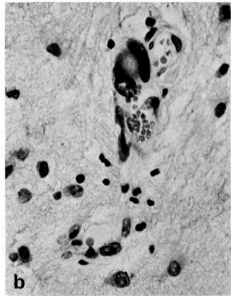

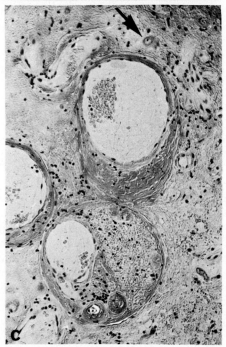

Fig. 9.40 Woman aged 55. Radiation necrosis. X-rays to pituitary fossa for chromophobe adenoma. Progressive neurological illness began 12 months after treatment and ended in death 5 months later. (*a*) Coronal section through the brain at the level of pituitary stalk, shows ill-defined areas of swelling and necrosis (outlined by arrows) affecting the hypothalamus and the amygdaloid nuclei. (*b*) cells with bizarre giant nuclei, possibly endothelial cells of blood vessels, at the edge of the necrotic regions. Astrocytes have enlarged nuclei and swollen cytoplasm. Haematoxylin and eosin. × 300. (*c*) Blood vessels in the necrotic, rather acellular area are tortuous, enlarged and some are thrombosed. Their walls show fibrinoid necrosis. A nerve cell (arrow) survives in the necrotic zone. Haematoxylin and eosin. × 75. (Reproduced by courtesy of the Editor, *Brain*.)

Damage caused by physical agents

X-irradiation
Cases have been reported in which therapeutic radiation to the scalp or neck for carcinoma, or

Müller and Wilcke 1965, Cobalt-60 beads; Kristensson, Molin and Sourander 1967, spinal cord). The symptoms of radiation necrosis do not appear until months after treatment, but may then progress rapidly to a fatal issue. In such cases the cortex in the damaged areas is swollen, yellow or brownish, tough and poorly demarcated from the underlying white matter which may also have an unduly firm consistency or may be cystic or necrotic (Fig. 9.40a). Microscopically, in cases of moderate severity there is disappearance of neurons in the cortex especially on the summits of convolutions with massive fibrillary gliosis spreading in from the surface. Near the centre of the lesion and in the path of the irradiation there are irregular or scattered areas of necrosis, which in most reports has affected white matter more than grey. Fibrinoid necrosis (Fig. 9.40c) or hyaline change of the walls of the blood vessels is a characteristic finding and thrombosis is frequently seen. The diseased vessels are surrounded by fibrinous or albuminous exudate which infiltrates the necrotic tissue. There is remarkably little cellular reaction to the necrosis. There is, however, an increased number of astrocytes in the surrounding tissue, and many are swollen and have large nuclei. The nuclei of the endothelial cells of blood vessels may also enlarge and become bizarre (Fig. 9.40b). Massive deposition of *amyloid* in the brain has also been reported after X-ray treatment for carcinoma of the scalp (Fischer and Holfelder 1930). Delayed necrosis of the brain, preferentially, of the white matter was produced 13 to 17 weeks after irradiation of the brain in monkeys (Haymaker, Brahim, Miguel and Call 1968).

The literature on the effects of irradiation of the brain of young or mature experimental animals is too extensive to be reviewed here (but see Haley and Snider 1962, 1964; Zeman 1968).

Laser-irradiation

If a laser beam of sufficient intensity is focused on the skull of an animal it will die instantaneously, death being due to a sudden rise in intracranial pressure due to vaporization of the brain under the bone which absorbs the energy (Hayes, Fox and Stein 1967). At lower intensities there is a circumscribed area of coagulation necrosis (Lampert, Fox and Earle 1966) surrounded by a zone of oedema.

α-particle radiation

The effects of this on the brain have proved interesting. Tissue is damaged according to the amount of energy absorbed and this is greatest at the greatest depth of particle penetration (Malis, Baker, Kruger and Rose 1960). Therefore irradiation with α-particles produces a thin straight line of necrosis with a zone of partial damage above it. A marked growth of nerve fibres, which become myelinated, takes place across the gap (Rose, Malis, Kruger and Baker 1960; Maxwell and Kruger 1964; Estable-Puig, de Estable, Tobias and Haymaker 1965). This is one of the few situations where regeneration or at least nerve growth can be studied in the adult central nervous system.

Ultra-sound

Focused ultra-sound waves may produce a circumscribed lesion in the brain especially in the white matter, the tissue in the path of the beam remaining apparently normal (Åstrom, Bell, Ballantine and Heidensleben 1961). The beam must be applied through a burrhole in the skull because the high ultrasonic absorption of bone results in much heat and secondary damage to surrounding tissues (Lynn and Putnam 1944). There is necrosis of the target area with fragmentation and severing of nerve fibres and blood vessels though with little haemorrhage. This kind of lesion has been used as an alternative to frontal leucotomy in patients. On post-mortem examination of 25 such cases, Nelson, Lindstrom and Haymaker (1959) found degrees of tissue damage varying from slight astrocytic reaction and questionable myelin damage to large areas of necrosis in the white matter surrounded by a zone of demyelination. In cases where the dura had been accidentally opened, laminar cortical necrosis was also seen. The central core of the lesion in the white matter was remarkable in that it sometimes showed no dissolution even several weeks after treatment.

References

Afra, D., Müller, W. & Wilcke, O. (1965) Spätveränderungen im menschlichen Gehirn nach intraoperativer Einlage von Co60-Perlen. *Acta Neuropathologica (Berlin)*, **4**, 299-311.

Anzelius, A. (1943) The effect of an impact on a spherical liquid mass. *Acta pathologica et microbiologica scandinavica*, Suppl. 48, 153-159.

Åstrom, K. E., Bell, E., Ballantine, H. T. & Heidensleben, E. (1961) An experimental neuropathological study of the effect of high-frequency focused ultrasound on the brain of the cat. *Journal of Neuropathology and Experimental Neurology*, **20**, 484-520.

Behrman, S., Mandybur, T. & McMenemey, W. H. (1962) Un cas de maladie Creutzfeld-Jacob à la suite d'un traumatisme cérébrale. *Revue Neurologique*, **107**, 453-459.

Bikeles (1895) quoted by Jakob (1913).

du Boulay, G. (1963) Distribution of spasm in the intracranial arteries after subarachnoid haemorrhage. *Acta radiologica n.s.* **1** (diagnosis), 257-266.

Brandenburg, W. & Hallervorden, J. (1954) Dementia pugilistica mit anatomischem Befund. *Virchows Archiv für pathologische Anatomie und Physiologie*, **325**, 680-709.

Browder, J. & Rabiner, A. M. (1951) Regional swelling of the brain in subdural hematoma. *Annals of Surgery*, **134**, 369-375.

Brown, W. J., Yoshida, N., Canty, T. & Verity, M. A. (1972) Experimental concussion. *American Journal of Pathology*, **67**, 41-57.

Burton, C., Velasco, F. & Dorman, J. (1968) Traumatic aneurysm of a peripheral artery. Review and case report. *Journal of Neurosurgery*, **28**, 468-474.

Cairns, H. (1952) Disturbances of consciousness with lesions of the brain-stem and diencephalon. *Brain*, **75**, 109-146.

Cairns, H., Calvert, C. A., Daniel, P. & Northcroft, G. B. (1947) Complications of head wounds, with especial reference to infection. *British Journal of Surgery*, War Surgery suppl. 1, 198-243.

Caveness, W. F. & Walker, A. E. (1966) *Head injury*, pp. 503-545, Lippincott, Philadelphia.

Caveness, W. F., Walker, A. E. & Ascroft, P. B. (1962) Incidence of post-traumatic epilepsy in Korean veterans as compared with those from world war I and world war II. *Journal of Neurosurgery*, **19**, 122-128.

Chason, J. L., Haddad, B. F., Webster, J. E. & Gurdjian, E. S. (1957) Alteration in cell structure following sudden increase in intracranial pressure. *Journal of Neuropathology and Experimental Neurology*, **16**, 102-107.

Christensen, E. & Husby, J. (1963) Chronic subdural hematoma in infancy. *Acta neurologica scandinavica*, **39**, 323-342.

Chusid, J. G. & de Gutiérrez-Mahoney, C. G. (1953) Ossifying subdural hematoma. *Journal of Neurosurgery*, **10**, 430-434.

Constantinides, J. & Tissot, R. (1967) Lésions neurofibrillaires d'Alzheimer généralisées sans plaques séniles. *Archives Suisses de Neurologie, Neurochirurgie et Psychiatrie*, **100**, 117-130.

Corsellis, J. A. N. & Brierley, J. B. (1959) Observations on the pathology of insidious dementia following head injury. *Journal of Mental Science*, **105**, 714-720.

Corsellis, J. A. N., Bruton, C. J. & Freeman-Browne, D. (1973) The aftermath of boxing. *Psychological Medicine*, **3**, 270-303.

Courtney, J. W. (1899) Traumatic cerebral edema: its pathology and surgical treatment—a critical study. *Boston Medical and Surgical Journal*, **140**, 345-348.

Courville, C. B. (1953) *Commotio Cerebri*, San Lucas Press, Los Angeles.

Courville, C. B. & Amyes, E. W. (1952) Late residual lesions of the brain consequent to dural hemorrhage. *Bulletin of the Los Angeles Neurological Society*, **17**, 163-176.

Crompton, M. R. (1964) Cerebral infarction following rupture of cerebral berry aneurysms. *Brain*, **87**, 263-280.

Crompton, M. R. (1970) Visual lesions in closed head injury. *Brain*, **93**, 785-792.

Crompton, M. R. (1971) Hypothalamic lesions following closed head injury. *Brain*, **94**, 165-172.

Crompton, M. R. & Layton, D. D. (1961) Delayed radionecrosis of the brain following therapeutic X-radiation of the pituitary. *Brain*, **84**, 85-101.

Daniel, P. M. & Strich, S. J. (1969) Histological observations on Wallerian degeneration in the spinal cord of the baboon, *Papio papio. Acta neuropathologica (Berlin)*, **12**, 314-328.

Denny-Brown, D. (1945) Cerebral concussion. *Physiological Reviews*, **25**, 296-325.

Denny-Brown, D. & Russell, W. R. (1941) Experimental cerebral concussion. *Brain*, **64**, 93-164.

Denst, J., Richey, T. W. & Neubuerger, K. T. (1958) Diffuse traumatic degeneration of the cerebral grey matter. *Journal of Neuropathology and Experimental Neurology*, **17**, 450-460.

Estable-Puig, J. F., de Estable, R. F., Tobias, C. & Haymaker, W. (1965) Degeneration and regeneration of myelinated fibers in the cerebral and cerebellar cortex following damage from ionizing particle radiation. *Acta neuropathologica (Berlin)*, **4**, 175-190.

Evans, J. P. & Scheinker, I. M. (1945) Histologic studies of the brain following head trauma. VI. Post-traumatic central nervous system changes interpreted in terms of circulatory disturbances. *Research Publications Association for Research in Nervous and Mental Diseases*, **24**, 254-273.

Faas, F. H. & Ommaya, A. K.   (1968) Brain tissue electrolytes and water content in experimental concussion in the monkey. *Journal of Neurosurgery*, **28**, 137-144.

Falconer, M. A. & Russell, D. S.   (1944) Experimental traumatic cerebral cysts in the rabbit. *Journal of Neurosurgery*, **1**, 182-189.

Fischer, A. W. & Holfelder, H.   (1930) Lokales Amyloid im Gehirn.   Eine Spätfolge von Röntgenbestrahlungen. *Deutsche Zeitschrift für Chirurgie*, **227**, 475-483.

Foerster, O. & Penfield, W.   (1930) Der Narbenzug am und im Gehirn bei traumatischer Epilepsie in seiner Bedeutung für das Zustandekommen der Anfälle und für die therapeutische Bekämpfung derselben. *Zeitschrift für die gesamte Neurologie und Psychiatrie*, **125**, 475-572.

French, J. D.   (1952) Brain lesions associated with prolonged unconsciousness. *Archives of Neurology and Psychiatry* (*Chicago*), **68**, 727-740.

Freytag, E.   (1963a) Autopsy findings in head injuries from blunt forces.   Statistical evaluation of 1,367 cases. *Archives of Pathology*, **75**, 402-413.

Freytag, E.   (1963b).   Autopsy findings in head injuries from firearms.   Statistical evaluation of 254 cases. *Archives of Pathology*, **76**, 215-225.

Friede, R. L.   (1960) Specific cord damage at the atlas level as a pathogenetic mechanism in cerebral concussion. *Journal of Neuropathology and Experimental Neurology*, **19**, 266-279.

Friede, R. L.   (1961) Experimental concussion acceleration. *Archives of Neurology* (*Chicago*), **4**, 449-462.

Gaupp, R.   (1933) Zweikernige Ganglienzellen in traumatischen Hirndefekten. *Zeitschrift für die gesamte Neurologie und Psychiatrie*, **149**, 122-128.

Girard, P. F., Tommasi, M. & Trillet, M.   (1963) Les lésions anatomiques de l'encéphalopathie post-traumatique (Comas prolongés et 'morts du cerveau'). *Acta neuropathologica* (*Berlin*), **2**, 313-327.

Goldsmith, W.   (1966) The physical processes producing head injuries in *Head Injury* (Eds. Caveness, W. F. & Walker, A. E.), pp. 350-382, Lippincott, Philadelphia.

Goldstein, F. P., Rosenthal, S. A. E., Garancis, J. C., Larson, S. J. & Brackett, C. E.   (1970) Varieties of growing skull fractures in childhood. *Journal of Neurosurgery*, **33**, 25-28.

Graham, D. I. & Adams, J. H.   (1971) Ischaemic brain damage in fatal head injuries. *Lancet*, **1**, 265-266.

Grahmann, H. & Ule, G.   (1957) Beitrag zur Kenntnis der chronischen cerebralen Krankheitsbildern bei Boxern.   (Dementia pugilistica und traumatische Boxer-Encephalopathie.) *Psychiatria et Neurologia* (*Basel*), **134**, 261-283.

Greenfield, J. G.   (1938) Some observations on cerebral injuries. *Proceedings of the Royal Society of Medicine*, **32**, 43-52.

Grimberg, L.   (1934) Paralysis agitans and trauma. *Journal of Nervous and Mental Diseases*, **79**, 14-42.

Groat, R. A., Rambach, W. A. & Windle, W. F.   (1945) Concussion of the spinal cord.   An experimental study and critique of the use of the term. *Surgery, Gynecology and Obstetrics*, **81**, 63-74.

Groat, R. A. & Simmons, J. Q.   (1950) Loss of nerve cells in experimental cerebral concussion. *Journal of Neuropathology and Experimental Neurology*, **9**, 150-163.

Groat, R. A., Windle, W. F. & Magoun, H. W.   (1945) Functional and structural changes in the monkey's brain during and after concussion. *Journal of Neurosurgery*, **2**, 26-35.

Gross, A. G.   (1958) A new theory on the dynamics of brain concussion and brain injury. *Journal of Neurosurgery*, **15**, 548-561.

Gurdjian, E. S. & Webster, J. E.   (1958) *Head Injuries*, Mechanisms, diagnosis and management, pp. 62-92, Little, Brown, Boston.

Gurdjian, E. S., Webster, J. E. & Lissner, H. R.   (1955) Observations on the mechanism of brain concussion, contusion, and laceration. *Surgery, Gynecology and Obstetrics*, **101**, 680-690.

Guthkelch, A. N.   (1971) Infantile subdural haematoma and its relationship to whiplash injuries. *British Medical Journal*, **2**, 430-431.

Güttinger, W.   (1950) Der Stosseffekt auf eine Flüssigkeitskugel als Grundlage einer physikalischen Theorie der Entstehung von Gehirnverletzungen. *Zeitschrift für Naturforschung*, **5a**, 622-628.

Haley, T. J. & Snider, R. S.   (1962) *Response of the Nervous System to Ionizing Radiation*.   *Proceedings of an International Symposium*, Academic Press, New York.

Haley, T. J. & Snider, R. S.   (1964) *Response of the Nervous System to Ionizing Radiation*.   *Proceedings of the 2nd International Symposium*, Little, Brown, Boston.

Hallervorden, J. & Quadbeck, G.   (1957) Die Hirnerschütterung und ihre Wirkung auf das Gehirn. *Deutsche Medizinische Wochenschrift*, **82**, 129-134.

Harnett, R. W. F., Paterson, J. R. S., Lowe, K. G., Stewart, I. M. & Uytman, J. D.   (1959) Treatment of cerebral fat embolism. *Lancet*, **2**, 762-764.

Hauser, G. (1900) Ueber einen Fall von Commotio cerebri mit bemerkenswerthen Veränderungen im Gehirn. *Deutsches Archiv für Klinische Medizin*, **65**, 433-448.

Hayes, J. R., Fox, J. L. & Stein, M. N. (1967) The effects of Laser irradiation on the central nervous system. 1. Preliminary studies. *Journal of Neuropathology and Experimental Neurology*, **26**, 250-258.

Haymaker, W., Brahim, M. Z. M., Miguel, J. & Call, N. (1968) Delayed radiation effects in the brains of monkeys exposed to X- and γ rays. *Journal of Neuropathology and Experimental Neurology*, **27**, 50-79.

Henn, R. H. E. & Spann, W. (1965) Untersuchungen über Häufigkeit der cerebralen Fettembolie nach Trauma mit verschieden langer Überlebenszeit. *Monatschrift für Unfallheilkunde*, **68**, 513-522.

Holbourn, A. H. S. (1943) Mechanics of head injuries. *Lancet*, **2**, 438-441.

Holbourn, A. H. S. (1944) The mechanics of trauma with special reference to herniation of cerebral tissue. *Journal of Neurosurgery*, **1**, 190-200.

Holbourn, A. H. S. (1945) The mechanics of brain injuries. *British Medical Bulletin*, **3**, 147-149.

Holbourn, A. H. S. (1956) Personal communication.

Hollander, D. & Strich, S. J. (1970) Atypical Alzheimer's disease with congophilic angiopathy presenting with dementia of acute onset in *Ciba Foundation Symposium. Alzheimer's Disease and Related Conditions* (Eds. Wolstenholme, G. E. W. & O'Connor, M.), pp. 105-124, Churchill, London.

Ingraham, F. D. & Matson, D. D. (1944) Subdural hematoma in infancy. *Journal of Pediatrics*, **24**, 1-37.

Ishii, S., Hayner, R., Kelly, W. A. & Evans, J. P. (1959) Studies of cerebral swelling. II. experimental cerebral swelling produced by supratentorial extradural compression. *Journal of Neurosurgery*, **16**, 152-166.

Jakob, A. (1913) Experimentelle Untersuchungen über die traumatischen Schädigungen des Zentralnervensystems (mit besonderer Berücksichtigung der Commotio cerebri und Kommotionsneurose). *Histologische und histopathologische Arbeiten über die Grosshirnrinde*, **5**, 182-358.

Jellinger, K. (1965) Protrahierte Formen der posttraumatischen Encephalopathie. *Beiträge zur gerichtlichen Medizin*, **23**, 65-118.

Jellinger, K. (1966) Läsionen des extrapyramidalen Systems bei akuten und prolongierten Komazuständen. *Wiener Zeitschrift für Nervenheilkunde*, **23**, 40-73.

Jellinger, K. & Seitelberger, F. (1970) Protracted post-traumatic encephalopathy. Pathology, pathogenesis and clinical implications. *Journal of the Neurological Sciences*, **10**, 51-94.

Jennett, W. B. (1962) *Epilepsy after Blunt Head Injuries*, Heinemann Medical, London.

Johnston, I. H., Johnston, J. A. & Jennett, B. (1970) Intracranial pressure changes following head injury. *Lancet*, **2**, 433-436.

Klatzo, I. (1967) Neuropathological aspects of brain edema. *Journal of Neuropathology and Experimental Neurology*, **26**, 1-14.

Klatzo, I., Piraux, A. & Laskowski, E. J. (1958) The relationship between edema, blood brain barrier and tissue elements in a local brain injury. *Journal of Neuropathology and Experimental Neurology*, **17**, 548-564.

Klintworth, G. K. (1965) The pathogenesis of secondary brainstem haemorrhages as studied in an experimental model. *American Journal of Pathology*, **47**, 525-536.

Köppen, M. (1900) Ueber Veränderungen der Hirnrinde unter einen subduralen Hämatom. *Archiv für Psychiatrie und Nervenkrankheiten*, **33**, 596-660.

Krauland, W. (1950) Über Hirnschäden durch stumpfe Gewalt. *Deutsche Zeitschrift für Nervenheilkunde*, **163**, 265-328.

Krauland, W. (1955) Verletzungen der A. carotis interna im Sinus cavernosus und Verletzungen der grossen Hirnschlagadern mit Berücksichtigung der Aneurysmenbildung in *Handbuch der speziellen pathologischen Anatomie und Histologie* (Eds. Lubarsch, O., Henke, F. & Rössle, R.), vol. 13, part III, pp. 170-176, Springer Verlag, Berlin.

Kristensson, K., Molin, B. & Sourander, P. (1967) Delayed radiation lesions of the human spinal cord. Report of 5 cases. *Acta neuropathologica (Berlin)*, **9**, 34-44.

Lampert, P. W., Fox, J. L. & Earle, K. M. (1966) Cerebral edema after LASER radiation. An electron microscopic study. *Journal of Neuropathology and Experimental Neurology*, **25**, 531-541.

Langfitt, T. W., Shawaluk, P. D., Mahoney, R. P., Stein, S. C. & Hedges, T. R. (1964) Experimental intracranial hypertension and papilledema in the monkey. *Journal of Neurosurgery*, **21**, 469-478.

Langfit, T. W., Tannanbaum, H. M. & Kassell, N. (1966) The etiology of acute brain swelling following experimental head injury. *Journal of Neurosurgery*, **24**, 47-56.

Lewin, W. (1949) Acute subdural and extradural haematoma in closed head injury. *Annals of the Royal College of Surgeons of England*, **5**, 240-274.

Lewin, W. (1968) Vascular lesions in head injuries. *British Journal of Surgery*, **55**, 321-331.

Lindenberg, R. (1964) Die Schädigungsmechanismen der Substantia nigra bei Hirntraumen und das Problem des posttraumatischen Parkinsonismus. *Deutsche Zeitschrift für Nervenheilkunde*, **185**, 637-663.

Lindenberg, R., Fisher, R. S., Durlacher, S. H., Lovitt, W. V. & Freytag, E. (1955) Lesions of the corpus callosum following blunt trauma to the head. *American Journal of Pathology*, **31**, 297-317.

Lindenberg, R. & Freytag, E. (1960) The mechanism of cerebral contusions. A pathologic-anatomic study. *American Journal of Pathology*, **69**, 440-469.

Lindenberg, R. & Freytag, E. (1969) Morphology of brain lesions from blunt trauma in early infancy. *American Journal of Pathology*, **87**, 298-305.

Lindsley, D. B. (1960) Attention, consciousness, sleep and wakefulness in *Handbook of Physiology* (Eds. Field, J., Magoun, H. W. & Hall, V. E.), Section 1, vol 3, pp. 1533-1593, American Physiological Society, Washington, D.C.

Lissner, H. R. & Evans, F. G. (1960) Experimental studies on the relation between acceleration and intra-cranial pressure changes in man. *Surgery, Gynecology and Obstetrics*, **111**, 329-338.

Loew, F. & Wüstner, S. (1960) Diagnose, Behandlung, und Prognose der traumatischen Hämatome des Schädelinneren. *Acta neurochirurgica*, Suppl. **8**, 1-158.

Louis, M. (1788) *Recueil d'observations d'Anatomie et de Chirurgie pour servir de base à la théorie des lésions de la tête par contre-coup* in *Œvres diverses de chirurgie*, vol. 2, pp. 13-37.

Lundberg, N., Troupp, H. & Lorin, H. (1965) Continuous recording of the ventricular-fluid pressure in patients with severe acute traumatic brain injury. *Journal of Neurosurgery*, **22**, 581-590.

Lynn, J. G. & Putnam, T. J. (1944) Histology of cerebral lesions produced by focused ultrasound. *American Journal of Pathology*, **20**, 637-649.

Malis, L. I., Baker, C. P., Kruger, L. & Rose, J. E. (1960) Effects of heavy, ionizing, monoenergetic particles on the cerebral cortex. I. Production of laminary lesions and dosimetric considerations. *Journal of Comparative Neurology*, **115**, 219-241.

Mawdsley, C. & Ferguson, F. R. (1963) Neurological disease in boxers. *Lancet*, **2**, 795-801.

Maxwell, D. S. & Kruger, L. (1964) Electron microscopy of radiation induced laminar lesions in the cerebral cortex of the rat in *Response of the Nervous System to Ionizing Radiation* (Eds. Haley, T. J. & Snider, R. S.), pp. 54-83, Little, Brown, Boston.

Mayer, E. Th. (1967) Zentrale Hirnschäden nach Einwirkung stumpfer Gewalt auf den Schädel. *Archiv für Psychiatrie und Nervenkrankheiten*, **210**, 238-262.

McKissock, W., Taylor, J. C., Bloom, W. H. & Till, K. (1960) Extradural haematoma. Observations on 125 cases. *Lancet*, **2**, 167-172.

McLaurin, R. L. & Tutor, F. T. (1961) Acute subdural hematoma. Review of ninety cases. *Journal of Neurosurgery*, **18**, 61-67.

McMenemey, W. H., Grant, H. C. & Behrman, S. (1965) Two examples of 'Presenile dementia' (Pick's disease and Stern-Garcin syndrome) with a history of trauma. *Archiv für Psychiatrie und Nervenkrankheiten*, **207**, 128-140.

McMillan, J. B. (1956) Emboli of cerebral tissue in the lungs following severe head injury. *American Journal of Pathology*, **32**, 405-415.

McTaggart, D. M. & Neubuerger, K. T. (1970) Cerebral fat embolism. Pathologic changes in the brain after survival of 7 years. *Acta Neuropathologica (Berlin)*, **15**, 183-187.

Mealey, J. (1968) Subdural hematoma in infancy. In *Pediatric Head Injuries*, pp. 166-201, Charles C Thomas, Springfield, Ill.

Miller, J. D. & Jennett, W. B. (1968) Complications of depressed skull fracture. *Lancet*, **2**, 991-995.

Minauf, M. & Schacht, L. (1966) Zentrale Hirnschäden nach Einwirkung stumpfer Gewalt auf den Schädel. II. Mitteilung. Läsionen im Bereich der Stammganglien. *Archiv für Psychiatrie und Nervenkrankheiten*, **208**, 162-176.

Morin, M. A. & Pitts, F. W. (1970) Delayed apoplexy following head injury ('traumatische Spät-Apoplexie'). *Journal of Neurosurgery*, **33**, 542-547.

Nelson, E., Lindstrom, P. L. & Haymaker, W. (1959) Pathological effects of ultrasound on the human brain. A study of 25 cases in which ultrasonic irradiation was used as a lobotomy procedure. *Journal of Neuropathology and Experimental Neurology*, **18**, 489-508.

Neubuerger, K. (1925) Ueber cerebrale Fett-und Luftembolie. *Zeitschrift für die gesamte Neurologie und Psychiatrie*, **95**, 278-318.

Neubuerger, K. T., Sinton, D. W. & Denst, J. (1959) Cerebral atrophy associated with boxing. *Archives of Neurology and Psychiatry (Chicago)*, **81**, 403-408.

Nevin, N. C. (1967) Neuropathological changes in the white matter following head injury. *Journal of Neuropathology and Experimental Neurology*, **26**, 77-84.

Nyström, S. (1960) A case of decortication following a severe head injury. *Acta psychiatrica scandinavica*, **35**, 101-112.

Ojemann, R. G., Fisher, C. M., Adams, R. D., Sweet, W. H. & New, P. F. J.   (1969) Further experience with 'normal' pressure hydrocephalus.   *Journal of Neurosurgery*, **31**, 279-294.

Ommaya, A. K.   (1966) Trauma to the nervous system.   *Annals of the Royal College of Surgeons of England*, **39**, 317-347.

Ommaya, A. K., Faas, F. & Yarnell, P.   (1968) Whiplash injury and brain damage.   *Journal of the American Medical Association*, **204**, 285-289.

Ommaya, A. K., Grubb, R. L. & Naumann, R. A.   (1971) Coup and contre-coup injury, observations on the mechanics of visible brain injuries in the rhesus monkey.   *Journal of Neurosurgery*, **35**, 503-516.

Ommaya, A. K. & Yarnell, P.   (1969) Subdural haematoma after whiplash injury.   *Lancet*, **2**, 237-239.

Oppenheimer, D. R.   (1968) Microscopic lesions in the brain following head injury.   *Journal of Neurology, Neurosurgery and Psychiatry*, **31**, 299-306.

Payne, E. E.   (1968) Brains of boxers.   *Neurochirurgia*, **11**, 173-188.

Peerless, J. S. & Rewcastle, N. B.   (1967) Shear injuries of the brain.   *Canadian Medical Association Journal*, **96**, 577-582.

Penfield, W.   (1927) The mechanism of cicatricial contraction in the brain.   *Brain*, **50**, 499-517.

Pennybacker, J. & Russell, D. S.   (1948) Necrosis of the brain due to radiation therapy.   Clinical and pathological observations.   *Journal of Neurology, Neurosurgery and Psychiatry*, **11**, 183-198.

Phillips, G.   (1954) Traumatic epilepsy after closed head injury.   *Journal of Neurology, Neurosurgery and Psychiatry*, **17**, 1-10

Phillips, J. Y.   (1955) Cerebral cortical damage incident to chronic subdural hematoma in infancy.   *Bulletin of the Los Angeles Neurological Society*, **20**, 30-36.

Pickles, W.   (1950) Acute general edema of the brain in children with head injuries.   *New England Journal of Medicine*, **242**, 607-611.

Polis, A.   (1894) Recherches expérimentales sur la commotion cérébrale.   *Revue de Chirurgie*, **14**, 273-319; 645-730.

Pudenz, R. H. & Shelden, C. H.   (1946) The Lucite calvarium.   A method for direct observation of the brain. II. Cranial trauma and brain motion.   *Journal of Neurosurgery*, **3**, 487-505.

Putnam, T. J. & Cushing, H.   (1925) Chronic subdural hematoma.   *Archives of Surgery (Chicago)*, **11**, 329-393.

Ramon y Cajal, S.   (1928) In *Degeneration and Regeneration of the Nervous System* (Translated May, R. M.), vol. 2, pp. 492-515.   Reprinted Hafner Publishing Co, New York, 1959.

Roberts, A. H.   (1969) *Brain Damage in Boxers*, Pitman Medical, London.

Rose, J. E., Malis, L. I., Kruger, L. & Baker, C. P.   (1960) Effects of heavy, ionizing, monoenergetic particles on the cerebral cortex.   II. Histological appearances of laminar lesions and growth of nerve fibers after laminar destructions.   *Journal of Comparative Neurology*, **115**, 243-296.

Rosenblath, W.   (1899) Über einen bemerkenswerthen Fall von Hirnerschütterung.   *Deutsches Archiv für klinische Medizin*, **64**, 406-427.

Russell, D. S. & Rubinstein, L. J.   (1971) *Pathology of Tumours of the Nervous System*, 3rd edition, p. 5, Edward Arnold, London.

Russell, W. R. & Schiller, F.   (1949) Crushing injuries to the skull: clinical and experimental observations.   *Journal of Neurology, Neurosurgery and Psychiatry*, **12**, 52-60.

Scagliosi, G.   (1898) Ueber die Gehirnerschütterung und die daraus im Gehirn und Rückenmark hervorgerufenen histologischen Veränderungen.   Experimentelle Untersuchungen.   *Virchows Archiv für pathologische Anatomie und Physiologie*, **152**, 487-525.

Schacht, L. & Minauf, M.   (1965) Zentrale Hirnschäden nach Einwirkung stumpfer Gewalt auf den Schädel. 1. Mitteilung.   Balkenläsionen.   *Archiv für Psychiatrie und Nervenkrankheiten*, **207**, 416-427.

Schmaus, H.   (1890) Beiträge zur pathologischen Anatomie der Rückenmarkserschütterung.   *Virchows Archiv für pathologische Anatomie und Physiologie*, **122**, 326-356; 470-495.

Schutta, H. S., Kassell, N. F. & Langfitt, T. W.   (1968) Brain swelling produced by injury and aggravated by arterial hypertension.   *Brain*, **91**, 281-294.

Sellier, K. & Unterharnscheidt, F.   (1963) Mechanik und Pathomorphologie der Hirnschäden nach stumpfer Gewalteinwirkung auf den Schädel.   *Hefte zur Unfallheilkunde*, **76**, 1-140.

Sights, W. P.   (1969) Ballistic analysis of shot gun injuries to the central nervous system.   *Journal of Neurosurgery*, **31**, 25-33.

Sjövall, H.   (1943) The genesis of skull and brain injuries.   *Acta pathologica et microbiologica scandinavica*, *Suppl.* **48**, 1-151.

Small, J. M. & Woolf, A. L.   (1957) Fatal damage to the brain by epileptic convulsions after a trivial head injury.   *Journal of Neurology, Neurosurgery and Psychiatry*, **20**, 293-301.

Smith, B.   (1963) Cerebral pathology in subarachnoid haemorrhage.   *Journal of Neurology, Neurosurgery and Psychiatry*, **26**, 535-539.

Spatz, H.   (1932) Die Erkennbarkeit der Rindenkontusion im Endzustand in anatomischer und klinischer Hinsicht.   *Zentralblatt für die gesamte Neurologie und Psychiatrie*, **61**, 514-515.

Spicer, E. J. F. & Strich, S. J.   (1967) Haemorrhages in posterior-root ganglia in patients dying from head injuries.   *Lancet*, **2**, 1389-1391.

Spillane, J. D.   (1962) Five boxers.   *British Medical Journal*, **2**, 1205-1210.

Strich, S. J.   (1956) Diffuse degeneration of the cerebral white matter in severe dementia following head injury.   *Journal of Neurology, Neurosurgery and Psychiatry*, **19**, 163-185.

Strich, S. J.   (1961) Shearing of nerve fibres as a cause of brain damage due to head injury.   A pathological study of twenty cases.   *Lancet*, **2**, 443-448.

Strich, S. J.   (1968) Notes on the use of the Marchi method for staining degenerating myelin in the peripheral and central nervous system.   *Journal of Neurology, Neurosurgery and Psychiatry*, **31**, 110-114.

Strich, S. J.   (1969) The pathology of brain damage due to blunt head injuries in *The Late Effects of Head Injury* (Eds. Walker, A. E., Caveness, W. F. & Critchley, M.). pp. 501-524, Charles C Thomas, Springfield, Ill.

Symonds, C.   (1962) Concussion and its sequelae.   *Lancet*, **1**, 1-5.

Tani, E. & Evans, J. P.   (1965) Electron microscopic study of brain swelling.   III. Alterations in the neuroglia and the blood vessels of the white matter.   *Acta neuropathologica (Berlin)*, **4**, 625-639.

Taylor, A. R.   (1967) Post-concussional sequelae.   *British Medical Journal*, **3**, 67-71.

Tomlinson, B. E.   (1964) In *Acute Injuries of the Head* (Ed. Rowbotham, G. F.), pp. 93-158, Livingstone, Edinburgh.

Tomlinson, B. E.   (1970) Brain-stem lesions after head injury.   *Journal of Clinical Pathology*, **23** (Suppl. Roy. Coll. Path.), **4**, 154-165.

Ule, G., Döhner, W. & Bues, E.   (1961) Ausgedehnte Hemisphärenmarkschädigung nach gedecktem Hirntrauma mit apallischem Syndrom und partieller Spätrehabilitation.   *Archiv für Psychiatrie und Nervenkrankheiten*, **202**, 155-176.

Unterharnscheidt, F.   (1963) Die gedeckten Schäden des Gehirns.   Experimentelle Untersuchungen mit einmaliger, wiederholter und gehäufter stumpfer Gewalteinwirkung auf den Schädel.   *Monographien aus dem Gesamtgebiet der Neurologie und Psychiatry*, **103**, 1-124.

Unterharnscheidt, F. & Higgins, L. S.   (1969) Traumatic lesions of brain and spinal cord due to non-deforming angular acceleration of the head.   *Texas Reports on Biology and Medicine*, **27**, 127-166.

Wacks, M. R. & Bird, H. A.   (1970) Massive gross pulmonary embolism of cerebral tissue following severe head trauma.   *Journal of Trauma*, **10**, 344-348.

Welte, E.   (1948) Über die Zusammenhänge zwischen anatomischem Befund und klinischem Bild bei Rindenprellungsherden nach stumpfen Schädeltrauma.   *Archiv für Psychiatrie und Nervenkrankheiten*, **179**, 243-315.

Wiener, L. M. & Nathanson, M.   (1962) The relationship of subdural hematoma to anticoagulant therapy.   *Archives of Neurology (Chicago)*, **6**, 282-286.

Windle, W. F.   (1948) Damage to myelin sheaths of the brain after concussion.   *Anatomical Record*, **100**, 725.

Windle, W. F. & Groat, R. A.   (1945) Disappearance of nerve cells after concussion.   *Anatomical Record*, **93**, 201-209.

Windle, W. F., Groat, R. A. & Fox, C. A.   (1944) Experimental structural alterations in the brain during and after concussion.   *Surgery, Gynecology and Obstetrics*, **79**, 561-572.

Winkelman, N. W.   (1942) Cerebral fat embolism.   A clinicopathologic study of two cases.   *Archives of Neurology and Psychiatry (Chicago)*, **47**, 57-76.

Witkowski, L.   (1877) Ueber Gehirnerschütterung.   *Virchows Archiv für pathologische Anatomie und Physiologie*, **69**, 498-516.

Wolman, L.   (1956) Pituitary necrosis in raised intracranial pressure.   *Journal of Pathology and Bacteriology*, **72**, 575-586.

Yamada, S., Kindt, G. W. & Youmans, J. R.   (1967) Carotid artery occlusion due to nonpenetrating injury.   *Journal of Trauma*, **7**, 333-342.

Zeman, W.   (1968) Histologic events during the latent interval in radiation injury in *The Central Nervous System. Some Experimental Models of Neurological Disease* (Eds. Bailey, O. T. & Smith, D. E.), pp. 184-200, Williams and Wilkins, Baltimore.

Zülch, K. J.   (1970) Gehirntumor und Trauma.   *Hefte zur Unfallheilkunde*, **107**, 33-44.

10

Malformations of the Nervous System, Perinatal Damage and Related Conditions in Early Life

Revised by H. Urich

Prenatal malformations

General considerations

Problems of classification

The act of birth marks no particular milestone in the development of the human brain and many years must elapse before approximate structural maturity is achieved. Although the term malformation thus includes in its scope anomalies originating in postnatal life, the latter can usually be more precisely classified on the basis of their aetiology. This is far from being the case in prenatal malformations. Deductions as to the pathogenesis of early malformations of the brain are apt to be fallacious, for the immature nervous system does not react to disease in the same way as adult tissue and parts may be absorbed without trace of neuroglial or connective tissue repair. Inflammatory reactions are not seen before the 6th month of fetal life (Eicke 1959). Moreover, it is known from observations on animals that the same anomaly may be produced both by genetic and environmental causes. Considerations such as these lead to the conclusion that, in the present state of knowledge, malformations of the nervous system are best classified by their morphological features alone. For detailed accounts of the subject the reader is referred to the monographs of Warkany (1971) and of Crome and Stern (1972).

The findings of experimental teratology

Much light has been thrown on the mechanisms of abnormal development by the study of experimentally induced malformations in animals. Since the observations of Hippel (1907) that irradiation of pregnant rabbits produces malformations of the eye in the offspring, a very large literature has grown up around the subject. The older reviews (Gruenwald 1947a, b, c; Willis 1958) have now been largely superseded by the work of Kalter (1968) whose monograph reviews in detail both malformations induced experimentally and those occurring spontaneously in a wide range of species. The following brief account of the various teratogenic agents is largely based on Kalter's work.

Vitamin deficiencies. A wide range of malformations can be obtained by feeding pregnant animals with diets deficient in specific vitamins, or by administering counteracting substances, such as inactive analogues, antimetabolites and antagonists. *Riboflavin deficiency* was one of the earliest teratological techniques used in mammals (Warkany and Nelson 1940). With rare exceptions it produced mainly skeletal malformations. However, addition of the riboflavin-antagonist galactoflavin produces a wider range of lesions, including hydrocephalus (Baird, Nelson, Monie, Wright and Evans 1955; Nelson, Baird, Wright and Evans 1956). In mice the hydrocephalus is associated with an enormous expansion of the 4th ventricle resembling the Dandy-Walker malformation in man (Kalter and Warkany 1957; Kalter 1963). *Folic acid deficiency* produces hydrocephalus in rats, either without an obvious obstruction in the cerebrospinal fluid pathway (Monie, Armstrong and Nelson 1961), or with aqueduct stenosis (Stempak 1965). Combined *vitamin B_{12}* and folic acid deficiency also produces hydrocephalus (Richardson and Hogan 1946). Exencephaly and eye anomalies can be caused by *pantothenic acid* deficiency (Boisselot 1949). *Vitamin A* deficiency was known to be teratogenic in pigs since the work of Hale (1933) but the first malformations of the central nervous system were induced in rabbits by Millen, Woollam and Lamming (1953). The hydrocephalus which ensued was present at birth in one series of experiments (Millen *et al.* 1953), but developed postnatally in another (Millen and Woollam 1956). In the latter group there was stenosis of the aqueduct which was fully patent in the congenital variety. The authors concluded that the hydrocephalus was caused by excessive production of cerebrospinal fluid and the aqueduct stenosis was a secondary phenomenon (Millen and Woollam 1958). Cerebral malformations are also induced occasionally by deficiencies of *vitamin E* (Cheng and Thomas 1953) and of *nicotinic acid* (Chamberlain and Nelson 1963).

Hypervitaminosis A. The teratogenic effect of an excessive intake of vitamin A was discovered by Cohlan (1953). Severe cerebral malformations, of which exencephaly was the most common, were produced with a high degree of consistency in rats (Cohlan 1954; Giroud and Martinet 1956) and subsequently in other species. These malformations presented excellent experimental models for the study of the morphogenesis of anencephaly.

Trypan blue. Gillman, Gilbert, Gillman and Spence (1948) reported that injection of pregnant rats with trypan blue produced a wide range of malformations in the offspring, including those of the central nervous system. The most common lesions are hydrocephalus and spina bifida, while exencephaly is relatively uncommon (Gillman, Gilbert, Spence and Gillman 1951). A hindbrain malformation resembling the Arnold–Chiari deformity in man has also been recorded (Gunberg 1956). The mechanism of action of trypan blue remained controversial for many years. Recently Beck, Lloyd and Griffiths (1967) adduced convincing evidence that its action is on the lysosomal enzymes in the epithelium of the yolk-sac blocking its histotrophic activity, particularly the uptake of protein.

Tissue antibodies. Malformations can be induced in fetal rats by injections of heterologous antisera against rat kidney (Brent, Averich and Drapiewski 1961), rat placenta (Brent 1967) and rat yolk-sac (Brent and Johnson 1967). The nephrotoxic serum is concentrated in the basement membrane of the maternal renal glomeruli, in the adrenal glands and in the visceral and parietal layers of the yolk-sacs, but not in the embryonic tissues (Slotnick and Brent 1966). The most common malformation caused by the apparent yolk-sac dysfunction is a non-obstructive hydrocephalus, the morphology of which was studied by Duckett, Brent and Jensch (1974).

Ionizing radiation. X-rays have been used for a long time as a teratogenic agent which can both be timed and dosed with considerable accuracy. The systematic studies of Hicks (1952, 1953*a*, *b*, 1954) still retain their validity. Pregnant rats were subjected to a single dose of ionizing radiation on the successive days of their 3 weeks' gestation and a timetable of predictable malformations constructed. Exposure prior to the 9th day did not affect the primitive neural tube, but a similar dose given on the 9th day led to severe head deformities and anencephaly. Stenosis of the aqueduct followed radiation on the 11th day and from the 13th to the 18th day various cortical and striatal disturbances and absence of the corpus callosum were brought about. Minor degrees of damage led to micrencephaly without obvious loss of nerve cells, while irradiation shortly before birth caused a cerebellar malformation with distortion of the granular layer. This work was considerably expanded and extended to other species by a number of workers. The effects of radiation can be modified by other factors. They are intensified by anoxia (Russell 1954), by thyroxine, insulin and cortisone (Woollam and Millen 1960) and mitigated by cysteamin (Wolff and Kirrmann 1954). The exact mechanism by which radiation induces malformations is still controversial. Hicks' view that the 'stage specificity' of the changes correlates well with phases of enhanced metabolic activity of the neuroblasts, associated with increased formation of nucleic acid and proteins, is probably an oversimplification as it does not explain the relative immunity of the primitive neuroepithelium in the first few days of embryonal life during which mitotic activity is intense. It is probable that the teratogenic activity of X-rays depends on the balance of destruction and repair processes. In the earliest stages of growth, destruction of a few cells can easily be compensated by the still totipotential remaining cells. With advancing differentiation this is no longer possible and the combination of destruction and partial repair leads to malformations.

Other chemical substances. Numerous drugs have now been tested for teratogenic properties and many have been found to induce occasional malformations of the central nervous system. These include alkylating substances, anti-metabolites, alkaloids, hypoglycaemic agents, anti-thyroid drugs, salicylates, antibiotics, anti-histamines, thalidomide and many others. Hydrocephalus has been induced in the offspring of pregnant rats by administration of *tellurium* between the 9th and 15th day of gestation (Duckett 1971, 1972).

Hypoxia. Experiments using diminished oxygen supply as the teratogenic agent are of interest as this factor may be concerned in human malformations. Owing to its ability to utilize anaerobic as well as aerobic sources of energy, the neuroblast is much more resistant to anoxia than the mature neuron. It is therefore not surprising that these experiments met with only limited success. Anoxia in chick embryos has been shown to lead to anencephaly, cyclopia and forking of the aqueduct (Muskett 1953). Ingalls, Curley and Prindle (1950, 1952) subjected pregnant mice to reduced atmospheric pressures and so produced a gradually increasing degree of hypoxia. Exencephaly or hydrocephalus appeared in a small number of offspring. Degenhardt (1954, 1960) observed two instances of exencephaly and one of cyclopia in the offspring of pregnant rabbits exposed to anoxia. Rats and hamsters are apparently less susceptible to the teratogenic effects of oxygen deprivation.

Infection. This is another subject of great interest in view of the undoubted teratogenic effect of some virus infections in man. It has been critically reviewed by Elizan and Fabiyi (1970). The two well-established human teratogenic viruses, rubella and cytomegalovirus, do not produce malformations in animals. A variety of developmental abnormalities can be produced in various species by viruses normally pathogenic to those species. Thus intrauterine infection with blue-tongue virus can produce hydranencephaly in sheep. Hydrocephalus and cerebellar hypoplasia can be similarly produced in pigs infected by the hog cholera virus. The rat virus, the HI virus of hamsters and the feline panleucopenia virus can all cause cerebellar hypoplasia in their respective species.

General conclusions. It may be concluded from this review of experimental teratology that several factors play a part in teratogenesis. Probably the most important is the time of injury, as widely disparate mechanisms operating at the same stage of development will produce similar end-results. Nevertheless, the nature of the noxa is of importance as some agents produce highly specific disorders. Genetic factors must also be taken into account. The susceptibility to noxious agents varies from species to species and from strain to strain within the same species. The common experience that in an exposed litter only some fetuses are affected and a proportion invariably escapes damage has also been attributed to genetic differences between littermates. This interplay between genetic and environmental factors may be of importance in human teratology.

Nutrition and brain growth. Variations in size of the brain as opposed to specific malformations have received little attention from experimental teratologists, but a considerable amount of evidence has accumulated to indicate that starvation may affect the growth of the brain. The adult brain is remarkably resistant to starvation (Donaldson 1911) but nutritional deprivation during the period of growth leads both to a reduction in brain size and abnormalities of behaviour (Winick and Noble 1966; Randt and Derby 1973). An analysis of the factors involved in brain growth reveals the great complexity of the problem (Dobbing 1970). Impairment of growth may be due to inhibition of cell division or interference with cell maturation. Cell division occurs in two phases, neuronal and glial. Multiplication of neuroblasts occurs early and is completed in fetal life, while the peak of proliferation of glial cells occurs much later and extends into postnatal life. Maturation involves development of cell processes, establishment of synaptic connections and myelination. The extent to which all these processes may be affected by nutrition or other exogenous factors offers a wide field for further research.

Aetiology

Despite intensive investigations the causation of prenatal malformations in man remains largely undetermined. The problem is complicated by the fact that the same type of structural anomaly may be produced both by genetic and exogenous causes. Some important factors have come to light in recent years which point the way to further fields of research.

Genetic factors. Very few cerebral malformations are caused by simple Mendelian inheritance and those are fully listed in McKusick's (1968) catalogue. The following conditions may be cited as examples. Some forms of microencephaly may be inherited as autosomal recessive traits, for instance the type which occurs in bird-headed dwarfs (Seckel 1960; Kloepfer, Platou and Hansche 1964; Harper, Orti and Baker 1967; McKusick, Mahloudji, Abbott, Lindenberg and Kepas 1967). A sex-linked variety of hydrocephalus, associated with stenosis of the aqueduct, has been reported by Bickers and Adams (1949) and by Edwards, Norman and Roberts (1961). Hereditary congenital facial paralysis is an example of dominant inheritance (van der Wiel 1957; Skyberg and van der Hagen 1965).

Epidemiological studies of common malformations, such as anencephaly, spina bifida and hydrocephalus, have revealed a high risk of recurrence of these conditions in the same families (Record and McKeown 1950; Carter, David and Laurence 1968). Detailed analysis of the data suggests the interplay of environmental and genetic factors, the latter probably polygenic in nature.

Finally, malformations have been reported in association with inborn errors of metabolism such as sudanophil leucodystrophy (Norman, Tingey, Valentine and Danby 1962) and maple syrup disease (Martin and Norman 1967). While these observations are too rare to exclude fortuitous association, the possibility of genetic links must be considered.

Cytogenetic abnormalities. The study of disordered chromosome patterns has thrown important light on congenital anomalies of the nervous system (for full reviews see Källén and Levan 1970; Crome and Stern 1972). The most important group of anomalies are the *trisomies*, in which an additional chromosome is present in one group. Trisomy in the G (21-22) group is commonly found in mongolism (Lejeune, Gautier and Turpin 1959). D (13-15) trisomy is associated with multiple congenital abnormalities (Patau, Smith, Therman, Inhorn and Wagner 1960) which include cyclopia and other forms of holoprosencephaly and arhinencephaly. Multiple anomalies also occur in E (17-18) trisomy (Edwards, Harnden, Cameron, Crosse and Wolff 1960) in which the CNS malformations are largely confined to the cerebellum (Norman 1966). *Translocations,* either of the D/G or the G/G type are found in cases of mongolism with 46 chromosomes (Polani, Briggs, Ford, Clarke and Berg 1960). *Deletions* of parts of one chromosome are often associated with mental subnormality; the best known is the 'cri de chat' syndrome associated with deletion of the short arm of the no. 5 chromosome (Lejeune, Lafourcade, Berger, Vialatte, Boeswillwald, Seringe and Turpin 1963). Abnormalities of *sex chromosomes* (Miller 1964) include Klinefelter's syndrome (XXY) and Turner's syndrome (XO) as well as a variety of more complex chromosomal combinations. Many of them are associated with mental retardation, but little is known of the structural changes in their brains. Most cases of Turner's syndrome who survive to adult life show no cerebral malformations. Cortical dysplasia and grey matter heterotopias were described in a mentally subnormal girl with the syndrome (Brun and Sköld 1968) and cerebellar malformations were found in a girl dying in infancy (Molland and Purcell 1975). However, most XO fetuses undergo spontaneous abortion (Carr 1967) and these often show gross malformation. *Mosaicism* in which an abnormal karyotype is found only in a proportion of cells, the remainder being normal, occurs in several conditions, such as Turner's syndrome or mongolism. These patients tend to be less severely affected than those who present chromosomal abnormalities in pure form.

Maternal age. Shuttleworth's (1909) original observation that mongoloid children are often born when their mothers approach the end of their reproductive period has been amply confirmed by detailed studies (Bleyer 1938; Penrose 1954). This applies only to the common trisomic type of mongolism, the rare translocation type being genetically determined and appearing at any age. A higher average maternal age was also found in a group of miscellaneous malformations (Pitt 1962) and in a series of mentally subnormal subjects from which mongolism was excluded (Åkesson 1966).

Maternal infections. The demonstration of a relationship between maternal infection during pregnancy and maldevelopment of the offspring has furnished additional evidence of the pathogenetic importance of environmental factors. It is well established that maternal infections other than syphilis may pass the placenta and interfere with development, and Gregg's (1941) original observations on the malign effect of rubella have been amply confirmed. Swan (1949) estimated that no fewer than 93% of the mothers of his 558 collected cases had been infected during the first four months of pregnancy. This selected group of patients, however, gives far too high an incidence. The Swedish survey of Lundström (1952) included mothers infected with rubella during the first four months of pregnancy and showed that the incidence of stillbirths, neonatal deaths, immaturity and malformations in this group was 17% compared with 6% in the controls. Greenberg, Pelliterri and Barton (1957) put the incidence at 12%. Transmission to the embryo may occur without overt disease in the mother. It is likely that the teratogenic virulence of the virus varies in different epidemics since there are numerous instances of maternal infection in early pregnancy without untoward consequences to the child (Landtman 1948). More recent observations on the effects of maternal rubella and other infections have been summarized by Knobloch and Pasamanick (1962).

In Swan's (1949) large series the commonest abnormalities were microcephaly, cardiac defects, deafness and cataract. Hydrocephalus, absent corpus callosum, mongolism, epilepsy and spastic syndromes were also represented. The deafness is due to defective development of the organ of Corti and is seldom total. The critical stage for the development of the cochlea is about a month later than that for the lens, so that cataract and deafness are not often found in the same individual (Ingalls 1950). Swan, however, noted that the time of the clinical onset of the maternal infection did not always coincide with the known stage of active differentiation of the affected organ in the offspring and suggested that these discrepancies might be due to variation in the proliferation of the virus or in the resistance of the cells to infection. Very few adequate examinations have been made of the micrencephalic brains following rubella embryopathy. Friedman and Cohen's (1947) case showed absence of the corpus callosum and anomalies of the cerebral cortex. In the two cases described by Mutrux, Wildi and Bourquin (1949) the gyral pattern was normal. The abnormal features were mild hydrocephalus, a small

corpus callosum and perivascular and marginal gliosis. Kappers (1959) examined a 6-week-old embryo, the mother's infection having taking place a month before miscarriage. The main pathological changes were deep infoldings of the hemispheric neuroepithelium, proliferation and rosette formations in the choroid plexus, endothelial thickening of vessel walls, and a defect in the roof of the rhombencephalon, probably due to necrosis and rupture. Töndury and Smith (1966) reviewed their experience of 57 fetuses aborted after maternal infections with rubella; 68% showed evidence of damage to various organs. In none was any direct disease found in brain cells, but endothelial damage with focal haemorrhages was seen in some. In 10 affected fetuses the width of the cerebral cortex was reduced in comparison with normal controls.

The evidence that other virus diseases are capable of causing malformations is less convincing, though on several occasions structural anomalies have been reported following maternal infections occurring in early pregnancy. Cerebral destruction resembling hydranencephaly has been reported in association with infective hepatitis in the mother (Kass 1951). Measles, mumps, varicella, infective mononucleosis, poliomyelitis and western equine encephalitis have all been incriminated, though the method of collecting these cases often makes aetiological deductions of doubtful value (Muller 1950). The same doubts arise when the possible teratogenic effect of Asian influenza is considered (Ingalls 1960).

Cytomegalic inclusion body disease (salivary gland virus encephalitis) may also involve the fetal nervous system and lead to hydrocephalus with widespread evidence of inflammation and periventricular calcifications. In Diezel's (1954) case the maternal infection was thought to have occurred in the 4th month of pregnancy, and the infant's brain showed the malformation of micropolygyria in addition to the usual destructive lesions. Several similar cases have now been recorded (Haymaker, Girdany, Stephens, Lillie and Fetterman 1954; Crome and France 1959; Bignami and Appicciutoli 1964). All these cases showed micrencephaly with extensive cortical microgyria, occasional cerebellar microgyria, subependymal calcifications and typical giant intranuclear inclusions, mainly in glial cells. Occasionally cases are encountered in older children which display all these features with the exception of inclusion bodies. These may well represent burnt-out cases of intrauterine cytomegalovirus infections though proof may be difficult to obtain.

Granulomatous meningo-encephalitis is another group of diseases which may attack the developing nervous system, usually in the later stages of fetal life (Wyatt and Tribby 1952). Of these toxoplasmosis (see p. 269) is the best known. A condition also characterized by hydrocephalus, periventricular calcifications, thickened leptomeninges and eccentric degenerative changes in the smaller blood vessels has been described as a separate disease by Sabin and Feldman (1948) on the grounds of the negative serological tests ('Sabin's non-toxoplasmic vascular encephalopathy').

Intra-uterine meningitis following staphylococcal infection is another very rare cause of congenital hydrocephalus (Crosby, Mosberg and Smith 1951). A comprehensive account of the prenatal and perinatal infections of the central nervous system has been given by Wolf and Cowen (1959).

Anoxia. In rare instances the fetus has survived damage due to carbon monoxide poisoning in the mother. Hallervorden (1949) reported the case of a child aged one year whose mother had attempted suicide by coal gas inhalation when five months pregnant. The child's brain showed not only softenings of the globus pallidus and putamen but extensive micropolygyria of the cerebral cortex. A somewhat different case was reported by Bankl and Jellinger (1967). A premature infant born six weeks after an episode of maternal carbon monoxide poisoning during the 24th week of pregnancy showed massive necrosis of the cerebral hemispheres with the exception of the inferior and medial aspects of the temporal lobes, also extensive patchy necrosis of the brainstem. Between the destroyed and preserved parts of the temporal cortex there was a zone of typical microgyria.

Lack of oxygen or other nutritional deficiency has been thought to follow faulty implantation of the ovum and to lead to various malformations. The evidence in favour of this theory is mainly based upon the finding that extrauterine gestation is associated with a greatly increased incidence of maldevelopments both in embryos (Mall 1908) and in viable babies (Suter and Wichser 1948).

Irradiation. Deep X-ray or radium therapy to the pelvis during the first four months of pregnancy has produced many cases of microcephaly (Murphy 1947). Anomalies of the eye (optic atrophy, choroidoretinitis, abnormal retinal pigmentation) are much commoner in these cases than in micrencephaly of genetic origin. Four histologically examined cases in which therapeutic irradiation or radium treatment has been carried out during pregnancy are quoted by Cowen and Geller (1960). Various anomalies of the eyes, cerebral hemispheres and thalamus were present in Johnson's (1938) cases. Courville and Edmundson (1958) reported microcephaly with diffuse loss of cortical nerve cells. Cerebellar microgyria with some structural disorientation were the main features of the cases of Miskolczy (1931) and of van Bogaert and Radermecker (1955). It is interesting to note that at autopsy three of these brains exhibited meningo-encephalitis. To these cases may be added that of Uiberrack (1942) which showed pachygyria of the cerebral cortex and defective development of the vermis. Studies on children exposed *in utero* to the atomic explosions at Hiroshima and Nagasaki revealed a relatively high incidence of microcephaly and mental retardation, but no specific malformations (Plummer 1952; Yamazaki, Wright and Wright 1954). Follow-up studies confirmed these observations (Wood, Johnson and Omori 1967; Miller 1968).

Maternal diabetes. Hoet, Gommers and Hoet (1960) have reviewed the evidence that disturbed carbohydrate metabolism and associated vitamin deficiencies are causal factors in malformations. Arhinencephaly has been reported in the offspring of diabetic mothers (Dekaban and Magee 1958; Dekaban 1959).

Drugs. The *thalidomide* tragedy has drawn attention to the teratogenic action of drugs in man. However, even children severely malformed by the action of thalidomide show no evidence of cerebral damage. Only exceptionally cerebral lesions were reported in association with aural and ocular anomalies (Horstmann 1966). *Aminopterin*, a folic acid antagonist, has been used to induce therapeutic abortions. However, in a few cases fetuses survived and showed gross cerebral malformations (Thiersch 1952).

Other environmental factors. The geographical distribution and seasonal incidence of some common malformations, revealed by epidemiological studies, prompted the search for environmental factors with a similar distribution in time and space. In a detailed study Renwick (1972) advanced the hypothesis that some toxic factor present in potatoes affected by the blight fungus *Phytophthora infestans* may have teratogenic potentialities. This hypothesis awaits experimental confirmation.

Pathogenesis

It is impossible to evolve a coherent theory of pathogenesis of the cerebral malformations in our present state of knowledge. The study of the end-stage of human maldevelopment can only lead to speculation on possible mechanisms unsupported by evidence. It is even impossible to determine the time at which the noxa must have operated to produce a given anomaly (the *determination period*). It is only permissible to speculate on the latest possible time at which the malformation may have been produced, in the light of our knowledge of the normal development of the human brain (the *termination period*). The determination period may precede the termination period by a variable span of time.

Further information can be obtained from detailed studies of fetuses which have undergone spontaneous abortion (Sternberg 1929; Dekaban and Bartelmez 1964; Brocklehurst 1969; Padget 1970). These studies are facilitated by the fact that a high percentage of malformed fetuses are aborted. In her large material Padget emphasized the importance of midline cleft formation in many malformations, even those in which ultimately no visible cleft remains. She adapted Yakovlev and Wadsworth's (1946) concept of cortical defects with 'sealed lips' or 'lips separated' to midline lesions, but did not support their emphasis on the distinction between developmental and destructive clefts. In her opinion, the mechanism by which the cleft is produced is immaterial to the subsequent development of the lesion, which ultimately depends on the balance of destructive and reparative processes.

Another source of valuable information is the examination of fetuses which have undergone therapeutic abortion because they were known to be exposed to a teratogenic agent. Our knowledge of the pathogenesis of the embryopathy of rubella is based on studies on such material (Kappers 1959; Tondury and Smith 1966).

The most detailed study is possible on animal material, both on experimental malformations and on those occurring spontaneously, particularly genetic ones where the affected strains can be bred at will. Important observations have been made in this field, to mention only the studies on the pathogenesis of anencephaly by Giroud and his associates (Giroud and Martinet 1956; Giroud 1959, 1960). In general, however, this immense field has remained largely untapped and awaits further investigation.

If any general conclusions are possible from these scattered observations, it is that teratogenic noxae act primarily by selective destruction of cells, necrosis of which has been observed repeatedly. Caution is, however, necessary in the interpretation of this phenomenon, as necrosis of groups of cells occurs in normal development, in remodelling of organs and removal of superfluous parts (Glücksman 1951). Even pathological tissue destruction is followed by repair processes of various degrees of effectiveness. In addition, destruction of parts of the embryonal structure removes the inductor and inhibitor influences on neighbouring cell groups. This may in some instances lead to arrest of normal processes, in others to excessive and uninhibited growth as observed by Patten (1952, 1953). Until the interaction of these processes is unravelled by a step-by-step analysis, the morphogenesis of individual malformations will remain largely speculative.

Cyclopia and arhinencephaly

In its most extreme form the cyclopian monster exhibits a centrally placed, diamond-shaped orbit containing a single globe showing various degrees of doubling of the intrinsic structures. There are also gross malformations of the mouth and nose, the latter being usually represented by a proboscis placed above the eye. The optic nerves are sometimes absent, one cause for this being that the nerve fibres have been prevented from growing back along the optic stalks because of the primary absence of the choroidal fissures (Gruenwald 1945). Owing to the failure of the anterior telencephalon to divide into two hemispheres, a single ventricle without a corpus callosum or septum pellucidum is formed. This 'holosphere' (Yakovlev 1959) is partially roofed by a rudimentary macrogyric cortex in which nine distinct cytoarchitectonic areas can be distinguished. The hippocampus, fascia dentata and subiculum occupy the entire circumference. The ventricle is closed behind by a thin membrane attached to the thalamus. The basal ganglia form unpaired protuberances in the floor of the holosphere. Except for the absence of the cortical projection systems the brainstem and cerebellum are normal. This concentration of primary anomalies in the forebrain region and in the face may be explained as the result of faulty induction by the prechordal mesenchyme. Similarly, the cyclopian eye is not the consequence of a fusion of anlagen, but of faulty induction (Adelmann 1930). The whole subject is well covered by Yakovlev's (1959) account which is based on the examination of 10 specimens.

In the less severe forms of cyclopia the eyes may be separate but microphthalmic, and a flattened nose is present (cebocephaly). The mildest variety is known as arhinencephaly and is often associated with hare-lip. As in the cyclops, the olfactory bulbs and tracts are absent and in the great majority of cases there is an unpaired ventricle. The longitudinal cerebral fissure may, however, be present, but the hemispheres are connected together in its depths not by a corpus callosum but by a plate of grey matter or by interdigitating gyri. The hippocampal formations have often been described as being unduly small in these brains, but in de Jong's (1927) case they were found to be larger than normal. The anterior commissure is absent. Hypertrophy of the basal ganglia was a feature of the arhinencephalic brain described by Goldstein and Riese (1925). Stewart's (1939) specimen was an example of the least severe variety of the condition; the hemispheres were fully separated and there was a complete corpus callosum although a distinctly small one. Unilateral absence of the olfactory tract, accompanied by similar cerebral anomalies, has also been described. Partial separation of the hemispheres, with a single ventricular cavity, can also occur in the presence of intact olfactory tracts and general intelligence is not necessarily reduced (Nathan and Smith 1950). An interesting point shown by some cases is that foramina may be present in the cribriform plate despite the absence of the olfactory bulbs—a fact consistent with the development of the olfactory nerves independently of their central connections.

The cerebellum may contain numerous and often massive heterotopic collections of nerve cells in its white matter (Norman 1966; Terplan, Sandberg and Aceto 1966). These will be discussed in conjunction with other cerebellar dysplasias (see p. 405).

Of the aetiological factors responsible for this group of malformations, trisomy of Group D (13-15) is the most important (Bühler, Bodis, Rossier and Stalder 1962; Miller, Pickard, Alkan, Warner and Gerald 1963). However, other chromosomal abnormalities have been observed, such as deletion of the short arm of no. 18 (Faith and Lewis 1964). In addition familial cases with normal karyotype also occur (Demyer, Zeman and Palmer 1963; Hintz, Menking and Sotos 1968).

Anencephaly

In this common maldevelopment the brain is either absent ('total anencephaly') or rudimentary ('partial anencephaly' or 'hemicrania') and there is an associated defect of the cranial vault and scalp. The frontal bones are absent above the supraciliary ridge, the parietal bones and the squamous part of the occipital bone are usually missing and the bones at the base of the skull are abnormally small (Marin-Padilla 1970). The cervical vertebrae are reduced in number and in rather more than half the cases there is a rachischisis, continuous with the cranial defect, which may reach the lumbar region (Nañagas 1925). In partial anencephaly the cerebellum and brainstem may be largely spared, but usually the brain is represented by a thin rudiment of highly vascular tissue containing elements of neurons, neuroglia and choroid plexus—the area cerebrovasculosa. The anterior pituitary may occasionally be identifiable, and its absence or hypoplasia is thought to be correlated with the extremely small adrenals which are a constant feature of the condition. The clinical and pathological features of anencephaly have been well presented by Thomas and Ajuriaguerra (1959). There is no doubt that part of the malformation is due to a disintegration of preformed portions of the brain, since in many specimens the eyes are normal though there may be no trace of the optic nerves. The primary defect appears to be defective closure of the anterior end of the neural tube. The process has been followed in rat embryos rendered anencephalic by excess of vitamin A

(Giroud 1959). Before the onset of degenerative changes the cellular growth of the various parts of the telencephalon is not greatly disturbed, except that development is distorted by the presence of an unclosed neural plate and the cerebral hemispheres are found beneath the everted diencephalon. Vogel and McClenahan (1952) have shown, by the method of injecting fusible metal, that major arteries do not penetrate the areas of cerebral malformation, but are often replaced by a number of slender abnormal branches rising from the internal carotid arteries. In cases in which the cerebellum and brainstem are involved, the vertebral system is also disorganized. The authors consider that anomalies of the major arteries occurring between the 3rd and 5th week of fetal life may be an important pathogenic factor in anencephaly. Vogel (1958) has reported anencephaly in one head of a conjoined double twin, again with striking vascular anomalies on that side. Whether these vascular abnormalities are solely responsible for the condition, however, remains doubtful, for Giroud (1960) has observed a normal arrangement of vessels in young anencephalic embryos.

Malformations of the spinal cord

Amyelia, or total absence of the spinal cord, is only found in association with anencephaly. An interesting feature of the condition is the occasionally independent development of many of the spinal ganglia, the posterior roots of which may be seen passing inwards towards the area medullo-vasculosa, as if in search of their non-existent spinal cord—a good example of the principle of 'self-determination' in the formation of the nervous system. The muscles of these monsters are well developed despite the absence of anterior spinal nerve roots.

Much commoner are the various forms of *myelodysplasia* associated with spina bifida. They represent a wide range of anatomical variants which have only recently been subjected to detailed studies (Talwalker and Dastur 1970; Emery and Lendon 1973; Rokos 1973). Their terminology is confused and the classical terms myelocele, meningomyelocele, meningocele and spina bifida occulta are only roughly descriptive and do not account for all the anatomical features. The anomalies which occur at the site of the spina bifida and those affecting the spinal cord

and its coverings above and below the main lesion may have to be considered separately.

Myelocele is the most severe of the malformations encountered at the site of the spinal cleft. It represents a situation in which the neural tube has failed to close (*myeloschisis*). The spinal cord forms a flat disc, often covered by a thin layer of highly vascular granulation tissue and presents on the surface as a raw, red, velvety area. This is usually surrounded by a zone devoid both of neural elements and of epidermis. Whether this is the result of secondary degeneration or is an essential feature of the lesion remains controversial. Rare instances occur where only one-half of a diastematomyelic cord remains open, the other being closed round its own central canal ('hemimyelocele', Duckworth, Sharrard, Lister and Seymour 1968). The disc of cord in myelocele may retain its normal relationship to the posterior surface of the vertebral bodies (*simple myeloschisis*) or may be separated from it and float on the dorsal surface of an arachnoid cyst (*cystic myelocele*). The granulation tissue which commonly forms on the surface of the raw area may become organized and epithelialized (*scarred myelocele*), a situation frequently confused with meningomyelocele. In all forms of myelocele the microscopic appearances are those of an opened neural tube, complicated by secondary destructive changes and coincidental developmental errors. The cord is represented by a flat disc in which the anterior horns and roots occupy a medial, the posterior horns and roots a lateral position. The posterior surface is covered with ependyma which is however hardly ever intact. Secondary degenerative changes in the exposed plaque of neural tissue lead to its breaking up into islands separated by glial scars. In addition, ectopic islands of neural tissue, consisting mainly of glia, but containing sparse neurons and aberrant ependymal canals, may be found outside the spinal cord. Posterior root ganglia may also be found occupying abnormal positions in the subarachnoid space. The *pathogenesis* of the lesion is still controversial. While most writers favour the theory of a primary failure of closure of the neural groove, developed by Lebedeff (1881) and von Recklinghausen (1886), others favour the rupture of a preformed neural tube from pressure of the cerebrospinal fluid. The latter view, originally proposed by Morgagni

(1761), was recently revived and developed by Gardner (1960, 1961, 1968). Rokos (1973) believes that the primary damage occurs at the neuroepidermal junction, thus removing the inductor influences of the epidermis on the closing neural tube. A simultaneous removal of the inhibitor influences may lead to the over-growth of neural elements, a phenomenon previously observed by Patten (1953).

Meningomyelocele is a group of conditions in which the subcutaneous hernial sac is lined by intact meninges and contains herniated parts of the spinal cord. Apart from the scarred myelo-celes, frequently and erroneously included in this group, two main types may be distinguished. In one the closed, but flattened and deformed ('winged') cord floats on the posterior surface of an arachnoid cyst separating it from the vertebral bodies. In the other the spinal cord keeps its anterior attachment to the vertebral bodies, but its central canal is grossly dilated and the thinned-out posterior part of the cord accompanies the meningeal hernia (*myelocystocele* or *meningo-myelocystocele*). Both myeloceles and meningo-myeloceles are associated with wide defects in the vertebral arches, often affecting several vertebrae. They are most common in the upper lumbar and lower thoracic regions, but may occasionally occur at higher levels.

By contrast *meningoceles*, which by definition consist only of herniation of the meninges, the spinal cord retaining its normal position within the spinal canal, tend to occur with small defects in the vertebral arches and are most common in the lower lumbar and sacral regions. In their detailed study Talwalker and Dastur (1970) found that all simple meningoceles were associated with a small defect confined to a single vertebral arch. Wider defects in a single arch were associated with tethering of nerve roots to the hernial neck, while defects in several arches were accompanied by tethering of the cord, this latter group forming a transition between meningoceles and meningo-myeloceles. Even among the meningoceles only a minority conformed to the definition of simple herniation of the meninges. Some contained aberrant neural tissue apparently unconnected with the spinal cord, others had fistulous openings leaking cerebrospinal fluid on to the surface and one was associated with a vascular hamar-toma.

Spina bifida occulta denotes a defect in a vertebral arch without herniation of the contents of the spinal canal. However, the neural tissues may show a variety of minor malformations which may manifest themselves clinically as a progressive neurological deficit, often becoming apparent only in adolescence or early adult life. Accounts of these malformations are to be found mainly in radiological (Gryspeerdt 1963) or surgical litera-ture (James and Lassman 1962; Till 1969). The lesions consist most commonly of fibrous bands tethering the cord to the edge of the bony defect. Other associated malformations include dia-stematomyelia and hydromyelia, and also a variety of hamartomas.

The spinal cord may be abnormal both above and below the area of spina bifida and the various forms of herniation (Emery and Lendon 1973). The most common abnormalities above the main lesion are duplication of the cord (diastematomyelia or diplomyelia), hydromyelia and syringomyelia. Duplication of the cord or of the central canal was also frequently found below the level of the hernia. In some instances no cord tissue is found caudal to the plaque.

Diastematomyelia. The spinal cord may divide into two halves, each of which undergoes sub-sequent modifications of structure. The extent of the duplication is usually limited to about 10 segments and of the 42 cases reviewed by Herren and Edwards (1940) only two occurred at a level higher than the midthoracic. This doubling of the cord is often seen adjoining the region affected by myeloschisis. More than half the cases are associated with spina bifida occulta. The cord usually shows an increasing degree of hydromyelia as the point of division is approached from higher levels. This dilation is succeeded first by a bi-furcation of the central canal, then by the appear-ance of a dorsal cleft, reinforced by the downward growth of a connective tissue septum which separates the cord into two halves. Each opposed medial surface of these two divisions of the cord has a fissure, containing branches of the anterior spinal artery and probably caused by their inroad during the course of development (Lichtenstein 1940). (Such clefts have often been thought to be the true anterior fissures of a double cord, but this theory would involve the assumption that each 'cord' had rotated through 90°.) Each new half of the cord possesses a posterior and an anterior horn with their roots. In certain instances, the anterior horn becomes secondarily divided into two parts, but the posterior roots remain unpaired. Very rarely, the two divisions of the cord, instead of lying laterally, are found in a dorsoventral position (Dominok 1962).

The two parts of the cord are often separated from each other by a fibrous septum or bony spur attached to the dorsal surface of the vertebral body. When this is present, each half of the

tapers rapidly towards the cranial end of the cord (Mackenzie and Emery 1971). Diverticula of the dilated central canal may dissect the cord both downwards and upwards forming syringo-myelic cavities. In a monograph devoted to the subject Staemmler (1942) classified hydromyelia into two types, one being a simple dilatation of a normally placed central canal, the other being due to incomplete fusion of the posterior columns

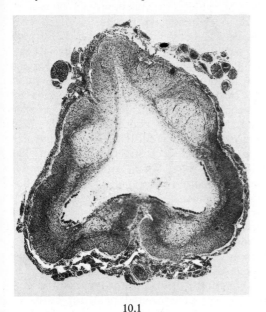

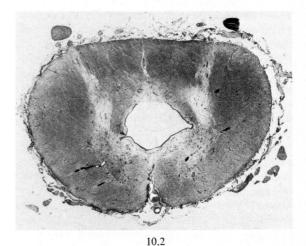

10.1   10.2

Fig. 10.1 Hydromyelia in a case of Arnold–Chiari malformation in a newborn child with early gliosis replacing lines of ependyma in the dorsal extension.
Fig. 10.2 Hydromyelia in a man aged 25 who died of poliomyelitis. Both hydromyelia and Chiari's type I deformity were clinically silent.

divided cord has its own dural sac. In the absence of a septum each has its own pial invest-ment, but the arachnoid and dura are shared (James and Lassman 1964). Diastematomelia by itself does not cause any disability and any associated neurological deficit is produced by pressure or traction either by the septum or associated fibrous bands. In reviewing his surgical experience of 37 cases Guthkelch (1974) reached the conclusion that the cause of pro-gressive spinal cord damage was repeated minor trauma resulting from spinal flexion, and not traction due to differential growth of the cord and vertebral column.

Hydromyelia frequently accompanies the major malformations of the spinal cord. It may extend upwards into the lower cervical segments but

and therefore a true dysraphic manifestation (Figs. 10.1 and 10.2).

Ectopic neural tissue. Islands of aberrant neural tissue, mainly consisting of glia, but sometimes containing sparse neurons and canals lined by ependyma, are common in all major dysraphic malformations. They have been described in various types of spina bifida (Talwalker and Dastur 1970; Rokos 1973), in anencephaly (Thomas and Ajuriaguerra 1959) and in occipital encephalocele (Karch and Urich 1972). Cooper and Kernohan (1951) devoted a detailed study to their structure and distribution.

Abnormalities of the filum terminale. The filum terminale in some cases of spina bifida may be abnormally short and thick, tethering the lower end of the cord to the sacrum. These abnormal fila may contain organized or disorganized cord elements, often with multiple ependymal tubules (Talwalker and Dastur 1970, 1974). Mere duplication of the central canal in the filum is probably a normal variant (Lendon and Emery 1970). Some of the thickened fila also contain an excessive amount of mesenchymal elements such as cartilage, bone or fibrofatty tissue (Talwalker and Dastur 1974). These must be considered akin to the spinal hamartomas.

Of the *hamartomas* associated with dysraphic malformations, *lipomas* are most common (Dubowitz, Lorber and Zachary 1965; Giuffré 1966). Their incidence and distribution was studied by Emery and Lendon (1969) who found most of them in the filum terminale, either in its intrathecal or its extrathecal portions, or in both. Dural fibrolipomas, either in the neighbourhood of the hernia or remote from it, formed the second largest group. An important though less numerous group are the 'leptomyelolipomas' of the region of the conus, which consist of a bizarre mixture of neural, meningeal and fibrofatty elements. Finally, lipomas may occur in the connective tissue septa separating the two halves of the diastematomyelia. Histologically the lipomas consist of lobules of adipose tissue separated by fibrous bands and septa. Occasionally they contain other mesenchymal elements such as smooth or striated muscle fibres (Taniguchi and Mufson 1950).

Another group of hamartomatous lesions is of dermal origin. Skin dimples or hairy tufts are not uncommon over spina bifida occulta. Occasionally deep skin-lined sinuses may lead into intraspinal *dermoid cysts* (List 1941*a*).

Endodermal hamartomas of various complexity, reproducing various parts of the alimentary and respiratory tracts, occur in cases of *anterior spina bifida* where there is a failure of fusion of the two halves of vertebral bodies (Willis 1958). The most common of these hamartomatous lesions are *enterogenous cysts* of the spinal canal, usually lying anterior to the spinal cord and lined with mucus-producing columnar epithelium (Harriman 1958).

Minor malformations of the spinal cord and status dysraphicus. In spina bifida occulta and also in cases without rachischisis the cord may exhibit a number of minor malformations. Although these anomalies do not usually give rise to neuro-

logical signs they have been considered of importance by some writers as forming an integral part of the syndrome of status dysraphicus. The conception of this condition as a morbid entity dates from the clinical observations of Fuchs (1909) who distinguished a group of individuals having in common some of the following features: spina bifida, syndactyly, trophic and vasomotor disturbances, sensory disturbances of syringomyelic type, sphincter weakness and skin anomalies such as naevi and hypertrichosis. This syndrome was elaborated by Bremer (1927), who noted the frequency of kyphosis and sternal deformities in the group and who also demonstrated abnormal glial proliferation and small cavities in the region of the dorsal septum in the spinal cords of some of these cases. Bremer stressed the familial concentration of these anomalies and considered that status dysraphicus was inherited as a distinctive constitutional disability. In more recent times this opinion has been supported by Benda (1952), who has described a similar clinico-pathological syndrome ('oligoencephaly') among feeble-minded mental defectives. Among these minor malformations may be mentioned the absence of the posterior septum or the presence of a cleft in this situation, anomalies of the central canal such as patency in adult life, and various distortions and asymmetries of the anterior and posterior horns of grey matter. These findings are important in so far as they indicate the developmental origin of the abnormalities seen elsewhere in the nervous system of these patients, but great care must be taken to exclude the presence of artefacts which may easily be produced by careless removal of the spinal cord (van Gieson 1892).

The Chiari malformations

In 1891 Chiari attempted a classification of cerebellar malformations frequently associated with hydrocephalus and subdivided them into three types. In a subsequent paper (1895) he gave further details and added more cases to his material. Since then a large literature has accumulated on the subject causing some conceptual and terminological confusion, which can be unravelled only by a detailed historical analysis. Only the main landmarks of the dispute can be mentioned here; for full historical reviews the reader is referred to the theses of

Peach (1964a), Brocklehurst (1968) and Rokos (1973).

Chiari type I malformation. In Chiari's original description the medulla was displaced downwards into the spinal canal and was covered on its dorsolateral aspects by peg-like processes arising from the cerebellar tonsils and neighbouring parts of the cerebellar hemispheres. These prolongations might be asymmetrical or unilateral and might reach only to the atlas, but in many cases they passed through the lower border of the axis so that their lower end was opposite the origin of the 3rd cervical nerve roots. Their tissue might be sclerosed or softened. As an example of this type he cited the case of a girl aged 17 in whom the malformation had caused no symptoms during life. There was some widening of the lateral and 3rd ventricles but no enlargement of the head. In his later report (1895) Chiari analysed his material of 14 cases. In seven of these the malformation was found in children under the age of 10 years, in one in the second decade and in six in adults. In one case only was it associated with a meningomyelocele.

There is still some uncertainty about the status of the type I malformation. There is no doubt that some cases so labelled represent only a severe grade of tonsillar herniation and pressure coning in cases of chronic hydrocephalus due to a variety of mechanisms. Another group is associated with bony malformations such as platybasia, achondroplasia, or the Klippel–Feil anomaly. In other cases the malformation of the posterior fossa structures is associated with syringomyelia. Finally there is a group of genuine cerebellar ectopias in which peg-shaped or finger-like protrusions, symmetrical or asymmetrical, are unassociated with displacements of the cerebellum as a whole (Fig. 10.3). These protrusions of the cerebellar hemispheres are connected by fibrovascular adhesions to the back and sides of the somewhat elongated lower medulla.

The relationship of the type I malformation to spina bifida is also controversial. In most cases there is no evidence of any spinal malformation (Chiari 1895; McConnell and Parker 1938; Greenfield 1958). Others associated this lesion with spina bifida in the lower lumbar or sacral region. Perhaps that is due to the widespread tendency to classify all mild cases surviving into adult life as examples of Chiari type I, some of

which may represent minimal degrees of the type II malformation. The main criterion of distinction remains the derivation of the ectopic cerebellar tissue, which in the type I malformation originates from the cerebellar hemisphere and not from the vermis. This applies even to cases in which a

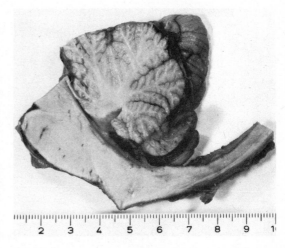

Fig. 10.3 Chiari type I malformation. The ectopic nodule of cerebellar tissue has no connection with the normal vermis.

unilateral protrusion descends in the midline thus mimicking a type II malformation on surgical exploration.

Chiari type II, or Arnold–Chiari malformation (Fig. 10.4). In Chiari's original description the protrusion of the lower parts of the cerebellum was associated with an elongation of the 4th ventricle which extended into the spinal canal. The malformation was illustrated by an example of a 6-month-old baby with fairly severe hydrocephalus (43 cm). In this case there were heterotopic nodules of grey matter, the size of beans, in the walls of the lateral ventricles. The cerebellum was small and the tentorium less vaulted than normal. The pons was elongated; its lower quarter lay below the level of the foramen magnum and was flattened from before backwards. The medulla lay entirely in the spinal canal and the lower cranial nerves were considerably elongated. Where the medulla joined the spinal cord there was a swelling the size of a bean which covered the upper 9 mm of the spinal cord and reached to the 5th cervical pair of nerve roots and the disc between the 4th and 5th cervical vertebrae. This swelling contained a pouch-like prolongation of the 4th ventricle. It was covered on its dorsal and lateral surfaces by flattened protrusions of cerebellar tissue arising from the amygdalae and the lower part of the vermis. The cervical cord was abnormally

the two halves rejoined to form a cylindrical band which ended opposite the first sacral vertebra.

In his subsequent analysis of seven cases of this type Chiari (1895) found an associated meningomyelocele or spina bifida in all cases.

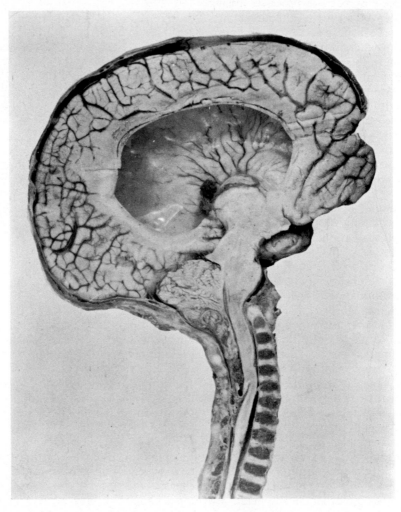

Fig. 10.4 Arnold–Chiari malformation and hydrocephalus in a 7-week-old infant. (By courtesy of Prof. Moncrieff and the photographic department, Mr D. Martin, Hospital for Sick Children.)

short (24 mm) and its roots were crowded together. The upper pairs of posterior roots appeared between the cervical cord and the overlying mass arising in the lower medulla. The thoracic cord contained a cylindrical cavity filled with clear serum. At the lower thoracic level the cord split into two halves and into a meningomyelocele at the junction of the thoracic and lumbar cord. Below the 5th lumbar segment

The malformation was always associated with hydrocephalus of congenital type.

Meanwhile Arnold (1894) gave detailed description of a similar case associated with meningomyelocele but without hydrocephalus. In fact, priority of the description of this malformation belongs to Cleland whose full account appeared in 1883.

Schwalbe and Gredig (1907) gave the name

Arnold–Chiari malformation to the Chiari type II lesion which they found to be always associated with meningomyelocele. The term was introduced to English readers by Russell and Donald (1935) who reported 10 similar cases. Despite some doubts about the importance of Arnold's contribution, the term is now generally accepted and is quite unexceptionable provided it is confined to the type II malformation. There is no justification whatever for distinguishing the cerebellar malformation as Arnold's deformity and the medullary malformation as Chiari's deformity (List 1941*b*; Lichtenstein 1942) as both authors gave full descriptions of both components.

There are now many excellent descriptions of the type II malformation and associated anomalies (Daniel and Strich 1958; Peach 1965*a* and others). It has become apparent that this malformation is less stereotyped than would appear from the early descriptions. Referring to the elongation of the 4th ventricle and the cerebellar component, Schwalbe and Gredig (1907) recognized five types of the Arnold–Chiari malformation: (1) a large part of the inferior vermis lies within the cavity of the elongated ventricle; (2) a similar protrusion of the vermis lies dorsal to the roof of the fourth ventricle; (3) the cerebellar protrusion is short and covers only the upper part of the elongated ventricle; (4) the elongated ventricle contains the displaced choroid plexus; (5) the elongated ventricle is roofed by a thick glial membrane only. The thick glial membrane forming the roof of the 4th ventricle is a constant feature of the malformation. It frequently obliterates the foramen of Magendie, in some instances giving rise to a cystic dilatation of the ventricle at the site of the foramen (Peach 1964*b*). The structure of the cerebellar tongue may vary considerably (Variend and Emery 1974). In some cases it shows approximately normal lobulation with only minor deviations in cortical cytoarchitecture. In others the lobules may be abnormally small or distorted and show depletion of cellular elements. Heterotopic masses of cerebellar cortical cells may be found in the underlying white matter. In extreme examples the cerebellar tissue is completely dysplastic and consists of a totally disorganized mass of cellular elements. The cerebellum above the level of the malformation is usually hypoplastic, roughly pyramidal in shape and may show minor degenerative changes (Aring 1938). The white matter of the lateral lobes may contain heterotopic foci of cortical

cells (Sandbank 1955). In some instances deep clefts, communicating with the 4th ventricle, extend into the white matter. Rarely the superior vermis is absent and the hemispheres are separated by a midline cleft. Finally, in an extreme example, the whole cerebellum was displaced downwards leaving a space filled with cerebrospinal fluid between its upper surface and the tentorium (Penfield and Coburn 1938).

The elongation of the medulla is also subject to considerable variations (Emery and Mackenzie 1973). These authors have classified the medullary deformity into five grades, of which only the two most severe ones are associated with the characteristic Z-shaped kink at the junction of the medulla and the spinal cord. The degree of shortening of the cervical cord and the angle at which the spinal nerve roots reach their intervertebral foramina depends on the degree of elongation of the medulla. It is worth emphasizing that the upward or horizontal direction of the spinal roots is confined to the cervical cord and becomes normal at thoracic levels. The dysplasias of the spinal cord associated with the Arnold–Chiari malformation have already been described (see p. 369).

Multiple anomalies have been found at the higher levels of the neuraxis. The tectum of the midbrain has a characteristic beaked appearance, the point consisting of the elongated and fused inferior colliculi and directed backwards and downwards. This anomaly, already observed by Cleland (1883), was described in detail by Feigin (1956). Stenosis or forking of the aqueduct and fusion of the thalami, with formation of a large massa intermedia, are common abnormalities in the ventricular system (Cameron 1957). In a detailed study of 100 cases Emery (1974) observed that the aqueduct was anatomically patent in all cases. It was severely shortened in almost all cases and compressed laterally in most. Some form of forking was present in about one-quarter of the cases. Dorsal displacement and angulation was associated with beaking of the tectum. He concluded that the aqueduct in many of these children was in a valve-like state, patency being dependent upon lateral compression of a flattened tube. Hydrocephalus, ranging from slight to extreme, is an almost constant feature of the Arnold–Chiari malformation. Other abnormalities also occur in the cerebral hemispheres. The most common is a derangement of convolutional pattern in which the cortex is folded into an excessive number of small gyri. This condition, best termed polygyria, differs from microgyria in its preservation of a normal cortical cytoarchitecture. Peach (1965a) found areas of true microgyria, with a four-layered cortex, in about one-half of his cases. This observation requires confirmation as regrettably few brains with this anomaly have been subjected to cytoarchitectural studies. Hetertopias of grey matter in the walls of the lateral ventricles (Chiari 1891) are uncommon.

Associated skeletal malformations include the almost invariably present spina bifida. In most cases the defect is thoracolumbar or lumbar, less commonly lumbosacral (Peach 1965b). High cervical defects are uncommon and cases showing this type of meningomyelocele are more accurately classified as Chiari type III. Low cervical or cervicothoracic lesions are exceedingly rare. Malformations of vertebral bodies are not infrequent, most commonly in the form of hemivertebrae.

The posterior fossa in the Arnold–Chiari malformation is small. The tentorium is displaced downwards and is attached close to the foramen magnum. It is hypoplastic and has an unusually wide incisura. The falx cerebri is also frequently hypoplastic. The bones of the vault of the skull are thin and frequently show multiple fenestration. This craniolacunia appears to be independent of the size of the head and the degree of hydrocephalus.

Two closely linked problems remain highly controversial. One is the occurrence of the Arnold–Chiari malformation in the absence of meningomyeloceles. There is only one well documented case of a typical Chiari type II deformity unassociated with spina bifida (Peach 1964c). This is obviously an exceptional occurrence, but the possibility of minor degrees of the deformity associated with sacral meningocele, spina bifida occulta or complete closure of the vertebral arches cannot be ruled out. Patients with this type of anomaly would be likely to survive to adult life, which leads to the problem of the Arnold–Chiari malformation in later life. A vast amount of mainly clinical literature has grown around this subject (Ogryzlo 1942; Gardner and Goodall 1950; Teng and Papatheodorou 1965; Carmel and Markesbery 1969 and many others). There is little doubt that most of these cases are examples of Chiari type I deformity and the use of the term Arnold–Chiari

is a misnomer. It is, however, difficult to exclude the possibility that some of these cases, however inadequately documented, may indeed represent minor degrees of the type II malformation.

The *pathogenesis* of the Arnold–Chiari malformation is the subject of many highly speculative theories, well reviewed by Brocklehurst (1971).

(1) The hydrodynamic theories originate from Morgagni (1761) who believed that the hydrocephalus, hydromyelia and meningomyelocele were all due to excessive accumulation of fluid within the neuraxis. In a greatly modified form this theory was revived by Gardner (1959), who maintains that the primary malformation of the roof of the 4th ventricle leads to hydrocephalus, the pressure of which is transmitted downwards into the central canal and leads to rupture of the previously closed neural tube. The main objection to this theory is that the events take place at a time before the choroid plexuses become active and when the ventricular system is still a closed, low-pressure cavity. That hydrocephalus may be instrumental in forcing the contents of the posterior fossa downwards was the view proposed by Chiari and still held in a modified form by Emery and his associates. A totally different version of the hydrodynamic theory was proposed by Cameron (1957). He held that the primary lesion was the failure of the neural tube to close, forming an open myelocele. This, far from leading to accumulation of fluid in the ventricular system, caused an excessive drainage of fluid and apposition of ependymal surfaces which became fused; hence the stenosis and forking of the aqueduct and the large massa intermedia.

(2) The second group comprises the traction theories. The starting point here again is the meningomyelocele where the cord is tethered to the walls of the hernia. As the spine grows faster than the cord the latter is subject to traction which may be transmitted to the brainstem (Lichtenstein 1942). It is difficult to reconcile this view with the shortening of the cervical cord, excessive elongation of the medulla leading to its doubling up on the cervical cord, and the displacement of the nerve roots confined to the cervical segments. Furthermore, fixation of the cord in spina bifida occulta, in spinal lipomas, etc., is not as a rule associated with malformations of the hind brain.

(3) The overgrowth theory (Barry, Patten and Stewart 1957) states that the primary fault is

excessive growth of neural tissue in relation to its craniovertebral encasement, beginning at the 4th week of development. At the lumbosacral level this prevents the vertebral arches from joining in the midline. At the cranial level the large brain displaces the tentorium downwards and causes herniation of the hind brain into the cervical canal. The situation becomes stabilized by adhesions, leading to further elongation and distortion during further development. Abnormal growth of the cerebellum and brainstem with failure of formation of the pontine flexure were put forward as a possible explanation of the hind brain malformation by Daniel and Strich (1958).

(4) The teratological theories are based on observations from experimental teratology, where a single insult may lead to destructive lesions affecting widely disparate areas of the neuraxis followed by repair and compensatory phenomena. Spina bifida can be produced in experimental animals by a variety of methods. There is, however, no exact experimental counterpart to the full picture of the Arnold–Chiari malformation. It is therefore of great interest that Rokos (1973) succeeded in producing hind brain malformations, approximating to the human situation, by mechanical damage to the roof-plate of the 4th ventricle in the chick embryo.

The hydrocephalus in the Arnold–Chiari malformation was thought by Russell and Donald (1935) to be the direct result of the downward displacement of the hind brain. The foramina for the exit of cerebrospinal fluid are thus situated within the spinal canal. As the cerebellar protrusions plug the foramen magnum, the cerebrospinal fluid is unable to reach the intracranial subarachnoid space and to be absorbed from there, but must be absorbed from the spinal canal. However, other factors, such as stenosis or forking of the aqueduct, and the occlusion of the foramen of Magendie may play an important part in causing hydrocephalus.

Chiari type III malformation. This is a rare malformation of which Chiari (1891) quoted only one example. It consists of a high cervical or occipitocervical meningomyelocele with herniation of the cerebellum through the bony defect. Further examples of this rare condition were described by Peach (1965a). These cases are related to occipital encephaloceles on one hand and to *iniencephaly* on the other. The latter is a malformation of

the neck in which the vertebral bodies are fused, their arches absent and a myeloschisis of the cervical cord is present. The open cord, however, does not present on the surface but is covered by prolapsed brain tissue, including the cerebellum, and externally by meninges and skin. The head is retroflexed and the occiput may be joined to the vertebrae of the lower spine (Gilmour 1941; Cimmino and Painter 1962).

The encephaloceles

Defects in the cranium with herniation of the meninges and brain are uncommon in comparison with anencephaly, spina bifida and the Chiari malformations. Their incidence is subject to considerable geographical variations. A concise review of the sites, incidence and contents of the various cranial herniae was published by Emery and Kalhan (1970).

Occipital encephaloceles. Occipital defects with herniation of the meninges and brain are the subject of an extensive clinical literature (Ingraham and Swan 1943; Fischer, Uihlein and Keith 1952; Cohn and Hamby 1953; Barrow and Simpson 1966; Lorber 1967). On the other hand, the pathology of the condition has received remarkably little attention. Admittedly minor degrees of herniation, in which only one or both occipital poles protrude through the bony defect, present no particular problems, but more severe examples are associated with a variety of complex malformations (Karch and Urich 1972).

The bony defect may be confined to the occipital squame or extend to the foramen magnum and involve the posterior arch of the atlas. The base of the skull may be deformed in that the anterior and middle fossae are abnormally small and the posterior fossa large and subdivided into two compartments by an abnormally low insertion of the tentorium. The upper compartment between the ridge of the petrous temporal bone and the tentorium is broad and shallow and contains parts of the cerebral hemispheres. The lower may be narrow and funnel-shaped and its contents vary according to the degree of herniation. The dural folds are also abnormal. The falx is displaced to follow the asymmetrical, oblique course of the sagittal fissure. The tentorium consists of two crescentic folds running from the apex of the petrous temporal bone to the margin of the occipital defect. The straight sinus is absent.

Herniation of the cerebral hemispheres is asymmetrical and as much as one-half of a hemisphere may be displaced into the hernial sac (Fig. 10.5). Hydrocephalus in the intracranial portion is uncommon, but it may occur in the protruding part if it contains a choroid plexus. The lateral ventricles tend to be narrow and their walls show a tendency to fusion when in apposition. Defects in the commissural system include absence of the anterior commissure, septum pellucidum and fornix. The corpus callosum can usually be identified.

An unusual form of occipital encephalocele in which the contents of the hernial sac consisted entirely of a cyst communicating with the lateral recess of the fourth ventricle ('posterior fossa ventriculocele') was described by Evrard and Caviness (1974). This was associated with an extensive cerebellar cortical defect, anomalies of the ipsilateral roof and brainstem nuclei, thalamic fusion and massive hydrocephalus with periventricular leucomalacia in the cerebral hemispheres.

Sincipital encephaloceles. Meningoceles and encephaloceles in the anterior part of the head

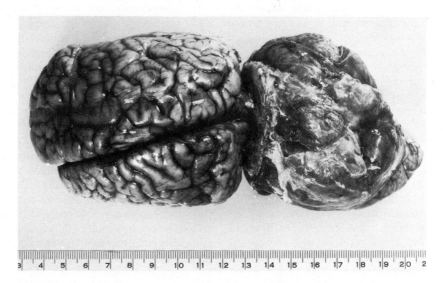

Fig. 10.5 Occipital encephalocele. Asymmetrical herniation of cerebral hemispheres.

The hernial sac in severe cases contains parts of the cerebellum and brainstem. Apart from elongation and distortion the structures of the hind brain may show various degrees of disorganization (Fig. 10.6). Midline clefts in the cerebellum are common and severe cortical malformations also occur. Superimposed on developmental errors are ischaemic changes due to strangulation of blood vessels in the hernial neck. Hydromyelia is common in the spinal cord. The brainstem and upper cervical cord are often surrounded by a rich venous plexus, perhaps representing persistence of the embryonic vascular network. Islands of aberrant neural tissue may be found in the neighbourhood of the brainstem and spinal cord.

are rare in Western Europe and North America, but are apparently common in South-east Asia. Suwanwela and Suwanwela (1972) analysed their own material collected in Bangkok, reviewed the literature and proposed a classification based on the site of the bony defect.

The most common variety falls into the fronto-ethmoidal group which may be subdivided into nasofrontal, naso-ethmoidal and naso-orbital types. The hernial sac presents in the region of the root of the nose and contains the frontal poles of the brain or larger parts of the frontal lobes. Associated defects include hydrocephalus and elongation of the brainstem and hypothalamus.

Of the rare defects in the cranial vault, the

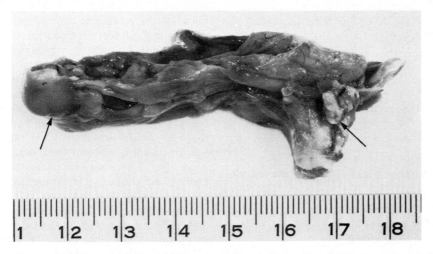

Fig. 10.6 Occipital encephalocele. Elongation and distortion of brainstem; cerebellar rudiments indicated by arrows. (Reproduced by courtesy of the Editor, *Journal of Neurological Sciences*.)

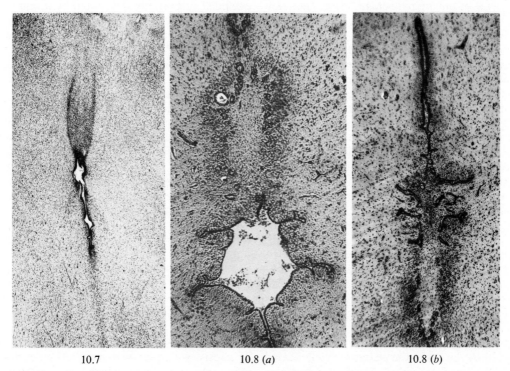

10.7	10.8 (*a*)	10.8 (*b*)

Fig. 10.7 Stenosis of the Sylvian aqueduct in stillborn hydrocephalic infant. Note the nucleus dorsalis which is a conspicuous feature of early life.

Fig. 10.8 (*a* and *b*) Gliosis of the aqueduct. In its dorsal part the outline of the aqueduct is indicated only by ependymal cells. The ventral part becomes a narrow, ependyma-lined slit.

interfrontal is most frequently seen. Defects in the anterior or posterior fontanelles, between the parietal bones and in the temporal region also occur.

Basal defects with intranasal meningoceles may be transethmoidal, transsphenoidal or spheno-ethmoidal.

Massive craniofacial clefts may involve either the vault and the upper part of the face, or the base and lower part of the face.

Aqueductal malformations leading to hydrocephalus

Obstructive hydrocephalus is commonly caused by narrowing or closure of the Sylvian aqueduct and four main types of this anomaly have been described by Russell (1949).

(1) Stenosis of the aqueduct may be said to be present when narrowing occurs without abnormal gliosis in the surrounding tissue (Fig. 10.7). The normal aqueduct varies considerably in cross-section at different levels. Two constrictions regularly occur, the first beneath the middle of the superior corpora quadrigemina, the second at the level of the intercollicular sulcus. Between these two narrowings the aqueduct shows a well-marked dilatation or ampulla. Woollam and Millen's (1953) measurements indicate that considerable differences in cross-section also occur between individual specimens at the same situation in the aqueduct; thus at the commencement of the ampulla the average cross-section in 10 cases was 0·9 mm² but the individual variation ranged from as little as 0·2 mm² up to 1·8 mm². In order to establish that stenosis is the cause of hydrocephalus it is therefore necessary to employ control sections made at different levels. According to Alvord (1961) the development of hydrocephalus is determined not only by a reduction in size of the aqueductal lumen but also by the length of the aqueduct, the viscosity of the CSF, and differences between the 3rd and 4th ventricles.

There is a rare hereditary variety of this condition. In the family described by Bickers and Adams (1949), congenital hydrocephalus was confined to seven males in two generations and a simple aqueductal stenosis was proved at autopsy in one of the siblings. In a similar case examined by the writer the pedigree also indicated inheritance by a sex-linked Mendelian recessive factor (Edwards, Norman and Roberts 1961).

(2) Forking of the aqueduct is present when two main channels of greatly reduced dimensions are found one behind the other in the midsagittal plane of the brainstem and separated by normal intervening tissue. The dorsal channel shows considerable branching and adjacent groups of ependymal cells may also form short tubules, while the ventral passage is usually a narrow slit. Serial sections show that each main channel may communicate with the other or may enter the ventricle independently or end blindly, but there is usually an aqueductal lumen of some sort to be seen, however functionally inadequate it may be. There may be associated maldevelopment of neighbouring structures, such as fusion of the corpora quadrigemina or of the oculomotor nuclei, and spina bifida is commonly present (Cameron 1957). The term 'atresia' is inappropriate for this condition (Russell 1949). In brains without hydrocephalus a secondary channel may occasionally be present for a short distance ventral to an aqueduct of normal appearance, but since the cross-section of the latter is not reduced there is no obstruction to the circulation of the cerebrospinal fluid.

(3) Septum formation. The aqueduct may be occluded or partially obstructed by a thin neuroglial membrane. This is usually found at the caudal end, but may also occur in the middle or upper third of the aqueduct. Certain of these cases are associated with granular ependymitis of the ventricular system suggestive of an infection during fetal life.

(4) Gliosis of the aqueduct. In this condition a narrowing of the aqueduct or its subdivision into two or more smaller channels is found, in conjunction with a well-marked proliferation of fibrillary glia. The surrounding zone of gliosis evidently marks out the area of the pre-existing aqueduct, since its peripheral edge is outlined by disorderly groups of ependymal cells (Fig. 10.8). The narrowed lumen itself has no ependymal lining. This gliotic stenosis may be present at only one part of the aqueduct, in which event the anterior part of the channel shows dilatation. Unlike cases of forking, the glial type of obstruction is not associated with other maldevelopments of the brainstem or elsewhere.

The pathogenesis of the gliosis is obscure. The condition appears to differ from the primary type of gliosis, with polypoid granulations projecting into the aqueduct, which has occasionally been reported in von Recklinghausen's disease (Laurence 1962). Russell (1949) has pointed out that whereas the ependyma is highly vulnerable and has little regenerative power, the subependymal glia is readily stimulated to proliferation. Bacterial toxins are thus conceivable pathogenetic agents. Granular ependymitis in the ventricular system below the level of the obstruction would be in favour of an infection. Gliosis of the aqueduct is usually associated clinically with an insidious onset of raised intracranial pressure in early life, but it may also occur in adults. The resulting hydrocephalus thus belongs in the majority of instances to the class of postnatal malformations.

This simple and clear-cut classification is, however, open to criticism. Drachman and Richardson (1961) reported a case which displayed features of both forking and gliosis. In reviewing the literature they concluded that too many mixed or intermediate cases occurred to support the validity of a separation into clear-cut types. They also expressed doubt whether congenital lesions could be confidently distinguished from acquired ones. Recently Williams (1973) advanced the interesting hypothesis that in some cases aqueduct stenosis could be the result of hydrocephalus, rather than its primary cause.

Dandy–Walker syndrome

The association of hydrocephalus with a posterior fossa cyst and hypoplasia of the cerebellar vermis was recognized as an entity by Dandy and Blackfan (1914) and confirmed by Taggart and Walker (1942). In this condition the cerebellar hemispheres are separated by an enlarged ventricle, the roof of which is represented by a thin, bulging membrane, consisting of neuroglia lined on the inside by ependyma and on the outside by pia arachnoid. This membrane arises from the brainstem in the same way as a normal roof, but laterally it is attached in a curved line to the ventromedial aspects of the lateral lobes (Fig. 10.9). The cerebellar folia facing the lumen of

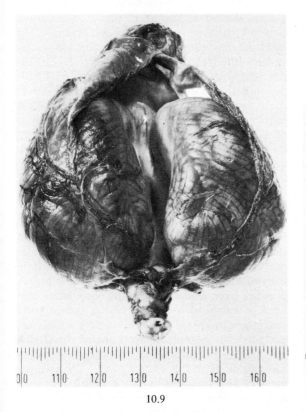

10.9

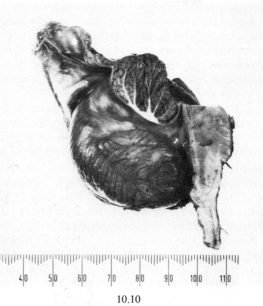

10.10

Figs. 10.9 and 10.10 Dandy–Walker malformation.
Fig. 10.9 Inferior surface of cerebellum showing defect in vermis and line of attachment of tent-like cyst.
Fig. 10.10 Sagittal section showing preservation of superior vermis and incorporation of rudiment of inferior vermis into cyst wall.

the cyst are lined by ependyma. Cerebellar tissue may extend into the roof membrane near the line of reflexion and isolated islands may be found more distally. The cyst may extend upward in a tent-like fashion through the tentorial incisura as far as the splenium of the corpus callosum. The cerebellar vermis is absent in some cases, but usually the superior vermis is well formed and the rudimentary inferior vermis is incorporated into the roofing membrane (Fig. 10.10). The fastigium is flattened. The choroid plexus is hypoplastic and situated at the caudal end of the ventricle. In many cases the foramen of Magendie is absent and in some the foramina of Luschka are also closed. In their detailed study of 28 cases Hart, Malamud and Ellis (1972) found the state of the foramina highly variable. Similarly the degree of hydrocephalus varied from barely detectable to extreme. There was no correlation between the degree of hydrocephalus and the size of the posterior fossa cyst, the extent of hypoplasia of the vermis or the patency or non-patency of the foramina. A variety of associated malformations of the brain was found in two-thirds of the cases and anomalies in other systems in one-quarter.

As a corollary of the enlargement of the posterior fossa, deformities occur in the skull, dural folds and venous sinuses. The skull is characteristically dolichocephalic with mainly occipital expansion (Benda 1954). The attachment of the tentorium is almost vertical and X-rays reveal the lateral sinuses and torcular in an abnormally elevated position in the parietal bones (Taggart and Walker 1942).

A similar malformation occurs spontaneously in mice as a hereditary condition (Brodal, Bonnevie and Harkmark 1944) or may be induced experimentally by feeding galactoflavin to pregnant mice (Kalter 1963). The observations on the pathogenesis of the lesions in affected animals have revealed that the malformations arise at an early stage and precede the development of the choroid plexuses and the opening of the roof foramina. This supports the views of Brodal and Hauglie-Hanssen (1959) who argued that in man the agenesis of the inferior vermis must precede, and cannot be dependent on, the formation of the foramina. This contradicts the opinion of previous writers who ascribed the condition to an atresia of the foramina of Magendie and Luschka (Gibson 1955). Gardner (1959) drew attention to several similarities between the Dandy–Walker and Arnold–Chiari malformations and postulated a similar pathogenetic mechanism based on his hydrodynamic theory. It is certainly possible that both conditions may be due to damage to the primitive roof plate of the 4th ventricle, though perhaps occurring in different stages of development.

The Dandy–Walker syndrome must be distinguished from other cysts in the posterior fossa. Gardner, Abdullah and McCormack (1957) have described arachnoid cysts lying above the foramen of Magendie and arising from a splitting of the membrane. In an adult case reported by Kramer (1954) arachnoid cysts incorporating malformed paraflocculi had occluded the lateral foramina and caused hydrocephalus. The various forms of posterior fossa cysts were reviewed by Alvord and Marcuse (1962), who added two cases in which large cysts lying on the superior surface of the cerebellum caused hydrocephalus by obstruction of the incisura tentorii. The structure of the cyst walls resembled that seen in the Dandy–Walker syndrome in that they consisted of a leptomeningeal and a glial component. The cysts did not communicate with the ventricular system and their apparent epithelial lining was interpreted as consisting of flattened glial cells and not true ependyma. The whole subject of these 'extra-axial cysts' of the posterior fossa requires further clarification, especially as cysts of a similar structure have also been described in the chiasmatic, interpeduncular and quadrigeminal plate cisterns (Harrison 1971).

Cerebral atrophy due to hydrocephalus

Characteristic changes take place in the wall of the hemispheres when a rise in intraventricular pressure causes an expansion of the brain within the yielding calvarium of the infant skull. Whereas pressure from without, as by the accumulation of fluid in subdural hygroma, causes compression but little atrophy of the brain unless vessels are occluded, in infantile hydrocephalus the stretch put upon the distended cerebral wall causes rapid thinning of the white matter. The enlargement of the ventricles is not a uniform process and depends not only upon the site of the block in the circulation of the cerebrospinal fluid but also on the duration of the hydrocephalus. In subarachnoid block, for example, the lateral ventricles are the first to enlarge, followed later by the 3rd ventricle, the aqueduct and 4th ventricle. The corpus callosum is elevated and thinned and the septum pellucidum fenestrated or destroyed. Extreme thinning of the floor of the 3rd ventricle is common and is associated with erosion of the clinoid processes, and damage to the hypothalamus may lead to infantilism or to precocious puberty. The atrophy of the periventricular white matter is due to ischaemia following the compression of capillaries by the rising intraventricular pressure (De 1950). The grey matter of the cortex is remarkably resistant, perhaps because of its rich blood supply, and Penfield and Elvidge (1932) have pointed out that since the axons of the unaffected cortical neurons must be preserved, the brunt of the atrophy has fallen upon the collaterals. Microscopically, the most obvious changes are first seen in the neuroglia. There is reduction in the numbers of oligodendroglial and astrocytic cells and the processes of the latter tend to become elongated and wavy. Macrophages are found in small numbers in the atrophied white matter and may lie in a linear band some distance from the ependymal surface, thus giving the impression that 'all the myelinated fibres at a certain depth had been simultaneously destroyed' (Penfield and Elvidge 1932). With the continued increase in the hydrocephalus the cerebral atrophy becomes severe, and eventually the wall of the hemisphere is reduced in places to a thin membrane. It is always the vertex which is most atrophied since it lacks the buttressing support of the basal ganglia. For this reason the axons of the motor neurons originating in the paracentral and upper parts of the precentral gyrus undergo a greater stretching than do those supplying the upper extremities, so that paraplegia is common in severe hydrocephalus while the arms retain a useful degree of function (Yakovlev 1947). More recently Weller and Wisniewski (1969) produced, in rabbits, progressive oedema of the periventricular white matter caused by seepage of cerebrospinal fluid through the damaged ependyma into the extracellular space of the cerebral parenchyma. This chronic oedema may account for some of the cerebral damage in hydrocephalus. These observations were amplified in young dogs (Weller, Wisniewski, Shulman and Terry 1971). In the early stages loss of ependyma was accompanied by severe oedema of the subependymal white matter. Tissue damage followed and in later stages was associated with proliferation of

fibrous astrocytes. At that time the oedema subsided and the ependyma was reconstituted, but remained abnormal in structure. In man, biopsies of white matter taken at the time of insertion of a ventricular shunt in five hydrocephalic infants revealed oedema in one case, gliosis in the other four (Weller and Shulman 1972). In cortical biopsies of hydrocephalic brains Struck and Hemmer (1964) found an increased extracellular space and alterations in cell organelles within neurons and glia.

Rupture of the ventricular wall may lead to the formation of smooth-walled, cystic cavities in the white matter. These diverticula may open into the subarachnoid space and lead to relief of symptoms. Tandon and Harkmark (1959) have described a case in which rupture of the suprapineal recess into the superior cistern had led to a temporary improvement in a patient with a tumour of the brainstem. Spontaneous rupture of the lamina terminalis has also been reported.

Malformations of the commissural system

The telencephalic commissures include the hippocampal, the anterior and the callosal. They all develop from the commissural plate, a thickening in the lamina terminalis, which acts as a bridge facilitating the passage of the interhemispheric fibres. The first fibres of the corpus callosum appear in the 3rd fetal month, after which this structure grows rapidly and expands mainly in a backward direction, achieving its adult position by the 5th month. For a full review of the embryology of the commissural system the reader is referred to the paper by Loeser and Alvord (1968).

Agenesis of the corpus callosum. This exists in three forms: total absence of the telencephalic commissures, absence of corpus callosum with preserved anterior and hippocampal commissures and partial absence of the posterior part of the corpus callosum (Loeser and Alvord 1968). When callosal fibres fail to cross the midline the medial part of the hemisphere develops in an abnormal manner. The cingulate gyrus is imperfectly formed or is displaced below the surface and in its place a number of radially placed convolutions are present (Fig. 10.11). This arrangement has been compared by Kirschbaum (1947) to the drawing-in of gyri around a porencephalic defect. Another abnormal, though inconstant, feature is the separation of the calcarine from the parieto-occipital fissure. The two halves of the body of the fornix are separated throughout their length. Between them protrudes the elevated membranous roof of the 3rd ventricle which is invariably enlarged. A typical septum pellucidum is necessarily absent, but this structure may be represented

the lateral ventricle. In cases in which the corpus callosum was completely missing the callosal bundle behaved in the same way. Moreover, as in one of Kirschbaum's cases, the fronto-occipital tract appeared as a separate structure thus disposing of an earlier theory that this tract may be the callosal bundle. It is not

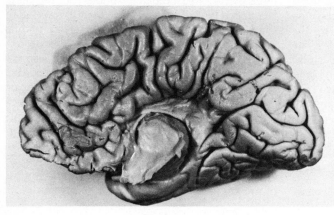

10.11

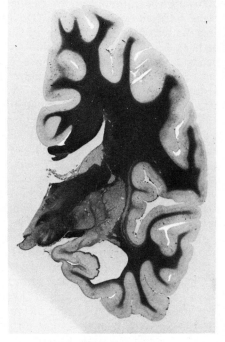

Fig. 10.11 Absent corpus callosum. Note the absence of the posterior part of the cingulate sulcus and the radiate arrangement of the sulci.

Fig. 10.12 Coronal section of a hemisphere showing the longitudinal callosal bundle.

10.12

by two laminae running obliquely in a dorso-lateral direction between the fornix and the bundle of Probst (1900). This is a prominent rounded bundle of myelinated fibres, running longitudinally above the body of the fornix (Fig. 10.12). It takes its origin from the white matter of the frontal pole, passes through the medial part of the roof of the lateral ventricle and merges with the white matter enclosing the posterior horn, reaching its largest diameter at about the level of the optic chiasma. The consensus of opinion is that this aberrant bundle is formed by uncrossed fibres of the corpus callosum. De Lange (1925) showed that, in a brain in which only the anterior half of the corpus callosum was present, an uncrossed bundle of fibres was continuous on either side posteriorly with the crossed part of the corpus callosum and formed the forceps major enclosing the posterior horn of

easy, however, to rule out the possibility that the bundle of Probst is a normal uncrossed component of the corpus callosum which has undergone hypertrophy and has become unmasked by the failure of the crossed fibres to develop. Some support is given to this theory by Becker's (1952) demonstration that a bundle of fibres, running in the anteroposterior direction and in close proximity to the corpus callosum, makes its appearance in newborn puppies after complete destruction of one hemisphere.

Absence of the corpus callosum is compatible with normal mentality. The cause of associated mental retardation must be sought elsewhere in the nervous system. An unduly small brain is often an associated anomaly. De Lange (1925) found a disordered cortical cytoarchitecture with an exceptionally thick granular layer in all cortical areas and absence of its normal three-layered subdivision in the calcarine cortex. Large grey matter heterotopias lining parts of the lateral ventricles were present in one of Kirschbaum's (1947) cases. Other associated abnormalities include lipomas, meningiomas, paraphyseal or arachnoid cysts filling the interhemispheric defect. In many of these complex malformations the longitudinal callosal bundle may be absent.

A group of patients has recently been reported in which otherwise asymptomatic agenesis of the corpus callosum was associated with relapsing spontaneous hypothermia. In the case studied by Noël, Hubert, Ectors, Franken and Flament-Durand (1973) this was ascribed to loss of nerve cells and gliosis in the premammillary area of the hypothalamus.

There is no evidence that genetic factors play a part in the aetiology of callosal malformations in man, but in mice a similar deformity may be inherited as a Mendelian recessive (King 1936). A developmental defect in vascularization in the territory of the anterior cerebral artery has been postulated (de Morsier and Mozer 1935; de Morsier 1951, 1952). This view was opposed by Marburg (1949) on the grounds that development of the corpus callosum precedes the differentiation of the individual cerebral arteries; moreover, a vascular process should lead to more widespread interference in the growth of the hemispheres than is in fact found. Loeser and Alvord (1968) suggest that commissural defects may relate to imperfect closure of the anterior neuropore with a resulting defective commissural plate.

The anterior commissure. Absence of the anterior commissure may be associated with agenesis of the corpus callosum in total absence of the telencephalic commissures. This was studied in detail by de Morsier (1954), who found only 12 cases in the literature. By contrast the anterior commissure, when present in callosal defects, may be larger than normal.

Absence of the anterior commissure is a constant feature of arhinencephaly (p. 367) even if parts of the corpus callosum are present. The commissure may also be absent in cases of trisomy 18 (Sumi 1970), and in some cases of occipital encephalocele (Karch and Urich 1972).

Malformations of the septum pellucidum. The septum pellucidum, although not a commissure, is embryologically part of the commissural system arising from the commissural plate. Originally it fills the space between the corpus callosum and the hippocampal fibre system and extends as far back as the hippocampal commissure. With the apposition of the latter structure and the body of the fornix to the corpus callosum the posterior part of the septum disappears. If it persists, it may contain a cavity, the *cavum Vergae*, or '6th ventricle'. The *cavum septi pellucidi* develops early in fetal life and is always present in premature infants but tends to obliterate or remain as a narrow slit in the fully developed brain. A large cavum, or '5th ventricle' is a fairly common anomaly, which may be congenital or acquired. The cava septi pellucidi and Vergae are the subject of a detailed study of Shaw and Alvord (1969). Most cava are asymptomatic and of no clinical significance. When very large they may cause pressure symptoms by obliteration of the foramina of Monro leading to hydrocephalus which may be intermittent. These large cava are sometimes called cysts of the septum pellucidum (Dandy 1931). It is possible that some of these cysts may be responsible for the 'bobble-head doll syndrome' (Benton, Nellhaus, Huttenlocher, Ojemann and Dodge 1966; Laurence 1966). The acquired variety of cavum is probably traumatic in origin (Corsellis, Bruton and Freeman-Browne 1973). In severe hydrocephalus the septum may be destroyed or fenestrated. Gross and Hoff (1959) described various anomalies of the septum which are often associated with prenatal porencephaly or heterotopic formations in the region of the insula and claustrum. These range from complete absence to hypoplasia. In one type of malformation the lateral ventricles are defective in their frontal horns and the corpus callosum partially fused with the caudate nuclei. The two laminae of the septum pellucidum are widely divergent and closely applied to the surfaces of the caudate nuclei, thus forming the boundaries of a single ventricular cavity. These maldevelopments are often associated with atrophy of the optic nerves and tracts ('dysplasie septo-optique', de Morsier 1956) which is attributed by Gross and Hoff to stretching of the nerves during the abnormal development of the brain rather than to a primary dysplasia.

Micrencephaly

The arbitrary brain weight of 900 g is usually accepted as the upper limit for micrencephaly in the adult. In the majority of instances the departure from normal standards is obvious enough and a brain weight even as low as 25 g has been recorded in an infant who survived four months (von Monakow 1926). The rudimentary cerebral cortex of this tiny brain possessed a recognizable area gigantopyramidalis and there were hypertrophied and uncrossed pyramidal tracts (Yakovlev and Wadsworth 1946; Minkowski 1955).

Destructive processes starting before birth usually lead to obviously malformed brains of small dimensions, as in porencephaly. Unless there is an associated hydrocephalus, little or no postnatal growth of the head occurs since the sutures tend to ossify prematurely. Widespread ulegyria follows arteritis of meningeal vessels (Figs. 10.13 and 10.14), but since the signs of meningitis in early infancy are easily overlooked it is often difficult to establish with certainty that the onset of an infection was prenatal, except in well-known conditions such as toxoplasmosis or syphilis (Laurence 1959).

Familial microcephaly. This type of small-headedness has long been recognized as a distinctive clinical entity and may be inherited as a Mendelian recessive. The small cranium with its receding forehead and superabundant, furrowed scalp contrasts strikingly with the more normal dimensions of the face with its prominent nose and large ears. The naked-eye appearance of the cerebrum is also highly characteristic. The brain, including the cerebellum which is often disproportionately large, usually weighs from 500 to 600 g. The convolutional pattern is greatly simplified and somewhat resembles that of the higher anthropoid apes (Conolly 1950), the gyri being relatively broad for the size of the brain (Fig. 10.15). The cortical nerve cells are usually well developed but there are numerous minor anomalies of architectonics including abnormal variations in the depth of individual layers—often in the direction of a marked reduction but sometimes tending towards undue thickness.

Nerve cells irregularly orientated or disproportionately large for the layer in which they are found may also be present and heterotopic aggregations, some of considerable size, are commonly seen in the subcortical white matter. By far the most striking histological abnormality, though one not peculiar to this form of micrencephaly, is the frequent grouping of the cortical nerve cells in columnar blocks separated from one another by acellular strips (Fig. 10.16). The latter are occupied by radially disposed bundles of myelinated fibres. Sometimes only the superficial nerve cells exhibit this clustering together and then an appearance is given which is reminiscent of the glomerular formations seen normally in the hippocampal gyrus. Myelination of the central white matter, basal ganglia and long fibre tracts is normal and the corpus callosum often appears unduly massive for such small hemispheres. The caudate nucleus also may be disproportionately large, even for a normal brain—an example of what von Monakow has termed 'hypergenesis'.

The micrencephalies, even the genetic ones, form a heterogeneous group (Cowie 1960). The appearance described above resemble closely these found by McKusick *et al.* (1967) in 'bird-headed dwarfs'. Another form of familial microcephaly associated with ocular symptoms and pigmentary atrophy of the retina was described by McKusick, Stauffer, Knox and Clark (1966).

Micrencephaly with cerebral calcification. Jervis (1954*b*) collected from the literature five examples of this condition and added two of his own. The brain is symmetrically reduced in size and weighs about half the normal. There is no obvious convolutional shrinkage but the lateral ventricles are somewhat enlarged. The most striking feature is the presence of very coarse and confluent mineral deposits which are sufficiently massive to be recognized macroscopically and visualized during life on X-rays of the skull. The putamen, globus pallidus, dentate nucleus and the deeper cortical layers are mainly affected by this change.

Smaller amounts of this substance, which is mainly calcium carbonate with an admixture of iron salts, are widespread throughout the brain, occurring free in the tissues or as droplets in the walls of vessels. After decalcification a strongly PAS-positive matrix is left behind. The loss of nerve cells sometimes seen in the cerebral cortex, thalamus and cornu Ammonis may well be a post-epileptic phenomenon. A conspicuous, patchy demyelination is found in the central white matter and the tegmentum of the midbrain, accompanied by a variable degree of fibrillary gliosis. The usual products of myelin breakdown are not in evidence. In Hallervorden's (1950) second case signs of an inflammatory process

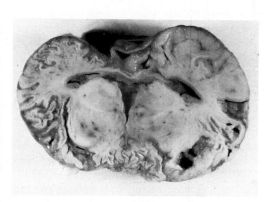

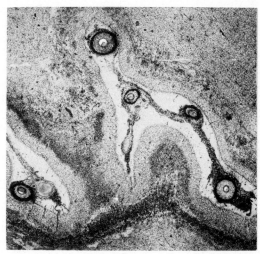

10.13

10.14

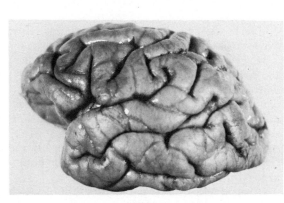

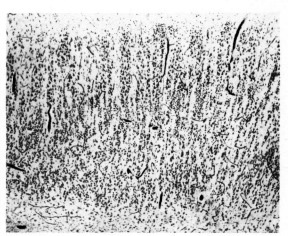

10.15

10.16

Fig. 10.13 Widespread ulegyria following post-meningitic vascular disease, probably prenatal in origin. From a 6-month-old infant. Brain weight 243 g.

Fig. 10.14 An area of ulegyria. The meningeal arteries show calcification of the elastica and intimal fibrosis.

Fig. 10.15 Familial microcephaly. Note the simple convolutional pattern with relatively broad gyri.

Fig. 10.16 The cerebral cortex shows typical columnar grouping of the nerve cells.

were present in the form of meningeal thickening and infiltrations, subintimal fibrosis of vessels, granular ependymitis and microglial rod cells in the cortex. A sibling of the patient had also suffered from micrencephaly with calcification.

Jervis calls attention to the close relationship of this condition to Fahr's 'non-arteriosclerotic cerebral calcification'. In one of his cases Jervis was able to exclude a general disturbance in calcium metabolism, as in the hypoparathyroidism which may be a feature of Fahr's disease. He inclines to the view that both the calcification and the patchy demyelination are due to circulatory disturbances and alterations in vascular permeability occurring in the course of an encephalitis of unknown origin, but the familial character of some of these cases is difficult to reconcile with this hypothesis. Calcifications of approximately the same distribution are found in a number of inflammatory and degenerative diseases (Erbslöh and Bochnik 1958) and it is evident that the aetiological factors concerned are multiple.

The writer has examined the brains of two siblings suffering from microcephaly, cerebral calcification, dwarfism, nerve deafness and retinitis pigmentosa, the clinical features of which were described by Neill and Dingwall (1950). Massive pericapillary calcifications were present in the putamina, thalami and in the cerebellar white matter superficial to the dentate nuclei. In the larger vessels the calcification was mainly in the adventitial coat. The deposits in the cerebral cortex were found mainly in the depths of the sulci in the arterial boundary zone regions and the granular layer of the calcarine cortex was also involved. Cerebellar atrophy was present and calcified Purkinje cells were a conspicuous feature. There was patchy demyelination of the centrum ovale and brainstem but this was not related to the calcifications nor was it perivascular (Figs. 10.17–10.22). The ventricles were denuded of ependyma, there was dense subependymal gliosis, and the choroid plexuses were atrophic. The latter findings suggested a specific degenerative process. A similar distribution of cortical calcifications has been noted in an adult case of Fahr's disease and supports the view that a vascular pathoclitic factor, possibly a peculiarity of capillary permeability, is concerned in the calcifying process (Norman and Urich 1960).

A further, apparently sporadic, case (Norman and Tingey 1966) showed similar lesions with marked micrencephaly (527 g), reduction of white matter, spotty demyelination, iron pigmentation of the globus pallidus and substantia nigra, and cerebellar cortical atrophy. Calcification was less extensive than in previous cases.

Moossy (1967) and Rowlatt (1969), in reporting two further typical cases, drew attention to the association of these lesions with the clinical syndrome of dwarfism, retinal atrophy and deafness originally described by Cockayne (1936, 1946). Subsequent case reports, reviewed by Guzzetta (1972), have emphasized the microcephaly, mental retardation, bird-like facies, butterfly dermatitis due to photosensitivity and progressive deterioration with terminal blindness, deafness and paralysis. The condition is inherited as an autosomal recessive.

The lesions of Cockayne's syndrome were confused in the past with those of Pelizaens–Merzbacher's disease owing to a similar pattern of demyelination (Horanyi-Hechst and Meyer 1939; Gerstl, Malamud, Hayman and Bone 1965). The similarities and differences between the two conditions are fully discussed by Seitelberger (1970). It is of interest that the demyelinating process may involve peripheral nerves as well as the central white matter (Moosa and Dubowitz 1970). This has been confirmed by electron-microscopic studies which showed severe degenerative changes in myelin sheaths with preservation of axons, also the presence of dense bodies in the cytoplasm of Schwann cells (Roy, Srivastava, Gupta and Mayekar 1973).

However, demyelination was not prominent in the case reported by Crome and Kanjilal (1971) where calcifying angiopathy was the predominant feature. Some diffuse pallor of myelin with focal accentuation was present, but the authors considered it secondary to the vascular lesions. They pointed out the variability of the findings in the reported cases and cast doubts on the homogeneity of the material.

Other atypical cases, the relationship of which with Cockayne's syndrome is more debatable, have been reported. D'Hoore and Gullotta (1971) described the case of a microcephalic girl of 7 months who showed extensive demyelination of the white matter with sudanophil products of breakdown and a tendency to cavitation, associated with widespread perivascular calcification. Martin, Deberdt, Philippart, Van Acker and Hooft (1971) examined the brain of one of three siblings described clinically by Hooft,

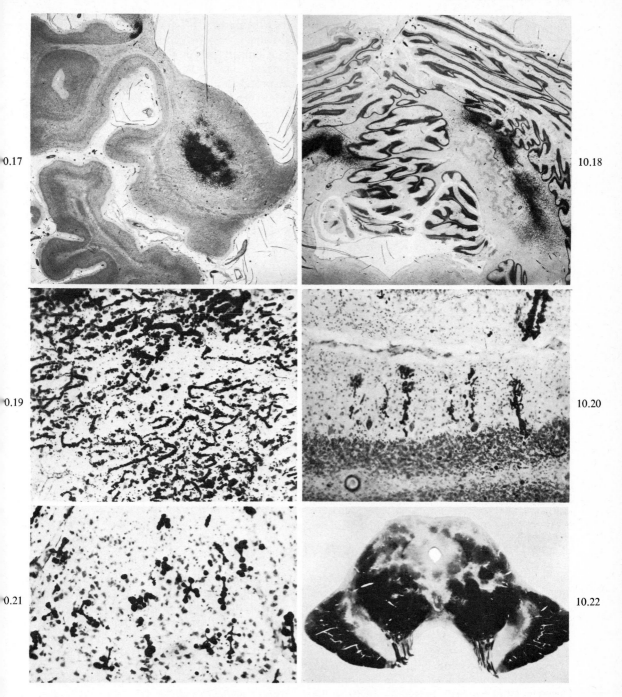

Figs. 10.17–10.22 Familial microcephaly with cerebral calcification.
Fig. 10.17 Calcified capillaries forming dense aggregations in the putamen and caudate nucleus. Note the calcification in the base of the second frontal gyrus. Carbol azure.
Fig. 10.18 Cerebellum showing calcifications in white matter dorsolateral to dentate nuclei. Carbol azure.
Fig. 10.19 Typical pericapillary calcifications. Carbol azure.
Fig. 10.20 Calcified dentrites of Purkinje cells. Carbol azure.
Fig. 10.21 Calcified microglial cells in cerebral grey matter. Carbol azure.
Fig. 10.22 Midbrain showing patchy demyelination of the tegmentum. Kultschitschy–Pal.

Hanwere and Acker (1968). The syndrome consists of microcephaly, peculiar facial appearance with large ears, mental retardation, progressive optic atrophy, spasticity and choreoathetosis. There was widespread demyelination of the white matter with a tigroid pattern in places, severe gliosis, atrophy of the optic pathways and degeneration of the granular layer of the cerebellum, but no calcification.

Megalencephaly

Excessive brain weights of the order 1600 to 2850 g have been recorded in individuals of normal or exceptional intelligence as well as in epileptics as irregularities of stratification, the presence of isolated cells or groups of cells of disproportionately large size (as in pachygyria) or heterotopias in the subcortical white matter. A disproportionate enlargement of the spinal cord due to blastomatous glial overgrowth has also been reported in megalencephaly of this type (Kastein 1940; Ferraro and Barrera 1935).

(2) In a second type of abnormally large brain the generalized increase in size is not associated with any neuroglial preponderance. In Wilson's (1934) case both grey and white matter were uniformly massive, but in the example recorded by Peter and Schluter (1927) the corpus callosum and centrum semi-ovale did not participate in

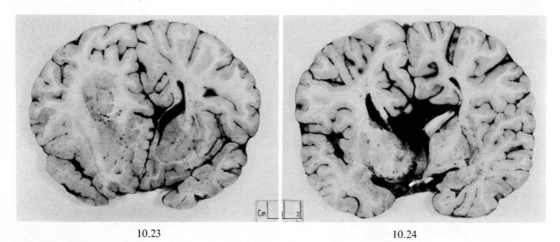

10.23   10.24

Fig. 10.23 Megalencephaly with multiple cerebral anomalies. Note the large heterotopias in the white matter on the left lobe and the longitudinal callosal bundle on the right side.
Fig. 10.24 A more posterior level showing absence of the corpus callosum, abnormal gyral pattern and polygyria in right temporal lobe.
From a child of 3 years with total brain weight of 1554 g (cerebellum 186 g).

and mental defectives (Jakob 1929). The term 'megalencephaly' has, however, a pathological connotation and should be reserved for heavy brains having additional structural anomalies, and of these three main varieties may be distinguished.

(1) First, megalencephaly may be associated with a diffuse overgrowth of the protoplasmic macroglia (Volland 1910; Schminke 1920; Hallervorden 1926; Weil 1933). As in tuberous sclerosis, a malignant transformation of the astrocytes may sometimes occur. Thus in Weil's cases (that of a 7-year-old child with a brain weight of 1856 g) the brainstem and cerebellum show abnormalities of an unspecific sort, such the general enlargement. In the latter case the depth of cerebral cortex was notably increased without there being obvious anomalies in cytoarchitectonics. In another case (Peter 1928) the cerebellum was disproportionately enlarged and the Purkinje cells showed various irregularities of alignment and size.

(3) In a third and heterogeneous group of cases, megalencephaly is an incidental feature of some other malformation or degenerative condition. Tuberous sclerosis may be associated with a heavy brain (Borremanns, Dykmans and van Bogaert 1933) and syringomyelia has also been reported (Benda 1952). In one of the writer's cases, that of a child of 3 years with a

brain weight of 1554 g, there were multiple congenital malformations (abnormal gyration of the cerebral cortex, massive heterotopias in one frontal lobe with partial atresia of the lateral ventricle, longitudinal callosal bundles, and an absent olfactory tract on the side of the heterotopic formations) (Figs. 10.23 and 10.24). Excessive brain weights have frequently been reported in the infantile form of amaurotic family idiocy (Aronson, Volk and Epstein 1955). In these cases there is always a great excess of fibrillary neuroglia in the cerebral white matter, often with status spongiosus and widespread absence of myelin. In view of these findings it is not surprising that megalencephaly has also been reported in late infantile metachromatic leucodystrophy and also in 'spongy degeneration of the white matter'.

Unilateral megalencephaly ('hemimegalencephaly'), in which the abnormality is confined to one hemisphere, has been reported repeatedly (Laurence 1964; Bignami, Palladini and Zappella 1967). In some cases this forms part of homolateral hemigigantism, in others it is an isolated lesion. In the case of Bignami et al. there was widening of the cortical ribbon, fusion of the molecular layers of adjacent cortical surfaces in some sulci and a striking hypertrophy of nerve cells in the cortex and striatum.

Porencephaly

The term porencephaly was originally introduced by Heschl (1859) to designate a congenital defect extending from the surface of the cerebral hemisphere into the subjacent ventricle. During the passage of years the name has lost any precise meaning it may have once possessed and it is now commonly used for any excavation or cystic cavity occurring in the brain of a young individual. It is an advantage to separate from such a heterogeneous group the cerebral softenings associated with birth injury or postnatal vascular lesions. There then remains a by no means uniform class of case properly labelled 'prenatal porencephaly'—the qualification prenatal being applicable to porencephaly associated with unequivocal signs of prenatal malformation elsewhere in the brain (Fig. 10.25). The prenatal porencephalies so defined may be usefully subdivided into two groups: those showing evidence of old destructive processes and those which are distortions of growth with no concomitant patho-

logical findings such as glial scarring or calcification.

The studies of Yakovlev and Wadsworth (1946) have thrown light on the morphogenesis of the latter sort of porencephaly. These authors have drawn attention to a special type of maldevelopment which is characterized by symmetrically placed clefts in the cerebral cortex, a condition named by them 'schizencephaly'. These clefts, which involve the whole depth of the cerebral wall, lie in the line of primary fissures and their walls may be fused together forming a 'pia-ependymal seam', the line of junction of the molecular layers being marked by a streak of myelinated fibres and by elements derived both from the pia mater and the ependymal layer. The heaped-up grey matter of these approximated walls is unduly thick and is unlaminated. Dense aggregations of poorly differentiated cells are arranged in nests and large neurons with heavy chromatin and sometimes with two nuclei may be present. In the depths of the line of fusion these nerve cell layers may become coterminous with heterotopic collections of ependymal matrix cells or they may even extend into the subjacent caudate nucleus. There is no sign that a destructive process has been at work and there is no hydrocephalus, although the occipital horns of the lateral ventricles often show the relative dilatation of 'colpocephaly'. Yakovlev and Wadsworth consider that these clefts arise at points of localized agenesis in the cerebral wall before the end of the second month, at a time prior to the closure of the roof of the prosencephalon and before the three layers of His have differentiated.

An entirely different appearance is given to the brain when this type of maldevelopment is complicated by hydrocephalus. Provided the cerebral wall in the region of the clefts is not protected by the buttressing effect of the basal ganglia and expansion may take place, the lips of the clefts open out and large bilateral gaps bridged over by a thin roofing membrane appear on the surface of the hemispheres. Thus at first sight an impression is given of gross cortical destruction, whereas in fact the brain wall has yielded to pressure at weak spots caused by limited areas of defective growth. Owing to the primary malformation having occurred so early in development, retrograde atrophy of the thalamus is not present. Parts of the original clefts with their pia-ependymal seams may be

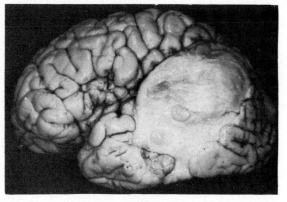

10.25

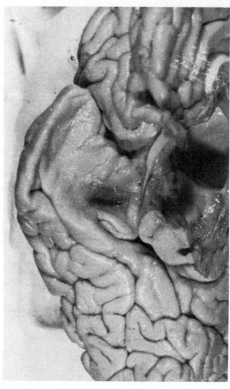

10.26

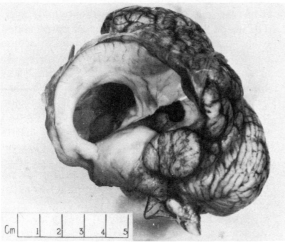

10.27

Cm | 1 | 2 | 3 | 4 | 5

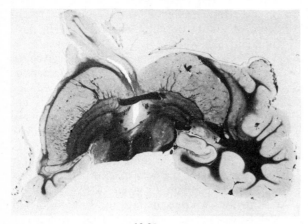

10.28

Fig. 10.25 Prenatal porencephaly. Note the islands of nervous tissue in the membranous wall of the expanded ventricle. There is a patch of micropolygyria in the upper bank of the Sylvian fissure. The condition was bilateral.

Fig. 10.26 Smooth depression in the undersurface of the temporal lobe caused by an arachnoidal cyst (which has been stripped off). The surrounding gyri are of normal pattern. A similar condition was present in the left temporal lobe.

Fig. 10.27 Bilateral and approximately symmetrical porencephaly of the frontoparietal areas. The cavities were roofed in by a thin membrane (as in hydranencephaly) which has been removed on the left side; much of the remaining cortex showed micropolygyria. Note the large basal ganglia forming the floor of the unpaired ventricle.
Fig. 10.28 Coronal section through the hypertrophied corpora striata which are abnormally rotated inwards. Part of the thin roofing membrane is seen attached to the preserved cortex on either side. Heidenhain's myelin.

found in the tissue lying at the margins of the defects and provide important evidence in support of this theory of the pathogenesis of the porencephaly.

In some specimens these large symmetrical defects in the cerebral wall occupy most of the frontal and parietal lobes. The contour of the brain is, however, preserved by a centrally placed arch of tissue which forms the superior attachment of the membranous covering of the ventricles and resembles in appearance the handle of a basket (Fig. 10.27). This remnant of grey matter was considered by Yakovlev and Wadsworth to represent the hypertrophied induseum griseum or hippocampal rudiment, but, in brains in which the pathological process has originated at a somewhat later date, the tissue is evidently derived from residual isocortex. In the brain examined in detail by Norman, Urich and Woods (1958) the preserved 'handle' of the basket-shaped brain contained grey matter derived from the cingulate gyrus. The putamina and caudate nuclei may be hypertrophied and are seen as prominent elevations in the floor of the single ventricular cavity (Fig. 10.28). In Yakovlev and Wadsworth's specimen (case 3) the thalamic projection fibres took an aberrant course, the majority entering the pyriform cortex while those from the medial nucleus ended in the caudate nucleus. In the writer's case the thalamic projection fibres all entered the striatum.

It is evident that the argument in favour of this type of malformation arising in embryonic life as the result of 'agenesis', and not at a later stage perhaps from a vascular lesion, largely depends upon the interpretation given to the pia-ependymal seam. This type of cleft formation is not always to be found in bilateral porencephaly of prenatal origin, as, for instance, in the typical 'basket-brain' described by Cohn and Neumann (1946). Wedge-shaped defects in the roofs of the posterior horns of the ventricles were present in the writer's case, but these were filled by neuroglial fibres, not by dysplastic grey matter, and there were signs of old necrotizing process elsewhere in the brain. In such cases the thin layer of tissue lying beneath the meninges and covering the cerebral defects resembles that found in hydranencephaly (p. 394) and may be interpreted as the atrophied and gliosed outer layer of a cortex which has undergone pathological change, possibly due to vascular lesions. No doubt the process of hydrocephalic stretching postulated by Yakovlev and Wadsworth applies equally to these encephaloclastic porencephalies, though they probably originate at a somewhat later date. It is certainly true that signs of old destructive lesions may sometimes be found at the margins of these foci where partially eroded tissue and much calcified debris may be present. The prenatal origin of the process, however, is shown by the radial arrangement of the marginal gyri and, more decisively, by micropolygyria. In the majority of instances it seems more reasonable to ascribe both the porus and microgyria to the action of a single pathological process, occurring about the third to the fifth fetal month, than to suppose that later softening has occurred in an area of cortical malformation (Schob 1930).

Arachnoid cysts. The varieties of porencephaly arising from a focal disturbance of growth in the developing wall of the hemisphere and exhibiting malformations in neighbouring and related structures must be distinguished from the deep indentations of the brain without cortical maldevelopment, commonly ascribed to the presence of arachnoid cysts. Starkman, Brown and Linnell (1958) reviewed the literature, added three cases of their own, all situated in the Sylvian fissure, and brought forward evidence that most of these intra-arachnoid collections of fluid may arise as congenital malformations of the leptomeninges. In one of Norman's cases both temporal poles were deformed by smooth-walled, roughly circular depressions, the floors of which became progressively thinned and atrophic as the centre was approached. There was no communication with the inferior horn of the lateral ventricle, but on one side the ependyma was exposed over one area (Fig. 10.26). These cavities were filled by cysts formed by a splitting of the arachnoid membrane, the outer layer of which formed the roof of the crater and preserved the normal contour of the temporal lobe. The surrounding cortex was normally convoluted and showed no malformation.

Anderson and Landing (1966) described nine further examples of arachnoid cysts, three in the classical Sylvian situation, three over the cerebral convexity and three parasagittal ones between the falx and the medial surface of the hemisphere. All presented with signs of raised intracranial pressure in infancy as opposed to some previously recorded asymptomatic cysts in adults found incidentally at autopsy. The cysts were apparently completely enclosed, did not communicate with the ventricular system or the subarachnoid space and contained either colourless fluid indistinguishable from cerebrospinal fluid or a xanthochromic one rich in protein.

A different interpretation of the Sylvian cysts was put forward by Robinson (1955, 1958, 1964). In his view the primary abnormality is a maldevelopment of the cerebral hemisphere affecting the temporal and, to a lesser extent, the frontal lobe ('the temporal lobe agenesis syndrome'). The cavity overlying the defect is therefore a form of external hydrocephalus, or perhaps an arachnoid diverticulum communicating with the basal cisterns, and not a true cyst. Robinson also drew attention to the deformity of the skull, consisting of an enlargement of the middle fossa with elevation of the lesser wing of the sphenoid and an outward bulge of the temporal squame. These bony changes are more conspicuous in children, predominantly boys, who present with signs of raised intracranial pressure than in symptom-free adults. These children are also prone to formation of subdural haematomas and hygromas even after trivial head injuries, which adds a further complicating factor.

Whatever the interpretation of the findings the mechanism of fluid accumulation under raised pressure in a totally or partially encysted space remains obscure. Williams and Guthkelch (1974) suggested that cerebrospinal fluid may be forced into arachnoid cysts communicating with the subarachnoid space by violent venous pulsations produced during coughing and straining, thus leading to their gradual expansion.

Ependymal cysts. Another rare condition to be distinguished from true porencephaly are cysts of the cerebral hemispheres lined with ependyma (Bouch, Mitchell and Maloney 1973). These occupy the white matter of the hemisphere and do not communicate either with the lateral ventricle, from which they are separated by a thin layer of tissue, or with the subarachnoid space. The cysts are smooth-walled and lined either with typical, cuboidal and ciliated, or atrophic, flattened ependyma. No trace of choroid plexus was found in any of the cysts. The cyst fluid showed a high protein content in the only case in which it had been examined (Jakubiak, Dunsmore and Beckett 1968). Although undoubtedly developmental in origin these cysts

remain silent for many years and present in later life with symptoms and signs of an expanding intracranial lesion.

Hydranencephaly

In this condition a prenatal destructive process has reduced the greater part of the cerebral hemispheres to membranous sacs. The lateral ventricles are enormously dilated but the infant's head is not enlarged at birth, though it may increase rapidly in size shortly afterwards. The affected areas are mainly those supplied by the internal carotid arteries, while those receiving blood from the vertebral system tend to be spared. The latter include the basal portions of the temporal and occipital lobes, the hippocampi and amygdaloid nuclei, brainstem and cerebellum. More rarely lesions also involve the midbrain, cerebellum or are unilaterally distributed. The wall of the membranous sac is composed only of two layers, the leptomeninges and a thin shell of gliosed tissue representing the remnants of the cortex, mainly its molecular layer. Blood pigment may be present in the meninges covering the sac-like hemispheres (Lange-Cosack 1944). There is no ependymal lining but the ventricular surface is smooth and covered by a narrow layer of condensed glial fibrils (the 'membrana gliae limitans'). These appearances distinguish hydranencephaly from congenital hydrocephalus, in which condition the atrophy mainly affects the white matter, and also from the bladder-like porencephalic brains due to extensive softening of the centrum semi-ovale. In this latter type of porencephaly the cortex may be largely reduced to a thin membrane but the ependymal wall of the ventricle is preserved and forms the inner boundary of the excavated hemisphere. The cortical destruction is never so uniform or so symmetrical as in hydranencephaly. There are, however, transitions between hydranencephaly and other encephalomalacias of early life (Norman et al. 1958) and in some cases there is anatomical evidence of an obstruction to the flow of CSF, thus linking the condition to fetal hydrocephalus. The classification of such cases presents difficulties (Crome and Sylvester 1958; Crome 1972).

Angiographic studies in hydranencephaly have given variable results. In the case described by Thelander, Shaw and Peel (1953) the vascular pattern was normal in both the arterial and venous phases. In that of Poser, Walsh and

Scheinberg (1955) the anterior cerebral arteries appeared rudimentary and the posterior cerebrals pursued an anomalous distal course.

In an unpublished case (quoted by Crome and Stern 1972) Barbara Smith observed splitting of the internal carotid artery within the sphenoid bone into a number of narrow and presumably inefficient channels. Fowler, Dow, White and Greer (1972) described a family in which five siblings showed evidence of hydranencephaly. Two of them were examined *post mortem* and both showed a remarkable anomaly of vascularization of the entire neuraxis consisting of endothelial hyperplasia with formation of 'glomeruloids'.

Pathogenesis. The distribution of the lesions in hydranencephaly suggests that some obstruction to the blood flow in the territories supplied by the internal carotid arteries has occurred in fetal life, though how this has been brought about is unknown. Pressure on the fetal neck by the cord or by amniotic bands, or even direct trauma, or infection in an attempt to procure abortion have been suggested (Lange-Cosack 1944; Fowler, Brown and Cabrera 1971), but do not carry conviction. Another suggestion is that the internal carotid arteries may be compressed against the sphenoid bones as a consequence of swelling of the fetal brain due to anoxia (Walsh and Lindenberg 1961). Thrombosis of the branches of the internal carotid arteries must also be considered as a possibility, for Becker (1949*b*) was able to produce softenings equivalent to hydranencephaly by injecting paraffin in olive oil into the carotid arteries of newborn puppies. The experiments of Vogel and McClenahan (1952) are also relevant. These workers occluded major cerebral arteries in 6-day-old chicks by electro-cauterization. Marked retardation in cortical development occurred and the forebrain in survivors often remained as a thin-walled cyst.

Hydranencephaly has also been produced in monkeys by ligating the carotid arteries and jugular veins in fetuses and then returning them to the uterus to complete the gestation (Myers 1969).

Pachygyria
(Lissencephaly, Agyria)

This variety of cerebral malformation has two essential features: a reduction in the number of secondary gyri and an increased depth of the grey matter underlying the smooth part of the cortex. In extreme instances the only indentation visible over the convexity and external aspect of the brain is a Sylvian fissure the course of which is shorter and more obliquely placed than normal (Fig. 10.29). Operculation is defective and the insula is exposed. It is more usual to find the primary fissures and a few sulci present to a limited extent. Thus in Greenfield and Wolfsohn's (1935) specimen the calcarine and parieto-occipital fissures and the Rolandic, olfactory and orbital sulci were represented by shallow grooves. The brain as a whole is usually small and under-weight ('microcephalia vera') but the lateral ventricles are relatively large, a relationship also present in the fetus and not due in the majority of cases to obstructive hydrocephalus. The term 'colpocephaly' has been applied to this condition by Yakovlev and Wadsworth (1946).

The hemispheric walls underlying the smooth parts of the cerebral cortex are composed of four main layers: (1) externally a molecular layer of normal proportions; (2) a layer of nerve cells which represents the true cortex and which may be shallower and more densely packed than is normal; (3) a much deeper and diffuse layer of grey matter in which the neurons tend to be arranged in broad columns separated by plume-like bundles of myelinated fibres which radiate from the deepest layer; (4) the fourth layer is a thin rind of white matter adjacent to the ventricle (Figs. 10.30, 10.31 and 10.32). A conspicuous feature of the second or cortical layer may be the presence of large cells with coarse tigroid bodies resembling giant cells of Betz, scattered irregularly throughout the layer or sometimes arranged in a superficial row (Fig. 10.34). In those parts of the brain where the primary fissures or sulci have been formed, the lamination of the cortex may be normal. The thin layer of central white matter and the fibres passing upwards from it towards the surface are well myelinated and often show dense fibrillary gliosis. Heterotopic islands of nerve cells of considerable size may also be present in the centrum semi-ovale (Fig. 10.35) and may bulge into the ventricular cavity giving a mammillated appearance to the ependymal surface (Fig. 10.38).

Lissencephaly ('smooth brain') and pachygyria may affect the central areas of the cortex in a symmetrical fashion as in the case of Fitzgerald (1940), in which absence of the pyramidal tracts

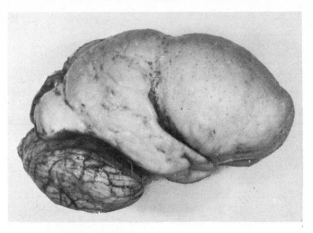

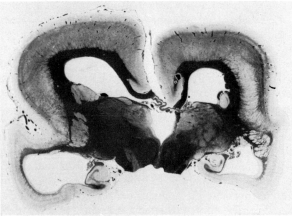

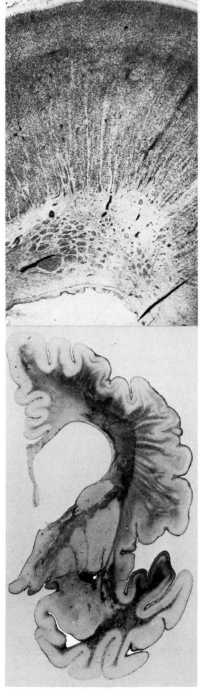

10.31

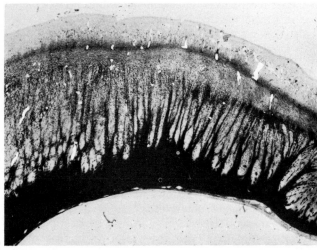

10.32

10.33

Fig. 10.29 Agyria and pachygyria. External appearance of brain.

Fig. 10.30 Section through the wall of the hemisphere shown in Fig. 10.23 to show the great depth of grey matter. Note the numerous heterotopias in the narrow white matter. Carbol azure.

Fig. 10.31 Coronal section of the brain in Fig. 10.23 to show the relative proportions of grey and white matter, and the well-developed thalami and cornua Ammonis. Heidenhain's myelin.

Fig. 10.32 Section through the hemispheric wall showing the plume-like radial fibres traversing the deeper layer of the grey matter. Kultschitsky–Pal method.

Fig. 10.33 Pachygyria. Upper bank of Sylvian fissure shows increased depth of grey matter and a few shallow sulci. There is generalized fibrous gliosis of white matter which was not associated with poverty of myelin. Holzer.

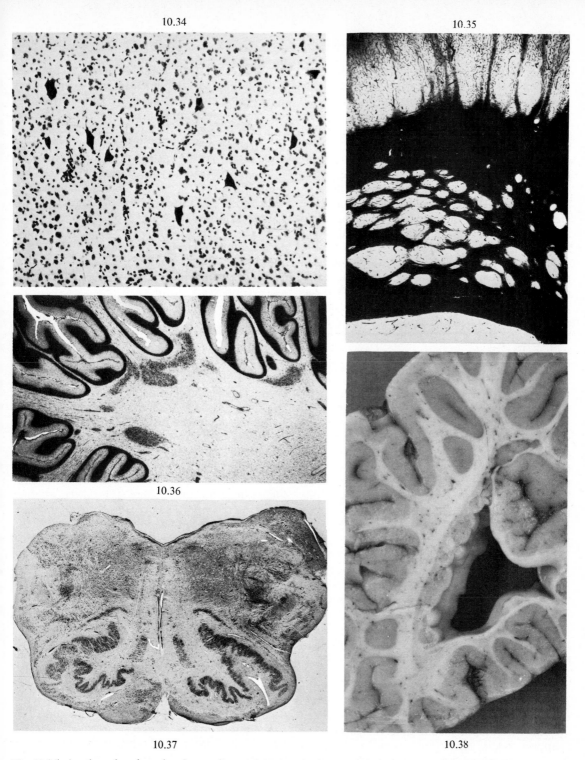

10.34

10.35

10.36

10.37

10.38

Fig. 10.34 Agyria and pachygyria. Large abnormal neurons in the pachygyric cortex. Carbol azure.

Fig. 10.35 Heterotopic islands of nerve cells in central white matter of agyric brain. Heidenhain's myelin.

Fig. 10.36 Heterotopic islands of nerve cells in the cerebellar white matter in a case of cerebral pachygyria. Carbol azure.

Fig. 10.37 Malformation of the inferior olives in a case of agyria. The dorsal cell band has lagged behind in its migration from the rhombic lip and has not been properly incorporated into the nucleus. Carbol azure.

Fig. 10.38 Another form of heterotopia—islands of nerve cells lie deep to the central white matter, having remained in the position of the original matrix layer. Note the characteristic bossed appearance of the ventricular wall.

was associated with spastic cerebral diplegia. Pachygyria is not uncommonly confined to one hemisphere and is then associated with a spastic hemiplegia. When only a small area of the cortical surface is involved, so that one or two broad gyri (macrogyria) are present, the condition has a superficial resemblance to tuberous sclerosis (Fig. 10.33) owing to the dense gliosis usually found in the affected cortex and also to the presence of large abnormal neurons in these areas. However, the bloated multinucleated neuroglial cells, bizarre giant cells and other features of Bourneville's disease are never seen.

The cerebellar cortex may also exhibit localized patches of agyria but in this case the disordered architecture ('cerebellar microgyria', p. 405) has no relation to any normal stage of development. As in the cerebrum, heterotopic islands of nerve cells are sometimes seen in the cerebellar white matter (Fig. 10.36).

The agyric cerebral cortex is a singularly clear-cut instance of a malformation explicable in terms of retardation of normal development, the structural pattern of the hemispheric wall having much in common with the fetal hemisphere at the third and fourth month. At this stage the neuroblasts as passing outwards from the germinal centres of the matrix towards their ultimate destination in the mantle layer. The zone of their passage, the intermediate zone of His, will eventually be filled by the myelinated fibres of the centrum semi-ovale. In pachygyria, however, a considerable proportion of the neuroblasts never reach the mantle layer and are left behind as a diffuse heterotopia which undergoes subsequent expansion by virtue of the continued maturation and growth of its constituent elements. The more superficial sheet of nerve cells, which, with its molecular layer ('marginal veil'), forms the true cortex, is more compactly arranged and may form shallow infoldings, though never showing normal lamination.

Evidence of retarded development may also be present in other parts of the brain. In several cases the inferior olives have been found broken up into heterotopic groups of cells lying in the restiform bodies and thus marking the path taken by the neuroblasts in their migration from the rhombic lip during the second month (Bruschweiler 1927, 1928; Greenfield and Wolfsohn 1935; de Lange 1939; Druckman, Chao and Alvord 1959; Miller 1963; Daube and Chou 1966). Less severe malformation of the olives was seen

in Walker's (1942) case in which the normal convolutions of the nucleus had been largely replaced by clumps of cells. A somewhat similar minor maldevelopment occurred in one of Norman's cases, the dorsal cell band of each olive being poorly convoluted and distinctly separated from the ventral portion (Fig. 10.37).

The olivary heterotopias, reviewed by Hanaway and Netsky (1971), may also occur in association with other cerebral malformations, such as the Dandy–Walker syndrome.

Lissencephaly usually occurs as a sporadic malformation, but some familial cases have been reported (Miller 1963; Reznik and Alberca-Serrano 1964).

Micropolygyria

The old-established name of microgyria is often loosely applied to any type of abnormally small convolutions, irrespective of whether this is the consequence of prenatal malformation or of a destructive process occurring at birth or in infancy. An excessive formation of secondary sulci may complicate the otherwise normal convolutional pattern of the brain and the small convolutions so formed, which may suitably be termed 'polygyria', do not necessarily exhibit gliosis or shrinkage. There is, however, another and a more important prenatal cortical anomaly now to be described which is known in the German literature as 'Microgyrie' and which may conveniently be referred to as 'micropolygyria' (Schob 1930) in order to avoid ambiguity.

The external aspect of this micropolygyric cortex (Fig. 10.39) does not usually give the impression of convolutional richness but rather of broad and irregular gyri the surfaces of which are wrinkled like a chestnut or finely bossed like morocco leather. It is only after section of the brain that the propriety of the name becomes apparent, for then one sees a wealth of small plications formed by bands of nerve cells lying deep to the surface (Fig. 10.40). The miniature convolutions are submerged because their molecular layers remain fused together and intervening sulci are not formed. Their 'crowns', however, project slightly above the general level of the brain surface, thus giving rise to the characteristic bossed appearance previously mentioned. The extent of the malformation varies considerably from brain to brain. It may be present only as

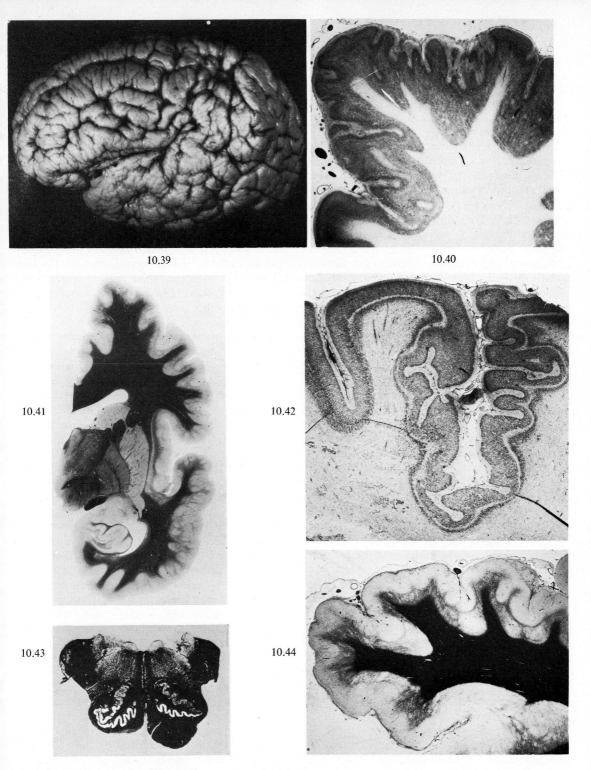

Fig. 10.39 Micropolygyria. 'Chestnut' appearance of brain.

Fig. 10.40 A common type of micropolygyric cortex. Miniature convolutions are found below the surface but are not exteriorized by sulci. Carbol azure.

Fig. 10.41 Coronal section of the hemisphere shown in Fig. 10.39. Note the micropolygyria in the unfissured temporal lobe. Kultschitsky–Pal method.

Fig. 10.42 The four-layered type of the micropolygyric cortex. Carbol azure.

Fig. 10.43 Hypertrophy of the right pyramid in a case of micropolygyria affecting only the cerebral cortex of the left side.

Fig. 10.44 The four-layered type of cortex stained for myelin.

a small patch, usually in the neighbourhood of the Sylvian fissure, or it may extend over much of the lateral cortical surface. The cingulate gyrus, calcarine cortex and hippocampus are spared. In some micropolygyric brains the Sylvian fissure takes an almost vertical course with gyri lying parallel to it on either side like the pleats of an accordion—the so-called 'carnivore' type of convolutional pattern. When the central convolutions are involved, the pyramidal tracts are absent or severely stunted and the clinical state of spastic diplegia is produced. Micropolygyria affecting only hemisphere (Fig. 10.41) is not uncommon and leads to a hemiplegia clinically indistinguishable from that following destructive lesions at birth. The pyramidal tract of the normal side may be hypertrophied and displace the inferior olive dorsally (Fig. 10.43). This phenomenon, which is also sometimes found in the sound pyramidal tract in cases of hemiplegia occurring at birth or in early postnatal life, is due to a relative increase in the number of fibres of large calibre at the expense of the fine fibres. The total number of axons in the hypertrophied pyramid does not exceed the normal. As in the agyric brain, the lateral ventricles are often larger than normal and the central white matter hypoplastic ('colpocephaly'). In some instances the thin hemispheric wall is not strong enough to resist even the normal pressure of the cerebrospinal fluid and a mild degree of hydrocephalus with enlargement of the head occurs.

The appearance of the nerve cell layers in micropolygyria usually varies in different parts of the cortex. The commonest pattern is a wavy, festoon-like arrangement of the nerve cell ribbon with non-separation of the molecular layers. These submerged 'gyri' may be relatively large with central cores of white matter pointing towards the surface like the fingers of a glove. Sometimes a more complex 'glandular' formation is seen in which tubular columns of cells ramify in tortuous plications. Yet another well-differentiated pattern shows a multifoliate structure somewhat resembling the structure of the normal cerebellar cortex though without the separation of the folia by sulci. It is not unusual to find sheets of nerve cells and their fused molecular layers heaped up one upon another so that the total depth of grey matter is greatly increased, and some of these deeper gyri may, in cross-section, be mistaken for heterotopias. Only in a minority of cases, however, is micropolygyria

associated with massive heterotopic collections of nerve cells in the periventricular white matter.

On microscopical examination there is usually no indication of differentiated lamination in the malformed areas, and a normal granular layer is never found. The nerve cells may be of immature type having a poorly developed cytoplasm compared with the size of the nucleus. There is no attempt at the formation of radial bundles and tangles of myelinated fibres may be present in sufficient density to suggest *état marbré*. The molecular layers commonly show abnormally dense strands of myelinated fibres running parallel to the surface. As in agyria, marked fibrillary gliosis of the whole white matter of the brain without any corresponding demyelination is a feature of some, but by no means all, micropolygyric brains.

Another pattern of abnormal cortex may be found in these brains, the four-layered type of micropolygyria. This deserves a rather more detailed description, because of the light it may throw upon the formal pathogenesis of the malformation. In this variant the grey matter consists of a molecular layer and two layers of nerve cells, separated from each other by an acellular strip containing myelinated fibres, which constitutes the third layer (Figs. 10.42 and 10.44). Bielschowsky (1923-4a) considered that only the outer two layers constituted the true cortex of the micropolygyric brain, the third layer being the analogue of the normal subsulcine or U fibres, while the rather vaguely demarcated fourth layer of nerve cells was heterotopic, representing as it were the stragglers of the main body of migrating neuroblasts which had arrived too late to be incorporated into the cortex proper. There is thus a marked resemblance between this variety of microgyric formation and the pachygyric cortex. In the latter, however, the heterotopic layer is much deeper and occupies most of the cerebral wall, thus indicating an earlier onset of the process of retardation in the neuroblast migration. Another link between the two conditions is that the same type of cerebellar malformation may be present in both. This so-called 'cerebellar microgyria' (p. 405) is characterized by the absence of a normal folial pattern; instead, the granular cells, molecular layers and Purkinje cells form a complex and anarchical arrangement beneath patches of smooth cerebellar cortex.

A different interpretation of the four-layered cortex has been put forward by Richman, Stewart and Caviness (1974). It is based on their own study of a case of circumscribed microgyria and on similar observations by Nieuwenhuijse (1913), Jacob (1940), Bertrand and Gruner (1955) and de Leon (1972). At the junction of the normal and microgyric cortex it was found that the cell-free layer was continuous with the middle laminae of the normal cortex and not with the U-fibres. The two cellular layers were in continuity with layers II and III and with layer VI respectively. The authors conclude that the four-layered cortex is the end-result of a post-migration lesion corresponding to the laminar necrosis of later life.

The four-layered type of cortex may not be present in brains showing widespread micro-polygyria and a mere slowing of neuronal migration cannot by itself explain the extremely varied and complex formations that are encountered (Crome 1952). One is thus forced back to the more general and vaguer conception of a disturbance in the relationship of factors governing the harmonious synthesis of the parts of a developing organ (Diezel 1954). Micropolygyria has been reported in cases in which fetal anoxia and fetal infection were certainly the responsible agents. Cytomegalic inclusion body disease is commonly associated with micropolygyria (Crome and France 1959). Hallervorden (1949) has reported the malformation in a child one year of age whose mother had attempted suicide by coal gas inhalation when five months pregnant. In addition to micropolygyria, the infant's brain showed softening of the globus pallidus and putamen. Interference with the blood supply of the developing cortex had evidently occurred in the latter case and this factor may well be of importance in others. In this connection it has been shown by de Morsier (1952) that the localization of various prenatal anomalies, including micropolygyria and heterotopias, may be strictly confined to the territories of the main cerebral arteries. The frequency of minor vascular malformations in the micropolygyric cortex has also been stressed by Bertrand and Gruner (1955). The meningeal network of vessels is very abnormal and instead of perforating branches of the usual size, numerous small vessels of varying dimensions penetrate the cortex obliquely. Vessels reaching the third layer of myelinated fibres tend to run along in the course of these fibres and supply the festoons of nerve cells from below, while the deepest cortical layer is supplied from the white matter. The anterior surface of the pons may show deep indentations from vessels pursuing an abnormal course, and the nuclei pontis are occasionally divided into lobules surrounded by myelinated fibres following the ramifications of these vessels. Similar vascular anomalies accompany the disordered cortical architecture of the cerebellum. These findings give some support to the original theory of pathogenesis put forward by Bielschowsky (1916-1918b). From this point of view, micropolygyria is essentially the outcome of an attempt to compensate for an initial disturbance of growth caused by abnormal vascularization of the cortical grey matter. A minor malformation of the cerebral cortex which may be found in micropolygyric or in otherwise normal brains is the condition of 'brain warts'. These are elevated nodular collections of fusiform and stellate neurons, usually in the superficial part of the crowns of gyri in the frontal lobes. There is often a central artery running up from the deeper layers and the myelinated fibres of the gyral core fan out to enclose the base of the nodule (Grcević and Robert 1960).

Cerebellar malformations

Agenesis. It is doubtful whether complete absence of the cerebellum occurs, since careful examination usually reveals a small nodule of recognizable cerebellar tissue (Stewart 1956). In a case of this sort examined by the writer the posterior columns throughout the spinal cord were separated by an ependyma-lined cleft, and uncrossed pyramidal tracts were seen as prominent bundles in the anterior columns. The latter malformation has been studied in detail by Verhaart and Kramer (1952). Absence of one hemisphere is much less rare (Figs. 10.45 and 10.46) and is associated with anomalies of the contralateral inferior olive (Fig. 10.47), which may take the form of atrophy rather than maldevelopment, as in Lichtenstein's (1943) case in which the foliated outline of the degenerated nucleus was clearly visible.

Hypoplasia. The small cerebellum frequently seen in mongols is an example of hypoplasia. A mild unilateral stunting in cerebellar growth is often found in brains showing malformation or long-standing destruction of large areas of the cerebral hemisphere of the opposite side. In many cases this may be ascribed simply to the loss of pontocerebellar fibres which form the bulk of the white matter of the cerebellar hemisphere. This condition is much commoner than crossed cerebellar atrophy (p. 409).

Palaeocerebellar aplasia. Partial or complete aplasia of the vermis is due to the failure of the two alar plates of the rhombencephalon to unite

nuclei (Lyssenkow 1931). In the condition described by Martin (1949, 1950) in which the neocerebellum as well as the rostral part of the vermis and the flocculi were severely underdeveloped, the dentate nuclei were represented by islands of nerve cells and the lateral vestibular nuclei were atrophied. Aplasia of the vermis with central cleft formation occurs in the dysraphic malformations, for instance in occipital

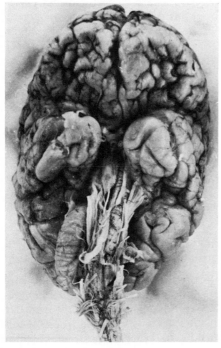

10.45

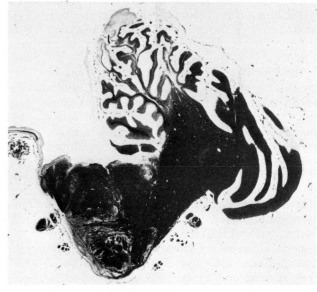

10.46

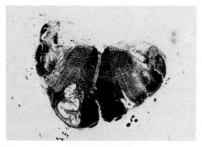

10.47

Figs. 10.45 and **10.46** Cerebellar agenesis; only a rudimentary right hemisphere is present. From a case of the Klippel–Feil deformity.

Fig. 10.47 Malformation of the inferior olives from the same case as Fig. 10.45. Note the small size of the olive contralateral to the cerebellar defect.

in the formation of the corpus cerebelli. The two halves of the cerebellum are separated by a midline cleft and the hemispheres and their peduncles are reduced in size. Various associated nuclear atrophies have been described, including those of the inferior olives, and of cuneate and arcuate

encephaloceles (Ostertag 1956; Karch and Urich 1972). Partial or complete agenesis of the vermis is a feature of the Dandy–Walker malformation (p. 381). A familial form of agenesis of the vermis was reported by Joubert, Eisenring, Robb and Andermann (1969). Only the inferior part of the vermis was absent in the familial cases described by de Haene (1955).

Ponto-neocerebellar hypoplasia. Brun (1917, 1918*a*, *b*) described under this title a cerebellum with hypoplastic, flattened, lateral lobes and well-developed vermis and flocculi (Figs. 10.48, 10.49 and 10.50). In these cerebellar hemispheres the mossy and climbing fibres are largely absent. The ventral part of the pons is unduly small and its transverse fibres and the nuclei pontis markedly reduced in numbers (Fig. 10.51). The dentate

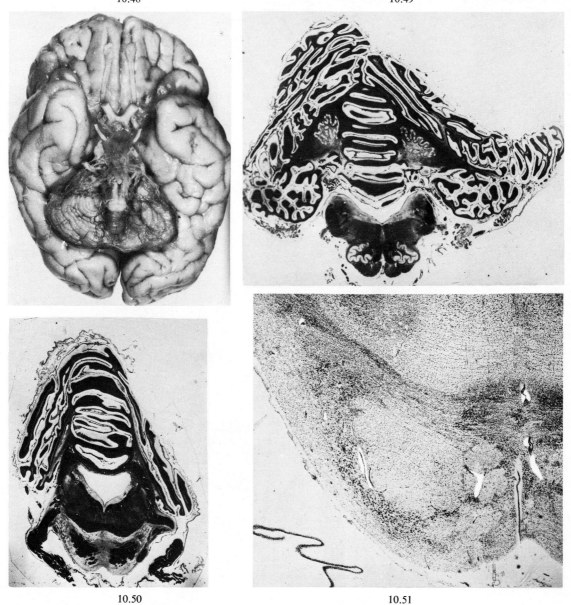

10.48

10.49

10.50

10.51

Figs. 10.48-10.51 Pontoneocerebellar hypoplasia.
Fig. 10.48 The cerebellum is small and flattened—'like a pressed fig'.
Fig. 10.49 Note the relatively large vermis and flocculi compared with the lateral lobes.
Fig. 10.50 Showing the poorly developed pes pontis and lateral lobes of cerebellum.
Fig. 10.51 The nuclei pontis are very poorly represented.

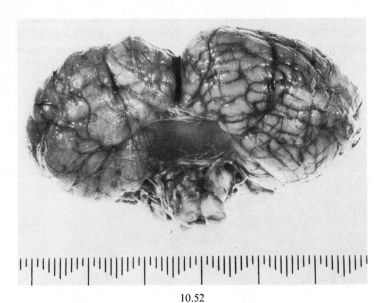

Figs. 10.52–10.54   Cerebellar pachygyria ('microgyria').

Fig. 10.52   Broad, irregular, asymmetrical gyri replacing normal pattern of lobules and folia.

10.52

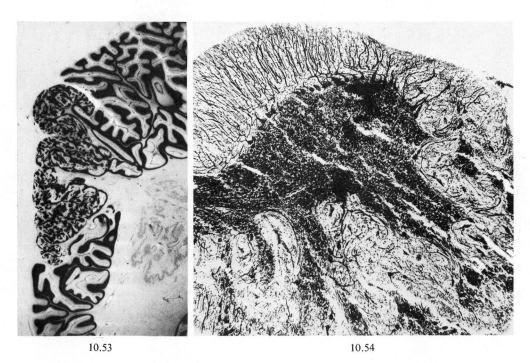

10.53   10.54

Fig. 10.53   The granular layer is disorganized.

Fig. 10.54   Showing transition between normal and malformed cerebellar cortices.   Cajal's silver nitrate pyridine method for the cerebellum.

nuclei are composed of isolated clumps of cells, a malformation also present in the cases of Brouwer (1924) and Biemond (1955). Biemond suggested that this malformation of the dentate nucleus may be the primary event, the other cerebellar changes being of a secondary character.

In this condition the small volume of the neo-cerebellum must be attributed to hypoplasia. The minor losses of Purkinje cells and patchy thinning of the granular layer in Biemond's case would not account for the great reduction in the size of the hemispheres. However, in other parts of the nervous system signs of a degenerative process may sometimes be found. Thus in an example of ponto-neocerebellar hypoplasia occurring in an infant of 3 months, the writer found both dentate nuclei almost completely degenerated and gliosed, except for the most dorsal convolutions (i.e. the part connected with the vermis) where groups of cells had survived. The original crenated outline of the nerve cell bands was, however, clearly distinguishable. This lesion was evidently related to the atrophy of the nucleus ventralis lateralis of each thalamus. A severe loss of nerve cells was also found in the inferior olives, particularly in the dorsal con-volutions, and this was also accompanied by marked fibrillary gliosis. The ventral pons was about half as thick as in the newborn and showed a great numerical reduction in its transverse fibres and in the nerve cells in the nuclei pontis. The remaining cells were often of small size, suggesting a retardation in development, but a heavy gliosis of the region was nevertheless seen. On the other hand, the small lateral lobes of the cerebellum showed no evidence of degeneration. In the brainstem certain nuclei with cerebellar connections were either absent or very poorly developed, their sites showing no traces of a destructive process (Norman and Urich 1958). Gross and Kaltenback (1959) have also noted the combination of malformation and system degeneration in their case.

Ponto-neocerebellar hypoplasia has been found associated with cerebral pachygyria in one instance (Kramer 1956). Cerebellar hypoplasia affecting predominantly the lateral lobes was also found in a case of Werdnig–Hoffmann's disease (Norman 1961a).

Cerebellar microgyria. In this condition the normal foliated lobules fail to develop over a variable extent of cortex, which thus presents a smooth and unconvoluted surface (Fig. 10.52). Microscopical examination reveals a complicated pattern of interlacing strands or islands of granular cells interspersed with relatively acellular strips representing the molecular layer (Fig. 10.53). These areas contain numerous displaced Purkinje cells which have a few arborizations and appears as retort-shaped forms when impregnated by silver (Fig. 10.54). They tend to orientate them-selves in the normal way at the junction of the aberrant molecular and granular layers and their cytons are often enclosed by normal basket fibres. Tangential fibres are seldom seen in these ectopic molecular layers, but numerous unmyelinated fibres are found passing in different directions. Since this malformation is generally associated with cerebral micropolygyria it has been called 'microgyria' of the cerebellum; but the name 'cerebellar agyria' would seem to be more appro-priate, since little or no suggestion is conveyed of miniature folia or of microgyric formations and this type of cerebellar anomaly may also be present in brains showing agyria (pachygyria) of the cerebral hemispheres (Walker 1942; Warner 1953). A cerebellar malformation of this type was found in the unique case described by van Bogaert and Radermecker (1955). The mother had been treated by radium for carcinoma of the cervix during the fifth month of pregnancy. Cerebellar microgyria also occurs in malformed brains due to intrauterine cytomegalovirus infec-tion (Bignami and Appicciutoli 1964).

Other cerebellar dystopias. Heterotopias of cor-tical cerebellar cells in the white matter and in the dentate nuclei are commonly found in trisomies (Norman 1966; Terplan, Sandberg and Aceto 1966; Terplan and Cohen 1968; Sumi 1970). They are found most commonly in trisomy D (13-15) but occur also in trisomy E (17-18) and occasionally in mongolism. Three distinct morphological forms can be recognized. One consists of islands of closely packed large, spherical or polygonal ganglion cells with well-developed Nissl bodies, situated in the subcortical white matter (Fig. 10.55). The cells are slightly larger than neonatal Purkinje cells and resemble the neurons of the dentate nucleus. This is the least specific form of cerebellar heterotopia which may be found in association with other mal-formations and also in apparently normal infants (Rorke, Riggs and Fogelson 1968). The second type consists of collections of small cells with

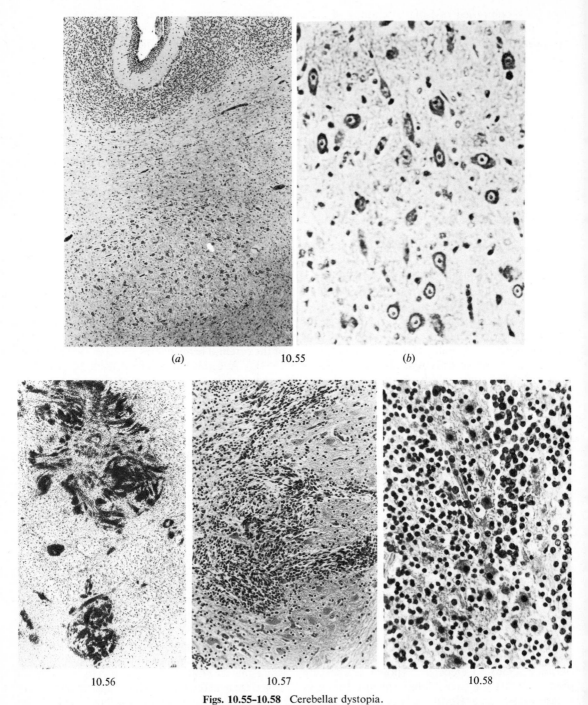

(a)   10.55   (b)

10.56   10.57   10.58

Figs. 10.55–10.58 Cerebellar dystopia.
Fig. 10.55 Island of large heterotopic cells in subcortical white matter. Klüver–Barrera. (a) ×50; (b) ×285.
Fig. 10.56 Low-power view of heterotopic aggregates of small cells in dentate nucleus (Trisomy D). Carbol azure. ×37·5.
Fig. 10.57 High-power view of similar heterotopia composed of cells of external granule type. H & E. ×112·5.
Fig. 10.58 Totally disorganized nodule of cerebellar tissue consisting of external and internal granules and of Purkinje cells (same case as Fig. 10.6). H & E. ×350.

darkly staining elongated nuclei, identical with those normally seen in the fetal external granular layer (Figs 10.56 and 10.57). In some cases there is an admixture of cells resembling those of the definitive granular layer. These heterotopic collections are seen most commonly in the neighbourhood of the dentate nuclei or in the deep white matter adjacent to the walls of the 4th ventricle. The third pattern consists of clear cut round or oval islands containing a mixture of large and small cells interspersed with strands of relatively acellular tissue and giving the impression of an abortive and disorganized three-layered cerebellar cortex.

In trisomy E these heterotopias tend to be less conspicuous and may be associated with minor cortical malformations. In one case the normal folia were replaced by tubular structures arranged round blood vessels in a small area of the lateral lobes (Norman 1966). Localized reversal of the granular and Purkinje cell layers has also been seen.

Various forms of cortical dystopia ranging from minor malformation to total disorganization with haphazard intermingling of all cortical elements may be found in the ectopic part of the cerebellar vermis in the Arnold–Chiari malformation. A totally disorganized spherical nodule of cerebellar tissue was also described in one case of occipital encephalocele (Karch and Urich 1972) (Fig. 10.58).

Congenital cerebellar atrophy

A distinction between cerebellofugal and cerebellopetal types of atrophy was first made by Bielschowsky (1920-21) who noted that in certain cases of amaurotic family idiocy the brunt of the destructive process had fallen upon the afferent elements, so that the granule cells, mossy fibres and climbing fibres had largely disappeared, whereas the cells of Purkinje were preserved. This distribution of lesions is thus the converse of what is found in the cerebello-olivary degeneration of later life in which the Purkinje cell layer is invariably the most severely affected part of the cortex.

Although this contrast is not an absolute one and 'pure' types are by no means the rule, this classification according to the predominant locality of the lesions is a useful one and is applicable to the two types of congenital cerebellar atrophy now to be described.

Congenital cerebellar atrophy of granular layer type.

The cerebellum is much diminished in size and shows shrinkage and sclerosis of the folia (Fig. 10.59). In some cases the vermis is much less affected (Ule 1952). Microscopically it is seen that the granule and Golgi cells are absent or very scanty over the greater part of the cortex and the mossy fibres have also disappeared (Fig. 10.60). The Purkinje cells, on the other hand, are numerous and very conspicuous partly because of the small size of the shrunken folia and also because the majority of the cells are scattered throughout the molecular layer (Fig. 10.60). These ectopic neurons are of anomalous shape, resembling retorts or spindles, and are devoid of basket or climbing fibres. The tangential fibres of the molecular layer are generally preserved but their descending branches, instead of forming distinct pericellular baskets, tend to be arranged in a thin, uniformly spaced, curtain which passes downwards to end in the denuded granular layer. As in other types of cerebellar disease the dendrites of the Purkinje cells often exhibit terminal club-shaped expansions which bear short filamentous processes (Fig. 10.61). It is, however, a characteristic feature of this condition that the radial branches of these 'asteroid bodies' often form a peculiarly dense brushwork (Fig. 10.62). When such a formation is attached to a dendritic stalk its origin is obvious, but similar asteroid bodies are often seen in isolation in the molecular layer, their fine radial fibres arranged around a central nuclear structure the peripheral portion of which is denser than the central. These dendritic swellings are not so coarse as the cactus-like formations in amaurotic idiocy and they do not contain lipid. They are best explained as a reaction to pathological change on the part of the damaged but surviving Purkinje cell and they exemplify what Bouman (1934) has called 'hyper-differentiation', to which category also belong the numerous axonal 'torpedoes' which are commonly seen in this and other cerebellar disorders. It is noteworthy that no case of granular atrophy has been accompanied by retrograde atrophy of the inferior olives.

A heavy fibrillary gliosis is seen in the molecular layer but gliosis is mild in the territory of the missing granules (Fig. 10.63). This neuroglial fibrosis is in part derived from the Bergmann astrocytes but the usual radial arrangement of the fibrils is replaced by a wilder, anisomorphic

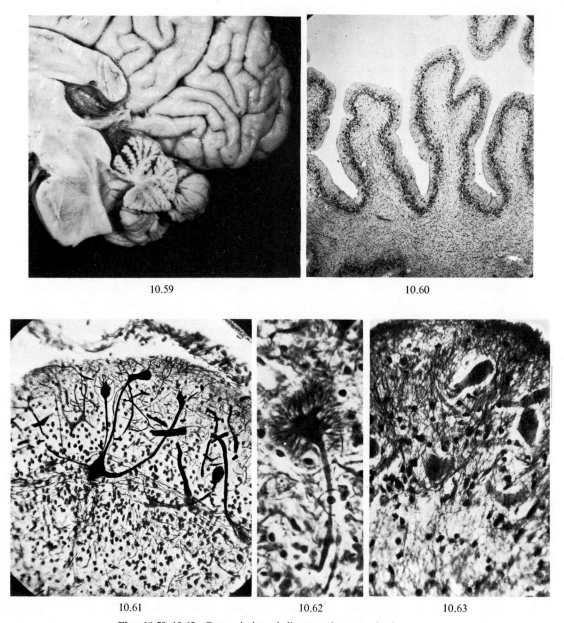

10.59   10.60

10.61   10.62   10.63

Figs. 10.59–10.63   Congenital cerebellar atrophy; granular layer type.

Fig. 10.59   Showing small size of cerebellum and shrinkage of dorsal vermis.

Fig. 10.60   Atrophy of the granular layer and preservation of the Purkinje cells many of which are present in the molecular layer.   Cresyl violet.

Fig. 10.61   Cactus-like expansions of the dendrites of the Purkinje cells.   Note the tangential fibres lying low in the molecular layer.   Cajal's silver nitrate pyridine method for the cerebellum.

Fig. 10.62   Dendritic expansion with fine terminal brushwork of fibres.   Bielschowsky.

Fig. 10.63   The fibrillary gliosis is mainly in the molecular level.   Heterotopic Purkinje cells are seen.   Holzer.

type of gliosis. It is unlikely that traction by gliosis is responsible for the grossly abnormal position of so many of the Purkinje cells, although it must be remembered that dislocation of previously normally aligned Purkinje cells into the molecular layer is a well-known phenomenon in diseases of the cerebellum (Schob 1921). A more probable explanation of the ectopic position of the cells is that, owing to the degeneration of the granular layer at a stage prior to the final organization of the cerebellar cortex, the migrating Purkinje cells have themselves been implicated in the pathological process. This view is supported by the observation that in folia where the Purkinje cells are in normal alignment there is always a well-formed granular layer.

The aetiology of this primary form of granular atrophy is unknown, though Norman (1940) thought that there was the likelihood of familial incidence in his cases. The condition is invariably associated with severe mental defect, though no characteristic pathological changes have been demonstrated in the cerebrum. From the clinical point of view there may be little evidence of ataxia, a feature shared by other cerebellar disorders of early life.

Congenital cerebellar atrophy with loss of Purkinje cells. One is on far less certain ground in placing this variety of cellular disease in the prenatal class and only rarely can the decision be taken with reasonable confidence. This hesitation arises from the well-known vulnerability of the Purkinje cells to the vascular disturbances associated with epilepsy which may lead to widespread destruction of these cells. Certainly, if lesions appropriate to epilepsy or birth injury are found elsewhere in the brain, the prenatal character of the cerebellar atrophy becomes improbable. There are, however, a few recorded cases in which cerebellar degeneration has evidently occurred very early in life and has led to a small cerebellum and widespread loss of Purkinje cells, especially in the hemisphere. In Scherer's (1933) case of a 2-year-old idiot the granular layer had also suffered slightly. Jervis (1950) described a familial case in which the granular layer showed widespread and severe rarefaction, but the substantial involvement of the Purkinje cells and the regular alignment of the survivors seems to put this case in a different category from that of primary granular layer degeneration.

A corollary to the degeneration of Purkinje cells is the presence of empty basket fibres. Axonal torpedoes and swollen dendritic 'antlers' may also be seen among the survivors. When the loss of Purkinje cells is considerable the dentate nucleus always shows characteristic changes in the form of a loss of myelinated fibres and an exceptionally heavy gliosis in the amiculum or 'fleece'. Secondary glial proliferation in the olives is found in long-standing cases but the amount of retrograde cell loss is very variable.

Cerebro-cerebellar atrophy. Lesions of one cerebral hemisphere sometimes lead to a degeneration of Purkinje and granular cells in the cerebellar hemisphere of the opposite side. With few exceptions, the cerebral lesions in the recorded cases have been extensive, have originated in early life and have taken several years to produce their effects. The cerebellar atrophy commonly involves the semilunar and quadrangular lobes and is usually distributed in a patchy way. The vermis and flocculus are rarely affected. There are two suggested pathways by which the chain of degeneration may reach the cerebellum from the cerebral cortex. The first, or antegrade way, is along the corticopontine tracts, the ipsilateral nucleus pontis and the opposite middle peduncle to the granular layer of the cerebellum and thence to the Purkinje cells. The second, or retrograde way, is from the precentral cortex (areas 4 and 6) to the ventrolateral nucleus of the thalamus, thence via the superior cerebellar peduncle to the opposite dentate nucleus and so the Purkinje cells and lastly to the granules. When the cerebral lesions are widespread it is not unusual to find both the thalamus and the cerebral peduncle degenerated, in which case it is only by determining whether the nucleus pontis or the dentate nucleus is the more affected that a conclusion can be reached as to which path may have been taken by the degenerative process. The most comprehensive account of the subject is that given by Verhaart and van Wieringen-Rauws (1950). From their review of 38 reported cases these authors conclude that cerebro-cerebellar atrophy is unpredictable, and even under apparently favourable conditions the barrier of the pontine or dentate nucleus may not be penetrated. There is, moreover, no sharp topographical relation between the cerebral and cerebellar lesions and the occurrence or extent of the latter may depend upon some innate tendency towards degeneration on the part of the cerebellum itself.

The tuberous sclerosis complex (Bourneville's disease)

The first recorded instance of patchy sclerosis of the cerebral cortex was given by von Recklinghausen (1862), whose case also showed multiple myomata in the heart. The name tuberous sclerosis was first applied to these cortical changes by Bourneville who described 10 cases in a series of papers published during the years 1880-1900. Although Bourneville had noted that facial and renal anomalies might be present, it was not until H. Vogt's paper of 1908 that the clinico-pathological syndrome was adequately delineated. Since the term 'tuberous sclerosis' applies only to one feature of a protean disorder, it is more precise to designate the condition 'the tuberous sclerosis complex' as suggested by Moulton (1942), unless the eponymous title of 'Bourneville's disease' is preferred. The term 'epiloia' was introduced by Sherlock (1911) to indicate the commonly encountered triad of adenoma sebaceum, epilepsy and mental deficiency. Recent reviews include those by Lagos and Gomez (1967) and by Donegani, Grattarola and Wildi (1972).

In the fully developed disease an extraordinary diversity of lesions may be encountered, brain, skin, kidneys, heart, bones and lungs being involved in characteristic ways. Many of these anomalies belong to the category of 'hamartoma', that is to say, they are congenital malformations with a potentiality for growth which does not exceed that of the normal tissue in which they are situated.

Central nervous system

The brain may be of normal weight but some reduction is common in low-grade defectives. Frank micrencephaly, as in one of Bielschowsky's (1923-24b) cases, is exceptional; so also is the very heavy brain recorded by Borremans et al. (1933). The convolutional pattern is usually within normal limits, although minor disturbances may be caused by the presence of the patho-gnomonic sclerotic patches or tubera in the gyri. When the leptomeninges are removed these tubera are easily distinguished by their pallor and stony-hard consistency which contrast with the appearance and feel of the neighbouring convolutions. There are two main varieties of tuber which have been named after Pellizzi (1901) who first described their points of difference. His first type is characterized by a hardening, blanching and widening of a gyrus, the crown of which is flattened and smooth (Fig. 10.66). The other variety is a rounded, flattened nodule, the surface of which is roughened and dimpled and which is sometimes slightly elevated above the level of the neighbouring gyri, from which it is superficially demarcated by a surrounding sulcus (Fig. 10.64). On microscopical examination, the sclerosed areas show an enormous increase in the number of astrocytic nuclei, the nerve cells being usually scanty or their lamination grossly disturbed. The histological picture is often dominated by groups of very large cells of bizarre shape, many of which exceed the size of giant Betz cells (Fig. 10.65). Their outlines are vague in Nissl preparations but a minority may suggest nerve cells by their pyramidal or spindle shape and the coarse tigroid bodies they contain. A much better demonstration of their morphology is obtained by metallic impregnation methods. The commonest form of abnormal cell in tuberous sclerosis is a large oval plump cell, rather like a swollen-bodied astrocyte, which often contains two or three peripherally placed nuclei with prominent nucleoli (Fig. 10.67). These cells do not possess processes. Many of the giant cells have a more obvious relationship either to neurons or to astrocytes. The neuronal derivatives may be shown by Bielschowsky's method to contain neurofibrils (Fig. 10.69), while the large glial types often stain well with Hortega's silver carbonate or Cajal's gold sublimate (Figs. 10.70 and 10.71). These giant cells are most numerous in the tubera, especially near the central umbilication. They are uncommon in the molecular layer and more frequent in the outer zone of the grey matter than in the deeper layers. Isolated examples may be found in any part of the cortex or subcortical white matter and in the latter situation substantial groups are often seen around blood vessels. In rare instances the majority of the large cells are to be found in the central cores of white matter where they show up as conspicuous heterotopias. Many of the large cells contain conspicuous vacuoles (Fig. 10.68) which have been shown to contain glycogen (Helmke 1937, Jacob 1964-65). Argentophilic globules, resembling those of Pick's disease, neurofibrillary tangles and granulovacuolar degeneration have been seen in the giant nerve cells by Hirano, Tuazon and Zimmermann (1968).

As might be expected from their very firm texture, the tubers exhibit a great proliferation of fibrillary astrocytes. The Holzer stain reveals dense fibrillary gliosis in the outer part of the molecular layer, particularly in the region of the central depression of the tuber where sheaves of coarse fibres form interlacing and brush-like patterns (Fig. 10.72). In comparison, the outer

Glial anomalies are not, however, confined to the tubers. A well-marked fibrillary gliosis may be present throughout the white matter of the brain; and in non-tuberous parts selective staining readily reveals atypical astrocytes.

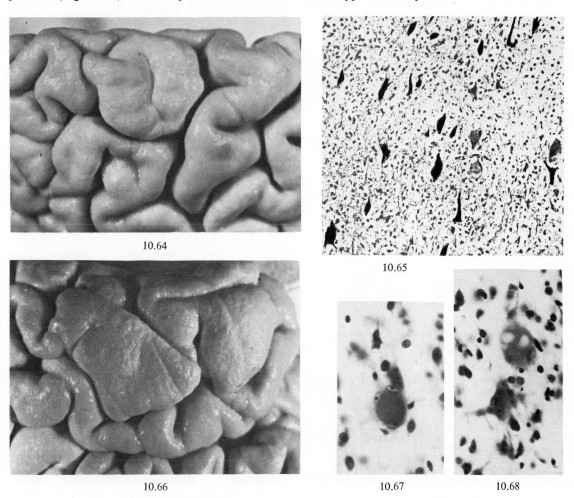

10.64

10.65

10.66

10.67   10.68

Figs. 10.64–10.68 Tuberous sclerosis.
Fig. 10.64 A cortical tuber (Pelizzi type 2).
Fig. 10.65 A group of giant cells in an area of tuberous sclerosis. Hortega's silver carbonate method for astrocytes.
Fig. 10.66 A cortical tuber (Pelizzi type 1).
Fig. 10.67 Multinucleated large glial cell of anomalous type. Carbol azure.
Fig. 10.68 Anomalous cell showing vacuolation. Carbol azure.

part of the grey matter is usually less gliosed, but a dense overgrowth of fibrils is usual in the deeper layers and in the adjoining white matter. Bundles of glial fibres connect these two zones of gliosis, passing through the less affected cortex in radial fashion. The central part of the cortex in such sclerosed gyri may occasionally show rarefaction of the tissues with status spongiosus.

Myelination is disturbed in the sclerotic convolutions, the cortex containing irregular tangles of fibres and the central cores and subcortical white matter showing patchy areas of rarefaction (Fig. 10.73). More sharply defined, circular areas devoid of myelin are caused by the presence of small fibrocellular tumours to be described later. Amyloid bodies and calcospherites are frequently

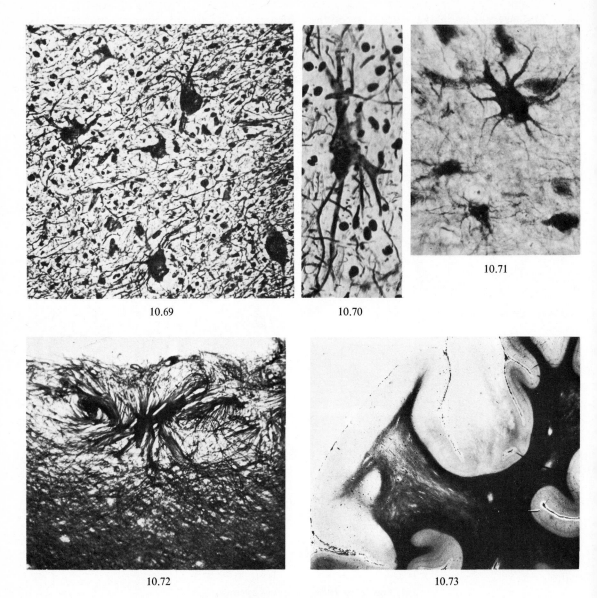

Figs. 10.69–10.73 Tuberous sclerosis.

Fig. 10.69 A group of large abnormal cells of neuronal type in an area of tuberous sclerosis. Bielschowsky.

Fig. 10.70 Giant cell of astrocytic type. Hortega's method for astrocytes.

Fig. 10.71 Giant astrocyte. Cajal's gold sublimate method.

Fig. 10.72 Sheaf-like bundles of neuroglial fibres in superficial part of a cortical tuber. Holzer.

Fig. 10.73 Myelin poverty in an area of neuroglial sclerosis. The flat margin of the central core of white matter lies beneath a cortical tuber and is a characteristic feature of myelin preparation. Heidenhain's myelin.

found in the tubers. In some cases massive calcification occurs and multiple 'brain stones' may be visible in X-rays of the skull (Yakovlev and Corwin 1939).

This account of the cellular abnormalities met with in the cerebral cortex applies in the main to other parts of the central nervous system. The cerebellar manifestations have been fully reviewed by van Bogaert, Paillas, Berard-Badier and Payan (1958). Tubers occur infrequently but heterotopic clusters of giant cells are not uncommon in the white matter. Monster cells in the layer of Purkinje cells are rare (Fig. 10.74). It is not unusual to find widespread loss of Purkinje cells and well-marked lobular atrophy, these changes being attributable to epilepsy. Giant cells and patchy glial overgrowth also occur in the basal ganglia and less frequently in the brainstem and spinal cord.

An important pathological feature of this disease is the presence of multiple small tumour-like nodules of a fibrocellular character. Their site of predilection is the sulcus terminalis from which they project into the lateral ventricle like the 'gutterings of a candle'. They are partially embedded in the substance of the thalamus or caudate nucleus and vary in size from a few millimetres to a centimetre or more in diameter (Fig. 10.75). They are also commonly seen beneath the ependyma of the lateral ventricles. In the cerebral cortex, nodules of similar type are usually found in the subcortical white matter just below the floor of a sulcus and they are also occasionally present in the cerebellum or brain-stem. Whatever may be their situation, these tumours show little variation in their structure and are composed of aggregations of large round or oval cells, intermingled with leashes or whorls of fibrillary glial tissue (Fig. 10.76). The nuclei of these large cells are often multiple, and elon-gated or irregularly lobulated forms lie at the periphery of the cell and may even entirely ring its margin. These cells may be seen to contribute long fleshy processes to the fibrous stroma of the tumour, the central parts of which often con-tain numerous blood vessels with greatly thickened walls. Fibrillary astrocytes, many of which are hyperplastic, also take part in the tumour and may predominate in the smaller subependymal nodules. Conspicuous iron-calcium deposits, either in the form of concentric spherules or larger confluent masses, are also a characteristic feature of these tumours and the neighbouring blood vessels may also show extensive calcifica-tion. Rings of collagen or reticulin may often be demonstrated around the concretions. When this calcification is sufficiently massive to show in X-ray photographs, the position of the nodules in relation to the lateral ventricles may be of diagnostic importance during life. It is also obvious that, if much increase takes place in the size of a nodule situated near the foramen of Monro or the opening of the aqueduct of Sylvius, the flow of cerebrospinal fluid may become ob-structed. Not only may a slow enlargement take

place during postnatal life but a malignant trans-formation of these tumours into astrocytomas or glioblastomas may occur. Diffuse infiltrative tumours of the hemisphere are a well-recognized complication of tuberous sclerosis. In the example recorded by Kufs (1949) the left cerebral hemi-sphere was generally enlarged and contained in the white matter a massive glioblastoma. An interesting feature of this case was that only in the hemisphere containing the tumour were there signs of tuberous sclerosis. In a smaller number of cases the tumour has contained numerous abnormal nerve cells in addition to glial derivates of a more or less primitive type, Globus (1938), in particular, has drawn attention to 'spongio-neuroblastomas' of this sort in tuberous sclerosis. In Jervis's (1954a) case the anomalous neurons were thought to be derived from normal elements which had undergone metaplasia.

Closely allied to these subependymal tumours are the retinal phakomata described by van der Hoeve (1921). Both the large nodular type which usually lies at the edge of the nerve head, and the smaller multiple, flattened forms that are present elsewhere in the fundus, have basically the same type of structure and primarily involve the nerve fibre layer of the retina. They are composed in varying proportions of glial fibres and vaguely outlined large cells with fleshy cyto-plasm which are probably abnormal forms of retinal neuroglia. Neuroglial fibrils are often present in whorls, recalling the appearance of the cerebral tumours, and calcifications or even ossification occurs at their centres. The larger tumours may be partially cystic and an associated angiomatous condition of the choroid has often been noted. The continued growth of these nodules may disorganize the eye, but it is not certain that true malignancy occurs. In Hall's (1946) case a small tumour mass was also found in the lens, but, as the author pointed out, this was probably heterotopic and not metastatic in origin.

Visceral anomalies
Heart. Batchelor and Mann (1945) reviewed 63 recorded instances of rhabdomyoma and found that tuberous sclerosis was an associated feature in half the cases, though this is probably a con-servative estimate. Rhabdomyomata may have three different distributions in the heart muscle: as a solitary tumour, usually at the apex of the left ventricle, as multiple small nodules and,

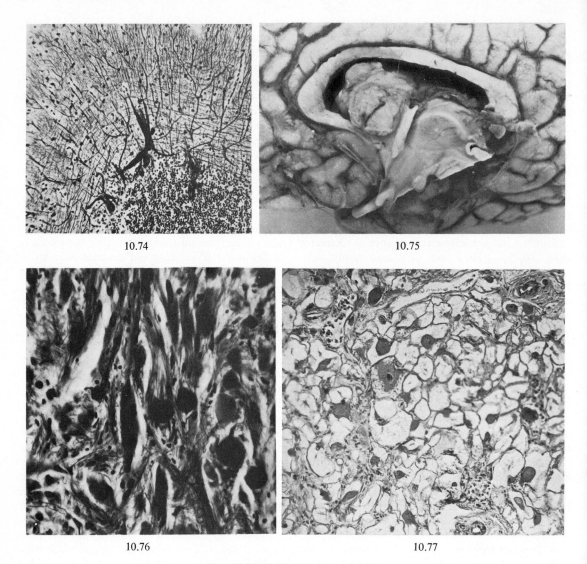

10.74

10.75

10.76

10.77

Figs. 10.74–10.77 Tuberous sclerosis.
Fig. 10.74 A large abnormal Purkinje cell from a case of tuberous sclerosis. Cajal's silver nitrate method for the cerebellum.
Fig. 10.75 A ventricular tumour of large size arising from the caudate nucleus. The usual glial nodules seen in this region in tuberous sclerosis are considerably smaller.
Fig. 10.76 A common type of ventricular tumour in tuberous sclerosis. Large oval cells are seen enmeshed in a neuroglial stroma. Hortega's method for astrocytes.
Fig. 10.77 Typical microscopic appearance of one of the multiple rhabdomyomatous nodules found in the tuberous sclerosis complex. H & E.

exceptionally, as a diffuse involvement of the myocardium as in Schminke's (1922) case. Multiple rhabdomyomata are by far the commonest finding. They present as small, rounded, pale areas, rarely exceeding a centimetre in diameter, projecting from, or flush with, the surface of the ventricular, papillary or auricular muscles. Micro-

scopically, the tumours are composed of a loose network of interlacing fibrils many of which possess the striations of skeletal muscle. These fibres may be seen to radiate from large rounded bodies with a granular, eosinophilic cytoplasm resembling the fetal heart muscle cells of Purkinje (Fig. 10.77). These elements, set against the spongy background of the tumour, suggested the appearance of spiders in their webs to Cesaris-Demel (1895) and have since his day been known as 'spider-cells'. They represent primitive striated muscle cells which have become grossly vacuolated by intracellular accumulations of glycogen. In later life these 'congenital nodular glycogen tumours', as Batchelor and Mann prefer to call them, undergo regressive changes, their mass decreasing in size and being finally largely replaced by connective tissue or fat (Steinbiss 1923) in which isolated cells of Purkinje type may still be found.

Apart from rhabdomyoma, cardiac anomalies are of rare occurrence in the tuberous sclerosis complex. Occasional stenosis of the great vessels has been reported (Rehder 1914; Schuster 1914; Critchley and Earl 1932), and in one case a large congenital diverticulum, lined by thick fibro-elastic tissue resembling that of the aorta, was found in the left ventricle (Norman and Taylor 1940). A feature of interest in this case was the presence of rhabdomyoma cells in the tissue adjoining the malformation.

Kidneys. Tumours are more commonly found in the kidneys in this condition than in any other organ, their frequency being estimated by Critchley and Earl (1932) as 80%. Whitish or yellow nodules, generally measuring less than 2 cm in diameter, are seen projecting from the surface or wholly embedded in the renal cortex. Cysts may also be present and in one of Inglis's (1950) cases glomeruli were demonstrated projecting into the walls of some of the smaller ones. Microscopically the solid parts of the tumour are composed of leashes of spindle-shaped cells, often with elongated nuclei, the sides of which are parallel and the ends blunt. An admixture with smaller, rounded cells may often be seen and bands of hyaline material may be found passing through the tumour. There is a very variable content of fat cells and blood vessels. The elongated tumour cells of the kidney have been generally considered to be of mesenchymal origin but Inglis (1950) has suggested that this type of tissue, as also the somewhat similar spindle-shaped cells of the lung nodules and other visceral tumours, are derived from Schwann cells.

Lungs. The rare pulmonary changes in tuberous sclerosis have been studied by Dawson (1954) and by Dwyer, Hickie and Garvan (1971). Unlike most of the visceral manifestations of tuberous sclerosis, the pulmonary variety leads to serious illness in adult life. The condition is commoner in women and often presents clinically as a pneumothorax. The outer surfaces of the lungs are covered by small subpleural cysts and much of the pulmonary tissue is replaced by cystic spaces embedded in a matrix composed in varying proportions of fibrous tissue, smooth muscle fibres and blood vessels. Compactly arranged nodules containing large muscle fibres are also a common feature.

Other organs, including the thyroid, liver, suprarenal, duodenum and ovary, have been reported to contain hamartomas of fibrocellular character.

Skin anomalies. Dawson (1954) has drawn attention to an early description of the highly characteristic feature of adenoma sebaceum which was given by Addison and Gull (1851) in the following words: 'a peculiar eruption extending across the nose and slightly affecting both cheeks. It consisted of shining tubercles varying in size to that of ordinary acne. They were of lightish colour with superficial capillary veins meandering over them giving them a faint rose tinge.' These pale nodules are usually known as the Balzer type of adenoma sebaceum, while the more vascular red type is named after Pringle. Microscopically the nodules consist of an overgrowth of the sebaceous glands, connective tissue and small blood vessels. Adenoma sebaceum is rarely present at birth and may not appear until puberty. An admixture of fibrous and angiomatous tissue also characterizes the subungual fibromata of the fingers and toes, a condition considered by many to be equal in importance to adenoma sebaceum in the clinical diagnosis of the tuberous sclerosis complex. Other skin lesions include shagreen patches, consisting of an irregular, faintly nodular, roughening, usually seen on the skin of the lower back. Depigmented or 'white' patches, clearly circumscribed, are another common feature. They may be present at birth or develop in early infancy and are the earliest manifestation of tuberous sclerosis (Gold and Freeman 1965). The skin lesions of tuberous sclerosis were fully reviewed by Butterworth and Wilson (1941).

Bones. There are not many recorded instances of bony anomalies associated with tuberous sclerosis, probably because few patients have been thoroughly examined radiologically. The calvarium may show a mottled appearance which is due to areas of increased density of both the inner table and the diploic trabeculae (Dickerson 1955). In Hall's (1946) case there was also hyperostosis of the petrous bones. Perhaps the commonest X-ray finding is the presence of small areas of rarefaction in the metacarpal and metatarsal bones. These lesions closely resemble those found in neurofibromatosis, but their relationship to any local neural abnormality is improbable since the rarefactions are due to a fibrous dysplasia of the bone (Dickerson 1955). Up to the present only one case of tuberous sclerosis has shown the peculiar condition of 'rheostosis', which is characterized by an irregular hyperostosis running down the shaft of a bone in one limb. The anomaly is regarded by Weber (1929) as the bony analogue of linear naevi.

Pathogenesis
The disease is inherited as a dominant and the mutation rate is high (Gunther and Penrose 1935). In considering the genetics of the condition incomplete forms of the disease must be taken into account. These are often overlooked in material collected mainly in institutions for the mentally retarded and epileptics. In Lagos and Gomez, (1967) series 38% of patients showing features of tuberous sclerosis were of average intelligence. The occurrence of incomplete forms and monosymptomatic 'formes frustes' has prompted the view that modifier genes may alter the expressivity of the simple dominant inheritance (Paulson 1967). The earlier writers, notably H. Vogt (1908) and Alzheimer (1904), regarded tuberous sclerosis as essentially the product of defective histogenesis and this view has been endorsed in more recent times by Schob (1930) and Globus (1932). The element of malformation is perhaps most obvious in the heterotopic collections of cells frequently seen in the subcortical white matter, though these are never so conspicuous a feature as in the grosser maldevelopments of micro- or pachygyria. The peculiar character of the giant cells, however, strongly suggests an earlier origin of the abnormalities than the time of the migration of neuroblasts, and it is considered probable that the disease exemplifies a primary defect of differentiation on the part of the primordial neuro-

epithelium (Globus 1932). Thus the sclerosis characteristic of the disorder is regarded as a primary anomaly of the neuroglia and it is perhaps surprising that genuine neoplasia is not more common when this background of disturbed balance of cellular growth is taken into account.

Much has been made of the so-called blastomatous features of tuberous sclerosis. Bielschowsky attempted to explain the multiple cerebral abnormalities of the condition as direct consequences of spongioblastic overgrowth. This theory, however, does not account satisfactorily for the large nerve cells which may be so conspicuous a feature of the disease. It is improbable that these are an expression of compensatory hypertrophy conditioned by the local glial overgrowth, since nerve cells of giant size are to be found in areas where the gliosis is relatively insignificant. The pathological findings outside the nervous system also provide substantial evidence in favour of the purely dysontogenetic nature of the disorder. In the heart the large muscle cells of the rhabdomyomata, while retaining an imprint of their embryonic prototype, possess none of the proliferative tendencies so often associated with cells of 'primitive' morphology. Rehder (1914) believed that these myoblasts are aberrant derivatives of primordial cells capable of forming both the specialized Purkinje fibres and the ordinary cells of the myocardium, a theory that at once suggests the analogous formation of giant cells in the brain from the indifferent cells of the matrix.

Bielschowsky (1914) emphasized the resemblances between the lesions of neurofibromatosis and tuberous sclerosis and proposed to classify the latter condition as the central form of von Recklinghausen's disease. However instructive such histological comparisons may be, the fact should not be lost sight of that tuberous sclerosis and von Recklinghausen's disease are genetically distinct conditions and any pathological affinities that they may possess are due to the influence of unrelated dominant genes upon the same embryonic layers (Borberg 1951). The same proviso applies to other conditions in which isolated features reminiscent of tuberous sclerosis may be found. Thus large abnormal neurons may be seen in certain cases of pachygyria in which there may also be a dense overgrowth of neuroglia. Giant cells of neuronal type and a deranged cortical architecture have also been reported in the brain of a case of Allbright's disease (Jervis and Schein 1951).

Encephalofacial angiomatosis (Sturge–Weber disease)

This neurocutaneous syndrome is characterized clinically, in its complete form, by naevus flammeus of the face, buphthalmos, hemiparesis of the contralateral limbs, epilepsy, mental defect and radiological evidence of intracranial calcifications. The latter sign is very rare below the age of 2 years. The clinical and pathological delineation of this disease has taken many years and many names have been attached to it in the course of time, but if an eponymous title is to be preferred the name of Sturge certainly deserves commemoration. Sturge was not only responsible in 1879 for the first clinical account of the essential features, but he also correctly deduced that an underlying naevoid condition of the brain was probably present in his patient. It was not, however, until nearly 20 years later that Kalischer (1897, 1901) recorded the first post-mortem examination and revealed the prophesied cerebral vascular anomaly. This patient was only 18 months old and the limited pathological examination showed no calcification. Weber (1922-23) described the typical gyriform radiographic contours of the cerebral calcifications, though according to Krabbe (1934) priority for their demonstration should be given to Wissing of Copenhagen. Krabbe (1934) himself made the important point that these calcifications occurred in the cortex and not in the meningeal vessels.

Somewhat similar curvilinear shadows of calcification are occasionally encountered in other conditions such as oligodendroglioma, brains injured by irradiation, lead encephalopathy (Lichtenstein 1954), Fahr's disease, or in the cases of progressive facial hemiatrophy reported by Merritt, Faber and Bruch (1937). The wide extent and uniform pattern of the phenomenon as seen in Sturge's disease is however virtually a pathognomonic picture.

It is advisable to limit the definition of Sturge's syndrome to cases showing at least two of the major signs, that is to say, facial naevus combined with either intracranial angioma or with angioma of the choroid of the eye (Louis-Bar 1944). This criterion rules out many superficially allied conditions such as spinal cord angiomas with cutaneous naevi of metameric distribution (Cobb 1915), cutaneous naevi associated with cerebellar symptoms (Louis-Bar 1941), and the familial non-calcifying meningeal angiomas of Divry and van Bogaert (1946). The inclusion of these and the other vaguely related naevoid states within the nosographic limits of the disease would be unjustified. The localization of the facial naevus is extremely important in the definition of the disease and only those cases in which it involves the supra-ocular region should be admitted. A complete record of the literature has failed to show a single case in which cerebral angiomatosis or gyriform calcification is present in association with a facial naevus limited to other areas of the face (Alexander and Norman 1960).

Neuropathological findings. The essential intracerebral anomaly is an excessive vascularity of the pia mater and in the majority of cases the occipital or parieto-occipital region of the brain is alone affected, the dura and skull being much more rarely involved. The majority of the meningeal vessels are of small venous type and lie in tortuous folds several layers deep in the subarachnoid space, giving a dark purple colour to the leptomeninges. The meningeal arteries frequently show conspicuous calcification of the subintimal layer (Fig. 10.80). This is an early manifestation and was present in a 3-month-old child examined by the writer. Groups of vessels with thick muscular coats but no elastic laminae may also be present among the superficial veins. Abnormal vessels rarely penetrate the cortex but an occasional abnormal convoluted vessel may be seen (Craig 1949) (Fig. 10.81). An unusual association of the Sturge–Weber syndrome with an intracerebral venous angioma in the contralateral hemisphere was reported by Norman (1963a). Beneath the hypervascularized meninges it is usual to find that extensive strips of the outer part of the cortex contain massive deposits of a crystalline material which imparts a gritty sensation on cutting with the knife. Microscopically, the molecular layer and outer part of the pyramidal cell layers are seen to be largely replaced by concretions, having the staining reaction of an iron-calcium mixture and varying in size from small spherules to enormous confluent masses of irregular outline (Fig. 10.78). In areas where these calcifications are less dense one can see the early stages of the process in the form of

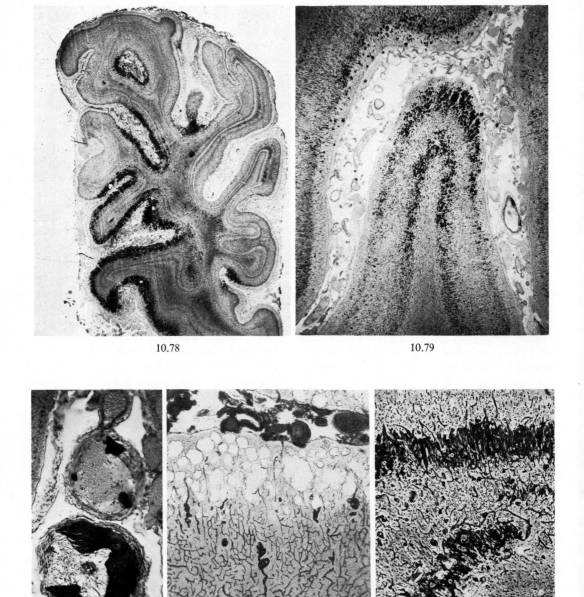

Figs. 10.78–10.82 Sturge–Weber's disease.

Fig. 10.78 Low-power view of section through occipital pole showing the venous angioma and dense calcifications mainly in the outer layers of the cortex. Carbol azure.

Fig. 10.79 The calcifications also affect the deeper cortical laminae. Carbol azure.

Fig. 10.80 Calcified meningeal arteries. Carbol azure.

Fig. 10.81 Abnormal convoluted blood vessels in the non-calcified layers of the cerebral cortex. Masson's trichrome.

Fig. 10.82 Adventitial fibrosis occasionally found in areas of laminar calcification. The calcium deposits are peculiarly dense and powdery in these areas. Gomori's reticulin.

granular incrustations of the walls of the smaller blood vessels.

Not only the outer cortical layers are affected, calcification may also pick out selectively the deeper laminae (Fig. 10.79). Scattered calcospherites and calcified capillaries are also common in the central cores of the affected gyri and in the subcortical white matter. Calcification of the larger veins may be present here. These changes in the white matter occur early in the disease, before there is any concentration of calcifications in the superficial layers of the cortex.

In some cases there is evidence of ischaemic cortical damage in addition to the destruction of tissue from the confluent growth of the calcifications. Laminar cortical necrosis with intense fibrosis of vessels and powdery calcium deposits of dystrophic type may be a prominent feature, particularly in the calcarine region (Fig. 10.82). After decalcification, an amorphous substance which stains positively with PAS remains behind. This represents the original perivascular colloidal matrix upon which the mineral salts have been deposited in successive layers (Mallory 1896).

Wohlwill and Yakovlev (1957) have described enlargement of the Gasserian ganglion in this condition. There was marked proliferation of the capsule cells and ectopic ganglion cells were present in the root. In one case a cavernous angioma was seen between the dural sheath and the nerve roots. The same authors have found angiomatous malformations in the lung, ovary and intestine in Sturge–Weber disease.

Chemical analysis of the brain shows that the mineral deposits are mainly composed of calcium phosphate and carbonate and that there is no excess of iron (Wachsmuth and Lowenthal 1950; Tingey 1955). The Prussian blue reaction given by the concretions is probably due to absorption of the available iron normally present in the tissues. Prolonged formalin fixation substantially increases the amount of iron found chemically.

Pathogenesis. It has been suggested that the Sturge–Weber disease is caused by partial chromosomal trisomy, but that in the majority of cases a translocated extra segment may not be demonstrable microscopically (Patau, Therman, Smith, Inhorn and Picken 1961). Certainly, there has been no reported familial instance of the true syndrome.

The combination of skin and pial angiomata is explicable in a general way as a malformation of the embryo's primitive vascular plexus, which precedes the formation of separate vessels for the supply of integument, skull and meninges. In the early stages of development the small telencephalic vesicle and the eye are closely approximated and the integument of the embryo's forehead might well share that part of the vascular plexus which supplies the occipital portions of the brain. The later anatomical separation of these two vascular territories occurs as the result of the subsequent growth backwards of the hemisphere. The embryological development of the blood vessels in relation to this syndrome has been well discussed by Thieffry, Arthuis, Faure and Lyon (1961). The rarity of dural and diploic hypervascularity remains an enigma. Kautsky (1949) developed the thesis that the vascular anomaly is primarily neurogenic in origin, but against the traditional view that the distribution of the facial naevus corresponds to one or more divisions of the trigeminal nerve several objections may be raised. Alexander in his monograph has pointed out how frequently these territories are transgressed and how often the naevus fails to reach the midline. Moreover, in some patients the philtrum is spared, the boundary of the naevus conforming to the defect of hare lip, and it seems probable that the distribution is determined in part by the layout of the fissures in the developing face (Alexander and Norman 1960).

The pathogenesis of the intracortical calcifications is also in doubt. As in all types of calcification the mineral deposits are laid down in a strongly PAS-positive polysaccharide matrix and it is generally held that some abnormality of permeability of the vessels is induced by the circulatory abnormalities conditioned by the meningeal angiomatosis. A case can be made for the importance of an angiomatous malformation formed by vessels of narrow calibre, since gyriform calcification is not found in association with the larger sized penetrating venous angiomas. Yet the angiomatosis in Divry and van Bogaert's (1946) case was not associated with calcification. One is forced to conclude that the rarity of overt malformation in the cortical vessels does not preclude some functional anomaly that may be a factor in the calcifying process. The building-up of crystalline hydroxylapatite in the larger concretions is probably a function of mesenchymal tissue (Bochnik 1953).

Mongolism (Down's syndrome)

The external appearance of the mongoloid brain is much more diagnostic than are the microscopical findings. The weight of the fully grown brain seldom exceeds 1200 g and is usually nearer the 1000 g level. The brain is abnormally rounded and short with a steeply rising, almost vertical occipital contour. The convolutional normalities of shape have been impressed on the developing brain by the retarded growth of the mongol skull and has pointed out that the crowns of gyri may be flattened, that the sagittally arranged sulci may show S-shaped distortion and that fibrous union may bind contiguous parts of the convolutions together.

Many microscopical anomalies have been described in mongolism but they are all shared

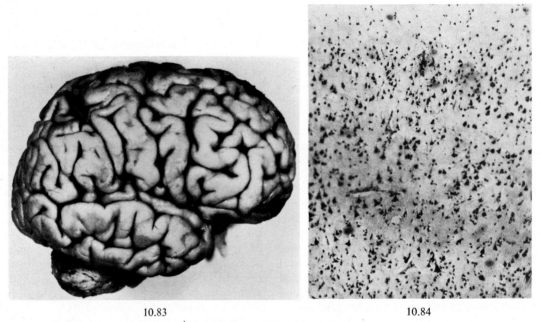

10.83   10.84

Figs. 10.83 and 10.84 Mongolism.

Fig. 10.83 Brain showing small cerebellum, flattened occipital contour and poorly developed superior temporal gyrus.
Fig. 10.84 Angular gyrus of a mongol showing diffuse loss of nerve cells in the third layer. Cresyl violet.

pattern usually shows no gross departure from normality, but there may be asymmetries on the two sides and the insula is often exposed on account of the poor development of the third frontal gyrus. Compared with the brain of a normal adult there is a poverty of secondary sulci, but the ape-like simplification of genetic micrencephaly is never found. Very characteristic of the mongol brain, though not peculiar to it, is narrowness of the superior temporal gyrus (Fig. 10.83). The anomaly is often bilateral and is present in about half the cases. Conspicuous smallness of the cerebellum and brainstem in comparison with the cerebrum as a whole is also a common feature (Crome, Cowie and Slater 1966).

Benda (1947) believes that most of these ab-

by other forms of severe oligophrenia. Davidoff (1928) reported patchy cerebral calcifications and a poverty of nerve cells in the third cortical layer of his cases (Fig. 10.84). In the writer's experience this finding is not very common, but irregularities of grouping certainly occur so that relatively acellular areas adjoin those which display an increased density due to the presence of clusters of small nerve cells. Systematic cell counts in random sections indicate that the nerve cells are, in fact, often increased on the average per unit area. This seeming paradox may be related to the small size of the brain as a whole, since, as a general rule, the more underdeveloped the state of the brain, the closer together are the cortical neurons. Benda (1947), however, believes that an active destruction of the nerve cells associated with anoxia and oedema takes place in mongols dying in infancy. The same author lays stress upon the poor myelination of the grey and white matter and has demonstrated a striking poverty of myelin in the subsulcine or U-fibres of the cortex. Meyer and Jones (1939) were the first to demonstrate a conspicuous fibrillary gliosis of the central white matter in many, but by no means all, mongols. There was often no corresponding pallor in myelin preparations, although patchy areas of demyelination were sometimes seen, as they were in Davidoff's cases. Benda has reported frequent minor malformations in the spinal cords of mongols and draws attention to a finding which he considers peculiar to the condition, namely the fusion of the columns of Clark, so that the nerve cells occupy a strip of grey matter lying behind the central canal. Except for undoubted signs of retarded or mildly perverted development, the mongol brain thus shows few pathological changes which cannot be explained on the basis of intercurrent disease. Whether such fortuitous lesions are in some way related to abnormal constitutional factors, such as general circulatory asthenia or endocrine anomalies, cannot be precisely determined at the present time. Certainly the frequent association of congenital heart disease is an important factor. Arterial and venous thromboses are well-known complications of Fallot's tetralogy, as are embolism and cerebral abscess due to detachment of vegetations from congenitally malformed or infected valves.

Middle-aged mongols often show clinical signs of premature senility and this may be reflected in the brain by the presence of senile plaques and Alzheimer's neurofibrillary change (Jervis 1948; Solitare and Lamarch 1966; Olson and Shaw 1969). In Malamud's (1972) series the brains of all mongoloids dying over the age of 40 showed lesions of this type in various degrees of severity. Ultrastructurally the neurofibrillary tangles are identical with those seen in typical cases of Alzheimer's disease (Schochet, Lampert and McCormick 1973).

Aetiology. Most, if not all, cases of Down's syndrome display various chromosomal abnormalities, such as trisomy G, D/G or G/G translocations or mosaicism. The additional chromosome in trisomy G is No. 21. The relative incidence of different chromosomal types has been remarkably constant in recorded series.

Trisomy G occurs in over 90% of cases, translocations in 2 to 4% and mosaicism in 2 to 3%. The incidence of trisomy increases with advancing maternal age, a relatively higher proportion of translocations occurs in children of younger mothers. Most familial cases are associated with translocations. The risk of a mother carrying a translocation chromosome producing another mongoloid child is somewhat less than the theoretical one in three in a D/G or G21/G22 translocation. In the rare G21/G21 translocation all children are invariably affected. For a full discussion on the cytogenetics of Down's syndrome the reader is referred to a series of articles by Polani and his collaborators (Hamerton, Giannelli and Polani 1965; Giannelli, Hamerton and Carter 1965; Polani, Hamerton, Giannelli and Carter 1965). The *pathogenesis* of the condition, or the mechanism by which an additional chromosome can cause a wide range of abnormalities with variable expressivity, has been the subject of abundant speculation, yet remains obscure.

Congenital facial palsy and ophthalmoplegia (Möbius' syndrome)

The clinical syndrome of congenital facial diplegia, often associated with ophthalmoplegia, multiple defects of muscles and skeletal deformity, has been fully reviewed by Henderson (1939) and by Dalloz and Nocton (1964). There have been few detailed pathological studies. Heubner (1900) reported complete absence of the nucleus of the abducens and diminished number of cells in that of the facialis. Spatz and Ullrich (1931) confirmed these findings and, in addition, described developmental anomalies in the nuclei of the oculomotor and trochlear nerves. The muscles supplied by the affected nerves may be absent and associated anomalies of the musculoskeletal system may be present in the extremities. When congenital unilateral facial paralysis is present in the absence of ophthalmoplegia the most likely cause is damage to the facial nerve at birth. The pathological findings in Rainy and Fowler's (1903) case can well be explained on this basis, as Stewart (1929–30) pointed out, since the Marchi stain revealed degeneration of the facial nerves throughout their course. Richter (1960), however, in an infant with unilateral facial palsy and congenital musculoskeletal anomalies who died at the age of 1 month, found only a few nerve cells in one facial nucleus and no sign of a degenerative process in the scanty intramedullary portion of the nerve. He considered the lesion to be due to developmental hypoplasia of the nucleus and not to secondary causes. The occurrence of genetically determined unilateral, as well as bilateral, cases (Skyberg and van der Hagen 1965) also militates against an exclusively traumatic aetiology.

Perinatal cerebral damage

In the previous editions of this book the term 'birth injury' was used in a broad sense to cover all types of lesion occurring during parturition. Birth in this context means the entire process of transition and adaptation from the intrauterine to the extrauterine environment and covers the whole perinatal period. The concept of injury, however, has to many readers retained its mechanical connotations and some writers prefer to draw a sharp distinction between mechanical trauma and anoxia, including in the latter category a variety of ischaemic lesions (Courville 1953, 1971; Towbin 1970). This apparently logical classification tends to obscure the complex interplay of the pathogenetic factors often involved.

Experience has shown that certain patterns of lesions recur in cases of presumed perinatal damage. The ascription of lesions found in long-term survivors to events occurring at birth is based on certain assumptions for which the evidence is largely circumstantial. In the first place it is worth emphasizing that no individual lesion or combination of lesions is pathognomonic of perinatal damage. Only in a proportion of cases is there historical evidence of untoward events at or around birth. In a higher proportion of cases a history may be discovered of circumstances conducive to cerebral damage, such as prematurity or postmaturity, unduly prolonged or precipitate labour, abnormal presentation or instrumental delivery. In the remaining cases the probability of damage at birth is still higher than either before or after. The protection afforded by the intrauterine environment renders cerebral damage unlikely, other than that due to placental insufficiency occurring in the immediate prenatal period. Postnatal damage occurring outside the perinatal period is usually well documented by a history of an illness from which a previously normal child emerged with a severe neurological handicap.

Confirmation that certain patterns of lesions commonly occur around birth may be obtained from the study of infants who died shortly after sustaining cerebral damage. The study of these acute lesions is far from complete and there are still many discrepancies between the patterns found in early and late cases. Surprisingly the significant damaging factors may be as difficult to unravel in the early lesions as in the late sequelae. Deductions as to pathogenesis of individual lesions therefore remain largely conjectural. Animal experiments have so far thrown little light on the human situation.

Intracranial haemorrhages

Subdural haemorrhage

If the fetal skull is subjected to severe anteroposterior compression, and particularly when the direction of this force is asymmetrical, the falx cerebri is stretched and in turn may pull upon one leaf of the tentorium cerebelli with sufficient tension to cause its rupture (Chase 1930). Tears in the free margin of the tentorium may involve veins draining into the Galenic system and blood from this source usually collects in an infratentorial situation. With more serious lacerations, rupture of the straight or transverse sinuses may occur with tearing of the great vein of Galen. These injuries are apt to take place during precipitate or breach deliveries. Tearing of the superior cerebral veins at their entrance into the sagittal sinus may follow excessive overriding of the parietal bones and is the commonest cause of chronic subdural haematomata (Guthkelch 1953). Rupture or thrombosis of the sinus itself has been a sequel of the overlapping of the parietal by the occipital bone (Craig 1938). This type of lesion has become less common with modern developments in obstetrics, in particular the use of elective caesarean section, but a significant incidence of subdural haematomata was still recorded in the British perinatal mortality survey (Butler and Bonham 1963).

Chronic subdural haematoma

Blood from a torn superior cerebral vein usually collects over the convexity of the hemisphere, lying above the level of the Sylvian fissure and sometimes extending from the frontal to the occipital poles. The haemorrhage may be bilateral. After clotting has taken place, organization leads to the formation of a thick outer layer adherent to the dura and composed of fibrous tissue containing numerous large sinusoidal vessels. The arachnoid surface of the haematoma becomes covered with a thin membrane composed of flattened connective tissue cells (Inglis 1946). Further haemorrhages may occur from the sinusoidal vessels of the dural membrane and a progressive expansion of the original lesion is brought about in this way or by osmosis (see Chapter 9). In long-standing cases calcification or ossification of the inner connective tissue layer may take place. Severe damage to the brain results not only from pressure upon the underlying tissues but also from compression of arteries against the edge of the tentorium, owing to displacement of the cranial contents (Lindenberg 1955). Pressure from these effusions may also interfere with the normal growth of the frontal lobes (Ingraham and Matson 1944). The enlargement of the head, seen in infants with large subdural effusions, may in part be due to a hydrocephalus of communicating type which follows obstruction of the subarachnoid space beneath the haematoma (Elvidge and Jackson 1949).

Subarachnoid haemorrhage

After severe leptomeningeal haemorrhage the surface of the brain is covered by a thin, easily detached, jelly-like layer of blood-stained meninges. In Craig's (1938) series of cases the parieto-occipital lobes were commonly affected and early softenings, oedema and microscopic haemorrhages were seen in the outer layers of the grey matter. Damage to the underlying cortex was emphasized by Dekaban (1962). These bleedings are generally regarded as asphyxial in origin and are very common in stillborn infants.

Intraventricular haemorrhage

Fatal intraventricular bleeding is almost exclusively found in premature infants (Ylppö 1919) and usually originates from the anterior terminal veins or, less often, from the choroidal veins. It is usually asphyxial in origin and may occur as a prenatal, natal or postnatal phenomenon. In the latter situation it is frequently associated with the respiratory syndrome of the newborn (Harrison, Heese and Klein 1968). It appears that prolonged anoxia, rather than single short episodes, is the major factor responsible for the bleeding.

Intracerebral haemorrhage

Large extravasations into the substance of the brain are unusual, but multiple petechial haemorrhages associated with congestion and oedema are not uncommon, and it is likely that these less lethal types of lesion may lead to neurological sequelae in survivors. Schwartz (1924, 1927) has described in detail the distribution of these haemorrhages and their subsequent evolution. He regards them as of venous origin, those in the cortex being related to the tributaries of the superior longitudinal sinus, while the more centrally placed haemorrhages occur in the drainage area of the great vein of Galen. Bilateral bleedings into the periventricular white matter of the frontoparietal and occipital regions are seen in the distribution of the anterior and posterior terminal veins and of the vena lateralis ventriculi. In the basal ganglia the most characteristic lesion is partial destruction of the head of the caudate nucleus and this may be accompanied by intraventricular haemorrhage. The thalamus also is often involved (Wald 1930), the putamen and globus pallidus rarely, though punctate bleedings are sometimes seen in the external segment of the latter.

Acute lesions of the cerebral parenchyma

Cortical lesions

Apart from haemorrhages, cortical infarction has been described in infants dying in the neonatal period. Dekaban (1962) reported bilateral haemorrhagic infarction of the occipital lobes which he suggested was the result of compression of the posterior cerebral arteries. Yates (1962) put forward the view that lesions of this type may be the result of damage to the vertebral arteries in the neck. Areas of haemorrhagic necrosis in cortical boundary zones occur in premature infants who die after prolonged hypoxia or circulatory failure (Smith 1974). The most common finding is destruction of cortical neurons which manifests itself in blanching of the cerebral cortex in Nissl preparations (Larroche 1968). It may be diffuse, laminar or patchy, often with accentuation in the depths of the sulci. An unusual variant is associated with survival of small clusters of neurons along the course of blood vessels. Neuronal damage may often be difficult to assess in cases of neonatal death. Karyorrhexis in the damaged cells may be a characteristic feature in the acute stage (Banker and Larroche 1962; Larroche 1968; Smith 1974). In his large series of 1152 cases of perinatal death Terplan (1967) found that these hypoxic brain changes occurred more frequently in full-term infants (37%) than in premature ones (13·9%).

that the small haemorrhages so often regarded by other investigators as the consequence of terminal asphyxia were only a minor indication of much more extensive damage which later led to widespread cavitation or neuroglial scarring. These progressive changes were most easily followed in the cerebral white matter in the drainage areas of the terminal veins. By the end of 24 hours the original haemorrhages were seen to be interspersed with yellowish-grey areas radiating from the region of the lateral ventricle towards the cortical grey matter. Liquefaction of the central zone then occurred and by the fourth day the texture of the peripheral tissues became loosened and fat-granule cells appeared. The stage of organization began at about the

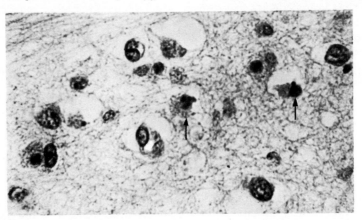

Fig. 10.85 Perinatal damage; karyorrhexis in nuclei pontis in acute anoxic lesion.

Cortical lesions of this type may be associated with similar changes in the basal ganglia and thalamus, and rarely in the brainstem, with the possible exception of the nuclei pontis where karyorrhexis is frequently seen (Fig. 10.85).

White matter lesions

Lesions in the white matter, particularly of periventricular distribution, have been the subject of many studies (Sehwartz 1924, 1927; Banker and Larroche 1962; De Reuck, Chattha and Richardson 1972). In Terplan's (1967) series these lesions were more common in premature than in full-term infants. The most detailed studies of these lesions and their evolution are those of Schwartz, who examined a large material derived not only from cases of immediately fatal birth injury but also from individuals who survived for periods of days, weeks, months and years. It was apparent

eighth day when the astrocytes at the margins of the cavity began to proliferate. After weeks or months, according to the size of the areas involved, fibrillary gliosis was well established and contained in its meshworks numerous groups of fat-granule cells (the stage of 'presclerosis'). Finally (the stage of sclerosis) the area was converted into a loose neuroglial scar.

When the tissues were more mature, or the vascular disturbances less intense, the general structure of the ground substance was preserved, and instead of liquefaction and cavity formation the process was one of destruction of axis cylinders and replacement by fibrillary neuroglia. The early stages were marked by the appearance of large numbers of lipid phagocytes, the so-called 'encephalitis' of Virchow. This is a pathological phenomenon associated with tissue breakdown and readily distinguishable from the normal increase in neuroglial cells which is always found in regions undergoing myelination (Roback and Scherer 1934).

Periventricular lesions in the newborn are not necessarily haemorrhagic. Banker (1961) describes as a frequent finding in premature infants the presence of coagulation necrosis, giving the macroscopic appearance of waxy or white streaks. In a later paper Banker and Larroche (1962) point out that these lesions tend to lie in the arterial boundary zones of the white matter. De Reuck, Chattha and Richardson (1972) also support the arterial origin of periventricular leucomalacia. They point out that these lesions often occur in the terminal territories of the ventriculopetal penetrating arteries, or in the boundary zone between the ventriculopetal and ventriculofugal arteries, either choroidal or striatal. It would seem that venous stasis may not be the only factor involved in their production.

A somewhat different lesion of the white matter was described by Courville (1960a) under the name of central haemorrhagic encephalopathy. Three infants dying during the first day of life after severe asphyxia and respiratory distress showed a diffuse, if somewhat irregular haemorrhagic infiltration of the white matter, sparing the cortex and the basal ganglia. The author suggested that this lesion might be a precursor of the cystic degeneration of the white matter.

A further feature of many infants dying during the neonatal period is massive oedema of the white matter (Veith 1962). The mechanism of this swelling and its significance in the pathogenesis of chronic cerebral damage remain obscure.

Late neuropathological sequelae of birth injury

The following varieties of long-standing lesion may be found singly or in combination with one another in the brains of patients suffering from cerebral palsy attributable to perinatal causes.

Cortex

Ulegyria (atrophic sclerosis; mantle sclerosis; sclerotic microgyria). In this condition the general convolutional pattern of the cortex is preserved but individual gyri or groups of gyri show varying degrees of shrinkage and sclerosis (Fig. 10.86). The most characteristic feature is the localized destruction of the lower parts of the walls of the convolution with relative sparing of its crown. The bulbous neuron-bearing crown and upper portion of the affected gyrus may be supported only by a narrow fibrous stalk from which all neural elements have disappeared ('mushroom' gyrus). Thus from the surface the uncut brain may have a deceptive appearance of normality since the greater part of the damage is hidden. In its minimal form this type of lesion expresses itself merely as a thinning of the grey matter in the depths of the sulci, and may easily be overlooked in myelin preparations, though the associated gliosis, which shows up as sharply defined, semilunar scars, is obvious enough in sections stained by Holzer's method (Figs. 10.91 and 10.92). The transition between the severely damaged and less affected regions tends to be abrupt, so that clear-cut complementary myelin and neuroglial pictures are the rule. The middle zone of the less affected cortical grey matter often shows a thin streak of laminar atrophy (Figs. 10.95 and 10.96), the margins of which contain abnormally dense aggregations of myelinated fibres. This phenomenon is termed 'hypermyelination' and collections of myelinated fibres in the form of plaques, networks, or whorls, are a common feature of ulegyria (Figs. 10.87 and 10.88). The white matter subjacent to the affected gyri usually shows considerable gliosis associated with a thinning of myelinated fibres or small cystic spaces. Lesions of the medullary core of the convolution vary from a thin linear strip of sclerosis, marking an area devoid of myelin, to gross cavitation. The most advanced stage of dissolution is seen in the 'hollow gyrus' the outline of which is maintained largely by the remaining molecular layer.

A condition resembling the 'granular atrophy' of the adult cortex may sometimes be present, both the walls of convolutions and their crowns presenting multiple small bosses due to the separation of islands of nerve cells by fibrillary neuroglia. The neuroglial fibres are sometimes arranged in dense bundles, slightly constricted in the middle and spreading out at both ends (the 'wheatsheaf' pattern). More commonly, the cortex shows narrow vertically disposed areas of clearing which correspond to the course of cortical branches of meningeal arteries. Sometimes one-half of a gyrus is destroyed and occasionally the whole convolution is represented as a thin leaf-like structure composed mainly of neuroglial fibres. The meninges covering sclerotic microgyria of this sort show fibrous thickening but are rarely adherent to the cortex. In these areas of ulegyria the small meningeal arteries

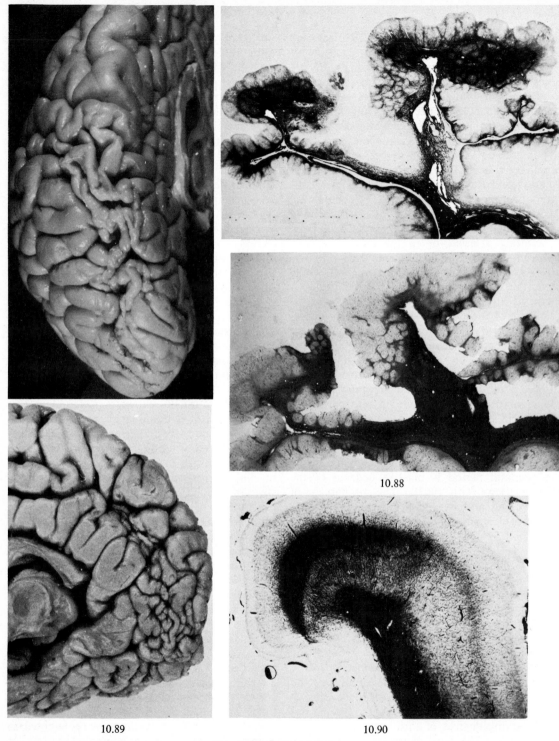

Figs. 10.86–10.90 Birth injury.

Fig. 10.86 Typical ulegyria of the superior parietal lobule.

Figs. 10.87 and **10.88** Hypermyelinated ulegyria. Note the linear streaks of necrosis in the central cores of the gyri. Corresponding Kultschitsky–Pal and Holzer preparations.

Fig. 10.89 Ulegyria of the calcarine cortex spreading a short distance along the lips of the cingulate sulcus.

Fig. 10.90 Hypermyelination of the stria of Gennari in an area adjoining partial destruction of the calcarine cortex. Heidenhain's myelin.

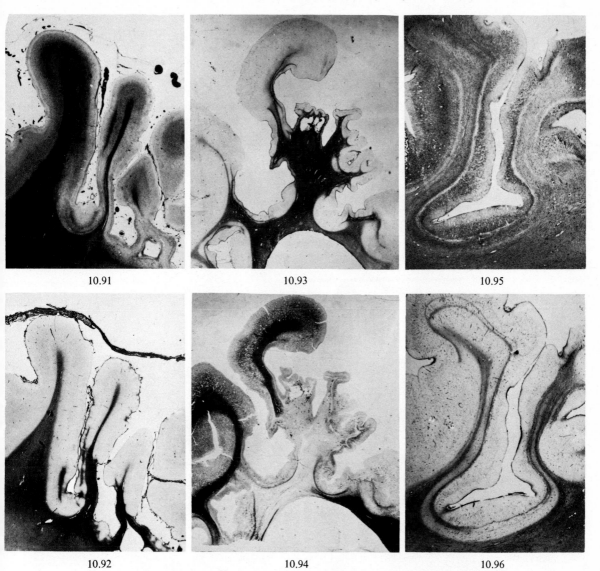

10.91   10.93   10.95

10.92   10.94   10.96

Figs. 10.91-10.96 Birth injury.
Figs. 10.91 and **10.92** Corresponding myelin and neuroglial preparations to show typical distribution of ulegyria in the central region. The precentral gyrus (on the left) is relatively intact. Heidenhain and Holzer.
Figs. 10.93 and **10.94** Cluster of small sclerotic microgyric formations (from the ulegyric area illustrated in Fig. 10.89. Kultschitsky–Pal and Holzer.
Figs. 10.95 and **10.96** Laminar loss of nerve cells and gliosis in the deeper part of the gyral walls and floor of a sulcus. Carbol azure and Holzer.

often show calcification of the elastica and thin eccentric plaques of subintimal fibrosis (Meyer 1949). These changes are more frequently seen in the depths of the sulci. In the atrophic grey matter it is usual to find considerable proliferation of the adventitial coats of the blood vessels, but connective tissue plays little or no part in the attempted repair of the encephalomalacia.

There are certain commonly recurring patterns in the distribution of these lesions. In the first place, ulegyria may be present in boundary zones between main arterial territories (Meyer 1953; Norman, Urich and McMenemey 1957). It is a characteristic feature of these lesions that both hemispheres may be involved in roughly symmetrical fashion. Thus the second frontal gyri

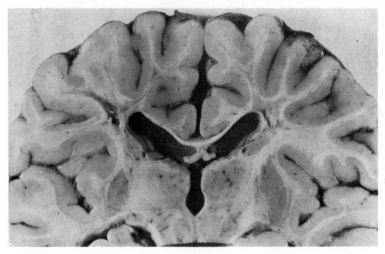

10.97

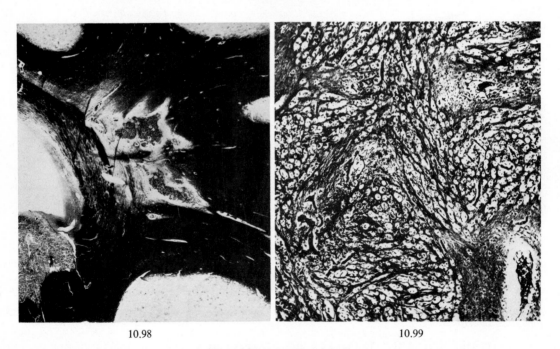

10.98   10.99

Figs. 10.97–10.99   Birth injury.

Fig. 10.97   Coronal section of the brain showing paraventricular softenings, more marked on the left.   The ventricles are dilated.   From a spastic idiot aged 4½ years, who showed bilateral *état marbré* of the medial thalamic nuclei.

Fig. 10.98   Paraventricular softening in an 8-month-old idiot.   Large aggregations of fat granule cells are still present.

Fig. 10.99   Microscopic appearances of area of softening shown in previous figure.   Fat granule cells are enmeshed in strands of fibrillary neuroglia.   (Schwartz's stage of 'presclerosis'.)   Hortega's method for astrocytes.

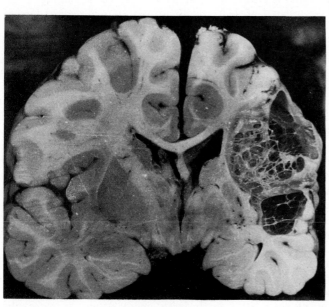

10.100

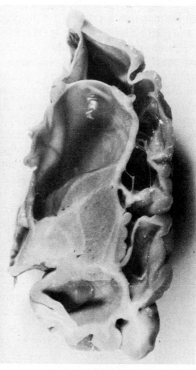

10.101

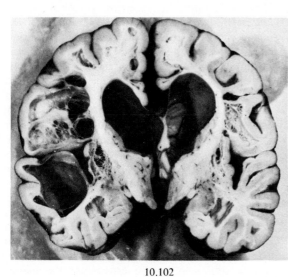

10.102

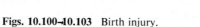

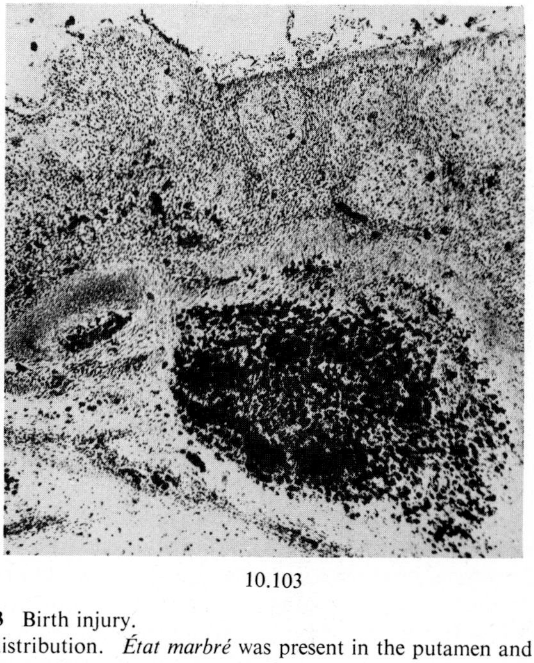

10.103

Figs. 10.100–10.103 Birth injury.
Fig. 10.100 Unilateral softening of middle cerebral arterial distribution. *État marbré* was present in the putamen and caudate nucleus of the affected side.
Fig. 10.101 Extensive cavitation of the central white matter ('central porencephaly'). The condition was bilateral. 8-month-old idiot. Twin birth; other twin dead *in utero* for several days.
Fig. 10.102 Cystic encephalomalacia of subcortical white matter. Note the bilateral softening of the putamina.
Fig. 10.103 Accumulations of fat granule cells in subcortical white matter (same brain as in Fig. 10.101). Scharlach R. and haematoxylin.

may be selectively involved, the lesions arching round the frontal pole and affecting a narrow strip of the orbital surface (Fig. 10.104). Boundary zone lesions of the parietal lobe reveal themselves most clearly as areas of atrophic sclerosis running in an anteroposterior direction through the upper part of the lobe and separated from the great longitudinal fissure for the greater part of their extent by a strip of preserved cortex. The middle temporal gyrus, lying between the main territories of the middle and posterior cerebral arteries, though theoretically at risk, has not yet been found affected in cases of birth injury.

Secondly, ulegyria may be limited to the fields of individual arterial branches. The territories supplied by the calcarine and posterior temporal branches of the posterior cerebral artery are often bilaterally involved (Norman and Urich 1962). The lips of the calcarine fissures are distorted by worm-like corrugations, which on section are seen to be clusters of miniature gyri arising from an atrophied parent stalk (Figs. 10.89, 10.93 and 10.94). This type of ulegyria has been termed 'vermiform atrophy' by Courville (1971). The remnants of the visual cortex often show a characteristic hypermyelination of the stria of Gennari (Fig. 10.90). Lesions referable to the middle cerebral artery may be extensive, in which event there is usually a large cystic softening in the Sylvian region which is fringed by ulegyria (Fig. 10.100); occasionally the areas affected are those supplied by the parietal branches in their more distal distribution (Norman 1961b). The post-central gyrus seems to be particularly vulnerable but the precentral gyrus often escapes damage or shows atrophy only in the depths of its posterior wall (Figs. 10.91 and 10.92).

When ulegyria is widespread, there is always a well-marked fibrillary gliosis of the whole of the centrum semi-ovale and an associated dilatation of the lateral ventricles. In such cases there is usually a slight general shrinkage of convolutions that are not obviously atrophied, except in so far as their central cores are rather narrow and gliosed. The number of subsidiary sulci is often increased in these areas and the impression of polygyria is given (Brouwer 1949). The whole of the corpus callosum is usually very thin but is nevertheless apparently well myelinated. *Cerebellar ulegyria* (Fig. 10.105) is much less common than its cerebral counterpart. The territory of the superior cerebellar artery is usually involved, with or without its branch to the dentate nucleus

(Norman and Urich 1962). As in the cerebral convolutions, the more deeply situated folia bear the brunt of the destructive process and boundary zone lesions may be present. Unlike the lobular atrophy of epilepsy, cystic softening may be present and there may be widespread ferrugination of Purkinje cells.

Sclerosis and cavitation of the centrum semi-ovale
A characteristic central lesion of birth trauma, almost its hallmark, is rarefaction or cavitation of the tissues adjoining the lateral angle of the lateral ventricle on one or, more often, on both sides (Fig. 10.97). Only in exceptional circumstances can this lesion be acquired in postnatal life. Banker and Larroche (1962) reported a case of a 9-week-old child in whom periventricular leucomalacia developed after cardiac surgery. When there are not obvious cystic spaces in this paraventricular region, a discoloration or puckering may be visible in the fresh specimen, while staining for myelin or for neuroglial fibres always reveals a much wider area of destruction than would have been anticipated from naked-eye inspection alone (Fig. 10.98). Even 8 months after birth large aggregations of macrophages may remain enmeshed in the loose glial scar (Fig. 10.99). This lesion is referred to in the French literature as 'sclérose cérébrale centro-lobaire' (Marie, Lyon and Bargeton 1959) and has sometimes been confused with that of a true demyelinating disease. A layer of intact myelinated fibres usually intervenes between the paraventricular softening and the ependyma, but, occasionally, a diverticulum is seen which communicates directly with the ventricle. The site of the original opening may show tags of remaining ependyma which distinguish this condition from other varieties of unilateral hydrocephalus.

In contrast to this more localized paraventricular softening of the white matter, a condition known as 'cystic degeneration' (Benda 1945) may be present. In such cases the greater part of the centrum semi-ovale is replaced by a series of trabeculated cavities (Figs. 10.101, 10.102 and 10.103) and the cortex itself may be converted into a thin rind by the erosion of the medullary cores of the gyri and the obliteration of the sulcal pattern. Extensive though this destruction is, these 'bladder-like' central porencephalies (Schwartz) of birth injury are found in brains showing a much greater amount of preserved or partially preserved cortex than is seen in prenatal hydranencephaly and there is often a tendency for the parieto-occipital areas to be predominantly affected. In a few cases with a history of birth injury there are changes in the superficial veins and arteries suggestive of old thrombosis (Crome 1958).

almost complete disappearance at some levels. More commonly, the residual damage is confined to the subependymal zone of the caudate nucleus where small cystic softenings may be seen (Schwartz 1949). In a few of these cases transventricular adhesions of fibrillary neuroglia may

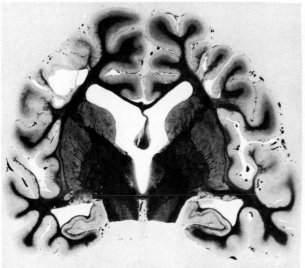
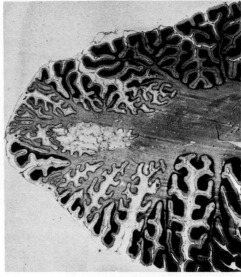

10.104   10.105

Figs. 10.104 and **10.105**   Birth injury.
Fig. 10.104   Boundary zone lesions of both second frontal convolutions.   Heidenhain's myelin.
Fig. 10.105   Boundary zone lesion of the semilunar lobules.   Carbol azure.

At the other end of the scale there are cases which show only minimal scarring and insignificant cortical lesions but considerable reduction in the bulk of the white matter. As a matter of fact, in many cases of perinatal damage, the centrum ovale and the corpus callosum appear to be reduced out of proportion to the cortical defects. This discrepancy is difficult to explain other than on disturbance of growth of the white matter. As the growth of the white matter continues well into the postnatal period and its cell population is largely derived from the periventricular matrix, it is possible that damage to this matrix may affect the postnatal growth and development of the hemispheric white matter (Lewis 1970).

Basal ganglia

Corpus striatum. The survivors of haemorrhage from the anterior terminal vein may show severe atrophy of the caudate nucleus, amounting to its

be found passing to the corpus callosum or septum pellucidum (Norman and McMenemey 1955). Cavitation of the putamina has also been described (Pfeiffer 1939) (Fig. 10.102).

État marbré (*status marmoratus*). This condition is frequently caused by birth injury, though not exclusively so, and is of considerable importance because of its association with the athetoid form of cerebral palsy. *État marbré* may be said to be present when myelinated nerve fibres are found in aggregations considerably in excess of what is normal for that particular region of the nervous system. In their typical form, as seen in the corpus striatum, these fibres are arranged in coarse networks or bundles which in myelin preparations resemble the veining of marble (Fig. 10.106). There is a tendency for these anomalous myelinated fibres to be more numerous around the large blood vessels and in one of the writer's cases dense rings of closely packed fibres surrounded some of the vessels of the medial

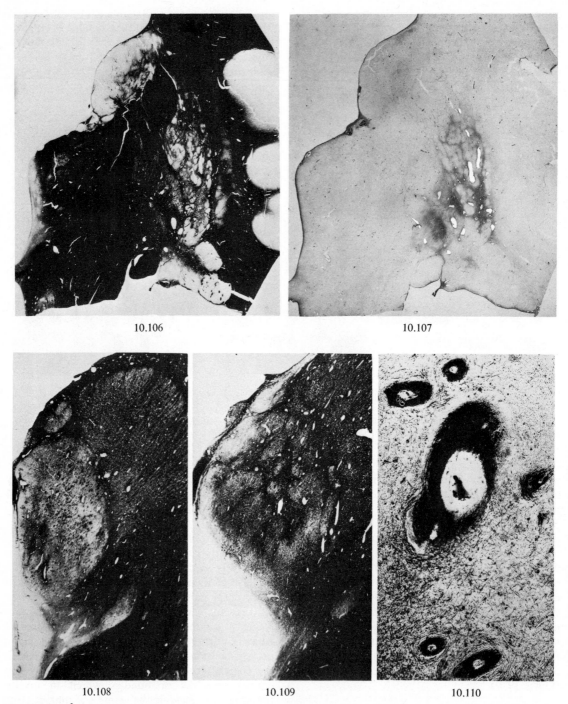

Fig. 10.106 *État marbré* of caudate nucleus and putamen.   Note the slight pallor of the outer segment of the globus pallidus.   Kultschitsky–Pal.

Fig. 10.107 Corresponding section to Fig. 10.106.   Gliosis of putamen and globus pallidus.   Holzer.

Fig. 10.108 Normal myelination of the dorsomedial nucleus of the thalamus.   Kultschitsky–Pal.

Fig. 10.109 *État marbré* of the dorsomedial nucleus of the thalamus (same brain as in Fig. 10.97).   Kultschitsky–Pal stain.

Fig. 10.110 Perivascular hypermyelination in dorsomedial nucleus of thalamus—an unusual form of *état marbré*.

thalamic nucleus and showed little or no spread to the intervening tissue (10.110). The normal myelinated fibre bundles of the putamen or caudate nucleus are not affected. The abnormal networks, together with the intervening and surrounding tissue, usually show a fibrillary gliosis of moderate degree (Fig. 10.107). As in the cerebral cortex, hypermyelination is not seen within an area of severe sclerosis though it may be present at the margins. The nerve cells of brain. The favoured sites of nerve cell loss are the ventrolateral part of the caudate nucleus, the dorsal and anterior part of the putamen, the thalamus, particularly its lateral nucleus, the external segment of the globus pallidus, the amygdaloid nucleus, the uncus and the h_2 segment of Ammon's horn, the inferior wall of the hippocampal gyrus, the cerebellar vermis and the walls of the Rolandic sulcus. These changes are usually bilateral. A characteristic depression

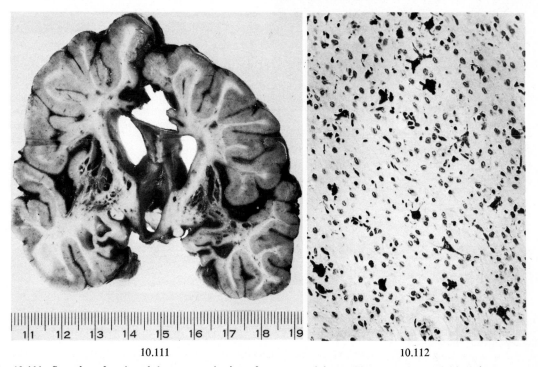

10.111   10.112

Fig. 10.111 Sequelae of perinatal damage; cavitation of putamen, globus pallidus and amygdaloid nucleus.
Fig. 10.112 Thalamic birth injury. Ferruginated neurons in area of neuronal loss and gliosis. Klüver–Barrera. × 185.

the affected part are usually conspicuously reduced in numbers, but the large neurons of the putamen and caudate nucleus appear to be less vulnerable and may be preserved in an otherwise devastated field. On the other hand, a few cases are on record in which gliosis and neuronal loss were not demonstrated (Alexander 1942; Carpenter 1955). In brains of apparently normal persons an increased density of myelinated fibres may often be seen in the most dorsal part of the putamen, but this is unaccompanied by gliosis or nerve cell loss, and cannot be regarded as pathological.

In many instances the marbling of the striatum is accompanied by lesions in other parts of the due to sclerotic atrophy is often seen in the paracentral lobules. The middle and posterior parts of the putamen are more severely affected than the anterior, the gliosis being denser and unaccompanied by marbling (Norman 1963b). A similar pattern of hippocampal, Rolandic and thalamic sclerosis has been observed in association with extensive cavitation of the putamen and globus pallidus which may represent a more severe degree of the same destructive lesion (Fig. 10.111).

État marbré is to be distinguished from *état fibreux* (C. and O. Vogt 1920), though these states may merge into each other in the birth-injured brain (Norman 1947). In *état fibreux* (*status fibrosus*) a diffuse loss of nerve cells with gliosis causes shrinkage of the tissues and a crowding together of the remaining myelinated fibres, so that the impression is given of an abnormally rich myelination of the area. The head of the caudate nucleus is markedly flattened and shows a superficial condensation of the myelinated fibres running along its inner and ventricular portion. In the putamen the usual

documented cases in which pallidal or palidoluysial atrophy has occurred in infants unaffected by neonatal jaundice. These are usually ascribed to asphyxia at birth, as in the well-known case of Scholz in which these lesions developed in an infant born in intact membranes (Meriwether, Hager and Scholz 1955). In the writer's experience post-asphyxial pallidoluysial atrophy is exceedingly rare and usually associated with widespread

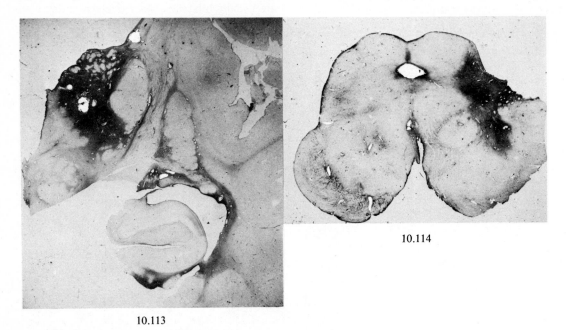

10.113

10.114

Fig. 10.113 Thalamic birth injury. The thalamus shows dense gliosis. Note the scar in the ventral wall of the hippo-campal gyrus (due to pressure by the edge of the tentorium), and the milder gliosis in the Sommer section and endplate of Ammon's horn. Holzer.
Fig. 10.114 Same brain as in Fig. 10.113. Glial scar in lateral part of midbrain probably due to local compression. Holzer.

site of the fibre increase is in the outer part of the nucleus adjoining the external capsule. This condition is usually attributable to post-epileptic encephalopathy.

Pallidal lesions. Loss of myelinated fibres in the globus pallidus, leading to striking pallor of this nucleus in sections stained for myelin, has been termed *état dysmyélinique* (*status dysmyelinisatus*) by C. and O. Vogt (1920). It is associated with loss of pallidal neurons and dense fibrillary gliosis and may occur in a variety of conditions, both in early and later life. In the perinatal context it is characteristic of the late sequelae of kernicterus. For fuller details of this now rare condition see 2nd edition, p. 397. There are, however, well-

lesions in other parts of the brain. The presence of ferruginated neurons in the globus pallidus may also help to distinguish these postasphyxial from posticteric cases.

Thalamic birth injury. Extensive retrograde atrophy of the thalamus is always found when widespread cortical or subcortical damage is present. Severe neuronal devastation, however, often occurs independently of cortical lesions. These direct effects on the thalamus may be difficult to distinguish from retrograde changes in some cases. The presence of ferruginated neurons (Fig. 10.112) favours direct damage, as does transgression of anatomical boundaries of individual nuclei and involvement of paraventricular and intralaminar cell groups. *État marbré* may be found in association with striatal marbling, or as an isolated phenomenon most commonly seen in the dorsomedial nucleus (Fig. 10.109). In interpreting these changes it must be borne in mind that there is normally a considerable variation in the myelin content of the dorsomedial nucleus (Fig. 10.108) (Alexander 1942), so that an associated loss of nerve cells should be demonstrated before the condition is regarded as pathological. It has been suggested that involvement of the thalami may be a factor of importance in the severe mental deficiency which is found in certain cases of athetosis (Norman 1947; Malamud 1950). Bilateral or unilateral damage to the thalamus, sometimes in the form of small cystic softenings, may be reasonably attributed to compression of the branches of the posterior cerebral arteries, particularly when they are associated with lesions in neighbouring parts of the brain, such as the geniculate bodies, Ammon's horn or midbrain (Walsh and Lindenberg 1961; Norman and Urich 1962 (Case 3)) (Figs. 10.113 and 10.114).

Pathogenesis of cerebral birth injury

Although conflicting opinions exist as to the importance or otherwise of birth injury as a cause of cerebral palsy, few would deny that there is ample opportunity for damage to the brain to occur during parturition. Several theories of pathogenesis have been put forward since the time of Little (1862), who suggested that 'capillary apoplexies' following asphyxia might be responsible for spastic birth palsies. The more important of these theories will be reviewed and their applicability to the lesions already described will be indicated. It is obvious that these pathogenetic mechanisms are not mutually exclusive.

Mechanical trauma. The effects of tearing of dural septa and veins during excessive moulding of the fetal head have already been mentioned. It is a debatable point whether less severe stress may also lead to significant lesions. A rise in the vertical diameter of the skull causes upward displacement of the apex of the tentorium, so that kinking of the great vein of Galen is likely to occur at its point of confluence with the less mobile straight sinus (Holland 1920, 1922). Le Gros Clark (1940) has drawn attention to the presence of a vascular structure resembling an arachnoid granulation, which may be found

above and behind the pineal gland and which, under circumstances just described, might facilitate obstruction of the vein of Galen. It is a plausible hypothesis that this mechanism, by causing severe congestion in the drainage area of the internal cerebral veins, may play a part in the production of bilateral lesions of the basal ganglia and central white matter. Whether this venous engorgement is brought about by the mechanism just described, or by asphyxial congestion, or by pressure differences as postulated by Schwartz (p. 436), it is undoubtedly true that in some fatal cases of birth injury the great vein of Galen has shown extraordinary dilatation (Turhan and Rössler 1942; Schwartz 1961).

Asphyxia. The intraventricular or subependymal haemorrhages arising from the anterior terminal veins in premature infants are commonly associated with severe asphyxia and it seems established that venous congestion from this cause may lead to the ultimate bursting of the vessel (Gröntoft 1954). Blood vessels in premature infants are fragile structures, as Ylppö (1919) showed in his classical paper, and the anatomical situation of the anterior terminal vein favours rupture since it lies beneath the ependyma and is embedded in the growth centres of the matrix which have not as yet disappeared. According to Gruenwald (1951), the walls of the veins lying in this undifferentiated tissue are thinner than those in the normal white matter. It is unnecessary to postulate mechanical trauma as a factor in this type of haemorrhage, since coincident tearing of the tentorium is rarely found in premature infants and similar terminal vein bleedings occur both in fetuses dead *in utero* and in infants succumbing to asphyxial attacks in postnatal life.

Asphyxial anoxaemia is thought by some writers to be of great pathogenetic significance in cerebral palsy (Wyllie 1951; Courville 1953). In infants asphyxiated at birth, but who have survived for two or three days, widespread 'areas of paling' may be found, especially in the striatum, globus pallidus, thalamus, nucleus subthalamicus, Ammon's horn and the amygdaloid nucleus. Homogenizing change in the Purkinje cells is also common. In such cases the cerebral cortex may escape except for paling and ischaemic nerve cell change in the central gyri. It is probable that extensive lesions of this sort are highly lethal but that the survivors will show the pattern of lesions associated with *état marbré* of the basal ganglia. In long-standing cases it is often difficult on histological grounds to distinguish between these anoxic lesions occurring at birth and those of a later, postepileptic encephalopathy, since most of the sites of predilection are common to both conditions (Weller and Norman 1955; Norman 1958). It would be equally difficult to differentiate between the residual lesions of perinatal anoxia and neonatal hypoglycaemia which is known to cause extensive neuronal necrosis (Anderson, Milner and Strich 1967). Little is known as yet about long-term effects in survivors of well-documented hypoglycaemic episodes in infancy. Banker (1967) reported her observations on three infants who survived the acute episode by a few months. All showed marked cerebral atrophy with large lateral ventricles, laminar neuronal loss in layers two and three, associated in places with *status spongiosus* and in one case with laminar calcification. Some loss of neurons was also found in the striatum and thalamus, but the cerebellum was normal in all three cases.

The calcification of the elastica and the eccentric subintimal fibrosis often seen in the walls of small meningeal arteries in areas of ulegyria are probably due to local anoxia (Meyer 1949).

Prenatal anoxaemia must also be taken into account since oxygen reserves are low in late fetal life. The hazards of even a normal birth may thus be aggravated and it is reasonable to suppose that what otherwise might have been reversible changes in the neurons may be converted into irreparable damage by the added stresses of labour. Interference with placental function probably accounts for some of the cases of cerebral palsy which follow caesarean section performed for placenta praevia (Clifford 1941). Schwartz noted as a rare finding that the pathological changes present in the central white matter of some of his neonatal cases were so advanced as to make it certain that the process had commenced before birth, and in a recently examined case the writer has seen extensive cystic degeneration of the brain in an infant who survived birth by only 24 hours. In two instances extensive cystic softening of the central white matter of the brain has been reported in infants of low birth weight whose mothers had suffered from severe anaemia in pregnancy. In both cases the treatment of the anaemia had caused serious reactions in the mother shortly before the onset of labour (Norman 1952; Sharpe and Hall 1953).

The relationship between fetal anoxia and lesions of the centrum semi-ovale and basal ganglia is most clearly demonstrated in infants who have survived the mother's attempted suicide by coal gas inhalation during late pregnancy (Maresh 1929; Neubürger 1935).

Interesting observations on the effects of chronic neonatal and infantile hypoxia were made by Brand and Bignami (1969). They studied the brains of infants with respiratory distress syndrome treated by prolonged positive pressure ventilator therapy. These infants developed interstitial pulmonary fibrosis as a result of oxygen toxicity and were subjected to prolonged hypoxia over several months. The lesions in the brains consisted of vascular proliferation and fibrillary gliosis. A marked increase in the number of small blood vessels, many of them dilated and tortuous, was found in the white matter of the cerebral hemispheres, cerebellum, brainstem and spinal cord. Fibrillary gliosis was most conspicuous in tracts undergoing active myelination during the period of hypoxia. These changes were unaccompanied by significant loss of nerve cells or demyelination.

Venous lesions: Schwartz's theory of venous stasis. Schwartz's (1924, 1927, 1961) studies on an unrivalled material convinced him that the great majority of cerebral birth injuries originated from venous lesions. In his view intense congestion of the venous sinuses and their tributaries could be brought about by blood being drawn into the presenting head after rupture of the membranes. It is generally admitted that the differential between intrauterine and atmospheric pressures is responsible for caput succedaneum or cephalhaematoma, but the novelty of Schwartz's theory was to ascribe intracerebral lesions to the same mechanism. From this standpoint birth injuries to the convexity of the cerebral cortex are to be related to circulatory stasis, thrombosis or haemorrhage in the drainage system of the superior longitudinal sinus, while lesions of the basal ganglia and centrum semi-ovale depend upon similar disturbances in the territory of the great vein of Galen.

This theory of the pathogenesis of cerebral birth injury was elaborated by Schwartz with great thoroughness and has exerted considerable influence. Bilateral ulegyria, spreading out from the margins of the great longitudinal fissure and involving the medial surface of the hemisphere as well as the upper part of the convexity, certainly suggests an antecedent sinus thrombosis and a number of cases are on record in which this pattern of lesions has been associated with obliteration of part of the superior longitudinal sinus (Norman 1936; Benda 1952). But it does not follow that lesions of a venous distribution are necessarily brought about by the mechanism postulated by Schwartz. Even with the Galenic lesions, which were so well described by Schwartz, the alternative mechanism of production described by Holland (p. 435) may carry greater conviction (Haller, Nesbit and Anderson 1956).

Compression of vessels in the depths of the sulci, whether by mechanical distortion of the brain substance or by the effect of oedema, is a likely explanation of the special vulnerability of the gyral wall so characteristic of ulegyria. The long narrow streaks of necrosis passing down the medullary cores of atrophic gyri into the central white matter (Fig. 10.87) are evidently related to the distribution of veins.

Cerebral oedema associated with venous engorgement is also a probable factor in the production of diffuse gliosis or confluent cavitation in the centrum semi-ovale. This problem of tissue anoxia due to venous stasis has been well discussed by Wolf and Cowen (1956), who have drawn attention to the occurrence of softenings in the cerebral white matter in infants suffering from cyanotic heart disease. Lindenberg (1963) believes that when white matter softenings occur in arterial boundary zones the two factors of venous congestion and systemic hypotension are involved, both being related to heart failure.

Arterial lesions. Granular atrophy of the cortex occurring in boundary zones between main arterial territories was first described by Lindenberg and Spatz (1939) in the brains of elderly individuals suffering from a form of obliterative endarteritis. Lesions of a similar distribution, for example those affecting the second frontal gyri, have since been reported in conditions associated with a severe fall in systemic blood pressure (Zülch 1954; Mettler, Cooper, Liss, Carpenter and Noback 1954; Adams, Brierley, Connor and Treip 1966). Lesions of 'watershed' distribution have also been produced by experimental hypotension in monkeys (Brierley and Excell 1966). The finding of boundary zone lesions in cases of birth injury (Meyer 1953) thus suggests that neonatal shock (asphyxia

pallida) has occurred. The mode of production of these lesions is not fully understood, but an explanation has been put forward based upon an analogy with an irrigation system supplying a series of fields with water. If there is a drop in the head of pressure it will be the last field which will suffer first (Zülch 1955). An important factor may be the presence of meningeal anastomotic channels between the major arterial territories, which may perhaps facilitate the short-circuiting of part of the peripheral vascular bed (Becker 1949a).

Lesions situated in the territory of individual arterial branches are brought about by a different mechanism. It is well known that in conditions of raised intracranial pressure displacement of the brain substance can stretch or compress arteries against the edge of the tentorium or the side of the foramen magnum, and it is thought that the same mechanism may be operative in head presentations associated with considerable cranial deformity. It has been suggested that, during birth, the uncus herniates into the incisura tentorii, causing compression of the anterior choroidal artery, and this may lead to ischaemia of the uncus and amygdaloid nucleus (Earle, Baldwin and Penfield 1953). Cerebral displacement may also cause temporary occlusion of branches of the posterior cerebral artery supplying the cornu Ammonis and adjacent parts of the temporal lobe, the thalamus (interpeduncular branches) or the calcarine cortex (Lindenberg 1955; Walsh and Lindenberg 1961). Lindenberg has brought forward evidence indicating that in states of raised intracranial pressure, such as may be brought about by oedema of the brain or by a subdural haematoma, branches of the middle cerebral artery may be compressed, the sites of predilection being at the limen insulae and at the posterior end of the Sylvian fissure.

It is an important consideration that lesions attributable to arterial compression have been found in brains also showing typical boundary zone lesions, since a low systemic blood pressure would clearly favour compression of the vessel wall (Norman *et al.* 1957). Indeed, without the intervention of this factor of reduced blood pressure, it might be difficult to conceive the soft brain tissue exerting sufficient force to occlude the lumen of an artery.

It is often difficult to assess the relative importance of these two closely associated factors. No doubt if ischaemic lesions lie in the territory of a vessel which can be kinked or compressed against a rigid structure like the tentorium it is unnecessary to ·stress the possible additional element of shock, but the situation is very different when compression by brain tissue alone is postulated. This applies to the bilateral patches of ulegyria often found in the upper part of the parietal lobes in cases of birth injury and these may well represent 'last field' lesions aggravated by local pressure. The remarkable symmetry of these lesions, and also of those of the calcarine cortex frequently associated with them, suggests the intervention of another pathogenetic factor besides compression, namely, a fall in systemic blood pressure below a critical level (Norman and Urich 1962). This theory of pathogenesis is greatly strengthened by analogous findings in cases of vascular disease in the adult. Hutchinson and Yates (1956, 1957) have shown that, in persons whose vertebral arteries in their cervical course are stenosed by atheroma, symmetrical infarction of the cerebellum and calcarine cortex may be precipitated by extraneous factors leading to a sudden fall in systemic blood pressure. Another factor operative at birth may be a local impediment to the flow of arterial blood in the vertebral arteries following intramural haematomata. Yates (1959) has demonstrated this lesion in a large number of infants dying in the perinatal period.

Pathogenesis of état marbré. The dense overgrowth of myelinated fibres present in areas of marbling was first thought to be a prenatal malformation by C. and O. Vogt (1920). More recently Alexander (1942) put forward the theory that *état marbré* of the corpus striatum was due to the aberrant ramification of the fibres of the frontopontine tracts. The writer has seen a few cases in which very coarse myelinated bundles have broken up the lateral thalamic nuclei into islands of nerve cells and in which there has been a great reduction in the size of the thalamus, striatum and globus pallidus on each side. Such findings suggest that in rare instances a prenatal disturbance of development may interfere with the normal growth of the thalamic projection fibres. The great majority of writers on the subject have followed Scholz (1924), who first suggested that the fibre overgrowth was the consequence of regenerative activity on the part of injured nerve cells. It is an incontestable fact that marbling of the cerebral cortex is very common at the margins of vascular lesions due

to birth injury; and in the adult similar formations may be seen as the sequel of carbon monoxide poisoning or in granular atrophy of the cortex associated with arterial hypertension. Widespread *état marbré* of the corpus striatum or thalamus, on the other hand, has no counterpart in the vascular lesions of adult life.

The view that *état marbré* was due to excessive myelination of regenerating or of pre-existing axons has always been open to some doubts largely due to the impossibility of demonstrating those axons by standard methods of silver impregnation. When Bignami and Ralston (1968) observed myelination of astroglial processes in long-term Wallerian degeneration in the spinal cord of the cat by means of electron-microscopy, they suggested that this process might explain the formation of hypermyelinated scars in *état marbré* and *plaques fibromyéliniques*. Borit and Herndon (1970) studied a case of marbling of the cortex and thalamus and found that many profiles of the myelinated fibres resembled astrocytic processes rather than axons. In view of the reservations which may be expressed about the interpretation of ultrastructural details in necropsy material these observations require further confirmation.

The great majority of cases of *état marbré* of the basal ganglia appear to follow birth injury, a few follow meningitis or a feverish illness in infancy (Malamud 1950) or are the sequels of nuclear jaundice or epilepsy. The relationship of *état marbré* of the corpus striatum and thalamus to birth injury has been amply demonstrated pathologically by cases in which these lesions have been found in association with typical birth injuries of the cerebral cortex or centrum semiovale (Benda 1945; Norman 1947; Sylvester 1960). In such cases the marbling of the basal ganglia is often asymmetrical and may be attributed to focal vascular lesions. The more usual symmetrical pattern of lesions described in the previous section is also evidently associated in many cases with a history of abnormal birth and neonatal distress, but the pathogenetic factor or factors responsible for this singularly stereotyped distribution are still obscure. Venous stasis in the Galenic system has been suggested as a likely factor, following Schwartz's early work (Norman 1947; Benda 1952; Schwartz 1961; Malamud 1962). Anoxia is strongly suggested by the involvement of so many areas known to be vulnerable in other conditions of clearer pathogenesis.

Some of the lesions in the hippocampus, particularly those in the resistant sector h_2 and in the inferior wall of the hippocampal gyrus, may be dictated by vascular compression due to anoxic brain swelling (Norman 1963). The often selective involvement of the cerebellar vermis and central gyri of the cerebral cortex are more difficult to explain, but have their counterparts in one or two of Windle's (1963) asphyxiated monkeys. The fact that symmetrical *état marbré* is usually a feature of full term infants may be of importance in this connection, since it is possible that by this time certain neurons are more dependent upon aerobic metabolism, especially the central gyri of the cerebral cortex which myelinate early. There is also reason to believe that an inherited factor may be operative in those few cases of striatal marbling in which another relative has suffered from athetosis. Up to the present, post-mortem examinations on both the athetoid members of the family have only been carried out in two instances. Koch (1949) recorded two identical twin idiots with double athetosis. One had striated marbling and slight pallidal demyelination, the other only pallidal changes and no *état marbré*, though in this last case the neuropathological investigation was by no means extensive. Van Bogaert (1950) has described the only example of *état marbré* verified in a brother and sister, both of whom showed thalamostriate marbling and cerebellar atrophy of lamellar type. Both patients were severe epileptics, a fact of possible pathogenetic significance. Van Bogaert explained the familial character of the disease on the basis of an inherited vascular anomaly which predisposed the individual to lesions of the type under discussion. He also pointed out that coincidental vascular lesions of a similar sort may occur in system degenerations and cited the example of *état marbré* appearing in the setting of familial myoclonus epilepsy (van Bogaert 1929).

Acute encephalopathies of vascular origin occurring in early life

The majority of cases belonging to this category conform clinically to the classical picture outlined by James Taylor (1905) in the following words: 'a child, hitherto healthy, suddenly becomes ill without any apparent cause, between the ages of 1 month and 6 years. The early symptoms are severe and consist of convulsions, fever, often vomiting and always coma. The limbs remain flaccid for some days, after which the flaccidity begins to lessen and the limbs become spastic.' It was to explain this mysterious form of infantile encephalopathy that Strümpell (1884) introduced his theory of a primary polio-encephalitis, but the intervening years have brought very little clinical evidence and no pathological confirmation of a relationship between anterior poliomyelitis and cerebral palsy of this type (Rothman 1931; Stewart 1948). No doubt this group of encephalopathies contains many examples of vascular thrombosis precipitated by sepsis or dehydration and there is the additional and highly important factor of the severe epilepsy which so often ushers in the illness and which in many cases appears to be responsible for much of the cerebral damage.

Sinus thrombosis. There is clinical evidence that partial thrombosis of the superior longitudinal sinus may lead to infantile hemiplegia (Mitchell 1952) or quadriplegia (Schlesinger and Welch 1952). The middle fifth of the sinus is the site of predilection for thrombosis and it is necessary for the clot to extend into the superior cerebral veins for a sufficient distance to obstruct the collateral circulation before haemorrhagic infarction of the cortex occurs (Bailey and Hass 1937). The veins open into the inferior angle of the lumen of the sinus and mural thrombosis in this situation will not interfere with the Pacchionian bodies which are mainly present in the upper angles of the cavity (Martin 1941). The anatomical variations in the arrangement of the superior longitudinal, lateral and straight sinuses are of considerable importance in understanding the clinical and pathological sequelae of the spread of thrombosis, particularly in cases of middle ear disease (Woodhall 1939).

There have been few adequate studies of the late neuropathological sequelae of infantile sinus thrombosis. One difficulty is that the sinus may completely recanalize and leave no residual sign of thrombosis. Another confusing point is the possibility that sinus thrombosis may have occurred in an infant whose brain has already been damaged from another cause, for example by birth injury. In cases of cerebral palsy supposedly due to sinus thrombosis, the gyral shrinkage and atrophy, with or without subcortical cystic degeneration, should occupy the region primarily affected by haemorrhage and oedema in the acute cases, that is, the upper part of the convexity including the medial surface. The intensity of the cerebral destruction should also shade off as the fissure of Sylvius is approached, unless thrombosis has spread to the Sylvian veins via the vein of Trolard. This type of distribution was found by the writer in a case of sinus thrombosis which had presumably occurred at birth or shortly afterwards (Norman 1936) and in an anatomically proved case of longitudinal sinus thrombosis which had led to unilateral cerebral atrophy (Dekaban and Norman 1958). In other cases, in which sinus thrombosis was inferred but not proved, there was marked demyelination and gliosis of the dorsal parts of the central white matter of the hemisphere in addition to the cortical ulegyria (Woolf 1955). In some instances the residual changes of an old venous thrombosis including a striking phlebectasia both within the areas of destruction and in the surrounding tissue. This may be seen both in the cerebrum and the cerebellum (Friede 1972).

Arterial lesions. Thrombosis of the middle cerebral artery is the commonest arterial lesion in acute infantile hemiplegia. Careful examination of the vessels has not often been carried out in these cases, but plaques of subintimal fibrosis associated with splitting of the internal elastic lamina have been noted in the middle cerebral trunk or in its branches by Bertrand and Bargeton (1955) in several hemispherectomy specimens. Mair (1952) has also reported similar findings. Opinion differs as to whether these changes should be regarded as the result of organization of thrombus, as seems probable, or as endarteritis following a previous infection. Certainly thrombosis of meningeal and larger arteries commonly follows arteritis in tuberculous or other forms of meningitis. In a case of healed pneumococcal meningitis of many years standing Smith, Norman and Urich (1957) found evidence of recanalization of the anterior and middle cerebral arteries at the base of the brain (Fig. 10.118). Almost complete destruction of the hemispheres had occurred in the areas supplied by these four vessels (Figs. 10.115 and 10.117). The bladder-like wall of the atrophied hemisphere consisted of four layers, the leptomeninges, the narrow gliotic cortical ribbon and a loose meshwork of connective tissue and blood vessels separated from the ventricle by a very thin layer of fibrous tissue, the 'membrana pia accessoria' (Fig. 10.116). The latter two layers are not found in prenatal

hydranencephaly and may be absent in parts of the cyst walls overlying old softenings in cases of birth injury.

Infantile atheroma is a possible rare cause of hemiplegia and the case reported by Ford and Schaffer (1927) may perhaps belong to this category. Dissecting aneurysm of the middle cerebral artery (see p. 140) is another rare cause of infantile hemiplegia (Norman and Urich 1957).

Embolism from congenital heart disease or thrombosis associated with polycythaemia are not uncommon complications of mongolism. Prenatal embolism of the internal carotid artery of obscure origin has been reported by Clark and Linell (1954). Cocker, George and Yates (1965) ascribed some of the obscure arterial obstructions to possible emboli derived from placental veins. Carmichael has suggested that a clot detached from the severed umbilical vein might under certain circumstances enter the arterial side of the circulation through the as yet unclosed foramen ovale. Neonatal paradoxical embolism of this sort would be favoured by states of asphyxia leading to a rise in pressure in the right auricle. These hypotheses could explain some of the mysterious cases of unilateral middle cerebral softenings, apparently present from birth, which are often vaguely ascribed to birth injury for want of a more plausible theory of pathogenesis.

Infantile encephalopathies of obscure origin

Under this title Lyon, Dodge and Adams (1961) reviewed a group of cases in which previously healthy infants or children suddenly become ill with fever, stupor or coma and, commonly but not invariably, convulsions. Respiratory difficulty and circulatory collapse often supervene and the patient may die within a few hours or days of the disease. Survivors may either recover completely or remain permanently handicapped both mentally and physically. The cerebrospinal fluid is usually under raised pressure but otherwise normal. The brains of children who die in the acute stage are swollen in most, but not all, cases. Microscopic changes are non-specific and consist either of hydropic degeneration or pyknosis of neurons, both of which are common agonal changes or may even be post-mortem artefacts. In long-term survivors with cerebral damage, the lesions conform to a postanoxic or postepileptic pattern. The authors discuss infection, fever, water and electrolyte imbalance, and hypoxia as

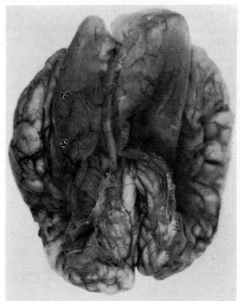

10.115

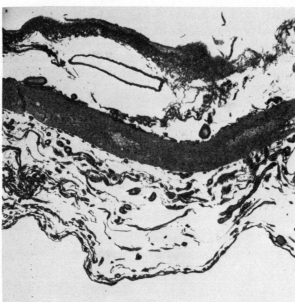

10.116

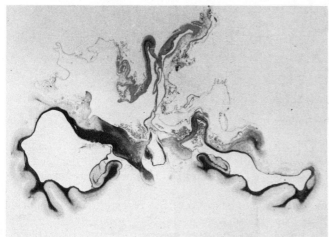

10.117

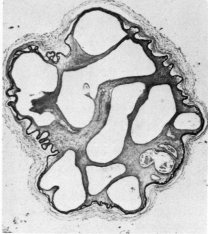

10.118

Figs. 10.115–10.118 Porencephaly.

Fig. 10.115 Superior surface of brain showing bladder-like remnants of frontal and parietal lobes. Case of arrested pneumococcal meningitis with thrombosis of anterior and middle cerebral arteries of both sides. Death at 12 years (11 years after the original illness).

Fig. 10.116 Structure of the membranous wall of the hemisphere. From without inwards (1) leptomeninges, (2) gliotic band of residual cortex, (3) meshwork of connective tissue and blood vessels derived from white matter and separated from the ventricle by (4) a thin layer of fibrous tissue, the 'pia accessoria'. Masson's trichrome.

Fig. 10.117 Coronal section of the brain showing preservation of areas supplied by the posterior cerebral arteries. Heidenhain's myelin.

Fig. 10.118 Middle cerebral artery in the subarachnoid space at base of brain (Fig. 10.115) showing recanalization. H & E.

possible aetiological factors without reaching definite conclusions. In their study of post-vaccinial encephalopathy in young infants Ehrengut, Ehrengut-Lange, Seitz and Weber (1972) put forward the view that these non-specific encephalopathies are the infantile equivalent of postinfective demyelinating encephalitis which does not occur before the age of 2 years. This relationship between infantile encephalopathy and the demyelinating or haemorrhagic encephalitides was already adumbrated by Brain, Hunter and Turnbull (1929).

A variant of this condition, associated with striking lipid infiltration of the liver and, to a

necropsy it is usual to find one hemisphere somewhat smaller than the other and its convolutions shrunken, especially in the temporal lobe where gyral atrophy may be pronounced (Figs. 10.119 and 10.120). Microscopically there are extensive pseudolaminar losses of nerve cells over large areas of the cerebral cortex, and these are not always confined to the macroscopically smaller hemisphere. The outer cortical layers are often diffusely affected so that the large pyramidal cells of the third layer form the most superficial part of the grey matter. Here and there, especially in the middle and inferior temporal gyri, the cortical cell losses may be more severe and almost

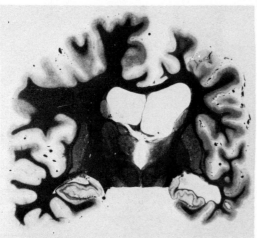

10.119   10.120

Figs. 10.119 and **10.120**   Post-epileptic encephalopathy.   Myelin and Holzer preparations of a brain showing post-epileptic hemiatrophy.

lesser extent, the kidneys ('white liver disease'), was described by Reye, Morgan and Baral (1963) (see p. 177).

It is still debatable what part, if any, these acute episodes play in the pathogenesis of the lesions to be described below.

Cerebral hemiatrophy
(Progressive lobar sclerosis of Schob)
In these cases the birth history and neonatal development are usually normal and the first sign of trouble is a severe fit or series of fits, usually experienced in early life, after which a persistent weakness of one side of the body is observed. The fits recur and, in apparent association with them, mental defect and hemiplegia or quadriplegia become established. At

the whole grey matter may be denuded. Even so, the sharply outlined areas of neuroglial scarring and severe myelin loss, which are characteristic of the ulegyria of birth injury, are never seen.

When the precentral gyrus is involved by laminar atrophy the deeper layers are usually well preserved and the pyramidal tract remains intact despite the contralateral spastic hemiparesis (Fig. 10.121). The condition of 'intracortical hemiplegia' (Spielmeyer 1906) or 'hemiplegia with intact pyramidal tracts' (Bielschowsky 1916-18a) has been attributed to the widespread laminal cell losses in the cortex, on account of which the cells of origin of the pyramidal tract no longer receive their normal afferent impulses. Penfield (1954) states that dexterous, voluntary movements are still possible after excision of the gyri surrounding the precentral gyrus. The 'patterned flow of impulses' received by the motor cortex cannot, therefore, be transcortical in origin as has often been assumed, but must

is usually the more affected and is macroscopically smaller.

Changes characteristic of epilepsy are almost invariably present in the cornu Ammonis, uncus and amygdaloid nucleus of the atrophied side

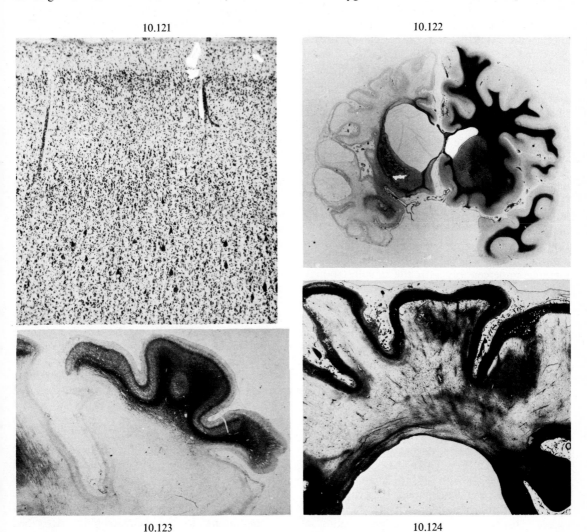

10.121

10.122

10.123

10.124

Fig. 10.121 Typical laminar atrophy of the outer layers of the motor cortex in epilepsy. Carbol azure.
Fig. 10.122 Hemiatrophy with status spongiosus. Note the shrinkage of left caudate nucleus and myelinised scar in putamen. Heidenhain's myelin.
Fig. 10.123 Same case as in Fig. 10.122 showing preservation of part of the visuosensory cortex. Kultschitsky–Pal.
Fig. 10.124 Part of the atrophied wall of the hemisphere showing dense gliosis of the superficial cortical layers and spongy state of the central white substance. PTAH.

depend upon the integrity of the thalamic connections.

In severely demented patients the cerebral cortex of both hemispheres may show laminar atrophy but even in these cases one hemisphere

and often also in the hippocampus of the less affected hemisphere. The cerebellum frequently shows a lobular atrophy mainly affecting the deeper folia. *État marbré* of the putamen may occur but seldom to the extent found after birth injury. The changes in the thalamus vary from small losses of nerve cells to massive atrophy. Since the centromedian nucleus is conspicuously exempt from pathological change unless the putamen has also been damaged, this thalamic atrophy appears to be largely retrograde from the cortex, an explanation first put forward by Bielschowsky (1916) and supported by Meyer, Beck and Sheppard (1955) in their case of severe cerebral damage following status epilepticus.

Hemiatrophy with status spongiosus. In the type of cerebral atrophy just described the pathological findings are consistent with a process of selective destruction of nerve cells occurring mainly in certain vulnerable regions of the nervous system. A much smaller number of cases is on record in which the lesions of the affected hemisphere are far more extensive and severe (Fig. 10.122). The leptomeninges are thickened and adherent to the underlying cortex, which is reduced to an outer rind of densely gliosed tissue of varying depth and an inner zone of loose neuroglial fibrils merging imperceptibly into the equally spongy, gliosed demyelinated centrum semi-ovale (Fig. 10.124). The cingulate gyrus and the calcarine area are the least affected parts of the cortex. The lateral ventricle of the atrophied side and the 3rd ventricle are dilated and the thalamus shrunken. Cases belonging to this group have been described by Siegmund (1923), Hallervorden (1939), Clark and Russell (1940) and Norman (1956). In Hallervorden's case the less affected hemisphere showed a small area of gyral *status spongiosus*, but with this exception the unilaterality of the cortical degeneration has been a remarkable feature. There has also been a clinical association with an initial bout of severe fits and these cases have shown the typical post-epileptic pattern of lesions outside the cerebral cortex. In Norman's case the preservation of part of the visuosensory cortex was striking (Fig. 10.123).

The pathogenesis of this extraordinary condition remains obscure, despite the obvious association with epilepsy. In Norman's case the internal carotid artery on the same side as the hemiatrophy showed a large *plaque* of subintimal fibrosis with splitting of the internal elastic membrane beneath it. These changes suggested an old mural thrombus and were only present at the level of the carotid syphon. While the cerebral findings were evidently not those of infarction, it is possible that the initial *status epilepticus* in this case might have been precipitated by embolism or severe arterial spasm. Hallervorden's (1930) theory of the effect of cerebral oedema due to serious transudation is a plausible explanation for the widespread spongy degeneration of the tissues. The same author attributed the common laminar lesions of the grey matter to oedema spreading along the more loosely constituted cortical layers. An abnormal permeability of the vessel walls could be induced by an infective process, but there is little to suggest encephalitis in the clinical histories of these cases, nor does the involvement of only one hemisphere favour such a conception.

Experiences from hemispherectomy

The operation of hemispherectomy was introduced by Krynauw (1950) for the treatment of infantile hemiplegia with uncontrollable epilepsy and behaviour disorders. The experience of the first 20 years was fully reviewed by Wilson (1970). This operation has yielded a large amount of material for the study of the pathology of infantile hemiplegia (Mair 1952; White 1961; Griffith 1967; Wilson 1970). The material consists of two different groups of cases. In one the hemiplegia was present since birth and the lesions are those of unilateral prenatal malformations or of perinatal damage. The other group consists of cases in which the condition developed postnatally, usually in the course of a febrile illness associated with predominantly unilateral convulsions and followed by hemiplegia and epilepsy. This sequence of events was called the 'H.H.E. syndrome' (hemiconvulsions, hemiplegia, epilepsy) by Gastaut, Poirier, Payan, Salamon, Toga and Vigouroux (1960). Two main groups of lesions were found in hemispherectomy specimens, some frankly vascular, either arterial or venous, others corresponding to the hemiatrophies described above. In the latter group many cases showed areas of more severe cortical destruction than those observed in the Schob type of hemiatrophy. These lesions were often associated with patchy rarefaction or cavitation of the white matter without reaching the total destruction of the Hallervorden type. It would appear that most cases of hemiatrophy occupy an intermediate position between the two classical types. Aguilar and Rasmussen (1960) emphasized the presence of inflammatory lesions in their material and suggested that encephalitis was an important cause of infantile hemiplegia with epilepsy. In other series, however, lesions of an infective nature were exceptionally rare. In general the study of hemispherectomy specimens has confirmed the wide range of lesions responsible for infantile hemiplegia already known from post-mortem studies (Norman 1962).

The post-hemispherectomy syndrome

The striking early successes of hemispherectomy for infantile hemiplegia have been marred by the appearance of late complications. After a trouble-free period with seizure relief lasting for some years, a period of insidious deterioration ensues. During this time there is evidence of repeated bleeding within the cerebrospinal fluid pathways, followed by the development of obstructive hydrocephalus leading to raised intracranial pressure, coma and death. The pathology of this syndrome was first reported by Ulrich, Isler and Vassalli (1965) and studied in detail by Oppenheimer and Griffith (1966). Bleeding occurs into the hemispherectomy cavity, the actual site of the haemorrhage remaining unidentified. At first the blood spreads freely over the cerebrospinal fluid pathway leading to haemosiderosis of the brain and spinal cord. The infiltration by iron pigment is most marked in the brainstem and spinal cord where it may extend to the depth of 3 mm. It also involves the tips of the cerebellar folia where it leads to a localized loss of cortical neurons. Over the remaining cerebral hemisphere the iron staining is patchy and variable. After some time the collection of blood, or blood-stained fluid, in the hemispherectomy cavity becomes encysted like a chronic subdural haematoma. The membrane is, however, not confined to the operation cavity but invests the lateral ventricle of the remaining hemisphere, so that the ventricular wall now consists of an inner collagenous layer adherent to a layer of proliferated subependymal glia in which are buried residual tubules and rosettes of the destroyed ependyma. Severe granular ependymitis also involves the lower parts of the ventricular system and may lead to gliosis and stenosis of the aqueduct. Adhesions may also form over the roof of the fourth ventricle and obliterate the foramina. All these factors contribute to the development of an obstructive hydrocephalus. After successful surgical treatment of these complications it has been observed that in some cases the inferior horn of the remaining lateral ventricle continues to expand. This localized hydrocephalus ('loculation of the temporal horn') is due to separation of the inferior horn with its choroid plexus by adhesions at the level of the vestibule (Falconer and Wilson 1969).

Alpers' disease
(poliodystrophia cerebri progressiva)

In a group of cases closely allied both clinically and pathologically to the post-epileptic encephalopathies, the claim has sometimes been made that the cerebral destruction is due to a primary degeneration of the grey matter. The illness usually starts in early life with convulsions. A progressive neurological condition characterized by spasticity, myoclonus and dementia ensues; this is often terminated by status epilepticus. Histological examination reveals extensive pseudo-laminar destruction of nerve cells in the cerebral cortex, usually most severe and accompanied by *status spongiosus* in the third and often the fifth layer. There is an increased activity of the microglial cells the processes of which contain neutral fat.

Degenerative changes are common in the striatum, thalamus and cerebellum, while in a few cases lesions in the globus pallidus, sub-thalamic nucleus and substantia nigra have been noted. One cerebral hemisphere may be particularly affected, as in the original case of Alpers (1931) whose name is often attached to this clinico-pathological syndrome.

In three cases, those of Alpers (1931), Christensen and Krabbe (1949) and Kramer (1953), minor developmental abnormalities in the form of 'immature' ganglion cells in the cerebral cortex were considered to be of pathological significance. Kramer also reported conspicuous groups of nerve cells in the white matter and underdevelopment of the cerebellar vermis and flocculi.

The disease may appear in a setting of apparent familial incidence, as in the brother and sister described by Ford, Livingstone and Pryles (1951), in both of whom the neuropathological examination revealed the characteristic lesions. In the family described by Kramer (1953), however, only one sibling showed the typical changes of progressive degeneration of the cortical grey matter, the other affected member being an idiot from birth with multiple cystic softenings in the brain. More recently Alpers (1960) has

Figs. 10.125 and **10.126**
Subtotal softening of the cerebral
hemispheres.

Fig. 10.125   Group of ferruginated neurons in cortical remnant.   Carbol azure.   × 185.

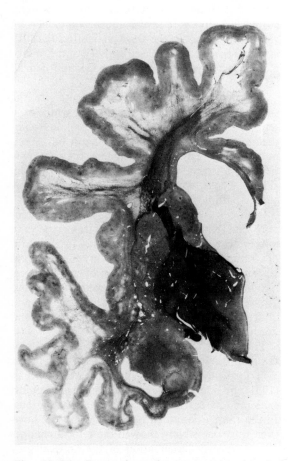

Fig. 10.126   Destruction of cortex and subcortical
white matter with preservation of deeper structures.
Kultschitsky–Pal.   × 1·65.

admitted seven other cases into this category:
those of Freedom (1927); Christensen and Krabbe
(1949); Ford *et al.* (1951: 3 cases); Kramer (1953);
and Jervis (1957).   Closely similar changes in the
grey matter, but accompanied by demyelination
in the centrum ovale or cerebellum have been
reported by De Jong and Bebin (1956); Löken
and Hörsdall (1961) and Liu and Sylvester (1960).
   Many more cases have been reported in recent
years and reviewed, among others, by Blackwood,
Buxton, Cumings, Robertson and Tucker (1963),
Christensen and Hojgaard (1964), Greenhouse
and Neubuerger (1964), Dreifuss and Netsky
(1964), Laurence and Cavanagh (1968) and
Jellinger and Seitelberger (1970).   It is apparent
that the eponym 'Alpers' disease' has been used
to cover a heterogeneous collection of cases
which are best divided with Jellinger and Seitelberger into three groups: (1) symptomatic, (2)
idiopathic, (3) atypical and unclassified.   The
first group includes cases of extensive perinatal
cortical damage (Courville 1960*b*) of post-
epileptic atrophy (Greenhouse and Neubuerger
1964) and possibly of an encephalitic process
(Dreifuss and Netsky 1964).   The second group
includes cases with normal birth, followed by
some delay in development and a steadily progressive neurological illness, characterized by
myoclonus, generalized convulsions, spasticity,
choreo-athetosis, progressive blindness and deafness, and profound mental deterioration.   Epileptic seizures usually follow the onset of the

illness but in some cases may be absent. A considerable proportion of these cases is familial, more than one sibling being affected, suggesting an autosomal recessive inheritance. The lesions are as a rule more severe than in postepileptic cases. The brains are strikingly microcephalic and the loss of cortical neurons is almost total, often accompanied by *status spongiosus* (Jellinger and Seitelberger 1970; Hopkins and Turner 1973). There is marked astrocytic gliosis, involving both the cortex and the greatly reduced white matter, as well as proliferation of phagocytic cells containing sudanophilic, anisotropic lipid. Crompton (1968), in reporting a non-familial case, drew attention to the similarity of appearance of the cortical lesions with those seen in Jakob–Creutzfeld's disease and spongiform encephalopathy of later life. The progressive nature of the process is well illustrated by comparison of biopsies, taken early in the course of disease, with post-mortem findings (Blackwood *et al.* 1963). Jellinger and Seitelberger (1970) believe that the initial changes consist of spongy transformation of the neuropil due to vacuolation of neuronal processes and hydropic swelling of astroglia. They suggest the term 'spongy glioneuronal dystrophy in infancy and childhood' to replace previous designations of the condition. However, even within the 'idiopathic' and familial group there appears to be considerable variation in the distribution of lesions. Laurence and Cavanagh (1968) emphasize the contrast between the almost total destruction of the cortex and the excellent preservation of the basal ganglia, brainstem and cerebellum. In other cases, however, the severity of cerebellar involvement was comparable with that of the cerebral cortex, and

lesions have also been reported in the globus pallidus, thalamus (other than retrograde degeneration) and in the substantia nigra. Outside the central nervous system some observers have recorded lesions in the liver: severe fatty infiltration (Jellinger and Seitelberger 1970) or cirrhosis (Blackwood *et al.* 1963; Wefring and Lamvik 1967; Hopkins and Turner 1973).

Alpers' disease must be distinguished from a small group of sporadic cases of *subtotal softening of the cerebral hemispheres* in infancy (Edinger and Fischer 1913; Jakob 1922, 1931; Schob 1929-1930; Courville 1960*c*). A fairly typical clinical history is that of an apparently normal birth, followed by epileptic seizures, irregular fluctuations in respiratory and cardiac rates, unresponsiveness to sensory stimuli and rapidly developing spasticity with opisthotonus. Death follows after a few months. At autopsy there is generalized atrophy of the cerebral hemispheres with softening of the cerebral cortex and white matter. In some cases the vertebro-basilar territory is better preserved than the carotid. Macroscopically there is an almost total loss of cortical neurons, with preservation of small groups of ferruginated cells in a dense glial stroma (Fig. 10.125). The white matter shows either total necrosis with cavitation and accumulation of lipid phagocytes, or may consist of a loose network of glia enclosing cystic spaces. In a case examined by the writers, sparse myelinated fibres were preserved in the periventricular white matter (Fig. 10.126). The basal ganglia, brainstem and cerebellum are usually remarkably well preserved. The lesions bear some similarity to those seen in the Hallervorden type of hemiatrophy, but are bilateral and symmetrical.

References

Adams, J. H., Brierley, J. B., Connor, R. C. R. & Treip, C. S. (1966) The effects of systemic hypotension upon the human brain. Clinical and neuropathological observations in 11 cases. *Brain*, **89**, 235-268.

Addison, T. & Gull, W. (1851) On a certain affection of the skin. Vitiligoidea alpha plana, beta tuberosa. *Guy's Hospital Reports 2nd series*, **7**, 256-276.

Adelmann, H. B. (1930) Problem of cyclopia. *Quarterly Review of Biology*, **11**, 161-182, 284-304.

Aguilar, M. J. & Rasmussen, T. (1960) Role of encephalitis in pathogenesis of epilepsy. *Archives of Neurology (Chicago)*, **2**, 663-676.

Åkesson, H. O. (1966) Condition at birth and mental deficiency. *Acta genetica (Basel)*, **16**, 283-304.

Alexander, G. L. & Norman, R. M. (1960) *The Sturge–Weber Syndrome*, Wright, Bristol.

Alexander, L. (1942) The diseases of the basal ganglia. *Research Proceedings of the Association for Research in Nervous and Mental Diseases*, **21**, 334-493.

Alpers, B. J. (1931) Diffuse progressive degeneration of grey matter of cerebrum. *Archives of Neurology and Psychiatry (Chicago)*, **25**, 469-505.

Alpers, B. J. (1960) Progressive cerebral degeneration of infancy. *Journal of Nervous and Mental Diseases*, **130**, 442-448.

Alvord, C. E. (1961) The pathology of hydrocephalus in *Disorders of the Developing Nervous System* (Eds. Fields and Desmond), pp. 343-419, Charles C. Thomas, Springfield, Ill.

Alvord, C. E. & Marcuse, P. M. (1962) Intracranial cerebellar meningoencephalocele (posterior fossa cyst) causing hydrocephalus by compression of the incisura tentorii. *Journal of Neuropathology and Experimental Neurology*, **21**, 50-69.

Alzheimer, A. (1904) Einiges über die anatomischen Grundlagen der Idiotie. *Zentralblatt für Nervenheilkunde*, **15**, 497-505.

Anderson, F. M. & Landing, B. H. (1966) Cerebral arachnoid cysts in infants. *Journal of Pediatrics*, **69**, 88-96.

Anderson, J. M., Milner, R. D. G. & Strich, S. J. (1967) Effects of neonatal hypoglycaemia on the nervous system: a pathological study. *Journal of Neurology, Neurosurgery and Psychiatry*, **30**, 295-310.

Aring, C. D. (1938) Cerebellar syndrome in adult with malformation of cerebellum and brain stem (Arnold–Chiari deformity) with note on occurrence of 'torpedoes' in cerebellum. *Journal of Neurology and Psychiatry*, **1**, 100-109.

Arnold, J. (1894) Myelocyste, Transposition von Gewebskeimen und Sympodie. *Beiträge zur pathologischen Anatomie und allgemeinen Pathologie*, **16**, 1-28.

Aronson, S. M., Volk, B. W. & Epstein, N. (1955) Morphologic evolution of amaurotic family idiocy. The protracted phase of the disease. *American Journal of Pathology*, **31**, 609-626.

Bailey, O. T. & Hass, G. M. (1937) Dural sinus thrombosis in early life: recovery from acute thrombosis of superior longitudinal sinus and its relation to certain acquired cerebral lesions in childhood. *Brain*, **60**, 293-314.

Baird, C. D. C., Nelson, M. M., Monie, I. W., Wright, H. V. & Evans, H. M. (1955) Congenital cardiovascular anomalies produced with the riboflavin antimetabolite galactoflavin in the rat. *Federation Proceedings*, **14**, 428.

Banker, B. Q. (1961) Cerebral vascular disease in infancy and childhood. *Journal of Neuropathology and Experimental Neurology*, **20**, 127-140.

Banker, B. Q. (1967) The neuropathological effects of anoxia and hypoglycemia in the newborn. *Developmental Medicine and Child Neurology*, **9**, 544-550.

Banker, B. Q. & Larroche, J. (1962) Periventricular leukomalacia of infancy. *Archives of Neurology (Chicago)*, **7**, 386-410.

Bankl, H. & Jellinger, K. (1967) Zentralnervöse Schäden nach fetaler Kohlenoxydvergiftung. *Beiträge zur pathologischen Anatomie und zur allgemeinen Pathologie*, **135**, 350-376.

Barrow, N. & Simpson, D. A. (1966) Cranium bifidum: investigation, prognosis and management. *Australasian Paediatric Journal*, **2**, 20-26.

Barry, A., Patten, B. M. & Stewart, B. H. (1957) Possible factors in the development of the Arnold–Chiari malformation. *Journal of Neurosurgery*, **14**, 285-301.

Batchelor, T. M. & Mann, M. E. (1945) Congenital glycogenic tumors of the heart. *Archives of Pathology*, **39**, 67-73.

Beck, F., Lloyd, J. B. & Griffiths, A. (1967) Lysosomal enzyme inhibition by trypan blue: a theory of teratogenesis. *Science*, **157**, 1180-1182.

Becker, H. (1949a) Über Hirngefässausschaltungen I. *Deutsche Zeitschrift für Nervenheilkunde*, **161**, 407-445.

Becker, H. (1949b) Über Hirngefässausschaltungen II. *Deutsche Zeitschrift für Nervenheilkunde*, **161**, 446-505.

Becker, H. (1952) Zur Faseranatomie des Stamm-und Riechhirns auf Grund von Experimenten an jugendlichen Tieren. *Deutsche Zeitschrift für Nervenheilkunde*, **168**, 345-383.

Benda, C. E. (1945) Late effects of cerebral birth injuries. *Medicine*, **24**, 71-110.

Benda, C. E. (1947) *Mongolism and Cretinism*, Grune and Stratton, New York.

Benda, C. E. (1952) *Developmental Disorders of Mentation and Cerebral Palsies*, Grune and Stratton, New York.

Benda, C. E. (1954) The Dandy–Walker syndrome or the so-called atresia of the foramen Magendie. *Journal of Neuropathology and Experimental Neurology*, **13**, 14-29.

Benton, J. W., Nellhaus, G., Huttenlocher, P. R., Ojemann, R. C. & Dodge, P. R. (1966) The bobble-head syndrome. Report of a unique truncal tremor associated with third ventricular cyst and hydrocephalus in children. *Neurology (Minneapolis)*, **16**, 725-729.

Bertrand, I. & Bargeton, E. (1955) Lésions vasculaires dans l'hémiplégie cérébrale infantile. *Excerpta medica (Amsterdam)*, Sect. VIII, 871-873.

Bertrand, I. & Gruner, J. (1955) Status verrucosus of cerebral cortex. *Journal of Neuropathology and Experimental Neurology*, **14**, 331-347.

Bickers, D. S. & Adams, R. D. (1949) Hereditary stenosis of the aqueduct of Sylvius as a cause of congenital hydrocephalus. *Brain*, **72**, 246-262.

Bielschowsky, M. (1914) Über tuberöse Sklerose und ihre Beziehungen zur Recklinghausenschen Krankheit. *Zeitschrift für gesamte Neurologie und Psychiatrie*, **26**, 133-155.

Bielschowsky, M. (1916-18a) Über Hemiplegie bei intakter Pyramidenbahn. *Journal für Psychologie und Neurologie (Leipzig)*, **22**, 225-266.

Bielschowsky, M. (1916-18b) Über Mikrogyrie. *Journal für Psychologie und Neurologie (Leipzig)*, **22**, 1-46.

Bielschowsky, M. (1920-21) Zur Histopathologie und Pathogenese der amaurotischen Idiotie mit besonderer Berücksichtigung der zerebellaren Veränderungen. *Journal für Psychologie und Neurologie (Leipzig)*, **26**, 123-199.

Bielschowsky, M. (1923-24a) Über die Oberflachengestaltung des Grosshirnmantels bei Pachygyrie, Mikrogyrie und bei normaler Entwicklung. *Journal für Psychologie und Neurologie (Leipzig)*, **30**, 29-75.

Bielschowsky, M. (1923-24b) Zur Histopathologie und Pathogenese der tuberösen Sklerose. *Journal für Psychologie und Neurologie (Leipzig)*, **30**, 167-199.

Biemond, A. (1955) Hypoplasia ponto-neocerebellaris, with malformation of the dentate nucleus. *Folia psychiatrica, neurologica et neurochirurgica Neerlandica*, **58**, 2-7.

Bignami, A. & Appicciutoli, L. (1964) Micropolygyria and cerebral calcification in cytomegalic inclusion disease. *Acta neuropathologica*, **4**, 127-137.

Bignami, A., Palladini, G. & Zappella, M. (1967) Unilateral megalencephaly with nerve cell hypertrophy: an anatomical and quantitative histochemical study. *Brain Research*, **9**, 103-114.

Bignami, A. & Ralston, H. J. III (1968) Myelination of fibrillary astroglial processes in long term Wallerian degeneration. The possible relationship to status marmoratus. *Brain Research*, **11**, 710-713.

Blackwood, W., Buxton, P. H., Cumings, J. N., Robertson, J. & Tucker, S. M. (1963) Diffuse cerebral degeneration in infancy (Alpers' disease). *Archives of Disease in Childhood*, **38**, 193-204.

Bleyer, A. S. (1938) Role of advancing maternal age in causing mongolism: study of 2822 cases. *American Journal of Diseases of Children*, **55**, 79-92.

Boisselot, J. (1949) Malformations foetales par insuffisance en acide pantothénique. *Archives Françaises de Pédiatrie*, **6**, 225-230.

Borberg, A. (1951) *Clinical and Genetic Investigations into Tuberose Sclerosis and Recklinghausen's Neurofibromatosis*, Munksgaard, Copenhagen.

Borit, A. & Herndon, R. M. (1970) The fine structure of plaques fibromyeliniques in ulegyria and in status marmoratus. *Acta neuropathologica (Berlin)*, **14**, 304-311.

Borremans, S., Dykmans, J. & van Bogaert, L. (1933) Etudes cliniques, généalogiques et histopathologiques sur les formes herédofamiliales de la sclérose tubéreuse. *Journal de Neurologie (Brussels)*, **33**, 713-746.

Bouch, D. C., Mitchell, I. & Maloney, A. F. J. (1973) Ependymal lined paraventricular cerebral cysts: a report of three cases. *Journal of Neurology, Neurosurgery and Psychiatry*, **36**, 611-617.

Bouman, L. (1934) Senile plaques. *Brain*, **57**, 128-142.

Bourneville, D. M. (1880-81) Sclérose tubéreuse des circonvolutions cérébrales: idiotie et épilepsie hémiplégique. *Archives de Neurologie (Paris)*, **1**, 81-91.

Bourneville, D. M. (1900) Idiotie et épilepsie symptomatiques de sclérose tubéreuse ou hypertrophique. *Archives de Neurologie (Paris)*, **10**, 29-39.

Brain, W. R., Hunter, R. D. & Turnbull, H. M. (1929) Acute meningoencephalomyelitis of childhood. *Lancet*, **1**, 221-227.

Brand, M. M. & Bignami, A. (1969) The effects of chronic hypoxia on the neonatal and infantile brain. A neuropathological study of five premature infants with the respiratory distress syndrome treated by prolonged artificial ventilation. *Brain*, **92**, 233-254.

Bremer, F. W. (1927) Die pathologisch-anatomische Begründung des Status dysraphicus. *Deutsche Zeitschrift für Nervenheilkunde*, **99**, 104-123.

Brent, R. L. (1967) The production of congenital malformations using tissue antisera. III. Placenta antiserum. *Proceedings of the Society for Experimental Biology and Medicine*, **125**, 1024-1029.

Brent, R. L., Averich, E. & Drapiewski, V. A. (1961) Production of congenital malformations using tissue antibodies. I. Kidney antisera. *Proceedings of the Society for Experimental Biology and Medicine*, **106**, 523-526.

Brent, R. L. & Johnson, A. (1967) The production of congenital malformations using tissue antisera. VII. Yolk sac. *Federation Proceedings*, **26**, 701.

Brierley, J. B. & Excell, B. J. (1966) The effects of profound systemic hypotension upon the brain of *M. Rhesus*: physiological and pathological observations. *Brain*, **89**, 269-298.

Brocklehurst, G.   (1968) The significance of the pathogenesis of spina bifida to its treatment.   M.Chir. Thesis, Cambridge.

Brocklehurst, G.   (1969) A quantitative study of a spina bifida fetus.   *Journal of Pathology and Bacteriology*, **99**, 205-211.

Brocklehurst, G.   (1971) The pathogenesis of spina bifida: a study of the relationship between observation, hypothesis and surgical incentive.   *Developmental Medicine and Child Neurology*, **13**, 147-163.

Brodal, A., Bonnevie, K. & Harkmark, W.   (1944) Hereditary hydrocephalus in the house mouse. II. The anomalies of the cerebellum: partial defective development of the vermis.   *Skrifter utgitt av det Norske Videnskapsakademi i Oslo*, **1**, No. 8, 1-42.

Brodal, A. & Haughlie-Hanssen, E.   (1959) Congenital hydrocephalus with defective development of the cerebellar vermis (Dandy–Walker syndrome).   *Journal of Neurology, Neurosurgery and Psychiatry*, **22**, 99-108.

Brouwer, B.   (1924) Hypoplasia ponto-neocerebellaris.   *Psychiatrische en Neurologische Bladen, Amsterdam*, **6**, 461-469.

Brouwer, B.   (1949) Traumatic changes in the brain after spontaneous delivery at full term.   *Proceedings of the Royal Society of Medicine*, **42**, 603-608.

Brun, A. & Sköld, G.   (1968) CNS malformations in Turner's syndrome. An integral part of the syndrome?   *Acta neuropathologica*, **10**, 159-161.

Brun, R.   (1917, 1918a, b) Zur Kenntnis der Bildungsfehler des Kleinhirns.   *Schweizer Archiv für Neurologie und Psychiatrie*, **1**, 61-123; **2**, 48-105; **3**, 13-88.

Bruschweiler, H.   (1927) Contribution à la connaissance de la microcephalia vera.   *Schweizer Archiv für Neurologie und Psychiatrie*, **21**, 246-282.

Bruschweiler, H.   (1928) Contribution à la connaissance de la microcephalia vera.   *Schweizer Archiv für Neurologie und Psychiatrie*, **22**, 73-121, 269-309.

Bühler, E., Bodis, L., Rossier, R. & Stalder, G.   (1962) Trisomie 13-15 mit Cebocephalie.   *Annales paediatrici (Basel)*, **199**, 198-205.

Butler, N. R. & Bonham, D. G.   (1963) *Perinatal Mortality. The first report of the British Perinatal Mortality Survey*, Livingstone, Edinburgh.

Butterworth, T. & Wilson, M.   (1941) Dermatologic aspect of tuberous sclerosis.   *Archives of Dermatology and Syphilology*, **43**, 1-41.

Cameron, A. H.   (1957) The Arnold–Chiari and other neuro-anatomical malformations associated with spina bifida.   *Journal of Pathology and Bacteriology*, **73**, 195-211.

Carmel, P. W. & Markesbery, W. R.   (1969) Arnold–Chiari malformation in an elderly woman.   *Archives of Neurology (Chicago)*, **21**, 258-262.

Carpenter, M. B.   (1955) Status marmoratus of thalamus and striatum associated with athetosis and dystonia.   *Neurology (Minneapolis)*, **5**, 139-146.

Carr, D. H.   (1967) Chromosome anomalies as a cause of spontaneous abortion.   *American Journal of Obstetrics and Gynecology*, **97**, 283-293.

Carter, C. O., David, P. A. & Laurence, K. M.   (1968) A family study of major central nervous system malformations in South Wales.   *Journal of Medical Genetics*, **5**, 81-106.

Cesaris-Demel, A.   (1895) Di un caso di rabdomioma multiplo del cuore.   *Archivio per le Scienze Mediche*, **19**, 129-157.

Chamberlain, J. G. & Nelson, M. M.   (1963) Multiple congenital abnormalities in the rat resulting from acute maternal niacin deficiency during pregnancy.   *Proceedings of the Society for Experimental Biology and Medicine*, **112**, 836-840.

Chase, W. H.   (1930) Anatomical study of subdural haemorrhage associated with tentorial splitting in newborn.   *Surgery, Gynecology and Obstetrics*, **51**, 31-41.

Cheng, D. W. & Thomas, B. H.   (1953) Relationship of time of therapy to teratogeny in maternal avitaminosis E.   *Proceedings of the Iowa Academy of Science*, **60**, 290-299.

Chiari, H.   (1891) Ueber Veränderungen des Kleinhirns infolge von Hydrocephalie des Grosshirns.   *Deutsche medizinische Wochenschrift*, **17**, 1172-1175.

Chiari, H.   (1895) Über die Veränderungen des Kleinhirns, des Pons, und der Medulla oblongata infolge von congenitaler Hydrocephalie des Grosshirns.   *Denkschriften der Akademie der Wissenschaften, Wien*, **63**, 71-116.

Christensen, E. & Hojgaard, K.   (1964) Poliodystrophia cerebri progressiva infantilis.   *Acta neurologica scandinavica*, **40**, 21-40.

Christensen, E. and Krabbe, K. H.   (1949) Poliodystrophia cerebri progressiva (infantilis): report of a case.   *Archives of Neurology and Psychiatry (Chicago)*, **61**, 28-43.

Cimmino, C. V. & Painter, J. W. (1962) Iniencephaly. *Radiology*, **79**, 942-944.

Clark, R. M. & Linnell, E. A. (1954) Case report: Prenatal occlusion of the internal carotid artery. *Journal of Neurology, Neurosurgery and Psychiatry*, **17**, 295-297.

Clark, W. E. le Gros (1940) Vascular mechanism related to great vein of Galen. *British Medical Journal*, **1**, 476.

Clark, W. E. le Gros & Russell, D. S. (1940) Atrophy of thalamus in case of acquired hemiplegia associated with diffuse porencephaly and sclerosis of left cerebral hemisphere. *Journal of Neurology and Psychiatry*, n.s. **3**, 123-140.

Cleland, J. (1883) Contribution to the study of spina bifida, encephalocele and anencephalus. *Journal of Anatomy and Physiology*, **17**, 257-292.

Clifford, S. H. (1941) Effects of asphyxia on newborn infant. *Journal of Pediatrics*, **18**, 567-578.

Cobb, S. (1915) Hemangioma of the spinal cord. *Annals of Surgery*, **62**, 641-649.

Cockayne, E. A. (1936) Dwarfism, with retinal atrophy and deafness. *Archives of Disease in Childhood*, **11**, 1-8.

Cockayne, E. A. (1946) Case reports: dwarfism with retinal atrophy and deafness. *Archives of Disease in Childhood*, **21**, 52-54.

Cocker, J., George, S. W. & Yates, P. O. (1965) Perinatal occlusion of the middle cerebral artery. *Developmental Medicine and Child Neurology*, **7**, 235-243.

Cohlan, S. Q. (1953) Excessive intake of Vitamin A during pregnancy as a cause of congenital anomalies in the rat. *Science*, **117**, 535-536.

Cohlan, S. Q. (1954) Congenital anomalies in the rat produced by the excessive intake of Vitamin A during pregnancy. *Pediatrics*, **13**, 556-567.

Cohn, G. A. & Hamby, W. B. (1953) Surgery of cranium bifidum and spina bifida: a follow-up report of 64 cases. *Journal of Neurosurgery*, **10**, 297-300.

Cohn, R. & Neumann, M. A. (1946) Porencephaly: clinicopathologic study. *Journal of Neuropathology and Experimental Neurology*, **5**, 257-270.

Conolly, C. J. (1950) *External Morphology of the Primate Brain*, Charles C. Thomas, Springfield, Ill.

Cooper, I. S. & Kernohan, J. W. (1951) Heterotopic glial nests in the subarachnoid space: histopathologic characteristics, mode of origin and relation to meningeal gliomas. *Journal of Neuropathology and Experimental Neurology*, **10**, 16-29.

Corsellis, J. A. N., Bruton, C. J. & Freeman-Browne, D. (1973) The aftermath of boxing. *Psychological Medicine*, **3**, 270-303.

Courville, C. B. (1953) *Cerebral Anoxia*, San Lucas Press, Los Angeles.

Courville, C. B. (1960a) Central hemorrhagic encephalopathy of early infancy. Report of three verified cases suggesting the genesis of infantile cystic degeneration in a paranatal anoxic disorder. *Neurology (Minneapolis)*, **10**, 70-80.

Courville, C. B. (1960b) Widespread softening of cerebral grey matter in infancy. *Bulletin of the Los Angeles Neurological Society*, **25**, 72-88.

Courville, C. B. (1960c) Syndrome of decorticate rigidity, convulsions and dementia occurring in early infancy. Review of literature and report of four verified cases with subtotal softening of forebrain. *Bulletin of the Los Angeles Neurological Society*, **25**, 1-17.

Courville, C. B. (1971) *Birth and Brain Damage*, Margaret Courville, Pasadena, Calif.

Courville, C. B. & Edmondson, H. A. (1958) Mental deficiency from intrauterine exposure to radiation. *Bulletin of the Los Angeles Neurological Society*, **23**, 11-20.

Cowen, D. & Geller, L. M. (1960) Long-term pathological affects of prenatal X-irradiation on the central nervous system of the rat. *Journal of Neuropathology and Experimental Neurology*, **19**, 488-527.

Cowie, V. (1960) The genetics and subclassification of microcephaly. *Journal of Mental Deficiency Research*, **4**, 42-47.

Craig, J. M. (1949) Encephalo-trigeminal angiomatosis (Sturge–Weber's disease) case report. *Journal of Neuropathology and Experimental Neurology*, **8**, 305-318.

Craig, W. S. (1938) Intracranial haemorrhage in new-born; study of diagnosis and differential diagnosis based upon pathological and clinical findings in 126 cases. *Archives of Disease in Childhood*, **13**, 89-124.

Critchley, M. & Earl, C. J. C. (1932) Tuberose sclerosis and allied conditions. *Brain*, **55**, 311-346.

Crome, L. (1952) Microgyria. *Journal of Pathology and Bacteriology*, **64**, 479-495.

Crome, L. (1958) Multilocular cystic encephalopathy of infants. *Journal of Neurology, Neurosurgery and Psychiatry*, **21**, 146-152.

Crome, L. (1972) Hydranencephaly. *Developmental Medicine and Child Neurology*, **14**, 224-226.

Crome, L., Cowie, V. & Slater, R. E.   (1966) A statistical note on cerebellar and brain-stem weight in mongolism. *Journal of Mental Deficiency Research*, **10**, 69-72.

Crome, L. & France, N. E.   (1959) Microgyria and cytomegalic inclusion disease in infancy. *Journal of Clinical Pathology*, **12**, 427-434.

Crome, L. & Kanjilal, G. C.   (1971) Cockayne's syndrome: case report. *Journal of Neurology, Neurosurgery and Psychiatry*, **34**, 171-178.

Crome, L. & Stern, J.   (1972) *Pathology of Mental Retardation*, 2nd Edition, Edinburgh and London, Churchill/ Livingstone.

Crome, L. & Sylvester, P. E.   (1958) Hydranencephaly (Hydrencephaly). *Archives of Disease in Childhood*, **33**, 235-245.

Crompton, M. R.   (1968) Alpers' disease. A variant of Creutzfeld–Jakob disease and subacute spongiform encephalopathy. *Acta neuropathologica (Berlin)*, **10**, 99-104.

Crosby, R. M. N., Mosberg, W. H. Jr. & Smith, G. W.   (1951) Intrauterine meningitis as cause of hydrocephalus. *Journal of Pediatrics*, **39**, 94-101.

Dalloz, J. C. & Nocton, F.   (1964) Le syndrome de Moebius. A propos de deux observations nouvelles. *Archives Françaises de Pédiatrie*, **21**, 1025-1047.

Dandy, W. E.   (1931) Congenital cerebral cysts of the cavum septi pellucidi (fifth ventricle) and cavum vergae (sixth ventricle). *Archives of Neurology and Psychiatry*, **25**, 44-66.

Dandy, W. E. & Blackfan, K. D.   (1914) Internal hydrocephalus—an experimental, clinical and pathological study. *American Journal of Diseases of Children*, **8**, 406-482.

Daniel, P. M. & Strich, S. J.   (1958) Some observations on the congenital deformity of the central nervous system known as the Arnold–Chiari malformation. *Journal of Neuropathology and Experimental Neurology*, **17**, 255-266.

Daube, J. & Chou, S. M.   (1966) Lissencephaly: two cases. *Neurology (Minneapolis)*, **16**, 179-191.

Davidoff, L. M.   (1928) Brain in mongolian idiocy; report of 10 cases. *Archives of Neurology and Psychiatry (Chicago)*, **20**, 1229-1257.

Dawson, J.   (1954) Pulmonary tuberous sclerosis and its relationship to other forms of disease. *Quarterly Journal of Medicine*, n.s. **23**, 113-145.

De, S. N.   (1950) A study of the changes in the brain in experimental internal hydrocephalus. *Journal of Pathology and Bacteriology*, **62**, 197-208.

Degenhardt, K. H.   (1954) Durch O$_2$-Mangel induzierte Fehlbildungen der Axialgradienten bei Kaninchen. *Zeitschrift für Naturforschung*, **93**, 530-536.

Degenhardt, K. H.   (1960) Cranio-facial dysplasia induced by oxygen deficiency in rabbits. *Biologia Neonatorum*, **2**, 93-104.

De Jong, R. N. & Bebin, J.   (1956) Clinical pathologic conference. *Neurology (Minneapolis)*, **6**, 208-217.

Dekaban, A. S.   (1959) Arhinencephaly in an infant born to a diabetic mother. *Journal of Neuropathology and Experimental Neurology*, **18**, 620-626.

Dekaban, A. S.   (1962) Cerebral birth injury. Pathology of haemorrhagic lesions. *Research Publications of the Association for Research in Nervous and Mental Diseases*, **39**, 196-227.

Dekaban, A. S. & Bartelmez, G. W.   (1964) Complete dysraphism in 14 somite human embryo. A contribution to normal and abnormal morphogenesis. *American Journal of Anatomy*, **115**, 27-41.

Dekaban, A. S. & Magee, K. R.   (1958) Occurrence of neurologic abnormalities in infants of diabetic mothers. *Neurology (Minneapolis)*, **8**, 193-200.

Dekaban, A. S. & Norman, R. M.   (1958) Hemiplegia in early life associated with thrombosis of the sagittal sinus and its tributary veins in one hemisphere. *Journal of Neuropathology and Experimental Neurology*, **17**, 461-470.

Demyer, W., Zeman, W. & Palmer, C. G.   (1963) Familial alobar holoprosencephaly (arhinencephaly) with median cleft lip and palate. Report of patient with 46 chromosomes. *Neurology (Minneapolis)*, **13** 913-918.

De Reuck, J., Chattha, A. S. & Richardson, E. P. Jr.   (1972) Pathogenesis and evolution of periventricular leukomalacia in infancy. *Archives of Neurology (Chicago)*, **27**, 229-236.

D'Hoore, E. & Gullotta, F.   (1971) Entmarkungsprozess mit Hirnverkalkungen bei einem mikrocephalen Säugling. Cockayne Syndrome? *Acta neuropathologica (Berlin)*, **18**, 311-316.

Dickerson, W. W.   (1955) Nature of certain osseous lesions in tuberous sclerosis. *Archives of Neurology and Psychiatry (Chicago)*, **73**, 525-529.

Diezel, P. B.   (1954) Mikrogyrie infolge cerebraler Speicheldrüsenvirusinfektion im Rahmen einer generalisierten Cytomegalie bei einem Säugling. Zugleich ein Beitrag zur Theorie der Windungsbildung. *Virchows Archiv für pathologische Anatomie und Physiologie*, **325**, 109-130.

Divry, P. & van Bogaert, L. (1946) Une maladie familiale caracterisée par une angiomatose diffuse cortico méningée non calcifiante et une démyelinisation progressive de la substance blanche. *Journal de Neurologie*, **9**, 41-54.

Dobbing, J. (1970) Undernutrition and the developing brain. *American Journal of Diseases of Children*, **120**, 411-415.

Dominok, G. W. (1962) Zur Frage der Diplomyelie. *Deutsche Zeitschrift für Nervenheilkunde*, **183**, 340-350.

Donaldson, H. H. (1911) The effect of underfeeding on the percentage of water, on the ether-alcohol extract, and on medullation in the central nervous system of the albino rat. *Journal of Comparative Neurology*, **21**, 139-145.

Donegani, G., Grattarola, F. R. & Wildi, E. (1972) Tuberous sclerosis: Bourneville disease in *Handbook of Clinical Neurology* (Eds. Vinken, P. J. & Bryun, G. W.), Vol. 14, pp. 340-389, North Holland Publishing Co., Amsterdam.

Drachman, D. A. & Richardson, E. P. (1961) Aqueductal narrowing, congenital and acquired. A critical review of the histologic criteria. *Archives of Neurology (Chicago)*, **5**, 552-559.

Dreifuss, F. E. & Netsky, M. G. (1964) Progressive poliodystrophy. The degeneration of cerebral grey matter. *American Journal of Diseases of Children*, **107**, 649-656.

Druckman, R., Chao, D. & Alvord, C. E. (1959) A case of atonic cerebral diplegia with lissencephaly. *Neurology (Minneapolis)*, **9**, 806-814.

Dubowitz, V., Lorber, J. & Zachary, R. B. (1965) Lipomas of the cauda equina. *Archives of Disease in Childhood*, **40**, 207-214.

Duckett, S. (1971) The morphology of tellurium-induced hydrocephalus. *Experimental Neurology*, **31**, 1-16.

Duckett, S. (1972) Teratogenesis of tellurium. *Annals of the New York Academy of Science*, **192**, 220-226.

Duckett, S., Brent, R. L. & Jensch, R. P. (1974) The morphology of immunologically induced hydrocephalus in the newborn rat. *Journal of Neuropathology and Experimental Neurology*, **33**, 365-373.

Duckworth, T., Sharrard, W. J. W., Lister, J. & Seymour, N. (1968) Hemimyelocele. *Developmental Medicine and Child Neurology*, *Suppl. 16*, 69-75.

Dwyer, J. M., Hickie, J. B. & Garvan, J. (1971) Pulmonary tuberous sclerosis. Report of three patients and a review of the literature. *Quarterly Journal of Medicine*, **40**, 115-125.

Earle, K. M., Baldwin, M. & Penfield, W. (1953) Incisural sclerosis and temporal lobe seizures produced by hippocampal herniation at birth. *Archives of Neurology and Psychiatry (Chicago)*, **69**, 27-42.

Edinger, L. & Fischer, B. (1913) Ein Mensch ohne Grosshirn. *Pflügers Archiv für die gesamte Physiologie des Menschen und der Tiere*, **152**, 535-561.

Edwards, J. H., Harnden, D. G., Cameron, A. H., Crosse, V. M. & Wolff, O. H. (1960) A new trisomic syndrome. *Lancet*, **1**, 787-790.

Edwards, J. H., Norman, R. M. & Roberts, J. M. (1961) Sex-linked hydrocephalus: report of a family with 15 affected members. *Archives of Disease in Childhood*, **36**, 481-485.

Ehrengut, W., Ehrengut-Lange, J., Seitz, D. & Weber, G. (1972) *Die post vakzinale Enzephalopathie*, Schattauer, Stuttgart.

Eicke, W. J. (1959) Les maladies inflammatoires de l'encéphale chez le foetus in *Malformations congénitales du Cerveau* (Eds. Heuyer, G., Feld, M. & Gruner, J.), pp. 81-92, Masson, Paris.

Elizan, T. S. & Fabiyi, A. (1970) Congenital and neonatal anomalies linked with viral infections in experimental animals. *American Journal of Obstetrics and Gynecology*, **106**, 147-165.

Elvidge, A. R. & Jackson, I. J. (1949) Subdural hematoma and effusion in infants; review of 55 cases. *American Journal of Diseases of Children*, **78**, 635-658.

Emery, J. L. (1974) Deformity of the aqueduct of Sylvius in children with hydrocephalus and myelomeningocele. *Developmental Medicine and Child Neurology*, **16**, *Suppl. 32*, 40-48.

Emery, J. L. & Kalhan, S. C. (1970) The pathology of exencephalus. *Developmental Medicine and Child Neurology*, **12**, *Suppl. 22*, 51-64.

Emery, J. L. & Lendon, R. G. (1969) Lipomas of the cauda equina and other fatty tumours related to neurospinal dysraphism. *Developmental Medicine and Child Neurology*, *Suppl. 20*, 62-70.

Emery, J. L. & Lendon, R. G. (1973) The local cord lesion in neurospinal dysraphism (meningomyelocele). *Journal of Pathology*, **110**, 83-96.

Emery, J. L. & Mackenzie, N. (1973) Medullo-cervical dislocation deformity (Chiari II deformity) related to neurospinal dysraphism (meningomyelocele). *Brain*, **96**, 155-162.

Erbslöh, F. & Bochnik, H. (1958) Symmetrische Pseudokalk-und Kalkablagerungen in Gehirn in *Handbuch der speziellen pathologischen Anatomie und Histologie* (Eds. Lubarsch, O., Henke, F. & Rössle, R.), Vol. 13, part 2B, pp. 1769-1809, Springer Verlag, Berlin.

Evrard, P. & Caviness, V. S. Jr. (1974) Extensive developmental defect of the cerebellum associated with posterior fossa ventriculocele. *Journal of Neuropathology and Experimental Neurology*, 33, 385-399.

Faith, S. A. & Lewis, F. J. W. (1964) Presumptive deletion of the short arm of chromosome 18 in a cyclops. *Human Chromosome Newsletter*, No. 14, p. 5.

Falconer, M. A. & Wilson, P. J. E. (1969) Complications related to delayed hemorrhage after hemispherectomy. *Journal of Neurosurgery*, 30, 413-426.

Feigin, I. (1956) Arnold–Chiari malformation with associated analogous malformation of mid-brain. *Neurology (Minneapolis)*, 6, 22-31.

Ferraro, A. & Barrera, S. E. (1935) Megalo-myelo-encephaly. *American Journal of Psychiatry*, 92, 509-526.

Fischer, R. G., Uihlein, A. & Keith, H. M. (1952) Spina bifida and Cranium bifidum: study of 530 cases. *Proceedings of the Mayo Clinic*, 27, 33-38.

Fitzgerald, P. A. M. F. (1940) *Contributions to Embryology*, No. 176, Carnegie Inst. of Washington.

Ford, R. R., Livingstone, S. & Pryles, C. V. (1951) Familial degeneration of the cerebral gray matter in childhood. With convulsions, myoclonus, spasticity, cerebellar ataxia, choreoathetosis, dementia and death in status epilepticus. Differentiation of infantile juvenile types. *Journal of Pediatrics*, 39, 33-43.

Ford, R. R. & Schaffer, A. J. (1927) Etiology of infantile acquired hemiplegia. *Archives of Neurology and Psychiatry (Chicago)*, 18, 323-347.

Fowler, M., Brown, C. & Cabrera, K. F. (1971) Hydrencephaly in a baby after an aircraft accident to the mother: case report and autopsy. *Pathology*, 3, 21-30.

Fowler, M., Dow, R., White, T. A. & Greer, C. H. (1972) Congenital hydrocephalus—hydrencephaly in five siblings with autopsy studies: a new disease. *Developmental Medicine and Child Neurology*, 14, 173-188.

Freedom, L. (1927) Über einen eigenartigen Krankheitsfall des jugendlichen Alters unter dem Symptomenbilde einer Littleschen Starre mit Athetose und Idiotie. *Deutsche Zeitschrift für Nervenheilkunde*, 96, 295-298.

Friede, R. L. (1972) Residual lesions of infantile cerebral phlebothrombosis. *Acta neuropathologica (Berlin)*, 22, 319-332.

Friedman, M. & Cohen, P. (1947) Agenesis of corpus callosum as a possible sequel to maternal rubella during pregnancy. *American Journal of Diseases of Children*, 73, 178-185.

Fuchs, A. (1909) Über den klinischen Nachweis kongenitaler Defektbildungen in den unteren Rückenmarksabschnitten (Myelodysplasie). *Wiener medizinische Wochenschrift*, 59, 2142-2147.

Gardner, W. J. (1959) Anatomic features common to Arnold–Chiari and Dandy–Walker malformations suggest common origin. *Cleveland Clinical Quarterly*, 26, 206-222.

Gardner, W. J. (1960) Myelomeningocele, the result of rupture of the embryonic neural tube. *Cleveland Clinical Quarterly*, 27, 88-100.

Gardner, W. J. (1961) Rupture of the neural tube: the cause of myelomeningocele. *Archives of Neurology*, 4, 1-7.

Gardner, W. J. (1968) Myelocele. Rupture of the neural tube? *Clinical Neurosurgery*, 15, 57-79.

Gardner, W. J., Abdullah, A. F. & McCormack, L. J. (1957) The varying expressions of embryonal atresia of the fourth ventricle in adults (Arnold–Chiari malformation, Dandy–Walker syndrome, 'arachnoid' cyst of the cerebellum, and syringomyelia). *Journal of Neurosurgery*, 14, 591-607.

Gardner, W. J. & Goodall, R. J. (1950) Surgical treatment of Arnold–Chiari malformation in adult. *Journal of Neurosurgery*, 7, 199-206.

Gastaut, H., Poirier, F., Payan, H., Salamon, G., Toga, M. & Vigouroux, M. (1959-60) H.H.E. Syndrome: hemiconvulsions, hemiplegia and epilepsy. *Epilepsia (Fourth Series)*, 1, 418-447.

Gerstl, B., Malamud, N., Hayman, R. B. & Bond, P. R. (1965) Morphological and neurochemical study in Pelizaeus–Merzbacher's disease. *Journal of Neurology, Neurosurgery and Psychiatry*, 28, 540-547.

Giannelli, F., Hamerton, J. L. & Carter, C. O. (1965) Cytogenetics of Down's syndrome (Mongolism) II. The frequency of interchange trisomy in patients born at a maternal age of less than 30 years. *Cytogenetics*, 4, 186-192.

Gibson, J. B. (1955) Congenital hydrocephalus due to atresia of foramen of Magendie. *Journal of Neuropathology and Experimental Neurology*, 14, 244-262.

Gillman, J., Gilbert, C., Gillman, T. & Spence, I. (1948) A preliminary report on hydrocephalus, spina bifida, and other congenital anomalies in the rat produced by trypan blue. *South African Journal of Medical Science*, 13, 47-90.

Gillman, J., Gilbert, C., Spence, I. & Gillman, T. (1951) A further report on congenital anomalies in the rat produced by trypan blue. *South African Journal of Medical Science*, 16, 125-135.

Gilmour, J. R. (1941) The essential identity of the Klippel–Feil syndrome and iniencephaly. *Journal of Pathology and Bacteriology*, 53, 117-131.

Giroud, A.   (1959) Morphogénèse d'anencéphalie in *Malformations congénitales du Cerveau* (Eds. Heuyer, G., Feld, M. & Gruner, J.), pp. 269-273, Masson, Paris.

Giroud, A.   (1960) Causes and morphogenesis of anencephaly in *Ciba Foundation Symposium on Congenital Malformations* (Eds. Wostenholme, G. E. W. & O'Connor, C. M.), pp. 199-212, Churchill, London.

Giroud, A. & Martinet, M.   (1956) Tératogénèse par hautes doses de Vitamine A en fonction des stades du developpement. *Archives d'Anatomie Microscopique et de Morphologie Experimentale*, 46, 77-99.

Giuffré, R.   (1966) Intradural spinal lipomas: review of the literature (99 cases) and report of an additional case. *Acta neurochirurgica*, 14, 69-95.

Globus, J. H.   (1932) Malformation in the central nervous system in *Cytology and Cellular Pathology of the Nervous System* (Ed. Penfield, W.), pp. 1147-1199, Hoeber, New York.

Globus, J. H.   (1938) Glioneuroma and spongioneuroblastoma, forms of primary neuroectodermal tumors of the brain. *American Journal of Cancer*, 32, 163-220.

Glücksman, A.   (1951) Cell death in normal vertebrate ontogeny. *Biological Reviews*, 26, 59-86.

Gold, A. P. & Freeman, J. M.   (1965) Depigmented nevi: the earliest sign of tuberous sclerosis. *Pediatrics*, 35, 1003-1005.

Goldstein, K. & Riese, W.   (1925) Klinische und anatomische Beobachtungen an einem vierjährigen riechhirnlosen Kinde. *Journal für Psychologie und Neurologie (Leipzig)*, 32, 291-311.

Grcević, N. & Robert, F.   (1960) Verrucose dysplasia of the cerebral cortex (Dysgénésie nodulaire disséminée of Morel and Wildi). *Journal of Neuropathology and Experimental Neurology*, 20, 399-411.

Greenberg, M., Pellitteri, O. & Barton, J.   (1957) Frequency of defects in infants whose mothers had rubella during pregnancy. *Journal of the American Medical Association*, 165, 675-678.

Greenfield, J. G.   (1958) *Neuropathology*, 1st Edition, Edward Arnold, London.

Greenfield, J. G. & Wolfsohn, J. M.   (1935) Microcephalia vera: study of 2 brains illustrating agyric form and complex microgyric form. *Archives of Neurology and Psychiatry (Chicago)*, 33, 1296-1316.

Greenhouse, A. H. & Neubuerger, K. T.   (1964) The syndrome of progressive neuronal poliodystrophy. *Archives of Neurology (Chicago)*, 10, 46-57.

Gregg, N. McA.   (1941) Congenital cataract following German measles in the mother. *Transactions of the Ophthalmological Society of Australia*, 3, 35-46.

Griffith, H. B.   (1967) Cerebral hemispherectomy for infantile hemiplegia in the light of the late results. *Annals of the Royal College of Surgeons of England*, 41, 183-201.

Gröntoft, O.   (1954) Intracranial haemorrhage and blood-brain barrier problems in new-born; pathologico-anatomical and experimental investigation. *Acta pathologica microbiologica scandinavica*, Suppl. C30 1-109.

Gross, H. & Hoff, H.   (1959) Sur les malformations ventriculaires depéndantes des dysgénésies commissurales in *Malformations Congénitales du Cerveau* (Eds. Heuyer, Feld, and Gruner), pp. 329-351, Masson, Paris.

Gross, H. & Kaltenback, E.   (1959) Über eine kombinierte progressive pontocerebellare Systematrophie bei einem Kleinkind. *Deutsche Zeitschrift für Nervenheilkunde*, 179, 388-400.

Gruenwald, P.   (1945) Absence of optic nerve in cyclopia. *Anatomical Record*, 91, 13-20.

Gruenwald, P.   (1947a) Mechanisms of abnormal development—causes of abnormal development in the embryo. *Archives of Pathology*, 47, 398-437.

Gruenwald, P.   (1947b) Embryonic development of malformation. *Archives of Pathology*, 47, 495-559.

Gruenwald, P.   (1947c) Postnatal developmental abnormalities. *Archives of Pathology*, 47, 648-664.

Gruenwald, P.   (1951) Subependymal cerebral hemorrhage in premature birth. *American Journal of Obstetrics and Gynecology*, 61, 1285-1292.

Gryspeerdt, G. L.   (1963) Myelographic assessment of occult forms of spinal dysraphism. *Acta radiologica*, 1D, 702-717.

Gunberg, D. L.   (1956) Spina bifida and the Arnold–Chiari malformation in the progeny of trypan blue injected rats. *Anatomical Record*, 126, 343-367.

Gunther, M. & Penrose, L. S.   (1935) The genetics of epiloia. *Journal of Genetics*, 31, 413-427.

Guthkelch, A. N.   (1953) Subdural effusions in infancy: 24 cases. *British Medical Journal*, 1, 233-239.

Guthkelch, A. N.   (1974) Diastematomyelia with median septum. *Brain*, 97, 729-742.

Guzzetta, F.   (1972) Cockayne–Neill syndrome in *Handbook of Clinical Neurology* (Eds. Vinken, P. J. & Bruyn, G. W.), Vol. 13, pp. 431-440, North Holland Publishing Co., Amsterdam.

Haene, A. de   (1955) Agénésic partielle du vermis de cervelet à caractère familial. *Acta neurologica psychiatrica belgica*, 55, 622-628.

Hale, F.   (1933) Pigs born without eyeballs. *Journal of Heredity*, 24, 105-106.

Hall, G. S.   (1946) A contribution to the study of melorheostosis: unusual bone changes associated with tuberose sclerosis. *Quarterly Journal of Medicine*, n.s. 12, 77-100.

Haller, E. S., Nesbitt, R. E. L. & Anderson, G. W.   (1956) Clinical and pathologic concepts of gross intra-cranial hemorrhage in perinatal mortality.   *Obstetrical and Gynecological Survey*, **11**, 179-204.

Hallervorden, J.   (1926) Der mikroskopische Hirnbefund in einem Falle von angeborener Hemihypertrophie der linken Körperhälfte einschliesslich des Gehirns.   *Deutsche Zeitschrift für Nervenheilkunde*, **89**, 28-30.

Hallervorden, J.   (1930) Eigenartige und nicht rubrizierbare Prozesse in *Handbuch der Geisteskrankheiten* (Ed. Bumke, O.), Vol. 11, pp. 1063-1107, Springer Verlag, Berlin.

Hallervorden, J.   (1939) Kreislaufstörungen in der Ätiologie des angeborenen Schwachsinns.   *Zeitschrift für die gesamte Neurologie und Psychiatrie*, **167**, 527-745.

Hallervorden, J.   (1949) Über eine Kohlenoxydvergiftung im Fetalleben mit Entwicklungsstörung der Hirnrinde.   *Allgemeine Zeitschrift für Psychiatrie*, **124**, 289-298.

Hallervorden, J.   (1950) Über diffuse symmetrische Kalkablagerungen bei einem Krankheitsbild mit Microcephalie und Meningoencephalitis.   *Archiv für Psychiatrie und Nervenkrankheiten*, **184**, 579-600.

Hamerton, J. L., Giannelli, F. & Polani, P. E.   (1965) Cytogenetics of Down's syndrome (Mongolism) I.   Data on a consecutive series of patients referred for genetic counselling and diagnosis.   *Cytogenetics*, **4**, 171-185.

Hanaway, J. & Metsky, M. G.   (1971) Heterotopias of the inferior olive; relation to Dandy–Walker malformation and correlation with experimental data.   *Journal of Neuropathology and Experimental Neurology*, **30**, 380-389.

Harper, R. C., Orti, E. & Baker, R. K.   (1967) Bird-headed dwarfs (Seckel's syndrome).   A familial pattern of developmental dental, skeletal, genital and central nervous system anomalies.   *Journal of Pediatrics*, **70**, 799-804.

Harriman, D. G. F.   (1958) An intraspinal enterogenous cyst.   *Journal of Pathology and Bacteriology*, **75**, 413-419.

Harrison, M. J. G.   (1971) Cerebral arachnoid cysts in children.   *Journal of Neurology, Neurosurgery and Psychiatry*, **34**, 316-323.

Harrison, V. C., Heese, H. de V. & Klein, M.   (1968) Intracranial haemorrhage associated with hyaline membrane disease.   *Archives of Disease in Childhood*, **43**, 116-120.

Hart, M. N., Malamud, N. & Ellis, W. G.   (1972) The Dandy–Walker syndrome.   A clinicopathological study based on 28 cases.   *Neurology (Minneapolis)*, **22**, 771-780.

Haymaker, W., Girdany, B. R., Stephens, J., Lillie, R. D. & Fetterman G. H.   (1954) Cerebral involvement with advanced periventricular calcification in generalized cytomegalic inclusion disease of the newborn.   *Journal of Neuropathology and Experimental Neurology*, **13**, 562-586.

Helmke, K.   (1937) Glykogenablagerung im Gehirn bei tuberöser Sklerose.   *Virchows Archiv für pathologische Anatomie und Physiologie*, **300**, 130-140.

Henderson, J. L.   (1939) The congenital facial diplegia syndrome: clinical features, pathology and aetiology.   *Brain*, **62**, 381-403.

Herren, R. Y. & Edwards, J. E.   (1940) Diplomyelia (duplication of spinal cord).   *Archives of Pathology*, **30**, 1203-1214.

Heschl, R.   (1859) Gehirndefect und Hydrocephalus.   *Vierteljahrschrift für praktikale Heilkunde*, **61**, 59-74.

Heubner, O.   (1900) Über angeborenen Kernmangel (infantiler Kernschwund, Moebius).   *Charité-annalen*, **25**, 211-243.

Hicks, S. P.   (1952) Symposium on cerebral palsy: some effects of ionizing radiation and metabolic inhibition on developing mammalian nervous system.   *Journal of Pediatrics*, **40**, 489-513.

Hicks, S. P.   (1953*a*) Developmental brain metabolism—effects of cortisone, anoxia, fluoroacetate, radiation, insulin and other inhibitors on the enbryo, newborn and adult.   *Archives of Pathology*, **55**, 302-327.

Hicks, S. P.   (1953*b*) Developmental malformations produced by radiation.   *American Journal of Roentgenology*, **69**, 272-293.

Hicks, S. P.   (1954) Mechanism of radiation anencephaly, anophthalmia, and pituitary anomalies repair in the mammalian embryo.   *Archives of Pathology*, **57**, 363-378.

Hintz, R. L., Menking, M. & Sotos, J. F.   (1968) Familial holoprosencephaly with endocrine dysgenesis.   *Journal of Pediatrics*, **72**, 81-87.

Hippel, E. von   (1907) Über experimentelle Erzeugung von angeborenen Star bei Kaninchen nebst Bemerkungen über gleichzeitig beobachteten Mikrophthalmus und Lidcolobom.   *Albrecht von Graefes Archiv für Ophthalmologie*, **65**, 326-360.

Hirano, A., Tuazon, R. & Zimmerman, H. M.   (1968) Neurofibrillary changes, granulo-vacuolar bodies and argentophilic globules observed in tuberous sclerosis.   *Acta neuropathologica (Berlin)*, **11**, 257-261.

Hoet, J. P., Gommers, A. & Hoet, J. J.   (1960) Causes of congenital malformations: role of prediabetes and hypothyroidism in *Ciba Foundation Symposium on Congenital Malformations* (Eds. Wolstenholme, G. E. W. & O'Connor, C. M.), pp. 219-235, Churchill, London.

Hoeve, J. Van Der (1921) Augengeschwülste bei der tuberösen Hirnsklerose (Bourneville). *Albrecht von Graefes Archiv für Ophthalmologie*, **105**, 880-889.

Holland, E. (1920) On cranial stress in the foetus during labour and on the effects of excessive stress on the intracranial contents; with an analysis of 81 cases of torn tentorium cerebelli and subdural cerebral haemorrhage. *Transactions of the Edinburgh Obstetrical Society*, **40**, 112-143.

Holland, E. (1922) On cranial stress in the foetus during labour and on the effects of excessive stress on the intracranial contents; with an analysis of 81 cases of torn tentorium cerebelli and subdural cerebral haemorrhage. *Journal of Obstetrics and Gynaecology of the British Empire*, **29**, 549-571.

Hooft, C., Hauwere, R. de, & Acker, K. G. van (1968) Familial non-congenital microcephaly, peculiar appearance, mental and motor retardation, progressive evolution to spasticity and athetosis. *Helvetica paediatrica acta*, **23**, 1-12.

Hopkins, I. J. & Turner, B. (1973) Spongy glio-neuronal dystrophy: a degenerative disease of the nervous system. *Journal of Neurology, Neurosurgery and Psychiatry*, **36**, 50-56.

Horanyi-Hechst, B. & Meyer, A. (1939) Diffuse sclerosis with preserved myelin islands: a pathological report on a case, with a note on cerebral involvement in Raynaud's disease. *Journal of Mental Science*, **85**, 22-28.

Horstmann, W. (1966) Hinweise auf zentralnervöse Schäden im Rahmen der Thalidomid-Embryopathie. Pathologisch-anatomische, elektrencephalographische und neurologische Befunde. *Zeitschrift für Kinderheilkunde*, **96**, 291-307.

Hutchinson, E. C. & Yates, P. O. (1956) The cervical portion of the vertebral artery: a clinico-pathological study. *Brain*, **79**, 319-331.

Hutchinson, E. C. & Yates, P. O. (1957) Carotico-vertebral stenosis. *Lancet*, **1**, 2-8.

Ingalls, T. H. (1950) Study of congenital anomalies by epidemiologic method, with consideration of retrolental fibroplasia as acquired anomaly of fetus. *New England Journal of Medicine*, **243**, 67-74.

Ingalls, T. H. (1960) Environmental factors in causation of congenital anomalies in *Ciba Foundation Symposium on Congenital Malformations* (Eds. Wolstenholme, G. E. W. & O'Connor, C. M.), pp. 51-67, Churchill, London.

Ingalls, T. H., Curley, F. J. & Prindle, R. A. (1950) Anoxia as a cause of fetal death and congenital defect in the mouse. *American Journal of Diseases of Children*, **80**, 34-45.

Ingalls, T. H., Curley, F. J. & Prindle, R. A. (1952) Experimental production of congenital abnormalities. Timing and degree of anoxia as factors causing fetal death and congenital abnormalities in the mouse. *New England Journal of Medicine*, **247**, 758-768.

Inglis, K. (1946) Subdural haemorrhage, cysts and false membranes: illustrating the influence of intrinsic factors in disease when development of the body is normal. *Brain*, **69**, 157-194.

Inglis, K. (1950) Neurilemmoblastosis. The influence of intrinsic factors in disease when development of the body is abnormal. *American Journal of Pathology*, **26**, 521-536.

Ingraham, F. D. & Matson, D. D. (1944) Subdural hematoma in infancy. *Journal of Pediatrics*, **24**, 1-37.

Ingraham, F. D. & Swan, H. (1943) Spina bifida and cranium bifidum: a survey of 546 cases. *New England Journal of Medicine*, **228**, 559-563.

Jacob, H. (1940) Die feinere Oberflächengestaltung der Hirnwindungen; die Hirnwarzenbildung und die Mikropolygyrie. *Zeitschrift für die gesamte Neurologie und Psychiatrie*, **170**, 64-84.

Jacob, H. (1964-65) Zentralnervöse Zell-und Gewebsdysfunctionen bei tuberöser Sklerose. *Archiv für Psychiatrie und Nervenheilkunde*, **206**, 208-227.

Jakob, A. (1922) Ein 10 Monate altes Kind ohne Neuhirn. *Zentralblatt für Neurologie*, **31**, 403.

Jakob, A. (1929) *Anatomie und Histologie des Grosshirns*, Vol. 1, pp. 42-49, Franz Deutick, Leipzig.

Jakob, A. (1931) Über ein dreieinhalb Monate altes Kind mit totaler Erweichung beider Grosshirnhemisphären (Kind ohne Grosshirn). *Deutsche Zeitschrift für Nervenheilkunde*, **117-119**, 240-265.

Jakubiak, P., Dunsmore, R. H. & Beckett, R. S. (1968) Supratentorial brain cysts. *Journal of Neurosurgery*, **28**, 129-136.

James, C. C. M. & Lassman, L. P. (1962) Spinal dysraphism: the diagnosis and treatment of progressive lesions in spina bifida occulta. *Journal of Bone and Joint Surgery*, **44**B, 828-840.

James, C. C. M. & Lassman, L. P. (1964) Diastematomyelia: a critical survey of 24 cases submitted to laminectomy. *Archives of Disease in Childhood*, **39**, 125-130.

Jellinger, K. & Seitelberger, F. (1970) Spongy glio-neuronal dystrophy in infancy and childhood. *Acta neuropathologica (Berlin)*, **16**, 125-140.

Jervis, G. A. (1948) Early senile dementia in mongoloid idiocy. *American Journal of Psychiatry*, **105**, 102-106.

Jervis, G. A. (1950) Early familial cerebellar degeneration (report of 3 cases in 1 family). *Journal of Nervous and Mental Diseases*, **111**, 398-407.

Jervis, G. A.   (1954a) Spongioneuroblastoma and tuberous sclerosis. *Journal of Neuropathology and Experimental Neurology*, **13**, 105-116.

Jervis, G. A.   (1954b) Microcephaly with extensive calcium deposits and demyelination. *Journal of Neuropathology and Experimental Neurology*, **13**, 318-329.

Jervis, G. A.   (1957) Degenerative encephalopathy of childhood (cortical degeneration, cerebellar atrophy, cholesterinosis of basal ganglia). *Journal of Neuropathology and Experimental Neurology*, **16**, 308-320.

Jervis, G. A. & Schein, H.   (1951) Polyostotic fibrous dysplasia (Albright's syndrome); report of case showing central nervous system changes. *Archives of Pathology*, **51**, 640-650.

Johnson, F. E.   (1938) Injury of the child by Roentgen ray during pregnancy. Report of a case. *Journal of Pediatrics*, **13**, 894-901.

Jong, H. de   (1927) Über Arhinencephalie mit Hypertrophien im Gehirn. *Zeitschrift für die gesamte Neurologie und Psychiatrie*, **108**, 734-770.

Joubert, M., Eisenring, J. J., Robb, J. P. & Andermann, F.   (1969) Familial agenesis of the cerebellar vermis. *Neurology (Minneapolis)*, **19**, 813-825.

Kalischer, S.   (1897) Demonstration des Gehirns eins Kindes mit Teleangiectasie der linksseitigen Gesichtskopfhaut und Hirnoberfläche. *Berliner Klinische Wochenschrift*, **34**, 1059.

Kalischer, S.   (1901) Ein Fall von Teleangiectasie (Angiom) des Gesichts und der weichen Hirnhaut. *Archiv für Psychiatrie und Nervenkrankheiten*, **34**, 171-180.

Källén, B. & Levan, A.   (1970) Chromosomes in man, with special reference to neuropathological disorders in *Neuropathology: Methods and Diagnosis* (Ed. Tedeschi, C. G.), pp. 547-582, Little, Brown, Boston.

Kalter, H.   (1963) Experimental mammalian teratogenesis, a study of galactoflavin induced hydrocephalus in mice. *Journal of Morphology*, **112**, 303-317.

Kalter, H.   (1968) *Teratology of the Central Nervous System.* University of Chicago Press, Chicago.

Kalter, H. & Warkany, J.   (1957) Congenital malformations in inbred strains of mice induced by riboflavin-deficient, galactoflavine containing diets. *Journal of Experimental Zoology*, **136**, 531-566.

Kappers, J. A.   (1959) Les malformations cérébrales consécutives à l'embryopathie rubéoleuse: à propos d'un cas chez un embryon de six semaines in *Malformations Congénitales du Cerveau* (Eds. Heuyer, G., Feld, M. & Gruner, J.), pp. 99-106, Masson, Paris.

Karch, S. B. & Urich, H.   (1972) Occipital encephalocele: a morphological study. *Journal of the Neurological Sciences*, **15**, 89-112.

Kass, A.   (1951) Congenital hydrocephalus in newborn infant-epidemic hepatitis in mother in second-third month of pregnancy. *Acta pediatrica*, **40**, 239-248.

Kastein, G. W.   (1940) Über Megalencephalie. *Acta neerlandica morphologiae normalis et pathologicae*, **3**, 249-277.

Kautsky, R.   (1949) Die Bedeutung der Hirnhautinnervation und ihrer Entwicklung für die Pathogenese der Sturge–Weber'schen Krankheit. *Deutsche Zeitschrift für Nervenheilkunde*, **161**, 506-525.

King, L. S.   (1936) Hereditary defects of the corpus callosum in the mouse; Mus musculus. *Journal of Comparative Neurology*, **64**, 337-363.

Kirschbaum, W.   (1947) Agenesis of the corpus callosum and associated malformations. *Journal of Neuropathology and Experimental Neurology*, **6**, 78-94.

Kloopfer, H. W., Platou, R. V. & Hansche, W. J.   (1964) Manifestations of a recessive gene for microcephaly in a population isolate. *Journal de Génétique Humaine*, **13**, 52-59.

Knobloch, H. & Pasamanick, B.   (1962) Mental Subnormality. *New England Journal of Medicine*, **266**, 1045-1051, 1092-1097 and 1155-1161.

Koch, G.   (1949) Athetose double bei eineiigen Zwillingen, Beitrag zur Erbpathologie der striären Erkrankungen. *Arzneimittel-Forschung*, **3**, 278-288.

Krabbe, K. H.   (1934) Facial and meningeal angiomatosis associated with calcifications of brain cortex: clinical and anatomo-pathologic contribution. *Archives of Neurology and Psychiatry (Chicago)*, **32**, 737-755.

Kramer, W.   (1953) Poliodysplasia cerebri. *Acta psychiatrica et neurologica scandinavica*, **28**, 413-427.

Kramer, W.   (1954) Malformation of the paraflocculus in man, with occlusion of the exit of the fourth ventricle. *Folia psychiatrica, neurologica et neurochirurgica Nèerlandica*, **57**, 298-307.

Kramer, W.   (1956) Dysgenetic gliosis of the brain—a case of macrogyria. *Journal of Neuropathology and Experimental Neurology*, **15**, 471-484.

Krynauw, R. A.   (1950) Infantile hemiplegia treated by removing one cerebral hemisphere. *Journal of Neurology, Neurosurgery and Psychiatry*, **13**, 243-267.

Kufs, H.   (1949) Über eine Spätform der tuberösen Hirnsklerose unter dem Bild des Hirntumors und andere abnorme Befunde bei dieser Krankheit. *Archiv für Psychiatrie und Nervenkrankheiten*, **182**, 177-186.

Lagos, J. C. & Gomez, M. R. (1967) Tuberous sclerosis: reappraisal of a clinical entity. *Mayo Clinic Proceedings*, **42**, 26-49.

Landtman, B. (1948) On the relationship between maternal conditions during pregnancy and congenital malformations. *Archives of Disease in Childhood*, **23**, 237-246.

Lange, C. de (1925) Brains with total and partial lack of corpus callosum and nature of longitudinal callosal bundle. *Journal of Nervous and Mental Diseases*, **62**, 449-476.

Lange, C. de (1939) Lissenzephalie beim Menschen. *Monatschrift für Psychiatrie und Neurologie*, **101**, 350-384.

Lange-Cosack, H. (1944) Die Hydranencephalie (Blasenhirn) als Sonderform der Grosshirnlosigkeit. *Archiv für Psychiatrie und Nervenkrankheiten*, **117**, 595-640.

Larroche, J. C. (1968) Nécrose cérébrale massive chez le nouveau-né. *Biologia neonatorum*, **13**, 340-360.

Laurence, K. M. (1959) The pathology of hydrocephalus. *Annals of the Royal College of Surgeons of England*, **24**, 388-401.

Laurence, K. M. (1962) Aqueduct gliosis and von Recklinghausen's disease. *Proceedings of the IVth International Congress of Neuropathology (Munich)*, pp. 353-357, Thieme, Stuttgart.

Laurence, K. M. (1964) A case of unilateral megalencephaly. *Developmental Medicine and Child Neurology*, **6**, 585-590.

Laurence, K. M. (1966) The bobble-head doll syndrome. *Developmental Medicine and Child Neurology*, **8**, 777-778.

Laurence, K. M. & Cavanagh, J. B. (1968) Progressive degeneration of the cerebral cortex in infancy. *Brain*, **91**, 261-280.

Lebedeff, A. (1881) Über die Entstehung der Anencephalie mit spina bifida bei Vögeln und Menschen. *Virchows Archiv für pathologische Anatomie und Physiologie*, **86**, 263-298.

Lejeune, J., Gautier, M. & Turpin, R. (1959) Étude des chromosomes somatiques de neuf enfants mongoliens. *Comptes Rendus Hebdomadaires des Séances de l'Académie des Sciences, Series D*, **248**, 1721-1722.

Lejeune, J., Lafourcade, J., Berger, R., Vialatte, J., Boeswillwald, M., Seringe, P. & Turpin, R. (1963) Trois cas de délétion partielle du bras court d'un chromosome 5. *Comptes Rendus Hebdomadaires des Séances de l'Académie des Sciences, Series D*, **257**, 3098-3102.

Lendon, R. G. & Emery, J. L. (1970) Forking of the central canal in the equinal cord of children. *Journal of Anatomy*, **106**, 499-505.

Leon, G. A. de (1972) Observations on cerebral and cerebellar microgyria. *Acta neuropathologica (Berlin)*, **20**, 278-287.

Lewis, P. D. (1970) Cell proliferation in the subependymal layer of the mammalian brain and its role in pathological processes. M.D. Thesis, Univ. of London.

Lichtenstein, B. W. (1940) Spinal dysraphism; spina bifida and myelodysplasia. *Archives of Neurology and Psychiatry (Chicago)*, **44**, 792-810.

Lichtenstein, B. W. (1942) Distant neuroanatomic complications of spina bifida (spinal dysraphism); hydrocephalus, Arnold–Chiari deformity, stenosis of aqueduct of Sylvius, etc., pathogenesis and pathology. *Archives of Neurology and Psychiatry (Chicago)*, **47**, 195-214.

Lichtenstein, B. W. (1943) Maldevelopments of cerebellum; pathologic study with remarks on associated degeneration of olivary bodies and pontine and dentate nuclei. *Journal of Neuropathology and Experimental Neurology*, **2**, 164-177.

Lichtenstein, B. W. (1954) Sturge–Weber Dimitri syndrome; cephalic form in neurocutaneous hemangiomatosis. *Archives of Neurology and Psychiatry (Chicago)*, **71**, 291-301.

Lindenberg, R. (1955) Compression of brain arteries as pathogenetic factor for tissue necroses and their areas of predilection. *Journal of Neuropathology and Experimental Neurology*, **14**, 223-243.

Lindenberg, R. (1963) Patterns of CNS vulnerability in acute hypoxaemia, including anaesthesia accidents in *C.I.O.M.S. Symposium on Selective Vulnerability of the C.N.S. in Hypoxaemia* (Eds. Schade, J. P. & McMenemey, W. H.), pp. 189-209, Blackwell Scientific, Oxford.

Lindenberg, R. & Spatz, H. (1939) Über die Thromboendarteritis obliterans der Hirngefässe (cerebrale Form der v. Winiwarter-Buergerschen Krankheit). *Virchows Archiv für pathologische Anatomie und Physiologie*, **305**, 531-557.

List, C. F. (1941a) Intraspinal epidermoids, dermoids and dermoid sinuses. *Surgery, Gynecology and Obstetrics*, **73**, 525-538.

List, C. F. (1941b) Neurologic syndromes accompanying developmental anomalies of occipital bone, atlas and axis. *Archives of Neurology and Psychiatry (Chicago)*, **45**, 577-616.

Little, W. J. (1862) On the influence of abnormal parturition, difficult labours, premature births, and asphyxia neonatorum, on the mental and physical condition of the child, especially in relation to deformities. *Transactions of the Obstetrical Society of London*, **3**, 293-344.

Liu, M. C. & Sylvester, P. E. (1960) Familial diffuse progressive encephalopathy. *Archives of Disease in Childhood*, **35**, 345-351.

Loeser, J. D. & Alvord, C. E. (1968) Agenesis of the corpus callosum. *Brain*, **91**, 553-570.

Löken, A. C. & Horsdal, O. (1961) Progressive degenerative encephalopathy of unusual type. A clinico-pathological study of a case characterized by widespread cortical atrophy and by spongy degeneration in the white matter and basal ganglia. *Journal of Neuropathology and Experimental Neurology*, **20**, 427-439.

Lorber, J. (1967) The prognosis of occipital encephalocoele. *Developmental Medicine and Child Neurology*, **13** (Suppl.), 75-86.

Louis-Bar, D. (1941) Sur un syndrome progressif comprenant des télangiectasies capillaires cutanées et conjonctivales symmétriques à disposition naevoïde et des troubles cérébelleux. *Confinia neurologica* (*Basel*), **4**, 32-42.

Louis-Bar, D. (1944) Les limites nosographiques de l'angiomatose encéphalo-trigéminée (Sturge–Weber–Krabbe). *Confinia neurologica* (*Basel*), **6**, 1-21.

Lundström, R. (1952) Rubella during pregnancy; its effects upon perinatal mortality, the incidence of congenital abnormalities and immaturity. A preliminary report. *Acta pediatrica*, **41**, 583-594.

Lyon, G., Dodge, P. R. & Adams, R. D. (1961) The acute encephalopathies of obscure origin in infants and children. *Brain*, **84**, 680-708.

Lyssenkow, N. K. (1931) Über aplasia palaeocerebellaris. *Virchows Archiv für pathologische Anatomie und Physiologie*, **280**, 611-625.

McConnell, A. A. & Parker, H. L. (1938) A deformity of the hind-brain associated with internal hydrocephalus. Its relation to the Arnold–Chiari malformation. *Brain*, 415-429.

Mackenzie, N. G. & Emery, J. L. (1971) Deformities of the cervical cord in children with neurospinal dysra-phism. *Developmental Medicine and Child Neurology*, Suppl. 25, 58-67.

McKusick, V. A. (1968) *Mendelian inheritance in man: catalogs of autosomal dominant, autosomal recessive and x-linked phenotypes*, 2nd Edition, The Johns Hopkins Press, Baltimore.

McKusick, V. A., Mahloudji, M., Abbott, M. H., Lindenberg, R. & Kepas, D. (1967) Seckel's bird-headed dwarfism. *New England Journal of Medicine*, **277**, 279-286.

McKusick, V. A., Stauffer, M., Knox, D. L. & Clark, D. B. (1966) Chorioretinopathy with hereditary micro-cephaly. *Archives of Ophthalmology*, **75**, 597-600.

Mair, W. E. P. (1952) Pathological changes in infantile hemiplegia: a report based on 17 hemispherectomies. *Proceedings of the 1st International Congress of Neuropathology* (*Rome*), Vol. 2, pp. 242-245, Rosenberg and Sellier, Torino.

Malamud, N. (1950) Status marmoratus: form of cerebral palsy following either birth injury or inflammation of central nervous system. *Journal of Pediatrics*, **37**, 610-619.

Malamud, N. (1962) Sequelae of perinatal trauma and postnatal disorders. Pattern of CNS vulnerability in neonatal hypoxemia. *Proceedings of the 4th International Congress of Neuropathology* (*Munich*), pp. 36-41, Thieme, Stuttgart.

Malamud, N. (1972) Neuropathology of organic brain syndromes associated with aging in *Aging and the Brain* (Ed. Gaitz, C. M.), pp. 63-87, Plenum Publ. Co., New York.

Mall, F. P. (1908) A study of the causes underlying the origin of human monsters. *Journal of Morphology*, **19**, 1-367.

Mallory, F. B. (1896) A contribution to the study of calcareous concretions in the brain. *Journal of Pathology and Bacteriology*, **3**, 110-117.

Marburg, O. (1949) So-called agenesia of corpus callosum (callosal defect). Anterior cerebral dysraphism. *Archives of Neurology and Psychiatry* (*Chicago*), **61**, 296-312.

Maresh, R. (1929) Über einen Fall von Kohlenoxydgasschädigung des Kindes in der Gebärmutter. *Wiener medicinische Wochenschrift*, **79**, 454-456.

Marie, J., Lyon, G. & Bargeton, E. (1959) La sclérose cérébrale centro-lobaire. A propos de l'étude anatomo-clinique d'un cas de diplégie spasmodique congenitale (Syndrome de Little). *Presse Médicale*, **67**, 2286-2289.

Marin-Padilla, M. (1970) Morphogenesis of anencephaly and related malformations. *Current Topics in Pathology*, **51**, 145-174.

Martin, F. (1949) Ueber eine vestibulo-cerebellare Entwicklungshemmung im Rahmen ausgedehnter osteo-neuraler Dysgenesien. *Acta psychiatrica et neurologica*, **24**, 207-222.

Martin, F. (1950) Ueber eine vestibulo-cerebellare Entwicklungshemmung im Rahmen ausgedehnter osteo-neuraler Dysgenesien. *Acta psychiatrica et neurologica*, **25**, 415-421.

Martin, J. J., Deberdt, R., Philippart, M., Van Acker, K. J. & Hooft, C. (1971) Peculiar dysmorphic syndrome with orthochromatic leucodystrophy. Discussion of its relationship with Cockayne's syndrome and Pelizaeus–Merzbacher's disease. *Acta neuropathologica (Berlin)*, **18**, 224-233.

Martin, J. K. & Norman, R. M. (1967) Maple syrup urine disease in an infant with microgyria. *Developmental Medicine and Child Neurology*, **9**, 152-159.

Martin, J. P. (1941) Thrombosis in superior longitudinal sinus following childbirth. *British Medical Journal*, **2**, 537-540.

Meriwether, L. S., Hager, H. & Scholz, W. (1955) Kernicterus: hypoxemia, significant pathogenic factor. *Archives of Neurology and Psychiatry*, **73**, 293-301.

Merritt, K. K., Faber, H. K. & Bruch, H. (1937) Progressive facial hemiatrophy; report of 2 cases with cerebral calcification. *Journal of Pediatrics*, **10**, 374-395.

Mettler, F. A., Cooper, I., Liss, H., Carpenter, M. & Noback, C. (1954) Patterns of vascular failure in central nervous system. *Journal of Neuropathology and Experimental Neurology*, **13**, 528-539.

Meyer, A., Beck, E. & Sheppard, M. (1955) Unusually severe lesions in brain following status epilepticus. *Journal of Neurology, Neurosurgery and Psychiatry*, **18**, 24-33.

Meyer, A. & Jones, T. B. (1939) Histological changes in brain in mongolism. *Journal of Mental Science*, **85**, 206-221.

Meyer, J.-E. (1949) Zur Ätiologie und Pathogenese des fetalen und frühkindlichen Cerebralschadens: anatomisch-statistiche Untersuchungen. *Zeitschrift für Kinderheilkunde*, **67**, 123-136.

Meyer, J.-E. (1953) Über die Lokalisation frühkindlicher Hirnschäden in arteriellen Grenzgebeiten. *Archiv für Psychiatrie und Nervenkrankheiten*, **190**, 328-341.

Millen, J. W. & Woollam, D. H. M. (1956) The effect of the duration of Vitamin A deficiency in female rabbits upon the incidence of hydrocephalus in their young. *Journal of Neurology, Neurosurgery and Psychiatry*, **19**, 17-20.

Millen, J. W. & Woollam, D. H. M. (1958) Vitamins and cerebrospinal fluid in *Ciba Foundation Symposium on the Cerebrospinal Fluid*, pp. 168-185, Churchill, London.

Millen, J. W., Woollam, D. H. M. & Lamming, G. E. (1953) Hydrocephalus associated with deficiency of Vitamin A. *Lancet*, **2**, 1234-1236.

Miller, J. Q. (1963) Lissencephaly in two siblings. *Neurology (Minneapolis)*, **13**, 841-850.

Miller, J. Q., Pickard, E. H., Alkan, M. K., Warner, S. A. & Gerald, P. S. (1963) A specific congenital brain defect (arhinencephaly) in 13-15 trisomy. *New England Journal of Medicine*, **268**, 120-124.

Miller, O. J. (1964) The sex chromosome anomalies. *American Journal of Obstetrics and Gynecology*, **90**, 1078-1139.

Miller, R. W. (1968) Effects of ionizing radiation from the atomic bomb on Japanese children. *Pediatrics*, **41**, 257-263.

Minkowski, M. (1955) Sur les altérations de l'écorce cérébrale dans quelques cas de microcéphalie. *Schweizer Archiv für Neurologie, Neurochirurgie und Psychiatrie*, **76**, 110-173.

Miskolczy, D. (1931) Ein Fall von Kleinhirnmissbildung. *Archiv für Psychiatrie und Nervenkrankheiten*, **93**, 596-615.

Mitchell, R. G. (1952) Venous thrombosis in acute infantile hemiplegia. *Archives of Disease in Childhood*, **27**, 95-104.

Molland, E. A. & Purcell, M. (1975) Biliary atresia and the Dandy–Walker anomaly, in a neonate with 45X Turner's syndrome. *Journal of Pathology*, **115**, 227-230.

Monakow, C. von (1926) Biologisches und Morphogenetisches über die Mikrocephalia vera. *Schweizer Archiv für Neurologie und Psychiatrie*, **18**, 3-39.

Monie, I. W., Armstrong, R. M. & Nelson, M. M. (1961) Hydrocephalus and other abnormalities in the rat young resulting from maternal pteroylglutamic acid deficiency from the 8th to 10th days of pregnancy. *Abstracts of the Teratological Society*, **1**, 8.

Moosa, A. & Dubowitz, V. (1970) Peripheral neuropathy in Cockayne's syndrome. *Archives of Disease in Childhood*, **45**, 674-677.

Moossy, J. (1967) The neuropathology of Cockayne's syndrome. *Journal of Neuropathology and Experimental Neurology*, **26**, 654-660.

Morgagni, G. B. (1761) *De Sedibus et Causis Morborum* (Transl. B. Alexander), Miller and Cadell, London, 1769.

Morsier, G. de (1951) Les syndromes vasculaires embryonnaires dans les malformations cérébrales. *Schweizer Archiv für Neurologie und Psychiatrie*, **67**, 440-443.

Morsier, G. de (1952) Les syndromes vasculaires embryonnaires dans les malformations cérébrales. *Proceedings of the 1st International Congress of Neuropathology (Rome)*, Vol. 2, pp. 213-234, Rosenberg and Sellier, Torino.

Morsier, G. de   (1954) Études sur les dysraphies crânio-encéphaliques.   *Schweizer Archiv für Neurologie, Neurochirurgie und Psychiatrie*, **74**, 309-361.

Morsier, G. de   (1956) Études sur les dysraphies crânio-encéphaliques, Part 3 (Agénésie de septum lucidum avec malformation du tractus optique. La dysplasic septo-optique).   *Schweizer Archiv für Neurologie, Neurochirurgie und Psychiatrie*, **77**, 267-292.

Morsier, G. de & Mozer, J. J.   (1935) Agénésie complète de la commissure calleuse et troubles du développement de l'hémisphère gauche avec hémiparésie droite et intégrité mentale. (Le syndrome embryonnaire précoce de l'artère cérébrale antérieure.)   *Schweizer Archiv für Neurologie und Psychiatrie*, **35**, 64-95.

Moulton, S. L.   (1942) Hamartial nature of the tuberous sclerosis complex and its bearing on the tumor problem.   *Archives of Internal Medicine*, **69**, 589-623.

Muller, H. C.   (1950) Congenital anomalies—Scope and incidence of congenital abnormalities.   *Pediatrics*, **5**, 320-324.

Murphy, D. P.   (1947) *Congenital Malformations*, 2nd Edition, Lippincott, Philadelphia.

Muskett, C. W.   (1953) Elektive Differenzierungsstörungen des Zentralnervensystems am Hühnchenkeim nach kurzfristigem Sauerstoffmangel.   *Beiträge zur pathologischen Anatomie und zur allgemeinen Pathologie*, **113**, 368-387.

Mutrux, S., Wildi, E. & Bourquin, J.   (1949) Contribution à l'étude clinique et anatomo-pathologique des troubles cérébraux de l'embryopathie rubéoleuse.   *Schweizer Archiv für Neurologie und Psychiatrie*, **64**, 369-383.

Myers, R. E.   (1969) Atrophic cortical sclerosis associated with status marmoratus in a perinatally damaged monkey.   *Neurology (Minneapolis)*, **19**, 1177-1188.

Nañagas, J. C.   (1925) A comparison of the growth of the body dimensions of anencephalic human fetuses with normal fetal growth as determined by graphic analysis and empirical formulae.   *American Journal of Anatomy*, **35**, 455-494.

Nathan, P. W. & Smith, M. C.   (1950) Normal mentality associated with maldeveloped 'rhinencephalon'.   *Journal of Neurology, Neurosurgery and Psychiatry*, **13**, 191-197.

Neill, C. A. & Dingwall, M. M.   (1950) A syndrome resembling progeria: a review of two cases.   *Archives of Disease in Childhood*, **25**, 213-223.

Nelson, M. M., Baird, C. D. C., Wright, H. V. & Evans, H. M.   (1956) Multiple congenital abnormalities in the rat resulting from riboflavin deficiency induced by the antimetabolite galactoflavin.   *Journal of Nutrition*, **58**, 125-134.

Neubürger, F.   (1935) Fall einer intrauterinen Hirnschädigung nach einer Leuchtgasvergiftung der Mutter.   *Beiträge zur gerichtlichen Medizin*, **13**, 85-95.

Nieuwenhuijse, P.   (1913) Zur Kenntnis der Mikrogyrie.   *Psychiatrische en neurologische bladen (Amsterdam)*, **17**, 9-53.

Noel, P., Hubert, J. P., Ectors, M., Franken, L. & Flament-Durand, J.   (1973) Agenesis of the corpus callosum associated with relapsing hypothermia—a clinico-pathological report.   *Brain*, **96**, 359-368.

Norman, R. M.   (1936) Bilateral atrophic lobar sclerosis following thrombosis of the superior longitudinal sinus.   *Journal of Neurology and Psychopathology*, **17**, 135-152.

Norman, R. M.   (1940) Primary degeneration of the granular layer of the cerebellum: an unusual form of familial cerebellar atrophy occurring in early life.   *Brain*, **63**, 365-379.

Norman, R. M.   (1947) État marbré of the corpus striatum following birth injury.   *Journal of Neurology and Psychiatry*, **10**, 12-25.

Norman, R. M.   (1952) Mental deficiencies.   *Proceedings of the 1st International Congress of Neuropathology (Rome)*, Vol. 2, pp. 276-282, Rosenberg and Sellier, Torino.

Norman, R. M.   (1956) La sclérose lobaire dans l'épilepsie et l'encéphalopathie de la naissance.   *Acta neurologica belgica*, **56**, 89-103.

Norman, R. M.   (1958) The pathogenesis of amygdaloid lesions in early life in *Temporal Lobe Epilepsy* (Eds. Baldwin, M. & Bailey, B.), p. 203, Charles C. Thomas, Springfield, Ill.

Norman, R. M.   (1961*a*) Cerebellar hypoplasia in Werdnig–Hoffmann disease.   *Archives of Disease in Childhood*, **36**, 96-101.

Norman, R. M.   (1961*b*) Hemiplegia due to birth injury in *Hemiplegic Cerebral Palsy in Children and Adults*, pp. 11-17, National Spastics Society, London.

Norman, R. M.   (1962) Neuropathological findings in acute hemiplegia in childhood with special reference to epilepsy as pathogenic factors.   *Little Club Clinics in Developmental Medicine*, **6**, 37-48.

Norman, R. M.   (1963*a*) Observations on the neuropathology of Sturge–Weber disease in *Les phakomatoses cérébrales*, pp. 471-481, S.P.E.I., Paris.

Norman, R. M. (1963b) Patterns of symmetrical brain damage in *C.I.O.M.S. Symposium on Selective vulnerability of the CNS in hypoxaemia* (Eds. Schade, J. P. & McMenemey, W. H.), pp. 243-249, Blackwell Scientific, Oxford.

Norman, R. M. (1966) Neuropathological findings in trisomies 13-15 and 17-18 with special reference to the cerebellum. *Developmental Medicine and Child Neurology*, **8**, 170-177.

Norman, R. M. & McMenemey, W. H. (1955) Transventricular adhesions in association with birth injury of caudate nucleus. *Journal of Neuropathology and Experimental Neurology*, **14**, 84-91.

Norman, R. M. & Taylor, A. L. (1940) Congenital diverticulum of left ventricle of heart in case of epiloia. *Journal of Pathology and Bacteriology*, **50**, 61-68.

Norman, R. M. & Tingey, A. H. (1966) Syndrome of micrencephaly, strio-cerebellar calcifications and leucodystrophy. *Journal of Neurology, Neurosurgery and Psychiatry*, **29**, 157-163.

Norman, R. M., Tingey, A. H., Valentine, J. C. & Danby, T. A. (1962) Sudanophil leucodystrophy in a pachygyric brain. *Journal of Neurology, Neurosurgery and Psychiatry*, **25**, 363-369.

Norman, R. M. & Urich, H. (1957) Dissecting aneurysm of the middle cerebral artery as a cause of acute infantile hemiplegia. *Journal of Pathology and Bacteriology*, **73**, 580-582.

Norman, R. M. & Urich, H. (1958) Cerebellar hyperplasia associated with systemic degeneration in early life. *Journal of Neurology, Neurosurgery and Psychiatry*, **21**, 159-166.

Norman, R. M. & Urich, H. (1960) The influence of a vascular factor on the distribution of symmetrical cerebral calcifications. *Journal of Neurology, Neurosurgery and Psychiatry*, **23**, 142-147.

Norman, R. M. & Urich, H. (1962) Birth injury due to compression of cerebral arteries in *London Conference on the Scientific Study of Mental Deficiency*, pp. 299-313, May and Baker, London.

Norman, R. M., Urich, H. & McMenemey, W. H. (1957) Vascular mechanisms of birth injury. *Brain*, **80**, 49-58.

Norman, R. M., Urich, H. & Woods, G. E. (1958) The relationship between prenatal porencephaly and the encephalomalacias of early life. *Journal of Mental Science*, **104**, 758-771.

Ogryzlo, M. A. (1942) The Arnold–Chiari malformation. *Archives of Neurology and Psychiatry*, **48**, 30-46.

Olson, M. I. & Shaw, C. M. (1969) Presenile dementia and Alzheimer's disease in mongolism. *Brain*, **92**, 147-156.

Oppenheimer, D. R. & Griffith, H. B. (1966) Persistent intracranial bleeding as a complication of hemispherectomy. *Journal of Neurology, Neurosurgery and Psychiatry*, **29**, 229-240.

Ostertag, B. (1956) Die Einzelformen der Verbildungen (einschliesslich Syringomyelie) in *Handbuch der speziellen pathologischen Anatomie und Histologie* (Eds. Lubarsch, O., Henke, F. & Rössle, R.), Vol. 13, pt. 4, Springer Verlag, Berlin.

Padget, D. H. (1970) Neuroschisis and human embryonic maldevelopment: new evidence of anencephaly, spina bifida and diverse mammalian defects. *Journal of Neuropathology and Experimental Neurology*, **29**, 192-216.

Patau, K., Smith, D. W., Therman, E., Inhorn, S. L. & Wagner, H. P. (1960) Multiple congenital anomaly caused by an extra chromosome. *Lancet*, **1**, 790-793.

Patau, K., Therman, E., Smith, D. W., Inhorn, S. L. & Picken, B. F. (1961) Partial trisomy syndrome. I: Sturge–Weber's disease. *American Journal of Human Genetics*, **13**, 287-298.

Patten, B. M. (1952) Overgrowth of the neural tube in young human embryos. *Anatomical Record*, **113**, 381-393.

Patten, B. M. (1953) Embryological stages in the establishing of myeloschisis with spina bifida. *American Journal of Anatomy*, **93**, 365-395.

Paulson, G. (1967) Changing concepts of tuberous sclerosis. *Developmental Medicine and Child Neurology*, **9**, 493-494.

Peach, B. (1964a) Arnold–Chiari malformation: its pathological anatomy and histology. M.D. Thesis, Manchester.

Peach, B. (1964b) Cystic prolongation of fourth ventricle: an anomaly associated with the Arnold–Chiari malformation. *Archives of Neurology (Chicago)*, **11**, 609-612.

Peach, B. (1964c) Arnold–Chiari malformation with normal spine. *Archives of Neurology (Chicago)*, **10**, 497-501.

Peach, B. (1965a) Arnold–Chiari malformation: anatomic features of 20 cases. *Archives of Neurology (Chicago)*, **12**, 613-621.

Peach, B. (1965b) Arnold-Chiari malformation: morphogenesis. *Archives of Neurology (Chicago)*, **12**, 527-535.

Pellizzi, G. B. (1901) Contributo allo studio dell'idiozia. *Rivista sperimentale di Freniatria e Medicina Legale delle Alienazioni Mentali*, **27**, 265-269.

Penfield, W.   (1954) Mechanisms of voluntary movement.   *Brain*, **77**, 1-17.

Penfield, W. & Coburn, D. F.   (1938) Arnold–Chiari malformation and its operative treatment.   *Archives of Neurology and Psychiatry (Chicago)*, **40**, 328-336.

Penfield, W. & Elvidge, A. R.   (1932) Hydrocephalus and the atrophy of cerebral compression in *Cytology and Cellular Pathology of the Nervous System* (Ed. Penfield, W.), pp. 1203-1217, Hoeber, New York.

Penrose, L. S.   (1954) Observations on the aetiology of mongolism.   *Lancet*, **2**, 505-509.

Peter, K.   (1928) Ein weiterer anatomischer Beitrag zur Frage der Megalencephalie und Idiotie.   *Zeitschrift für gesamte Neurologie und Psychiatrie*, **113**, 298-312.

Peter, K. & Schlüter, K.   (1927) Ueber Megalencephalie als Grundlage der Idiotie.   *Zeitschrift für die gesamte Neurologie und Psychiatrie*, **108**, 21-40.

Pfeiffer, F.   (1939) Ein besonderer Fall von 'status marmoratus'.   *Psychiatrisch-neurologische Wochenschrift*, **41**, 409-412.

Pitt, D. B.   (1962) A study of congenital malformations Parts I and II.   *Australian and New Zealand Journal of Obstetrics and Gynaecology*, **2**, 23-30; 82-90.

Plummer, C.   (1952) Anomalies occurring in children exposed in utero to atomic bomb in Hiroshima.   *Pediatrics*, **10**, 687-693.

Polani, P. E., Briggs, J. H., Ford, C. E., Clarke, C. M. & Berg, J. M.   (1960) A mongol girl with 46 chromosomes.   *Lancet*, **1**, 721-724.

Polani, P. E., Hamerton, J. L., Giannelli, F. & Carter, C. O.   (1965) Cytogenetics of Down's syndrome (Mongolism), III.   Frequency of interchange trisomies and mutation rate of chromosome interchanges.   *Cytogenetics*, **4**, 193-206.

Poser, C. M., Walsh, F. C. & Scheinberg, L. C.   (1955) Hydranencephaly, case report.   *Neurology (Minneapolis)*, **5**, 284-289.

Probst, M.   (1900) Experimentelle Untersuchungen über die Schleifenendigung, die Haubenbahnen, das dorsale Längsbündel und die hintere Commissur.   *Archiv für Psychiatrie und Nervenkrankheiten*, **33**, 1-57.

Rainy, H. & Fowler, J. S.   (1903) Congenital facial diplegia due to nuclear lesion.   *Review of Neurology and Psychiatry*, **1**, 149-155.

Randt, C. T. & Derby, B. M.   (1973) Behavioral and brain correlations in early life nutritional deprivation.   *Archives of Neurology (Chicago)*, **28**, 167-172.

Recklinghausen, F. von   (1862) Ein Herz von einem Neugeborenen, welches mehrere, theils nach aussen, theils nach den Höhlen prominirende Tumoren (Myomen) trug.   *Monatschrift für Geburtshilfe und Gynäkologie*, **20**, 1-2.

Recklinghausen, F. von   (1886) Untersuchungen über die spina bifida.   Teil 2 (über die Art und die Entstehung der spina bifida ihre Beziehung zur Rückenmarks- und Darmspalte).   *Virchows Archiv für pathologische Anatomie und Physiologie*, **105**, 296-330.

Record, R. G. & McKeown, T.   (1950) Congenital malformations of central nervous system; maternal reproductive history and familial incidence.   *British Journal of Social Medicine*, **4**, 26-50.

Rehder, H.   (1914) Ein Beitrag zur Kenntnis der sogenannten Rhabdomyome des Herzens.   *Virchows Archiv für pathologische Anatomie und Physiologie*, **217**, 174-184.

Renwick, J. H.   (1972) Hypothesis: anencephaly and spina bifida are usually preventable by avoidance of a specific but unidentified substance present in certain potato tubers.   *British Journal of Preventive and Social Medicine*, **26**, 67-88.

Reye, R. D. K., Morgan, G. & Baral, J.   (1963) Encephalopathy and fatty degeneration of the viscera: a disease entity in childhood.   *Lancet*, **2**, 749-752.

Reznik, M. & Alberca-Serrano, R.   (1964) Forme familiale d'hypertélorisme avec lissencéphalie se présentant cliniquement sous forme d'une arrieration mentale avec épilepsie et paraplégie spasmodique.   *Journal of the Neurological Sciences*, **1**, 40-58.

Richardson, R. L. & Hogan, A. G.   (1946) Diet of mother and hydrocephalus in infant rats.   *Science*, **106**, 644.

Richman, D. P., Stewart, R. M. & Caviness, V. S. Jr.   (1974) Cerebral microgyria in a 27-week fetus.   An architectonic and topographic analysis.   *Journal of Neuropathology and Experimental Neurology*, **33**, 374-384.

Richter, R. B.   (1960) Unilateral congenital hypoplasia of the facial nucleus.   *Journal of Neuropathology and Experimental Neurology*, **19**, 33-41.

Roback, H. N. & Scherer, H. J.   (1934) Über die feinere Morphologie des frühkindlichen Gehirns unter besonderer Berücksichtigung der Gliaentwicklung.   *Virchows Archiv für pathologische Anatomie und Physiologie*, **294**, 365-413.

Robinson, R. G. (1955) Intracranial collections of fluid with local bulging of the skull. *Journal of Neurosurgery*, **12**, 345-353.

Robinson, R. G. (1958) Local bulging of the skull and external hydrocephalus due to cerebral agenesis. *British Journal of Radiology*, n.s. **31**, 691-700.

Robinson, R. G. (1964) The temporal lobe agenesis syndrome. *Brain*, **87**, 87-106.

Rokos, J. (1973) Pathogenesis of congenital malformations of the central nervous system with special reference to spina bifida and Arnold–Chiari malformation. M.D. Thesis, Univ. Birmingham.

Rorke, L. B., Riggs, H. E. & Fogelson, M. H. (1968) Cerebellar heterotopia in infancy. *Journal of Neuropathology and Experimental Neurology*, **27**, 140.

Rothman, P. E. (1931) Polioencephalitis. *American Journal of Diseases of Children*, **42**, 124-132.

Rowlatt, U. (1969) Cockayne's syndrome. Report of a case with necropsy findings. *Acta Neuropathologica (Berlin)*, **14**, 52-61.

Roy, S., Srivastava, R. N., Gupta, P. C. & Mayekar, G. (1973) Ultrastructure of peripheral nerve in Cockayne's syndrome. *Acta Neuropathologica (Berlin)*, **24**, 345-349.

Russell, D. S. (1949) *Observations on the Pathology of Hydrocephalus*. Special Report Series, Medical Research Council, No. 265, HMSO, London.

Russell, D. S. & Donald, C. (1935) Mechanism of internal hydrocephalus in spina bifida. *Brain*, **58**, 203-215.

Russell, L. B. (1954) The effects of radiation on mammalian prenatal development in *Radiation Biology* (Ed. Hollander, A.), Vol. 1, pt. 2, pp. 861-918, McGraw-Hill, New York.

Sabin, A. B. & Feldman, H. A. (1948) Chorioretinopathy associated with other evidence of cerebral damage in childhood. A syndrome of unknown aetiology separable from congenital toxoplasmosis. *Journal of Pediatrics*, **35**, 296-309.

Sandbank, V. (1955) Le syndrome d'Arnold–Chiari. *Revue Neurologique*, **93**, 529-563.

Scherer, H. J. (1933) Beiträge zur pathologischen Anatomie des Kleinhirns; genuine Kleinhirnatrophien. *Zeitschrift für die gesamte Neurologie und Psychiatrie*, **145**, 335-405.

Schlesinger, B. & Welch, R. G. (1952) Quadraplegia complicating gastroenteritis. *Gt. Ormond Street Journal*, **3**, 14-19.

Schminke, A. (1920) Zur Kenntnis der Megalencephalie. *Zeitschrift für die gesamte Neurologie und Psychiatrie*, **56**, 154-180.

Schminke, A. (1922) Kongenitale Herzhypertrophie bedingt durch diffuse Rhabdomyombildung. *Beiträge für pathologische Anatomie*, **70**, 513-515.

Schob, F. (1921) Weitere Beiträge zur Kenntnis der Friedreichähnlichen Krankheitsbilder. *Zeitschrift für die gesamte Neurologie und Psychiatrie*, **73**, 188-238.

Schob, F. (1929-30) Totalerweichung beider Grosshirnhemisphären bei einem zwei Monate alten Saügling. *Journal für Psychologie und Neurologie (Leipzig)*, **40**, 365-381.

Schob, F. (1930) Pathologische Anatomie der Idiotie in *Handbuch der Geisteskrankheiten* (Ed. Bumke, O.), Vol. 11, pp. 779-995, Springer Verlag, Berlin.

Schochet, S. S., Lampert, P. W. & McCormick, W. F. (1973) Neurofibrillary tangles in patients with Down's syndrome: a light and electron microscopic study. *Acta neuropathologica (Berlin)*, **23**, 342-346.

Scholz, W. (1924) Zur Kenntnis des Status marmoratus (infantile partielle Striatumsklerose). *Zeitschrift für die gesamte Neurologie und Psychiatrie*, **88**, 355-382.

Schuster, P. (1914) Beiträge zur Klinik der tuberösen Sklerose des Gehirns. *Deutsche Zeitschrift für Nervenheilkunde*, **50**, 96-132.

Schwalbe, E. & Gredig, M. (1907) Über Entwicklungsstörungen des Kleinhirns, Hirnstamms und Halsmarks bei Spina bifida. *Beiträge für pathologische Anatomie*, **40**, 132-194.

Schwartz, P. (1924) Erkrankungen des Zentralnervensystems nach traumatischer Geburtsschädigung. *Zeitschrift für die gesamte Neurologie und Psychiatrie*, **90**, 263-468.

Schwartz, P. (1927) Die traumatischen Schädigungen des Zentralnervensystems durch die Geburt. *Ergebnisse der inneren Medizin und Kinderheilkunde*, **31**, 165-373.

Schwartz, P. (1949) Sub-ependymal cysts of caudate nucleus; typical cerebral birth injury. *Harefuah*, **37**, 168-170.

Schwartz, P. (1961) *Birth injuries of the Newborn*, Karger, New York.

Seckel, H. P. G. (1960) *Bird-headed Dwarfs: Studies in Developmental Anthropology including Human Proportions*, Charles C. Thomas, Springfield, Ill.

Seitelberger, F. (1970) Pelizaeus-Merzbacher Disease in *Handbook of Clinical Neurology* (Eds. Vinken, P. J. & Bruyn, G. W.), Vol. 10, pp. 150-202, North-Holland, Amsterdam.

Sharpe, O. & Hall, E. C. (1953) Renal impairment, hypertension and encephalomalacia in an infant surviving severe intrauterine anoxia. *Proceedings of the Royal Society of Medicine*, **46**, 1063-1065.

Shaw, C.-M. & Alvord, E. C.   (1969) Cava septi pellucidi et Vergae: their normal and pathological states. *Brain*, **92**, 312-224.

Sherlock, E. B.   (1911) *The Feebleminded*, Macmillan, London.

Shuttleworth, G. E.   (1909) Mongolian imbecility.   *British Medical Journal*, **2**, 661-665.

Siegmund, H.   (1923) Die Entstehung von Porencephalien und Sklerosen aus geburtstraumatischen Hirn-schädigungen.   *Virchows Archiv für pathologische Anatomie und Physiologie*, **241**, 237-276.

Skyberg, D. & Van Der Hagen, C. B.   (1965) Congenital hereditary unilateral facial palsy in four generations. *Acta paediatrica scandinavica, Suppl.* **159**, 77-79.

Slotnick, V. & Brent, R. L.   (1966) The production of congenital malformations using tissue antisera.   V. Fluorescent localization of teratogenic antisera in the maternal and fetal tissue of the rat.   *Journal of Immunology*, **96**, 606-609.

Smith, H. V., Norman, R. M. & Urich, H.   (1957) The late sequelae of pneumococcal meningitis.   *Journal of Neurology, Neurosurgery and Psychiatry*, **20**, 250-259.

Smith, J. F.   (1974) *Pediatric Neuropathology*, McGraw-Hill, New York.

Solitare, G. B. & Lamarche, J. B.   (1966) Alzheimer's disease and senile dementia as seen in mongoloids: neuropathological observations.   *American Journal of Mental Deficiency*, **70**, 840-848.

Spatz, H. & Ullrich, O.   (1931) Klinischer und anatomischer Beitrag zu den angeborenen Beweglichskeitdefekten im Hirnnervenbereich.   *Zeitschrift für Kinderheilkunde*, **51**, 579-597.

Spielmeyer, W.   (1906) Hemiplegie bei intakter Pyramidenbahn (intrakortikale Hemiplegie).   *Münchener medizinische Wochenschrift*, **53**, 1404-1407.

Staemmler, M.   (1942) *Hydromyelie, Syringomyelie und Gliose* (Monographien aus dem Gesamtgebiete der Neurologie und Psychiatrie no. 72), Springer Verlag, Berlin.

Starkman, S. P., Brown, T. C. & Linnell, E. A.   (1958) Cerebral arachnoid cysts.   *Journal of Neuropathology and Experimental Neurology*, **17**, 484-500.

Steinbiss, W.   (1923) Zur Kenntnis der Rhabdomyome des Herzens und ihrer Beziehungen zur tuberösen Gehirnsklerose.   *Virchows Archiv für pathologische Anatomie und Physiologie*, **243**, 22-38.

Stempak, J. G.   (1965) Etiology of antenatal hydrocephalus induced by folic acid deficiency in the albino rat. *Anatomical Record*, **151**, 287-295.

Sternberg, E.   (1929) Über Spaltbildungen des Medullarohres bei jungen menschlichen Embryonen, ein Beitrag zur Entstehung der Anencephalie und der Rachischisis.   *Virchows Archiv für pathologische Anatomie und Physiologie*, **272**, 325-374.

Stewart, R. M.   (1929-30) Congenital facial diplegia.   *Jorunal of Neurology and Psychopathology*, **10**, 317-322.

Stewart, R. M.   (1939) Arhinencephaly.   *Journal of Neurology and Psychiatry*, **2**, 303-312.

Stewart, R. M.   (1948) Infantile cerebral hemiplegia; clinical features and pathological anatomy.   *Edinburgh Medical Journal*, **55**, 488-505.

Stewart, R. M.   (1956) Cerebellar agenesis.   *Journal of Mental Science*, **102**, 67-77.

Struck, G. & Hemmer, R.   (1964) Elektronenmikroskopische Untersuchungen an der menschlichen Hirnrinde beim Hydrocephalus.   *Archiv für Psychiatrie und Nervenkrankheiten*, **206**, 17-27.

Strümpell, A.   (1884) Ueber die acute Encephalitis der Kinder (Polioencephalitis acuta, cerebrale Kinder-lähmung).   *Jahrbuch für Kinderheilkunde*, **22**, 173-178.

Sturge, W. A.   (1879) A case of partial epilepsy, apparently due to a lesion of one of the vaso-motor centres of the brain.   *Transactions of The Clinical Society of London*, 162-167.

Sumi, S. M.   (1970) Brain malformations in the trisomy 18 syndrome.   *Brain*, **93**, 821-830.

Suter, M. & Wichser, C.   (1948) Fate of living viable babies in extrauterine pregnancies.   *American Journal of Obstetrics and Gynaecology*, **55**, 489-495.

Suwanwela, C. & Suwanwela, N.   (1972) A morphological classification of sincipital encephalomeningoceles. *Journal of Neurosurgery*, **36**, 201-211.

Swan, C.   (1949) Rubella in pregnancy as aetiological factor in congenital malformation, still birth, miscarriage and abortion.   *Journal of Obstetrics and Gynaecology of the British Empire*, **56**, 341-363, 591-605.

Sylvester, P. E.   (1960) Marbling and perinatal anoxia.   *Acta paediatrica*, **49**, 338-344.

Taggart, J. K. & Walker, A. E.   (1942) Congenital atresia of the foramina of Luschka and Magendie.   *Archives of Neurology and Psychiatry (Chicago)*, **48**, 583-612.

Talwalker, V. C. & Dastur, D. K.   (1970) 'Meningoceles' and 'meningomyeloceles' (ectopic spinal cord). Clinicopathological basis of a new classification.   *Journal of Neurology, Neurosurgery and Psychiatry*, **33**, 251-262.

Talwalker, V. C. & Dastur, D. K.   (1974) Ectopic spinal cord (myelomeningocele) with tethering: a clinico-pathological entity.   *Developmental Medicine and Child Neurology*, **16**, Suppl. 32, 159-160.

Tandon, M. S. & Harkmark, W.   (1959) Spontaneous ventriculocisternostomy with relief of obstructive hydro-
cephalus.   *Neurology (Minneapolis)*, **9**, 699-703.
Taniguchi, T. & Mufson, J. A.   (1950) Intradural lipoma of the spinal cord.   *Journal of Neurosurgery*, **7**,
584-586.
Taylor, J.   (1905) *Paralysis and Other Diseases of the Nervous System in Childhood and Early Life*, J. & A.
Churchill, London.
Teng, P. & Papatheodorou, C.   (1965) Arnold-Chiari malformation with normal spine and cranium.   *Archives
of Neurology (Chicago)*, **12**, 622-624.
Terplan, K. L.   (1967) Histopathologic brain changes in 1152 cases of the perinatal and early infancy period.
Biologia Neonatorum, **11**, 348-366.
Terplan, K. L. & Çohen, M. M.   (1968) Cerebellar changes in association with 'partial' trisomy 18.   *American
Journal of Diseases of Children*, **115**, 179-184.
Terplan, K. L., Sandberg, A. A. & Aceto, T.   (1966) Structural anomalies in the cerebellum in association with
trisomy.   *Journal of the American Medical Association*, **197**, 557-568.
Thelander, H. E., Shaw, E. B. & Peel, J. J.   (1953) Angiography in case of hydranencephaly.   *Journal of
Pediatrics*, **42**, 680-686.
Thieffry, S., Arthuis, M., Faure, C. & Lyon, G.   (1961) in *18th Congrès de l'Association des Pédiatres de langue
française*, Rapport II, Karger, Basel.
Thiersch, J. B.   (1952) Therapeutic abortions with a folic acid antagonist.   4-aminopteroylglutamic acid
administered by the oral route.   *American Journal of Obstetrics and Gynaecology*, **63**, 1298-1304.
Thomas, A. & Ajuriaguerra, J. de   (1959) Étude anatomo-clinique de l'anencéphalie in *Malformations congéni-
tales du cerveau* (Eds. Heuyer, G., Feld, M. & Gruner, J.), pp. 207-267, Masson, Paris.
Till, K.   (1969) Spinal dysraphism.   A study of congenital malformations of the lower back.   *Journal of Bone
and Joint Surgery*, **51**B, 415-422.
Tingey, A. H.   (1955) Iron and calcium in Sturge-Weber disease.   *Journal of Mental Science*, **102**, 178-180.
Töndury, G. & Smith, D. W.   (1966) Fetal rubella pathology.   *Journal of Pediatrics*, **68**, 867-879.
Towbin, A.   (1970) Neonatal damage of the central nervous system in *Neuropathology: Methods and Diagnosis*
(Ed. Tedeschi, C. G.), pp. 609-653, Little, Brown, Boston.
Turhan, B. & Rossler, R.   (1942) Schädigung der vena magna Galeni durch Geburtstrauma.   *Monatschrift für
Psychiatrie und Neurologie*, **105**, 228-234.
Uiberrack, F.   (1942) Demonstration eines Falles von Ganglienzellerkrankung bei einem Fetus nach Röntgen-
bestrahlung der Mutter.   *Zentralblatt für Pathologie*, **80**, 187.
Ule, G.   (1952) Kleinhirnrindenatrophie vom Körnertyp.   *Deutsche Zeitschrift für Nervenheilkunde*, **168**
195-226.
Ulrich, J., Isler, W. & Vassalli, L.   (1965) L'effet d'hémorrhagies leptoméningées répétées sur le système nerveux
(La sidérose marginale du système nerveux central).   *Revue Neurologique*, **112**, 466-471.
Van Bogaert, L.   (1929) Sur une variété non décrite d'affection familiale.   L'épilepsie myoclonique avec
choréo-athétose (État marbré du strié avec dégénérescence cortico-olivaire).   *Revue Neurologique*, **36**,
385-414.
Van Bogaert, L.   (1950) Sur une athétose double (état marbré) chez un frère et une soeur.   *Monatschrift für
Psychiatrie und Neurologie*, **120**, 169-205.
Van Bogaert, L., Paillas, J. E., Berard-Badier, M. & Payan, H.   (1958) Étude sur la sclérose tuberéuse de
Bourneville à forme cérébelleuse.   *Revue Neurologique*, **98**, 673-689.
Van Bogaert, L. & Radermecker, M. A.   (1955) Une dysgénésie cérébelleuse chez un enfant du radium.   *Revue
Neurologique*, **93**, 65-82.
Van Der Weil, H. J.   (1957) Hereditary Congenital facial paralysis.   *Acta genetica et statistica medica*, **7**,
348.
Van Gieson, I.   (1892) A study of the artefacts of the nervous system.   The topographical alterations of the
gray and white matters of the spinal cord caused by autopsy bruises, and a consideration of heterotopia of
the spinal cord.   *New York Medical Journal*, **56**, 337-346, 365-379, 421-437.
Variend, S. & Emery, J. L.   (1974) The pathology of the central lobes of the cerebellum in children with myelo-
meningocele.   *Developmental Medicine and Child Neurology*, **16**, Suppl. 32, 99-106.
Veith, G.   (1962) Der perinatale Hirnschaden im Rahmen der Neugeborenen-Pathologie.   *Proceedings of the
IVth International Congress of Neuropathology*, Vol. III, pp. 6-11, Thieme, Stuttgart.
Verhaart, W. J. C. & Kramer, W.   (1952) The uncrossed pyramidal tract.   *Acta psychiatrica neurologica
scandinavica*, **27**, 181-200.
Verhaart, W. J. C. & Van Wieringen-Rauws, G. A.   (1950) On cerebrocerebellar atrophy.   *Folia psychiatrica,
neurologica, neurochirurgica neerlandica*, **53**, 481-501.

Vogel, F. S. (1958) The association of vascular anomalies with anencephaly. A post-mortem study of nine cases in one of which unilateral anencephaly was present in a conjoined double monster. *American Journal of Pathology*, **34**, 169-175.

Vogel, F. S. & McClenahan, J. L. (1952) Anomalies of major cerebral arteries associated with congenital malformations of the brain, with special reference to the pathogenesis of anencephaly. *American Journal of Pathology*, **28**, 701-711.

Vogt, C. & Vogt, O. (1920) Zur Lehre der Erkrankungen des striären Systems. *Journal für Psychologie und Neurologie (Leipzig)*, **25**, Suppl. 3, 627-846.

Vogt, H. (1908) Zur Pathologie und pathologischer Anatomie der verschiedenen Idioţieformen. II. Tuberöse Sklerose. *Monatschrift für Psychiatrie und Neurologie*, **24**, 106-150.

Volland, F. (1910) Über Megalencephalie. *Archiv für Psychiatrie und Nervenheilkunde*, **47**, 1228-1252.

Wachsmuth, N. & Lowenthal, A. (1950) Détermination chimique d'éléments minéraux dans les calcifications intracérébrales de la maladie de Sturge–Weber. *Acta Neurologica Psychiatrica Belgica*, **50**, 305-313.

Wald, A. (1930) Systematische Untersuchungen über geburtstraumatische Veränderungen der basalen Ganglien bei Neugeborenen und Säuglingen und ihre Bedeutung für die sogenannten angeborenen Erkrankungen der basalen Ganglien. *Zeitschrift für Kinderheilkunde*, **49**, 375-397.

Walker, A. E. (1942) Lissencephaly. *Archives of Neurology and Psychiatry (Chicago)*, **48**, 13-29.

Walsh, F. B. & Lindenberg, R. (1961) Hypoxia in infants and children: a clinical-pathological study concerning the primary visual pathways. *Bulletin of the Johns Hopkins Hospital*, **108**, 100-145.

Warkany, J. (1971) *Congenital Malformations: Notes and Comments*, Year Book Publishers, Chicago.

Warkany, J. & Nelson, R. C. (1940) Appearance of skeletal abnormalities in the offspring of rats reared on a deficient diet. *Science*, **92**, 383-384.

Warner, F. J. (1953) The histogenetic principle of microgyria and related cerebral malformations. *Journal of Nervous and Mental Diseases*, **118**, 1-18.

Weber, F. P. (1922-23) Right-sided hemihypotrophy resulting from right-sided congenital spastic hemiplegia, with a morbid condition of the left side of the brain, revealed by radiograms. *Journal of Neurology and Psychopathology*, **3**, 134-139.

Weber, F. P. (1929) A note on the association of extensive haemangiomatous naevus of the skin with cerebral (meningeal) haemangioma, especially cases of facial vascular naevus with contralateral hemiplegia. *Proceedings of the Royal Society of Medicine*, **22**, 431-442.

Wefring, K. W. & Lamvig, J. O. (1967) Familial progressive poliodystrophy with cirrhosis of the liver. *Acta paediatrica (Uppsala)*, **56**, 295-300.

Weil, A. (1933) Megalencephaly with diffuse glioblastomatosis of the brain stem and the cerebellum. *Archives of Neurology and Psychiatry (Chicago)*, **30**, 795-809.

Weller, R. O. & Shulman, K. (1972) Infantile hydrocephalus: clinical, histological and ultrastructural study of brain damage. *Journal of Neurosurgery*, **36**, 255-265.

Weller, R. O. & Wisniewski, H. (1969) Histological and ultrastructural changes with experimental hydrocephalus in adult rabbits. *Brain*, **92**, 819-828.

Weller, R. O., Wisniewski, H., Shulman, K. & Terry, R. D. (1971) Experimental hydrocephalus in young dogs: histological and ultrastructural study of the brain tissue damage. *Journal of Neuropathology and Experimental Neurology*, **30**, 613-626.

Weller, S. D. V. & Norman, R. M. (1955) Epilepsy due to birth injury in one of identical twins. *Archives of Disease in Childhood*, **30**, 453-459.

White, H. H. (1961) Cerebral hemispherectomy in the treatment of infantile hemiplegia. *Confinia Neurologica*, **21**, 1-50.

Williams, B. (1973) Is aqueduct stenosis a result of hydrocephalus? *Brain*, **96**, 399-412.

Williams, B. & Guthkelch, A. N. (1974) Why do central arachnoid pouches expand? *Journal of Neurology, Neurosurgery and Psychiatry*, **37**, 1085-1092.

Willis, R. A. (1958) *The Borderland of Embryology and Pathology*, Butterworth, London.

Wilson, P. J. E. (1970) Cerebral hemispherectomy for infantile hemiplegia. A report of 50 cases. *Brain*, **93**, 147-180.

Wilson, S. A. K. (1933-34) Megalencephaly. *Journal of Neurology and Psychopathology*, **14**, 193-216.

Windle, W. F. (1963) Selective vulnerability of the CNS of rhesus monkeys to asphyxia in *C.I.O.M.S. Symposium on Selective Vulnerability of the CNS in Hypoxaemia* (Eds. Schade, J. P. & McMenemey, W. H.), pp. 251-255, Blackwell Scientific, Oxford.

Winick, M. & Noble, A. (1966) Cellular response in rat during malnutrition at various ages. *Journal of Nutrition*, **89**, 300-306.

Wohlwill, F. & Yakovlev, P. I.   (1957) Histopathology of meningo-facial angiomatosis (Sturge–Weber's disease). Report of four cases. *Journal of Neuropathology and Experimental Neurology*, **16**, 341-364.

Wolf, A. & Cowen, D.   (1956) The cerebral atrophies and encephalomalacias of infancy and childhood. *Research Publications of the Association for Research in Nervous and Mental Diseases*, **34**, 199-330.

Wolf, A. & Cowen, D.   (1959) Perinatal infections of the central nervous system. *Journal of Neuropathology and Experimental Neurology*, **18**, 191-243.

Wolff, E. & Kirrmann, J. M.   (1954) L'influence protectrice de la cysteamine contre l'action tératogène des irradiations localisées. *Comptes Rendus des Séances de la Société de Biologie et de ses Filiales*, **148**, 1629-1631.

Wood, J. W., Johnson, K. G. & Omori, Y.   (1967) In utero exposure to the Hiroshima atomic bomb. An evaluation of head size and mental retardation. Twenty years later. *Pediatrics*, **39**, 385-392.

Woodhall, B.   (1939) Anatomy of the cranial blood sinuses with particular reference to the lateral. *Laryngoscope*, **49**, 966-1010.

Woolf, A. L.   (1955) The pathology of acute infantile cerebral diplegia. *Journal of Mental Science*, **101**, 610-628.

Woollam, D. H. M. & Millen, D. W.   (1953) Anatomical considerations in the pathology of stenosis of the cerebral aqueduct. *Brain*, **76**, 104-112.

Woollam, D. H. M. & Millen, J. W.   (1960) The modification of the activity of certain agents exerting a deleterious effect on the development of the mammalian embryo in *Ciba Foundation Symposium on Congenital Malformations* (Eds. Wolstenholme, G. E. W. & O'Connor, C. M.), pp. 158-172, Churchill, London.

Wyatt, J. P. & Tribby, W. W.   (1952) Granulomatous encephalomyelitis in infancy. *Archives of Pathology*, **53**, 103-120.

Wyllie, W. G.   (1951) The cerebral palsies of infancy in *Modern Trends in Neurology* (Ed. Feiling, A.), pp. 129-148, Butterworth, London.

Yakovlev, P. I.   (1947) Paraplegias of hydrocephalics (A clinical note and interpretation). *American Journal of Mental Deficiency*, **51**, 561-576.

Yakovlev, P. I.   (1959) Pathoarchitectonic studies of cerebral malformations. III. Arrhinencephalies (holotelencephalies). *Journal of Neuropathology and Experimental Neurology*, **18**, 22-55.

Yakovlev, P. I. & Corwin, W.   (1939) A roentgenographic sign in cases of tuberous sclerosis of brain (multiple 'brain stones'). *Archives of Neurology and Psychiatry*, **42**, 1030-1037.

Yakovlev, P. I. & Wadsworth, R. C.   (1946) Schizencephalies. A study of the congenital clefts in the cerebral mantle. I. Clefts with fused lips. II. Clefts with hydrocephalus and lips separated. *Journal of Neuropathology and Experimental Neurology*, **5**, 116-130 and 169-206.

Yamazaki, J. N., Wright, S. W. & Wright, P. M.   (1954) Outcome of pregnancy in women exposed to atomic bomb in Nagasaki. *American Journal of Diseases of Children*, **87**, 448-463.

Yates, P. O.   (1959) Birth trauma to the vertebral arteries. *Archives of Disease in Childhood*, **34**, 436-441.

Yates, P. O.   (1962) Perinatal injury to the neck and extracranial cerebral arteries. *Proceedings of the IVth International Congress of Neuropathology (Munich)*, Vol. III, pp. 20-23, Thieme, Stuttgart.

Ylppö, A.   (1919) Pathologisch-anatomische Studien bei Frühgeborenen. *Zeitschrift für Kinderheilkunde*, **20**, 212-431.

Zülch, K. J.   (1954) Mangeldurchblutung an der Grenzzone zweier Gefässgebiete als Ursache bisher ungeklärter Rückenmarksschädigungen. *Deutsche Zeitschrift für Nervenheilkunde*, **172**, 81-101.

Zülch, K. J.   (1955) Kreislaufstörungen an der Grenzlinie von Hirn- und Rückenmarksgefässen. *Proceedings of the 2nd International Congress of Neuropathology, London*, Vol. 2, pp. 613-615, Excerpta Medica, Amsterdam.

11

Demyelinating Diseases

D. R. Oppenheimer

The term 'demyelinating disease' is conventionally given to a group of diseases of the central nervous system characterized by large or small foci of myelin breakdown, followed by fibrous gliosis. The term originated from the discovery that in multiple (or disseminated) sclerosis axons remain relatively intact in the demyelinated areas. It is to this type of disease, affecting larger or smaller blocks of central nervous tissue, that the term should be restricted; that is, it should not be used to cover conditions such as the leucodystrophies, in which there is a defect in myelin formation; or for toxic/metabolic conditions, such as subacute combined degeneration of the cord, or cerebral oedema, in which it seems that myelin breakdown precedes axon destruction; or for peripheral neuropathies, in which the process of demyelination affects internodal segments of individual nerve fibres. A strict verbal definition of demyelinating disease is not at present possible, but in practice the term is used to cover multiple sclerosis and allied diseases.

During the past 30 years there has been much dispute concerning what conditions are, in fact, allied to multiple sclerosis. The separation of the leucodystrophies (see p. 541) is now generally accepted, but the relationship between multiple sclerosis and various acute encephalomyelopathies, characterized by perivenous destructive lesions, remains obscure. The subject is discussed on p. 491. Another condition, apparently unrelated to any of these, in which demyelination of central nervous tissue is a conspicuous feature, is central pontine myelinolysis (see p. 495).

Multiple sclerosis
(*Disseminated sclerosis*)

The lesions of multiple sclerosis were recognized and illustrated by Carswell (1838) and Cruveilhier (1835-42); but to Charcot (1877) must be given the credit for first recognizing the characteristic pathological feature of the disease—demyelination without destruction of axons. He was specially impressed by the firm texture of the lesions, which led him to give the disease the name *sclérose en plaques*. The term *sclerosis* has been universally preserved, with the descriptive adjectives *disseminated, multiple, insular* or *diffuse*; but it must be remembered that early lesions are by no means sclerotic (they are, if anything, softer than normal central nervous tissue), and

that glial scarring is not, as Charcot thought, a primary process. The term *plaque* is still commonly used to describe the lesions, although it suggests a flat disc rather than the spherical, ovoid, or other solid forms which the lesions take.

Since Charcot's description, multiple sclerosis has come to be recognized as one of the commonest organic diseases of the central nervous system throughout the temperate zones. Its clinical manifestations are very variable, not only in the symptoms and signs, which depend on the situation of the lesions, but also in the time course and progression of the disease. At one extreme there are *formes frustes* (recognized by Charcot) in which one or two neurological episodes in early life are followed by a lifelong remission. Occasionally, old lesions may be found at necropsy in cases with no history of neurological disease. At the other extreme there are fulminating cases, with rapid progression to death, without remissions. Between these extremes there is a continuum, with no clear dividing lines; nevertheless, it is convenient to classify the disease into a few broad types. Using the names of early investigators as eponyms, one may distinguish, first, a classical, or *Charcot type*, in which the onset of the disease is usually in the third or fourth decade of life, there are neurological remissions and relapses, and at necropsy lesions of various ages are found. The second type (generally called acute multiple sclerosis) was described by *Marburg* in 1906. Here, the illness takes a more rapid and fatal course, and all or nearly all the lesions are found to be recent. In the *Schilder* type (named after Schilder's (1912) description of a case) the clinical course is likewise more rapid than in the classical type; clinically the picture is dominated by progressive loss of 'higher' functions, and pathologically by massive demyelinative lesions in the cerebral hemispheres, with or without small lesions elsewhere. The type described by *Balò* (1928) is a fulminating condition, in which the diagnosis is made by the necropsy finding of laminated shells of demyelination, separated by layers of more or less intact myelin. In the type named after *Dévic* (1894) the brunt of the disease falls on the optic nerves and spinal cord. These varieties will be described in more detail below. Compared with the Charcot type, the other four types are rare, tending to occur in a younger age group, and the lesions are generally more severe and rapidly fatal. The clinical, epidemiological and pathological aspects of multiple sclerosis are very fully treated in two monographs (McAlpine, Compston and Lumsden 1955; McAlpine, Lumsden and Acheson 1972), and in volume 9 of the *Handbook of Clinical Neurology* (Vinken and Bruyn 1970). The pathology is exhaustively reviewed by Peters (1958, 1968).

Lesions in typical (Charcot type) cases

In cases coming to necropsy after an illness of several years, findings outside the central nervous system are either unrelated to the disease, or are secondary to it. Secondary features, seen in many chronic cases, include flexion contractures at elbows, hips and knees; emaciation, often with pressure sores; and chronic cystitis and pyelonephritis due to loss of bladder control. Naked eye examination may show little on the external surface of the brain that is characteristic of the disease. In some cases grey, slightly depressed areas, usually asymmetrical and sharply outlined, may be seen on the ventral surface of the pons (Fig. 11.1). In many cases there is some general shrinkage of the cerebral hemispheres, with widening of the sulci and slight or moderate enlargement of the ventricles. The surface of the spinal cord may show greyish, slightly

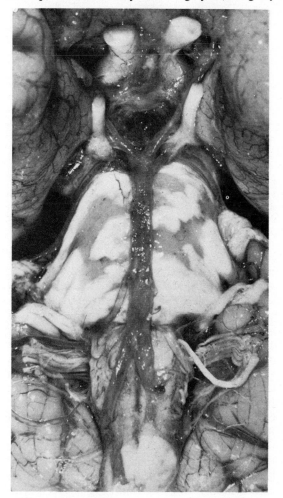

Fig. 11.1 Multiple sclerosis. Man, aged 40. 11-year history. Superficial lesions in pons. Leptomeninges have been removed.

depressed, areas, often extending over several segments, and in severe cases there may be obvious shrinkage of a large stretch of the cord. The apparent incidence of optic nerve involvement increases if the intraorbital portions of the nerves are routinely examined.

On section of the brain the lesions are usually obvious (Fig. 11.2). They appear as grey patches, with more or less sharply outlined edges, scattered irregularly through grey and white matter. The smaller lesions, only a few millimetres across, appear as circular or oval grey spots, at the

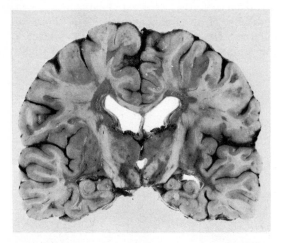

Fig. 11.2 Multiple sclerosis. Case as in Fig. 11.1. Coronal slice of fixed brain, showing large and small areas of demyelination. Many of the smaller lesions are perivascular. The largest ones are paraventricular.

centre of which a dilated blood vessel may often be seen. The larger ones are generally irregular in shape, with a lobulated outline. Recent lesions tend to be pinkish in colour, whereas older ones are grey and even gelatinous. The increased firmness in the older lesions, which originally gave rise to the use of the term 'sclerosis', is only appreciable in the unfixed brain. In general, lesions in white matter are more easily seen than those in grey matter, owing to contrast of colour. In the brainstem, they are nearly always present, but may be hard to detect, partly because of fixation artefacts resulting in blotchy discoloration of the tissues, and partly because it is here that so-called 'shadow plaques' are most frequent (see below). In slices of the cerebral hemispheres care is needed to avoid confusion between areas of demyelination in the centrum ovale and isolated areas of deeply-lying cortex. In sections of the cord, it is usually possible to see clear-cut areas

of demyelination; but in a severe or long-standing case, the outlines may be blurred by the effects of diffuse long tract degeneration. The lesions are often elongated in the long axis of the cord.

Distribution of lesions

From case to case, there are large variations; for instance, a case with extensive lesions in the spinal cord and optic nerves may show only a few small lesions in the cerebral hemispheres. In the brain, the lesions tend to be roughly— but only roughly—symmetrical, and it is rare to find extensive lesions on one side only. Lesions are very commonly found abutting on the lining of the ventricular system, in particular at the lateral angles of the lateral ventricles (including the inferior horns) and in the floor of the aqueduct and 4th ventricle. These periventricular 'plaques' may appear small in a coronal slice; but they are often continuous, extending from the tips of the posterior horns to the tips of the anterior and inferior horns, or from the aqueduct to the central canal. Small lesions confined to the cerebral cortex, or straddling the junction of cortex and white matter, are common but easily missed on naked-eye inspection. There is no site of predilection for the more centrally placed lesions, but there is a tendency for lesions in the cerebral white matter to stop short of the cortex, leaving about a millimetre of subcortical myelin intact. In the spinal cord there is often a similar tendency to spare a thin rim of subpial white matter; some lesions, however, appear to have spread inwards from the pial surface of the brainstem and cord.

Histology of lesions

The microscopic appearance of the lesions depends on their chronicity, and on their severity, i.e. destructiveness. In general, the more destructive lesions are found in the rarer forms of the disease. Taking the milder lesions first, their evolution in time can be followed both from a study of individual plaques for which there is clinical 'dating', and by observing the transition zone at the edge of an actively expanding plaque. A detailed description of the successive histological and chemical changes is given by Seitelberger (1960).

In the first few days, the lesions are hard to detect. They consist of structural changes (irregular bubbly expansions and altered staining reactions) in the myelin sheath, and microglial proliferation. During the ensuing weeks, the microglia becomes phagocytic, and can be seen to contain both fragments of myelin and globules of sudanophilic material. Mingled with them are large reactive astrocytes, and extracellular fragments of myelin and sudanophil lipid. Axis cylinders often display irregular thickenings, and an increased affinity for silver, without the fragmentation seen in early Wallerian degeneration. The most striking negative feature, which distinguishes a plaque of multiple sclerosis from an ischaemic infarct is that the bodies of nerve cells within the lesions appear perfectly normal (Fig. 11.19).

At the end of a few weeks—that is, at the time when the clinical signs would normally be remitting—the typical lesion is readily seen in sections stained for myelin as an unstained area with a smooth clearly defined edge. In cell stains, the area is more cellular than normal (Figs. 11.3 and 11.5), the additional cells being astrocytes and microglial phagocytes, with the greatest concentration at the edge of the lesion. Recognizable oligodendrocytes have largely or completely disappeared. There is often some lymphocytic

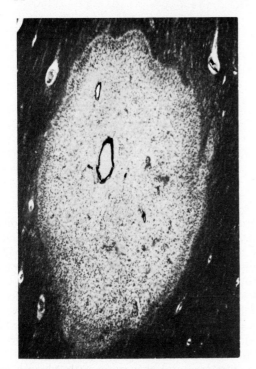

Fig. 11.3 Multiple sclerosis. Fresh perivenous lesion, showing great cellularity. Klüver-Barrera stain for myelin and cells. × 35.

cuffing of small vessels within or around the lesion; but this feature is not prominent in the early stages, and is often more conspicuous in older lesions. Fibrillar gliosis has started, but is not conspicuous.

After about six months, fibrillar gliosis is well advanced. The amount of sudanophilic lipid has decreased, and lipid phagocytes are seen congregating around small blood vessels, through the walls of which the material is presumably transferred to the blood stream. Reactive astrocytes are less in evidence. Finally, the lipid is disposed of, most of the glial cells disappear, and the area thenceforward consists of axis cylinders, nerve cells (if the lesion is in grey matter), and blood vessels, in a feltwork of glial fibrils. A good Holzer preparation will now appear as a negative image of the myelin preparation (Fig. 11.4). At the edge of the lesion, myelin sheaths come to an abrupt termination. Here, too, there is a persisting excess of small glial cells (Fig. 11.5). Frozen sections stained for fat will often show local accumulations of intra- and extracellular lipid at the border of the lesion, indicating continued activity of the demyelinating process. It is in this way that the larger plaques, with their irregular contours, develop.

Although preservation of axons is the rule in early lesions, there is commonly a partial destruction of axons, leading to Wallerian degeneration, in long-standing lesions. This can often be seen, for instance, in silver impregnations of old periventricular plaques with concomitant atrophy of the central white matter and of the corpus callosum. Wallerian degeneration is likewise responsible for some of the atrophy of the spinal cord seen in chronic cases, and for diffuse pallor of the long tracts of the cord in myelin stains.

Shadow plaques
In sections stained for myelin, some lesions do not show the total absence of myelin and the clear-cut outlines of the typical plaque. The reasons for this are various. The lesion may be an early one, in which the myelin is not yet completely broken down, but shows an impaired staining reaction; or some fibres in the area are demyelinated, while others are not; or else there is a uniform partial destruction of myelin sheaths. Chronic 'shadow plaques' of the last two kinds are relatively common in the brainstem, where it may be difficult to define the outlines, or even be

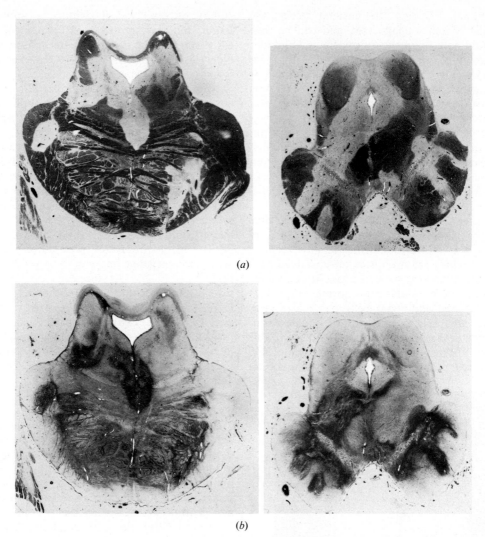

(a)

(b)

Fig. 11.4 Multiple sclerosis. Woman, aged 42. 6-year history. Chronic lesions in midbrain and pons stained (a) for myelin and (b) for glial fibres. Holzer.

certain of the presence, of a lesion from the myelin stain alone. In such instances, the plaque may show up clearly in the Holzer stain (Fig. 11.6), in which it is seen that a heavy gliosis can result from a partial demyelination. Not infrequently, 'shadow' areas are seen at the edge of a completely demyelinated area, or surrounding it in the form of a halo.

Fine structure of plaques
Reports on this are at present scanty, but there is a detailed account of the electron-microscopic appearances in three old, inactive lesions by

Périer and Grégoire (1965). Their main finding was of a very large extracellular space traversed by naked axons and condensed glial fibrils. The cells identified in the centre of the lesions were protoplasmic astrocytes. At the edges a few oligodendrocytes, reactive astrocytes and microglial cells were present. Normal-looking axons were seen running into, or out of, myelin sheaths which retained their normal structure up to their abrupt terminations. Preliminary accounts of the ultrastructural changes in early plaques are given by Lumsden (1970a). From these, it seems probable that the extracellular space described above results from the disruption of water-logged astrocytes (Figs. 11.7 and 11.8).

Lesions in severe and atypical cases

There appears to be a continuous variation from the typical, relatively indolent, lesions described above to the more severe and destructive ones. In these, the tempo of the process is quicker, liferate, and take on monstrous forms, with multiple nuclei; their appearance in small biopsy specimens may even give rise to a mistaken diagnosis of glioma. The affected tissue swells (Fig. 11.10); and in cases with a few months' survival the sharp edges of the lesions may be blurred by a combination of Wallerian degeneration and a post-oedematous spongy state (Fig. 11.11). Lesions of this severe type may be the

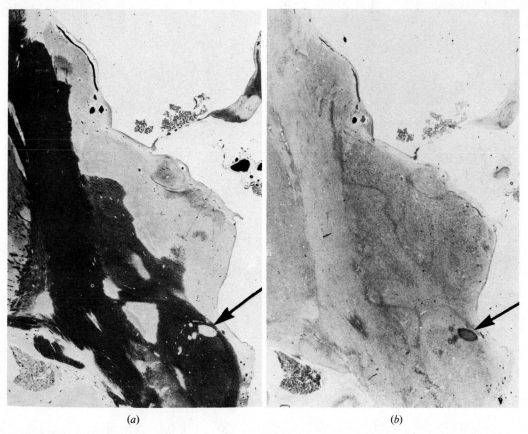

(a)   (b)

Fig. 11.5 Multiple sclerosis. Case as in Fig. 11.1. There is a fresh, cellular plaque in the red nucleus (arrows). The larger lesions have active, cellular margins. (a) Myelin, (b) Nissl.

and there are additional histological features. In the first place, axis cylinders may be destroyed, and even, in the most fulminating lesions, nerve cell bodies. In such cases, the lesion may be difficult to distinguish from an ischaemic infarct. Secondly, the cellular reaction is more intense, and acquires a more 'inflammatory' look, with extensive cuffing of vessels by lymphocytes and occasionally by plasma cells (Fig. 11.9). The myelin is broken down rapidly, and lipid phagocytes appear at an early stage. Astrocytes pro-

sole evidence of the disease in a case of death during the first episode; or they may be found coexisting with the more typical indolent lesions. They are characteristic of some of the rarer forms of multiple sclerosis, which are described below.

Marburg type (*Acute multiple sclerosis*)
Marburg in 1906 described three cases dying from an acute or subacute illness, with evidence of multiple lesions in the central nervous system. The lesions proved to be those of multiple

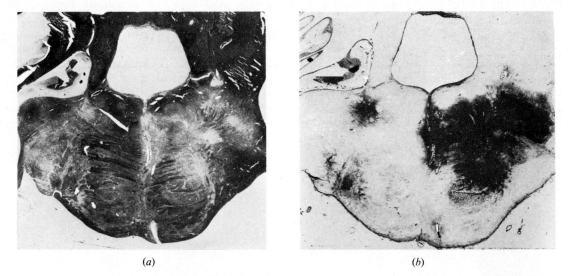

(a)   (b)

Fig. 11.6 Multiple sclerosis. Male, aged 56. 'Shadow plaques' in pons, stained (a) for myelin, (b) for glial fibres.

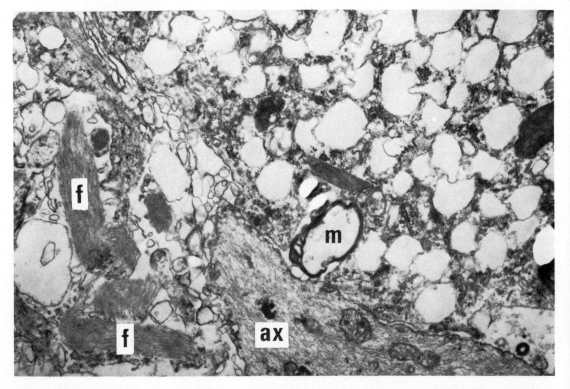

Fig. 11.7 Multiple sclerosis. Electronmicrograph from human necropsy material. Early lesion, showing a demyelinated axon (ax) bordered by a macrophage filled with myelin debris (m) and by glial fibres (f).   × 21,000. (Reproduced by the kindness of Dr S. Aparicio.)

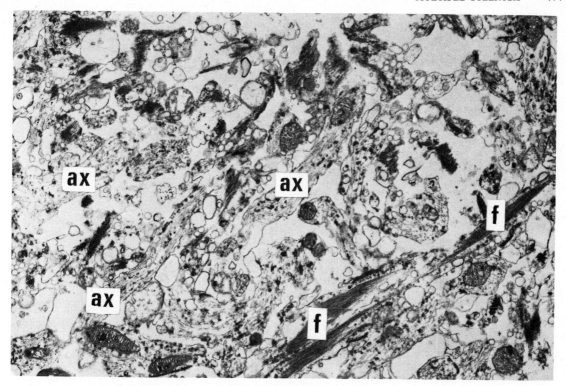

Fig. 11.8 Multiple sclerosis. Electronmicrograph from human necropsy material. Chronic lesion, showing demyelinated axons (ax), glial fibres (f) and a copious extracellular space. × 9000. (Reproduced by the kindness of Dr S. Aparicio.)

sclerosis, of the severe variety, most or all of them of recent origin. Such cases are sometimes labelled 'acute disseminated encephalomyelitis', but this term should be avoided, as it causes confusion between the acute form of multiple sclerosis and a different condition, which is described later in this chapter, namely, perivenous encephalomyelitis.   The relationship between the Marburg type of the disease and the classical Charcot type is discussed at length by Peters (1958). The differences, he claims, are mainly quantitative—more destruction, more 'inflammatory' features and a more florid cellular picture. No constant qualitative difference has been identified. Clinically, the Marburg type is relatively commoner in younger patients. The onset is often preceded by a feverish illness, which may be a banal virus infection; and the illness itself may be accompanied by a fever. The same clinical features are found in the Schilder and Dévic types, described below.

Schilder type (*Schilder's cerebral sclerosis: Schilder's disease: Sudanophilic diffuse sclerosis*).

Schilder in 1912 described the case of a 14-year-old girl, dying after a progressive neurological illness lasting 19 weeks, in which he found large, clear-cut areas of demyelination in both hemispheres, as well as a number of smaller lesions resembling plaques of multiple sclerosis. He regarded the disease as a juvenile variant of multiple sclerosis, and labelled it 'encephalitis periaxialis diffusa', by analogy with 'encephalitis periaxialis scleroticans disseminata'—Marburg's (1906) term for multiple sclerosis. Unfortunately, Schilder in subsequent papers (1913 and 1924) used the same term to describe two cases in which the pathology was clearly of a different type, and which were probably causes of a familial leucodystrophy and of subacute sclerosing encephalitis respectively (Lumsden 1951). Following this, confusion arose, and the term 'Schilder's disease' was used to cover many different conditions, particularly in children, in which widespread damage occurs in the cerebral hemispheres. The term 'diffuse sclerosis' which originally denoted no more than the finding of widespread gliosis, from whatever cause, came to be used

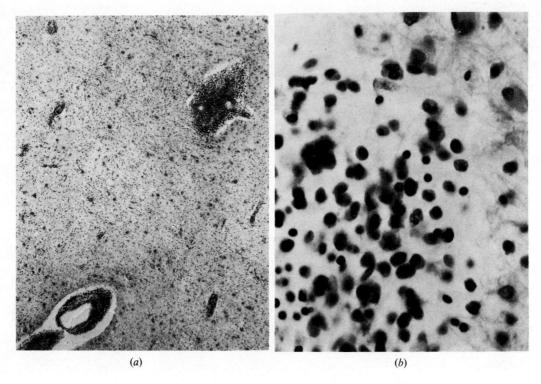

(a)   (b)

Fig. 11.9 Multiple sclerosis. (a) Acute lesion in white matter, with intense vascular cuffing, microglial proliferation and astrocytic hypertrophy. H and E. × 35. (b) Detail of vascular cuff, showing mixed cells, including many plasma cells. H and E. × 560.

improperly as the name of a disease, and as a synonym for 'Schilder's disease'. Clinical descriptions of 'diffuse sclerosis' and 'Schilder's disease' still tend to be based on the unsorted series of cases used by earlier authors.

This confusion was greatly lessened by Poser and van Bogaert (1956), who showed that after exclusion of cases of leucodystrophy, subacute encephalitis, post-epileptic encephalopathy and other conditions causing diffuse brain damage, there remained a group of cases, corresponding to Schilder's description of 1912, in which the lesions were essentially those of multiple sclerosis, usually of the severe variety, showing giant plaques in the hemispheres with or without typical smaller plaques elsewhere. Points of distinction from the leucodystrophies are that the lesions, though usually bilateral, are not symmetrical, and have the clear-cut boundaries, and the tendency to spare a rim of subcortical white matter, characteristic of multiple sclerosis. Furthermore, the condition is not familial. Poser (1957) analysed 105 such cases in the literature, and divided them

into 33 'pure' cases, in which the only lesions were large, usually bilateral, patches of demyelination in the cerebral hemispheres, and 72 cases of 'transitional' type, in which such lesions were combined with multiple smaller plaques. He found that the 'pure' type is preponderantly a disease of childhood, extremely rare after the age of 40, whereas the age of onset in the 'transitional' type corresponds closely with that of multiple sclerosis in general. The clinical course is variable, but there is a tendency for 'pure' cases to take an acute or subacute progressive course, with mental disturbances, blindness and deafness, whereas an episodic course, with remissions, is common in 'transitional' cases. In fact, no firm line separates such cases from the not uncommon instances of the Charcot type with very extensive involvement of the cerebral white matter (Fig. 11.12). In acute cases, with large destructive lesions, there is often a considerable degree of cerebral oedema, and the favoured clinical diagnosis tends to be of brain tumour or of encephalitis.

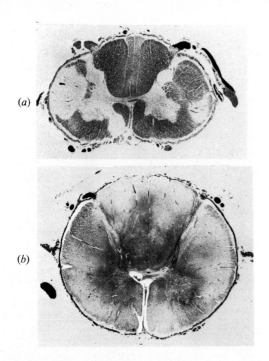

(a)

(b)

Fig. 11.10 Multiple sclerosis. Myelin-stained sections from sixth cervical level (*a*) showing chronic clear-cut lesions. × 4. (*b*) From a 25-year-old woman with 20-month history, dying with acute lesions throughout the brain and cord. The cord is swollen, and circular in cross-section, and the outlines of lesions are blurred by oedema.

Balò type (*Concentric sclerosis*)

This is a rare pathological curiosity, interesting mainly because of the clue which it may provide to the pathogenesis of plaques. It is characterized by zones of demyelination separated by narrow bands of preserved myelin, either in a concentric pattern (Fig. 11.13) or in the form of irregular blocks (*Landkartenherde*) (Fig. 11.14). Balò, in 1928, gave a detailed description of such a lesion in a man of 33 dying after a 10-week illness marked by progressive right hemiplegia and aphasia. The brain showed multiple plaques of acute demyelination, some of which had a concentrically laminated structure, the demyelinated laminae being separated by bands of preserved myelin. Both types of laminae were broader at the periphery of the lesions than at the centre, and the outer edge of each myelinated lamina was sharply defined, whereas the inner edge was more diffuse. The lesions stopped short of the immediately subcortical white matter. As Balò pointed out, similar cases had already

been described, by Marburg in 1906 and by Barré, Morin, Dragonesco and Reys in 1926—the first as a case of acute multiple sclerosis and the second as one of Schilder's disease. Since Balò's report, over 30 further case reports have appeared (for a recent review, see Courville 1970). In most cases the illness has been acute and rapidly progressive, and has occurred mainly in the

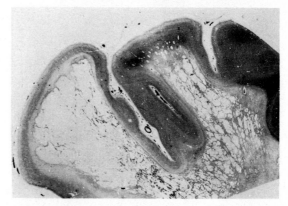

Fig. 11.11 Multiple sclerosis, Schilder type. Girl aged 12, dying after 5 months' illness. Post-oedematous spongy degeneration of white matter. On the right there is some preserved subcortical myelin. Myelin. × 1·6.

second and third decades of life. Two cases, however, have been described of older patients in whom the illness was of longer duration, and the lesions, though laminated, were of a different type, with bands of loose, spongy tissue alternating with bands of dense fibrous gliosis, with complete loss of myelin but partial preservation of axons. Grčević (1960) was uncertain whether this should be regarded as a chronic form of the Balò lesion, and coined the term *Concentric lacunar leukoencephalopathy*. In the case reported by Currie, Roberts and Urich in 1970, similar lesions were combined with lesions of the Dévic type of multiple sclerosis, described below.

Dévic type (*Neuromyelitis optica, neuropticomyelitis*)

The combination of visual failure with paraplegia, due to lesions in the optic nerves and spinal cord, is not uncommon in the chronic forms of multiple sclerosis. The term *Dévic's syndrome* is used when these two symptoms are severe, and occur within a few days or weeks of each other. The syndrome can arise from various causes: for example, it may be due to an acute perivenous

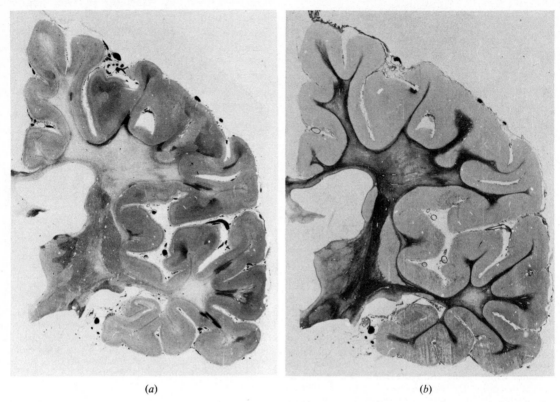

(a)   (b)

Fig. 11.12 Multiple sclerosis, Schilder ('transitional') type.   Woman aged 25, dying after protracted illness with remissions and relapses.   All levels of brain and cord severely affected.   Cerebral hemisphere, stained (a) for myelin, (b) for glial fibres.

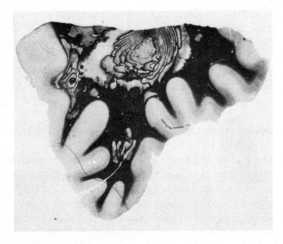

Fig. 11.13 Multiple sclerosis, Balò type.   Concentric demyelination in subcortical white matter.   Myelin.

encephalomyelitis; but the commonest necropsy findings in such cases are those of acute multiple sclerosis, with scattered fresh lesions and some of earlier date, and with a preponderance of damage in the optic nerves and the upper thoracic segments of the cord.

The clinical syndrome was described by Allbutt in 1870.   Dévic (1894) and his pupil Gault (1895) collected 16 cases, and several pathological descriptions were published before the end of the century.   Since then, over 300 cases, with and without necropsy, have been published.   The subject has been reviewed by Stansbury (1949), Peters (1958) and Cloys and Netsky (1970). Since patients showing the syndrome do not always die in the acute phase, relatively little is known about the pathology in the more benign cases.   The fatal cases can be roughly arranged into four groups according to the pathology:

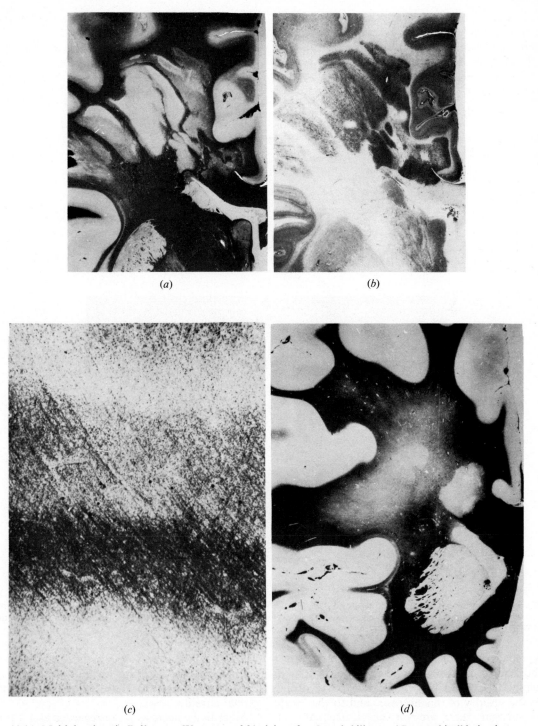

(a)

(b)

(c)

(d)

Fig. 11.14 Multiple sclerosis, Balò type. Woman aged 21, dying after 5 weeks' illness. 'Geographical' lesion in centrum ovale, stained (a) for myelin, (b) for cells (Nissl). Areas of complete demyelination are separated from bands of preserved myelin by a band of partial demyelination. (c) Myelin stain, showing these three stages. The direction of the bands is unrelated to the course of the nerve fibres. × 45. (d) Myelin stain, showing fresh lesions in frontal white matter, with surrounding oedema.

1. The optic nerves are partly or wholly demyelinated. In milder cases, the lesions are indistinguishable from those of acute multiple sclerosis; in the more severe ones, there is destruction of axons, and occasionally central liquefaction of the chiasm. In addition, a longish

The rest of the brain and cord appear normal apart from Wallerian degeneration.

2. The lesions described above are combined with plaques of acute multiple sclerosis in other areas, or with massive lesions, of Schilder type, in the cerebral hemispheres (Fig. 11.17).

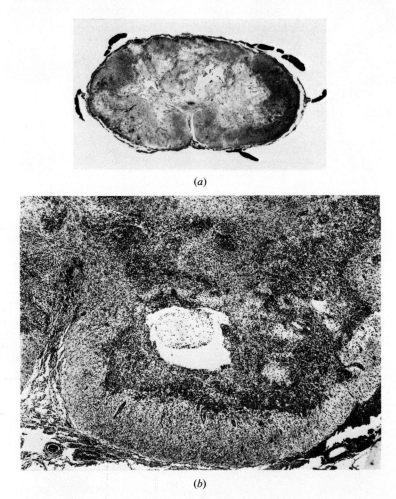

(a)

(b)

Fig. 11.15 Multiple sclerosis, Dévic type. Woman, aged 56. (a) Low power and (b) higher power views of a severely destructive lesion in the cervical cord, associated with a previous attack of retrobulbar neuritis with residual demyelination of one optic nerve.

segment of the spinal cord (most often the upper thoracic) is more or less necrotic, with loss of nerve cells and axons (Fig. 11.15). According to the severity of this necrosis, and to the length of survival, there are varying degrees of connective tissue reaction. With long survival, there may be invasion of the necrotic cord by myelinated fibres of peripheral nerve type derived from the posterior root ganglia (Fig. 11.16).

3. The lesions are simply those of acute or chronic multiple sclerosis, without necrosis.

4. The lesions are those of perivenous encephalomyelitis.

Since tissue necrosis is not regarded as a feature of multiple sclerosis, even in its severe forms, some authors have held that this finding in the first two groups justifies the use of the term *Dévic's disease* as something other than, though perhaps

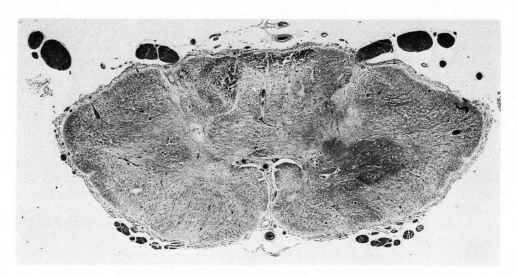

Fig. 11.16 Multiple sclerosis, Dévic type. Woman aged 35, dying after a 15-year illness, with remissions and relapses. Necropsy findings: demyelination of optic nerves and necrosis of the thoracic cord. Section from seventh cervical segment, showing mixture of necrosis and Wallerian degeneration, and invasion of posterior columns by myelinated nerve fibres from the posterior roots. Myelin.

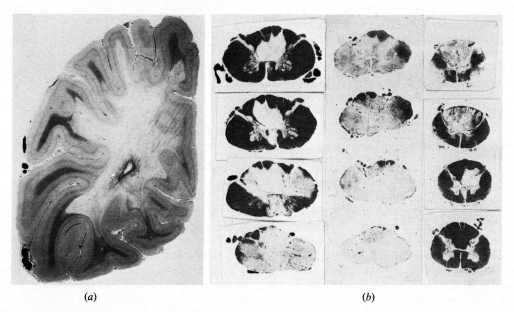

(a)   (b)

Fig. 11.17 Multiple sclerosis, mixed Schilder and Dévic type. (a) Left occipital lobe. Mallory's PTAH. (b) Cord, C6 to T5 and T11 to L2. The intervening thoracic segments were completely demyelinated. Myelin. (Case reported by Greenfield 1950.)

allied to, multiple sclerosis. This view ignores the possibility of secondary circulatory effects resulting from a primary demyelinating process. It has been mentioned already that acute severe lesions in the brain are accompanied by cerebral swelling. The same applies to the spinal cord (Fig. 11.10). Swollen spinal cords have been repeatedly observed at laminectomy in cases of the Dévic syndrome. The pial covering of the cord is a cylindrical tube, elliptical in cross-section in the cervical region, circular in the thoracic. Expansion within a fully stretched pia can only take place by expulsion of blood, and eventually by forcing of softened cord tissue upwards or downwards into less congested segments, producing an ascending level of paralysis, and the necropsy finding—common in cases of acute cord swelling—of a plug of necrotic tissue intruding into the base of the posterior columns. The same principle can be applied to the optic nerves, which in addition have to traverse a bony foramen.

Whether there are special factors favouring a selective simultaneous demyelination of the cord and the optic nerves is uncertain. It should be mentioned that necrosis of the cord has been found in patients with multiple sclerosis, without corresponding lesions in the optic nerves. A number of cases of so-called *acute necrotic myelopathy* (Hughes 1966) are probably examples of acute demyelination, resulting in oedema, circulatory stasis and necrosis. The very high protein levels and cell counts in the cerebrospinal fluid in such cases are probably a direct result of tissue necrosis, and do not rule out a diagnosis of multiple sclerosis.

Relation between lesions and symptoms

There are obvious difficulties in relating the lesions in an individual case to the patient's clinical history. There is at present no way of telling whether a demyelinated axon in a histological or electron-microscopical preparation was capable of transmitting nerve impulses during life. One can only assume that *some* demyelinated axons transmit impulses, from the fact that a total transverse demyelination can sometimes be observed in an optic nerve from a patient who was not blind in the relevant eye, or a total transverse demyelination of the spinal cord from a patient who could walk. Remission of symptoms is most simply accounted for by supposing that

conduction is blocked at the time of acute demyelination, and resumed at a later stage. Some of the permanent disabilities typical of the later stages of the disease may be attributed to axon degeneration, which certainly occurs. Whether other factors, such as overgrowth of glial fibres, also interfere with conduction, or with synaptic mechanisms, is not known. It is also not known to what extent, if any, recovery of function is helped by remyelination (see Harrison, McDonald and Ochoa 1972). An experimental approach to these problems has recently been devised (McDonald and Sears 1970a, b) in which demyelinative lesions, resembling those of multiple sclerosis, are produced by injections of diphtheria toxin into the spinal cord, and nervous conduction through the lesions is studied. The subject has been reviewed by McDonald (1974).

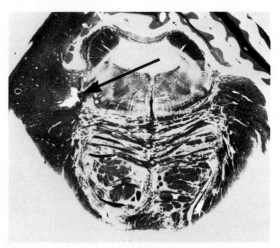

Fig. 11.18 Pons, from a woman of 57 with history of right trigeminal neuralgia. At necropsy a single lesion, typical of multiple sclerosis, was found in the entering root of the right trigeminal nerve (arrow). Myelin.

Many of the symptoms of multiple sclerosis, for instance localized numbness, loss of vision in one eye, or weakness of upper motor neuron type, can be simply related to loss of function in well-recognized pathways. Others, such as spontaneous paraesthesiae or trigeminal neuralgia, are less easily explained. In the case of trigeminal neuralgia, a plaque has often been observed in the region of the entering root of the relevant nerve (Fig. 11.18) (see White and Sweet 1969), but there is no obvious reason why such a lesion should give rise to recurrent paroxysms of pain.

Conversely, there is no known clinical manifestation of lesions in the most characteristic situation, in the lateral walls of lateral ventricles. (Considering the frequency with which these lesions involve the optic radiations, it is surprising that homonymous hemianopia is regarded as a rare feature of the disease.) There is, however, a good correlation between large lesions of the cerebral white matter (as seen in Fig. 11.12) and overall dementia.

Theories of aetiology and pathogenesis

There are several major problems, still awaiting a satisfactory answer, which must be considered separately if confusion is to be avoided. The first concerns the fundamental nature of the disorder, which renders the patient liable, over several decades, to recurrent bouts of demyelination. The second is the question how the disorder is acquired, and who is therefore at risk. The third, and most neglected, question concerns the local and temporary determinants of the appearance of a lesion in a particular site at a particular time. A fourth question is what determines whether a lesion is mild and of limited extent or severe and rapidly progressive.

The nature of the disease

Repeated attempts to incriminate an infective organism in multiple sclerosis have been unsuccessful, and some of these are discussed in detail by Prineas (1970). Field (1969) has suggested that multiple sclerosis may belong to the group of so-called 'slow virus' diseases represented in man by Kuru and Jakob–Creutzfeldt disease, but in view of the dissimilarity, both clinical and pathological, between Jakob–Creutzfeldt disease and multiple sclerosis, it would be surprising if this suggestion were confirmed. The search for consistent biochemical abnormalities in multiple sclerosis patients has also been inconclusive (see discussion by Bernsohn and Barron 1970; Lumsden 1972). There is, however, one fairly constant change in the body fluids, which provides a valuable diagnostic tool; that is, an elevation of the level of immunoglobulin (IgG) in the cerebrospinal fluid (Kabat, Freedman, Murray and Knaub 1950; see Tourtellotte 1970). It has long been suspected (Marburg 1906; Hallervorden and Spatz 1932-33) that the lesions of multiple

sclerosis are caused by a myelinolytic substance diffusing from the blood or cerebrospinal fluid, or both. Support for the diffusion theory comes not only from histological observations, but also from Broman's (1947) demonstration of 'leaky' veins in multiple sclerosis plaques, using supravital perfusions of trypan blue. The observation (Bornstein 1963; Raine, Hummelgard, Swanson and Bornstein 1973) that sera from patients with multiple sclerosis are able to destroy myelin in tissue culture has revived interest in the idea of a myelinotoxic substance. Lumsden (1971) claims that such a substance can be demonstrated by immunofluorescence in the active portions of plaques, that complement is involved, and that the substance is an immunoglobulin. The part, if any, played by cellular hypersensitivity remains obscure (see Behan, Behan, Feldman and Kies 1972).

The acquisition of the disease

The main evidence on this comes from epidemiological studies (see Acheson 1972). Broadly speaking, the disease is common in the temperate zones, and rare in the tropics, but the distribution of risk cannot be attributed solely to climate or latitude. It seems that an individual's chance of developing the disease depends on where he spent his childhood; that is, an emigrant from a high-risk to a low-risk area retains the high risk, and vice versa. Dean (1970) claims that the facts could be explained by supposing that a common virus infection, causing trivial symptoms followed by lifelong immunity in infants, is liable to cause multiple sclerosis if the infection occurs around the age of 15. This might suggest either a 'latent' virus disease analogous to subacute sclerosing panencephalitis, or, more plausibly (Sibley and Foley 1965), an immunological disorder resulting from the infection, somewhat analogous, on present theories, to post-infective encephalomyelitis (see below). A further piece of evidence linking virus infection with multiple sclerosis is the finding (Adams and Imagawa 1962; see Prineas 1970) of raised anti-measles antibodies in the serum and cerebrospinal fluid of a high proportion of multiple sclerosis patients. The significance of this observation is still uncertain. McDermott, Field and Caspary (1974) claim to have shown that there is an antigenic similarity between measles virus and the encephalitogenic factor (see p. 489) of central myelin.

Local and temporary determinants of plaque formation

Knowledge of the factors causing clinical episodes, due to the appearance of new plaques or the extension of old ones, is at present scanty, although some knowledge would be of the greatest value in the clinical management of established cases. The available evidence is partly clinical and partly histological. McAlpine (1955) gives a list of factors which can reasonably be suspected of provoking clinical episodes. The list includes

to be related either to venules or to an ependymal or pial surface (for detailed studies of these relationships see Dow and Berglund 1942; Fog 1950, 1965). If the view is accepted that the lesions are due to a myelinolytic substance, it is natural to suppose that the perivenous lesions, at any rate, result from a local breakdown of the blood–brain barrier, allowing the toxic substance temporary access to nervous tissue. In that case, any of the numerous causes of barrier breakdown might be the provoking factor. Among such

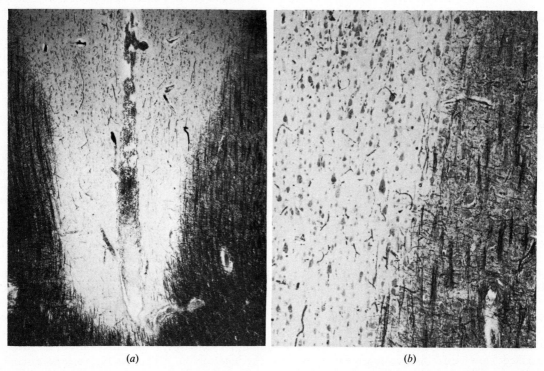

(a)   (b)

Fig. 11.19 Multiple sclerosis. (a) A perivenous lesion in cerebral cortex. The central vein is dilated, but not thrombosed. × 35. (b) Detail from edge of lesion, showing preservation of cortical neurons. × 200. Klüver–Barrera stain for myelin and cells.

poor health, fatigue, acute infection, trauma, allergic conditions, exposure to cold, and emotional upsets. It is hard to see what these have in common, apart from possible effects on blood flow in the central nervous system. The most convincing examples of the effect of trauma are cases in which localized trauma to the body has been followed, after an interval, by evidence of demyelination of an area of brainstem or spinal cord directly innervating the traumatized part. The main histological evidence is in the distribution of lesions. In general, lesions tend

causes are direct trauma and inflammation. Regarding the effects of trauma, knowledge is still at the anecdotal stage. There are reports, such as that of Russell (1946), strongly suggesting that minor head injuries and surgical procedures may have unexpectedly disastrous results in patients with multiple sclerosis. There is also evidence (Brain and Wilkinson 1957) that in patients having the not infrequent combination of multiple sclerosis and cervical spondylosis lesions are concentrated in the cervical cord, in the region where it is in contact with a spondylotic bar. As for the effect of inflammation, it is difficult to decide how to regard an inflammatory focus associated with a plaque. In a case I examined personally (Oppenheimer 1962), a young man with mild symptoms of multiple sclerosis was treated with intrathecal tuberculin. The ensuing aseptic meningitis did not subside in the usual manner. The patient's neurological state worsened rapidly and led to death in 10 months. There were some chronic plaques in the spinal cord; but the brain contained many fresh plaques of the severe type. Some were perivenous, but there was an unusually high proportion of surface plaques, many of them clearly associated with patches of heavy lymphocytic infiltration of the pia mater. In another case, also following intrathecal tuberculin therapy, there was a small meningitic focus in a Sylvian fissure. On each side of this, in the temporal and frontal opercula, there were small, fresh 'kissing' plaques in the cortex.

Theories associating the formation of plaques with vascular abnormalities include Putnam's (1937) view that thrombosis in small veins is a causal factor. Experimental work, and examination of serial sections of small plaques, have failed to support this theory. In general, any theory incriminating a local circulatory deficiency must face the objection that the lesions of multiple sclerosis do not resemble infarcts. In an anoxic lesion, the most vulnerable element is the nerve cell body, whereas in the typical plaque nerve cell bodies are conspicuously preserved (Fig. 11.19).

Factors determining the severity of lesions

Very little is known about this. Relevant facts are that in countries such as Japan, where multiple sclerosis is rare, the disease tends to be of severe type, with rapid progression; that the severe forms of the disease tend to be related to a feverish illness (see Peters 1958); and that some patients with a remitting history may end up with an acute, severe illness. In such cases, there is sometimes a suspicion that a second pathological process—cerebral oedema, for instance, or a mild 'allergic' encephalomyelitis—may be the precipitating factor. In considering the aetiology of a rare disease (and the severe forms of multiple sclerosis are rare) it must be remembered that two different pathological processes may coexist and interact. This has to be borne in mind when discussing the relation between multiple sclerosis and the encephalomyelopathies which are dealt with in the next section.

Perivenous encephalomyelitis

(*Acute disseminated encephalomyelitis: acute perivascular myelinoclasis*)

In this group of conditions the clinical onset is usually acute, with signs of multiple lesions in the central nervous system; the illness is nearly always monophasic, and is usually followed by a good recovery. If it is not fatal, the residual disabilities, if any, are not progressive, and recurrences are very rare. The lesions consist of narrow perivascular sleeves of tissue destruction, with inflammatory reaction.

Cases of this type are conveniently classified as follows:

1. Those in which the disease occurs with, or shortly after, a specific infection—in particular, measles and vaccinia.

2. Those in which it occurs spontaneously, or in the course of a non-specific respiratory infection.

3. Those in which the disease appears to be an allergic reaction to the administration of some extract of central nervous tissue. In humans, this has occurred most commonly as a complication of anti-rabies immunization.

4. To the above should probably be added a fourth group of cases, in which the disease is fulminating, nearly always fatal, and characterized by multiple small intracerebral haemorrhages.

These four varieties will be discussed separately.

Post- or para-infectious encephalitis. Post-vaccinial encephalomyelitis

Encephalomyelitis as a sequel to acute infectious disease was described at various times during the eighteenth and nineteenth centuries, but the characteristic pathological changes were not recognized until 1926, when Turnbull and McIntosh reported on seven fatal cases of encephalitis which had occurred in the London area following vaccination against smallpox. They described, as characteristic lesions, widespread perivascular infiltration of both grey and white matter by mononuclear cells, including plasma cells, and zones of perivascular softening in the white matter. About the same time post-vaccinial encephalomyelitis became a cause for anxiety in Holland, where 139 cases with 41 deaths were reported during the three-year period in 1924-26. A full pathological report on these cases was given by Bouman and Bok (1927).

As soon as the pathological picture of post-vaccinial encephalomyelitis became recognized, and epidemiological features of this group of conditions, reference may be made to the reviews by Miller, Stanton and Gibbons (1956), de Vries (1960) and Croft (1969). Briefly, the onset in post-vaccinial cases is usually 8 to 15 days following vaccination; in post-morbillar cases the onset usually follows the rash in less than a week, but may accompany or even precede it. The cerebrospinal fluid may contain extra cells and protein, but the findings are variable, and not diagnostic.

Morbid anatomy

The following description applies to cases of para-infectious encephalomyelitis, with death in the early stages, regardless of the nature of the primary infection. On naked-eye inspection,

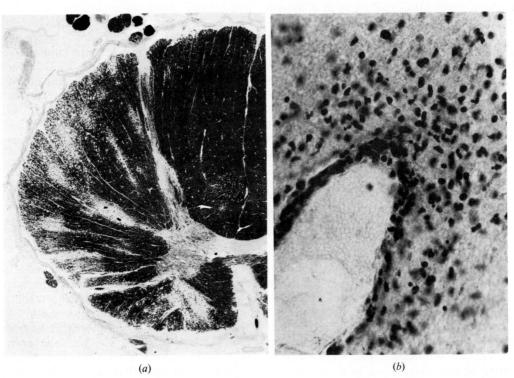

(a) (b)

Fig. 11.20 Perivenous encephalomyelitis. (a) Thoracic cord in a case of post-influenzal myelitis (Case 2 of Greenfield 1930). Myelin. (b) Post-morbillar encephalitis. Zone of cellular infiltration around a cerebral vessel. Nissl.

cases were reported with similar lesions following measles (Brock 1926), varicella (Glanzmann 1927), influenza (Greenfield 1930) and smallpox (Glanzmann 1927, Marsden and Hurst 1932). The latter cases were associated with the mild form of variola (alastrim) which was common in Great Britain at that time. For the clinical apart from congestion and a variable amount of cerebral oedema, the brain and spinal cord may appear normal. On the cut surface it may be possible to trace narrow greyish zones around the small veins in the white matter. Stained sections of the affected areas (Fig. 11.20) show congestion and inflammatory 'cuffing' of small veins, the exudate being composed mainly of lymphocytes and plasma cells, with an admixture of neutrophils in the early stages. At a somewhat later stage, there is proliferation of adventitial cells, and new reticulin fibres are formed. Surrounding these vessels, in a zone one or two millimetres wide, there is tissue destruction, in which it has often been observed that myelin breakdown is more extensive than axonal fragmentation. It is this observation which has led to the inclusion of perivenous encephalitis among the demyelinating diseases. The zones of destruction follow the course of small veins, and of their tributaries, for long distances. In places they may become confluent, but do not take the globoid or ellipsoid shape characteristic of the small perivenous plaques of multiple sclerosis. Within the zone, and for a short distance beyond it, there is a great proliferation of microglial cells, which soon become phagocytic. Astrocytes show reactive enlargement, and at a later stage there are perivascular sleeves of fibrous gliosis. A feature distinguishing the lesions from small perivenous plaques of multiple sclerosis is that the cellular infiltration is most intense at the centre of the lesion, rather than at the edge (cf. Fig. 11.3).

The distribution of lesions as between cerebrum, brainstem, cerebellum and spinal cord is very variable, but is generally symmetrical on the two sides. Lesions in white matter are more conspicuous, but grey matter is not immune. Nerve cells close to perivenous lesions normally appear healthy, but may show some chromatolysis, attributable to destruction of their axons. Meningeal exudate is usually slight, but lymphocytic cuffing of scattered pial venules may be seen.

There are few reports on the residual lesions in cases examined a year or more after recovery. The usual finding is of adventitial thickening of veins with collagen and reticulin, with a surrounding zone of rarefaction and fibrous gliosis (Malamud 1939) (Fig. 11.24).

'Spontaneous' cases

Lesions indistinguishable from those of para-infectious encephalitis are not uncommonly found in cases where there has been no proved antecedent viral infection. As with post-morbillar and post-vaccinial cases, attempts to isolate a virus from brain or cerebrospinal fluid have been unsuccessful.

Perivenous encephalitis, wherer para-infectious or 'spontaneous', appears to be rare in small children. The clinical diagnosis of 'virus encephalitis' or of 'post-infectious encephalitis' is commonly made in infants dying after an illness lasting a few days, with convulsions, coma and high fever; but the usual necropsy findings in such cases are of an acutely swollen brain, showing 'hypoxic' damage but without inflammatory changes, and an enlarged, fatty liver. This condition, generally known as *acute 'toxic' encephalopathy*, is discussed in Chapter 4. De Vries (1960) points out that this is the characteristic neurological complication of vaccination against smallpox in infants. He was unable to discover any instances of perivenous encephalitis following vaccination under the age of 2 years.

'Allergic' encephalomyelitis

'Neuroparalytic accidents' following anti-rabies treatment by injection of emulsions of nervous tissue have been known since the last century. In fatal cases, the lesions have generally been of the perivascular type described above, mainly in the spinal cord, but in some cases involving the brain or optic nerves (Bassoe and Grinker 1930; Stuart and Krikorian 1930, 1933). The theory that the virus of rabies, in its altered form, was responsible for the lesions was rendered improbable by the discovery that similar effects could be produced in animals by injections of sterile extracts of central nervous tissue (Rivers and Schwentker 1935; Ferraro and Jervis 1940). The lesions of this *experimental allergic encephalomyelitis* varied with the species of experimental animals, but in general corresponded closely with those of acute perivenous encephalomyelitis in humans (Roizin and Kolb 1959). It was subsequently found that the condition could be induced by injection of a suspension of the animal's own brain (Kabat, Wolf and Bezer 1947); that the effect was greatly enhanced by the use of Freund's and other 'adjuvants'; that the most active constituent of the crude brain extract (the so-called *encephalitogenic factor*) was a basic protein (Kies and Alvord 1959) or polypeptide (Lumsden, Robertson and Blight 1966) common to a number of animal species; and that the disease could be transferred to a healthy animal by injection of lymphocytes from an affected animal (Paterson 1960). The relevance of the experimental condition to human diseases is discussed later in this chapter. The analogous condition of *experimental allergic neuritis* is dealt with in Chapter 16.

On section (Fig. 11.21), numerous small haemorrhages are seen, mainly in the cerebral white matter and corpus callosum, but sometimes involving the brainstem and cerebellum. The cortex and basal ganglia are usually spared. The

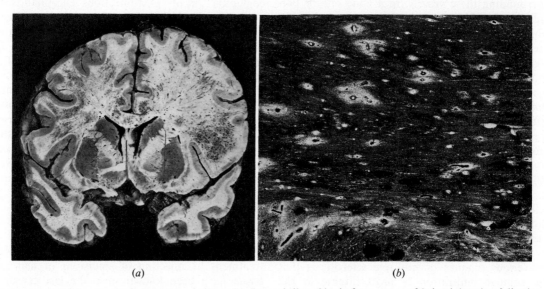

(a)   *(b)*

Fig. 11.21 Acute haemorrhagic leucoencephalitis. (*a*) Coronal slice of brain from a case of 3 days' duration following a respiratory infection (Case 10, Greenfield 1950). (*b*) Section of corpus callosum from same case, showing perivascular myelin loss and haemorrhages. Myelin.

Acute haemorrhagic leucoencephalitis (*Acute necrotizing haemorrhagic encephalopathy*)

Various forms of 'haemorrhagic encephalitis' and 'brain purpura' have been described from the end of the last century onwards. Weston Hurst (1941) described two cases of what he regarded as a distinct condition, which has been accepted as such by most subsequent writers (Adams, Cammermeyer and Denny-Brown 1949; Greenfield 1950; Crawford 1954). Clinically the disease is of abrupt onset, with pyrexia and rapidly developing coma, and is usually fatal within a few days. In some cases the onset is preceded by non-specific upper respiratory infection. The cerebrospinal fluid usually shows raised protein levels and high cell counts, including many neutrophil leucocytes; but no definite diagnostic test is known. The disease appears to affect predominantly young males.

Morbid anatomy

The brain is congested and swollen. In some cases a creamy subarachnoid exudate is seen.

lesions are sometimes, but not always, symmetrical, and may include larger areas of confluent haemorrhage. The more affected areas of white matter are soft and oedematous. The naked eye appearance is mimicked by some cases of cerebral fat embolism. Histological examination shows that the disease extends beyond the haemorrhagic areas. The lesions are of five main types, which are associated in varying proportions. (1) Necrosis of vessel walls, with fibrinous exudation into and through the wall and into the neighbouring tissue (Fig. 11.22). The small veins are most often affected in this manner, but small necrotic arteries are sometimes seen (Crawford 1954). (2) Oedema, which is essentially perivascular, but tends to become confluent and to affect fairly large areas. (3) Exudation of neutrophil leucocytes in the early stages, and later of mononuclear cells. In some very early lesions the exudate of polymorphonuclear cells may be the only change. (4) Zones of perivascular tissue destruction. These are seen round many vessels, and not only round the venules showing fibrinous exudate in their walls. There is a moderate excess of microglial cells in these zones, but this is usually less than that seen in para-infectious encephalitis. In cases dying after several days of illness most of these cells have become lipid phagocytes. Mitoses are common in them at all stages. (5) Haemorrhages of ball or ring type, or larger. Some of these are related to necrotic venules. The ring haemorrhages are

from experimental work. Some animals with experimental encephalitis show necrosis of vessel walls and haemorrhages alongside the more usual lesions. Levine and Wenk (1965) have produced, in rats, a hyperacute form of experimental encephalitis which they consider to be a close analogue of acute haemorrhagic leucoencephalitis. Their method involves the use of pertussis vaccine

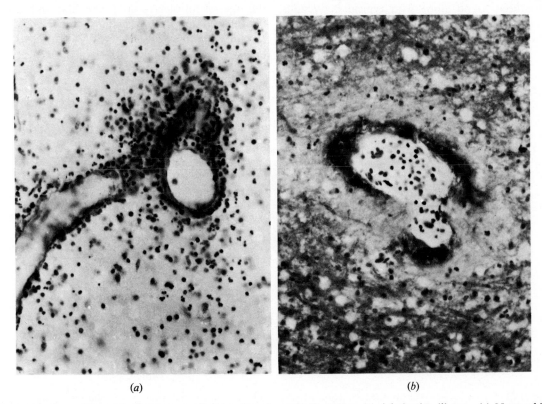

(a)   (b)

Fig. 11.22 Acute haemorrhagic leucoencephalitis. Female, aged 43, dying with fulminating illness. (a) Neutrophils cuffing a small intracerebral vein and infiltrating surrounding tissue. Nissl. × 300. (b) Fibrinous infiltration of venule and surrounding rarefaction. Phosphotungstic acid/hematoxylin. × 300.

usually centred on a thrombosed capillary round which there is a narrow zone of necrotic tissue.

Although the features of vessel wall necrosis, haemorrhage, and polymorphonuclear exudation would seem to separate this condition from the usual forms of perivenous encephalomyelitis, cases of intermediate type, with features of both conditions, have been described by Russell (1955). She considered that the two diseases formed a continuum, of which acute haemorrhagic leucoencephalitis represented the most severe and destructive form; and that both conditions had an 'allergic' basis. This view has received support

along with the conventional adjuvants. These authors suggest that whereas in the usual experimental condition the reaction is mainly cell-mediated, in the hyperacute form there is in addition a circulating humoral antibody.

The relationship between multiple sclerosis and perivenous encephalomyelitis

At first sight there is very little in common between these two conditions. Typically, the first is an episodic, remitting, but on the whole progressive disease, with large and small lesions occurring at different times in scattered areas of the CNS, while the second is a monophasic, non-relapsing, acute illness with diffuse lesions which follow the course of small veins. The main evidence for a relationship between the two comes from observations on atypical, 'transitional' cases with features of both conditions.

First, there are acute fatal cases where lesions resembling plaques of acute multiple sclerosis have been found along with typical perivenous lesions (Fig. 11.23). Van Bogaert in 1932 described the case of a girl of 12 who developed

logical disease after receiving 17 or 18 injections of anti-rabies vaccine prepared from animal spinal cord tissue. One of these showed merely the familiar lesions of a perivenous myelitis. The other eight showed a combination of perivenous lesions with a number of well-defined areas of myelin destruction, indistinguishable from the lesions of acute multiple sclerosis. In the following year Jellinger and Seitelberger (1958) described the case of an elderly man who had undergone treatment for paralysis agitans in the form of repeated injections of sterile calf's brain extract.

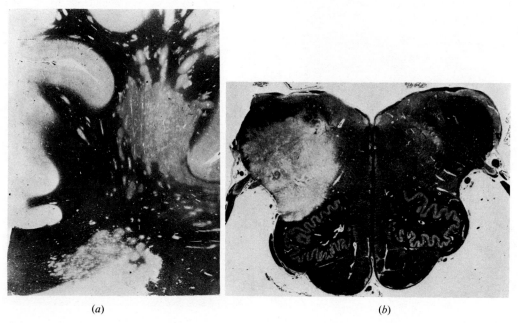

(a)   (b)

Fig. 11.23 'Mixed' case. Woman, aged 33, dying after 5-day illness. (a) Frontal white matter, showing perivenous encephalitis. Myelin. (b) Medulla, showing a lesion indistinguishable from acute multiple sclerosis. Myelin. (Reproduced by courtesy of Dr J. T. Hughes.)

an acute cerebrospinal disorder following chicken-pox, and died 16 days later. Both types of lesion were found in the brain. Döring (1941) described cases in which he felt that no clear line could be drawn between acute multiple sclerosis, of the Marburg type, and the perivenous type of encephalitis. He and Pette (1942) were early proponents of the view that multiple sclerosis and perivenous encephalitis were parts of a continuous spectrum of disease, for which they used the general term *demyelinating encephalitis.*

The most striking report of a 'mixed' pathology of this kind is that of Uchimura and Shiraki (1957). They described nine cases dying of acute neuro-

Here too there were multiple small perivenous lesions, combined with large fresh paraventricular 'plaques' indistinguishable from acute multiple sclerosis.

Secondly, there are rare cases in which a chronic or subacute illness, suggestive of multiple sclerosis, has been followed by the finding of sleeve-like perivenous lesions showing signs of continuing activity. In a case described by Oppenheimer (1966), a young man, after vaccination against smallpox, developed a subacute, relapsing and remitting illness, with dementia, amaurosis, and later tetraplegia. This progressed to death after 18 months. The lesions were all of perivenous

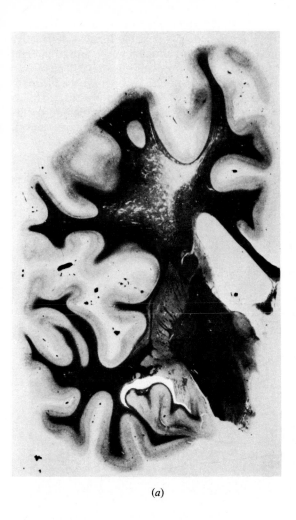

(a)

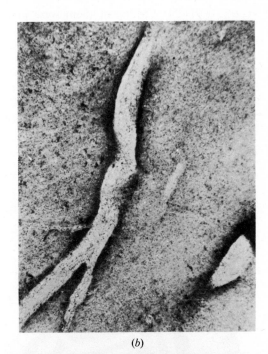

(b)

Fig. 11.24 Perivenous encephalitis. Subacute progressive case, with remissions and relapses. (*a*) Confluent lesions in centrum ovale. Myelin. × 35. (*b*) and (*c*) Fibrous scarring of small veins, with surrounding gliosis. PTAH. × 120.

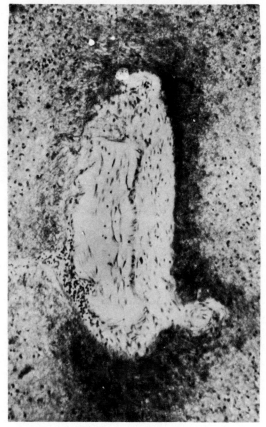

(c)

type (Fig. 11.24). Many of them were inactive and showed merely fibrous and glial scarring around the affected vessels; but in the centrum ovale on both sides the lesions were active and confluent, with considerable destruction of axons, and resulting degeneration of the pyramidal tracts. In another case (unpublished) the illness started at the age of 10, and took a progressive course,

A point to remember in discussing cases of this kind is that it is possible for two destructive processes to occur simultaneously, and to interact with each other, producing a 'mixed' picture in which it is impossible to distinguish the morphological features of the two processes. Unless both processes are of reasonably common occurrence, cases of this kind will be rare; and it

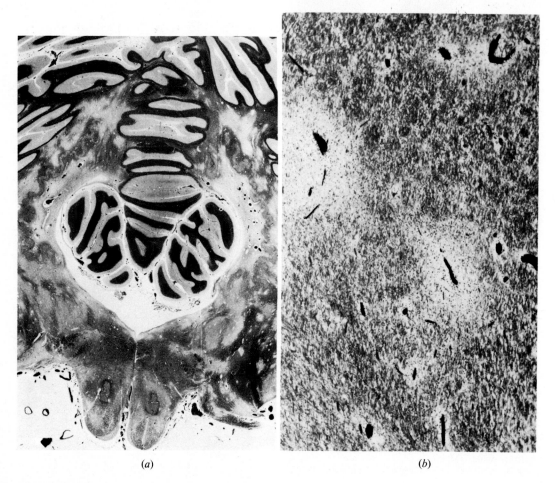

(a)   (b)

Fig. 11.25 Perivenous encephalitis. Girl, aged 15, dying after 5-year illness, with remissions and relapses. (a) Medulla and cerebellum, showing confluent lesions. Myelin. (b) Perivenous lesions in internal capsule. Myelin. × 60.

with partial remissions and relapses, ending in death at age 15, the final state being one of blindness, dementia and tetraparesis. Here again the pattern of lesions was perivenous, with spreading demyelination and cerebral atrophy, but no clear-cut plaques (Fig. 11.25). Nerve cells were spared, and there was only a mild degree of axonal damage, with consequent Wallerian degeneration.

appears that cases linking multiple sclerosis with perivenous encephalitis are indeed rare. The problem has not been solved; meanwhile it is safer and wiser to regard these two diseases not as parts of a continuous spectrum but as separate entities, both of which probably involve some disorder of immune mechanisms. Finding an answer to the problem of their relationship would be of great practical importance. Hitherto, no convincing analogue for multiple sclerosis has been found in natural or experimental diseases affecting animals other than man. Perivenous encephalitis has a convincing analogue in experimental allergic encephalitis, which is easily produced in the laboratory; but it remains uncertain what relevance this experimental work has to multiple sclerosis. Present-day knowledge of the immunopathology of these two conditions is summarized by Mackay, Carnegie and Coates (1973).

Demyelination in other diseases

There are various conditions, unrelated either to multiple sclerosis or to perivenous encephalitis, in which myelin breakdown is found to be in excess of axon destruction. Lumsden (1970*b*) has reviewed an assortment of these. Some are known to be due to toxic or metabolic causes, and are considered in Chapter 4. In addition, there are two recognized diseases, both of obscure aetiology, and in both of which demyelination is a prominent feature. These are central pontine myelinolysis, which is considered here, and progressive multifocal leucoencephalopathy (see p. 314).

anatomical structures, or to blood vessels. Axonal disruption and loss of nerve cells, when present, occurred in the most central part of the lesion, and the impression was of a process beginning near the raphe and spreading outwards. In one case, there were also characteristic changes of Wernicke's encephalopathy and polyneuropathy; with this exception, the nervous system showed

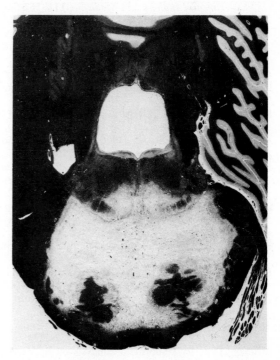

Fig. 11.26 Central pontine myelinolysis. Woman, aged 47, dying after a 2 months' illness. Myelin stain, showing lesion in pons, with partial sparing of pyramidal bundles.

Central pontine myelinolysis

Adams, Victor and Mancall in 1959 reported the presence of a symmetrical patch of demyelination in the centre of the pons in four adult patients. Three of them were chronic alcoholics, and all of them were in a state of severe malnutrition, with dehydration. Clinical disturbances (in particular, bulbar paralysis and flaccid tetraplegia) attributable to the pontine lesion had appeared between 2 and 4 weeks before death. The lesions, though differing in size, were similar in their site and histological appearance. On slicing the brainstem they were seen as laterally symmetrical areas of grey softening in the central part of the upper and middle pons, impinging on the tegmentum but not reaching the pial or ventricular surfaces. Histologically they showed a sharply defined area of myelin breakdown, with relatively good preservation of nerve cells and axis cylinders. The affected tissue was packed with phagocytes containing Sudanophil lipids. There were many reactive astrocytes, but oligodendrocytes had disappeared. There was no thrombosis or significant vascular disease, and only in one case was there some vascular cuffing by lymphocytes. The lesions appeared to be unrelated to neuro-

no other specific changes. Adams *et al.* (1959) recognized the disease as a demyelinative condition, distinguished from multiple sclerosis by its constant, solitary situation and by its lack of relation to vessels. They attributed the condition to malnutrition, but were unable to assign a specific cause.

Since then, little has been added either to the pathological description or to the understanding of the causes of this disease. Cases have been described occurring in childhood (Adams 1962), and in a few cases there have been lesions in other parts of the central nervous system (Mathieson and Olszewski 1960). In a few, there has been at least partial sparing of cortico-bulbar and corticospinal tracts (Fig. 11.26). In every case, the condition has appeared as a complication of some systemic disease, most commonly a severe and protracted one. An analysis by Paguirigan and Lefken (1969) lists 70 published cases, of which half were in alcoholics; in both the alcoholic and non-alcoholic group, about half were malnourished and dehydrated. The condition has not so far been reproduced in experimental animals.

References

Acheson, E. D.   (1972) The epidemiology of multiple sclerosis in *Multiple Sclerosis: A Reappraisal* (Eds. McAlpine, D., Lumsden, C. E. & Acheson, E. D.), 2nd edition, chapters 1 and 2, Churchill Livingstone, Edinburgh & London.

Adams, J. H.   (1962) Central pontine myelinolysis in *Proceedings of the 4th International Congress of Neuropathology* (Ed. Jacob, H.), Vol. 3, pp. 303-308, Thieme, Stuttgart.

Adams, J. M. & Imagawa, D. T.   (1962) Measles antibodies in multiple sclerosis. *Proceedings of the Society of Experimental Biology and Medicine*, **111**, 562-566.

Adams, R. D., Cammermeyer, J. & Denny-Brown, D.   (1949) Acute necrotizing hemorrhagic encephalopathy. *Journal of Neuropathology and Experimental Neurology*, **8**, 1-29.

Adams, R. D., Victor, M. & Mancall, E. L.   (1959) Central pontine myelinolysis. *Archives of Neurology and Psychiatry (Chicago)*, **81**, 154-172.

Allbutt, T. C.   (1870) On the ophthalmoscopic signs of spinal disease. *Lancet*, **1**, 76-78.

Balò, J.   (1928) Encephalitis periaxialis concentrica. *Archives of Neurology and Psychiatry (Chicago)*, **19**, 242-264.

Barré, J. A., Morin, V., Draganesco, S. & Reys, L.   (1926) Encéphalite periaxiale diffuse. *Revue Neurologique*, **2**, 541-557.

Bassoe, P. & Grinker, R. R.   (1930) Human rabies and rabies vaccine encephalomyelitis. *Archives of Neurology and Psychiatry (Chicago)*, **23**, 1138-1160.

Behan, P. O., Behan, W. M. H., Feldman, R. G. & Kies, M. W.   (1972) Cell-mediated hypersensitivity to neural antigens. Occurrence in humans and non-human primates with neurological diseases. *Archives of Neurology and Psychiatry (Chicago)*, **27**, 145-152.

Bernsohn, J. & Barron, K. D.   (1970) Chemical pathology of multiple sclerosis in *Handbook of Clinical Neurology* (Eds. Vinken, P. J. & Bruyn, G. W.), Vol. 9, pp. 310-319, North Holland Publishing Co., Amsterdam.

Bornstein, M. B.   (1963) A tissue-culture approach to demyelinative disorders. *National Cancer Institute Monographs*, **11**, 197-214.

Bouman, L. & Bok, S. T.   (1927) Die Histopathologie der Encephalitis post vaccinationem. *Zeitschrift für die gesamte Neurologie und Psychiatrie*, **111**, 495-510.

Brain, R. & Wilkinson, M.   (1957) The association of cervical spondylosis and disseminated sclerosis. *Brain*, **80**, 456-478.

Brock, J.   (1926) Ueber Systematik und Klinik meningoencephaler Krankheitszustände im Kindesalter. *Zeitschrift für Kinderheilkunde*, **40**, 552-572.

Broman, T.   (1947) Supravital analysis of disorders in the cerebral vascular permeability. II. Two cases of multiple sclerosis. *Acta Psychiatrica et Neurologica Scandinavica*, Suppl. **46**, 58-71.

Carswell, R.   (1838) *Pathological Anatomy. Illustrations of Elementary Forms of Disease.*   Chapter on 'Atrophy', Plate IV, Longman, Orme, Brown, Green & Longman, London.

Charcot, J. M.   (1877) *Lectures on the Diseases of the Nervous System* (Trans. G. Sigerson).   London: the New Sydenham Society, 1st series, lecture 6 (delivered 1868).

Cloys, D. E. & Netsky, M. G.   (1970) Neuromyelitis optica in *Handbook of Clinical Neurology* (Eds. Vinken, P. J. & Bruyn, G. W.), Vol. 9, pp. 426-436, North Holland Publishing Co., Amsterdam.

Courville, C. B.   (1970) Concentric sclerosis in *Handbook of Clinical Neurology* (Eds. Vinken, P. J. & Bruyn, G. W.), Vol. 9, pp. 437-451, North Holland Publishing Co., Amsterdam.

Crawford, T. (1954) Acute haemorrhagic leucoencephalitis. *Journal of Clinical Pathology*, **7**, 1-9.

Croft, P. B. (1969) Para-infectious and post-vaccinal encephalomyelitis. *Postgraduate Medical Journal*, **45**, 392-400.

Cruveilhier, J. (1829-42) *Anatomie pathologique du corps humain*, Vol. 2, livraison 52; Plate 2, Baillière, Paris.

Currie, S., Roberts, A. H. & Urich, H. (1970) The nosological position of concentric lacunar leucoencephalopathy. *Journal of Neurology, Neurosurgery and Psychiatry*, **33**, 131-137.

Dean, G. (1970) The multiple sclerosis problem. *Scientific American*, **223**, 40-46.

Dévic, M. E. (1894) Myélite subaiguë compliquée de névrite optique. *Bulletin Médical (Paris)*, **8**, 1033.

de Vries, E. (1960) *Postvaccinal Perivenous Encephalitis*, Elsevier, Amsterdam.

Döring, G. (1941) Zur Pathologie und Klinik der Entmarkungsencephalomyelitis. *Deutsche Zeitschrift für Nervenheilkunde*, **153**, 73-139.

Dow, R. S. & Berglund, G. (1942) Vascular pattern of lesions of multiple sclerosis. *Archives of Neurology and Psychiatry (Chicago)*, **47**, 1-18.

Ferraro, A. & Jervis, G. A. (1940) Experimental disseminated encephalopathy in the monkey. *Archives of Neurology and Psychiatry (Chicago)*, **43**, 195-209.

Field, E. J. (1969) Slow virus infections of the nervous system. *International Review of Experimental Pathology*, **8**, 129-239.

Fog, T. (1950) Topographic distribution of plaques in the spinal cord in multiple sclerosis. *Archives of Neurology and Psychiatry (Chicago)*, **63**, 382-414.

Fog, T. (1965) The topography of plaques in multiple sclerosis. *Acta Neurologica Scandinavica (Suppl 15)*, **41**, 1-161.

Gault, F. (1895) De la neuromyélite optique aiguë. Thesis, University of Lyon.

Glanzmann, E. (1927) Die nervösen Komplikationen der Varizellen, Variola und Vakzine. *Schweizerische Medizinische Wochenschrift*, **57**, 145-154.

Grčević, N. (1960) Concentric lacunar leukoencephalopathy. *Archives of Neurology (Chicago)*, **2**, 266-273.

Greenfield, J. G. (1930) Acute disseminated encephalomyelitis as sequel to 'influenza'. *Journal of Pathology and Bacteriology*, **33**, 453-462.

Greenfield, J. G. (1950) Encephalitis and encephalomyelitis in England and Wales during the last decade. *Brain*, **73**, 141-166.

Hallervorden, J. & Spatz, H. (1932-33) Ueber die konzentrische Sklerose. *Archiv für Psychiatrie und Nervenkrankheiten*, **98**, 641-701.

Harrison, B. M., McDonald, W. I. & Ochoa, J. (1972) Remyelination in the central diphtheria toxin lesion. *Journal of the Neurological Sciences*, **17**, 293-302.

Hughes, J. T. (1966) *Pathology of the Spinal Cord*, Lloyd-Luke, London.

Hurst, E. W. (1941) Acute haemorrhagic leucoencephalitis: a previously undefined entity. *Medical Journal of Australia*, **2**, 1-6.

Jellinger, K. & Seitelberger, F. (1958) Akute tödliche Entmarkungsencephalitis nach wiederholten Hirntrockenzelleninjektionen. *Klinische Wochenschrift*, **36**, 437-441.

Kabat, E. A., Freedman, D. A., Murray, J. P. & Knaub, V. (1950) A study of a crystalline albumin, gamma globulin and total protein in the cerebrospinal fluid of 100 cases of multiple sclerosis and in other diseases. *American Journal of Medical Science*, **219**, 55-64.

Kabat, E. A., Wolf, A. & Bezer, A. E. (1947) The rapid production of acute disseminated encephalomyelitis in rhesus monkeys by injection of heterologous and homologous brain tissue with adjuvants. *Journal of Experimental Medicine*, **85**, 117-130.

Kies, M. W. & Alvord, E. C. (1959) Encephalitogenic activity in guinea pigs of water soluble protein fractions of nervous tissue in '*Allergic*' *Encephalomyelitis* (Eds. Kies, M. W. & Alvord, E. C.), pp. 293-299, Thomas, Springfield, Ill.

Levine, S. & Wenk, E. J. (1965) A hyperacute form of allergic encephalomyelitis. *American Journal of Pathology*, **47**, 61-88.

Lumsden, C. E. (1951) Fundamental problems in the pathology of multiple sclerosis and allied demyelinating diseases. *British Medical Journal*, **1**, 1035-1043.

Lumsden, C. E. (1970a) The neuropathology of multiple sclerosis in *Handbook of Clinical Neurology* (Eds. Vinken, P. J. & Bruyn, G. W.), Vol. 9, pp. 217-309, North Holland Publishing Co., Amsterdam.

Lumsden, C. E. (1970b) Pathogenetic mechanisms in the leucoencephalopathies in anoxic-ischaemic processes, in disorders of the blood and in intoxications in *Handbook of Clinical Neurology* (Eds. Vinken, P. J. & Bruyn, G. W.), Vol. 9, pp. 572-663, North Holland Publishing Co., Amsterdam.

Lumsden, C. E. (1971) The immunogenesis of the multiple sclerosis plaque. *Brain Research*, **28**, 365-390.

Lumsden, C. E.   (1972) In *Multiple Sclerosis: A Reappraisal* (Eds. McAlpine, D., Lumsden, C. E. & Acheson, E. D.), 2nd edition, Part III, Churchill Livingstone, Edinburgh & London.

Lumsden, C. E., Robertson, D. M. & Blight, R.   (1966) Chemical studies on experimental allergic encephalomyelitis. *Journal of Neurochemistry*, **13**, 127-162.

McAlpine, D., Compston, N. D. & Lumsden, C. E.   (1955) *Multiple Sclerosis*, Livingstone, Edinburgh & London.

McAlpine, D., Lumsden, C. E. & Acheson, E. D.   (1972) *Multiple Sclerosis: A Reappraisal*, 2nd edition, Churchill Livingstone, Edinburgh & London.

McDermott, J. R., Field, E. J. & Caspary, E. A.   (1974) Relation of measles virus to encephalitogenic factor, with reference to the aetiopathogenesis of multiple sclerosis. *Journal of Neurology, Neurosurgery and Psychiatry*, **37**, 282-287.

McDonald, W. I.   (1974) Pathophysiology in multiple sclerosis. *Brain*, **97**, 179-196.

McDonald, W. I. & Sears, T. A.   (1970*a*) Focal experimental demyelination in the central nervous system. *Brain*, **93**, 575-582.

McDonald, W. I. & Sears, T. A.   (1970*b*) The effects of experimental demyelination on conduction in the central nervous system. *Brain*, **93**, 583-598.

Mackay, I. R., Carnegie, P. R. & Coates, A. S.   (1973) Immunopathological comparisons between experimental autoimmune encephalomyelitis and multiple sclerosis. *Clinical and Experimental Immunology*, **15**, 471-482.

Malamud, N.   (1939) Sequelae of postmeasles encephalomyelitis. A clinicopathologic study. *Archives of Neurology and Psychiatry (Chicago)*, **41**, 943-954.

Marburg, O.   (1906) Die sogenannte 'akute multiple Sklerose'. *Jahrbuch für Psychiatrie und Neurologie*, **27**, 211-312.

Marsden, J. P. & Hurst, E. W.   (1932) Acute perivascular myelinoclasis ('acute disseminated encephalomyelitis') in smallpox. *Brain*, **55**, 181-225.

Mathieson, G. & Olszewski, J.   (1960) Central pontine myelinolysis with other cerebral changes. *Neurology (Minneapolis)*, **10**, 345-354.

Miller, H. G., Stanton, J. B. & Gibbons, J. L.   (1956) Para-infectious encephalomyelitis and related syndromes. *Quarterly Journal of Medicine*, **25**, 427-505.

Oppenheimer, D. R.   (1962) Observations on the pathology of demyelinating diseases. D.M. Thesis, University of Oxford.

Oppenheimer, D. R.   (1966) A case of so-called demyelinating encephalitis. *Neuropatologica Polska*, IV, Suppl., pp. 717-721.

Paguirigan, A. & Lefken, E. B.   (1969) Central pontine myelinolysis. *Neurology (Minneapolis)*, **19**, 1007-1011.

Paterson, P. Y.   (1960) Transfer of allergic encephalomyelitis in rats by means of lymph node cells. *Journal of Experimental Medicine*, **111**, 119-136.

Périer, O. & Grégoire, A.   (1965) Electron microscopic features of multiple sclerosis lesions. *Brain*, **88**, 937-952.

Peters, G.   (1958) Chapters on multiple sclerosis and other demyelinating conditions in *Handbuch der speziellen pathologischen Anatomie und Histologie* (Eds. Lubarsch, O., Henke, F. & Rössle, R.), Vol. XIII/2A, Springer Verlag, Berlin.

Peters, G.   (1968) Multiple sclerosis in *Pathology of the Nervous System* (Ed. Minckler, J.), Vol. 1, pp. 821-843, McGraw-Hill, New York.

Pette, H.   (1942) *Die akut entzündlichen Erkrankungen des Nervensystems*, Thieme, Leipzig.

Poser, C. M.   (1957) Diffuse-disseminated sclerosis in the adult. *Journal of Neuropathology and Experimental Neurology*, **16**, 61-78.

Poser, C. M. & Van Bogaert, L.   (1956) Natural history and evolution of the concept of Schilder's diffuse sclerosis. *Acta Psychiatrica et Neurologica Scandinavica*, **31**, 285-331.

Prineas, J. W.   (1970) The etiology and pathogenesis of multiple sclerosis in *Handbook of Clinical Neurology* (Eds. Vinken, P. J. & Bruyn, G. W.), Vol. 9, pp. 107-160, North Holland Publishing Co., Amsterdam.

Putnam, T. J.   (1937) Evidences of vascular occlusion in multiple sclerosis and 'encephalomyelitis'. *Archives of Neurology and Psychiatry (Chicago)*, **37**, 1298-1321.

Raine, C. S., Hummelgard, A., Swanson, E. & Bornstein, M. B.   (1973) Multiple Sclerosis; serum-induced demyelination *in vitro*. *Journal of the Neurological Sciences*, **20**, 127-148.

Rivers, T. M. & Schwentker, F. F.   (1935) Encephalomyelitis accompanied by myelin destruction experimentally produced in monkeys. *Journal of Experimental Medicine*, **61**, 689-702.

Roizin, L. & Kolb, L. C.   (1959) Considerations on the neuropathologic pleomorphism and histogenesis of the lesions of experimental allergic encephalomyelitis in non-human species in '*Allergic*' *Encephalomyelitis* (Eds. Kies, M. W. & Alvord, E. C.), pp. 5-57, Thomas, Springfield, Ill.

Russell, D.·S.   (1946) The problem of demyelination. *London Hospital Gazette*, **49**, May Clinical Supplement.

Russell, D. S.   (1955) The nosological unity of acute haemorrhagic leucoencephalitis and acute disseminated encephalomyelitis. *Brain*, **78**, 369-376.

Schilder, P.   (1912) Zur Kenntnis der sogenannte diffuse Sklerose. *Zeitschrift für die gesamte Neurologie und Psychiatrie*, **10**, 1-60.

Schilder, P.   (1913) Zur Frage der Encephalitis diffusa. *Zeitschrift für die gesamte Neurologie und Psychiatrie*, **15**, 358-376.

Schilder, P.   (1924) Die Encephalitis periaxialis diffusa. *Archiv für Psychiatrie und Nervenkrankheiten*, **71**, 327-356.

Seitelberger, F.   (1960) Histochemistry of demyelinating diseases proper, including allergic encephalomyelitis in *Modern Scientific Aspects of Neurology*, (Ed. Cumings, J. N.), pp. 146-187, Arnold, London.

Sibley, W. A. & Foley, J. M.   (1965) Infection and immunization in multiple sclerosis. *Annals of the New York Academy of Sciences*, **122**, 457-468.

Stansbury, F. C.   (1949) Neuromyelitis optica (Dévic's disease). *Archives of Ophthalmology*, **42**, 292-335 and 465-501.

Stuart, G. & Krikorian, K. S.   (1930) Fatal neuroparalytic accident of anti-rabies treatment. *Lancet*, **1**, 1123-1125.

Stuart, G. & Krikorian, K. S.   (1933) Neuroparalytic accidents complicating antirabic treatment. *British Medical Journal*, **1**, 501-504.

Tourtellotte, W. W.   (1970) Cerebrospinal fluid in multiple sclerosis in *Handbook of Clinical Neurology* (Eds. Vinken, P. J. & Bruyn, G. W.), Vol. 9, pp. 324-382, North Holland Publishing Co., Amsterdam.

Turnbull, H. M. & McIntosh, J.   (1926) Encephalomyelitis following vaccination. *British Journal of Experimental Pathology*, **7**, 181-222.

Uchimura, I. & Shiraki, H.   (1957) A contribution to the classification and the pathogenesis of demyelinating encephalitis. *Journal of Neuropathology and Experimental Neurology*, **16**, 139-208.

van Bogaert, L.   (1932) Histopathologische Studie über die Encephalitis nach Windpocken. *Zeitschrift für die gesamte Neurologie und Psychiatrie*, **140**, 201-217.

Vinken, P. J. & Bruyn, G. W.   (1970) *Handbook of Clinical Neurology, vol. 9. Multiple Sclerosis and other demyelinating diseases*, North Holland Publishing Co., Amsterdam.

White, J. C. & Sweet, W. H.   (1969) *Pain and the Neurosurgeon*, Chapter 5, Thomas, Springfield, Ill.

12

Inborn Lysosomal Enzyme Deficiencies

L. Crome and J. Stern

The theory that storage disorders were due to lysosomal hydrolase deficiencies was first formulated by Hers (1965) in relation to glycogenesis. This theory has since been eagerly exploited and developed, so that many metabolic disorders can now be considered from this viewpoint (Hers and van Hoof 1973). As far as the central nervous system is concerned they fall into four main groups: (1) the lipidoses, most of which are in fact sphingolipidoses; (2) the mucopolysaccharidoses; (3) the mucolipidoses and (4) a miscellaneous array of insufficiently clarified lipid storage disorders and related conditions. Although the lysosomal origin of some disorders contained in the above groups is unproved or even unlikely, all will be considered below because they pose similar pathological, clinical and diagnostic problems and have to be differentiated from each other. With few exceptions all present in infancy or childhood with progressive dysfunction of the central nervous system, i.e. mental retardation or dementia, paralysis and epilepsy. Most are familial, being usually transmitted as recessive Mendelian traits. Some typical diseases, such as Hurler's syndrome, are easily recognizable clinically but in most the diagnosis has to be reached by a collective effort of clinicians and laboratory workers. The basic pathogenetic processes entail progressive accumulation of adventitious material containing an excess or disproportion of lipids, mucopolysaccharides and some other substances. The storage may involve primarily neurons—neurolipidoses, or white matter—leucodystrophies (Hers and van Hoof 1970).

All inborn lysosomal enzyme deficiencies are rare and few estimates have been made of their true incidence; some are quoted in the text*. In our experience mucopolysaccharidoses are more prevalent than the sphingolipidoses, occurring perhaps in the order of 1 : 100,000 of live births (McKusick, Howell, Hussells, Neufeld and Stevenson 1972). According to O'Brien (1973) the heterozygote frequency of Tay–Sachs disease (p. 507) is 0·026 for Jews in the USA and 0·0029 for non-Jews. Ellis (1974) states that one person in 30 is a heterozygote for Tay–Sachs disease among Ashkenazi Jews. This would amount to an incidence at conception of 1 : 3600. We quote the above estimates without endorsing their validity. In particular, it seems to us impossible to identify biologically Gentiles and Jews, whether Ashkenazi or not (Crome and Stern 1972).

Since neural tissue contains 50 to 70% of lipids in the dried white matter and 30 to 40% in the grey matter it is understandable why lipids should loom large in the classification of these disorders, particularly since recognition and measurement of the other constituents of the stored material, such as proteins, remain difficult and inconclusive. Moreover, many of the missing enzymes have been recognized in recent years; most are concerned with the metabolism of the sphingolipids and/or glycosaminoglycans.

* We are indebted to Dr Rosemary Stephens for figures of patients seen at Great Ormond Street Hospital for Sick Children in London since 1964. G_{M1} gangliosidosis—18; G_{M2}—54; globoid cell leucodystrophy—24; Niemann–Pick disease—10; ophthalmoplegic lipidosis—14; Gaucher's disease—10; Fabry's disease—16; metachromatic leucodystrophy—48; Batten's disease—80. In $3\frac{1}{2}$ years there were 55 cases of mucopolysaccharidoses: Sanfilippo's—21; Hunter's—11; Hurler's—3; Hurler–Scheie compound—1; Morquio—3 and Maroteaux–Lamy—4.

Sphingolipidoses

The chief lipids of myelin are cerebrosides, cholesterol and phospholipids—especially sphingomyelin. The nerve cell and its processes contains less phospholipids and more ganglioside. Salient aspects of these substances will next be considered.

Sphingolipids

Sphingolipids occupy a key position in the storage diseases of the nervous system. This group of compounds comprises the sphingomyelins, cere-

called *ceramide*. In the *sphingomyelins* ceramide is linked via the terminal (C_1) carbon to phosphorylcholine (Fig. 12.2). Sphingomyelin is, therefore, a sphingolipid and phospholipid. In the *cerebrosides* ceramide is linked to a hexose, usually galactose. Cerebrosides are therefore sphingolipids and glycolipids but not phospholipids (Fig. 12.3). If the galactose moiety is esterified in position 3 with a sulphate group a *sulphatide* is formed (Fig. 12.4).

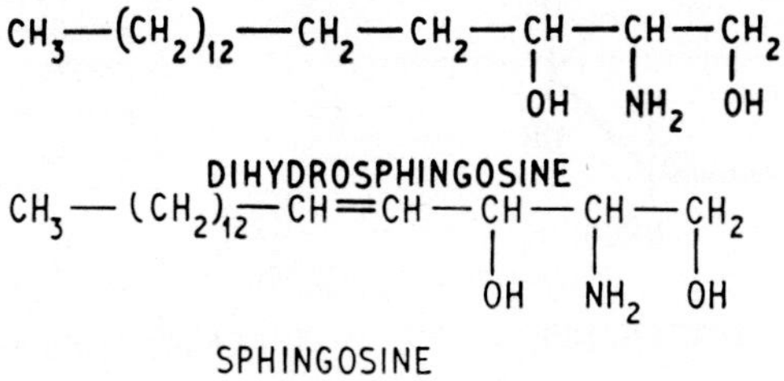

Fig. 12.1 Sphingosine and dihydrosphingosine.

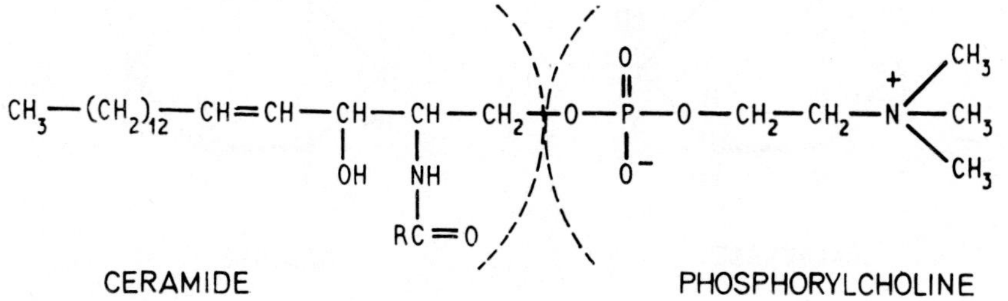

Fig. 12.2 Sphingomyelin.

brosides, sulphatides and gangliosides. All, as the name implies, contain either sphingosine—an unsaturated amino alcohol—or sometimes dihydrosphingosine (Fig. 12.1).

Sphingosine in which one of the hydrogens of the amino group is replaced by a fatty acid is

The most complex sphingolipids are the gangliosides (Figs. 12.5 and 12.6). They may contain for each molecule a ceramide (acylsphingosine) up to four hexoses and three molecules of N-acetylneuraminic acid (sialic acid, NANA). The hexoses may be galactose, glucose or

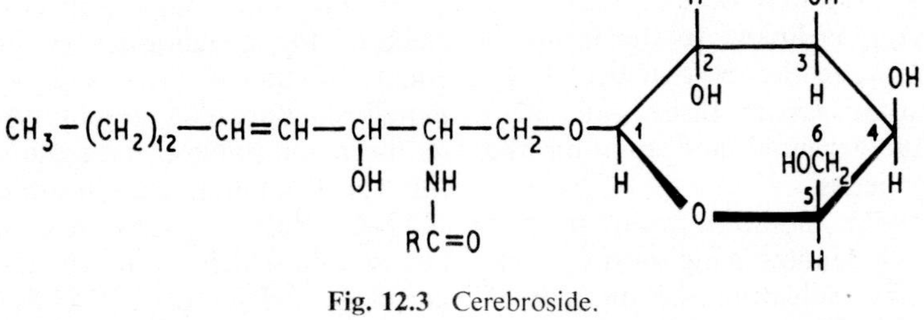

Fig. 12.3 Cerebroside.

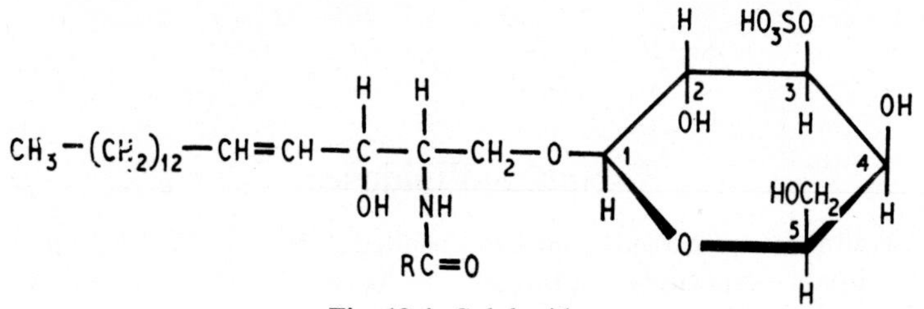

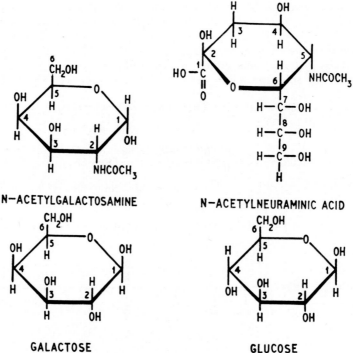

Fig. 12.4 Sulphatide.

N-ACETYLGALACTOSAMINE

N-ACETYLNEURAMINIC ACID

GALACTOSE

GLUCOSE

Fig. 12.5 Constituents of ganglioside.

N-acetylgalactosamine. The structure of the most important monosialoganglioside, G_{M1} is as follows:

ceramide–glucose–galactose–N–acetylgalatosamine–galactose
|
NANA

the sialic acid is linked to carbon 3 of the galactose. Disialogangliosides carry an additional sialic acid group, which in G_{D1a} is linked to the terminal galactose, and in G_{D1b} to the sialic acid of G_{M1}. The trisialoganglioside carries three sialic acid groups, one on the terminal and two on the middle galactose moieties.

In the Svennerholm notation used in this chapter the letter G denotes ganglioside. This is followed by letters indicating the number of

sialic acid residues: A—none, M (mono)—one, D (di)—two, and T (tri)—three. The number after the letter indicates the order in which the compounds separate on thin layer chromatography. G_{M1} and G_{A1} have four hexose groups, G_{M2} and G_{A2} three, G_{M3} and G_{A3} two. The sequence of the hexose groups is constant (Fig. 12.6). G_{T1}, G_{D1a}, G_{D1b} and G_{M1} account for the bulk of the gangliosides of human brain, but small amounts of G_{M2}, G_{M3} and of the asialogangliosides are also present. Asialogangliosides, as the name implies, have the same structure as the corresponding gangliosides, except for the NANA residue. *Globoside* is a ceramide tetrahexoside in which the third hexose is an α-linked galactose (while the ganglioside series has a

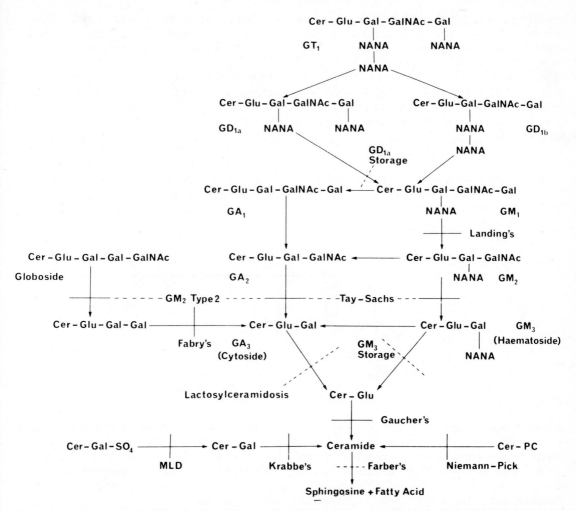

Fig. 12.6 Metabolic relationship of sphingolipids. (Adapted from Raine, 1970.) Solid bars represent proven and broken lines probable enzyme defects. Cer—ceramide; Glu—glucose; Gal—galactose; GalNAc—N-acetylgalactosamine; NANA—N-acetylneuraminic acid; SO_4—sulphate; PC—phosphorylcholine; MLD—metachromatic leucodystrophy. All glycosidic linkages are β except for the third hexose of globoside which is α-linked. GT_1, GD_{1B} and GM_1 are major gangliosides of human brain. GM_2 type 2 = Sandhoff's disease.

β-linked N–acetylgalactosamine as the third hexose):

ceramide–glucose–galactose–galactose–N–acetylgalactosamine

The brain lipids also contain *cholesterol* (Fig. 12.7) which may be esterified in position 3 with fatty acids. Cholesterol esters are virtually absent from normal white matter but often appear in large amounts in demyelinating tissue.

In brain *fatty acids* occur mainly as constituents of phospholipids and sphingolipids, seldom, except in pathological condition, as triglycerides, cholesterol esters or free fatty acids. The nomenclature of the fatty acids is confusing, even to

biochemists, because of its bewildering mixture of conventions, trivial names and systematic names. The nomenclature is based on the straight hydrocarbon chain having the largest number of carbon atoms: that is carbon atoms in branched chains are not counted. The position of substituents is usually defined by counting from the carboxyl group the carbon which is given the number 1. Substituents on the 2nd carbon occupy the α-position, those on carbon 3 the β-position and so on, substituents on the terminal carbon being in the ω position. For unsaturated fatty acids (fatty acids with double bonds), the number of carbon atoms and double bonds respectively is indicated by figures separated by a colon. Thus stearic acid, a saturated fatty acid (without double bonds), is designated $18:0$, palmitic acid is $16:0$. Linoleic acid is $18:2$ (18 carbon atoms, 2 double bonds) and linolenic acid $18:3$ (3 double bonds). All isomers with 18 carbons and 2 double bonds are called linoleic acid and the position of the double bonds is indicated thus:

$$\Delta 9, 12 - 18:2 \text{ or } 18:2^{\Delta 9,12}$$

in this case the double bonds would be at carbons 9 and 12 (counting from the carboxyl end). Similarly, isomer $\Delta 6, 9 - 18:2$ would have the

synaptic membranes. Grey matter sphingomyelin is characterized by a higher ratio of C_{18} to C_{24} acids than white matter sphingomyelin.

Synthesis of sphingolipids

Sphingosine is synthesized in brain from palmityl CoA and serine, with manganese and pyridoxal phosphate as cofactors, and esterified to form ceramide. The bulk of sphingomyelin is probably formed by the transfer of phosphorylcholine from cytidine diphosphate choline to ceramide but some may be formed by transfer of phosphorylcholine to sphingosine followed by esterification of the sphingosine moiety. Theoretically,

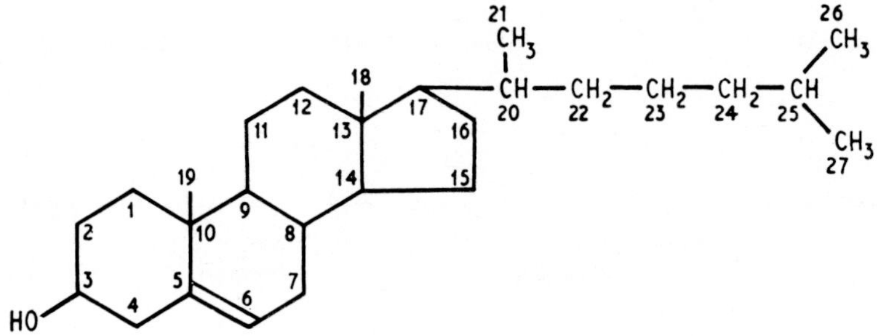

Fig. 12.7 Structure of cholesterol.

double bonds at carbons 6 and 9. Sometimes it is convenient to refer to the position of double bonds by counting from the terminal methyl group. The position is then indicated by ωx or $(n-x)$, where n is the number of carbon atoms in the chain and x the number of the carbons from the terminal methyl group. Sometimes it is the distance of the double bond from the methyl end of the chain which determines physiological activity. Thus some essential fatty acids are $\omega 6$, 9. Mammals cannot introduce double bonds into the $\omega 3$ and $\omega 6$ positions.

Long chain fatty acids in brain contain from 14 to 26 carbon atoms; derivatives of stearic acid with 18 and lignoceric acid with 24 carbons are prominent. Variations in fatty acid composition of lipids in different parts of the brain tend to differ with the nature of the membranes of which they are constituents. In membranes derived from glial cells longer chain fatty acids predominate as, for example, in the sphingomyelins, cerebrosides and sulphatides of myelin. In neuronal membranes, on the other hand, the shorter chain fatty acids are more prominent, as in the gangliosides which form part of the

galactocerebroside can be formed by the transfer of galactose from uridine diphosphate galactose to ceramide or by the transfer of galactose to sphingosine followed by esterification by acyl-CoA. At the time of writing the former mechanism seems favoured.

Biosynthesis of sulphatide is brought about by the action of active sulphate on galacterocerebroside.

The first step in the biosynthesis of ganglioside is the formation of glucosyl ceramide from uridine diphosphate glucose and ceramide, catalysed by a glucosyl transferase. Similar enzymes catalyse the stepwise addition of further monosaccharide units, while the source of sialic acid is cytidine monophosphate–N–acetylneuraminic acid. The precise order in which the above reactions proceed remains to be determined. It should be pointed out that it is not impaired synthesis of the sphingolipids which is the primary metabolic aberration in the lipidoses and leucodystrophies, but defects in their degradation by lysosomal hydrolases, and these will now be briefly considered. These observations are also relevant to the mucopolysaccharidoses (see below).

Degradation of sphingolipids

Lysosomes were discovered by the Nobel laureate C. de Duve and colleagues in the course of studies on the properties and intracellular location of particle-bound acid phosphatase. This enzyme, together with other hydrolases of maximum activity at acid pH, was found to be contained within the cytoplasm in organelles, surrounded by a membrane, which de Duve called *lysosomes*. Their role is the disposal of unwanted matter of both extra- and intracellular origin. The membrane prevents premature contact between the enzymes and their substrates. The name *primary lysosomes* is given to the organelles which have not yet been involved in digestive activity; they become *secondary lysosomes* once they are engaged in the catabolism of substrates.

Extracellular material is engulfed by *endocytosis* and a vacuole, (*hetero*)*phagosome*, forms around the ingested material. Fusion then occurs between the phagosome and the lysosome and digestion of the exogenous material can proceed. Degradation of excess intracellular material is carried out by an analogous process, *autophagy*. Vacuoles referred to as *autophagosomes* are formed and contain intracellular constituents such as mitochondria, endoplasmic reticulum and glycogen, and subsequently fuse with lysosomes. The sequestered cytoplasmic material is broken down in the same way as that of extracellular origin. Hetero- and autophagosomes are the equivalent in the cell of the digestive system of higher organisms. Autophagy is a continuous process in normal cells; its rate may be increased or decreased in certain physiological or pathological conditions. Indigestible residues may form *residual* or *dense bodies*, which may in some cases be extruded from the cell by exocytosis. Some residual bodies seem to lose hydrolytic activity, others may fuse with newly formed endocytic vacuoles and participate in a second act of digestion. Residual bodies are prominent in storage diseases, in which there is apparently no mechanism for their extrusion.

Enzyme defects have been identified at virtually every one of the catabolic steps of sphingolipid metabolism illustrated in Fig. 12.6 and Table 12.1. In nearly every case this is followed by the intralysosomal accumulation of molecules which require the missing enzyme for their degradation, with, on occasions, a spill-over into the cytoplasm, and almost invariable hypertrophy of the lysosomes. Storage is progressive, starting in some cases before birth. The rate of accumulation of stored substances is a function of the quantity of material that has to be degraded in the course of cellular activity. This will vary from tissue to tissue and is a factor in the extent of individual organ involvement. The stored material will be heterogeneous if the bond resistant to hydrolysis occurs in more than one type of molecule. Further, some substances not directly involved in the underlying disease process may be trapped in the cell by physicochemical interaction with the primary stored material. The effect of the inborn lysosomal defect on the activity of other lysosomal enzymes is variable. The activity of some is reduced, perhaps due to the inhibitory action of the stored materials; the activity of others may, contrariwise, be enhanced sometimes several fold. The mechanism of this phenomenon is not understood. In brain, one cannot ignore the possible effect of mechanical distortion of cells on their metabolic activity during the later stages of excessive storage.

In inborn lysosomal disorders enzyme deficiency may be complete in some cases, in others as much as 30% or even more of average enzyme activity may be preserved. This is not, of course, unexpected. Mutations can result in complete inactivation of the enzyme affected, but also in enzymes with altered kinetic properties, or decreased stability, or simply in a low level of a qualitatively normal enzyme. Some examples are given in Table 12.1. Owing to variations in techniques, values reported by different centres are not always strictly comparable. Further complications are introduced by the existence of isoenzymes of differing activity and substrate specificity. An example is provided by the lysosomal β-galactosidases. In G_{M1} gangliosidosis the missing enzyme occurs in the form of three isoenzymes of comparatively low specificity (p. 527). Deficiency of the enzyme may be demonstrated with artificial substrates, and in addition to G_{M1} ganglioside, a compound resembling keratan sulphate, is also stored (p. 519). In the variant of this disorder, G_{M1} gangliosidosis type II, the activity pattern of the isoenzymes is different, as is the course of the disease (p. 528). In contrast, the missing β-galactosidases of Krabbe's leucodystrophy (p. 546) is much more specific and deficiencies can only be demonstrated with the natural substrates of the enzyme.

Too close a correlation must not be expected between the reduction in enzyme activity and

Table 12.1 *Lysosomal hydrolase activity as percentage of normal in patients with lipid storage diseases* (Adapted from Brady 1973 and Hers 1973)

Disorder	Enzyme	Tissue %	Peripheral blood cells %	Fibroblasts %	Page reference
Gaucher's					
Infantile form	Glucocerebrosidase	Spleen 0 to 9	3 to 4	4 to 5	513
Adult form	Glucocerebrosidase	Spleen 12 to 44	13 to 28	10 to 30	513
Niemann–Pick's					
Infantile form	Sphingomyelinase	Liver 0 to 7	ND	6·5	514
Adult form	Sphingomyelinase	Liver 15 to 20	17	10	514
Tay–Sachs	G_{M2} hexosaminidase A	Brain 0 to 2	—	0 to 10	507
Sandhoff's	G_{M2} hexosaminidase A	Brain 10	—	—	512
	G_{M2} hexosaminidase B	Brain undetectable	—	—	512
Krabbe's	Galactocerebrosidase	Brain 4 to 11	2	11	546
Metachromatic leucodystrophy	Sulphatidase	Kidney 1	11	2·6	549
Fabry's					
Affected males	Ceramide trichexosidase	Intestine 1	1	10	516
Carrier females	Ceramide trichexosidase	Intestine 26	10	57	516
Lactosylceramidosis	Lactosylceramidase*	Liver 15 to 20	—	10 to 15	516
Generalized gangliosidosis	G_{M1} galactosidase	Brain 5	5·6	5·6	527
	G_{M1} galactosidase	Liver 0 to 2	—	—	527

* See comment on p. 516

the severity of the disease. As in other inborn errors this will be affected not only by the general genetic make-up of patients but also by their enhanced vulnerability to other adverse factors such as infections, intercurrent illness associated with dehydration, acidosis or similar metabolic stress. The brain seen by the pathologist may have been injured by the underlying disorder and by any exacerbating factor as well as the terminal illness.

Aspects of classification

A pathologist trying to identify a case of lipidosis soon comes up against problems of classification. To understand the somewhat confusing terminology one must approach it historically. The first condition recognized in this series, known as Tay–Sachs disease or now as G_{M2} gangliosidosis, was described in 1881 by Tay, a London ophthalmologist, and its character more fully established by Sachs (1887) in New York. A few other conditions were identified later: the congenital, the late infantile (in contrast to the Tay–Sachs, which is a disease of early infancy) also referred to as the Bielschowsky type, one affecting still older children referred to as the juvenile or Spielmeyer–Vogt type, and the adult or the Kufs type. The late infantile and the

juvenile variants are sometimes referred to as 'amaurotic family idiocy' or Batten's or Batten–Mayou type. This constituted the first phase of classification, based on the age of onset and clinicopathological features. Other lipid storage disorders, such as Niemann–Pick's disease, Gaucher's disease and gargoylism or Hurler's disease, Hunter's disease and others were added later to a list that is still being enlarged.

The second phase, from the mid-thirties, was a period of the chemical identification of the stored substances. Thus, Tay–Sachs disease proved to be a gangliosidosis, Niemann–Pick's disease a sphingomyelinosis and Gaucher's disease a cerebrosidosis. The stored lipid in Batten's disease has not yet been satisfactorily analysed but is related to ceroid or lipofuscin (p. 531). It then became known that an excess of sphingolipid was also present in some of the mucopolysaccharidoses and some of these conditions are referred to as mucolipidoses (Spranger and Wiedemann 1970). Later still an excess of sphingolipid was observed in certain leucodystrophies, i.e. metachromatic leudodystrophy and globoid cell leucodystrophy, in both of which storage is mainly in the white matter.

The third, contemporary, stage began with the recognition of the missing enzymes in some of these conditions. While promising to be definitive this classification is still incomplete and does not fit in completely with previous categories. It was also found that lack of several distinct enzymes may result in a clinically similar condition, as is the case with the G_{M2} gangliosidoses or some mucopolysaccharidoses, while, on the other hand, lack of the same enzyme may produce heterogeneous results. At present, authors continue to use terms based on all three stages of classification and some confusion is therefore inevitable.

The sphingolipidoses have been reviewed by many eminent workers in this field. Those requiring a full list of sources can be referred, for example, to the reviews by Volk, Adachi and

isoenzymes can split globoside and G_{A2} (the asialoganglioside of G_{M2}), but only hexosaminidase A will cleave G_{M2} ganglioside. For details of the biochemistry of human hexosaminidases, readers are referred to Suzuki and Suzuki (1973) and Shrivastava and Beutler (1974).

G_{M2} gangliosidosis (*Tay–Sachs disease*)

The originally described variant of G_{M2} gangliosidosis is caused by hexosaminidase A deficiency. Ceramide trihexoside, which is an asialo derivative of G_{M2}, is also stored in neural tissue. The condition is transmitted as a Mendelian recessive trait.

Signs commence in early infancy. The picture is one of lassitude, mental deterioration, loss of

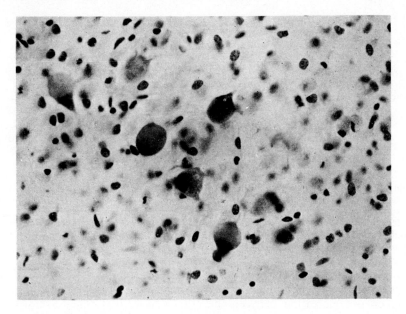

Fig. 12.8 The cortex in lipidosis. There is marked neuronal loss and the few remaining nerve cells show distension, nuclear displacement, and disappearance or powdering of the Nissl substance. Cresyl violet. × 412.

Schneck (1972) and by Suzuki and Suzuki (1973) and Sandhoff (1974).

G_{M2} gangliosidoses

These are conditions caused by hexosaminidase deficiency. The enzyme occurs in two forms, A and B, and one or both were found to be deficient in the three variants of the G_{M2} gangliosidosis while in the fourth, of which only one case has been published in detail, both hexosaminidases were apparently normal (Sandhoff 1969; Sandhoff and Jatzkewitz 1972). Both

vision, hyperacusis (i.e. an exaggerated motor response to sound), convulsions, increasing weakness, spasticity and paralysis. Contrasted with the leucodystrophies (white matter diseases), grey matter diseases, of which G_{M2} gangliosidosis is one, often commence with fits and mental regression. Retinoscopy may reveal a cherry-red spot. While the retinogram remains unaffected, the EEG deteriorates rapidly after birth and the visual evoked responses also disappear by the age of 16 months (Pampiglione, Privett and Harden 1974). A proportion of lymphocytes in the peripheral blood may be vacuolated and some polymorphs show basophilic granulation, but these are not reliable diagnostic criteria. The children usually die before their fifth year.

On naked-eye inspection the brain is, depending on the duration of the disease, normal in size, micrencephalic or excessively large—megalencephalic. Such enlargement is thought to be due to neuronal swelling and astrocytic hyperplasia. It is usually firm or, indeed, indurated; there

black. In the youngest patients, however, the granules may not be sudanophil at all. They are invariably PAS positive, Luxol fast blue positive, may be metachromatic with toluidin blue and cresyl violet, and usually show strong acid phosphatase activity. Neuraminic acid may be detected by a positive Bial test which is, however, not always reliable. On electron microscopy the granules appear as concentrically

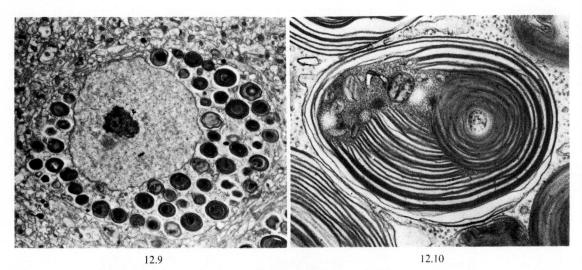

12.9   12.10

Fig. 12.9 Tay–Sachs disease. Small, rounded cortical neurons with displaced normal nucleus, and cytoplasm filled with numerous membranous cytoplasmic bodies (MCBs). Between the latter are normal cytoplasmic components. The surrounding neuropil seems normal. × 4600.
Fig. 12.10 Tay–Sachs disease. An MCB from a cortical neuron. The higher magnification reveals the lamellar structure with an approximate periodicity of 50 nm × 39,000. (Figs 12.9 and 12.10 by courtesy of Dr R. D. Terry and the Editor of *Journal of Neuropathology and Experimental Neurology*.)

may be ulegyria, with narrowing of the cortical ribbon, together with discoloration and blurring of the normally crisp demarcation between the grey and white matter. The centrum semiovale may be oedematous or show a greyish discoloration from myelin loss. The optic nerves are usually reduced in size and the cerebellum and brainstem are often small and atrophic.

Histologically, the characteristic feature is ubiquitous enlargement of neurons, particularly the larger ones, caused by accumulation of adventitious material in their cytoplasm. The nuclei are displaced sideways or into the apical dendrites, and the Nissl substance becomes powdery or disappears entirely (Fig. 12.8). The staining of the stored material is somewhat variable; it is usually finely granular and sudanophil in frozen sections, staining a faint dullish red with Sudan III or IV and greyish with Sudan

laminated cytoplasmic structures referred to as membranous cytoplasmic bodies (MCBs) (Figs. 12.9 and 12.10). They average about 1 μm in diameter. These bodies have been found not only in the central nervous system but wherever the neurons are distended, i.e. the retina, myenteric plexuses and autonomic nerve ganglia. They have also been observed in an immature form in affected fetuses (Adachi, Torii, Schneck and Volk 1971). On light microscopy apical dendrites and axis cylinders may display a number of localized swellings (Fig. 12.11). These are particularly well demonstrated by silver impregnation of the cerebellum where the axonal swellings of the Purkinje cells assume the form of so-called 'torpedo bodies' (Fig. 12.37). As neurons perish, glial cells proliferate (Figs. 12.12 and 12.13). Many lipid macrophages appear in the grey and white matter and some contain the same material

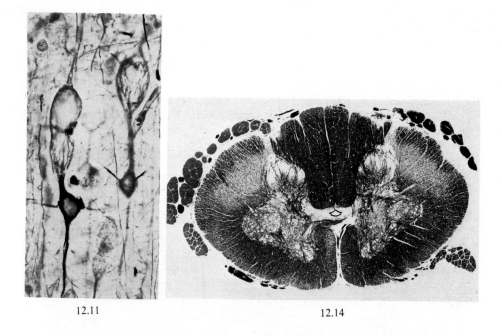

12.11

12.14

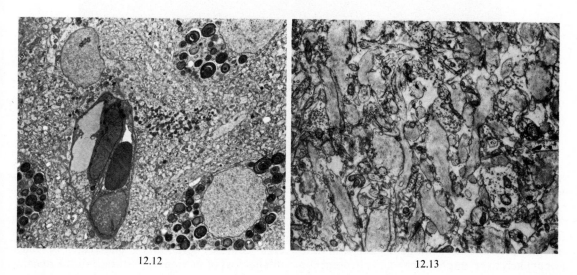

12.12

12.13

Fig. 12.11 Distension of apical dendrites in Tay–Sachs disease (Bielschowsky silver impregnation).

Fig. 12.12 Tay–Sachs disease. Portion of three cortical neurons, each with MCBs, are apparent near the edges. The central portion is a branching small vessel, probably capillary, over the top of which is draped an astrocyte containing numerous smaller inclusions. The neuropil is still intact. × 2550.

Fig. 12.13 Tay–Sachs disease. This is the neuropil in the late stage in which there is extensive astrocytic gliosis and a marked increase in the extracellular space. The irregular elongate outlines containing delicate filaments are astrocytic processes. × 7500. (Figs. 12.12 and 12.13 by courtesy of Dr R. D. Terry and the Editor of *Journal of Neuropathology and Experimental Neurology*.)

Fig. 12.14 Pyramidal tract degeneration in Tay–Sachs disease.

as the neurons while most show deposition of brighter red sudanophil neutral fats and cholesterol esters.   Further, there is an associated astrocytosis and fibrous gliosis while another consequence of neuronal loss is secondary myelin loss, especially of the long descending tracts (Fig. 12.14) (cf. Fardeau and Lapresle 1963). Such myelin loss may be extensive and severe enough to suggest leudodystrophy as in the case

particularly marked gliosis and atrophy in the granular layer and of the mossy and climbing fibres, the Purkinje cells being relatively well preserved (Figs. 12.15 and 12.36), and that this contrasted with the more usual 'centrifugal' type of atrophy in most other conditions, in which Purkinje cells are the first to vanish.   As already mentioned, Purkinje cells may show localized axonal and dendritic swellings.

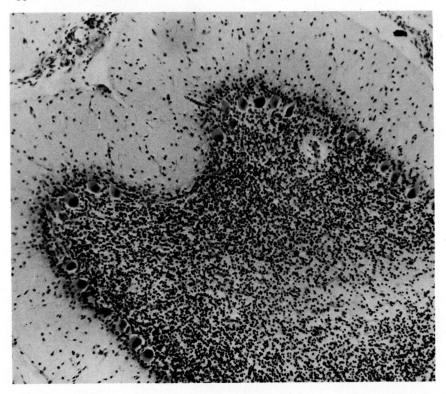

Fig. 12.15 'Centripetal' cerebellar atrophy in a case of juvenile Tay–Sachs disease.   Purkinje cells are distended but are nevertheless well preserved.   There is some perceptible loss of the granular layer.   Cresyl violet.   × 160.

of lipidosis reported by Haberland and Brunngraber (1970).   Myelin loss in G_{M2} gangliosidosis and probably in other storage disorders, is however unlikely to be simply a secondary phenomenon and there is evidence that myelin anabolism is directly interfered with by the metabolic aberrations (Haberland, Brunngraber, Witting and Brown 1973).

The cerebellum is often atrophic; Purkinje cells and granules are usually depleted.   Bielschowsky (1920-21) has pointed out, however, that in the late infantile cases, some of which might now be regarded as juvenile gangliosidosis (p. 512), cerebellar atrophy was 'centripetal' in type with

Retinal degeneration may be a conspicuous feature of the disease.   Retinal nerve and glial cells contain adventitious material.   In older infants loss of neurons and storage in the remaining ones may be associated with gradually increasing retinal pigmentation.   The fovea may be widened, a gap being present in the inner nuclear layer while the outer one can also be deficient in this region.   It has been suggested by Greenfield, Aring and Landing (1955) that degeneration may commence in the region of the fovea and spread from there outwards, although isolated lesions may also be found peripherally.   Several other reports on retinal changes have been published

(Mossakowski 1964; Manshot 1968). The red colour of the cherry-red spot seems to be caused by the choroid shining more brightly through the atrophic, thinned retina (Duke and Clark 1962). The whitish halo around the cherry-red spot has been said to be caused by the accumulated lipids in the densely arranged nerve cells around the fovea (Wolter and Allen 1964). However, the cherry-red spot may well be absent and, in older cases, atrophy may appear as diffuse clinically as it is histologically, the choroid showing through over a wide area. The cherry-red spot is, however, by no means pathognomonic of G_{M2} gangliosidosis. It has been observed, for

tension in the spiral ganglia as well as secondary inflammatory change (Boies 1963; Kelemen 1965).

Involvement of the myenteric plexuses is of special diagnostic importance since it provides a ready means of certain diagnosis of a storage disorder. Both the Meissner and Auerbach plexuses are affected, showing distension of nerve cells by the characteristically staining storage material (Fig. 12.16). Nerve cells in other autonomic, visceral and retroperitoneal ganglia are also affected (see p. 559).

Demyelinating peripheral nerve neuropathy has been reported in Tay–Sachs disease by Kristensson, Olsson and Sourander (1967).

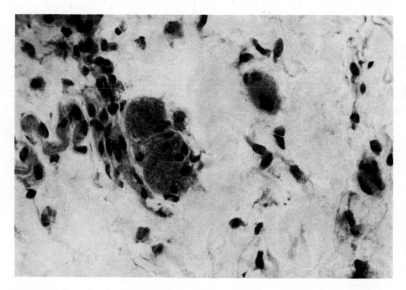

Fig. 12.16 Tay–Sachs disease. Distended neurons of the Meissner plexus in a rectal biopsy. The cytoplasm is filled with granular sudanophil material. Cryostat section stained with Sudan III and haematoxylin. ×400.

example, in cases of mucopolysaccharidosis (Titarelli, Giagheddu and Spadetta 1963), Niemann–Pick's disease (Goldstein and Wexler 1931), ceroid-lipofuscinosis (Vogt–Spielmeyer type) and G_{M1} gangliosidosis (p. 528).

Electroretinography may be useful in the differential diagnosis of the neurolipidoses. The principle is that electrical activity is generated only by the outer nuclear layer so that it is reduced if that layer is affected, as, say, in ceroid-lipofuscinosis, and tends to stay normal in degenerative conditions involving only the ganglion cell layer, such as Tay–Sachs disease (Carr and Gouras 1966) (see also p. 564).

The inner ears of Tay–Sachs patients have shown a number of anomalies, including neuronal dis-

Somatic tissues show no specific macroscopic change in Tay–Sachs disease but this is not to say that they remain entirely unaffected by the enzyme deficiency. A Swedish team (Eeg-Olofson, Kristensson, Sourander and Svennerholm 1966) have shown that in a typical case G_{M2} was present in excess in some somatic tissues. G_{M2} has also been found in the spleen and liver by Svennerholm (1966) and it is not at all unusual on microscopy to find distension of a few reticulo-endothelial cells in the liver and spleen giving the characteristic staining reactions. Inclusion bodies were seen in liver cells by Volk, Adachi, Schneck, Saifer and Kleinberg (1969). Storage of gangliosides was demonstrated in tissue cultures of non-neuronal cells of a case of Tay–

Sachs disease by Batzdorf, Sarlieve, Gold and Menkes (1969).

Juvenile G$_{M2}$ gangliosidosis

A few children manifest G$_{M2}$ gangliosidosis relatively late, i.e. from 2 to 6 years, and its progress is slower (*Bernheimer–Seitelberger disease*). Early signs include loss of speech, mental retardation, progressive spasticity and seizures. Optic atrophy and retinitis pigmentosa are present in some cases (O'Brien, Okada, Ho, Fillerup, Veath and Adams 1971). Cherry-red spots may occur but megalencephaly does not develop. The condition may

Total hexosaminidase deficiency (*Sandhoff disease*)

In this variant of gangliosidosis (also known as Sandhoff–Jatzkewitz–Pilz disease) both hexosaminidases A and B are absent while lipid globoside is increased in various viscera, especially the kidney (Krivit, Desnick, Lee, Moller, Wright, Sweeley, Snyder and Sharp 1972; Okada, McCrea and O'Brien 1972). It has become obvious that there is considerable heterogeneity in the enzymic activity (or lack of it) in reported cases. This is stressed particularly by Vidailhet, Neimann, Grignon, Hartemann, Philippart, Paysant, Nabet and Floquet (1973) and Fontaine, Résibois, Tondeur, Jonniaux, Farriaux, Voet, Maillard

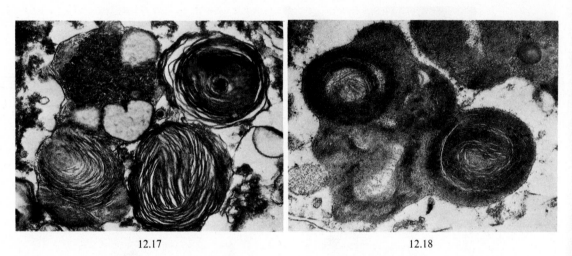

12.17   12.18

Fig. 12.17 Juvenile G$_{M2}$ gangliosidosis. Membranous cytoplasmic bodies often coexist with lipofuscin.   × 31,500. (By courtesy of Dr K. Suzuki.)

Fig. 12.18 Juvenile G$_{M2}$ gangliosidosis. Large irregular inclusions consisting of several MCBs with or without lipofuscin or other type of inclusions are present in the same neuron.   × 31,500. (By courtesy of Dr K. Suzuki and the Editor of *Neurology*.)

be associated with *partial* or *profound* deficiency of hexosaminidase A (Brett, Ellis, Haas, Ikonne, Lake, Patrick and Stephens 1973). On examination, the brain is usually atrophic, neurons showing the same changes as in the infantile variant. It has been said that neuronal distension appears to be more conspicuous in the subcortical formations of the grey matter than in the cerebral cortex. On electron-microscopy neurons show many abnormal inclusions, some like MCBs, and also poorly defined lamellar structures, lipofuscin bodies, membranovesicular bodies and large, up to 15 µm, conglomerations formed by all the above inclusions (Figs. 12.17 and 12.18) (Suzuki, Suzuki, Rapin, Suzuki and Ishii 1970).

and Loeb (1973). In a later case partial activity of hexosaminidase B was preserved in the serum and plasma (Spence, Ripley, Embil and Tibbles 1974). The clinical picture closely resembles that of Tay–Sachs disease; so do the pathological changes, even though the authors reporting the first two cases have stressed the unusually marked myelin loss in the cerebral hemispheres and conspicuous reactive gliosis. PAS-positive material was present in liver cells, Kupffer cells, some histiocytes and renal tubular cells (Suzuki, Jacob, Suzuki, Kutty and Suzuki 1971). Histiocytes with vacuolated cytoplasm may be present in the lungs, spleen, lymph glands and bone marrow. One child, aged 2½ years, examined *post mortem*

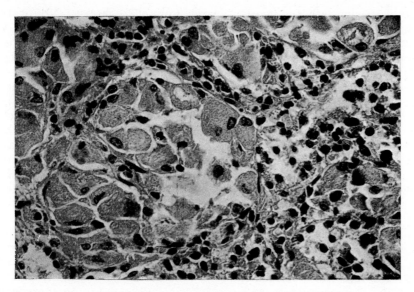

Fig. 12.19   Adventitious cells in the spleen in a case of Gaucher's disease.   Haematoxylin and eosin.   × 400.

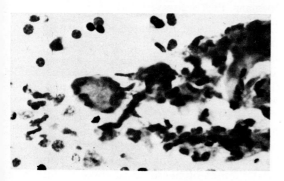

Fig. 12.20   A perivascular cell from cerebral white matter.

by Dolman, Chang and Duke (1973), showed a grossly enlarged brain (1690 g) with a small and indurated cerebellum, shrunken optic nerves and bright yellow dorsal root ganglia.   The endocardium of the atria and of the mitral and tricuspid valves was thickened and opaque.   The histological findings were much as in Tay–Sachs disease, but the neuronal lipids were perhaps more sudanophil than in other cases.   The authors were particularly impressed by conspicuous vacuolation of pancreatic acinar cells.   Lipid granules were present in many tissues, particularly in the endothelium, smooth muscle and fibroblasts. These granules stained deep blue with Luxol fast blue and orange with Sudan IV (see also p. 563).

Congenital and fetal manifestations

Tay–Sachs disease may be neonatal or, indeed, fetal in onset.   The diagnosis in fetal cases is established by lack of hexosaminidase A and increase of G_{M2} in cultured amniotic cells. G_{M2} ganglioside is also increased in the brain and the neurons show inclusions of granular amorphous material and loose membranous structures (Schneck, Friedland, Valenti, Adachi, Amsterdam and Volk 1970; Adachi et al. 1971; Schneck, Amsterdam and Volk 1974).   Abnormal membrane-bound bodies containing delicate membranous structures have been seen in some neurons of a 12-week-old fetus (Percy, McCormick, Kaback and Herndon 1973; Adachi, Schneck and Volk 1974), but lysosomes are not formed before this stage so that earlier inclusions are not membrane-bound (see also p. 562).

Gaucher's disease

Gaucher's disease is primarily a storage disorder of the reticulo-endothelial system, neural tissues being seldom heavily implicated.   The main stored substance is glucosylceramide but other sphingolipids, such as lactosylceramide and G_{M3} ganglioside may also accumulate, albeit to a lesser degree.   The enzymic deficiency is of glucocerebrosidase (β-glucosidase).   In the more common adult form of the disease the clinical picture is dominated by splenomegaly and hyper-splenism, i.e. anaemia and leucopenia. However, when the disease affects infants or children they may also show mental retardation, opisthotonos, paralysis, spasticity and convulsions. Charac-teristic X-ray appearances such as flask-shaped enlargement of the lower ends of the femora and/or bone erosion are seen as a rule in older patients but may also be present in infants (Jackson and Simon 1965). The skin and con-junctiva may show focal yellowish brown pig-mentation. Serum acid phosphatase is raised. In early life the disease may assume either an infantile form which is rapidly fatal or, more rarely, a subacute juvenile one which runs a more protracted course. There is evidence that these forms are genetically distinct, only one of them recurring in the same affected families. Prenatal onset has been reported by Drukker, Sachs and Gatt (1970). Transmission is as a Mendelian recessive trait but in a few cases it was said to have been as a Mendelian dominant. The condition has been fully reviewed by Fredrick-son and Sloan (1972b).

The spleen is greatly enlarged, the liver less so; lymph nodes show varying degrees of enlarge-ment or may be normal in size due to the presence of numerous Gaucher cells which may also be present in the bone marrow and in many other organs (Fig. 12.19). The brain is reduced in size in the 'cerebral' cases and may present recognizable atrophy and sclerosis of the grey matter.

The typical Gaucher cell is a large macrophage of 20 to 100 μm diameter with a central or eccentric small, sometimes multiple, nucleus and a wrinkled cell cytoplasm which contains granules or fibrils. The stored substance is invariably PAS-positive, Luxol fast blue negative and weakly sudanophil. It is positive for acid phosphatase. On electron-microscopy Gaucher cells contain hollow helical tubules of 200 to 300 nm diameter. A whole group of these tubules is usually found within a membrane-limited space. Cerebroside may be histo-chemically demonstrable in neurons but there is no neuronal distension akin to that of the other sphingolipidoses. If affected, the brain shows merely a non-specific severe patchy loss of nerve cells while a few may, as mentioned, contain glyco-lipid and cerebroside (Adams 1965). Neuronal storage with distension of the cells is not a constant or conspicuous feature and is more marked in the juvenile form of the disease. Neuronal loss may be apparent in the cerebral cortex as well as in subcortical formations. What is much more striking in some of these cases is proliferation of histiocytes in the adventitia of blood vessels in the white matter and the transformation of a few of these into typical Gaucher cells (Fig. 12.20). Other perivascular macrophages contain PAS-positive fibrils. Moreover, a few histiocytes storing adventitious material may make their appearance in the grey matter of the brain (Minauf, Stögman and Krepler 1970; Levin and Hoenig 1972). The electron-microscopical in-clusions (Gaucher bodies) have sometimes been seen within neurons of the 'cerebral' cases (Adachi, Wallace, Schneck and Volk 1967). The sural nerve of a patient examined by Bischoff, Reutter and Wegmann (1967) presented an accumulation of a lipid-containing substance, predominantly in Schwann cells and, to a lesser extent, in axons.

Niemann–Pick's disease

The lipids stored in this disorder contain great excess of sphingomyelin, cholesterol and, less constantly, of other phospholipids such as lyso-bisphosphatidic acid and of glucosylceramide (Dacremont, Kint, Carton and Cocquyt 1974. A generally accepted classification is that of Crocker (1961). Type A, the 'classical' form, starts in early infancy and is associated with neuronal lipidosis; type B exhibits only visceral lipidosis; type C runs a milder course and has a later onset of neurological involvement; type D refers only to the so-called Nova Scotia variant which is similar to type C but was believed, albeit on inconclusive evidence, to be genetically distinct. In type D excess of cholesterol is greater than that of sphingomyelin. Other forms have been reported and Pilz (1970), for example, dis-tinguishes five forms. The enzymic defect in Niemann–Pick's disease, types A and B, is that of sphingomyelinase but deficiency of this enzyme in types C and D has not been definitely estab-lished. A few adults have shown sphingomyelin accumulation without neurological involvement and with no sphingomyelinase deficiency. The condition has been diagnosed in a fetus whose tissue-culture grown amniotic cells lacked sphingo-myelinase (Epstein, Brady, Schneider, Bradley and Shapiro 1971) (see also p. 560 et seq.).

The cerebral form of the disease, which is the most common one, may be, in accordance with

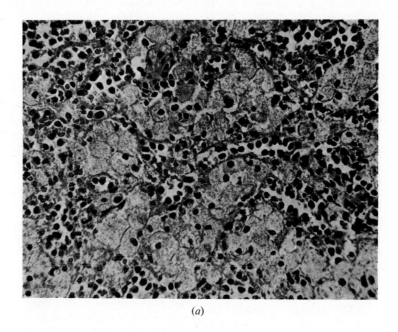

(a)

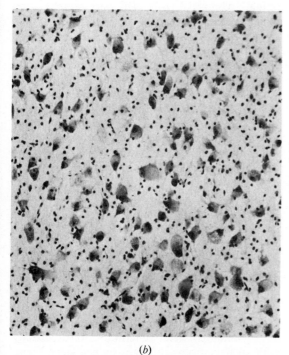

(b)

Fig. 12.21 Niemann–Pick's disease. (a) The spleen shows characteristic 'foam' cells. Haematoxylin and eosin. ×200. (b) The cerebral cortex. Nerve cells are ballooned and the nuclei displaced. Changes are essentially as in Tay–Sachs disease.

the time of onset, infantile, late infantile, juvenile or adolescent. Unlike G_{M2} gangliosidosis all forms are dominated by marked enlargement of lymph glands, liver and spleen. The patients suffer from anaemia, thrombocytopenia and occasionally jaundice. As in other lipidoses the cytoplasm of some lymphocytes is vacuolated. One such case examined by Heyne, Kemmer, Simon and Kasper (1974) revealed on electron-microscopy a botryoid accumulation of these vacuoles which contrasted with more sparsely scattered cytoplasmic vacuolation in a case of Landing's disease and one of Batten's disease also examined by them. The cherry-red spot of the retina may be present in the infantile cases and the skin may show patches of hyper-pigmentation. Paralysis, epilepsy and mental retardation set in. Type B cases survive longer than the others and show, of course, no neuro-logical or mental involvement.

The most striking features are the enlargement of lymph glands, particularly abdominal ones, and splenomegaly. The spleen is greatly en-larged, Malpighian bodies are not visible and the pulp may show yellowish areas of discolora-tion. The brain may be reduced in size and indurated. The cerebral ventricles are enlarged and the cerebellum is sclerotic. On histological examination, the characteristic feature is the presence of clusters and sheets of 'foam' cells in many somatic tissues (Fig. 12.21a). These cells measure 20 to 90 μm, are usually round and filled with mulberry-like lipid droplets which dissolve on paraffin processing leaving the cyto-plasm vacuolated. In frozen preparations they are sudanophil and stain unspecifically for un-saturated fatty acids and phospholipids; many are birefringent. It is possible to demonstrate sphingomyelin in them histochemically by the Baker method. Besides the foam cells, many tissues, especially those of older patients, show an excess of ceroid pigment (p. 533). Although foam cells are the hallmark of Niemann–Pick's disease they are by no means pathognomonic; similar cells (at least on light microscopy) are also seen to occur in many other metabolic and infective conditions such as lipogranulomatosis (p. 537). Letterer–Siwe disease, G_{M1} ganglio-sidosis, Wolman's disease and histiocytosis. On electron-microscopy one finds residual body in-clusions containing fine lamellar structures and closely packed granules of moderate density (Volk, Wallace and Aronson 1968; Pilz 1970).

The distended neurons in the cerebral cases show changes similar to those in G_{M2} gangliosidosis (Fig. 12.21b). Neuronal loss is often accom-panied by glial proliferation, phagocytosis of sudanophil debris and loss of myelin. Foam cells have been observed in the meninges. On electron-microscopy the lipid-laden neurons may contain concentric lamellar inclusions enveloped by single membranes (Suzuki and Suzuki 1973). Other electron-microscopical studies in this disease are by Volk and Wallace (1966) and Wallace, Lazarus and Volk (1967). The retinal changes in Niemann–Pick's disease have been described by Goldstein and Wexler (1931) and Rintelen (1936). All aspects of Niemann–Pick's disease are reviewed by Fredrickson and Sloan (1972a). A condition that may prove to be a variant of the disease is discussed on p. 538.

Lactosylceramidosis

We know of only one reported case of lacto-sylceramidosis. The female infant suffered from mental regression, hypotonia, cerebellar ataxia and spasticity. She presented with hepatospleno-megaly and reddish macular discoloration of the retina. Abnormal foam cells were present in the bone marrow. She died at the age of 4 years (Dawson, Matalon and Stein 1971). Excessive lactosylceramide was found in erythrocytes, plasma, bone marrow, brain, liver and in the urinary deposits. In addition, an excess of glucocerebroside was present in the liver. The missing enzyme in this case was initially thought to be lactosyl cerebroside galactosidase, but this was not borne out in subsequent studies. While, therefore, lactosylceramidosis is theoretically possible, an authenticated case has yet to be reported.

Fabry's disease

Fabry's disease usually presents in adolescence with the appearance of keratotic papules and macules (angiokeratomata) upon the lower part of the body and limbs. Other symptoms and signs include burning pain in the limbs, bouts of fever, vasomotor and other autonomic disturb-ances, impaired renal function, corneal opacity, with such neurological signs as headache, hemi-paraesthesia, paralysis, aphasia, ataxia, nystagmus and disturbances of consciousness. Death ensues ultimately from renal failure or from cerebral or cardiac complications. The condition is transmitted as a sex-linked recessive trait, but heterozygous females may show partial involvement, particularly corneal opacity. The missing enzyme is ceramide trihexosidase (α-galactosyl hydrolase) and an intermediate level of this enzyme activity has been found in the female carriers of the disease. The stored substance is galactosylgalactosylglucosyl ceramide. Mapes, Anderson, Sweeley, Desnick and Krivit (1970) have shown that, at least in principle, enzyme replacement by plasma infusion of this enzyme is feasible and might be used to delay the accumulation of ceramide trihexosamide in the tissues.

Pathological examination may show enlargement of the heart as well as the skin lesions already mentioned. Histologically, the skin lesions are angiokeratomata and telangiectases (Frost, Spaeth and Tanaka 1966). Birefringent granules of the adventitious lipid are present in endothelial cells and histiocytes within the lesions and these are PAS-positive and sudanophil. Such granules are present in many other tissues and in the urinary deposit. Foam cells are found in the bone marrow, other parts of the reticuloendothelial system and most other tissues. The cytoplasm of the glomerular cells of the kidney may be vacuolated. Eosinophil and sudanophil granules are present in renal glomeruli, distal tubules and loops of Henle. Osmiophilic laminated glycolipid bodies up to 12 μm in diameter are present in glomerular epithelial cells

and can be demonstrated in the urine (Duncan 1970). Lipid storage has been observed in the epithelial cells of bronchi, in muscle, lungs, bone marrow, spleen and lymph glands. In the central nervous system lipid storage is seen in the neurons which are said to be particularly associated with the autonomic innervation, such as the dorsal nuclei of the vagi, reticular formation, hypothalamic nuclei, substantia nigra, amygdaloid nuclei, parts of the thalami, the nuclei of the cuneate and gracile columns and the intermediolateral columns of the spinal cord. The affected neurons are ballooned. Their cytoplasm contains foamy, sudanophil, PAS-positive, birefringent material. Similar material is present in glial and endothelial cells within the affected areas. Peripheral nerves show some loss of myelin and of axis cylinders; adventitious granular material is present in the perineurium. Similar deposits are present in autonomic nerves and ganglia. On electron-microscopy the inclusions are seen to be of single-membrane-bound dense granules. Regular lamellar patterns may be present within the inclusions. Lattice-like and concentric lamellar structures have also been observed.

Further information on the disease is available in the reports of Bischoff, Fierz, Regli and Ulrich (1968), Tondeur and Résibois (1969), Christensen Lou and Reske-Nielsen (1971), Volk, Adachi and Schneck (1972), Sweeley, Krivit, Klionsky and Desnick (1972) and Haebara, Hazama and Amano (1974).

Disorders of glycosaminoglycan metabolism

The mucopolysaccharidoses and mucolipidoses are disorders caused by deficiencies of enzymes concerned in the metabolism of the glycosaminoglycans. As a result excessive amounts or abnormal proportions of the compounds accumulate in the tissues and may be excreted in the urine. Some of these disorders may also be associated with sphingolipidosis of the brain. The missing enzymes in the two main groups are different, and there is as a rule no abnormal urinary excretion of mucopolysaccharides in cases of mucolipidosis as there is in the mucopolysaccharidoses yet the clinical distinction between them can be tenuous.

Besides the deficiency of the main enzyme in each condition, there are often quantitative changes in other hydrolases. For example, in the Hurler syndrome, a condition caused by lack of α-L-iduronidase, there is also reduced activity of β-galactosidase, and an increase in that of β-glucuronidase, α-fucosidase, N-acetyl-β-hexosaminidase and acid phosphatase. Some enzymes may be occasionally increased, for example α-galactosidase, α-arabinosidase and arylsulphatase A (Den Tandt and Giesberts 1973). Since hydrolases split linkages of compounds and not particular moieties as such, several substances with similar linkages may be affected by lack of an enzyme and the stored material need not be chemically homogeneous.

Study of these conditions has passed through the usual stages of progress. It commenced with the recognition of Hunter's syndrome in 1917 and Hurler's syndrome in 1919. Four other main variants were identified later. During this period the stored adventitious material was analysed by a number of workers. The final stage

nomenclature has been introduced for these compounds but the old names are still widely used (Table 12.2). A notation likely to come into increasing use is one by McKusick (1972): MPS I H—Hurler's syndrome; MPS I S—Scheie's syndrome; MPS I H/S—Hurler-Scheie syndrome; MPS II A—Hunter's syndrome, severe; MPS II B—Hunter's syndrome, mild; MPS III A—Sanfilippo's syndrome A; MPS III B—Sanfilippo's

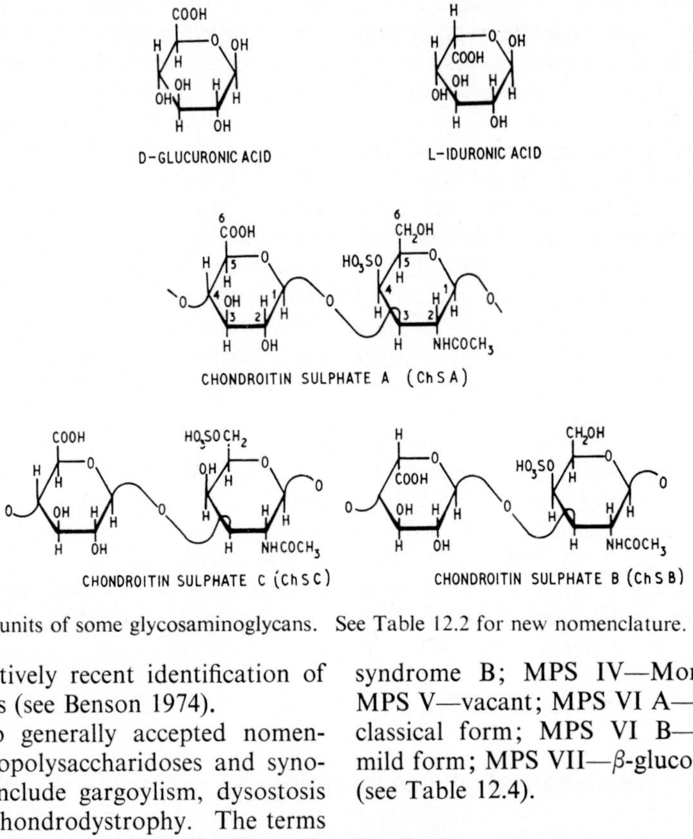

Fig. 12.22 Repeating units of some glycosaminoglycans. See Table 12.2 for new nomenclature.

came with the relatively recent identification of the missing enzymes (see Benson 1974).

There is still no generally accepted nomenclature of the mucopolysaccharidoses and synonyms still in use include gargoylism, dysostosis multiplex and lipochondrodystrophy. The terms MPS I (for Hurler's disease), MPS II (for Hunter's syndrome), MPS III (Sanfilippo's syndrome), MPS IV (Morquio syndrome), MPS V (Scheie's) and MPS VI (Maroteux–Lamy) are still widely used in the United States of America.

Glycosaminoglycans

The glycosaminoglycans (mucopolysaccharides) are macromolecules of repeating units of hexosamine and hexuronic acid (Fig. 12.22). Many of these compounds are present in a variety of animal tissues, particularly in the cornea, blood vessels and cartilage, where they are important constituents of the ground substance. A new

syndrome B; MPS IV—Morquio's syndrome; MPS V—vacant; MPS VI A—Maroteaux–Lamy, classical form; MPS VI B—Maroteaux–Lamy, mild form; MPS VII—β-glucoronidase deficiency (see Table 12.4).

Synthesis

The starting point for the synthesis of the glycosaminoglycans are the uridine diphosphate glucose (UDP) derivatives of glucuronate, iduronate, xylose, N-acetylglucosamine, N-acetylgalactosamine and galactose, the molecular constituents which make up the finished biopolymer. Polymerization starts with the synthesis of the linkage region which is, for example, of the form

glucuronate–galactose–galactose–xylose–O–serine

The xylose is covalently linked to protein via serine. Synthesis proceeds by the stepwise addition of UDP sugars by glycosyl transferases.

Chondroitin sulphate consists of about 40 disaccharide units, hyaluronic acid of several thousands. The precise process whereby polymerization is terminated is not as yet understood. As in the case of the sphingolipids sulphation is brought about by active sulphate (3'-phospho-adenosine-5'-phosphosulphate). Generally, several glycosaminoglycan chains are attached to the

Table 12.2   Nomenclature of Mucopolysaccharides

Former name	New Name
Acid mucopolysaccharide	Acidic glycosaminoglycan
Chondroitin sulphate A	Chondroitin-4-sulphate
Chondroitin sulphate B	Dermatan sulphate
Chondroitin sulphate C	Chondroitin-6-sulphate
Heparitin sulphate	Heparan sulphate
Corneal keratosulphate	Keratan sulphate I
Skeletal keratosulphate	Keratan sulphate II
Chondromucoprotein	Proteoglycan or protein-polysaccharide.

protein molecule which forms the core of the glycosaminoglycan-protein complex called *proteoglycan*. The protein core may bear more than one type of pendant polysaccharide. The principal glycosidic and sulphate linkages in glycosaminoglycans implicated in the mucopolysaccharidoses are shown in Table 12.3. It will be noted that keratan sulphate, although classed as a mucopolysaccharide, does not contain hexuronic acid. The structure of chondroitin-4-sulphate and chondroitin-6-sulphate differs only in the position of the sulphate group. In dermatan sulphate iduronic acid is the principal uronic acid but some glucuronic acid is also present; heparan sulphate contains more glucuronic than iduronic acid. Fuller accounts of the biochemistry of the mucopolysaccharides are by McKusick (1972) and Dorfman and Matalon (1972).

Degradation

It has been known for a long time that patients with mucopolysaccharidoses accumulate in their tissues and excrete in the urine an excess of glycosaminoglycans but the biochemical basis of the disorders defied numerous investigators. Only when it was discovered that the genetic defect could be demonstrated in cultured cells from patients did progress become more rapid. Skin fibroblasts synthesize, secrete, re-ingest, accumulate and degrade acid glycosaminoglycans. From experiments in which fibroblasts were cultured in

media containing labelled sulphate it could be concluded that secretion, initial accumulation and biosynthesis were not significantly different in cells from patients with mucopolysaccharidoses and in controls. On the other hand, whereas in normal fibroblasts the incorporation of labelled material reaches a maximum in one to two days and then levels off, in cells from patients the initial rate is maintained linearly for up to a week. Furthermore, normal fibroblasts can ingest labelled proteoglycans by pinocytosis; these are taken up by lysosomes and eventually degraded. While the rate of uptake is similar for control and patients' fibroblasts, degradation of ingested material is defective in patients' cells (see also p. 562).

A remarkable discovery was then made about cells from a different genotype. The culture medium in which such cells had been grown, or even extracts of concentrates of urine, could correct the storage abnormality of Hurler or Hunter fibroblasts—a form of 'replacement therapy' for fibroblasts (Neufeld and Cantz 1971). The substance responsible for this

DERMATAN SULPHATE

HEPARAN SULPHATE

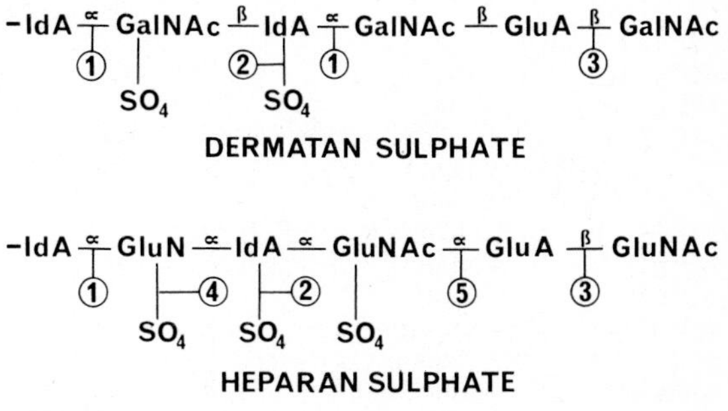

Fig. 12.23 Summary of the enzymic defects of the mucopolysaccharidoses: IdA—iduronic acid; GalNAC—N-acetylgalactosamine; GluA—glucuronic acid; GluN—glucosamine; GluNAC—N-acetylglucosamine; SO$_4$—sulphate. Defects of degradation in position 1—Hurler's and Scheie's diseases; in 2—Hunter's disease; in 3—glucuronidase deficiency; in 4—Sanfilippo A disease; in 5—Sanfilippo B disease.

phenomenon was called '*corrective factor*'. Using cross-correction experiments it was then established that Hurler cells could correct Hunter cells but not Scheie cells, suggesting that the Hurler and Scheie syndromes lacked the same factor. By the same technique, fibroblasts from two clinically indistinguishable cases of the Sanfilippo syndrome did show cross-correction, proving the genetic heterogeneity of the disorder. A distinct corrective factor was also demonstrated

Table 12.3 *Glycoside and sulphate linkages of acidic glycosaminoglycans.*
(Adapted from Dorfman and Matalon, 1972 and Benson, 1974)

	Glycosidic	Sulphate	Linkage to protein
Chondroitin 4- and 6-sulphate	β-N-acetylgalactosamine β-glucuronic acid	Galactosamine-O-SO₄	Gal–Gal–Xyl–Ser
Dermatan sulphate	β-N-acetylgalactosamine α-iduronic acid β-glucuronic acid	Galactosamine-O-SO₄ Iduronic acid-O-SO₄	Gal–Gal–Xyl–Ser
Heparan sulphate	α-N-acetylglucosamine β-glucuronic acid α-iduronic acid	Glucosamine-O-SO₄ Iduronic acid-O-SO₄ Glucosamine-N-SO₄	Gal–Gal–Xyl–Ser
Keratan sulphate I (corneal)	β-N-acetylglucosamine β-galactose	Galactosamine-O-SO₄ Galactose-O-SO₄.	GluNAc–AspNH₂
Keratan Sulphate II (skeletal)	β-N-acetylglucosamine β-galactose	Glucosamine-O-SO₄ Galactose-O-SO₄	GalNAc–Ser GalNAc–Thr

Gal—galactose; Glu—glucose; Xyl—xylose; GalNAc—N-acetylgalactosamine; GluNAc—N-acetylglucosamine; SO₄—sulphate; Ser—serine; AspNH₂—asparagine; Thr—threonine.

Table 12.4 *The mucopolysaccharidoses*

	Syndrome	Genetics	Mental retardation	Excess urinary MPS	Enzyme affected
MPS I H	Hurler	Recessive	+ + +	DS and HS	α-L-iduronidase
MPS I S	Scheie	Recessive	+ −	DS and HS	α-L-iduronidase
MPS II A	Hunter A	Sex-linked	+ + +	DS and HS	Sulphoiduronate sulphatase
MPS II B	Hunter B	Sex-linked	+	DS and HS	Sulphoiduronate sulphatase
MPS III A	Șanfilippo A	Recessive	+ + +	HS	Heparan N-sulphatase
MPS III B	Sanfilippo B	Recessive	+ + +	HS	α-acetylglucosaminidase
MPS IV	Morquio	Recessive	+ −	KS	?
MPS V	Vacant				
MPS VI A	Maroteaux–Lamy classical	Recessive	+ −	DS	Arylsulphatase B
MPS VI B	Maroteaux–Lamy mild	Recessive	−	DS	Arylsulphatase B
MPS VII	β-Glucuronidase deficiency	Recessive	+ + +	Excess MPS ?	β-glucuronidase

MPS—mucopolysaccharide; DS—dermatan sulphate; HS—heparan sulphate; KS—keratan sulphate.

for the Maroteaux–Lamy syndrome. The corrective factors when purified were found to be proteins by their molecular weight, lability to heat and alkaline pH. It was then postulated that the corrective factors are lysosomal hydrolases and this was confirmed when suitable substrates for the assay of these enzymes became available. In the mucopolysaccharidoses lysosomal proteases seem not to be deficient. An excellent review of this field is by Neufeld and Cantz (1973).

The sites of genetically determined defects of glycosaminoglycan degradation are shown in Fig. 12.23 and Tables 12.3 and 12.4. Iduronic acid residues occur both in dermatan sulphate and heparan sulphate and this explains the accumulation of both of the mucopolysaccharides in the Hurler and Scheie syndromes. Similarly, sulphoiduronate linkages occur both in dermatan sulphate and, to a lesser extent, in heparan sulphate. The deficiency in sulphoiduronate sulphatase explains the accumulation of both these glycosaminoglycans in Hunter's syndrome. The Hurler and Scheie syndromes appear to be mutations at the same genetic locus, the latter giving rise to much less severe clinical manifestation. By analogy with the haemoglobinopathies C and S, McKusick *et al.* (1972) have postulated genetic compounds of intermediate severity and the existence of such a genotype has been confirmed (Danes 1974).

Hurler's disease

Hurler's disease may be taken as a paradigm of the mucopolysaccharidoses because it is possibly the commonest, was one of the first to be described and is associated with all the clinical and pathological features of the group, i.e. the typical facies (gargoylism), profound skeletal deformities—dysostosis multiplex, cerebral sphingolipidosis engendering severe mental retardation, and urinary excretion of glycosaminoglycans. The condition is due to lack of α-L-iduronidase, and excess of dermatan sulphate and of heparan sulphate is found in the urine. According to Dekaban and Constantopoulos (1973), the glycosaminoglycan level of the cerebrospinal fluid is considerably raised in the Hurler, Hunter and Sanfilippo syndromes but not in the Scheie syndrome. The main clinical signs are mental retardation, dwarfism, dorsal kyphosis with tendency to gibbus formation, short neck, a large dolichocephalic head (Fig. 12.24), coarse hair, thick low-set ears, hirsutism, lumbar kyphosis, a tendency towards flexion contractures with limitation of joint movements, claw-like hands, hepatosplenomegaly, cardiac defects, inguinal and umbilical herniae,

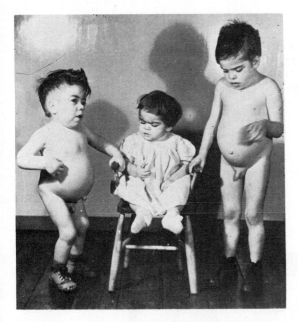

Fig. 12.24 Three unrelated patients with Hurler's disease showing the characteristic facies and abdominal distension.

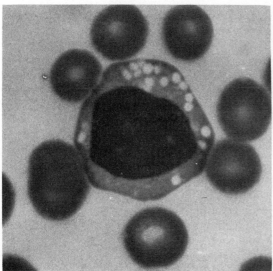

12.25   12.26

Fig. 12.25 A lymphocyte of a case of Hurler's syndrome with cytoplasmic vacuolation. May–Grunewald–Giemsa. (By courtesy of Dr Ursula Mittwoch.)
Fig. 12.26 Metachromatic inclusions in a case of Hurler's syndrome. May–Grunewald–Giemsa.

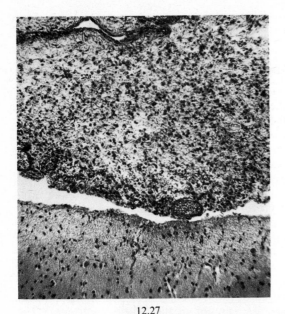

12.27

Fig. 12.27 Thickened leptomeninges in Hurler's syndrome, showing excess of fibroblasts, 'clear' cells and collagen.

Fig. 12.28 The occipital lobe in a case of Hurler's syndrome. Many small pits are present in the white matter. These are caused by tissue rarefaction around blood vessels.

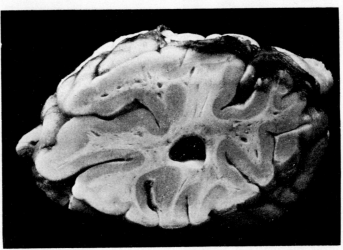

12.28

corneal opacity and frequent deafness. It is inherited as a Mendelian recessive trait. Its incidence may be of the order of 1 in 100,000. The characteristic facial and skeletal features are not usually recognizable in the first year. A Hurler-like appearance in an infant under 6 months suggests G_{M1} gangliosidosis or I-cell disease rather than Hurler's syndrome (Spranger 1973). Basophil metachromatic inclusions may be present in polymorph leucocytes—Alder or Reilly bodies—and the cytoplasm of lymphocytes is vacuolated, the vacuoles containing demonstrable metachromatic material (Figs. 12.25 and 12.26). Similar metachromatic inclusions are usually found in histiocytes of the bone marrow —Buhot cells (see also p. 560 *et seq.*).

The brain is usually reduced in size but not as much as in some of the other sphingolipidoses. The leptomeninges are often opaque and may in some cases be greatly thickened (Fig. 12.27). It is uncertain whether the thickening of the skull (see below) may damage the brain or pituitary by compression. Some authors have held that the thickening of the meninges with resulting impermeability may cause hydrocephalus, but in our experience and contrary to many published statements this is rare in this disease. On the other hand, moderate compensatory ventricular dilatation secondary to atrophy of the surrounding brain is quite common. On the cut surface the cerebral cortex seems normal, the white matter is somewhat firm and may often show characteristic pits or larger lacunae around blood vessels (Fig. 12.28). Such cavitation may be gross, as in the case reported by Norman, Urich and France (1959).

Although storage of adventitious material is demonstrable in most neurons the course of the cellular material is faintly sudanophil, strongly PAS and alcian blue positive and often metachromatic, i.e. staining red with cresyl violet or thionin in an acid solution. The perivascular pitting corresponds histologically to marked rarefaction and reticulation, the lacunae being traversed by a few stout collagenous trabeculae and finer remnants of the glial framework. Enclosed in the meshes of the trabeculae are occasional lipid-containing macrophages, the spaces being otherwise empty (Fig. 12.30). Although frequent in Hurler's disease, this change

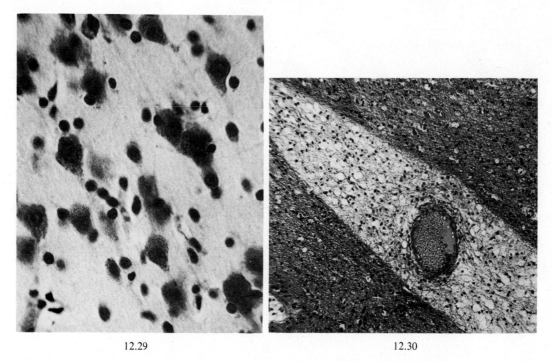

12.29   12.30

Fig. 12.29 Cortical neurons in Hurler's syndrome are distended and contain granular material in their cytoplasm. Cresyl violet.   × 400.)

Fig. 12.30 Perivascular rarefaction in the white matter of a case of Hurler's syndrome.

disease is slower than in the other lipidoses and hence many neurons survive to the end even in the more protracted cases. Correspondingly, there is less replacement gliosis and less demyelination although some will indeed be in evidence at all levels of the CNS. As in the other lipidoses, the larger cells show the storage more conspicuously. They display ballooning of cytoplasm (Fig. 12.29), displacement of the nucleus into the axis hillock and of neurofibrils towards the cell margin together with powdering or disappearance of the Nissl substance. The intra-

is not really specific and may be encountered in other unrelated conditions.

As stated, storage is generalized and the subcortical formations are as affected as the cerebral cortex. As in other lipidoses the dendrites of Purkinje cells may exhibit round or oval swellings (Fig. 12.31) containing the adventitious material, but the cerebellum shows relatively little atrophy. Some fibrous gliosis may be demonstrated in the white matter of the cerebrum and elsewhere. The walls of many small arteries at all levels of the CNS are thickened.

The ultrastructure of the adventitious material has been studied repeatedly (Aleu, Terry and Zellweger 1965; Loeb *et al.* 1968; van Hoof 1973). Rather pleomorphic, transversely striated 'zebra bodies' have been observed and these are believed to be analogous to the membranous cytoplasmic bodies of Tay–Sachs disease (Fig. 12.32). Neuronal cytoplasm also contains granular zones, small concentric membranous bodies and vacuoles, while larger vacuoles are present in the cytoplasm of perithelial cells. Some astrocytes show lamellar inclusions resembling the neuronal ones.

The conspicuous somatic changes in Hurler's disease are due not to sphingolipid but to glucosaminoglycan storage. Thus, for example, Constantopoulos, Louie and Dekaban (1973) found

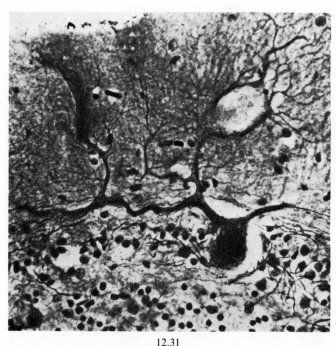

12.31

Fig. 12.31 An oval lipid-containing swelling of a Purkinje cell dendrite in the molecular layer of the cerebellum. Bielschowsky silver impregnation. × 475.

Fig. 12.32 Hurler's disease. Intracytoplasmic inclusions (zebra bodies) in the neurons of Hurler's disease. They consist of alternate electron-dense and lucent compact lamellae which are loosely packed in some areas.   × 50,000. (By courtesy of Dr Suzuki.)

Fig. 12.33 Adventitious 'clear' cells in the corneal Bowman's capsule in a case of Hurler's syndrome. Haematoxylin and eosin. × 550.

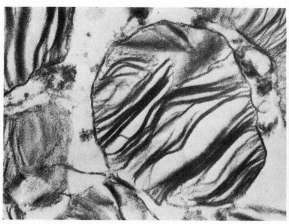

12.32

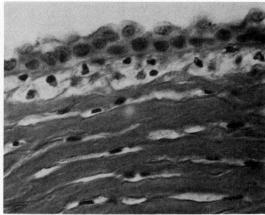

12.33

that the kidney of affected individuals contained 10 times the amount of mucopolysaccharide compared with normal controls, a 15- to 50-fold increase in dermatan sulphate and a 3- to 5-fold increase in heparan sulphate. In addition, there was a marked shift towards smaller molecules in the molecular weight distribution.

At necropsy the pathologist will observe the characteristic external appearances described above and will then be impressed, on removing the calvarium, by the thickness of the bones and the peculiar clay-like greasy material in the bones of the skull which will tend to clog his saw. Many other bones, such as the vertebrae and metacarpals, are misshapen. The characteristic bony changes are perhaps best seen in the skull bones and vertebrae. These show widespread osteoid tissue and new coarse woven bone formation and the presence of mosaic and arrest lines in bony trabeculae. The epiphyses and epiphyseal cartilage plates of long bones show defective cartilage proliferation and bone formation. The marrow may contain granular histiocytes—so-called Buhot cells. A tell-tale feature is the occurrence, in the fibrous tissue surrounding bony trabeculae and bone marrow, as in connective tissues elsewhere, of so-called 'clear cells', that is histiocyte or fibroblast-like cells with vacuolated 'clear' cytoplasm in which metachromatic glycosaminoglycan granules may be demonstrated if precautions are taken not to dissolve them out in aqueous fixatives (Lagunoff, Ross and Benditt 1962). Similar granules are present in the vacuoles of some leucocytes, particularly lymphocytes (p. 521). The liver and spleen are considerably enlarged. Both liver and Kupffer cells are enlarged and their cytoplasm is vacuolated, but this is not a very specific finding. Needle biopsies of the liver have been studied by Callahan, Hackett and Lorincz (1967), who found osmium fixation followed by plastic embedding of their material to be particularly useful in displaying the cell vacuoles. It should be mentioned that liver histology by light microscopy is scarcely distinctive enough to confirm the diagnosis in doubtful cases but it may exclude other conditions. The ultrastructure of liver cells has also been studied by a number of other authors (van Hoof and Hers 1964; Callahan and Lorincz 1966; Loeb *et al.* 1968). Numerous membrane-bound cytoplasmic vacuoles, some containing granular precipitate, are frequently found and similar vacuoles are seen in other tissues. The lamellar structures which are occasionally present are probably gangliosides. Smaller and less common vacuoles present a lipid-like appearance. The enlarged spleen also contains 'clear' cells which in frozen tissue are PAS-positive and metachromatic with toluidine blue. Storage of the adventitious material, wherever it may occur in connective tissues, seems to provoke fibrosis and this is particularly evident in fasciae, endocardium, the walls of blood vessels and the meninges. Fibrosis is conspicuous in the endocardium where it results in thickening and shortening of the chordae tendineae and the margins of the heart valves leading to incompetence. The coronaries are likewise thickened and their lumina constricted. The heart is usually enlarged. Heart failure is a common result of these changes (see also Henderson, MacGregor, Thannhauser and Holden 1952; Berenson and Greer 1963; Lorincz 1965; Krovetz, Lorincz and Schiebler 1965; Okada, Rosenthal, Scaravelli and Lev 1967).

The corneal opacity is caused by 'clear cells' arranged in one or more layers, appearing first in Bowman's capsule (Fig. 12.33) which may be displaced by these cells and then in other parts of the cornea. In stained sections these cells have small dark nuclei and barely visible colourless granules in their cytoplasm.

Other mucopolysaccharidoses

Hunter's syndrome is the only disorder in this series inherited as a Mendelian sex-linked trait. Clinical and pathological changes are much as in the Hurler's syndrome but neuronal storage and mental deterioration may not set in in the milder form of this disease. Many of the patients are deaf but clouding of the cornea is said not to occur. In a case of this disorder studied by Goldberg and Duke (1967) abnormal glycosaminoglycans were in fact present in the corneal epithelium, sclera, iris and ciliary body. The retina showed pigment atrophy. The adventitious material in Hunter's syndrome, as in the Hurler's syndrome, contains dermatan and heparan sulphates. The missing enzyme is sulphoiduronate sulphatase. The condition may be somewhat more common than the Hurler syndrome according to McKusick (1972).

The *Sanfilippo syndrome* occurs in two forms: A—due to deficiency of heparan N-sulphatase

(Kresse and Neufeld 1972) and B—due to deficiency of α-N-acetyl glucosaminidase (O'Brien 1972b). The disorder is characterized by relatively mild somatic and skeletal changes in the presence of severe mental retardation which sets in, as reported by Rampini (1969), after initial apparently normal development. McKusick (1972) believes the syndrome to be less common than the Hurler or Hunter syndromes but this may not be so everywhere.

In the *Scheie syndrome* (Scheie, Hambrick and Barness 1962) the adventitious substances are dermatan and heparan sulphates and the missing enzyme is α-L-iduronidase. Mental retardation may be slight or absent and in other respects the condition resembles a mild Hurler's syndrome but with severe corneal opacity. Aortic regurgitation and retinitis pigmentosa have been reported in some cases. Joint contractures and corneal clouding may appear between 3 and 6 years of age. Its incidence in British Columbia has been estimated at 1 in 500,000 births (Lowry and Renwick 1971).

The *Maroteaux–Lamy syndrome* (polydystrophic dwarfism) also resembles Hurler's disease but for its slower course and milder or entirely absent mental retardation. The stored substance is dermatan sulphate. Arylsulphatase B deficiency has been reported in tissues of these patients by Stumpf, Austin, Crocker and La France (1973), a finding not yet confirmed by other workers. This condition has been fully reviewed by Spranger, Koch, McKusick, Natzschka, Wiedemann and Zellweger (1970).

The stored substance in the *Morquio syndrome* is keratan sulphate but the missing enzyme has not been identified. It is indeed likely that this syndrome is not homogeneous and comprises several genetic and clinical disorders (Danes and Grossman 1969; McKusick 1969; Norman and Pischnotte 1972). Its incidence may be of the order of 1 in 40,000 births (McKusick 1972). Its clinical features include retardation of growth, generalized spondyloepiphyseal dysplasia, kyphosis, pigeon chest, and in some cases corneal opacities and aortic regurgitation. The liver may be enlarged. A dangerous but preventable complication is atlanto-occipital dislocation with spinal cord compression. Spinal cord compression may likewise develop in the lower spine at the site of the gibbus. It should be noted that the patient's appearance is usually normal at birth in contrast to other congenital skeletal dysplasias with which the condition may be otherwise confused. Intelligence is as a rule normal. The excessive urinary excretion of keratan sulphate may cease in some patients as they grow older. The only detailed neuropathological report of a case is by Gilles and Deuel (1971). The brain showed mild ventricular dilatation with shrinkage of the thalami. Some neuronal loss was present in the cerebral cortex and was very marked in the thalami. Sudanophil material was present in the neurons of certain areas, such as the thalami and parts of the hippocampus. On electron-microscopy inclusions somewhat similar to those in Hurler's disease were seen. These far-reaching changes are difficult to reconcile with the prevailing view of intelligence remaining normal in the Morquio syndrome but the authors cite instances of retarded mental development in some previously reported cases. Furthermore, numerous 'transitional' cases with features of both Hurler's and Morquio's syndromes have been described, and these are mentally retarded. Their condition has been referred to as *Morquio–Ulrich's disease* (Dyggve, Melchior and Clausen 1962; Kaufman, Rimoin and McAlister 1971).

β-Glucuronidase deficiency is, at the time of writing, the latest mucopolysaccharidosis to be discovered (Sly, Quinton, McAlister and Rimoin 1973; Spranger 1973). Only two cases have been described. The patients suffered from retardation of growth, hepatosplenomegaly and hip dysplasia. Both cases showed protrusion of the sternum. There was slight excess of glycosaminoglycans in the urine. Granular inclusions were present in circulating polymorphs. Virtual absence of lysosomal β-D-glucuronidase was demonstrated in leucocytes and cultures of skin fibroblasts. The parents of one patient also showed a certain deficiency of the enzyme. Skin fibroblast cultures of this case were studied by Hall, Cantz and Neufeld (1973), who reported excessive accumulation and lengthened turnover time of the sulphated glycosaminoglycans in these cells. The pathological changes of this condition are not yet known.

Atypical mucopolysaccharidoses

Many reports have appeared of cases of mucopolysaccharidosis that do not fit into any of the above categories. Spranger (1973), for example, mentions some resembling both the Hurler and the Scheie syndromes which may have been caused by a Hurler mutation on one gene and an allelic Scheie mutation on another—the *Hurler–Scheie compound*. In the case reported by Winchester, Grossman, Lim and Danes (1969) coarsened facial features suggestive of Hurler's disease and peripheral corneal opacities were associated with progressive deformities of joints resembling rheumatoid arthritis. Gross mental retardation was absent and there was no excess of mucopolysaccharides in the urine. Further cases of the *Winchester syndrome* have been reported by Hollister, Rimoin, Lachman, Cohen, Reed and Westin (1974), who found no evidence of lysosomal storage in their patients. Other patients presented Hurler syndrome-like features in association with extrapyramidal signs, and in another group of patients Hurler syndrome-like features were associated with excessive urinary excretion of chondroitin sulphate. Two siblings described by Horton and Schimke (1970) showed multiple soft tissue contractures with fine corneal opacities, and excreted mucopolysaccharides, mainly heparan and dermatan sulphates, in the urine. Their intelligence remained unaffected. These particular cases have been regarded as examples of the Hurler–Scheie compound. Chondroitin 4-sulphaturia and chondroitin 6-sulphaturia have

also been described. For a recent review see van Hoof (1974).

Under the name of *geleophisic dwarfism* ('focal' mucopolysaccharidosis) Spranger, Gilbert, Tuffli, Rossiter and Opitz (1971) described cases of small stature, bone dysplasia, some mental retardation and, as far as could be ascertained, focal rather than generalized deposition of mucopolysaccharides (mainly dermatan sulphate). Spranger *et al.* (1971) believe that the variant described by Esterly and McKusick (1971) under the name of *stiff skin syndrome* belongs to the same group. No mucopolysaccharides were excreted in the urine of these cases. Three siblings studied by Altay and Say (1973) excreted dermatan and heparan sulphate in the urine but were not mentally retarded. They were dwarfed and suffered from bone dysplasia affecting the vertebrae and bones at the hip joints. There was corneal clouding but no characteristic facies of Hurler's syndrome. There is no doubt that further deviant cases and syndromes within the group will be defined more accurately in the future but not enough is known of their pathology to warrant further discussion here. For further references see Groover, Burke, Gordon and Berdon (1972) and Spranger (1973).

The mucolipidoses

The mucolipidoses are a group of disorders characterized by an association of mucopolysaccharidosis with neuronal and visceral storage of sphingolipids and/or glycolipids (Spranger and Wiedemann 1970). In all but one of these conditions (infantile sulphatidosis, Austin type) there is no urinary excretion of mucopolysaccharides. As far as is known, all are transmitted as Mendelian recessive traits. For a review of these disorders see van Hoof (1974).

G$_{M1}$ gangliosidosis

G$_{M1}$ *gangliosidosis Type I* was the first of the mucolipidoses to be described and may perhaps be taken as a paradigm for the group. The original report was by Landing, Silverman, Craig, Jacoby, Lahey and Chadwick (1964) and the condition is often referred to as Landing's disease, generalized gangliosidosis, pseudo-Hurler's disease

or, incorrectly, as Tay–Sachs disease with visceral involvement—the latter term should be reserved for the variant of Tay–Sachs disease with visceral storage of globoside and deficiency of hexosaminidases A and B (see p. 512). As the name implies, the adventitious substance contains an excess of G$_{M1}$ ganglioside in neural tissue. There is also a lesser increase of its asialo derivatives and of lactosylceramide and glucocerebroside. In the somatic tissues the stored material contains galactose-rich polysaccharides. Glycoproteins are also increased. The basic enzymic deficiency in the disease is of ganglioside β-galactosidases. Such deficiency has been demonstrated in the brain, liver, cultured fibroblasts and leucocytes. The latter can therefore be used in the diagnosis of the condition (Singer, Nankervis and Schafer 1972) (see also p. 560 *et seq.*).

The patients show changes of Hurler's disease which set in, however, at an earlier age than in that condition. Signs include rapid mental deterioration, dysostosis multiplex, paralysis, blindness and epilepsy with hepatosplenomegaly and alveolar ridge hypertrophy. About half of the reported cases have shown cherry-red retinal spots. Few children survive beyond the second year. Foam cells, resembling those of Niemann–Pick's disease are present in some tissues, and vacuolated lymphocytes may be found in the peripheral blood. The eyes show storage of glycosaminoglycans in the cornea and of gangliosides in the nerve cells of the retina (Emery, Green, Wyllie and Howell 1971).

To the naked eye the brain shows little change while other organs resemble those of early Hurler's disease, splenohepatomegaly being particularly conspicuous. Histologically, neuronal

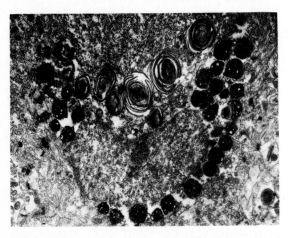

Fig. 12.34 G_{M1} gangliosidosis. Neuronal and glial inclusions in the cerebral cortex. Neuronal inclusions are identical with membranous cytoplasmic bodies (MCBs) of infantile G_{M2} gangliosidosis (Tay–Sachs disease). × 3750. (By courtesy of Dr K. Suzuki and the Editor of *Journal of Neuropathology and Experimental Neurology*.)

lipidosis is accompanied by secondary gliosis and myelin loss, again as in Hurler's disease. Among reported visceral changes are vacuolation of liver cells and the presence in all organs of foam cells containing sudanophil, PAS and Alcian blue positive metachromatic granules. Cells in the proximal tubules and glomeruli of the kidney are distended and vacuolated. Keratan sulphate-like material is stored in the liver and spleen.

On electron-microscopy, affected nerve cells contain MCB-like lamellar bodies measuring 0·3 to 3 μm in diameter (Fig. 12.34). Small glial cells contain different membrane-bound inclusions

consisting of myelin-like figures and straight or curved lamellae. Pleomorphic abnormal inclusions are present in larger astrocytes (Suzuki, Suzuki and Chen, 1968). Histiocytes in the liver and spleen are filled with interwoven bundles of fine tubular structures about 200 Å in diameter. The vacuoles within liver cells, which are such a prominent feature on light microscopy, are surrounded by a single membrane and contain amorphous material.

G_{M1} *gangliosidosis type II*, also known as *Derry's disease*, has its clinical onset later than type I. Patients show mental and neurological regression with spasticity and epilepsy beginning at 6 to 18 months and they die between the ages of 3 and 10 years. They display no external signs of Hurler's disease, visceromegaly or cherry-red spots of the retina. Ocular changes in this condition have been described by Emery *et al.* (1971). Foam cells are present in the bone marrow. Definite though mild skeletal abnormalities have been observed. Abnormal neuronal storage of G_{M1} ganglioside occurs as in type I but it accumulates very little or not at all in the somatic tissues. In contrast to type I, only two of the β-galactosidase isoenzymes, B and C, are said to be inactive, isoenzyme A being normal (O'Brien *et al.* 1971), but this is not the complete enzymological explanation (cf. Suzuki and Suzuki 1973, 1974*a*; Chou, Kaye and Nadler 1974).

The brain is atrophic. The tissues, apart from the already mentioned slight skeletal changes, are normal. Histological changes in neural tissues are as in type I. There is neurolipidosis with secondary gliosis and myelin loss. In spite of the apparent macroscopic normality, foam cells are present in many tissues (including the colonic mucosa). On electron-microscopy findings are essentially as in type I (Fig. 12.34). Both types of G_{M1} gangliosidosis are reviewed by O'Brien (1972*a*).

Fucosidosis

Very few cases of fucosidosis have so far been reported, but at least one presented a clinical and radiological picture somewhat akin to Hurler's disease. The stored mucopolysaccharides and glycolipids in the liver and brain contain an excess of fucose. No abnormality of brain gangliosides has come to light. The condition appears to be due to lack of α-fucosidase. Urinary mucopolysaccharides are normal but the chloride and sodium of the saliva and sweat may be elevated. Histological examination shows that liver and Kupffer cells are distended by a sudanophil substance and PAS-positive material may be found in many tissues. Neurons are distended by material which, on electron-microscopy, shows round structures with reticular and lamellar formations. For further information readers are referred to the original reports (Durand, Borrone and Della Cella 1969; Loeb, Tondeur, Jonniaux, Mockel-Pohl and Vamos-Hurwitz 1969; Dawson and Spranger 1971). An instance of this condition in a juvenile has been reported by Patel, Watanabe and Zeman (1972). In addition to severe mental retardation, hypotonia, kyphoscoliosis and pigeon chest, this patient showed angiokeratoma corporis diffusum and anhydrosis.

Mannosidosis

At the time of writing we know of only six certain and two possible cases of mannosidosis (Autio, Nordén, Öckerman, Riekkinen, Rapola and Louhimo 1973). The patients have only vague signs of Hurler's disease. They are mentally retarded, have impaired speech and coarse facial features. They are prone to intercurrent infection; some have had lens opacities, a degree of deafness, Hurler-like vertebrae and umbilical herniae. The skull is thickened. The main laboratory findings are vacuolation of a large proportion of lymphocytes (30% in one case) and coarse granulation of polymorphs. The urine contains an excess of a mannose-rich fraction. The diagnosis should be based on actual isolation of mannose-rich carbohydrates rather than on the total mannose content of the urine (Tsay, Dawson and Matalon 1974). Biopsy of the liver has shown cellular vacuolation as in other mucopolysaccharidoses. On electron-microscopy storage vacuoles bound by a single membrane are seen in liver and Kupffer cells. Nearly all vacuoles contain electron-opaque globules. Tubular structures, electron-dense aggregates, membrane fragments and myelin figures are frequent. α-Mannosidase activity in the liver is low; it is also abnormally low in leucocytes but not in plasma or urine. Many tissues contain an excess of mannose. Post-mortem findings have been reported in one case (Kjellman, Gamstorp, Brun and Palmgren 1969). The brain showed neuronal loss and lipidosis, the cerebellum was grossly atrophic and loss of myelin was widespread,

especially in the centrum semiovale where it was accompanied by extensive gliosis.

Mucosulphatidosis

Cases of mucosulphatidosis combine the clinical and pathological features of metachromatic leucodystrophy (p. 549) with certain signs of Hurler's disease. The condition is also referred to as infantile sulphatidosis, Austin type (cf. Rampini, Isler, Baerlocher, Bischoff, Ulrich and Plüss 1970; Murphy, Wolfe, Balazs and Moser 1971). Mental and neurological progress of the affected infants is slow. Regression sets in with seizures, paralysis and, often, blindness and deafness. The patients die between the ages of 4 and 12 years. They do not look like cases of Hurler's disease, have no corneal opacity and present few if any of the characteristic skeletal anomalies, although mild dysostosis, minor changes in the vertebrae and metacarpals as well as pigeon chest may be present. Abnormal granulation may be seen in the polymorphs, lymphocytes and myeloid cells of the bone marrow. Plasma cells contain vacuoles and inclusions resembling those in Buhot cells. Urine, unlike that in other mucolipidoses, does contain mucopolysaccharides such as dermatan sulphate and heparan sulphate, but their overall excretion is often only two to four times the normal so that the toluidine blue test may be negative. An excess of sulphatide is also excreted. As in metachromatic leucodystrophy, biopsy of the sural nerve shows myelin degeneration with metachromasia.

The adventitious material stored in the brain, peripheral nerves and kidney is, as in metachromatic leucodystrophy, sulphatide. Other sulphated compounds are also increased in the liver, kidney and plasma but not the brain. The grey matter shows a moderate increase of total gangliosides, particularly G_{M2} and G_{M3}. The enzymic deficiency is not only of arylsulphatase A, as in simple metachromatic leucodystrophy, but also of arylsulphatases B and C. It is hence a *multiple sulphatase deficiency*.

The pathological findings are as in the classical forms of metachromatic leucodystrophy (p. 549). In addition there is a variable amount of neuronal loss, the remaining neurons being ballooned and containing PAS-positive but non-metachromatic material. Liver cells, Kupffer cells and many splenic cells are vacuolated as in Hurler's disease.

Metachromasia may be demonstrated in these cells if care is taken with the histological processing.

Mucolipidosis I

Mucolipidosis I, also known as lipomucopolysaccharidosis, was first described by Spranger, Wiedemann, Tolksdorf, Graucob and Caesar (1968). The patients show some clinical evidence of Hurler syndrome with slow mental and neurological regression. Features of dysostosis multiplex may be detected radiologically. Peripheral lymphocytes are vacuolated and the bone marrow contains characteristic foam cells. Mucopolysaccharides are not excreted in the urine. Biopsy of the sural nerve has shown metachromatic myelin degeneration. Nerve cells in the myenteric plexuses are ballooned. The brain shows neuronal lipidosis (Berard, Toga, Bernard, Dubois, Mariani and Hassoun 1968). The findings in the liver biopsies of six cases, including two of their own, are discussed by Freitag, Blümcke and Spranger (1971). Liver and Kupffer cells are distended and contain vacuoles. An occasional foam cell may be present. The main feature on electron-microscopy is the presence of numerous membrane-bound vacuoles in the sinusoids and in liver cells, Kupffer cells, fibroblast-like cells and endothelial cells. The vacuoles contain myelin-like figures, dense bodies with a homogeneous appearance, small clear vesicles, and occasional tubular and paracrystalline structures.

No enzymic defect has so far been identified in this condition but because of the elevated level of β-galactosidase in the liver, van Hoof and Hers (1968) have referred to it as 'mucopolysaccharidosis gal+'.

Mucolipidosis II

Mucolipidosis II is often referred to as 'I-cell disease' on account of inclusions seen on phase or electron-microscopy in fibroblast tissue culture cells grown from these csaes. The patients suffer from skeletal malformation, gingival hyperplasia, hepatosplenomegaly, herniae, and develop physical and mental retardation associated with an appearance suggestive of Hurler's disease. Dysostosis multiplex is present and lymphocytes may be vacuolated. Rapola, Autio, Aula and Nanto (1974) have visualized by electron-microscopy numerous inclusions in peripheral blood lymphocytes similar to those of the fibroblasts. Cultured fibroblasts store dermatan sulphate, hyaluronic acid, G_{D2} and other lipids. The nature of the substances stored in the tissues has not been established. Although the specific enzyme deficiency also remains obscure, multiple deficiencies in lysosomal hydrolases have been demonstrated in tissues, but the enzymes deficient in tissues are present in excess in the serum. What may be a variant of the disease has been described by Tondeur, Vamos-Hurwitz, Mochel-Pohl, Dereume, Cremer and Loeb (1971). Further information may be obtained in the reports of Leroy, de Mars and Opitz (1969), Leroy, Spranger, Feingold, Opitz and Crocker (1971), Hanai, Leroy and O'Brien (1971), Walbaum, Demaene, Scharfman, Farriaux, Tondeur, Vamos-Hurwitz, Kint and van Hoof (1973) and Dacremont, Kint and Coquyt (1974).

Mucolipidosis III

Mucolipidosis III (pseudopolydystrophy) is an alternative designation for the pseudo-Hurler dystrophy of Maroteaux and Lamy. It was Spranger and Wiedeman (1970) who suggested that this condition was indeed a mucolipidosis, but until storage of sphingolipid is actually demonstrated it may be better to regard it as a mucopolysaccharidosis without mucopolysacchariduria. Indeed, McKusick (1969) considers that mucolipidosis I and II also fall into the same category.

Some workers regard the cerebrosidoses, including Gaucher's disease (p. 513) as variants of the mucolipidoses. There is little doubt, moreover, that further mucolipidoses will soon be identified. Berman, Livni, Shapira, Merin and Levij (1974) have reported on a child with corneal opacities and some mental retardation. The bone marrow contained weakly PAS-positive lipid and macrophages. Electron-microscopy of the liver and conjunctiva revealed many membranous lamellar cytoplasmic structures, single membrane bound vacuoles and fibrogranular material. Histochemical study indicated an excess of lipid and, possibly, of mucopolysaccharides.

Miscellaneous neurolipidoses and glycogenosis

Batten's disease

Batten's disease or *ceroid lipofuscinosis* is one of the lipidoses in which the adventitious material is not a ganglioside and contains, as far as can be ascertained, no excess of other sphingolipids. The condition was previously referred to according to age of onset by a variety of chiefly eponymous names, such as *Bielschowsky's* type, *Bielschowsky–Jansky's*, *Spielmeyer–Vogts*, *Spielmeyer–Sjögren's*, *Batten's disease*, *Batten–Mayou's* or simply as *amaurotic family idiocy*; however, not all the cases so described suffered from the condition to be considered here. According to some workers (Zeman and Siakotos 1973), Kufs' disease (p. 533) is a variant of the same disorder while Dekaban and Herman (1974) have likewise proposed its subdivision into three or four variants on clinical and pathological grounds. An infantile subgroup has been delineated by the clinical and electrophysiological course of the disorder by Santavuori, Haltia, Rapola and Raitta (1973). The patients of this subgroup (Finnish or infantile type) survive for a number of years in a decerebrate state after a progressively rapid deterioration of the EEG, electroretinogram and visual evoked responses (VER). That the condition in these cases is indeed ceroid lipofuscinosis has been confirmed histologically by Haltia, Rapola, Santavuori and Keränen (1973). The electron-microscopical picture is distinct and the brain shows gross atrophy. The tendency in London is to retain the name of Batten's disease for the group and subdivide it into early infantile (Santavuori type), late infantile (Bielschowsky type) and juvenile (Spielmeyer type).

The late infantile and juvenile conditions usually present with progressive dementia, which may be slower than in the other lipidoses, grand mal or myoclonic epilepsy, blindness and increasing motor disability. Inspection of the fundus often discloses retinal atrophy with or without pigmentation. At some stage in the course of the disease younger patients display a characteristic EEG high-voltage discharge in response to a low-rate light flicker (Pampiglione 1968) while the electroretinogram shows gradual disappearance of responses in step with the degeneration of the outer retinal layers. A proportion of lymphocytes in juvenile cases are vacuolated, and hypergranulation of leucocytes has also been considered useful not only in the detection of patients but also of heterozygotes (Donahue, Watanabe and Zeman 1968; Merritt, Smith,

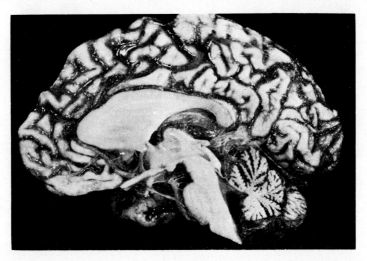

Fig. 12.35 The brain of a 4-year-old child with Batten's disease. It weighed 400 g and shows generalized atrophy with particularly well-marked cerebellar sclerosis.

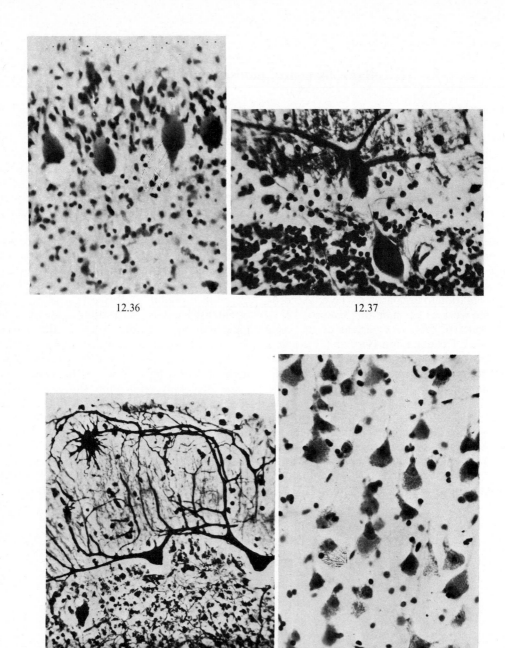

12.36

12.37

12.38

12.39

Figs 12.36-12.39 Batten's disease.

Fig. 12.36 'Centripetal' form of cerebellar degeneration. The Purkinje cells are relatively well preserved while the granular layer has almost entirely vanished.

Fig. 12.37 Axonal 'torpedo' in an axon of a Purkinje cell.

Fig. 12.38 A 'cactus-like' body—a form of dendritic expansion of Purkinje cells (this also occurs in some other forms of cerebellar atrophy. Cajal's silver nitrate pyridine method.

Fig. 12.39 Cortical nerve cells.

Strouth and Zeman 1968; Witzleben, Smith, Nelson, Monteleoni and Livingston 1971).

Transmission in familial cases is Mendelian recessive but it is quite unlikely that the condition is genetically (or chemically) homogeneous. Dominant transmission was observed by Boehme, Cottrell, Leonberg and Zeman (1971) but the patients in this series were of an older age group (p. 534).

Depending on the duration and severity of the disease, the brain shows varying degrees of atrophy and sclerosis (Fig. 12.35) affecting all formations. The ventricles are correspondingly enlarged. The optic nerves are usually thin and gliotic.

On histological examination there is in advanced cases marked neuronal depletion with parallel gliosis and myelin loss. The cerebellum may show selective atrophy of the granular layer (Fig. 12.36) (p. 510). As in other forms of cerebellar degeneration, axons of Purkinje cells may show 'torpedo' bodies (Fig. 12.37) and their dendrites may have 'cactus'-like expansions (Fig. 12.38). The surviving nerve cells are distended by the adventitious material (Fig. 12.39). Prior to staining, this substance is golden brown in colour and autofluorescent. It is insoluble in the usual fat solvents, is strongly sudanophil and PAS-positive. It is stored at all levels of the central nervous system and in the autonomic nerve ganglia. Variable amounts of it are also present in somatic tissues (Kristensson, Rayner and Sourander 1965). Large quantities have been seen, for example, in the thyroid (Dayan and Trickey 1970). The retina shows loss of cells in all layers and, often, an excess of pigment in the deeper layers and in the choroid (Fig. 12.40).

In recent years electron-microscopical study of the stored material and affected cells has been vigorously pursued. Not all cases have shown the same changes but it has emerged that the bulk of the material is held within lysosomes and takes the diverse forms of multi-locular bodies, curvilinear bodies, structures with a 'fingerprint pattern', multilamellar cytosomes, and so on. The inclusions are often mixed. Attempts to establish clinical and nosological categories by the type of ultrastructure have so far proved inconclusive. For further information see Zeman (1971), Towfighi, Baird, Gambetti and Gonatas (1973), Zeman and Siakotos (1973), Dekaban and Herman (1974) and Pellissier, Hassoun, Gambarelli, Tripier, Roger and Toga

(1974). Ebhardt, Cervos-Navarro and Rey Pias (1974), as well as Schwendemann and Colmant (1974) report that characteristic electron-microscopical changes can be observed not only in neurons but also in macrophages and other cells of the rectal mucosa. This is important since, for diagnosis, it is sufficient to obtain a suction biopsy of the rectal mucosa (see p. 559).

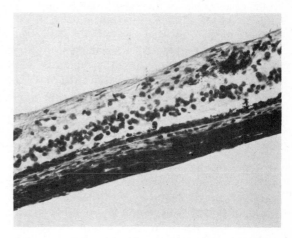

Fig. 12.40 The retina in a case of Batten's disease. Marked cellular loss and some pigmentation are present in all layers.

The stored material is a lipopigment, ceroid, akin to or identical with the lipofuscin which accumulates throughout life in all animal cells. It is rather insoluble, chemically inert, and therefore difficult to analyse. According to Zeman (1974) the pigment contains two fractions differing in physicochemical properties; one (ceroid) is less inert than the other (lipofuscin). He believes that essential steps in the formation of ceroid are peroxidation of polyunsaturated fatty acids followed by cross-linking of reactive breakdown products of fatty acid peroxides to protein. The total amount of lipid in neural tissue is not usually increased. The nature of the enzymatic defect (or defects) remains unknown. Some reduction in the leucocyte peroxidase activity has been demonstrated by Armstrong, Dimmitt, Grider, Van Wormer and Austin (1973), Armstrong, Dimmitt and Van Wormer (1974) and Patel, Koppang, Patel and Zeman (1974).

Kufs' disease

Kufs' disease is a rather vaguely defined non-gangliosidotic neurolipidosis and is regarded by some as the adult form of ceroid-lipofuscinosis (p. 531). Symptoms commence in adolescence or early adult life with insidious dementia, epilepsy that may be myoclonic, cerebellar dysfunction and pareses. Regression is usually slow. A few of the reported cases have been familial and a disorder resembling Kufs' disease described by Boehme *et al.* (1971) affected 11 individuals in four generations of the same family and thus appeared to be dominant in transmission.

Not all the reported cases have shown unequivocal neurolipidosis; the changes in some were marginal. Nor has the lipidosis been ubiquitous; only certain levels and regions were affected. The storage material is ceroid or ceroid-like, as in Batten's disease, but it is by no means certain that it was identical in all the recorded cases (cf. Seitelberger and Nagy 1958). Another reported change has been the presence in some of the distended neurons of a homogeneous colourless structure having in silver preparations the features of Alzheimer's neurofibrillary change (Löken and Cyvin 1954). There may be focal neuronal depletion in the cerebral and cerebellar cortices. The autonomic plexuses also show storage of the adventitious substance according to Roizin, Slade, Hermida and Asao (1962), who described it as a complex lipid consisting of phospholipids with traces of glycolipids and cerebrosides. On electron-microscopy the cytoplasm is seen to contain lysosome-like organelles and osmiophilic bodies, some showing concentric central or peripheral lamination (Kornfeld 1971). Other lamellar structures have been described in necropsy material by Escolá Picó (1964).

In the case reported by Chou and Thompson (1970) neuronal lipid storage was most marked in the diencephalon and mesencephalon. Electron-microscopy showed lipofuscin-laden bodies, 0·5 to 1·2 μm in diameter, and miniature membranous cytoplasmic bodies.

Visceral storage has been reported in this condition. For further details and references to Kufs' disease readers are referred to Fine, Barron and Hirano (1960), De Vries (1968) and Zeman and Siakotos (1973).

Congenital amaurotic family idiocy

This variant of neurolipidosis is usually referred to as the *Norman and Wood type* or *congenital amaurotic family idiocy*. It was first described in three siblings by Norman and Wood (1941)

and then by Brown, Corner and Dodgson (1954). No precise neurochemical or enzymological methods were then available and it is therefore impossible to be certain of the true nature of the adventitious substance. The disorder was present at birth and the oldest infant died at 7 weeks. On pathological examination there was external hydrocephalus, the brains being very small. Surviving nerve cells in the cerebral cortex were ballooned and filled with sudanophil, PAS-positive material (Fig. 12.41). Fibrous gliosis was widespread and sudanophil debris and some

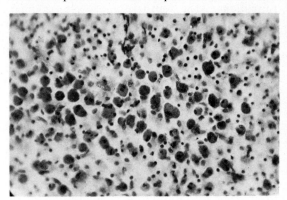

Fig. 12.41   Congenital amaurotic idiocy (Norman and Wood). Distended neurons in the cerebral cortex.

doubly refractile cholesterol esters were found in the centrum semiovale, some of the cholesterol esters encrusting the bodies of astrocytes. The cerebellum was likewise severely involved. Small groups of lipid-containing macrophages were present in the liver, spleen and lymph glands. Chemical analysis in one case showed slight excess of ganglioside in the cortex and of cholesterol in the white matter.

At the time the condition seemed quite distinct from any of the sphingolipidoses but it is now known that the latter may also be congenital and that ganglioside and cells containing adventitious material can be found in somatic tissues in some cases. While the tinctorial qualities of the stored material in the Norman and Wood cases were indeed unlike those usually found in early Tay–Sachs disease only further experience can show whether they constitute a really separate condition.

Atypical neurolipidoses

All neurolipidoses are rare and since modern methods of their identification are new and still somewhat esoteric it is not surprising that many cases do not fit neatly into any of the delineated syndromes. Such cases have been described for example by Kidd (1967), Elfenbein (1968), Elfenbein and Cantor (1969), De Leon, Kaback, Elfenbein, Percy and Brady (1969) and Pellissier, Gambarelli, Hassoun and Toga (1974). The cases described by Kidd (1967) and by Elfenbein (1968) may be instances of the so-called sea-blue histiocyte syndrome (p. 538). A case of possible G_{M3} gangliosidosis has been reported by Pilz, Sandhoff and Jatzkewitz (1966). Another case of G_{M3} lipidosis has been recorded by Max, Maclaren, Brady, Bradley, Rennels, Tanaka, Garcia and Cornblath (1974).

Wolman's disease

Wolman's disease is a storage disorder of the reticuloendothelial system, the adventitious material consisting of triglycerides (chiefly with oleic acid) and cholesterol esters (Lake and Patrick 1970). It is due to a deficiency of acid esterase. The disorder presents in infants with vomiting, diarrhoea and failure to thrive. Hepatosplenomegaly and abdominal enlargement are present from birth and the patients die rather rapidly, often before the age of 6 months. A characteristic radiological feature is punctate calcification of the adrenals. Some lymphocytes are vacuolated and droplets of lipid can be demonstrated in their cytoplasm. Understandably, there is variability in the clinical manifestation (Patrick and Lake 1973). Acid esterase deficiency has also been found in individuals with relatively mild symptoms and lipidosis, so-called *cholesterol ester storage disease* (Burke and Schubert 1971; Sloan and Fredrickson 1972). Wolman's disease appears to be transmitted as a Mendelian recessive trait. Patrick and Lake (1969) suggest that assay of acid *p*-nitrophenyl esterase in peripheral leucocytes may be useful in the detection of heterozygotes.

The main pathological findings are enlargement of the liver and spleen, frequent ascites and calcification of the adrenals. The liver may be yellowish orange in colour. The brain is as a rule normal on naked-eye examination.

Foam cells are present in the liver, spleen and lamina propria of the gut, particularly of the small intestine. These cells contain cholesterol and cholesterol esters as well as free fatty acids and triglycerides. Besides, foam cells the spleen

and lymph glands may contain cholesterol ester crystals. Smooth muscle cells, neurons in the myenteric and other autonomic ganglia and some cells of the serosa and submucosa of the gut contain sudanophil material. The adrenals show necrosis with calcium deposition in the deeper cortical layers. Many of the surviving cells in these layers are distended and contain anisotropic crystals.

The brain is not always abnormal but several authors have observed certain neuropathological changes. Lipid deposition in some neurons of the brainstem and a few Purkinje cells, as well as the leptomeninges and choroid plexuses, was reported by Kahana, Berant and Wolman (1968). Appearances akin to sudanophil leucodystrophy were seen by Guazzi et al. (1968). Perivascular foam cells and retarded myelination were reported by Crocker, Vanter, Neuhauser and Rosowsky (1965) and Marshall et al. (1969).

Electron-microscopy of foam cells shows osmiophilic droplets of neutral fat (Lough, Fawcett and Wiegenberg 1970). Some inclusions present dense peripheral margins around lucent centres, others are adjacent to or situated within lysosomes. Somewhat similar changes have been reported by Lake and Patrick (1970). All lipid depositions show an intact membrane associated with acid phosphatase, indicating a lysosomal origin.

Aspartylglycosaminuria

The first cases of aspartylglycosaminuria were discovered in England. One patient was a woman aged 30 who was severely subnormal and suffered from periodic attacks of mania. Her subnormal and similarly affected brother had short episodes of loss of consciousness but not mania (Pollitt, Jenner and Merskey 1968). Since then most of the cases have been reported from Finland from where the disease has been reviewed by Autio (1972). All patients have shown mental retardation and, allegedly, characteristic facies. About half of them have skin lesions such as large naevi, acne and dermatitis caused by photosensitivity. Lymphocytes show vacuolation. The disease is transmitted as a Mendelian recessive trait.

The patients excrete aspartylglycosamine in the urine. Other compounds present in the urine consist of a combination of aspartylglycosamine, N-acetylneuraminic acid and hexosamine while there are also substances containing uronic acid (Palo and Savolainen 1972). Some of these compounds were found in the brain and liver of a patient. It seems likely that the disorder is caused by lack of aspartylglycosamine amidase. Electron-microscopy showed many enlarged lysosomes in all tissues examined (Arstila, Palo, Haltia, Riekkinen and Autio 1972). Some contained granular electronlucent material. Other, smaller lysosomes contained dense material. In the brain the larger lysosomes were most numerous in neurons but were also present in other cells. In the brain of a case coming to necropsy Haltia and Palo (1974) found large vesicles in the neurons which contained no demonstrable lipid or carbohydrate.

Kinky hair disease

The condition with the strange name of kinky hair disease was first observed by Menkes, Alter, Steigleder, Weakley and Sung (1962) in five males in two generations of the same family. The patients had erect, undulating, colourless white hair, showing pili torti, monilethrix and trichlorrhexis nodosa, and were severely mentally retarded. Pathological examination revealed focal degeneration of the cerebral cortex and basal ganglia, secondary degeneration of the white matter and cerebellar atrophy. A further nine cases were reported by Aquilar, Chadwick, Okuyama and Kamoshita (1966) and the biochemical findings in these by O'Brien and Sampson (1966). The chemical change may involve dokosahexaenoic acid (22 : 6) (see, however, Lou, Holmer, Reske-Nielsen and Vagn-Hansen 1974). It was suggested by Danks, Stevens, Campbell, Gillespie, Walker-Smith, Blomfield and Turner (1972) that intestinal copper absorption may be at fault, and this is endorsed by Bourgeois, Galy, Baltassat and Béthenod (1974). Reske-Nielsen, Lou and Vagn-Hansen (1974) suggest that the genetic defect might be one of intracellular copper transport. The incidence of the disease in Melbourne has been estimated at 1 to 35,000 live births.

The pathology of the condition has been studied by Aquilar et al. (1966), Ghatak, Poon, Hirano and French (1969), French, Sherard, Lubell, Brotz and Moore (1972), Vagn-Hansen, Reske-Nielsen and Lou (1973) and Vuia and Heye (1974). It appears that large arteries inside and outside the skull show tortuosity and degenerative changes such as intimal fibrosis and splitting of the internal elastic lamina, and that some of the degenerative lesions in the brain may be secondary. The brain shows areas of cerebral necrosis. The white matter was reduced in volume and presented some cavitation in one of the cases which also showed degeneration of Clarke's columns and the spinocerebellar tracts (Ghatak et al. 1969). The cerebellum shows some changes in all its layers. Some Purkinje cells present in silver preparations cactus-like dendritic sprouting and proliferation. On electron-microscopy of Purkinje cells in formalin-fixed necropsy material, Vuia and Heye (1974) noted proliferation of mitochondria which contained osmiophilic inclusions. In the case reported by Vagn-Hansen et al. (1973) the most serious degenerative changes were seen in the white matter of the cerebral hemispheres and the authors suggest that the condition is related to the leucodystrophies.

Hand–Schüller–Christian disease

Hand–Schüller–Christian disease occupies a dubious nosological space encroached on three sides by infection, neoplasm and metabolic disorder. It is closely related to or is indeed an instance of fortuitous distribution of lesions in such conditions as histiocytosis X, eosinophil granuloma and Letterer–Siwe disease. For a discussion of the theoretical and practical problems involved in the classification of these disorders readers are referred to one of many reviews, such as that of Vogel and Vogel (1972). Lysosomes may be involved in the pathogenesis of the condition so that it is reasonable to consider it here, albeit briefly, since the nervous system is affected relatively rarely and then only as part of more widely disseminated changes.

The characteristic features are granulomatous lesions, large and small, scarce or numerous, in many tissues, particularly bones. Because of this variability of distribution it is difficult to outline a typical clinical picture; Vogel and Vogel (1972) point out that the triad sometimes regarded as characteristic—exophthalmos, diabetes insipidus and granulomata of the skull bones, will be encountered in only one of ten patients. Mental retardation is not usual in this condition and other neurological or mental symptoms are likewise rare. Some cases, however, show lesions in the brain and other parts of the central nervous system (Chiari 1933; Teilum 1942; Feigin 1956). The typical lesions are granulomata, containing histiocytes, xanthomatous cells, foam cells, lymphocytes, eosinophils and occasional multinucleated giant cells. The part of the brain involved more frequently than the rest is the hypothalamus (Henschen 1931; Cureton 1949). Areas of myelin loss with astrocytosis may surround the granulomatous nodules and also be scattered elsewhere in the central nervous system. The material in the foam cell is sudanophil and some of it is also birefringent. It probably consists mainly of cholesterol esters.

Farber's disease (lipogranulomatosis)

Lipogranulomatosis, first described by Farber (1952) and Farber, Cohen and Uzman (1957), is a disorder in which disseminated granulomatous lesions are associated with neuronal lipidosis. The disease starts in infancy with hoarseness, restriction of joint movements, swelling of joints and an outcrop of subcutaneous nodules, especially near joints. Physical and mental development is retarded. On pathological examination there is diffuse and nodular granulomatous infiltration of the skin and periarticular tissues, most of the cells being lymphocytes, histiocytes and foam cells. Distended neurons give sphingolipid-like staining reactions (Crocker, Cohen and Farber 1967). The only reported electron-microscopical studies were of the liver and subcutaneous nodules (Rampini and Clausen 1967; Hers and van Hoof 1969). The liver cells showed osmiophilic deposits surrounding electron-lucent material in a granular matrix. There were also clear vacuoles as in the mucopolysaccharidoses. The Kupffer cells contained dense bodies with an osmiophilic matrix and some miniscule tubular structures. The latter, somewhat similar to the curvilinear bodies sometimes found in cases of Batten's disease, were much more abundant in the histiocytes of the dermis.

On chemical analysis Clausen and Rampini (1970) found an increase of glucose- and galactosamine-containing glycolipids in the brain and liver although total glycolipids were only slightly raised. Prensky, Ferreira, Carr and Moser (1967) reported on a large increase of ceramide in the liver, lung and kidney. Cera-

midase deficiency has been demonstrated by Sugita, Dulaney and Moser (1972). The condition may yet come to be viewed as one of the mucolipidoses.

Cerebrotendinous xanthomatosis

Cerebrotendinous xanthomatosis is a rare familial disease first described by van Bogaert, Scherer and Epstein (1937). The clinical picture is of some mental retardation, slowly progressing cerebellar dysfunction and myoclonus. It starts in adolescence and terminates with bulbar paralysis in adult life. A few patients have been hypercholesterolaemic, a point of contrast with Hand–Schüller–Christian disease (Giampalmo 1954), but others were not. Among the reported manifestations of the disease are xanthomata of the tendons and lungs with xanthelasma of the eyelids. Although the stored substance looks like cholesterol it was established that it contains cholestanol, a derivative of cholesterol (Menkes 1970). Cholesterol side chain degradation appears to be incomplete (Setoguchi, Salen, Tint and Mosbach 1974).

Xanthomatous deposits containing the crystalline sterol are present in many tissues, e.g. tendons, bones, lungs and the brain. Lesions in the somatic tissues show foam cells, crystalline needle-shaped structures (or clefts in paraffin sections), lymphocytes, histiocytes and some foreign body giant cells. In the brain the concentration of cholestanol is increased and lesions take the form of myelin loss with possible cystic necrosis which is particularly well marked in the centre of the cerebellum and superior cerebellar peduncles. Foam cells and 'sterol' clefts are also present in the demyelinated areas. Numerous lipid-laden macrophages and foreign body giant cells surround blood vessels and the 'sterol' clefts. Other changes include loss of myelin from portions of the lateral and posterior columns of the spinal cord which may also show 'sterol' clefts and foam cells. The brainstem shows loss of myelin from the pyramids, transverse pontine fibres and hila of the inferior olives. The substantia nigra, red nuclei and basal ganglia may likewise be affected.

In a child with progressive psychomotor degeneration who died at the age of 4 years, Jervis (1957) discovered diffuse cortical degeneration akin to Alpers' disease, marked atrophy of the cerebellum and degeneration of the basal ganglia with accumulation of large amounts of lipids consisting mainly of cholesterol.

The sea-blue histiocyte syndrome

This condition derives its name from the presence in the bone marrow, spleen and liver of large histiocytes, 20 to 60 μm in diameter, with an eccentric nucleus and a cytoplasm that contains numerous coarse granules staining sea-blue or bluish-green with the Wright–Giemsa stain. This stored material is a PAS-positive, frequently sudanophil lipid. It is autofluorescent. The syndrome is characterized by hepatosplenomegaly, macular abnormalities of the eyes, pulmonary infiltration and thrombocytopenia. Focal pigmentation of the skin has been noted in some cases. Transmission is probably as a Mendelian recessive trait but no enzyme defect has so far been identified. The concentration of sphingomyelin and other phospholipids in the spleen is increased. The course of the disease in adults has been benign and no necropsy findings have been published. Changes in biopsy material from the liver, spleen and lymph glands have been reported, however, by Silverstein and Ellefson (1972) while the electron-microscopy of the sea-blue histiocyte has been described by Lynn and Terry (1964). Before the recent delineation of the syndrome (Sawitsky, Rosner and Chodsky 1972) similar cases were being described under a variety of headings, such as unidentified reticuloendothelial cell storage disease, adult Niemann–Pick's disease, lipid storage disease and ceroid pigmentophagia.

It should be mentioned that sea-blue histiocytes are also found in other conditions, e.g. in the jejunal mucosa of cases of Wolman's disease and in 'acquired' sea-blue histiocytoses, e.g. in granulocytic leukaemia, and after administration of certain drugs (Yamamoto, Adachi, Kitani, Shinji, Seki, Nasu and Nishikawa 1971).

A quite different form of the disorder has been described by Neville, Lake, Stephen and Sanders (1973). They studied a series of nine children aged between 1 and 8 years. The main signs were ataxia, dementia, fits and rigidity. After the age of 5 years, all developed a vertical supranuclear ophthalmoplegia. Some presented with neonatal jaundice, hepatosplenomegaly and transient failure to thrive. The liver and spleen were only moderately enlarged or, in older patients, entirely impalpable. A previously unknown form of neuronal lipid storage was also present, but the brain sphingomyelin was normal. The spleen contained numerous foam cells with a very high concentration of sphingomyelin and this contrasted with the liver which showed few foam cells and only mildly raised sphingomyelin. Sphingomyelinase activity was normal. Numerous foam cells and occasional sea-blue histiocytes were present in the bone marrow—the latter, probably, an incidental finding. A suitable name for the condition would be *ophthalmoplegic lipidosis* (Lake—personal communication). Because of the striking neurological signs of the disease, changes might be expected in the central nervous system, but none has been reported so far. The disorder may yet prove to be a variant of Niemann-Pick's disease (p. 516).

Generalized glycogenosis

At least seven inborn errors are known at various sites of the glycogen metabolic pathway (Fig. 12.42). Structurally normal or abnormal glycogen accumulates in most of these disorders. The brain is not usually involved. An exception is *glycogenosis type II* or *Pompe's disease*. Hers (1973) uses the term Pompe's disease to designate the infantile variant, dominated by cardiomegaly; he referred to *all* forms, including the infantile, juvenile and adult, as glycogenosis type II. The main clinical features of Pompe's disease are muscular weakness and, as mentioned, cardiac enlargement (Fig. 12.43) with ultimate heart failure causing dyspnoea and cyanosis. Intelligence may remain normal but some cases have been mentally retarded. The usual presenting signs in the late infantile and juvenile cases are difficulty in walking and increasing muscular dystrophy. Myopathy is also the main trouble of adult patients.

The enzymatic defect of the condition is in acid α-glucosidase (acid maltase) activity while that of some other lysosomal enzymes, such as α-galactosidase and N-acetyl β-hexosaminidase is often increased. The accumulated glycogen is chemically normal. Transmission is as a Mendelian recessive trait. Hers and de Barsy (1973) estimate its incidence in the Belgian population at 1 : 150,000 births.

The most conspicuous change at necropsy of the children is the enlarged globular heart, the cut surface of which is pale and somewhat glassy

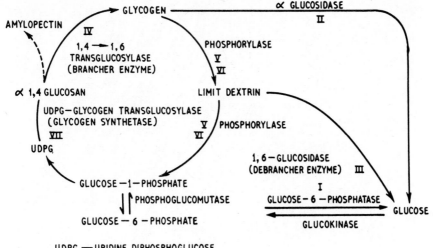

UDPG — URIDINE DIPHOSPHOGLUCOSE

Fig. 12.42 The metabolism of glycogen.

in texture. Glycogen may be demonstrated by pouring iodine over it. The brain is usually normal in appearance. Skeletal muscle, the tongue and the diaphragm may be thickened. The liver may also be slightly enlarged.

The histological hallmark of the disease is the presence of large amounts of intracellular glycogen in all the affected tissues, such as muscle, heart, liver and brain. It is noteworthy, however, that the glycogen content of various muscles can be very uneven. The glycogen gives the usual staining reactions, i.e. it is PAS and Best carmine positive, but much of it is dissolved in the course of fixation and histological processing, leaving the cytoplasm in paraffin-embedded sections

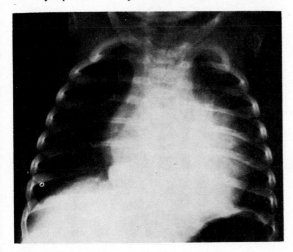

Fig. 12.43 Globular enlargement of the heart in a child with generalized glycogenosis.

vacuolated and largely empty. In advanced cases the cells are converted to little more than miniature empty bags. In haematoxylin and eosin preparations the heart presents a characteristic lace-like pattern, the endocardium being sometimes fibro-elastotic (Fig. 12.44), the liver is plant-like, and the brain is superficially like that of a lipidosis, much glycogen being demonstrable in both neurons and glial cells. Some glycogen is easily lost in histological processing of the brain as of other tissues so that many neurons show uneven vacuolation, some being entirely empty (Figs. 12.45 and 12.46). There may be a variable amount of neuronal loss, some formations being much more affected than others (Martin, Barry, van Hoof and Palladini 1973), and the white matter shows fine fibrous gliosis (Fig. 12.47). On chemical analysis there is in the white matter a marked deficiency in total phospholipids, cholesterol and cerebrosides. The peripheral nervous system is also involved in the storage. Nerve cells in the dorsal root ganglia, myenteric plexuses and the Schwann cells of peripheral nerves show glycogen deposition.

Besides glycogen some muscle cells contain basophilic metachromatic substances staining with mucicarmine, alcian blue and toluidin blue (Schnabel 1971). These are hyaluronidase and diastase resistant. They are possibly mucopolysaccharides and their presence confirms the general rule that lysosomal deposits are not chemically homogeneous (see p. 505). However, they disappear on digestion with amylase (Martin *et al.* 1973).

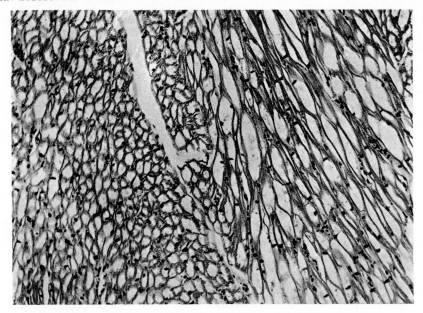

Fig. 12.44 The myocardium in generalized glycogenosis. Haematoxylin and eosin. × 150.

A good deal of work has gone into the electron-microscopy of the glycogenoses, mainly liver and muscle, and the findings are summarized by Hers and de Barsy (1973). Glycogen accumulation has a dual localization. Part of it is freely dispersed throughout the cytoplasm and the rest is contained within vacuoles of varying sizes and shapes. Some of these vacuoles are enveloped by unit membranes. They are probably lyso-somes altered by storage. It was shown by Hug, Garancis, Schubert and Kaplan (1966) that, while much of the dispersed glycogen disappears during starvation and after adrenaline administration, vacuolar glycogen remains unaltered.

Lysosome-derived residual bodies characteristic of type II glycogenosis have been found by Hug, Schubert and Soukup (1972) in uncultured amniotic cells obtained by amniocentesis, the

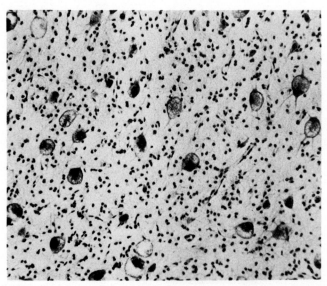

Fig. 12.45 The basal ganglia in a case of generalised glycogenosis. The nerve cells are distended and show irregular vacuolation, some appearing entirely empty. Haematoxylin and eosin. × 120.

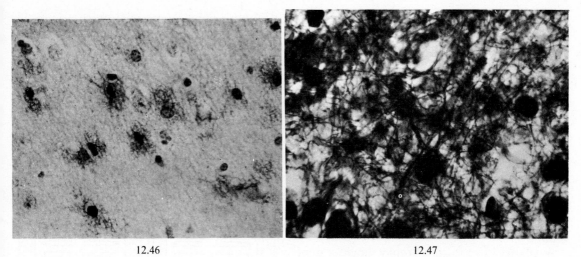

12.46   12.47

Fig. 12.46 Glycogen deposition in astrocytes in a case of generalized glycogenosis. PAS with haematoxylin after treatment with diastase. × 300.
Fig. 12.47 Fine fibrous gliosis and astrocytic hyperplasia in the white matter of a case of generalized glycogenosis. Holzer. × 1000.

diagnosis being later confirmed enzymologically. A rapid diagnostic method of prenatal diagnosis in such cases has thus become possible (see p. 562).

For histological details on the pathology of Pompe's disease readers are referred to the case reports of Crome, Cumings and Duckett (1963), Mancall, Aponte and Berry (1965), Dincsoy, Dincsoy, Kessler, Jackson and Sidbury (1965), Hernandez, Marchesi, Goldring, Kissane and Hartmann (1966), Bordiuk, Legato, Lovelace and Blumenthal (1970) and Martin *et al.* (1973).

It should be mentioned that *incidental* brain damage may occur in other forms of glycogenosis. Hypoglycaemia may, for example, be responsible for such damage in cases of von Gierke's disease. Another disorder in which the brain may be involved is glycogen synthetase deficiency (Lewis, Spencer-Peet and Stewart 1963; Parr, Teree and Larner 1965). In these cases mental retardation is one of the symptoms. The findings in the brain of one of them were thought to be consistent with diffuse non-specific degeneration of the cerebral white matter of a kind usually found after prolonged hypoglycaemia or anoxia. Glycogen was not demonstrated in the liver, muscle, kidney or adrenals of this case.

Occasionally, no enzyme deficiency is demonstrable in glycogen storage disease. Briggs and Haworth (1964) described a case of 'idiopathic glycogen storage disease', otherwise resembling von Gierke's disease, but without glucose-6-phosphatase deficiency. Spencer-Peet, Norman, Lake, McNamara and Patrick (1971) found that 6 of 23 children with hepatic glycogen storage disease had none of the known enzyme defects. Again, in a child studied by Résibois-Grégoire and Dourov (1966), glycogen deposition was confined to the brain. Glycogen was not seen in the lysosomes and the condition was therefore probably not Pompe's disease. The enzymatic defect was not identified.

Leucodystrophies

It seems reasonable to discuss under the single heading of leucodystrophy, an array of disorders at least two of which, globoid cell leucodystrophy and metachromatic leucodystrophy, are at the same time storage diseases with known enzymatic defects. These can thus be classed, as is frequently done, with other sphingolipidoses. All leucodystrophies show certain pathological similarities, i.e. widespread and often symmetrically bilateral degeneration and/or failure of myelin formation of the central nervous system. The arcuate fibres in the affected regions tend to be spared, as initially are the axis cylinders. In older patients the external margins of the demyelinated areas may, however, fall short of the arcuate fibres and the cerebral cortex. Peripheral nerves usually show segmental demyelination (p. 701). As a reflection of the above changes the disorders are clinically 'white matter diseases' with early symptoms that are motor rather than mental, in contrast to 'grey matter diseases', and a course dominated by progressive paralysis and ataxia rather than dementia and epilepsy, even though in the youngest patients the disease may well also manifest itself by total lack of mental development.

A typical case of leucodystrophy should seldom be missed by the pathologist. The brain is usually reduced in size and weight and the convolutions may be narrowed, while their number and pattern remain normal. Palpation of the hardened white matter through the overlying soft cortex often invokes the familiar metaphor of a mailed fist in a velvet glove. On the cut surface the ventricles are frequently dilated and large areas of the white matter are greyish or bluish with the subcortical zone tending to retain its normal colour. These appearances may, however, vary in the different disorders and to some extent from case to case, while ensuing breakdown of tissue or calcification may further modify the macroscopic picture.

Some cases of leucodystrophy occur sporadically but in most disorders there is evidence of Mendelian recessive transmission, while adrenoleucodystrophy (p. 544) seems to be restricted to males.

The biochemistry of demyelination

The metabolic pathways in the biosynthesis of most myelin lipids are now reasonably well understood (Davison and Peters 1970). The myelin sheath is formed by the spiral winding of the external membrane of the Schwann cell or oligodendrocyte around the nerve axon. Myelin contains lipids and proteins in the ratio of 4 : 1, salts and approximately 40% water. The lipid molecules form bimolecular leaflets which combine into regular multimolecular aggregates (Fig. 12.48). The stability of myelin has been attributed to the nature of its fatty acids which are mainly saturated and of long chain length (19 to 26 carbon atoms). Protein (20 to 30% of dry weight) and polysaccharide molecules can attach themselves to the bimolecular leaflets (Sjöstrand 1963; O'Brien

1970) but cannot, apparently, penetrate into the centre of the myelin membrane. Myelin may be regarded as a simplified type of membrane which lacks some of the proteins characteristic of other membranes. Once formed, most of the myelin sheath undergoes only very slow turnover (Cuzner, Davison and Gregson 1965). Awareness of this relative stability prompted some workers to formulate as a corollary the theory of 'vulnerable periods'

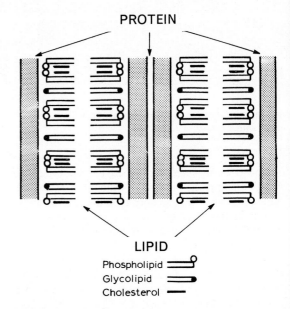

Fig. 12.48 Structure of myelin.

of brain development *during myelination* when 'dysmyelination' could easily occur. It is now realized, however, that there is, on the other hand, a small rapidly metabolizing component of myelin which includes the phosphoinositides in the form of their calcium and magnesium salts. This component plays a part in controlling the permeability of certain areas of the nerve membrane to univalent ions (Dawson 1966). More recent work indicates that the turnover of myelin proteins (Smith 1972) and of cholesterol (Spohn and Davison 1972) is also more rapid than was previously believed.

In the early stages of demyelination the regular lamellar pattern is loosened (Adams and Leibowitz 1969). This may be brought about by diverse factors, such as inflammation, immuno-pathological processes, anoxia or ischaemia. Often demyelination occurs in a sequential manner so that outer lamellae are split off first. Lysophosphatides form from phosphatides by the removal of a fatty acid molecule, and esterified cholesterol appears. The lysophosphatides are cytolytic and may induce or facilitate further demyelination. However, the brain also contains enzymes for the detoxication and reacylation of the lysophosphatides. The transfer of fatty acid from lecithin to cholesterol has been demonstrated in plasma (Glomset 1962), and a similar mechanism may well operate in the brain. Cholesterol is an essential component of myelin. It enhances lipid compaction and probably contributes to the highly organized alignment of the lipid molecules in the myelin sheath. Esterified cholesterol is much less suitable as a membrane constituent. The Marchi method for detecting degenerating myelin is based on differences in the staining properties of free and esterified cholesterol. As demyelination proceeds, there is a concomitant loss of phospholipids (including sphingomyelin, free cholesterol and cerebrosides) and an increase in esterified cholesterol. In certain inflammatory conditions, such as haemorrhagic virus encephalitis and inclusion body encephalitis, there is also a raised mucopolysaccharide level, demonstrable by the raised total hexosamine (Cumings 1965a).

Any factor interfering with the metabolism of the oligodendrocytes or reducing their viability may retard myelination or favour disintegration of the already formed myelin sheath. For example, X-irradiation of 2-day-old rats results in smallness of oligodendroglia and a reduction in the amount of formed myelin (Schjeide, Lin and De Vellis 1968). If, as appears likely, the process of myelin formation involves the aggregation of lipid and protein molecules, it is clearly important that during myelination the right lipids and proteins are synthesized in proper order and proportions. Interference with the synthesis of myelin proteins and lipids at this stage due to a deficiency of essential metabolites, enzymes or cofactors could result in a structurally imperfect myelin sheath ('*dysmyelination*', see below). Such a sheath may be abnormally vulnerable and prone to degenerate prematurely. This occurs in Refsum's disease, and perhaps also in at least some of the leucodystrophies as well as in some metabolic disorders with extra-cerebral enzyme deficiencies, such as phenylketonuria, in which toxic levels of metabolites may interfere with brain metabolism or inhibit the passage across the blood–brain barrier of essential metabolites which cannot be synthesized in the brain.

Aetiology and pathogenesis

Because of the frequent familial incidence of the leucodystrophies, mostly with evidence of recessive or sex-linked transmission, it has long been suspected that they are caused by inborn errors of metabolism and this has been confirmed in two of the conditions. Leaving aside demyelination due to extra-cerebral metabolic errors such as phenylketonuria, and environmental causes such as virus leucoencephalitis, non-Wallerian primary demyelination of the leucodystrophies may in theory be the result of three pathogenetic processes. It could, first, be a primary mechanism, the metabolic defect directly causing degeneration of already formed myelin. Second, the defect may operate *ab initio* preventing correct myelination. Third, there could be a combination of these two mechanisms: myelin is formed imperfectly and is hence more liable to break down. Much has been written on this subject (cf. Poser 1962; Seitelberger 1970) but we are not in a position to summarize or recapitulate here the diverse published views. It may be said, however, that some authors (Poser 1962) regard leucodystrophies as *dysmyelinating* diseases caused by inborn errors of metabolism that interfere with the proper anabolism of myelin. This is in contrast to the *demyelinating* diseases characterized by degeneration of initially well-formed myelin. This view is not fully accepted by all authors.

Classification

Classification of the leucodystrophies has presented and still presents some difficulty and no unanimity has yet been achieved in the designation of the various forms of these disorders. The previously used generic term, Schilder's disease, has been largely abandoned since most conditions can now be classified with greater precision. Some workers still employ that term for rather vaguely defined non-familial cases which also show certain features of multiple sclerosis (see p. 551), designating all other conditions as leucodystrophies. The latter are often divided into sudanophil, metachromatic, Krabbe's (or globoid cell) type, Alexander's, and leucodystrophies with mixed sudanophil and 'prelipoid' products of myelin degeneration. The sudanophil group is further subdivided into adrenoleucodystrophy, simple storage type,

Pelizaeus–Merzbacher type, Seitelberger (connatal) type and Löwenberg–Hill type. Most workers also include among the leucodystrophies the so-called spongiform type of diffuse sclerosis (spongiform encephalopathy or Canavan's sclerosis). We shall conform here to the above classification. For a very full discussion of the leucodystrophies readers can be referred to the handbook edited by Vinken and Bruyn (1970) and to Ulrich (1971).

Sudanophil leucodystrophy

Sudanophil leucodystrophy is the commonest and 'simplest' of the group. It mainly affects infants or children although many adult cases have also been described. In familial cases transmission is as a Mendelian recessive trait. The clinical picture is dominated by increasing paralysis, ataxia, blindness, mental retardation or dementia which may in adults be associated with psychotic symptoms. Frequently there is optic atrophy or pallor of optic discs. CSF protein may be raised and peripheral nerves usually show segmental demyelination.

At necropsy there is at times considerable reduction of brain weight, shrinkage of gyri and diminution in the size of the brainstem and cerebellum. Shrinkage of pyramids exposes the inferior olives very conspicuously upon the anterior surface of the medulla. The white matter of the cerebrum and cerebellum is greyish in tinge and may be indurated or, contrariwise, rarefied or irregularly cystic. Arcuate fibres tend to be spared. Histologically, the condition is characterized by widespread demyelination of the white matter (Fig. 12.49) and the presence in the demyelinated parts of the white matter of distinctly sudanophil products of myelin breakdown (Fig. 12.50), and the process is therefore sometimes referred to as 'simple storage' or, because of the staining properties of the debris, as 'orthochromatic' (contrasted with 'metachromatic' demyelination) (Peiffer 1959b). The sudanophil substances are found mainly within macrophages and astrocytes, but extracellular granules or globules are likewise in evidence. In later stages there is more fibrous gliosis and less sudanophil storage (Fig. 12.51). Nerve cells are usually well preserved as are the axis cylinders (Fig. 12.52) until the process is well advanced, when they also perish. However, there may be secondary loss of neurons in subcortical formations, such as the basal ganglia. 'Prelipoid' substances are absent. (This term is used in respect of substances that stain weakly or not at all with the Sudan dyes.) The electron-microscopy by Nelson, Osterberg, Blaw, Story and Kozak (1962) of a biopsy of the brain of a case of sudanophil leucodystrophy yielded no essentially novel data.

Chemically, the sudanophil material consists mainly of cholesterol esters; hexosamine may also be increased. No definite enzymatic deficiency has yet been identified and it seems unlikely that the condition will prove to be homogeneous (see below).

It may be difficult or impossible to distinguish sudanophil leucodystrophy histologically from massive bilateral demyelination that occurs in some other conditions such as phenylketonuria (Crome 1962). Similar changes may develop in cases of severe head injury (p. 333) and in subacute sclerosing panencephalitis (p. 313). The condition has been described in association with meningeal angiomatosis (Guazzi and Martin 1967; Bruens, Guazzi and Martin 1968; van Bogaert 1970). Under the tentative heading of cerebrohepatorenal syndrome, Passarge and McAdams (1967) described a familial disorder comprising sudanophil leucodystrophy, craniofacial deformity vaguely suggestive of Down's syndrome, renal cysts and hepatomegaly with micronodular cirrhosis of the liver in one of the cases. Leucodystrophy was associated with microcephaly and pachygyria in two siblings reported by Norman, Tingey, Valentine and Danby (1962) and Norman, Tingey, Valentine and Hislop (1967). Sudanophil degeneration of the white matter, particularly one resembling Pelizaeus–Merzbacher disease, i.e. tigroid in appearance (p. 553), has been observed in some cases of Cockayne's syndrome (Seitelberger 1970).

Adrenoleucodystrophy

Considerable interest is being taken in the association of sudanophil leucodystrophy with adrenal atrophy or hypoplasia—adrenoleucodystrophy. The condition is restricted to males and is probably transmitted as a sex-linked recessive trait. Patients show the usual leucodystrophic signs of neurological deterioration and evidence of adrenal failure, such as cutaneous pigmentation and arterial hypotension. ACTH stimulation tests usually reveal evidence of primary adrenocortical failure and there is often

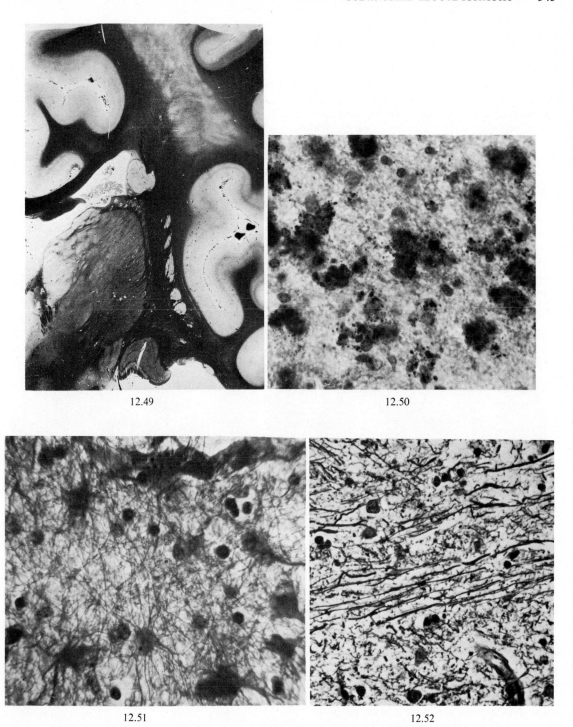

12.49

12.50

12.51

12.52

Figs 12.49-12.52 Sudanophil leucodystrophy.
Fig. 12.49 The centrum semiovale. There is widespread demyelination stopping short of the arcuate fibres. Heidenhain–Woelcke method.
Fig. 12.50 Sudanophil extra- and intracellular debris. Sudan III and haematoxylin. × 450.
Fig. 12.51 Fibrous gliosis. Holzer. × 560.
Fig. 12.52 Some axis cylinders remain in a totally demyelinated area. Bielschowsky's silver impregnation. × 400.

a low 24-hour urine 17–OH–steroid excretion. The CSF protein is raised. Electroencephalography shows diffuse slowing. The most reliable diagnostic test is adrenal biopsy in the opinion of Schaumburg, Powers, Raine, Suzuki and Richardson (1975). The histological changes in the adrenal are, according to them, mostly restricted to the zona reticularis and fasciculata. The main feature is atrophy and presence of ballooned cortical cells, many of which have a striated cytoplasm and vacuoles. A minority of cases show lymphocytic infiltration of the adrenal and scarring (Figs. 12.53a and b). Ballooning of cells is also not a constant or ubiquitous

brain are essentially those of sudanophil leucodystrophy with some associated 'inflammatory' changes in the white matter. Inclusions similar to those seen by electron-microscopy in cells of the adrenal can also be detected in the macrophages within the white matter of the brain. It has been suggested by Schaumburg et al. that adrenoleucodystrophy is a lipid storage disease caused by an error in membrane sterol metabolism. Richardson (1975) makes the challenging statement that all previously reported male cases of Schilder's disease were in reality cases of adrenoleucodystrophy, while those in females and in males without adrenal atrophy were cases of

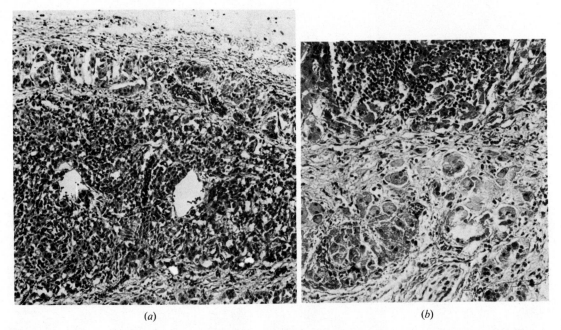

(a)   (b)

Fig. 12.53 Adrenoleucodystrophy. (a) 'Pseudolaminar' atrophy of the adrenal without marked lymphocytic infiltration. Haematoxylin and eosin. × 110. (b) Atrophy of the adrenal with lymphocytic infiltration and distension of some cells. Haematoxylin and eosin. × 160.

change and the atrophy is often 'pseudolaminar'. The adrenal medulla is not affected by the atrophy and has indeed appeared hypertrophied to a few authors. Such appearances are however likely to prove spurious. On electron-microscopy the cytoplasm shows linear or occasionally twisted lamellar accumulation. The individual lamellae show a trilaminar structure consisting of paired electron-dense leaflets separated by an electron-lucent space. Somewhat similar inclusions have been seen in the Schwann cells of a peripheral nerve by Schaumburg et al. (1975) and in the interstitial cells of the testes. Changes in the

multiple sclerosis. Earlier case reports of adrenoleucodystrophy are by Turkington and Stempfel (1966), Gordon and Marsden (1966), Hoefnagel, Brun, Ingbar and Goldman (1967), Forsyth, Forbes and Cumings (1971) and Schaumburg, Powers, Suzuki and Raine (1974). The condition has been reviewed by Blaw (1970).

Globoid cell leucodystrophy

Globoid cell leucodystrophy, also known as *Krabbe's disease* and *galactosylceramide lipidosis*, is usually a disorder of infants, but it may also occur in older patients (Dunn, Lake, Dolman and Wilson 1969; Crome, Hanefeld, Patrick and Wilson 1973). Clinical features include spasticity progressing to total decerebration with hyperextension of body and legs and flexion at the elbows. Mental development is retarded or entirely absent. The patients have frequent episodes of pyrexia. Seizures may commence a little later and there may be excessive responses to stimuli. Motor nerve conduction time is delayed and segmental demyelination has been reported in peripheral nerves (Lake 1968; Sourander and Olsson 1968; Joosten, Krijgsman, Gabreëls-Festen, Gabreëls and Baars 1974). The CSF usually contains a gross excess of protein, with an increase of albumin and α_2-globulin and a decrease in the β and γ fractions (Hagberg, Sourander and Svennerholm 1963). On chemical analysis, the affected white matter shows a loss of galactocerebroside and a greater loss of sulphatide. It contains a significant excess of glucocerebroside, and galactosyl-glucosylceramide. In absolute terms all lipids are reduced in the white matter but myelin lipids are affected more than the phospholipids (Vanier and Svennerholm 1974). The missing enzyme has been identified as galactocerebroside β-galactosidase (Suzuki and Suzuki 1974b).

The cerebrum and cerebellum are small. The white matter of the centrum semiovale and of the cerebral gyri is shrunken and so is the corpus callosum. The affected parts are indurated and discoloured but the arcuate fibres are well preserved.

Histological examination reveals a profound or even total lack of myelin in the white matter, the intact arcuate fibres standing out prominently in sections stained for myelin (Fig. 12.54). The demyelinated areas show great overgrowth of glial cells and fibres but the characteristic feature is the presence of so-called globoid cells, which are often arranged in densely packed clusters (Fig. 12.55). These may also be found in the spinal cord and optic nerves. The globoid cells are usually very evident but may be difficult to find in some lesions, particularly those affected by dense fibrous gliosis and thus presumably of longer duration. On the other hand globoid cells may be present in other conditions, although not usually in clusters (Gulotta, Heyer, Tropitzsch, Homer and Citoler 1970; Crome and Zapella 1963). Globoid cells are spherical bodies, measuring 20 to 25 μm in diameter, and have single or multiple nuclei and a faintly granular basophilic cytoplasm. They stain faintly with the Sudan dyes and strongly with PAS. On electronmicroscopy they are seen to possess many pseudopods and two types of abnormal inclusions: (1) moderately dense, straight or curved hollow tubules with an irregularly crystalloid crosssection and (2) right-handed twisted tubules reminiscent of the abnormal inclusions in Gaucher's disease (Fig. 12.56). Electronmicroscopical changes have been seen already in a 22-week-old fetus (Suzuki, Schneider and Epstein 1971; Ellis, Nielsen, McCulloch and Schneider 1974). The peripheral nerves also show abnormal tubular inclusions similar to those in the globoid cells, and these are present in histiocytes and Schwann cells (Suzuki and Suzuki 1973). Besides the globoid cells smaller 'epithelioid' cells, 10 to 20 μm in diameter, are often grouped around blood vessels. Globoid cells are thought to be modified macrophages and it seems certain that they evolve by enlargement of the 'epithelioid' cells. We have, for example, been able to demonstrate β-glucuronidase in both types of cell (Hanefeld and Crome 1971). Other histochemical parameters also seem identical in both types of cells (Volk, Adachi and Schneck 1972). The bulk of the stored material in the globoid cells is galactocerebroside and this is exclusively a constituent of myelin. So-called myelin bodies, eosinophil non-nucleated structures of 40 to 60 μm diameter are also occasionally found in the white matter.

The cerebral cortex shows little apparent change but focal neuronal loss may occur. Likewise, Purkinje cells and granules may be depleted in the cerebellum.

As mentioned, peripheral nerves show segmental demyelination. On electron-microscopy Bischoff and Ulrich (1969) found, however, that axons and myelin sheaths were generally spared. Osmiophilic substance and groups of irregularly arranged needle-shaped structures were seen in cavities derived from vesicular organelles of Schwann cells and histiocytes. In necropsy material Hogan, Gutmann and Chou (1969) observed marked increase of collagen and evidence of segmental demyelination. (Inclusions similar to those in the globoid cells of the brain are found in the cytoplasm of histiocytes, in collagen and around blood vessels (Suzuki and Grover 1970a). Globoid cells were never found in peripheral nerves.)

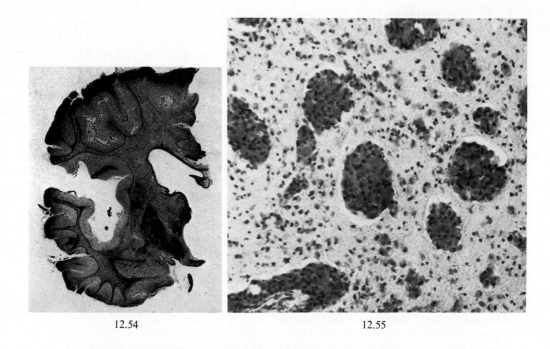

12.54   12.55

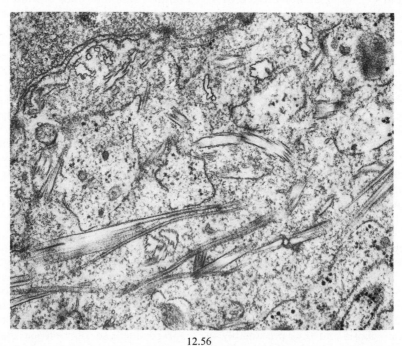

12.56

Fig. 12.54 Cerebral hemisphere in a case of Krabbe's leucodystrophy. There is generalized lack of myelin in the white matter but the arcuate fibres are spared. Heidenhain–Woelcke method for myelin.

Fig. 12.55 Tightly packed clusters of globoid cells in a case of Krabbe's leucodystrophy. In the lower left corner is a blood vessel surrounded by epithelioid cells. Haematoxylin and eosin. × 230.

Fig. 12.56 Globoid cell leucodystrophy. Scattered intracytoplasmic inclusions in a globoid cell. Both tubular and crystalloid structures are clearly seen. × 375,000. (By courtesy of Dr K. Suzuki and Masson et Cie., Paris.)

It is of interest that a globoid cell reaction can be produced in the white matter of animals by the intracerebral injection of natural or synthetic cerebrosides such as cerebron or kerasin (Austin and Lehfeldt 1965; Olsson, Sourander and Svennerholm 1966; Suzuki 1970). A condition analogous to globoid cell leucodystrophy occurs in dogs (Fletcher, Kurtz and Low 1966; Hirth and Nielsen 1967; Fletcher, Kurtz and Stadlan 1971; Suzuki, Tadashi, Fletcher and Suzuki 1974).

Metachromatic leucodystrophy (sulphatidosis)

In metachromatic leucodystrophy sulphatides are stored in the central nervous system, chiefly in the white matter, as well as in many somatic tissues. The condition occurs in two enzymatically distinct forms: *arylsulphatase A deficiency* and *multiple sulphatase deficiency*, the latter being considered with the mucolipidoses on p. 529. The clinical picture of the classical form, arylsulphatase A deficiency, is in the main that of all leudodystrophies, motor loss and dysfunction appearing earlier and being more prominent than epilepsy and mental retardation. The course of the disease tends to be more protracted than in some other leucodystrophies. It is transmitted as a Mendelian recessive trait. By age of onset the disease may be infantile, late infantile, juvenile or adult (Pilz 1970). These variants are probably genetically distinct, with the same one recurring in the affected families. Stumpf and Austin (1971) have adduced evidence favouring a qualitative difference of the enzyme abnormality in the late infantile and juvenile forms of the disorder. Existence of a congenital form is regarded as dubious.

The condition is diagnosed by the demonstration of aryl sulphatase deficiency in leucocytes, urine or cultured fibroblasts. The urine usually contains an excess of sulphatides. Nerve conduction time is increased and repeated EEG recording may help in the early diagnosis of the condition (Fullerton 1964; Mastropaolo, Pampiglione and Stephens 1971). It is to be noted, however, that some metachromatic material can be seen in the peripheral nerves of normal children (Olsson and Sourander 1969). What is characteristic of metachromatic leucodystrophy is, according to the authors, its presence partly in Schwann cells and partly in perivascular phago-cytes. Axis cylinders and the myelin sheaths are damaged (see also p. 562 *et seq.*).

The clinical picture in adults, unlike that in children, is usually one of psychosis, e.g. schizophrenia (Betts, Smith and Kelly 1968).

The incidence of the leucodystrophies as a group has not been worked out, these diseases not being notifiable in this country and many cases, moreover, remaining undiagnosed. Gustavson and Hagberg (1971) have estimated that the late infantile form of metachromatic leucodystrophy occurs in 1 : 40,000 births in northern Sweden.

The brain may show little reduction in size; it may indeed be large for age, but in most cases there will be some micrencephaly, and the cerebral ventricles will then be correspondingly widened. The convolutions show occasional ulegyria. On the cut surface the white matter may be ivory white in colour and show faint striation or granularity (Fig. 12.57). In other instances it may be greyish in colour. Demyelination and the sparing of the arcuate fibres are more obvious in the formalin-fixed than in the fresh specimen.

The characteristic histological features are extensive loss of myelin, cellular and fibrous gliosis and the presence of brown intra- and extracellular metachromatic material after staining with cresyl violet or thionin in an acidified solution. (Pseudoisocyanine is recommended for the demonstration of sulphatides by Harzer and Benz 1973.) A striking finding is the occurrence of conspicuous intra- and extracellular spherical coarsely granular structures 20 to 30 μm in diameter laden with this metachromatic material (Fig. 12.58); their staining reactions are those of sulphatides. They are PAS positive, Sudan black positive and Bial negative (for sialic acid). While most of the material is found in the white matter some is also demonstrable in certain groups of neurons both in the cerebral cortex and, even more so, in subcortical formations. It may also be found in peripheral nerves and myenteric plexuses but not in the neurons of these plexuses. It is constantly present in the kidney (hence the diagnostic metachromasia test on urine), and often in the liver, gall bladder, pancreas, lymph glands, adrenals and ovaries. In somatic tissues the bulk of the metachromatic material appears in the form of coarse, homogeneous irregularly sized globules with only a small proportion of the substance assuming the shape of discrete

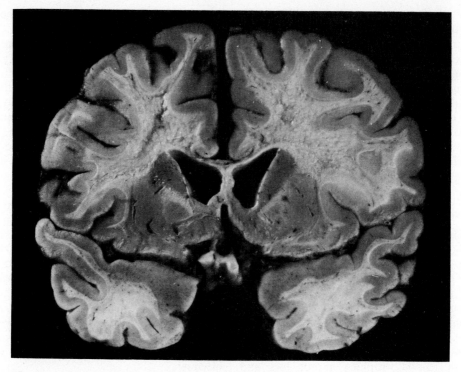

Fig. 12.57 Metachromatic leucodystrophy.   Coronal section through the brain shows granularity and slight discoloration of the white matter, the arcuate fibres remaining preserved.

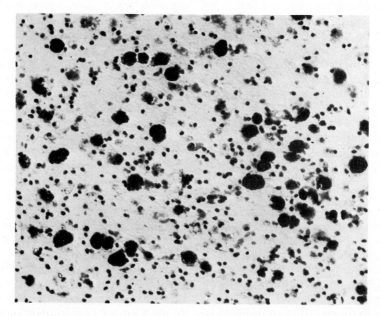

Fig. 12.58 Metachromatic bodies in the white matter (thionin, mounted in microil).

fine granules. Storage is at times so bulky as to render stained sections strikingly brown even to the naked eye. The staining is, however, rather erratic and often impermanent, while some of the substance can also be dissolved in the course of the histological processing. It must be searched for in fresh frozen preparations. According to some authors (Norman, Urich and Tingey 1960) another type of granular material, staining

with dark and light bands. Concentric membranes may also be present. Smaller inclusions are granular (Fig. 12.59). The abnormal inclusions may likewise be found in the Schwann cells of the peripheral nerves (Aurebeck, Osterberg, Blaw, Chou and Nelson 1964; Grégoire, Perier and Dustin 1966; Résibois-Grégoire 1967; Terry 1971; Haberland, Brunngraber, Witting and Daniels 1973). Storage appears to take

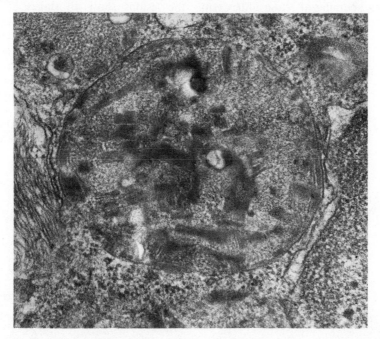

Fig. 12.59 Metachromatic leucodystrophy. A cortical glial cell contains a large, round, membrane-bound aggregate of lamellar and granular metachromatic material. Smaller aggregates appear to be floating free in the cytoplasm. × 41,250. (By courtesy of Dr R. D. Terry and the North Holland Publishing Co.)

like myelin, may be scattered among the metachromatic particles. It has not been present in our cases.

Some cases of metachromatic leucodystrophy show concomitant absence of oligodendroglia in the white matter. It was therefore suggested by Brain and Greenfield (1950) that these constituted a distinct variant of metachromatic luecodystrophy —due to primary degeneration of the oligodendroglia. This view is not now accepted, since *most* advanced cases show such oligodendroglial loss.

As mentioned, there is as a rule marked astrocytosis in the affected areas as well as loss of axis cylinders.

Electron-microscopy shows inclusions in neurons and glial cells of a lamellar pattern

place in Schwann cells related to normal myelin segments rather than in those undergoing demyelination and remyelination (Webster 1962; Cravioto, O'Brien, Landing and Finck 1966; Terry, Suzuki and Weiss 1966).

Schilder's disease

The name *Schilder's disease* or *diffuse cerebral sclerosis* at first covered all recognized cases of leucodystrophy, but since most of these can now be classified more accurately, it has become rather difficult to define criteria for the continued use of the original term. It has even been suggested that further use of this term is no longer justified (Richardson 1975) (p. 546). Nevertheless, other authors have used it for cases showing large, not necessarily quite symmetrical, areas of de-myelination in the centrum semiovale, often accompanied by smaller plaques of myelin loss, which are unlike the diffuse lesions of the leuco-dystrophies. The pathology of such cases would thus represent a stage between the leucodys-trophies and such distinct conditions as dis-seminated encephalomyelitis and multiple sclerosis (cf. Poser and van Bogaert 1956). The disorder is said to be entirely sporadic, affecting adolescents and adults rather than infants or children. It may

greyish or yellowish discoloration, and these may, depending on the degree and duration of the process, be soft or indurated. The arcuate fibres are usually spared. The corpus callosum, brain-stem and cerebellum may also show demyelina-tion. While the larger lesions have somewhat blurred edges those of the small ones are crisp and indistinguishable from the plaques of mul-tiple sclerosis. When examined histologically, the lesions show all stages of orthochromatic demyelination with release of sudanophil debris, which are at first engulfed in macrophages. Older lesions show greater astrocytosis and fibrous gliosis. Axonal damage is usually rather severe. A characteristic feature of Schilder's disease is said to be perivascular lymphocytic infiltration in the affected white matter. This, however, is not always present and is, contrariwise, often encountered in indubitable cases of leucodys-

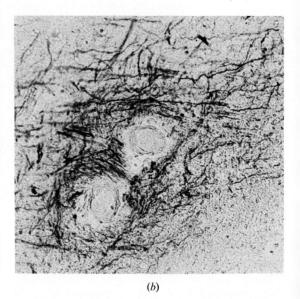

(a)   (b)

Fig. 12.60 Pelizaeus–Merzbacher disease. (a) Profound demyelination of the white matter with sparing of islets of myelin. (b) A surviving perivascular islet of myelin in the midst of widespread demyelination.

assume a variety of clinical forms, being pseudo-tumourous in some cases, or presenting as psychosis or paralysis. In other instances it can, like multiple sclerosis, be episodic in its course (Lhermitte 1950).

The brain may show little external change although some micrencephaly and ulegyria develop in more protracted instances. On sectioning, the white matter shows large and small areas of

trophy. The grey matter is usually free from inflammatory change. If searched for, plaques of demyelination resembling multiple sclerosis are often found elsewhere in the central nervous system. On electron-microscopy of two cases regarded as instances of Schilder's disease, Suzuki and Grover (1970b) found the changes in astrocytes to be like those reported in sudano-phil leucodystrophy. The degeneration of myelin appeared to be primary, as in multiple sclerosis. A further case has been studied biochemically and histologically by Hogan, Joseph, Hurt and Krigman (1972).

Pelizaeus–Merzbacher disease

The characteristics of Pelizaeus–Merzbacher leucodystrophy are its relatively protracted course and prevalence in males, amounting perhaps to sex-linkage; on histological examination there is frequent but not quite invariable sparing of myelin islets in the midst of the degenerating white matter (tigroid demyelination).

The clinical and pathological aspects of the disease have been fully discussed by Seitelberger (1970). It usually presents in infancy with motor dysfunction, such as nystagmus, tremor and ataxia. Some optic discs are pale and retinal pigmentation may set in later. Mental retardation becomes evident and later still spasticity sets in and there may be occasional athetoid movements.

The brain is often reduced in size, especially the brainstem and cerebellum, and the ventricles are then dilated. Stained sections show widespread myelin loss with preservation of irregularly shaped and sized, often perivascular, islets of myelin (Figs. 12.60a and b). Higher magnification, however, reveals that, in spite of general preservation of the islets, individual myelin fibres within them show certain evidence of degeneration, such as pallor of staining, varicosities and fragmentation. The decay of myelin follows an orthochromatic course: sudanophil debris appears but may be sparse, possibly because of the slow progression of the disease. Axis cylinders tend to be preserved and fibrous gliosis is usually patchy but considerable. The cerebellum is often atrophic. Neurochemical studies have revealed a reduction of total lipids in keeping with the degree of demyelination.

It must be mentioned that considerable individual variations have been observed both in the clinical course and pathological picture of the disease.

Seitelberger's leucodystrophy

This condition, which Seitelberger (1970) regards as a congenital variant of Pelizaeus–Merzbacher's disease, is characterized by prevalence in males, total lack of psychomotor progress and very extensive demyelination. Few cases have been reported: Seitelberger lists 13. The patients die at an earlier age than those with classical Pelizaeus–Merzbacher's disease, in general before the age of 10 years. It must be said, however, that there is no consensus on the definition of the Pelizaeus–Merzbacher syndrome. For example, in a case reported by Schneck, Adachi and Volk (1971) neurochemical and morphological findings were in keeping with myelin aplasia rather than demyelination while another case of a 3-month-old boy regarded as an instance of Pelizaeus–Merzbacher's disease (Watanabe, Patel, Goebel, Siakotos, Zeman, De Meyer and Dyer 1973) showed normal myelin sheaths but oligodendroglial change.

The brain shows generalized atrophy and the white matter of the centrum semiovale and the corpus callosum is thin and discoloured. Histological examination shows that demyelination is greatly advanced (Fig. 12.61) but a few micro-islets of surviving myelin may nevertheless be present. Nerve cells and axis cylinders tend to be well preserved. Sudanophil products of myelin degradation are scarce. The cerebellum may show loss of nerve cells, demyelination and astrocytosis. The occurrence of concomitant cerebral malformation—microgyria—has been reported. As in the Pelizaeus–Merzbacher disease, the white matter shows a reduction of total lipids on chemical examination. In a case that might have been of this kind, Adachi, Schneck, Volk and Torii (1970) found on electron-microscopy only occasional sheaths with few lamellar formations in the white matter; cortical neurons were normal.

Seitelberger draws attention to the reported occurrence of some cases resembling both the congenital and the classical form of Pelizaeus–Merzbacher's disease. He lists these separately as 'transitional' forms. None of these has been familial. A possible instance of this condition is reported by Liaño, Ricoy, Diáz-Flores and Gimeno (1974).

Löwenberg–Hill leucodystrophy

This form of leucodystrophy presents at a much later age than the syndromes already discussed and the patients show psychotic features rather than mental retardation. However, a few of the reported cases have been dwarfed and microcephalic (Lüthy and Bischoff 1961). Most were

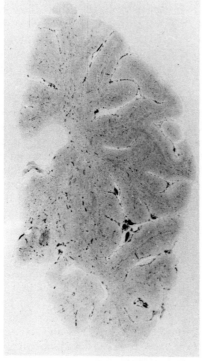

(a)

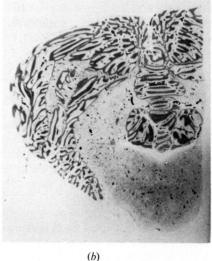

(b)

Fig. 12.61 Seitelberger type of leuco-dystrophy. Complete absence of stainable myelin in (a) the cerebral hemisphere and (b) in the cerebellum and brainstem. Heidenhain's method for myelin.

males and the transmission could have been simple dominant.

The brains of patients with the Löwenberg–Hill leucodystrophy are small and show diffuse demyelination with preservation of some myelin islets which are said, however, not to be as crisply outlined as in the classical form of Pelizaeus–Merzbacher's disease. Degradation products are scarce and axis cylinders tend to be well preserved. Fibrous gliosis is seen in the demyelinated areas. Arcuate fibres are spared.

Leucodystrophy with mixed sudanophil and pre-lipoid debris

In certain cases of diffuse demyelination not all the breakdown products are sudanophil; some are PAS-positive without being metachromatic. A number of these cases have, in addition, shown scattered granules of light-brown pigment which sometimes stained positively for iron (Diezel 1955; Diezel and Richardson 1957; Peiffer 1959a). Reported cases have differed widely in age and clinical presentation and do not seem to constitute a genetically or metabolically homogeneous group.

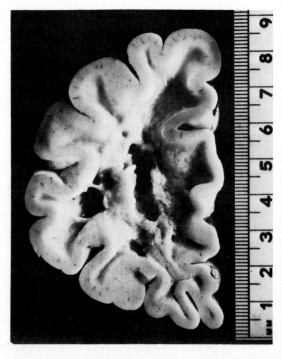

Fig. 12.62 Coronal block of the frontal lobe from a case of Alexander's leucodystrophy.

The Alexander type of leucodystrophy

This condition, first described by Alexander (1949), commences in infancy or later childhood, the clinical picture being of progressive dementia, paralysis and epilepsy. With onset before the union of the cranial sutures the patients become

deep to the external and internal surfaces of the brain. Rosenthal fibres are irregularly shaped elongated or rounded hyaline eosinophil bodies staining black with the myelin stains (Fig. 12.63), and deep purple with Mallory's phosphotungstic acid haematoxylin. They are PAS-negative and not sudanophil. Their precise nature has not

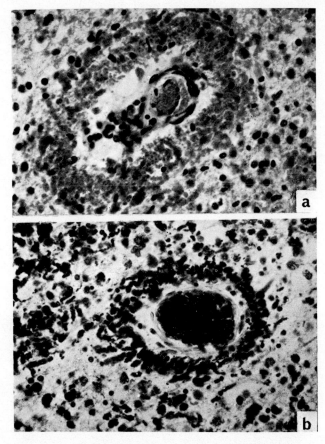

Fig. 12.63 Rosenthal fibres in a case of Alexander's leucodystrophy are particularly dense and numerous around a blood vessel. (*a*) Haematoxylin and eosin. × 400. (*b*) Heidenhain–Woelcke. × 400.

megalencephalic. All reported cases have been sporadic. The large brain shows a somewhat indurated, uniformly white, cortical ribbon. The subjoining white matter is discoloured and may be loosened in texture, soft, jelly-like, collapsed or broken down (Fig. 12.62). Histological examination reveals diffuse demyelination and rarefaction of the white matter with little or no sparing of the arcuate fibres. The distinctive feature is the presence throughout the central nervous system of innumerable Rosenthal fibres arranged most densely around blood vessels and

been established but it is obvious that they contain or consist mainly of proteins. They also occur, albeit in smaller numbers, in many other conditions associated with reactive or neoplastic astrocytosis. Some areas of the cerebral cortex in Alexander's disease show fibrous gliosis and there may be diffuse neuronal loss both in the cerebral cortex and subcortical formations.

On electron-microscopy Rosenthal fibres appear first as dense round osmiophilic structures merging with thickened glial fibrils.

Further details of the condition will be found

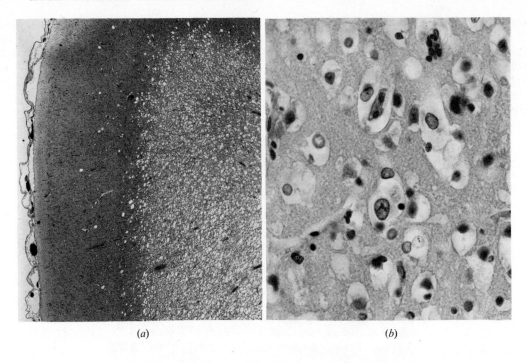

(a)   (b)

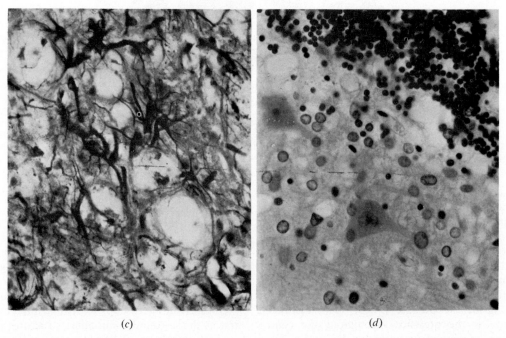

(c)   (d)

Fig. 12.64 Spongiform leucodystrophy. (a) Low-power view of the cortex and white matter. (b) Deeper layers of the cortex. (c) White matter.   × 400.   (d) Cerebellar cortex with large vesicular astrocytic nuclei.   × 400.

in case reports, such as those by Vogel and Hallervorden (1962), Herndon and Rubinstein (1968), Schochet, Lampert and Earle (1968) and Herndon, Rubinstein, Freeman and Mathieson (1970).

Spongiform leucodystrophy

Non-specific spongiform degeneration or rarefaction of neural tissue, the status spongiosus of German authors, is a relatively common neuropathological finding in diverse conditions. It has been regarded by some as a consequence of long-standing widespread or localized brain oedema. On histological examination, tissue sections, especially of the white matter, show rarification, displaying countless vacuoles which coalesce into grosser cavities (Fig. 12.64). Such spongiform degeneration may be associated with lack of myelination, demyelination or gliotic change. In some children spongiform degeneration of the white matter is the sole ascertainable pathological change. Such cases, especially if familial, have been named *spongiform leucodystrophy* or, less appropriately, *Canavan's type of diffuse sclerosis*. Three forms of the condition have been described, a congenital, an infantile and a juvenile. The infantile cases were often Jewish. They showed severe mental retardation, enlargement of the head and hypotonia followed by spastic paralysis. The CSF protein was sometimes raised. The condition tended to be transmitted as a Mendelian recessive trait. In addition to the status spongiosus the cerebral cortex of these cases (and subcortical grey matter) shows numerous enlarged, bare vesicular astrocytic nuclei resembling Alzheimer II cells. Although there is considerable variation in the extent and position of the demyelination and spongiform change, the part most affected is the centrum semiovale where the white matter may be converted into a loose meshwork of bare glial and axonal fibres. The arcuate fibres are often involved and the degeneration may extend into the deeper layers of the cerebral cortex where Alzheimer II cells are particularly numerous. The basal ganglia may be affected. In the cerebellum there is frequently an oedematous space (lamina dissecans) between the granular and molecular layers, Purkinje cells being displaced outwards. Spongiform leucodystrophy has been fully described in a monograph by van Bogaert and Bertrand (1967) and has been recently reviewed by Adachi, Schneck, Cara and Volk (1973). For a detailed description, including characteristic electron-microscopical data, readers are referred to the case reports of two siblings by Kolkmann, Rana and Nützendel (1971). Most of the infantile cases die in infancy but more chronic ones surviving into later childhood are known to occur (Adachi and Volk 1968). No specific enzyme deficiency has been identified as a cause of the leucodystrophy, and, indeed, the condition is probably not homogeneous. A somewhat similar disorder, sometimes associated with retinitis pigmentosa, has been reported in older children. This was first described by Kearns and Sayre (1958) and about 20 cases have been recently reviewed by Tridon, Martin, Vidailhet, Floquet, Philippart and Neimann (1974). None was familial.

Spongiform leucodystrophy, a disease primarily of the white matter, is not to be confused with 'spongy degeneration of the grey matter' which may also occur in children (Janota 1974).

Comparative medicine

Since human lysosomal enzymopathies affecting the brain are rather rare, search for animal models is of special interest. A few instances have already been cited in the text and we summarize here some of the available information.

Lipidosis has been reported in dogs. The clinical and pathological pictures in these animals resemble those in human neurolipidosis (Hagen 1953; Ribelin and Kintner 1956; Diezel, Koppang and Rossner 1965). Excessive accumulation of lipofuscin suggestive of ceroid lipofuscinosis has been observed in mutant mice by O'Steen and Nandy (1970). G_{M2} gangliosidosis has been described in German short-hair pointers by Karle and Schiefer (1967).

A condition resembling gargoylism occurs in cattle, the affected calves being known as 'snorter dwarf cattle'. Their urine shows an abnormal pattern of mucopolysaccharide excretion and some of the lesions resemble human ones (Lorincz

1960-61). Mannosidosis has been described in Angus cattle (Whitten and Walker 1957; Jolly 1970, 1971; Hocking *et al.* 1972). G_{M1} gangliosidosis in Friesian calves has been reported by Donnelly, Sheahan and Rogers (1973). A condition of neurovisceral storage, possibly analogous to human mucopolysaccharidosis has been reported in two of three newborn goats by Hartley and Blakemore (1973).

A condition analogous to globoid cell leucodystrophy occurs in dogs (Fletcher, Kurtz and Low 1966; Hirth and Nielsen 1967; Fletcher, Kurtz and Stadlan 1971), and a syndrome resembling metachromatic leucodystrophy in mink (Andersen and Palludan 1968). Analysis of lipids in the demyelinated brains of mutant mice has been reported by Baumann, Jacque, Pollet and Harpin (1968) and Jacque, Harpin and Baumann (1969).

Reviews of degenerative neurological disorders in animals have been published by Howell (1970), Herschkowitz (1973) and Jolly and Blakemore (1973).

Laboratory diagnosis

Readers of the earlier sections of this chapter will have no doubt come to appreciate the special problems and difficulties of diagnosing diseases due to inborn lysosomal enzyme deficiencies. Closely similar clinical patterns may be shared by a number of distinct syndromes. Even such a unique clinical picture as that of gargoylism may, for example, be the result of different enzymopathies. Thorough clinical evaluation of the patient does, of course, narrow down the search for a diagnosis but is never sufficient to confirm it. Pathologists not fully familiar with paediatric neurology may be helped by one of many useful and succinct reviews covering this subject, such as those by Wilson (1972) or Noronha (1974). We have ourselves indicated salient clinical features in outlining each of the syndromes. In this concluding part we discuss briefly relevant laboratory procedures and possibilities. These are haematological, biochemical, enzymological, histopathological and electrophysiological. Rapid recent progress in all these fields, especially enzymology, has brought with it the possibility of identifying almost all the known lysosomal enzyme defects in living patients. Moreover some conditions can be diagnosed even before birth in fetuses, while some heterozygotes can likewise be identified by appropriate tests.

Histopathology

Our work has been mainly with light microscopy. We realize that in some circumstances electron-microscopy can supply diagnostic data that would not be otherwise forthcoming. It has therefore been our practice to set aside in certain cases portions of biopsies for this purpose, fix these by appropriate methods and despatch them, with prior agreement, to some of the slowly increasing number of our colleagues with facilities for electron-microscopy. Nevertheless, it is probably still true that light microscopy will, in combination with relevant non-histopathological methods, supply the diagnosis in all but a few exceptional cases.

One of the first questions to be answered is which tissue to obtain as biopsy. The ones usually considered are brain, liver, peripheral nerve, gut, lymph glands and skin.

The stage has been reached where most conditions can be diagnosed without resort to *brain biopsy*, which raises a difficult ethical problem. However, a biopsy can always be obtained when craniotomy is performed to exclude some focal condition, such as subdural haematoma, brain abscess or tumour. It may also be resorted to when all else fails, and in conditions which cannot be conclusively identified in any other way. This is true particularly of some leucodystrophies, e.g. spongiform leucodystrophy (p. 557), Alexander's disease (p. 555) or sudanophil leucodystrophy (p. 544). The surgeon will excise with minimum damage to the biopsy material a small portion of the cortex *and* white matter from one of the 'silent' areas, e.g. agranular frontal lobe. This must be divided into at least three parts: for light- and electron-microscopy, for biochemistry and for enzymology. Some workers also keep a little deep-frozen material for histochemical tests but we have not found histo-chemistry to be crucial. It is important to obtain instructions on the initial handling of the material from the specialists who are to examine it. If these are followed, it is astonishing how much information can be extracted from very small specimens by multi-disciplinary study.

A needle biopsy of the *liver* is a relatively simple and safe clinical procedure. Unfortunately, histological changes due to lysosomal enzyme deficiencies are often non-specific. Vacuolation of liver and Kupffer cells and its electron-microscopical counterpart of enlarged membrane-bound lysosomes with or without identifiable residual bodies, is very common in all the muco-polysaccharidoses and mucolipidoses. On the other hand, liver biopsy can be diagnostic, almost in itself, in Wolman's disease (p. 535), Niemann–Pick's disease (p. 514), Gaucher's disease (p. 513) and generalized glycogenosis. Not entirely specific but nevertheless diagnos-tically valuable changes may be seen in other disorders, such as Batten's disease and the gangliosidoses. Part of the biopsy can be deep-frozen and used for biochemical analysis to determine the possible presence of adventitious storage material, such as sphingomyelin or ganglioside: a slight excess of this substance may be found in the liver even in primary neuro-lipidoses, such as G_{M2} gangliosidosis (p. 507). Granulomatous lesions may be found in Hand–Schüller–Christian disease and other conditions affecting the brain secondarily or incidentally (p. 536).

Since its inception *intestinal biopsy* has become one of the most useful methods of investigating storage diseases (Bodian and Lake 1963). Most of these are generalized conditions involving autonomic nerves and ganglia, particularly the myenteric plexuses of Meissner and Auerbach, situated respectively in the intestinal submucosa and between the two layers of the muscularis. When so affected, the nerve cells in these plexuses are distended and give the characteristic staining reactions of the lipidoses, metachromatic leuco-dystrophy and Batten's disease. The distribution of pathological changes may not be uniform at all levels of the intestinal tract. It has been suggested that such distribution patterns may vary in the different lipidoses (Kamoshita and Landing 1968). If so, it would be theoretically possible to obtain 'false positive' results in rectal biopsies but we have not experienced this diffi-culty. On the other hand, a superficial suction biopsy of the rectal mucosa may contain few if any nerve cells and it is, furthermore, difficult to cut serial sections of it by cryostat. However, it has been reported that in Batten's disease characteristic *electron-microscopical* changes ap-pear not only in neurons (Duckett, Cracco, Lublin and Scott 1974) but also in other cells of the rectal mucosa and submucosa (p. 533). Should this be confirmed of this and other storage diseases, as is likely, the scope and value of suction as opposed to full-thickness rectal biopsy will be considerably enlarged. As matters stand, a full-thickness rectal biopsy taken high enough to get past the hypoganglionic lower segment of the viscus may cause considerable bleeding. In our laboratory we recommend appendicectomy as a substitute, this being a less painful and less dangerous operation. The appendix is, of course, richly endowed with nerve cells and the laparotomy enables the surgeon to obtain, if required, other material for examina-tion, e.g. lymph glands or a specimen of the liver.

Characteristic foam cells are present in the lamina propria of the gut in cases of Wolman's disease (p. 535) but care must be taken to dis-tinguish these from muciphages which are also distended and vacuolated PAS-positive histio-cytes that are often normally present in the lamina propria of the colon and rectum.

Peripheral nerve biopsy, almost invariably of the sural nerve, has been coming into increasing use. The chief changes looked for in lysosomal enzymopathies are segmental demyelination, which is present in almost all leucodystrophies, and storage of adventitious material. Segmental de-myelination may be seen in teased nerve fibres. In axonal (Wallerian) degeneration both axis cylinders and myelin sheaths degenerate con-currently. Fibres regenerating after such de-generation show abnormally short internodal lengths. Segmental degeneration involves, on the other hand, only some internodal segments of the myelin sheaths, axis cylinders remaining initially intact. Fibres which have regenerated following this mode of degeneration show variable internodal lengths. A number of techniques have been used to demonstrate the above changes. For example, the method recommended by McLeod Walsh and Little (1969) involves fixation in 10% formalin and subsequent staining in 1% osmic acid (other workers use Sudan black). The nerve is then macerated in two parts of glycerol to one of water for 24 hours. Single fibres are teased out under the dissecting microscope and cleaned and mounted in clove oil.

Adventitious substance can be demonstrated in peripheral nerves both by light- and electron-microscopy. Such substances are most conspicuous in the mucopolysaccharidoses and metachromatic leucodystrophy (p. 549), but storage can also be seen, especially with the aid of an electron microscope, in many other disorders. This is so in ceroid lipofuscinosis (p. 531), globoid cell leucodystrophy (p. 546). Gaucher's disease (p. 513) and Fabry's disease (p. 516). Metachromatic myelin degeneration has been reported in mucolipidosis I. Demyelination of peripheral nerves has also been reported in G_{M2} gangliosidosis but this may not be a constant finding.

Examination of enlarged *lymph glands* may be diagnostic in cases of Gaucher's disease, Niemann–Pick's disease, G_{M1} lipidosis, and of lymphoma or granulomatous conditions, such as Hand–Schüller–Christian disease. As with brain tissue it is advisable to submit the material to both histopathological and chemical examination. The same applies to examination of the spleen, if it is removed entirely or submitted to biopsy.

Histopathological examination of the *skin* is diagnostic in Fabry's disease (p. 516), the diagnosis being confirmed by the chemical demonstration of ceramide trihexoside in the urine and the presence of laminated bodies in renal cells seen on electron-microscopy of the urinary deposit (Desnick, Dawson, Desnick, Sweeley and Krivit 1971; Duncan 1970).

Haematological manifestations

Examination of blood and bone marrow films is of considerable help in the diagnosis of the mucopolysaccharidoses, particularly in conjunction with urinary screening tests. Basophilic granules in the cytoplasm of polymorphonuclear leucocytes, so-called Reilly–Alder bodies, were the first haematological abnormality described in gargoylism. Unfortunately, they are not constant. Mucopolysaccharide inclusions and vacuoles in the cytoplasm of lymphocytes are a much more regular finding. These inclusions stain metachromatically with toluidine blue (Fig. 12.26). Such inclusions have not been observed in the majority of lipidoses, but they do occur in some of the mucolipidoses (Table 12.5). They

are soluble in aqueous, particularly, saline solutions, so that vacuolated cells result when they are removed. Examination of the stained blood films is thus a very useful diagnostic procedure. The method is straightforward but certain precautions are necessary. In our laboratories the method of Mittwoch (1963) has proved satisfactory in detecting MPS I, II and III. Not all the lymphocytes contain inclusions, in fact the proportion may be as low as 1 to 2%.

Vacuolation of lymphocytes is much more difficult to interpret. It has been reported in the mucolipidoses, juvenile Tay–Sachs disease, Niemann–Pick's and Gaucher's disease, as well as in the mucopolysaccharidoses, but not by all observers. The significance of slighter involvements of lymphocytes, regarded by some workers as an indication of heterozygosity, is dubious. It should be emphasized that vacuoles may be regarded as pathological only if sharply defined, as if punched into the cytoplasm.

Abnormalities in the cells of the bone marrow have been reported in several of the storage disorders. For example, histiocytes with numerous variably sized metachromatic inclusions and Buhot cells, that is plasma cells or histiocytes with ring-like bodies within big clear vacuoles, are seen characteristically in the Hurler, Hunter and Sanfilippo syndromes. Characteristic cells are found in the bone marrow in Niemann–Pick's, Gaucher's and Wolman's diseases, as well as G_{M1}, types I and II.

Biochemical tests on urine

Over 40 years ago Fölling in Norway devised a simple urinary screening test which proved of great help in the detection of phenylketonuria. This encouraged clinical chemists to propose straightforward procedures for the identification of patients with other genetic metabolic diseases, including the storage disorders. Provided regard is paid to the limitations of any simple screening procedure, and provided results are confirmed by more specific and precise tests, results will be valuable.

Urinary screening has been widely applied to the detection of the mucopolysaccharidoses. The polyanionic glycosaminoglycans excreted in excess in urine can be stained by a number of basic dyes such as toluidine blue, alcian blue or azure A, when urine is spotted on filter paper. Acidic glycosaminoglycans form insoluble complexes

Table 12.5 *Haematological manifestations in mucopolysaccharidoses, mucolipidoses and sphingolipidoses*

Disease	Blood	Bone marrow	Splenomegaly
Hurler's	Abnormal granulations in lymphocytes	Buhot cells and abnormal reticular	+
Hunter's	(Mittwoch–Gasser cells) and granulocytes	cells	+
Sanfilippo's	(Reilly–Alder anomaly)		(+)
Morquio's	Abnormal granulations in lymphocytes and		(+)
Scheie's	granulocytes comparatively rare		(+)
Maroteaux–Lamy's	Abnormal granulations often large and numerous		(+)
G_{M1} gangliosidosis I	Vacuolated lymphocytes	Histiocytic foam cells	+
Fabry's	—	Foam cells	(+)
Sandhoff's	—	—	(+)
Fucosidosis	Vacuolated lymphocytes, some with abnormal granulations	—	+
Mannosidosis	Vacuolated lymphocytes	Vacuolated lymphoid cells; inclusion bodies in granulocytes	(+)
Mucosulphatidosis	Abnormal granulations in lymphocytes and granulocytes	Buhot cells	(+)
Mucolipidosis I	Vacuolated lymphocytes	Foam cells	
I-cell disease	Vacuolated lymphocytes	Cells resembling osteoblasts	
Farber's	Impaired digestion of bacteria by leucocytes	Foam cells	+
Gaucher's	Occasional Gaucher cells	Gaucher cells, histiocytes	+
Niemann–Pick's	Occasional foam cells; vacuolated lymphocytes	Foam cells	+
Wolman's	Sudanophilic lipid in vacuolated lymphocytes	Foam cells	+

when solutions of acid albumin or detergents such as cetyltrimethylammonium chloride or cetylpyridinium chloride are added to urine. The resulting turbidity may be used as a measure of the concentration of the glycosaminoglycans, or the precipitate may be spun down and analysed chemically for its content of uronic acid. Detailed instructions on how to carry out some of the above tests are given by Thomas and Howell (1973), a critical assessment of the various techniques by Lewis, Kennedy and Raine (1973) and a review of glycosaminoglycan in infancy and childhood by Pennock, White, Murphy, Charles and Kerr (1973).

Of the dyes, alcian blue is now preferred to toluidine blue because of the lower specificity of the latter. Alcian blue may also be used to measure the urinary glycosaminoglycans colorimetrically (Whiteman 1973).

For most procedures 24-hour specimens of urine are recommended. Whiteman expresses his results as a glycosaminoglycan : creatinine ratio. In the widely used acid albumin turbidity test it is essential to dialyse the urine and to include a urine blank. Bacterial degradation of the glycosaminoglycans must be guarded against when collecting specimens.

Electrophoresis of urine concentrates on cellulose acetate yields characteristic patterns which are often helpful in pointing to a more precise diagnosis (Lewis, Kennedy and Raine 1973). In carrying out electrophoretic experiments it must be remembered that the urinary glycosaminoglycans excreted in excess in the mucopolysaccharidoses are partially degraded, and that their electrophoretic properties are not necessarily identical with those of standards prepared from animal tissues.

Urine has not been widely used in investigations of the sphingolipidoses. However, urinary deposit is an excellent source of exfoliated cellular elements and can be used for chemical analysis. The feasibility of this approach has been demonstrated by Desnick *et al.* (1971) but their methods are perhaps too complex for use in a routine laboratory (Table 12.6). Fortunately the sphingolipids in the urinary sediment are sufficiently stable for specimens to be posted to specialized centres. Comparatively simple tests for the assay of urinary arylsulphatase A for the diagnosis of metachromatic leucodystrophy, and of β-galactosidase for Landing's disease have been described by Thomas and Howell (1973). It is likely that assay of arylsulphatase will replace

Table 12.6 *Urinary sediment analysis in the diagnosis of disorders of the glycosphingolipids*
(Desnick *et al.* 1971)

Disease	Accumulated lipid	Relative increase times normal
Krabbe's leucodystrophy	Gal–Cer	77
Gaucher's disease		
Adult type	Glu–cer	5 to 15
Infantile type	Glu–cer	11
Lactosyl ceramidosis (see p. 516)	Gal–Clu–Cer	2
Fabry's disease	Gal–Gal–Glu–Cer	10 to 200
Sandhoff's disease	NAcGal–Gal–Gal–Glu–Cer	30
Metachromatic leucodystrophy	HSO_3–3–Gal–Cer	20 to 80

tests for the diagnosis of metachromatic leuco-dystrophy based on the rather capricious meta-chromasia of urinary cells when stained with cresyl violet.

Enzyme assays

Measurement of deficient enzyme is the only definitive way of establishing the diagnosis in a patient or, in favourable circumstances, the heterozygous status of a relative. Initially, labelled *natural* substrates had to be used and this made the tests very laborious. Fortunately, it is now possible to use a number of synthetic substrates for fluorimetric and spectrophoto-metric assays, e.g. in Fabry's disease (Brewster, Whaley and Kane 1974). When, as in Niemann–Pick's or Krabbe's disease and in some of the mucopolysaccharidoses, such substrates are not yet available, they are being actively sought.

In some disorders, of which Tay–Sachs disease is an example, the enzyme defect is only unmasked after separation of the isoenzymes by electro-phoresis (Westwood and Raine 1974), heat in-activation (O'Brien 1973) or pH inactivation (Saifer and Perle 1974).

Enzyme defects are usually ascertainable in leucocytes, fibroblasts and, occasionally, in the serum or even urine. Lysosomal enzymes are reasonably stable: cultured skin fibroblasts may be stored frozen at low temperatures, and this also applies, albeit to a somewhat lesser extent, to leucocytes. Acetone powder extracts have also been used successfully. It is therefore possible to send samples to reference centres regardless of distance.

Antenatal diagnosis

A remarkable development of the past decade has been the diagnosis of inherited metabolic disease in fetuses by amniocentesis. Amnio-centesis is usually performed at 14 to 18 weeks by the transabdominal route. It is advisable to identify the position of the placenta by ultra-sound to avoid a bloody tap. The fluid itself, uncultured and cultured cells have all been used in the diagnosis.

Amniotic fluid may be regarded, with some reservations, as fetal urine and tested at once for adventitious material such as excess of glyco-saminoglycans or sulphatide, and lack of enzyme activity, such as of hexosaminidase A in Tay–Sachs disease (Epstein, Brady, Schneider, Bradley and Shapiro 1971) or of α-glucosidase in Pompe's disease. While amniotic fluid itself is recom-mended by some authorities for the diagnosis of the adrenogenital syndrome it is unlikely to be widely used in lysosomal disorders, since it contains a number of constituents—cellular, mucoid and proteinaceous—of both maternal and fetal origin. This makes the interpretation of results extremely hazardous, with the possi-bility of both false positives and false negatives (Neufeld 1972).

Similar disadvantages attach, in most cases, to uncultured cells, some of which may also be of maternal origin. Again, if only one of two or more isoenzymes are deficient, assay of enzyme activity must be preceded by some fractionation or isolation procedures. When working with uncultured cells both the quantity and quality of the material available are likely to be inade-quate, but there is the advantage that results are obtained quickly.   At present it is considered essential to confirm any such results by enzyme assay on cultured cells from the same sample (Melancon and Nadler 1973).

Methods for the culture of amniotic fluid cells are now well worked out; a detailed description will be found, for example, in the review by Melancon and Nadler (1973).   Cultured cells may be examined by enzyme assay, morphologically by light, phase contrast or electron-microscopy, measurement of uptake of labelled substrate, cross correction studies (p. 519) and chemical analysis of stored metabolites.

Table 12.7   *Enzyme assays on cultured cells offered by specialized centres in the UK**

Disease	Enzyme deficiency
Fabry's disease	Ceramide trihexosidase
Fucosidosis	α-fucosidase
Gaucher's disease	Glucocerebrosidase
Krabbe's disease	Galactocerebrosidase
Landing's disease	G_{M1} galactosidase
Mannosidosis	α-mannosidase
Metachromatic leuco- dystrophy	Sulphatidase
MPS I (Hurler)	α-iduronidase
MPS II (Hunter)	Sulphoiduronate sulphatase
MPS III A (Sanfilippo)	Heparan sulphamidase
MPS III B (Sanfilippo)	α-acetylglycosaminidase
MPS I (Scheie)	α-iduronidase
MPS VI (Maroteaux– Lamy)	Arylsulphatase B
Niemann–Pick's disease	Sphingomyelinase
Pompe's disease	α-glucosidase (acid)
Refsum's disease	Phytanic acid α-oxidase
Sandhoff's disease	G_{M2} hexosaminidase A and B
Tay–Sachs disease	G_{M2} hexosaminidase A
Wolman's disease	Acid esterase

In most centres several of the above techniques are used concurrently and consecutively and diagnosis has usually been reliable.   Many of the procedures are, however, specialized and elaborate so that only a few laboratories, who are engaged in research on a particular disorder, are likely to be able to help.   For further details see Dorfman (1972), Harvey (1973) and Milunsky (1973).

Assays of lysosomal enzymes offered by centres in the United Kingdom are listed in Table 12.7. The Clinical Genetics Society publishes a list of

centres willing to carry out these assays.*   They emphasize that it is important to communicate early with the laboratory concerned to find out the current status of expertize in the field, the reliability of any diagnosis, the form in which material is to be submitted, and what biochemical, family and obstetric information is required.   In general, it is desirable that material should be sent to at least two centres who should know of each other.   All results should be ultimately confirmed on the fetus or infant.   An instance of successful joint investigation is the antenatally diagnosed case of Sanfilippo A syndrome (Harper *et al.* 1974).

Biochemical analysis of brain tissue

Before the advent of assays for specific lysosomal enzymes, biochemical analysis of brain tissue, obtained by biopsy or at necropsy, was indispensable in the diagnosis of the neurolipidoses.   In the United Kingdom this approach was closely associated with the name of the late Professor J. N. Cumings at the National Hospital, Queen Square.   Comparatively simple biochemical techniques in conjunction with histological examination were most effective in the differential diagnosis of patients with progressive dementia (Blackwood and Cumings 1959; Cumings 1965*a*, *b*).

Biopsy specimens and necropsy specimens removed within a few hours of death are frozen in dry ice and transported and stored in the frozen state until examined.   Analytical techniques include solvent extraction, usually with mixtures of methanol and chloroform, partition dialysis, thin layer chromatography on silica gel, and column chromatography on florisil and DEAE cellulose columns.   Fatty acid profiles are often determined by gas liquid chromatography of the methyl esters of the fatty acids.   Examples of these techniques will be found, for example, in various symposia (Aronson and Volk 1967; Bernsohn and Grossman 1971; Volk and Aronson 1972).   Today the major contribution of postmortem biochemical analysis of brain tissue is in research rather than diagnosis in which its place has increasingly been taken by enzyme assays on more readily available blood, urine or skin fibroblasts.   Brain biopsies for diagnostic purposes are nowadays hardly ever justified (p. 558).

* List available from Dr K. M. Laurence, The Welsh National School of Medicine, Heath Park, Cardiff.

Table 12.8 *Electrophysiological Investigations*

Disease	EEG	ERG	VEP	Nerve conduction
Tay–Sachs disease	Abnormal	Normal	Disappears	
Batten's disease				
Santavuori (type)	Abnormal	Disappears	Disappears	
Bielschowsky (type)	Abnormal	Disappears	Abnormal	
Spielmeyer (type)	Abnormal	Disappears	Disappears	
Leucodystrophy				
Krabbe's	Abnormal	Normal	May disappear	Abnormal
Metachromatic	Abnormal	Normal	May disappear	Abnormal
Mucopolysaccharidoses	Mild abnormality	Possible mild abnormality	Possible mild abnormality	
Fabry's disease	Abnormal			Abnormal

Electrophysiology*

Electroencephalography (EEG), studies of the visual system by means of electroretinography (ERG) (p. 511) and cortical visual evoked potentials (VEP), as well as peripheral nerve function tests can all provide valuable diagnostic information. The particular combinations of abnormalities will depend upon the distribution of the lesions of the various diseases within the nervous system.

EEG abnormalities will vary according to the stage of the disease at which the recording is made. The EEG changes at different stages of Tay–Sachs disease, Batten's disease and the leucodystrophies have been well documented (Pampiglione, Privett and Harden 1974; Santavuori, Haltia and Rapola 1974; Harden and Pampiglione 1975; Mastropaolo, Pampiglione and Stephens 1971; Wilson, Lake and Dunn 1969. Changes in Fabry's disease have been reported by Visser and de Groot (1970).

A simple technique for recording the ERG and VEP in small children and babies was described by Harden and Pampiglione (1970) and their experience of the evolution of the abnormalities of the evoked wave forms during the course of various progressive neurometabolic diseases in 82 patients with a verified diagnosis has been described in detail (Harden and Pampiglione 1975). These tests readily distinguish patients with retinal involvement or involvement of the cortical pathways.

Impaired function of the peripheral nerves can be diagnosed by measurements of the conduction velocity of motor and sensory fibres with reference to the normal values at different ages through childhood (Gamstorp 1963; Gamstorp and Shelburne 1965). Diseases causing most slowing of conduction velocity are those with segmental demyelination, notably the leucodystrophies (Fullerton 1964; Dunn, Lake, Dolman and Wilson 1969).

Characteristic patterns of the abnormalities in the storage diseases have been summarized in Table 12.8.

* We are indebted for these data to Dr Ann Harden and Dr Ruth Harris.

References

Adachi, M., Schneck, L., Cara, J. & Volk, B. W.   (1973) Spongy degeneration of the central nervous system (van Bogaert and Bertrand type, Canavan's disease). A review. *Human Pathology*, 4, 331-347.

Adachi, M., Schneck, L. & Volk, B. W.   (1974) Ultrastructural studies of eight cases of fetal Tay–Sachs disease. *Laboratory Investigation*, 30, 102-112.

Adachi, M., Schneck, L., Volk, B. W. & Torii, J.   (1970) Histochemical, ultrastructural and biochemical studies of a case with leucodystrophy due to congenital deficiency of myelin. *Journal of Neuropathology and Experimental Neurology*, 29, 149-150.

Adachi, M., Torii, J., Schneck, L. & Volk, B. W.   (1971) The fine structure of fetal Tay–Sachs disease. *Archives of Pathology*, 91, 48-54.

Adachi, M. & Volk, B. W.   (1968) Protracted form of spongy degeneration of the central nervous system (van Bogaert and Bertrand type), *Neurology (Minneapolis)*, 18, 1084-1092.

Adachi, M., Wallace, B. J., Schneck, L. & Volk, B. W.   (1967) Fine structure of central nervous system in early infantile Gaucher's disease. *Archives of Pathology*, 83, 513-526.

Adams, C. W. M.   (1965) *Neurohistochemistry*, Elsevier, Amsterdam.

Adams, C. W. M. & Leibowitz, S.   (1969) The general pathology of demyelinating diseases in *The Structure and Function of Nervous Tissue* (Ed. Bourne, G. H.), Vol. III, pp. 310-382, Academic Press, New York.

Aleu, F. P., Terry, R. D. & Zellweger, H.   (1965) Electronmicroscopy of two cerebral biopsies in gargoylism. *Journal of Neuropathology and Experimental Neurology*, 24, 304-317.

Alexander, W. S.   (1949) Progressive fibrinoid degeneration of fibrillary astrocytes. *Brain*, 72, 373-381.

Altay, C. & Say, B.   (1973) Case report. Three siblings with atypical mucopolysaccharidosis. *Acta paediatrica scandinavica*, 62, 73-76.

Andersen, H. A. & Palludan, B.   (1968) Leucodystrophy in mink. *Acta Neuropathologica (Berlin)*, 11, 347-360.

Aquilar, M. J., Chadwick, D. L., Okuyama, K. & Kamoshita, S.   (1966) Kinky hair disease. *Journal of Neuropathology and Experimental Neurology*, 25, 507-522.

Armstrong, D., Dimmitt, S., Grider, L., van Wormer, D. & Austin, J.   (1973) Deficient leucocyte peroxidase activity in the Batten–Spielmeyer–Vogt syndrome. *Transactions of the American Neurological Association*, 98, 3-10.

Armstrong, D., Dimmitt, S. & van Wormer, D. E.   (1974) Studies in Batten disease. I. Peroxidase deficiency in granulocytes. *Archives of Neurology (Chicago)*, 30, 144-152.

Aronson, S. M. & Volk, B. W.   (1967) *Inborn Disorders of Sphingolipid Metabolism*, Pergamon, Oxford.

Arstila, A. W., Palo, J., Haltia, M., Riekkinen, P. & Autio, S.   (1972) Aspartylglucosaminuria I: Fine structural studies on liver, kidney and brain. *Acta Neuropathologica (Berlin)*, 20, 207-216.

Aurebeck, G., Osterberg, K., Blaw, M., Chou, S. & Nelson, E.   (1964) Electronmicroscopic observations on metachromatic leucodystrophy. *Archives of Neurology (Chicago)*, 11, 273-288.

Austin, J. H. & Lehfeldt, D.   (1965) Studies in globoid (Krabbe) leucodystrophy. III. Significance of experimentally-produced globoid-like elements in rat white matter and spleen. *Journal of Neuropathology and Experimental Neurology*, 24, 265-289.

Autio, S.   (1972) Aspartylglucosaminuria. *Journal of Mental Deficiency Research*, Monograph No. 1.

Autio, S., Nordén, N. E., Öckerman, P.-A., Riekkinen, P., Rapola, J. & Louhimo, T.   (1973) Mannosidosis: clinical, fine-structural and biochemical findings in three cases. *Acta paediatrica scandinavica*, 62, 555-565.

Batzdorf, U., Sarlieve, L. L., Gold, V. A. & Menkes, J. H.   (1969) Demonstration of stored ganglioside in cultured cells from brain biopsy. *Archives of Neurology (Chicago)*, 20, 650-652.

Baumann, N. A., Jacque, C. M., Pollet, S. A. & Harpin, M. L.   (1968) Fatty acid and lipid composition of the brain of a myelin deficient mutant, the 'Quaking' mouse. *European Journal of Biochemistry*, 4, 340-344.

Benson, P. F.   (1974) Enzyme defects of glycosaminoglycan degradation in the mucopolysaccharidoses. *Developmental Medicine and Child Neurology*, 16, 534-539.

Berard, M., Toga, M., Bernard, P., Dubois, P., Mariani, R. & Hassoun, H.   (1968) Pathological findings in one case of neuronal and mesenchymal storage disease. Its relationship to lipidoses and mucopolysaccharidoses. *Pathologia europaea*, 3, 172-183.

Berenson, G. S. & Greer, J. C.   (1963) Heart disease in the Hurler and Marfan syndrome.   *Archives of Internal Medicine*, **111**, 58-69.

Berman, E. R., Livni, N., Shapira, E., Merin, S. & Levij, I. S.   (1974) Congenital corneal clouding with abnormal systemic storage bodies: a new variant of mucolipidosis.   *Journal of Pediatrics*. **84**, 519-526.

Bernsohn, J. & Grossman, H. J.   (1971) *Lipid Storage Diseases: Enzymatic Defects and Clinical Implications*, Academic Press, New York.

Betts, T. A., Smith, W. T. & Kelly, R. E.   (1968) Adult metachromatic leucodystrophy (sulphatide lipidosis) simulating acute schizophrenia.   Report of a case.   *Neurology (Minneapolis)*, **18**, 1140-1142.

Bielschowsky, M.   (1920-21) Zur Histopathologie und Pathogenese der amaurotischen Idiotie mit besonderer Berücksichtigung der zerebellaren Veränderungen.   *Journal für Psychologie und Neurologie (Leipzig)*, **26**, 123-199.

Bischoff, A., Fierz, V., Regli, F. & Ulrich, I.   (1968) Peripher-neurologische Störungen bei der Fabryschen Krankheit (Angiokeratoma corporis diffusum universale).   *Klinische Wochenschrift*, **46**, 666-671.

Bischoff, A. Reutter, F. W. & Wegmann, T.   (1967) Erkrankung des peripheren Nervensystems beim Morbus Gaucher.   *Schweizerische medizinische Wochenschrift*, **97**, 1139-1146.

Bischoff, A. & Ulrich, J.   (1969) Peripheral neuropathy in globoid cell leukodystrophy (Krabbe's disease). Ultrastructural and histochemical findings.   *Brain*, **92**, 861-870.

Blackwood, W. & Cumings, J. N.   (1959) Diagnostic cortical biopsy.   A histological and chemical study. *Lancet*, **2**, 23-24.

Blaw, M. E.   (1970) Melanodermic type leukodystrophy in *Handbook of Clinical Neurology* (Eds. Vinken, P. J. & Bruyn, G. W.), Vol. 10, pp. 128-133, North Holland Publishing Co., Amsterdam.

Bodian, M. & Lake, B. D.   (1963) The rectal approach to neuropathology.   *British Journal of Surgery*, **50**, 702-714.

Boehme, D. H., Cottrell, J. C., Leonberg, S. C. & Zeman, W.   (1971) A dominant form of neuronal ceroid-lipofuscinosis.   *Brain*, **94**, 745-760.

Bogaert, L. van   (1970) Familial type of orthochromatic leucodystrophies with diffuse leptomeningeal angiomatosis in *Handbook of Clinical Neurology* (Eds. Vinken, P. J. & Bruyn, G. W.), Vol. 10, pp. 120-127, North Holland Publishing Co., Amsterdam.

Bogaert, L. van & Bertrand, I.   (1967) *Spongy Degeneration of the Brain in Infancy*, North Holland Publishing Co., Amsterdam.

Bogaert, L. van, Scherer, H. J. & Epstein, E.   (1937) *Une Forme Cérébrale de la Cholestérinose Généralisée*, Masson, Paris.

Boies, L. R.   (1963) Tay–Sachs disease in its relation to otolaryngology.   *Archives of Otolaryngology*, **77**, 166-173.

Bordiuk, J. M., Legato, M. J., Lovelace, R. E. & Blumenthal, S.   (1970) Pompe's disease.   Electromyographic, electron microscopic and cardiovascular aspects.   *Archives of Neurology (Chicago)*, **23**, 113-119.

Bourgeois, J., Galy, G., Baltassat, P. & Béthenod, M.   (1974) Maladie de Menkes.   Étude du métabolisme du cuivre dans une observation personelle.   *Pédiatrie*, **29**, 573-594.

Brady, R. O.   (1973) The abnormal biochemistry of inherited disorders of lipid metabolism.   *Federation Proceedings*, **32**, 1660-1667.

Brain, W. R. & Greenfield, J. G.   (1950) Late infantile metachromatic leucoencephalopathy with primary degeneration of the interfascicular oligodendroglia.   *Brain*, **73**, 291-317.

Brett, E. M., Ellis, R. B., Haas, L., Ikonne, J. U., Lake, B. D., Patrick, A. D. & Stephens, R.   (1973) Late onset G_{M2}-gangliosidosis clinical, pathological, and biochemical studies on eight patients.   *Archives of Disease in Childhood*, **48**, 775-785.

Brewster, M. A., Whaley, S. A. & Kane, A. C.   (1974) Variables in the laboratory diagnosis of Fabry's disease by measurement of methylumbelliferyl-α-galactosidase.   *Clinical Chemistry*, **20**, 383-386.

Briggs, J. N. & Haworth, J. C.   (1964) Liver glycogen disease.   Report of a case of hyperuricemia, renal calculi and no demonstrable enzyme defect.   *American Journal of Medicine*, **36**, 443-449.

Brown, N. J., Corner, B. D. & Dodgson, M. C. H.   (1954) A second case in the same family of congenital familial cerebral lipidosis resembling amaurotic family idiocy.   *Archives of Disease in Childhood*, **29**, 48-54.

Bruens, J. H., Guazzi, G. C. & Martin, J. J.   (1968) Infantile form of meningeal angiomatosis with sudanophilic leucodystrophy associated with complex abiotrophies.   Study of a second family.   *Journal of the Neurological Sciences*, **7**, 417-425.

Burke, J. A. & Schubert, W. K.   (1971) Deficient activity of acid lipase in cholesterol-ester storage disease. *Journal of Laboratory and Clinical Medicine*, **78**, 988-989.

Callahan, W. P., Hackett, R. L. & Lorincz, A. E.   (1967) New observations by light microscopy on liver histology in the Hurler's syndrome. A needle biopsy study of 11 patients using plastic embedded tissue. *Archives of Pathology*, **83**, 507-512.

Callahan, W. P. & Lorincz, A. E. (1966) Hepatic ultrastructure in the Hurler syndrome. *American Journal of Pathology*, **48**, 277-298.

Carr, R. E. & Gouras, P. (1966) Clinical electroretinography. *Journal of the American Medical Association*, **198**, 173-176.

Chiari, H. (1933) Über Veränderungen im Zentralnervensystem bei generalisierter Xantomatose vom Typus Schüller–Christian. *Virchows Archiv für pathologische Anatomie*, **288**, 527-553.

Chou, L., Kaye, C. I. & Nadler, H. L. (1974) Brian β-galactosidase and G$_{M1}$ gangliosidosis. *Pediatric Research*, **8**, 120-125.

Chou, S. M. & Thompson, H. G. (1970) Electron microscopy of storage cytosomes in Kufs' disease. *Archives of Neurology (Chicago)*, **23**, 489-501.

Christensen Lou, H. O. & Reske-Nielsen, E. (1971) The central nervous system in Fabry's disease. *Archives of Neurology (Chicago)*, **25**, 351-359.

Clausen, J. & Rampini, S. (1970) Chemical studies in Farber's disease. *Acta neurologica scandinavica*, **46**, 313-322.

Constantopoulos, G., Louie, M. & Dekaban, A. E. (1973) Acid mucopolysaccharides (glycosaminoglycans) in normal human kidneys and in kidneys of patients with mucopolysaccharidoses. *Biochemical Medicine*, **7**, 376-388.

Cravioto, H., O'Brien, J. S., Landing, B. H. & Finck, B. (1966) Ultrastructure of peripheral nerve in metachromatic leucodystrophy. *Acta Neuropathologica (Berlin)*, **7**, 111-124.

Crocker, A. C. (1961) The cerebral defect in Tay–Sachs disease and Niemann–Pick disease. *Journal of Neurochemistry*, **7**, 69-80.

Crocker, A. C., Cohen, J. & Farber, S. (1967) The 'lipogranulomatosis' syndrome; review with report of patient showing milder involvement in *Inborn Disorders of Sphingolipid Metabolism* (Eds. Aronson, S. M. & Volk, B. W.), pp. 485-503, Pergamon, Oxford.

Crocker, A. C., Vanter, G. F., Neuhauser, E. B. D. & Rosowsky, A. (1965) Wolman's disease: three new patients with a recently described lipidosis. *Pediatrics*, **35**, 627-640.

Crome, L. (1962) The association of phenylketonuria with leucodystrophy. *Journal of Neurology, Neurosurgery and Psychiatry*, **25**, 149-153.

Crome, L., Cumings, J. N. & Duckett, S. (1963) Neuropathological and neurochemical aspects of generalized glycogen storage disease. *Journal of Neurology, Neurosurgery and Psychiatry*, **26**, 422-430.

Crome, L., Hanefeld, F., Patrick, D. & Wilson, J. (1973) Late onset globoid cell leucodystrophy. *Brain*, **96**, 841-848.

Crome, L. & Stern, J. (1972) Disorders of gestation in *Pathology of Mental Retardation*, 2nd Edn., pp. 62-63, Churchill Livingstone, Edinburgh & London.

Crome, L. & Zapella, M. (1963) Schilder's disease (sudanophilic leucodystrophy) in five male members of one family. *Journal of Neurology, Neurosurgery and Psychiatry*, **26**, 431-438.

Cumings, J. N. (1965a) Cerebral lipid biochemistry in the demyelinations in *Biochemical Aspects of Neurological Disorders* (Eds. Cumings, J. N. & Kremer, M.), pp. 229-251, Blackwell Scientific, Oxford.

Cumings, J. N. (1965b) Some lipid diseases of the brain. *Proceedings of the Royal Society of Medicine*, **58**, 21-28.

Cureton, R. J. R. (1949) A case of intracerebral xanthomatosis with pituitary involvement. *Journal of Pathology and Bacteriology*, **61**, 533-540.

Cuzner, M. C., Davison, A. N. & Gregson, N. A. (1965) Chemical and metabolic studies of rat myelin of the central nervous system. *Annals of the New York Academy of Science*, **122**, 86-94.

Dacremont, G., Kint, J. A., Carton, D. & Cocquyt, G. (1974) Glucosylceramide in plasma of patients with Niemann–Pick disease. *Clinica chimica Acta*, **52**, 365-367.

Dacremont, G., Kint, J. A. & Coquyt, G. (1974) Brain sphingolipids in I-cell disease (mucolipidosis II). *Journal of Neurochemistry*, **22**, 599-602.

Danes, B. S. (1974) In vitro confirmation of genetic compound of the Hurler and Scheie compounds. *Lancet*, **1**, 680.

Danes, B. S. & Grossman, H. (1969) Bone dysplasias, including Morquio's syndrome, studied in skin fibroblast cultures. *American Journal of Medicine*, **47**, 708-720.

Danks, D. M., Stevens, B. J., Campbell, P. E., Gillespie, J. M., Walker-Smith, J., Blomfield, J. & Turner, B. (1972) Menkes' kinky-hair syndrome. *Lancet*, **1**, 1100-1103.

Davison, A. N. & Peters, A. (1970) *Myelination*, Thomas, Springfield, Ill.

Dawson, G., Matalon, R. & Stein, A. O. (1971) Lactosylceramidosis: lactosylceramide galactosyl hydrolase deficiency and accumulation of lactosylceramide in cultured skin fibroblasts. *Journal of Pediatrics*, **79**, 423-429.

Dawson, G. & Spranger, J. W. (1971) Fucosidosis: a glycosphingolipidosis. *New England Journal of Medicine*, **285**, 122.

Dawson, R. M. C. (1966) Phosphoinositides in nervous tissue. *Biochemical Journal*, **98**, 19P.

Dayan, A. D. & Trickey, R. J. (1970) Thyroid involvement in juvenile amaurotic family idiocy (Batten's disease). *Lancet*, **2**, 296-297.

Dekaban, A. S. & Constantopoulos, G. (1973) Mucopolysaccharidoses. Relation of elevated cerebral spinal fluid to mental retardation. *Archives of Neurology* (*Chicago*), **28**, 385-388.

Dekaban, A. S. & Herman, M. M. (1974) Childhood, juvenile and adult cerebral lipidoses. Are they different nosological entities? *Archives of Pathology*, **97**, 65-73.

De Leon, G. A., Kaback, M. M., Elfenbein, I. B., Percy, A. K. & Brady, R. O. (1969) Juvenile dystonic lipidosis. *Johns Hopkins Hospital Medical Journal*, **125**, 62-77.

Den Tandt, W. R. & Giesberts, M. A. H. (1973) Deficiency of lysosomal enzymes in storage diseases. *Biochemical Medicine*, **7**, 441-451.

Desnick, R. J., Dawson, G., Desnick, S. J., Sweeley, C. C. & Krivit, W. (1971) Diagnosis of glycosphingolipidoses by urinary-sediment analysis. *New England Journal of Medicine*, **284**, 739-744.

De Vries, E. (1968) A case of the adult form of amaurotic idiocy, diagnosed during life as Huntington's chorea. *Psychiatria, Neurologia, Neurochirurgia, Netherlands*, **71**, 203-209.

Diezel, P. B. (1955) Histochemische Untersuchungen an den Globoidzellen der familiären infantilen diffusen Sklerose vom Typus Krabbe. (Zugleich eine differentialdiagnostische Betrachtung der zentralnervösen Veränderung beim Morbus Gaucher.) *Virchows Archiv für pathologische Anatomie*, **327**, 206-228.

Diezel, P. B., Koppang, N. & Rossner, J. A. (1965) Fermenthistochemische und elektronenmikroskopische Untersuchungen an der juvenilen amaurotischen Idiotie des Hundes. *Deutsche Zeitschrift für Nervenheilkunde*, **187**, 720-736.

Diezel, P. B. & Richardson, E. P. (1957) Histochemical and neuropathological studies in leukodystrophy (degenerative diffuse cerebral sclerosis, Scholz, Bielschowsky and Henneberg type). *Journal of Neuropathology and Experimental Neurology*, **16**, 130-131.

Dincsoy, M. Y., Dincsoy, H. P., Kessler, A. D., Jackson, M. A. & Sidbury, J. B. (1965) Generalized glycogenosis and associated endocardial fibroelastosis. Report of 3 cases with biochemical studies. *Journal of Pediatrics*, **67**, 728-740.

Dolman, C. L., Chang, E. & Duke, R. J. (1973) Pathologic findings in Sandhoff disease. *Archives of Pathology*, **96**, 272-275.

Donahue, S., Watanabe, I. & Zeman, W. (1968) Morphology of leucocytic hypergranulation in Batten's disease. *Annals of the New York Academy of Science*, **155**, 847-859.

Donnelly, W. J. C., Sheahan, B. J. & Rogers, T. A. (1973) G_{M1} gangliosidosis in Friesian calves. *Journal of Pathology*, **111**, 173-179.

Dorfman, A. (1972) *Antenatal Diagnosis*, University of Chicago Press, Chicago.

Dorfman, A. & Matalon, R. (1972) The mucopolysaccharidoses in *The Metabolic Basis of Inherited Disease*, (Eds. Stanbury, J. B., Wyngaarden, J. B. & Fredrickson, D. S.), 3rd edn., pp. 1218-1272, McGraw-Hill, New York.

Drukker, A., Sachs, M. I. & Gatt, S. (1970) The infantile form of Gaucher's disease in an infant of Jewish Sephardic origin. *Pediatrics*, **45**, 1017-1023.

Duckett, S., Cracco, J., Lublin, F. & Scott, T. (1974) Electron microscopical diagnosis of lipidosis with the use of rectal biopsy. *American Journal of Diseases of Children*, **127**, 704-705.

Duke, J. R. & Clark, D. B. (1962) Infantile amaurotic familial idiocy (Tay–Sachs disease) in the negro race. *American Journal of Ophthalmology*, **53**, 800-805.

Duncan, C. (1970) The renal lesion of angiokeratoma corporis diffusum (Fabry's disease): report of three cases including some electronmicroscopic findings. *Pathology*, **2**, 9-14.

Dunn, H. G., Lake, B. D., Dolman, C. L. & Wilson, J. (1969) The neuropathy of Krabbe's infantile cerebral sclerosis. *Brain*, **92**, 329-344.

Durand, P., Borrone, C. & Della Cella, G. (1969) Fucosidosis. *Journal of Pediatrics*, **75**, 665-674.

Dyggve, H. V., Melchior, J. C. & Clausen, J. (1962) Morquio–Ulrich's disease. An inborn error of metabolism? *Archives of Disease in Childhood*, **37**, 525-534.

Ebhardt, G., Cervós-Navarro, J. & Rey Pias, J. M. (1974) Alterations in non nervous cells of rectum mucosa in storage disease in *VIIth International Congress of Neuropathology*, Abstracts, p. 77, Akadémiai Kiadó, Budapest.

Eeg-Olofson, L., Kristensson, K., Sourander, P. & Svennerholm, L.   (1966) Tay–Sachs disease.   A generalised metabolic disorder.   *Acta paediatrica scandinavica*, **55**, 546-562.

Elfenbein, I. B.   (1968) Dystonic juvenile idiocy without amaurosis.   A new syndrome.   Light and electron microscopic observations of cerebrum.   *Johns Hopkins Medical Journal*, **123**, 205-221.

Elfenbein, I. B. & Cantor, H. E.   (1969) Late infantile amaurotic idiocy with multilamellar cytosomes: an electron microscopic study.   *Journal of Pediatrics*, **75**, 253-264.

Ellis, R. B.   (1974) Carrier detection and prenatal diagnosis of Tay–Sachs disease.   *Proceedings of the Royal Society of Medicine*, **67**, 1257.

Ellis, W. G., Nielsen, S. L., McCulloch, J. R. & Schneider, E. L.   (1974) Globoid cell development in globoid cell leukodystrophy (Krabbe's disease): an ultrastructural comparison of fetal, early infantile and late infantile lesions.   *Journal of Neuropathology and Experimental Neurology*, **53**, 568.

Emery, J. M., Green, W. R., Wyllie, R. G. & Howell, R. R.   (1971) G_{M1}-gangliosidosis.   Ocular and pathological manifestations.   *Archives of Ophthalmology*, **85**, 177-187.

Epstein, C. J., Brady, R. O., Schneider, E. L., Bradley, R. M. & Shapiro, D.   (1971) *In utero* diagnosis of Niemann–Pick disease.   *American Journal of Human Genetics*, **23**, 533-535.

Escola Picó, J.   (1964) Über die Ultrastruktur der Speichersubstanzen bei Spätfällen von familiärer amauro-tischen Idiotie.   *Acta Neuropathologica (Berlin)*, **3**, 309-318.

Esterly, N. B. & McKusick, V. A.   (1971) Stiff skin syndrome.   *Pediatrics*, **47**, 360-369.

Farber, S. (1952) A lipid metabolic disorder—disseminated lipogranulomatosis—a syndrome with similarity to, and important differences from, Niemann–Pick and Hand–Schüller–Christian disease.   *American Journal of Diseases of Children*, **84**, 499-500.

Farber, S., Cohen, J. & Uzman, L. L.   (1957) Lipogranulomatosis.   A new lipo-glyco-protein storage disease *Journal of Mount Sinai Hospital*, **24**, 816-837.

Fardeau, M. & Lapresle, J.   (1963) Maladie de Tay–Sachs avec atteinte importante de la substance blanche.   A propos de deux observations anatomo-cliniques.   *Revue neurologique*, **109**, 157-175.

Feigin, I.   (1956) Xanthomatosis of nervous system.   *Journal of Neuropathology and Experimental Neurology*, **15**, 400-416.

Fine, D. I. M., Barron, K. D. & Hirano, A.   (1960) Central nervous system lipidosis in an adult with atrophy of the cerebellar granular layer; a case report.   *Journal of Neuropathology and Experimental Neurology*, **19**, 355-369.

Fletcher, T. F., Kurtz, H. J. & Low, D. G.   (1966) Globoid cell leukodystrophy (Krabbe type) in the dog.   *Journal of the American Veterinary Medical Association*, **149**, 165-172.

Fletcher, T. F., Kurtz, H. J. & Stadlan, E. M.   (1971) Experimental Wallerian degeneration in peripheral nerve of dogs with globoid cell leukodystrophy.   *Journal of Neuropathology and Experimental Neurology*, **30**, 593-602.

Fontaine, G., Résibois, A., Tondeur, M., Jonniaux, G., Farriaux, J. P., Voet, W., Maillard, E. & Loeb, H.   (1973) Gangliosidosis with total hexosaminidase deficiency: clinical, biochemical and ultrastructural studies and comparison with conventional cases of Tay–Sachs disease.   *Acta Neuropathologica (Berlin)*, **23**, 118-132.

Forsyth, C. C., Forbes, M. & Cumings, J. N.   (1971) Adrenocortical atrophy and diffuse cerebral sclerosis.   *Archives of Disease in Childhood*, **46**, 273-284.

Fredrickson, D. S. & Sloan, H. R.   (1972a) Sphingomyelin lipidoses: Niemann–Pick disease in *Metabolic Basis of Inherited Disease* (Eds. Stanbury, J. B., Wyngaarden, J. B. & Fredrickson, D. S.), 3rd Edn., pp. 783-807, McGraw-Hill, New York.

Fredrickson, D. S. & Sloan, H. R.   (1972b) Glucosyl ceramide lipidoses: Gaucher's disease in *Metabolic Basis of Inherited Disease* (Eds. Stanbury, J. B., Wyngaarden, J. B. & Fredrickson, D. S.), 3rd Edn., pp. 730-759, McGraw-Hill, New York.

Freitag, F., Blümcke, S. & Spranger, J. W.   (1971) Hepatic ultrastructure in mucolipidosis I (lipomucopoly-saccharidosis).   *Virchows Archiv für pathologische Anatomie, Abt. B, Zellpathologie*, **7**, 189-204.

French, H. J., Sherard, E. S., Lubell, H., Brotz, M. & Moore, C.   (1972) Trichopoliodystrophy.   A report of a case and biochemical studies.   *Archives of Neurology (Chicago)*, **26**, 229-244.

Frost, P., Spaeth, G. L. & Tanaka, Y.   (1966) Fabry's disease: glycolipid lipidosis.   Skin manifestations.   *Archives of Internal Medicine*, **117**, 440-446.

Fullerton, P. M.   (1964) Peripheral nerve conduction in metachromatic leucodystrophy (sulphatide lipidosis).   *Journal of Neurology, Neurosurgery and Psychiatry*, **27**, 100-105.

Gamstorp, I.   (1963) Normal conduction velocity of ulnar, median and peroneal nerves in infancy, childhood and adolescence.   *Acta paediatrica (Uppsala)*, *Suppl. 146*, 68-78.

Gamstorp, I. & Shelburne, S. A.   (1965) Peripheral sensory conduction in ulnar and median nerves of normal infants, children and adolescents.   *Acta paediatrica scandinavica*, **54**, 309-313.

Ghatak, N. R., Poon, T. P., Hirano, A. & French, J. (1969) Kinky hair disease. Neuropathologic findings and electron microscopic study of skeletal muscle. *Journal of Neuropathology and Experimental Neurology*, **28**, 157.

Giampalmo, A. (1954) Les lipidoses cholestériniques du système nerveux. *Acta neurologica belgica*, **54**, 786-808.

Gilles, F. H. & Deuel, R. K. (1971) Neuronal cytoplasmic globules in the brain in Morquio's syndrome. *Archives of Neurology (Chicago)*, **25**, 293-403.

Glomset, J. A. (1962) The mechanism of the plasma cholesterol esterification reaction: plasma fatty acid esterase. *Biochimica et biophysica Acta (Amsterdam)*, **65**, 128-135.

Goldberg, M. F. & Duke, J. R. (1967) Ocular histopathology in Hunter's syndrome. Systemic mucopolysaccharidosis type II. *Archives of Ophthalmology*, **77**, 503-512.

Goldstein, I. & Wexler, D. (1931) Niemann–Pick disease with cherry-red spots in the macula: ocular pathology. *Archives of Ophthalmology*, **5**, 704-716.

Gordon, N. & Marsden, H. B. (1966) Diffuse cerebral sclerosis and adrenal atrophy. *Developmental Medicine and Child Neurology*, **8**, 719-723.

Greenfield, J. G., Aring, C. D. & Landing, B. H. (1955) Clinical pathologic conference. *Neurology (Minneapolis)*, **5**, 732-739.

Grégoire, A., Périer, O. & Dustin, P. (1966) Metachromatic leucodystrophy, an electron microscopic study. *Journal of Neuropathology and Experimental Neurology*, **25**, 617-636.

Groover, R. V., Burke, E. C., Gordon, H. & Berdon, W. E. (1972) The genetic mucopolysaccharidoses. *Seminars in Hematology*, **9**, 371-402.

Guazzi, G. C. & Martin, J. J. (1967) La forme infantile de la leucodystrophie soudanophile avec angiomatose méningée non calcifiante. *Acta neurologica belgica*, **67**, 463-474.

Guazzi, G. C., Martin, J. J., Philippart, M., Roels, H., Van der Eecken, H., Vrints, L., Delbeke, M. J. & Hooft, C. (1968) Wolman's disease. *European Neurology*, **1**, 334-362.

Gulotta, F., Heyer, R., Tropitzsch, G., Hormes, R. & Citoler, P. (1970) Ungewöhnliche orthochromatische Leucodystrophie bei drei Geschwistern. *Neuropädiatrie*, **2**, 173-186.

Gustavson, K.-H. & Hagberg, B. (1971) The incidence and genetics of metachromatic leucodystrophy in Northern Sweden. *Acta paediatrica scandinavica*, **60**, 585-590.

Haberland, C. & Brunngraber, E. G. (1970) Early infantile neurolipidosis with failure of myelination. *Archives of Neurology (Chicago)*, **23**, 481-488.

Haberland, C., Brunngraber, E., Witting, L. & Brown, B. (1973) The white matter in G_{M2} gangliosidosis. A comparative histopathological and biochemical study. *Acta Neuropathologica (Berlin)*, **24**, 43-55.

Haberland, C., Brunngraber, E., Witting, L. & Daniels, A. (1973) Juvenile metachromatic leucodystrophy. Case report with clinical, histopathological, ultrastructural and biochemical observations. *Acta Neuropathologica (Berlin)*, **26**, 93-106.

Haebara, H., Hazama, F. & Amano, S. (1974) Neural involvement in Fabry's disease in *VIIth International Congress of Neuropathology*, Abstracts, p. 121, Akadémiai Kiadó, Budapest.

Hagberg, B., Sourander, P. & Svennerholm, L. (1963) Diagnosis of Krabbe's infantile leucodystrophy. *Journal of Neurology, Neurosurgery and Psychiatry*, **26**, 195-198.

Hagen, L. O. (1953) Lipid dystrophic changes in central nervous system in dogs. *Acta pathologica et microbiologica scandinavica*, **33**, 22-35.

Hall, C. W., Cantz, M. & Neufeld, E. F. (1973) β-glucuronidase deficiency mucopolysaccharidosis: studies in cultured fibroblasts. *Archives of Biochemistry and Biophysics*, **155**, 32-38.

Haltia, M. & Palo, J. (1974) Aspartylglycosaminuria: a generalised storage disease in *VIIth International Congress of Neuropathology*, Abstracts, p. 122, Akadémiai Kiadó, Budapest.

Haltia, M., Rapola, J. Santavuori, P. & Keränen, A. (1973) Infantile type of so-called neuronal ceroid-lipofuscinosis. Part 2. Morphological and biochemical studies. *Journal of the Neurological Sciences*, **18**, 269-285.

Hanai, J., Leroy, J. & O'Brien, J. S. (1971) Ultrastructure of cultured fibroblasts in I-cell disease. *American Journal of Diseases of Children*, **122**, 34-38.

Hanefeld, F. & Crome, L. (1971) Histochemistry of Krabbe's disease. *Lancet*, **1**, 195.

Harden, A. & Pampiglione, G. (1970) Neurophysiological approach to disorders of vision. *Lancet*, **1**, 805-809.

Harden, A. & Pampiglione, G. (1975) VEP/ERG/EEG studies in progressive neurometabolic 'storage' diseases in *Proceedings of the International Symposium on Cerebral Evoked Potentials in Man*, Brussels, 1974.

Harper, P. S., Laurence, K. M., Parkes, A., Wusteman, F. S., Kresse, H., Von Figura, K., Ferguson-Smith, M. A., Duncan, D. M., Logan, R. W., Hall, F. & Whiteman, P. (1974) Sanfilippo A disease in the fetus. *Journal of Medical Genetics*, **11**, 123-132.

Hartley, W. J. & Blakemore, W. F. (1973) Neurovisceral storage and dysmyelogenesis in neonatal goats. *Acta Neuropathologica (Berlin)*, **25**, 325-333.

Harvey, D. (1973) Biochemical aspects of prenatal diagnosis. *British Journal of Hospital Medicine*, **10**, 591-594.

Harzer, K. & Benz, H. V. (1973) Quantitative Metachromasie mit Pseudoisocyanin: Eine neue Methode zur Bestimmung von Sulfatiden sowie ihre Anwendung bei der Diagnose der Metachromatischen Leukodystrophie (Sulfatid-Lipidose). *Zeitschrift für klinische Chemie und klinische Biochemie*, **11**, 471-475.

Henderson, J. L., MacGregor, A. R., Thannhauser, S. J. & Holden, R. (1952) The pathology and biochemistry of gargoylism. A report of three cases with a review of the literature. *Archives of Disease in Childhood*, **27**, 230-253.

Henschen, F. (1931) Über Christians Syndrom und dessen Beziehungen zur allgemeinen Xanthomatose. *Acta paediatrica (Uppsala)*, **12** (*Suppl. 6*), 1-93.

Hernandez, A., Marchesi, V., Goldring, D., Kissane, J. & Hartmann, A. F. (1966) Cardiac glycogenosis. Hemodynamic, angiocardiographic, and electron microscopic findings—report of a case. *Journal of Paediatrics*, **68**, 400-412.

Herndon, R. M. & Rubinstein, L. J. (1968) Leucodystrophy with Rosenthal fibers (Alexander's disease): a histochemical and electron microscopic study. *Neurology (Minneapolis)*, **18**, 300.

Herndon, R. M., Rubinstein, L. J., Freeman, J. M. & Mathieson, G. (1970) Light and electron microscopic observations on Rosenthal fibers in Alexander's disease and in multiple sclerosis. *Journal of Neuropathology and Experimental Neurology*, **29**, 524-551.

Hers, H. G. (1965) Inborn lysosomal diseases. *Gastroenterology*, **48**, 625-633.

Hers, H. G. (1973) The concept of inborn lysosomal disease in *Lysosomes and Storage Diseases* (Eds. Hers, H. G. & van Hoof, F.), pp. 148-171. Academic Press, New York and London.

Hers, H. G. & De Barsy, T. (1973) Type II glycogenosis (acid maltase deficiency) in *Lysosomes and Storage Diseases* (Eds. Hers, H. G. & van Hoof, F.), pp. 197-216, Academic Press, New York and London.

Hers, H. G. & van Hoof, F. (1969) Genetic abnormalities of lysosomes in *Lysosomes in Biology and Pathology*, (Eds. Dingle, J. T. & Fell, H. B.), Vol II, pp. 19-40, North Holland Publishing Co., Amsterdam.

Hers, H. G. & van Hoof, F. (1970) The genetic pathology of lysosomes. *Progress in Liver Disease*, **3**, 185-205.

Hers, H. G. & van Hoof, F. (1973) *Lysosomes and Storage Diseases*, Academic Press, New York and London.

Herschkowitz, N. N. (1973) Genetic disorders of brain development: animal models in *Biology of Brain Dysfunction* (Ed. Gaull, G. E.), Vol. 2, pp. 151-184, Plenum Press, New York and London.

Heyne, K., Kemmer, Ch., Simon, Ch. & Kasper, J. M. (1974) Struktur und diagnostische Bedeutung von Leukozyten bei Neurolipidosen. *Kinderärztliche Praxis*, **42**, 216-222.

Hirth, R. S. & Nielsen, S. W. (1967) A familial canine globoid cell leukodystrophy (Krabbe type). *Journal of Small Animal Practice*, **8**, 569-575.

Hocking, J. D., Jolly, R. D. & Batt, R. D. (1972) Deficiency of mannosidase in Angus cattle. An inherited lysosomal storage disease. *Biochemical Journal*, **128**, 69-78.

Hoefnagel, D., Brun, A., Ingbar, S. H. & Goldman, H. (1967) Addison's disease and diffuse cerebral sclerosis. *Journal of Neurology, Neurosurgery and Psychiatry*, **30**, 56-60.

Hogan, C. R., Gutmann, L. & Chou, S. M. (1969) The peripheral neuropathy of Krabbe's (globoid) leukodystrophy. *Neurology (Minneapolis)*, **19**, 1094-1100.

Hogan, E. L., Joseph, K. C., Hurt, J. P. & Krigman, M. R. (1972) Schilder's diffuse sclerosis: a biochemical and ultrastructural study of myelinoclastic demyelination. *Acta Neuropathologica (Berlin)*, **20**, 85-95.

Hollister, D. W., Rimoin, D. L., Lachman, R. S., Cohen, A. H., Reed, W. B. & Westin, G. W. (1974) The Winchester syndrome: a nonlysosomal connective tissue disease. *Journal of Pediatrics*, **84**, 701-709.

Horton, W. A. & Schimke, R. N. (1970) A new mucopolysaccharidosis. *Journal of Pediatrics*, **77**, 252-258.

Howell, J. McC. (1970) Diseases affecting myelination in domestic animals in *Myelination* (Eds. Davison, A. N. & Peters, A.), pp. 199-228, Thomas, Springfield, Ill.

Hug, G., Garancis, J. C., Schubert, W. K. & Kaplan, S. (1966) Glycogen storage disease, types 2, 3, 8 and 9. A biochemical and electronmicroscopic analysis. *American Journal of Diseases of Children*, **111**, 457-474.

Hug, G., Schubert, W. K. & Soukup, S. (1972) Type II glycogenosis: ultrastructure of amniotic fluid cells in *Antenatal Diagnosis* (Ed. Dorfman, A.), pp. 165-172, University of Chicago Press, Chicago.

Jackson, D. C. & Simon, G. (1965) Unusual bone and lung changes in a case of Gaucher's disease. *British Journal of Radiology*, **38**, 698-700.

Jacque, C. M., Harpin, M. L. & Baumann, N. A. (1969) Brain lipid analysis of a myelin deficient mutant, the quaking mouse. *European Journal of Biochemistry*, **11**, 218-224.

Janota, I. (1974) Spongy degeneration of grey matter in 3 children. Neuropathological report. *Archives of Disease in Childhood*, **49**, 571-575.

Jervis, G. A. (1957) Degenerative encephalopathy of childhood. Cortical degeneration, cerebellar atrophy, cholesterinosis of basal ganglia. *Journal of Neuropathology and Experimental Neurology*, **16**, 308-320.

Jolly, R. D. (1970) Diagnosis and control of pseudolipidosis of Angus calves. *New Zealand Veterinary Journal*, **18**, 228-229.

Jolly, R. D. (1971) The pathology of the central nervous system in pseudolipidosis of Angus calves. *Journal of Pathology*, **103**, 113-121.

Jolly, R. D. & Blakemore, W. F. (1973) Inherited lysosomal storage diseases: an essay in comparative medicine. *Veterinary Record*, **92**, 391-400.

Joosten, E. M. G., Krijgsman, J. B., Gabreëls-Festen, A. A. W. M., Gabreëls, F. J. M. & Baars, P. E. C. (1974) Infantile globoid cell leucodystrophy: some remarks on clinical, biochemical and sural nerve biopsy findings. *Neuropädiatrie*, **5**, 191-209.

Kahana D., Berant, M. & Wolman, M. (1968) Primary familial xanthomatosis with adrenal involvement (Wolman's disease). Report of a further case with nervous system involvement and pathogenetic considerations. *Pediatrics*, **42**, 70-76.

Kamoshita, S. & Landing, B. H. (1968) Distribution of lesions in myenteric plexus and gastrointestinal mucosa in lipidoses and other neurologic disorders of children. *American Journal of Clinical Pathology*, **49**, 312-318.

Karle, E. & Schiefer, B. (1967) Familial amaurotic idiocy in male German shorthair pointers. *Pathologia veterinaria*, **4**, 223-232.

Kaufman, R. L., Rimoin, D. L. & McAlister, W. H. (1971) The Dyggve–Melchior–Clausen syndrome. *Birth Defects: Original Article Series* (Ed. Bergsma, D.), Vol. 7, pp. 144-149, The National Foundation—March of Dimes, New York.

Kearns, T. P. & Sayre, G. P. (1958) Retinitis pigmentosa, external ophthalmoplegia and complete heart block. *Archives of Ophthalmology* **60**, 183.

Kelemen G. (1965) Tay–Sachs Krankheit und Gehörorgan. *Zeitschrift für Laryngologie und Rhinologie*, **44**, 728-738.

Kidd, M. (1967) An electronmicroscopical study of a case of atypical cerebral lipidosis. *Acta Neuropathologica (Berlin)*, **9**, 70-78.

Kjellman, B., Gamstorp, I., Brun, A. & Palmgren, G. (1969) Mannosidosis: a clinical and histopathological study. *Journal of Pediatrics*, **75**, 366-373.

Kolkmann, F.-W., Rana, B. N. & Nützenadel, W. (1971) Zur Frage der Beziehungen zwischen Morbus Canavan (infantile spongiöse Neurodystrophie van Bogaert-Bertrand) und Pelizaeus-Merzbachersche Krankheit. Kasuistischer, feinstruktureller und zytochemischer Beitrag. *Neuropädiatrie*, **2**, 305-324.

Kornfeld, M. (1971) Electron microscopic observation of neurovisceral thesaurismosis in an adult (Kufs type of amaurotic family idiocy with visceral involvement). *Journal of Neuropathology and Experimental Neurology*, **30**, 144.

Kresse, H. & Neufeld, E. F. (1972) The Sanfilippo A corrective factor. Purification and mode of action. *Journal of Biological Chemistry*, **247**, 2164.

Kristensson, K., Olsson, Y. & Sourander, P. (1967) Peripheral nerve change in Tay–Sachs and Batten–Spielmeyer–Vogt disease. *Acta pathologica et microbiologica scandinavica*, **70**, 630-632.

Kristensson, K., Rayner, S. & Sourander, P. (1965) Visceral involvement in juvenile amaurotic idiocy. *Acta Neuropathologica (Berlin)*, **4**, 421-424.

Krivit, W., Desnick, R. J., Lee, I., Moller, J., Wright, F., Sweeley, C. C., Snyder, P. D. & Sharp, H. L. (1972) Generalised accumulation of neutral glycosphingolipids with G_{M2} ganglioside accumulation in the brain. *American Journal of Medicine*, **52**, 763-770.

Krovetz, L. J., Lorincz, A. E. & Schiebler, G. L. (1965) Cardiovascular manifestations of the Hurler syndrome: hemodynamic and angiocardiographic observations in 15 patients. *Circulation*, **31**, 132-141.

Lagunoff, D., Ross, R. & Benditt, E. P. (1962) Histochemical and electron microscopic study in a case of Hurler's syndrome. *American Journal of Pathology*, **41**, 273-286.

Lake, B. D. (1968) Segmental demyelination of peripheral nerves in Krabbe's disease. *Nature (London)*, **217**, 171-172.

Lake, B. D. & Patrick, A. D. (1970) Deficiency of E600 resistant acid esterase activity with storage of lipids in lysosomes. *Journal of Pediatrics*, **76**, 262-266.

Landing, B. H., Silverman, F. N., Craig, J. M., Jacoby, M. D., Lahey, M. E. & Chadwick, D. L. (1964) Familial neurovisceral lipidosis. *American Journal of Diseases of Children*, **108**, 503-522.

Leroy, J. G., De Mars, R. I. & Opitz, J. M.   (1969) I-cell disease in *Birth Defects, Original Series* (Eds. Bergsma, D. & McKusick, V. A.), Vol. 5, pp. 174-184, National Foundation—March of Dimes, New York.

Leroy, J. G., Spranger, J. W., Feingold, M., Opitz, J. M. & Crocker, A. C.   (1971) I-cell disease: a clinical picture. *Journal of Pediatrics*, **79**, 360-365.

Levin, S. & Hoenig, E. M.   (1972) Astrocytic gliosis of vascular adventitia and arachnoid membrane in infantile Gaucher's disease. *Journal of Neuropathology and Experimental Neurology*, **31**, 147-157.

Lewis, G. M., Spencer-Peet, J. & Stewart, K. M.   (1963) Infantile hypoglycaemia due to inherited deficiency of glycogen synthetase in liver. *Archives of Disease in Childhood*, **38**, 40-48.

Lewis, P. W., Kennedy, J. F. & Raine, D. N.   (1973) The laboratory diagnosis of the mucopolysaccharidoses in *S.S.I.E.M. Symposium No. 11*, to be published.

Lhermitte, F.   (1950) *Les Leucoéncephalites*, Flammarion, Paris.

Liaño, H., Ricoy, J. R., Diáz-Flores, L. & Gimeno, A.   (1974) A sporadic case of presumed Pelizaeus–Merzbacher disease. *European Neurology*, **11**, 304-316.

Loeb, H., Jonniaux, G., Résibois, A., Cremer, N., Dodian, J., Tondeur, M., Grégoire, P. E., Richard, J. & Cieters, P.   (1968) Biochemical and ultrastructural studies in Hurler's syndrome. *Journal of Pediatrics*, **73**, 860-874.

Loeb, H., Tondeur, M., Jonniaux, G., Mockel-Pohl, S. & Vamos-Hurwitz, E.   (1969) Biochemical and ultrastructural studies in a case of mucopolysaccharidosis 'F' (fucosidosis). *Helvetica paediatrica acta*, **24**, 519-537.

Löken, K. & Cyvin, K.   (1954) A case of clinical juvenile amaurotic idiocy with the histological picture of Alzheimer's disease. *Journal of Neurology, Neurosurgery and Psychiatry*, **17**, 211-215.

Lorincz, A. E.   (1960-61) Heritable disorders of acid mucopolysaccharide metabolism in humans and snorter calf cattle. *Annals of the New York Academy of Science*, **91**, 644-658.

Lorincz, A. E.   (1965) Hurler's syndrome in *Medical Aspects of Mental Retardation* (Ed. Carter, C. H.), pp. 628-650, Thomas, Springfield, Ill.

Lou, H. C., Holmer, G. K., Reske-Nielsen, E. & Vagn-Hansen, P.   (1974) Lipid composition in gray and white matter of the brain in Menkes disease. *Journal of Neurochemistry*, **22**, 377-381.

Lough, J., Fawcett, J. & Wiegenberg, B.   (1970) Wolman's disease. An electron microscopic, histochemical and biochemical study. *Archives of Pathology*, **89**, 103-110.

Lowry, R. B. & Renwick, D. H. G.   (1971) The relative frequency of the Hurler and Hunter syndromes. *New England Journal of Medicine*, **284**, 221.

Lüthy, F. & Bischoff, A.   (1961) Die Pelizaeus–Merzbachersche Krankheit. Ihre Zuordnung zu den Leukodystrophien an Hand von drei eigenen Fällen. *Acta Neuropathologica (Berlin)*, **1**, 113-134.

Lynn, R. & Terry, R. D.   (1964) Lipid histochemistry and electron microscopy in adult Niemann–Pick disease. *American Journal of Medicine*, **37**, 987-994.

McKusick, V. A.   (1969) The nosology of the mucopolysaccharidoses. *American Journal of Medicine*, **47**, 730-747.

McKusick, V. A.   (1972) The mucopolysaccharidoses in *Heritable Disorders of Connective Tissue*, 4th Edn., pp. 521-686, Mosby, St Louis.

McKusick, V. A., Howell, R. R., Hussells, I. E., Neufeld, E. F. & Stevenson, R. E.   (1972) Allelism, non-allelism and genetic compounds among the mucopolysaccharidoses. *Lancet*, **1**, 993-996.

McLeod, J.G., Walsh, J.C. & Little, J.M.   (1969) Sural nerve biopsy. *Medical Journal of Australia*, **2**, 1092-1096.

Mancall, E. L., Aponte, G. E. & Berry, R. G.   (1965) Pompe's disease (diffuse glycogenosis) with neuronal storage. *Journal of Neuropathology and Experimental Neurology*, **24**, 85-96.

Manshot, W. A.   (1968) Retinal histology in amaurotic idiocies and tapeto-retinal degenerations. *Ophthalmologica*, **156**, 28-37.

Mapes, C. A., Anderson, R. L., Sweeley, C. C., Desnick, R. J. & Krivit, R.   (1970) Enzyme replacement in Fabry's disease, an inborn error of metabolism. *Science*, **169**, 987-989.

Marshall, W. C., Ockenden, B. G., Fosbrooke, A. S. & Cumings, J. N.   (1969) Wolman's disease. A rare lipidosis with adrenal calcification. *Archives of Disease in Childhood*, **44**, 331-341.

Martin, J. J., Barry, T., van Hoof, F. & Palladini, G.   (1973) Pompe's disease: an inborn lysosomal disorder with storage of glycogen. A study of brain and striated muscle. *Acta Neuropathologica (Berlin)*, **23**, 229-244.

Mastropaolo, C., Pampiglione, G. & Stephens, R.   (1971) E.E.G. studies in 22 children with sulphatide lipidosis (metachromatic leucodystrophy). *Developmental Medicine and Child Neurology*, **13**, 20-31.

Max, S. R., Maclaren, N. K., Brady, R. O., Bradley, R. M., Rennels, M. B., Tanaka, J., Garcia, J. H. & Cornblath, M.   (1974) G_{M3} (haematoside) sphingolipodystrophy. *New England Journal of Medicine*, **291**, 929-931.

Melançon, S. B. & Nadler, H. L.   (1973) Prenatal diagnosis of genetic disorders leading to mental retardation in *Methods of Neurochemistry* (Ed. Fried, R.), Vol. 5, pp. 1-57, Dekker, New York.

Menkes, J. H.   (1970) Cerebrotendinous xanthomatosis in *Handbook of Clinical Neurology* (Eds. Vinken, P. J. & Bruyn, G. W.), Vol. 10, pp. 532-541, North Holland Publishing Co., Amsterdam.

Menkes, J. H., Alter, M., Steigleder, G. K., Weakley, D. R. & Sung, J. H.   (1962) A sex-linked recessive disorder with retardation of growth, peculiar hair and focal cerebral and cerebellar degeneration.   *Pediatrics*, **29**, 764-779.

Merritt, A. D., Smith, S. A., Strouth, J. C. & Zeman, W.   (1968) Detection of heterozygotes in Batten's disease.   *Annals of the New York Academy of Science*, **155**, 861-867.

Milunsky, A.   (1973) *The Prenatal Diagnosis of Hereditary Disorders*, Thomas, Springfield, Ill.

Minauf, M., Stögman, W. & Krepler, P.   (1970) Zur Beteiligung des Zentralnervensystems beim infantilen Morbus Gaucher.   Klinik und Neuropathologie.   *Archiv für Kinderheilkunde*, **181**, 85-97.

Mittwoch, U.   (1963) The demonstration of mucopolysaccharide inclusions in the lymphocytes of patients with gargoylism.   *Acta haematologica (Basel)*, **29**, 202-207.

Mossakowski, J.   (1964) Morphology and histochemistry of retinal lesions in the infantile (Tay–Sachs) and late infantile (Bielschowsky) forms of amaurotic idiocy.   *Polish Medical Journal*, **3**, 142-155.

Murphy, J. V., Wolfe, H. J., Balazs, E. A. & Moser, H. W.   (1971) A patient with deficiency of arylsulfatase A, B, C and steroid sulfatase, associated with storage of sulfatide, cholesterol sulfate and glycosaminoglycans in *Lipid Storage Disease: Enzymatic Defects and Clinical Implications* (Eds. Bernsohn, J. & Grossman, H. J.), pp. 67-110, Academic Press, New York.

Nelson, E., Osterberg, K., Blaw, M., Story, J. & Kozak, P.   (1962) Electron microscopic and histochemical studies in diffuse sclerosis (sudanophilic type).   *Neurology (Minneapolis)*, **12**, 896-909.

Neufeld, E. F.   (1972) Mucopolysaccharidoses in *Antenatal Diagnosis* (Ed. Dorfman, A.), pp. 217-228, University of Chicago Press, Chicago.

Neufeld, E. F. & Cantz, M. J.   (1971) Corrective factors for inborn errors of mucopolysaccharide metabolism.   *Annals of the New York Academy of Science*, **179**, 580-587.

Neufeld, E. F. & Cantz, M.   (1973) The mucopolysaccharidoses studied in cell culture in *Lysosomes and Storage Diseases* (Eds. Hers, H. G. & van Hoof, F.), pp. 262-275, Academic Press, New York and London.

Neville, B. G. R., Lake, B. D., Stephen, R. & Sanders, M. D.   (1973) A neurovisceral storage disease with vertical supranuclear ophthalmoplegia, and its relationship to Niemann–Pick disease.   A report of nine patients.   *Brain*, **96**, 97-120.

Norman, M. E. & Pischnotte, W. O.   (1972) Morquio's disease.   *American Journal of Diseases of Children*, **124**, 719-722.

Norman R. M. Tingey, A. H., Valentine, J. C. & Danby, T. A.   (1962) Sudanophil leucodystrophy in a pachygyric brain.   *Journal of Neurology, Neurosurgery and Psychiatry*, **25**, 363-369.

Norman, R. M., Tingey, A. H., Valentine, J. C. & Hislop, H. J.   (1967) Sudanophil leucodystrophy: a study of intersib variation in the form taken by the demyelinating process.   *Journal of Neurology, Neurosurgery and Psychiatry*, **30**, 75-82.

Norman, R. M., Urich, H. & France, N. E.   (1959) Perivascular cavitation of the basal ganglia in gargoylism.   *Journal of Mental Science*, **105**, 1070-1077.

Norman, R. M., Urich, H. & Tingey, A. H.   (1960) Metachromatic leucoencephalopathy: a form of a lipidosis.   *Brain*, **83**, 366-380.

Norman, R. M. & Wood, N.   (1941) A congenital form of amaurotic family idiocy.   *Journal of Neurology, Neurosurgery and Psychiatry*, **4**, 175-190.

Noronha, M. J.   (1974) Cerebral degenerative disorders of infancy and childhood.   *Developmental Medicine and Child Neurology*, **16**, 228-241.

O'Brien, J. S.   (1970) Lipids and myelination in *Developmental Neurology* (Ed. Himwich, W. A.), pp. 262-286, Thomas, Springfield, Ill.

O'Brien, J. S.   (1972a) G_{M1} Gangliosidosis in *The Metabolic Basis of Inherited Disease* (Eds. Stanbury, J. B., Wyngaarden, J. B. & Fredrickson, D. S.), 3rd Edn., pp. 639-662, McGraw-Hill, New York.

O'Brien, J. S.   (1972b) Sanfilippo syndrome: profound deficiency of alpha-acetylglucosaminidase activity in organs and skin fibroblasts from type-B patients.   *Proceedings of the National Academy of Sciences (Washington)*, **69**, 1720.

O'Brien, J. S.   (1973) Tay–Sachs disease: from enzyme to prevention.   *Federation Proceedings*, **32**, 191-199.

O'Brien, J. S., Okada, S., Ho, M. W., Fillerup, D. L., Veath, M. L. & Adams, K.   (1971) Ganglioside storage diseases.   *Federation Proceedings*, **30**, 956-969.

O'Brien, J. S. & Sampson, E. L.   (1966) Kinky hair disease: II. Biochemical studies.   *Journal of Neuropathology and Experimental Neurology*, **25**, 523-530.

Okada, S., McCrea, M. & O'Brien, J. S. (1972) Sandhoff's disease (G_{M2} gangliosidosis type 2): clinical, chemical and enzyme studies in five patients. *Pediatric Research*, **6**, 606-615.

Okada, R., Rosenthal, I. M., Scaravelli, G. & Lev, M. (1967) A histopathologic study of the heart in gargoylism. *Archives of Pathology*, **84**, 20-30.

Olsson, Y. & Sourander, P. (1969) The reliability of the diagnosis of metachromatic leucodystrophy by peripheral nerve biopsy. *Acta paediatrica scandinavica*, **58**, 15-24.

Olsson, Y., Sourander, P. & Svennerholm, L. (1966) Experimental studies on the pathogenesis of leucodystrophies. I. The effect of intracerebrally injected sphingolipids in the rat's brain. *Acta Neuropathologica (Berlin)*, **6**, 153-163.

O'Steen, W. K. & Nandy, K. (1970) Lipofuscin pigment in neurons of young mice with a hereditary central nervous system defect. *American Journal of Anatomy*, **128**, 359-366.

Palo, J. & Savolainen, H. (1972) Thin layer chromatographic demonstration of aspartylglucosamine and a novel acidic carbohydrate in human tissues. *Journal of Chromatography*, **65**, 447-450.

Pampiglione, G. (1968) Some inborn metabolic disorders affecting cerebral electrogenesis in *Some Recent Advances in Inborn Errors of Metabolism* (Eds. Holt, K. S. & Coffey, V. P.), pp. 80-100, Livingstone, Edinburgh.

Pampiglione, G., Privett, G. & Harden, A. (1974) Tay–Sachs Disease: neurophysiological studies in 20 children. *Developmental Medicine and Child Neurology*, **16**, 201-208.

Parr, J., Teree, T. M. & Larner, J. (1965) Symptomatic hypoglycaemia, visceral fatty metamorphosis, and aglycogenosis in an infant lacking glycogen synthetase and phosphorylase. *Pediatrics*, **35**, 770-777.

Passarge, E. & McAdams, A. J. (1967) Cerebro-hepato-renal syndrome. *Journal of Pediatrics*, **71**, 691-702.

Patel, V., Koppang, N., Patel, B. & Zeman, W. (1974) Paraphenylene diamine mediated peroxidase deficiency in English Setters with neuronal ceroid lipofuscinosis. *Laboratory Investigation*, **30**, 366-368.

Patel, V., Watanabe, I. & Zeman, W. (1972) Deficiency of α-L-fucosidase. *Science*, **176**, 426-427.

Patrick, A. D. & Lake, B. D. (1969) Deficiency of an acid lipase in Wolman's disease. *Nature (London)*, **222**, 1067-1068.

Patrick, A. D. & Lake, B. D. (1973) Wolman's disease in *Lysosomes and Storage Diseases* (Eds. Hers, H. G. & van Hoof, F.), pp. 453-473, Academic Press, New York and London.

Peiffer, J. (1959a) Über die metachromatischen Leukodystrophien (Typ Scholz). *Archiv für Psychiatrie und Zeitschrift für die gesamte Neurologie*, **199**, 386-416.

Peiffer, J. (1959b) Über die nicht metachromatischen Leukodystrophien. *Archiv für Psychiatrie und Zeitschrift für die gesamte Neurologie*, **199**, 417-436.

Pellisier, J. F., Gambarelli, D., Hassoun, J. & Toga, M. (1974) Atypical juvenile neurolipidosis: electron microscopic study of a brain biopsy in *VIIth International Congress of Neuropathology, Abstracts*, p. 240, Akadémiai Kiadó, Budapest.

Pellissier, J. F., Hassoun, J., Gambarelli, D., Tripier, M. F., Roger, J. & Toga, M. (1974) Ceroid-lipofuscinose neuronale. Étude ultrastructurelle de deux biopsies cérébrales. *Acta Neuropathologica (Berlin)*, **28**, 353-359.

Pennock, C. A., White, F., Murphy, D., Charles, R. G. & Kerr, H. (1973) Excess glycosaminoglycan excretion in infancy and childhood. *Acta paediatrica scandinavica*, **62**, 481-491.

Percy, A. K., McCormick, U. M., Kaback, M. M. & Herndon, R. M. (1973) Ultrastructure manifestations of G_{M1} and G_{M2} gangliosidosis in fetal tissues. *Archives of Neurology (Chicago)*, **28**, 417-419.

Pilz, H. (1970) Clinical, morphological and biochemical aspects of sphingolipidoses. *Neuropädiatrie*, **1**, 383-427.

Pilz, H., Sandhoff, K. & Jatzkewitz, H. (1966) Eine Gangliosidwechselstörung mit Anhäufung von Ceramidlactosid, Monosialo-ceramid, Lactosid und Tay–Sachs Gangliosid im Gehirn. *Journal of Neurochemistry*, **13**, 1273-1282.

Pollitt, R. J., Jenner, F. A. & Merskey, H. (1968) Aspartylglycosaminuria. An inborn error of metabolism associated with mental defect. *Lancet*, **2**, 253-255.

Poser, C. M. (1962) Concept of dysmyelination in *Cerebral Sphingolipidoses* (Eds. Aronson, S. M. & Volk, B. W.), pp. 141-164, Academic Press, New York.

Poser, C. M. & Bogaert, L. van (1956) Natural history and evolution of the concept of Schilder's diffuse sclerosis. *Acta psychiatrica scandinavica*, **31**, 285-331.

Prensky, A. L., Ferreira, G., Carr, S. & Moser, H. W. (1967) Ceramide and ganglioside accumulation in Farber's lipogranulomatosis. *Proceedings of the Society for Experimental Biology and Medicine*, **126**, 725-728.

Raine, D. N. (1970) Biochemical relationships in the neuronal sphingolipidoses. *Developmental Medicine and Child Neurology*, **12**, 348-356.

Rampini, S.   (1969) Das Sanfilippo-Syndrom (polydystrophe Oligophrenie, HS-Mukopolysaccharidose). Bericht über 8 Fälle und Literaturübersicht. *Helvetica paediatrica acta*, **24**, 55-91.

Rampini, S. & Clausen, J.   (1967) Farbersche Krankheit (disseminierte Lipogranulomatose). Klinisches Bild und Zusammenfassung der chemischen Befunde. *Helvetica paediatrica acta*, **22**, 500-515.

Rampini, S., Isler, W., Baerlocher, K., Bischoff, A., Ulrich, J. & Plüss, H. J.   (1970) Die Kombination von metachromatischer Leukodystrophie und Mukopolysaccharidose als selbständiges Krankheitsbild (Mukosulfatidose). *Helvetica paediatrica acta*, **25**, 435-552.

Rapola, J., Autio, S., Aula, P. & Nanto, V.   (1974) Lymphocyte inclusions in I-cell disease. *Journal of Pediatrics*, **85**, 88-92.

Résibois-Grégoire, A.   (1967) Electron microscopic studies on metachromatic leucodystrophy. II. Compound nature of the inclusions. *Acta Neuropathologica (Berlin)*, **9**, 244-253.

Résibois-Grégoire, A. & Dourov, N.   (1966) Electron microscopic study of a case of cerebral glycogenosis. *Acta Neuropathologica (Berlin)*, **6**, 70-79.

Reske-Nielsen, E., Lou, H. C. & Vagn-Hansen, P. L.   (1974) Menkes' disease. A hypothesis with recommendations for future investigations. *Acta Neuropathologica (Berlin)*, **28**, 361-363.

Ribelin, W. E. & Kintner, L. D.   (1956) Lipodystrophy of the central nervous system in a dog. A disease with similarities to Tay–Sachs disease of man. *Cornell Veterinarian*, **46**, 532-537.

Richardson, E. P.   (1975) Schilder's disease—what is it? *Journal of Neuropathology and Experimental Neurology*, in press.

Rintelen, F.   (1936) Die Histopathologie der Augenhintergrundsveränderungen bei Niemann–Pickscher Lipoidose; zugleich zur Frage der Beziehungen zwischen Tay–Sachsscher Idiotie und Niemann–Pickscher Lipoidose. *Archiv für Augenheilkunde*, **109**, 332-345.

Roizin, L., Slade, W., Hermida, H. & Asao, H.   (1962) Comparative histologic, histochemical and electron microscopic studies of rectal biopsies in a case of adult hereditary cerebromacular degeneration in *Cerebral Sphingolipidoses* (Eds. Aronson, S. M. & Volk, B. W.), pp. 57-72, Academic Press, New York.

Sachs, B.   (1887) On arrested cerebral development with special reference to its cortical pathology. *Journal of Nervous and Mental Disease*, **14**, 541-553.

Saifer, A. & Perle, G.   (1974) Automated determination of serum hexosaminidase A by pH inactivation for detection of Tay–Sachs disease heterozygotes. *Clinical Chemistry*, **20**, 538-543.

Sandhoff, K.   (1969) Variation of β-N-acetylhexosaminidase pattern in Tay–Sachs disease. *FEBS Letters*, **4**, 351-354.

Sandhoff, K.   (1974) Sphingolipidoses. *Journal of Clinical Pathology*, **27**, *Suppl.* (*Royal College of Pathologists*), **8**, 94-105.

Sandhoff, K. & Jatzkewitz, H.   (1972) The chemical pathology of Tay–Sachs disease in *Sphingolipids, Sphingolipidoses and Allied Disorders* (Eds. Volk, B. W. & Aronson, S. M.), pp. 305-319, Plenum Press, New York.

Santavuori, P., Haltia, M., Rapola, J. & Raitta, C.   (1973) Infantile type of so-called neuronal ceroidlipofuscinosis. Part 1. A clinical study of 15 patients. *Journal of the Neurological Sciences*, **18**, 257-267.

Santavuori, P., Haltia, M. & Rapola, J.   (1974) Infantile type of so-called neuronal ceroid-lipofuscinosis. *Developmental Medicine and Child Neurology*, **16**, 664-667.

Sawitsky, A., Rosner, F. & Chodsky, S.   (1972) The sea-blue histiocyte syndrome, a review: genetic and biochemical studies. *Seminars in Hematology*, **9**, 285-297.

Schaumburg, H. H., Powers, J. M., Suzuki, K. & Raine, C. S.   (1974) Adreno-leukodystrophy (sex-linked Schilder disease). *Archives of Neurology (Chicago)*, **31**, 210-213.

Schaumburg, H. H., Powers, J. M., Raine, C. S., Suzuki, K. & Richardson, E. P.   (1975) *Archives of Neurology (Chicago)*, in press.

Scheie, H. G., Hambrick, G. W. & Barness, L. A.   (1962) A newly recognised Forme Fruste of Hurler's disease (gargoylism). *American Journal of Ophthalmology*, **53**, 753-769.

Schjeide, O. A., Lin, R. I. S. & De Vellis, J.   (1968) Molecular composition of myelin synthesized subsequent to irradiation. *Radiation Research*, **33**, 107-128.

Schnabel, R.   (1971) Zur Histochemie der mucopolysaccharidartigen Substanzen (basophile Substanzen) in der Skelettmuskulatur bei neuromuskulärer Glykogenose (Typ II). *Acta Neuropathologica (Berlin)*, **17**, 169-178.

Schneck, L., Adachi, M. & Volk, B. W.   (1971) Congenital failure of myelinization: Pelizaeus–Merzbacher Disease? *Neurology (Minneapolis)*, **21**, 817-824.

Schneck, L., Amsterdam, D. & Volk, B. W.   (1974) Antenatal diagnosis and therapeutic trends in sphingolipidoses. *Journal of the American Medical Association*, **228**, 615-618.

Schneck, L., Friedland, J., Valenti, C., Adachi, M., Amsterdam, D. & Volk, B. W.   (1970) Prenatal diagnosis of Tay–Sachs disease. *Lancet*, **1**, 582-584.

Schochet, S. S., Lampert, P. W. & Earle, K. M. (1968) Alexander's disease. A case report with electron microscopic observations. *Neurology (Minneapolis)*, **18**, 543-549.

Schwendemann, G. & Colmant, H. (1974) Bioptic studies on ceroid-lipofuscinosis: light and electron microscopic observations in *VIIth International Congress of Neuropathology*. Abstracts, p. 275, Akadémiai Kiadó, Budapest.

Seitelberger, F. (1970) Pelizaeus–Merzbacher disease in *Handbook of Clinical Neurology* (Eds. Vinken, P. J. & Bruyn, G. W.), Vol. 10, pp. 150-202, North Holland Publishing Co., Amsterdam.

Seitelberger, F. & Nagy, K. (1958) Zur Histopathologie und Klinik der Spätform von amaurotischer Idiotie. *Deutsche Zeitschrift für Nervenheilkunde*, **177**, 577-596.

Setoguchi, T., Salen, G., Tint, G. S. & Mosbach, E. H. (1974) A biochemical abnormality in cerebrotendinous xanthomatosis. Impairment of bile acid biosynthesis associated with incomplete degradation of the cholesterol side chain. *Journal of Clinical Investigation*, **53**, 1393-1401.

Shrivastava, K. & Beutler, E. (1974) Studies on human β-D-N-acetylhexosaminidases. III. Biochemical genetics of Tay–Sachs and Sandhoff's disease. *Journal of Biological Chemistry*, **249**, 2054-2057.

Silverstein, M. N. & Ellefson, R. D. (1972) The syndrome of the sea-blue histiocyte. *Seminars in Hematology*, **9**, 299-307.

Singer, H. S., Nankervis, G. A. & Schafer, I. A. (1972) Leukocyte beta-galactosidase activity in the diagnosis of generalized G_{M1} gangliosidosis. *Pediatrics*, **49**, 352-361.

Sjöstrand, F. S. (1963) The structure and formation of the myelin sheath in *Mechanisms of Demyelination* (Eds. Rose, A. S. & Pearson, C. M.), pp. 1-43, McGraw-Hill, New York.

Sloan, H. R. & Fredrickson, D. S. (1972) Enzyme deficiency in cholesteryl ester storage disease. *Journal of Clinical Investigation*, **51**, 1923-1926.

Sly, W. S., Quinton, B. A., McAlister, W. & Rimoin, D. L. (1973) Beta glucuronidase deficiency. Report of clinical, radiologic and biochemical features of a new mucopolysaccharidosis. *Journal of Pediatrics*, **82**, 249-257.

Smith, M. E. (1972) The turnover of myelin proteins. *Neurobiology*, **2**, 35-40.

Sourander, P. & Olsson, Y. (1968) Peripheral neuropathy in globoid cell leucodystrophy (Morbus Krabbe). *Acta Neuropathologica (Berlin)*, **11**, 69-81.

Spence, M. W., Ripley, B. A., Embil, J. A. & Tibbles, J. A. R. (1974) A new variant of Sandhoff's disease. *Pediatric Research*, **8**, 628-637.

Spencer-Peet, J., Norman, M. E., Lake, B. D., McNamara, J. & Patrick, A. D. (1971) Hepatic glycogen storage disease. Clinical and laboratory findings in 23 cases. *Quarterly Journal of Medicine*, **40**, 95-114.

Spohn, M. & Davison, A. N. (1972) Cholesterol metabolism in myelin and other subcellular fractions of rat brain. *Journal of Lipid Research*, **13**, 563-570.

Spranger, J. W. (1973) Morphological aspects of the mucopolysaccharidoses in *S.S.I.E.M. Symposium No. 11*, to be published.

Spranger, J. W., Gilbert, E. F., Tuffli, G. A., Rossiter, F. P. & Opitz, J. M. (1971) Geleophysic dwarfism—a 'focal' mucopolysaccharidosis? *Lancet*, **2**, 97-98.

Spranger, J. W., Koch, F., McKusick, V. A., Natzschka, J., Wiedemann, H.-R. & Zellweger, H. (1970) Mucopolysaccharidosis VI (Maroteaux–Lamy's disease). *Helvetica paediatrica acta*, **25**, 337-362.

Spranger, J. W. & Wiedemann, H.-R. (1970) The genetic mucolipidoses. *Neuropädiatrie*, **2**, 3-16.

Spranger, J. W., Wiedemann, H.-R., Tolksdorf, M., Graucob, E. & Caesar, R. (1968) Lipomucopolysaccharidose. Eine neue Speicherkrankheit. *Zeitschrift für Kinderheilkunde*, **103**, 285-306.

Stumpf, D. & Austin, J. (1971) Metachromatic leukodystrophy (MLD). IX. Qualitative and quantitative differences in urinary arylsulfatase A in different forms of MLD. *Archives of Neurology (Chicago)*, **24**, 117-124.

Stumpf, D. A., Austin, J. H., Crocker, A. C. & La France, M. (1973) Mucopolysaccharidosis type VI (Maroteaux–Lamy syndrome). I. Sulfatase B deficiency in tissues. *American Journal of Diseases of Children*, **126**, 747-755.

Sugita, M., Dulaney, J. T. & Moser, H. W. (1972) Ceramidase deficiency in Farber's disease (lipogranulomatosis). *Science*, **178**, 1100-1102.

Suzuki, K. (1970) Ultrastructural study of experimental globoid cells. *Laboratory Investigation*, **23**, 612-619.

Suzuki, K. & Grover, W. D. (1970a) Krabbe's leukodystrophy (globoid cell leukodystrophy): an ultrastructural study. *Archives of Neurology (Chicago)*, **22**, 385-396.

Suzuki, K. & Grover, W. D. (1970b) Ultrastructural and biochemical studies of Schilder's disease. I. Ultrastructure. *Journal of Neuropathology and Experimental Neurology*, **29**, 392-404.

Suzuki, Y., Jacob, J. C., Suzuki, K., Kutty, K. M. & Suzuki, K. (1971) G_{M2}-gangliosidosis with total hexosaminidase deficiency. *Neurology (Minneapolis)*, **21**, 313-328.

Suzuki, K., Schneider, E. L. & Epstein, C. J. (1971) In utero diagnosis of globoid cell leukodystrophy (Krabbe's disease). *Biochemical and Biophysical Research Communications*, **45**, 1363-1366.

Suzuki, K. & Suzuki, K. (1973) Disorders of sphingolipid metabolism in *Biology of Brain Dysfunction* (Ed. Gaull, G. E.), Vol. 2, pp. 1-73, Plenum Press, New York.

Suzuki, Y. & Suzuki, K. (1974*a*) Glycosphingolipid β-galactosidases. IV. Electrofocussing characterization in G_{M1}-gangliosidoses. *Journal of Biological Chemistry*, **249**, 2113-2117.

Suzuki, Y. & Suzuki, K. (1974*b*) Glycosphingolipid β-galactosidases. II. Electrofocussing characterization of the enzymes in human globoid cell leucodystrophy (Krabbe's disease). *Journal of Biological Chemistry*, **249**, 2105-2108.

Suzuki, K., Suzuki, K. & Chen, G. C. (1968) Morphological, histochemical and biochemical studies on a case of systemic late infantile lipidosis (generalised gangliosidosis). *Journal of Neuropathology and Experimental Neurology*, **27**, 15-38.

Suzuki, K., Suzuki, K., Rapin, I., Suzuki, Y. & Ishii, N. (1970) Juvenile G_{M2}-gangliosidosis. Clinical variant of Tay-Sachs disease or a new disease. *Neurology (Minneapolis)*, **20**, 190-204.

Suzuki, Y., Tadashi, M., Fletcher, T. F. & Suzuki, K. (1974) Glycosphingolipid β-galactosidases. III. Canine form of globoid cell leucodystrophy; comparison with the human disease. *Journal of Biological Chemistry*, **249**, 2109-2112.

Svennerholm, L. (1966) The patterns of gangliosides in mental and neurological disorders. *Biochemical Journal*, **98**, 20P.

Sweeley, C. C., Krivit, W., Klionsky, B. & Desnick, R. J. (1972) Fabry's disease: glycosphingolipid lipidosis in *The Metabolic Basis of Inherited Disease* (Eds. Stanbury, J. B., Wyngaarden, J. B. & Fredrickson, D. S.), 3rd Edn., pp. 633-687, McGraw-Hill, New York.

Tay, W. (1881) Symmetrical changes in the region of the yellow spot in each eye of an infant. *Transactions of the Ophthalmological Society of the U.K.*, **1**, 155-157.

Teilum, G. (1942) Zerebrale und viscerale Xanthomatose mit Diabetes insipidus. *Beiträge zur pathologischen Anatomie und zur allgemeinen Pathologie*, **106**, 460-481.

Terry, R. D. (1971) Some morphologic aspects of the lipidoses in *Lipid Storage Diseases: Enzymatic Defects and Clinical Implications* (Eds. Bernsohn, J. & Grossman, H. J.), pp. 3-25, Academic Press, New York.

Terry, R. D., Suzuki, K. & Weiss, M. (1966) Biopsy study in three cases of metachromatic leucodystrophy, *Journal of Neuropathology and Experimental Neurology*, **25**, 141-143.

Thomas, G. H. & Howell, R. R. (1973) *Selected Screening Tests for Genetic Metabolic Diseases*, Year Book Medical Publishers, Chicago.

Titarelli, R., Giagheddu, M. & Spadetta, V. (1963) Reperto oftalmoscopico tipico di malattia di Tay–Sachs in soggetto adulto con sindrome mioclonica. *Rivista oto-neuro-oftalmologica*, **38**, 610-616.

Tondeur, M. & Résibois, A. (1969) Fabry's disease in children, an electron microscopic study. *Virchows Archiv für pathologische Anatomie. Abt. B. Zellpathologie*, **2**, 254-339.

Tondeur, M., Vamos-Hurwitz, E., Mockel-Pohl, S., Dereume, J. P., Cremer, N. & Loeb, H. (1971) Clinical, biochemical and ultrastructural studies in a case of chondrodystrophy presenting the I-cell phenotype in tissue culture. *Journal of Pediatrics*, **79**, 366-378.

Towfighi, J., Baird, H. W., Gambetti, P. & Gonatas, N. K. (1973) The significance of cytoplasmic inclusions in late infantile and juvenile amaurotic idiocy. *Acta Neuropathologica (Berlin)*, **23**, 32-42.

Tridon, P., Martin, J.-J., Vidailhet, M., Floquet, J., Philippart, M. & Neimann, N. (1974) Spongiose cérébrale juvénile. *Pédiatrie*, **29**, 235-247.

Tsay, G. C., Dawson, G. & Matalon, R. (1974) Excretion of mannose-rich complex carbohydrate by a patient with α-mannosidase deficiency (mannosidosis). *Journal of Pediatrics*, **84**, 865-868.

Turkington, R. W. & Stempfel, R. S. (1966) Adrenocortical atrophy and diffuse cerebral sclerosis (Addison–Schilder's disease). *Journal of Pediatrics*, **69**, 406-412.

Ulrich, J. (1971) *Die zerebralen Entmarkungskrankheiten im Kindesalter*, Springer Verlag, Berlin.

Vagn-Hansen, P. L., Reske-Nielsen, E. & Lou, H. C. (1973) Menkes' disease—a new leucodystrophy? A clinical and neuropathological review together with a new case. *Acta Neuropathologica (Berlin)*, **25**, 103-119.

van Hoof, F. (1973) Mucopolysaccharidoses in *Lysosomes and Storage Diseases* (Eds. Hers, H. G. & van Hoof, F.), pp. 217-259, Academic Press, New York and London.

van Hoof, F. (1974) Mucopolysaccharidoses and mucolipidoses. *Journal of Clinical Pathology*, **27**, Suppl. (*Royal College of Pathologists*), **8**, 64-93.

van Hoof, F. & Hers, H. G. (1964) L'ultrastructure des cellules hépatiques dans la maladie de Hurler (gargoylisme). *Comptes rendus hebdomadaires des séances de l'Académie des sciences, Série D, Sciences Naturelles, Paris*, **259**, 1281-1283.

van Hoof, F. & Hers, H. G.   (1968) The abnormalities of lysosomal enzymes in mucopolysaccharidoses. *European Journal of Biochemistry*, **7**, 34-44.

Vanier, M. T. & Svennerholm, L.   (1974) Chemical pathology of Krabbe's disease. I. Lipid composition and fatty acid pattern of phosphoglycerides in brain.   II. Composition of cerebroside sulphatide and sphingomyelins in the brain.   *Acta paediatrica scandinavica*, **63**, 494-506.

Vidailhet, M., Neimann, N., Grignon, G., Hartemann, P., Philippart, M., Paysant, P., Nabet, P. & Floquet, J.   (1973) Maladie de Sandhoff (gangliosidose G $_{M2}$, de Type 2).   *Archives françaises de Pédiatrie*, **30**, 45-60.

Vinken, P. J. & Bruyn, G. W.   (1970) *Handbook of Clinical Neurology*, North Holland Publishing Co., Amsterdam.

Visser, S. L. & De Groot, W. P.   (1970) EEG and EMG in Fabry's disease.   *Electroencephalography and Clinical Neurophysiology*, **28**, 427.

Vogel, F. S. & Hallervorden, J.   (1962) Leukodystrophy with diffuse Rosenthal fibre formation.   *Acta Neuropathologica (Berlin)*, **2**, 126-143.

Vogel, J. M. & Vogel, P.   (1972) Idiopathic histiocytosis: a discussion of eosinophilic granuloma, the Hand–Schüller–Christian syndrome, and the Letterer–Siwe syndrome.   *Seminars in Hematology*, **9**, 349-369.

Volk, B. W., Adachi, M., Schneck, L., Saifer, A. & Kleinberg, W.   (1969) G $_5$-ganglioside variant of systemic late infantile lipidosis.   Generalised gangliosidosis.   *Archives of Pathology*, **87**, 393-403.

Volk, B. W., Adachi, M. & Schneck, L.   (1972) The pathology of sphingolipidoses.   *Seminars in Hematology*, **9**, 317-348.

Volk, B. W. & Aronson, S. M.   (1972) *Sphingolipids, Sphingolipidoses and Allied Disorders*, Plenum Press, New York.

Volk, B. W. & Wallace, B. J.   (1966) The liver in lipidoses: An electron microscopic and histochemical study.   *American Journal of Pathology*, **49**, 203-225.

Volk, B. W., Wallace, B. J. & Aronson, S. M.   (1968) Some ultrastructural and histochemical aspects of lipidoses.   *Pathologia europaea*, **3**, 200-217.

Vuia, O. & Heye, D.   (1974) Neuropathological aspects in Menkes' kinky hair disease (trichopoliodystrophy).   *Neuropädiatrie* **5**, 329-339.

Walbaum, R., Demaene, Ph., Scharfman, W., Farriaux, J. P., Tondeur, M., Vamos-Hurwitz, E., Kint, J. A. & van Hoof, F.   (1973) La mucolipidose de type II (I-cell disease).   *Archives françaises de Pédiatrie*, **30**, 577-592.

Wallace, B. J., Lazarus, S. S. & Volk, B. W.   (1967) Electron microscopic and histochemical studies of viscera in lipidoses in *Inborn Disorders of Sphingolipid Metabolism* (Eds. Aronson, S. M. & Volk, B. W.), pp. 107-120, Pergamon Press, New York.

Watanabe, I., Patel, V., Goebel, H. H., Siakotos, A. N., Zeman, W., De Meyer, W. & Dyer, J. S.   (1973) Early lesions of Pelizaeus—Merzbacher disease: electron microscopic and biochemical study.   *Journal of Neuropathology and Experimental Neurology*, **32**, 313-333.

Webster, H. de F.   (1962) Schwann cell alterations in metachromatic leucodystrophy: preliminary phase and electron microscopic observations.   *Journal of Neuropathology and Experimental Neurology*, **21**, 534-541.

Westwood, A. & Raine, D. N.   (1974) Separation of three isoenzymes of N-acetyl-β-D-hexosaminidase from human tissues by cellulose acetate membrane electrophoresis.   *Journal of Clinical Pathology*, **27**, 913-915.

Whiteman, P.   (1973) The quantitative determination of glycosaminoglycans in urine with alcian blue 8GX.   *Biochemical Journal*, **131**, 343-350.

Whittem, J. H. & Walker, J.   (1957) 'Neuropathy' and 'pseudolipidosis' in Aberdeen-Angus calves.   *Journal of Pathology and Bacteriology*, **74**, 281-293.

Wilson, J.   (1972) Investigation of degenerative disease of the central nervous system.   *Archives of Disease in Childhood*, **47**, 163-170.

Wilson, J., Lake, B. D. & Dunn, H. G.   (1969) Krabbe's neurodystrophy.   Some genetic and pathogenetic considerations.   *Journal of the Neurological Sciences*, **10**, 563-575.

Winchester, P., Grossman, H., Lim, W. N. & Danes, B. S.   (1969) A new acid mucopolysaccharidosis with skeletal deformities simulating rheumatoid arthritis.   *American Journal of Roentgenology*, **106**, 121-129.

Witzleben, C. L., Smith, K., Nelson, J. S., Monteleoni, P. L. & Livingston, D.   (1971) Ultrastructural studies in late-onset amaurotic idiocy: lymphocyte inclusions as a diagnostic marker.   *Journal of Pediatrics*, **79**, 285-293.

Wolter, J. R. & Allen, R. J.   (1964) Retinal neuropathology of late infantile amaurotic idiocy.   *British Journal of Ophthalmology*, **48**, 277-284.

Yamamoto, A., Adachi, S., Kitani, T., Shinji, Y., Seki, K., Nasu, T. & Nishikawa, M.   (1971) Drug-induced lipidosis in human cases and in animal experiments—accumulation of an acid glycerophospholipid.   *Journal of Biochemistry (Tokyo)*, **69**, 613-615.

Zeman, W.,   (1971) Morphologic approaches to the nosology of nervous system defects in *Birth Defects: Original Article Series* (Ed. Bergsma, D.), Vol. 7, No. 1, pp. 23-30, *National Foundation*—March of Dimes, New York.

Zeman, W.   (1974) Studies in the neuronal ceroid-lipofuscinoses. *Journal of Neuropathology and Experimental Neurology*, **33**, 1-12.

Zeman, W. & Siakotos, A. N.   (1973) The neuronal ceroid-lipofuscinoses in *Lysosomes and Storage Diseases* (Eds. Hers, H. G. & van Hoof, F.), pp. 519-551, Academic Press, New York and London.

13

The Hypothalamus and Pituitary Gland

P. M. Daniel and C. S. Treip

The pathology of the hypothalamus and of the pituitary gland are described in a single chapter, since the two regions are physiologically interdependent and may be jointly spoken of as the hypothalamic-pituitary axis. Some acquaintance with the anatomy (Daniel 1966a) and physiology (Harris 1960) of the hypothalamus and of the pituitary gland is necessary for the study of pathological processes in this region; the chapter has accordingly been prefaced by brief outlines of these topics. From the practical point of view, it is pertinent to note that both the hypothalamus and the pituitary are readily damaged during the removal of the brain at necropsy; care must therefore be taken in carrying out this procedure. In particular, traction on the optic nerves should be avoided. Similarly, the infundibular process (posterior lobe) of the pituitary can easily be damaged or destroyed when the gland is taken out; ideally it should be dissected out within its dural capsule, and removed with the dorsum sellae attached.

The earlier literature on the pathology of the hypothalamus is relatively inaccessible, the most comprehensive survey being that by Orthner (1955). Other reviews have been published by Bauer (1954), Herzog (1955), Orthner (1961) and Sheehan (1968).

Anatomy of the hypothalamus

The hypothalamus is one of the most primitive parts of the central nervous system and has complex and extensive connections (Clark 1938; Rioch, Wislocki and O'Leary 1940; Nauta and Haymaker 1969; Raisman 1970; Daniel and Prichard 1975). Its boundaries are poorly defined, but may be said roughly to comprise the lateral walls and base of the lower part of the 3rd ventricle, below the level of the hypothalamic sulcus. The *rostral* boundary is a coronal plane lying slightly anterior to the optic chiasma while the *caudal* boundary lies immediately posterior to the mamillary bodies. The lateral boundaries are more difficult to define; at various coronal levels the following structures may be found situated laterally: the lowermost portion of the thalamus, the internal capsule, the globus pallidus, the ansa lenticularis, and the optic tract. Below, the parts of the grey matter which make up the walls and floor of the 3rd ventricle form, in man, a funnel-shaped structure, the infundibulum or tuber cinereum, which is clearly visible as a protuberance at the base of the brain and is prolonged downwards as the pituitary stalk, ending in the pituitary gland. The neural tissue of the stalk and the infundibular process of the pituitary gland make up the neurohypophysis (Fig. 13.28). Myelinated fibres, apart from a few well-defined tracts, are rarely seen in the hypothalamus.

Nuclear topography of the hypothalamus

The *supraoptic nucleus* is well defined and overlies the rostral extremity of the optic tract just caudal to the optic chiasma (Fig. 13.1). Its neurons are large (Fig. 13.2a, b) in comparison with those of the surrounding hypothalamic nerve cells and have prominent, often eccentric nuclei, with conspicuous nucleoli (Fig. 13.2b). These cells stand out because the Nissl granules are not scattered evenly throughout the perikaryon, but are collected peripherally, leaving a clear perinuclear zone. This appearance superficially resembles the central chromatolysis which may be seen when the axon of a nerve cell is damaged,

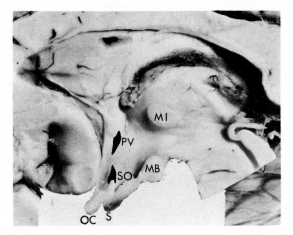

Fig. 13.1 View of the wall of the 3rd ventricle to show sites of supraoptic (SO) and paraventricular (PV) nuclei. MB, mamillary body; MI, massa intermedia; OC, optic chiasma; S, pituitary stalk.

and may give rise to diagnostic difficulties. (Similar appearances are seen in the cells of many hypothalamic nuclei.) The number of magnocellular neurons in the human supraoptic nucleus varies between 50,000 and 76,000 cells (Rasmussen 1938; Maccubbin and Van Buren 1963; Morton 1970).

The *paraventricular nucleus* lies close beneath the ependymal lining of the third ventricle, parallel to its lateral wall and dorsal and caudal to the supraoptic nucleus (Figs. 13.1, 13.2*a*). The large cells, some 30,000 to 54,000 in number (Maccubbin and Van Buren 1963), are similar

to those of the supraoptic nucleus; there are also many small neurons.

The *mamillary bodies* are composed of two nuclear masses, the *mamillary nuclei*, each about 5 mm in diameter and enclosed within a capsule of myelinated nerve fibres. Each mamillary nucleus is divided into a large medial and a small lateral portion (Clark 1938); there is, in addition, a laterally and inferiorly situated nucleus intercalatus, composed of large, dark, angular nerve cells.

The three nuclei so far described, supraoptic, paraventricular and mamillary, are easily identified histologically, being clearly demarcated from the adjacent regions of the hypothalamus. The remaining hypothalamic nuclei are less well defined. A number of them have been identified only in fetal material, since some hypothalamic nuclei, particularly the ventromedial, are better demarcated in the fetus than in the adult.

The grey matter forming the walls of the 3rd ventricle in the region above the tuber cinereum is divided into *ventromedial* and *dorsomedial hypothalamic nuclei*. These two nuclei, composed of small, uniform nerve cells with poorly staining cytoplasm, are found in the medial part of the hypothalamus between the attachment of the tuber cinereum and the paraventricular nucleus. Above the mamillary nucleus lies the *posterior*

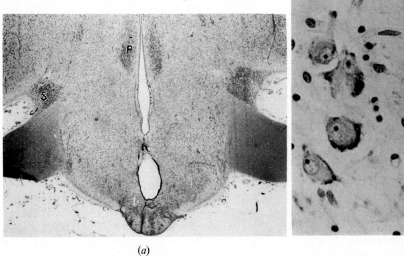

(*a*)   (*b*)

Fig. 13.2 (*a*) Coronal section through hypothalamus, showing site of supraoptic (S) and paraventricular (P) nuclei. Luxol fast blue. Nissl. ×6. (*b*) Cells of supraoptic nucleus with eccentric nuclei and peripherally arranged Nissl substance. Nissl. ×400.

hypothalamic nucleus, also situated medially and not sharply outlined.

All the nuclei so far described lie adjacent to the cavity of the 3rd ventricle. The region lateral to the anterior column of the fornix which does not contain easily identifiable cell masses is the *lateral hypothalamic area*, through which passes the ill-defined *medial forebrain bundle*, a major connecting group of tracts to and from the hypothalamus.

Finally, in the lowermost part of the lateral hypothalamic area there are well-defined nuclei, the *tuberal nuclei*, which have been identified only in man. The cells have a characteristic appearance, being small and lightly staining and with eccentric nuclei (Clark 1938).

Blood supply of the hypothalamus

The vascular supply of the hypothalamus derives from small arteries arising from the circle of Willis (Dawson 1958; Daniel 1966*a*, *b*). The finer vascular pattern of the nuclear masses resembles that seen elsewhere in the grey matter of the brain and the blood supply of the tracts is similar to that of white matter elsewhere. However, Finley (1940) showed that the supraoptic and paraventricular nuclei have a far richer capillary blood supply than any other of the hypothalamic nuclei. There is a sparse connection, by means of capillary vessels, between the territory of the hypothalamus proper and that of the neural tissue of the pituitary gland (Duvernoy 1972).

Connections of the hypothalamus

Many connections of the hypothalamic nuclei are still unclear, but certain known pathways are important in the understanding of the function of the hypothalamic region (Raisman 1966, 1970; Nauta and Haymaker 1969; Daniel and Prichard 1975). As a generalization it may be said that afferent fibres reach the lateral hypothalamus, while the cells of the medial hypothalamus are largely efferent. Most of the nerve fibres of the hypothalamus are non-myelinated, so that the few myelinated bundles stand out clearly. Of these, the *mamillothalamic tract* forms an efferent connection between the hypothalamus and the anterior nucleus of the thalamus; the latter nucleus sends nerve fibres as a projection to the cingulate gyrus (Meyer, Beck and McLardy 1947), so that by way of the hypothalamus the hippocampus of the temporal lobe projects on to the cingulate cortex. The hypothalamus is also connected to the dorsomedial nucleus of the thalamus by the extensive *periventricular system* of non-myelinated nerve fibres, lying immediately beneath the ependymal lining of the 3rd ventricle. The dorsomedial nucleus of the thalamus projects upon the prefrontal cortex in a point to point manner (Meyer *et al.* 1947). 'One fact which stands out very strongly is that, by way of the anterior or dorsomedial nuclei of the thalamus, the greater part of the cortex of the frontal lobe must be regarded as a projection area receiving the products of activity of the hypothalamus in the same way that the visual cortex is the projection area for retinal activities, or the auditory cortex for cochlear activities' (Clark 1948).

No well-defined fibre tracts are connected to the ventromedial and dorsomedial hypothalamic nuclei, but these nuclei are thought to have connections with the other hypothalamic nuclei by means of the periventricular system of nerve fibres and the medial forebrain bundle. The ventromedial and dorsomedial nuclei also probably have connections with the subthalamic region, the premamillary hypothalamic area and the nuclei of the thalamus.

The axons of the nerve cells of the supraoptic nucleus form a tract of fine, mainly non-myelinated fibres which pass through the rostral part of the tuber cinereum to run downwards in the neural part of the pituitary stalk into the infundibular process (the neural or posterior lobe of the pituitary gland). The axons of the paraventricular nucleus take a curved course (convex rostrally) towards the tuber cinereum and pass near to or through the supraoptic nucleus (Christ 1966) on their way to the infundibular process. These two sets of fibres together form the *hypothalamo-neurohypophysial tract*. Although the influence of this tract on water metabolism has long been known (Fisher, Ingram and Ranson 1938), the work of Scharrer and Scharrer (1954) and Bargmann (1954) threw new light on the activities of the specialized cells of the supraoptic and paraventricular nuclei. Neurosecretory material, stainable by the Gömöri chrome alum haematoxylin method, and representing a carrier or precursor of antidiuretic hormone, is produced by the cells of these two nuclei and passes along the nerve fibres of the hypothalamo-neurohypophysial tract to the infundibular process (see review by Sloper 1966). Occasional small beadlike swellings are seen along some of the nerve fibres forming the tract. In addition, the colloid masses (Herring bodies), which stain with chrome alum haematoxylin and are found in the infundibular process, appear to be swellings at or near the ends of nerve fibres of the tract. Many fine non-myelinated fibres end near the vessels of the primary capillary beds (Green 1951) and the finding of neurosecretory material at these endings (Rinne 1960) makes it very probable that some of these nerve fibres are derived from the neurosecretory cells of the supraoptic and paraventricular nuclei (Szentágothai, Flerkó, Mess and Halász 1968).

Functions of the hypothalamus

Some of the information available on the functions of the hypothalamus is derived from the study of pathological conditions in man (Besser 1974), but by far the greater part is the result of work on experimental animals.

The functions of the hypothalamus may be divided into four main groups of activities: (1) control of endocrine function through the neurohypophysis and pars distalis; (2) control of feeding and drinking; (3) control of autonomic function; (4) relationship with emotional stability.

Control of endocrine activity
Neurohypophysis. It is generally believed that the neurohypophysial hormones or their analogues are formed in the supraoptic and paraventricular nuclei and pass down the nerve fibres of the supraoptico-neurohypophysial tract to the neurohypophysis. Here the hormones (vasopressin and oxytocin) are stored or released into the circulation as needed. It is thought (Jewell and Verney 1957) that an osmo-receptor mechanism operates in the hypothalamus to control the water balance of the body.

Pars distalis. For many years the anterior pituitary (pars distalis) was thought to control the endocrine system by means of servomechanisms operating via the circulatory system, independently of the central nervous system. However, Hinsey (1937) had suggested that hypothalamic substances (neurohumors) entered the primary capillary plexus of the hypophysial portal system and thus reached the adenohypophysial sinusoids and parenchymal cells, to influence the production of adenohypophysial hormones. Experimental confirmation of this

theory was provided by the pituitary transplantation experiments of Harris and Jacobsohn (1952). From another standpoint discrepancies in the simple feedback theory of, for example, release of adrenocorticotrophic hormone (ACTH), had led investigators to seek other mechanisms of anterior pituitary control. Much of the earlier evidence for a neurohumoral (hypothalamic) control of adenohypophysial secretion is summarized in Harris' (1955) monograph. McCann and Porter (1969) define the criteria for proof of neurohumoral regulation of adenohypophysial function as '(1) the demonstration of secretory elements in the brain that elaborate a substance(s) within diffusion distances of the primary capillary plexus of the hypophysial portal vessels; (2) the identification and characterization, using biological, chemical and physical criteria, of this substance in hypophysial portal vessel blood; and (3) the demonstration that hypophysial portal vessel blood containing this substance(s) on entering the sinusoids of the anterior pituitary affects its cells in such a way as to cause them to alter the rate of release of at least one trophic hormone.'

McCann and Porter's criteria have largely been fulfilled and much experimental evidence in favour of hypothalamic neurohumoral production has been demonstrated over the past 20 years (Locke and Schally 1972; Blackwell and Guillemin 1973). The cell bodies concerned with the production of hypothalamic neurohumors appear to lie either in the basal tuberal, the paraventricular or the suprachiasmatic regions. The substances themselves are known as 'releasing factors' and it is by negative feedback at the hypothalamic rather than at the adenohypophysial level that they are released, though some feedback probably also occurs at the pituitary level. For the most part the neurohumors are stimulatory to adenohypophysial secretion (e.g. corticotrophin releasing factor, thyrotrophin releasing factor) but there are also inhibitory factors (e.g. prolactin inhibiting factor). There appears to be at least one factor for each pituitary hormone. Many of the factors have been purified and some synthesized.

Control of feeding and drinking
The lateral hypothalamus and the ventromedial nucleus of the hypothalamus are regions associated with the control of feeding behaviour (Kennedy 1966) though such control is not exclusively hypothalamic (Brobeck 1960). Some

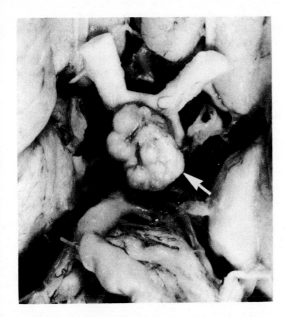

Fig. 13.3 Hamartoma (arrow) involving the tuber cinereum and hypothalamus.

patients with tumours or other lesions of the hypothalamic region become obese and hyperphagic. Thirst also appears to be under hypothalamic control, as the aphagia which occurs after experimental lesions of the lateral hypothalamus may be accompanied by permanent adipsia (Teitelbaum and Epstein 1962; Fitzsimons 1966). Fitzsimons (1972) considers that not only the hypothalamus but also the whole of the limbic system, including the amygdaloid nucleus, may control drinking and also its motivation.

Our experience of human disease, however, suggests that most clinical cases of abnormal thirst are associated with lesions primarily involving the neurosecretory system.

Control of autonomic functions

It has been found (Downey, Mottram and Pickering 1964) that thermosensitive receptors are present in the hypothalamus (as well as in other sites). Single neuron recordings from the anterior hypothalamus show that certain thermosensitive neurons increase their rate of firing with a rise of local temperature (Hardy, Hellon and Sutherland 1964). It has also been known since the work of Vogt (1954) that the anterior hypothalamus contains a high concentration of catecholamines (Shute and Lewis 1966) and indoleamines, which are largely located in neurons. Injection of these amines into the cerebral ventricles causes changes of temperature (Feldberg and Myers 1965), although the relationship of the thermoreceptor neurons to the amine-secreting neurons is not clear. In human disease there is an association between lesions within and around the 3rd ventricle and disturbances of thermoregulation.

The involvement of the hypothalamus in the

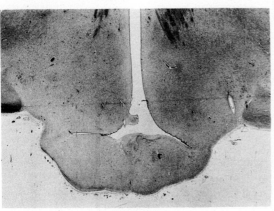

(a)

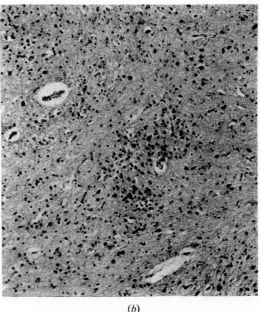

(b)

Fig. 13.4 (a) Coronal section through the hypothalamus showing a hamartoma expanding the floor of the 3rd ventricle and adjacent parts of the hypothalamus. Haematoxylin and eosin. × 4. (b) Groups of small, uniform cells are found in this hamartoma. Haematoxylin and eosin. × 80.

control of cardiovascular responses can be demonstrated by the eliciting of vasodilatation in skeletal muscle by electrical stimulation of the hypothalamus (Abrahams, Hilton and Zbrozyna 1964). Such vasodilatation in muscle occurs physiologically as part of the preparation for flight or attack. In man similar vasodilatation may accompany feelings of anxiety, which have also been induced by electrical stimulation of the medial hypothalamus (for references, see Hilton 1966).

Relationship with emotional stability

Because of its connections with the limbic system, the frontal lobes and the reticular formation of the brainstem, the hypothalamus is also associated with emotion (Smythies 1970). The anatomical associations are, however, complex and it is difficult to relate lesions of the limbic and other systems which may have caused emotional disturbance to changes in the hypothalamus.

Diseases of the hypothalamus

Congenital malformations

Hamartoma is the commonest malformation of the hypothalamus. Hamartomas are found either attached by a pedicle to the tuber cinereum or mamillary bodies, or as ill-defined masses infiltrating these structures (Figs. 13.3, 13.4*a*). They are usually not more than 1 cm in diameter, but may occasionally reach a much larger size (Lange-Cosack 1951). The pituitary gland is usually normal. The histological pattern (Fig. 13.4*b*) is one of groups of small cells (Schmidt, Hallervorden and Spatz 1958) scattered in a haphazard fashion through glial tissue in which there may be myelinated nerve fibres; the arrangement of the cells is not reminiscent of a nuclear formation (Driggs and Spatz 1940; Lange-Cosack 1951). Ependymal rests may be present (Schmidt *et al.* 1958). According to Lange-Cosack, hamartomas may be divided into those containing neurons and myelinated nerve fibres and those without these components. Interest in these lesions is centred chiefly on their association with sexual dysfunction, most commonly precocious puberty (Le Marquand and Russell 1934-1935; Weinberger and Grant 1941; Lange-Cosack 1951; Northfield and Russell 1967), although it may be difficult to determine whether precocious puberty had occurred when cases of hypothalamic hamartoma are examined in later life (Wolman

and Balmforth 1963). The mechanism whereby precocious puberty is produced is obscure.

Driggs and Spatz (1940) considered that the malformation showed hyperneurosecretion, a view supported by Wolman and Balmforth (1963) but opposed by Northfield and Russell (1967). Recent work on hypothalamic releasing factors suggests that visible neurosecretion may not be the substance responsible for gonadotrophic stimulation (McCann and Porter 1969). A more plausible explanation of the action of the hypothalamic hamartoma may be that the lesion disturbs the normal prepubertal hypothalamic inhibition of gonadotrophic activity (Donovan and Van der Werff ten Bosch 1965). Other varieties of hamartoma may be lipomatous nodules (Orthner 1961, case 13), or, occasionally, the type associated with tuberose sclerosis (Krabbe 1922).

Infective and inflammatory diseases of the hypothalamus

Pyogenic infections. The base of the brain is involved in purulent meningitis, but hypothalamic symptoms are seldom seen, perhaps because of the short duration of the acute disease. Purulent ventriculitis (pyocephalus) extending into the 3rd ventricle will impinge on hypothalamic structures and the disturbances of temperature regulation and the coma that may occur in these circumstances may be of hypothalamic origin. Meningitis and rupture of a cerebral abscess are the commonest causes of pyocephalus. Endocrine symptoms are seldom noticed because of the

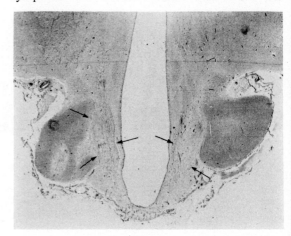

Fig. 13.5 Widespread infarction of the lower hypothalamus (arrows) and optic tract caused by septic emboli in a case of septicaemia. Haematoxylin and eosin. × 5·5.

usually short duration and fatal outcome of this condition. Direct involvement of the deeper structures of the hypothalamus by pyaemic abscess is rare. Occasionally widespread cerebral infarction, which may be septic, occurs as a complication of cerebral abscess associated with meningitis and may involve the hypothalamus (Fig. 13.5), causing disturbances of electrolyte metabolism.

of the pituitary, but not the infundibular process, are affected, it seems probable that spread has occurred from the diencephalon via the primary capillary bed into the long portal vessels of pars distalis. When, however, microorganismal infection cannot be presumed with certainty, but the

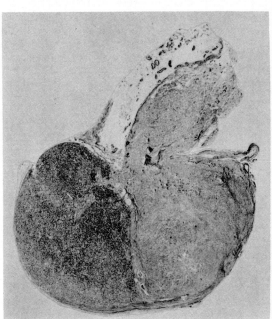 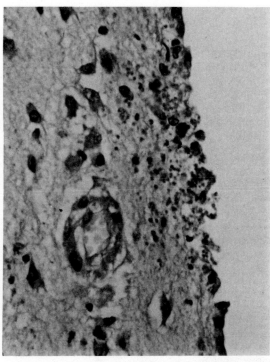

13.6	13.7

Fig. 13.6 Gagel type of granuloma. Sagittal section of pituitary showing enlargement of stalk and infundibular process. Haematoxylin and eosin. × 5·5.

Fig. 13.7 Infection by toxoplasma involving the ependyma of the 3rd ventricle, near the paraventricular nucleus. Haematoxylin and eosin. × 480.

Chronic inflammatory conditions involving the hypothalamus

The causes of these lesions are numerous (Orthner 1961). Giant cell granuloma (Rickards and Harvey 1954), sarcoidosis (Scadding 1967), syphilis, tuberculosis (Smith and Daniel 1947), cryptococcal infection, non-lipid reticulo-endotheliosis (Hewer and Heller 1949), lipidoses such as Hand–Schüller–Christian disease or histiocytosis-X (Kepes and Kepes 1969), and the so-called Gagel (1941) type of granuloma, in which the lesion is restricted to the neurohypophysis and hypothalamic floor, may all occur. These lesions may be very localized, as in the Gagel type, or may spread throughout the hypothalamo-neurohypophysial system. Thus, where the basal diencephalon and pars distalis

involvement of arterial walls by granuloma suggests the possibility of haematogenous spread, both pars distalis and pars nervosa may be affected, presumably via the internal carotid artery (Wilke 1956). If there is no evidence either of an infecting microorganism or of disease of neighbouring structures, such as the dura mater and bony sinuses, the question of aetiology must remain open, as a granulomatous histological pattern can be evoked by many different stimuli.

Non-specific granulomas include giant-cell granuloma and the localized Gagel type (Orthner 1961, cases 3, 4, 5). The hypothalamus proper in the Gagel type may contain little granulomatous tissue, although the pituitary stalk and the infundibular process may be involved (Fig. 13.6). Cellular constituents include neutrophils, lymphocytes and plasma cells, but not giant cells. If the hypothalamo-neurohypophysial tract is interrupted (as shown by clinical evidence such as diabetes insipidus), there is loss of neurons in the supraoptic and paraventricular nuclei, with glial replacement and loss of neurosecretory material. Orthner (1961) considers this lesion to be a localized form of encephalitis, but in the absence of clinical or other evidence of encephalitis this contention is difficult to uphold.

1956). The severity of the clinical picture depends on the degree of involvement of the pituitary gland and hypothalamus; the commonest symptom is diabetes insipidus (Rickards and Harvey 1954). In a personally observed case the patient, a man aged 33 years, with a 3½-year history, had a severe hypothalamic-pituitary syndrome, including hypogonadism, adrenal hypocorticalism, hypothyroidism and diabetes insipidus. The pathological changes were correspondingly extensive, with sarcoid lesions involving the major hypothalamic nuclei, the pituitary stalk and both

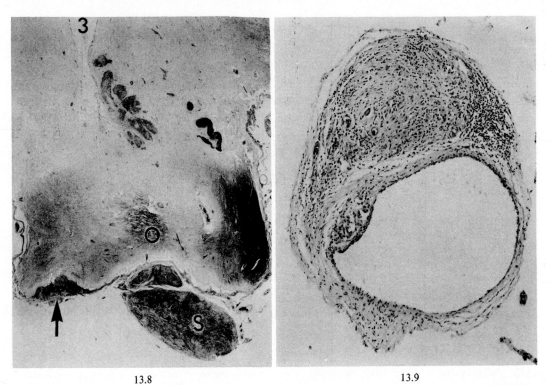

13.8   13.9

Fig. 13.8 Case of sarcoidosis. Coronal section in the plane of the optic chiasma. The pituitary stalk (S) is replaced and expanded by granulomatous tissue. There is a small plaque of this tissue (arrow) on the under aspect of the optic chiasma (O) and foci are seen to the right of the lower part of the 3rd ventricle (3). Luxol fast blue. Nissl. × 6·5.

Fig. 13.9 Sarcoidosis of meningeal vessels. Note granulomatous infiltration of medial and intimal coats of a small artery supplying the hypothalamus. Haematoxylin and eosin. × 75.

In specific chronic infections of the nervous system such as toxoplasmosis the lesions may be very widespread; for example, spread may occur through the ventricular system producing discrete ependymal lesions (Fig. 13.7), as well as into pars distalis of the pituitary. Sarcoidosis usually involves initially the meninges, but may spread into neighbouring brain, tracking along blood vessels (Wilke 1956; Kraemer and Paarmann

lobes of the pituitary gland (Fig. 13.8). A striking feature of this case was the presence of medial and intimal sarcoid lesions (Fig. 13.9) suggesting a haematogenous spread of the disease.

Vascular lesions of the hypothalamus

Vascular lesions of the hypothalamus are usually secondary to a more generalized cerebrovascular disease or accident, such as intracerebral or, more commonly, subarachnoid haemorrhage. Crompton (1963) has described the hypothalamic lesions associated with the rupture of berry aneurysms. Hypothalamic lesions occurred in about 60% of Crompton's cases and were most common with aneurysms of the anterior and posterior communicating arteries. Areas of ischaemic necrosis (up to 5 mm across) were the commonest finding and were often accompanied by infarcts elsewhere in the brain. Small haemorrhages were also seen, often in the supraoptic and paraventricular nuclei; occasionally they

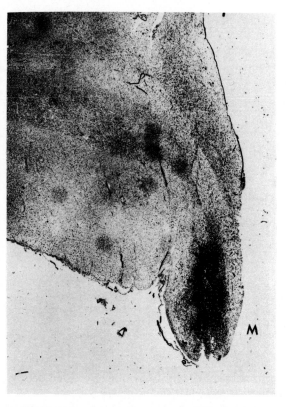

Fig. 13.10 Wernicke's disease. Note haemorrhages in the mamillary body (M). Haematoxylin and eoxin. × 5.

became confluent and destroyed the nuclei. Massive haemorrhage destroying the hypo-thalamus was the least common complication of ruptured aneurysm. Crompton considered that the haemorrhages in the hypothalamus were the result of venous back pressure caused by bleeding into the chiasmatic cistern. Hypo-thalamic infarction may occur in head injury

and is sometimes extensive (Figs. 13.13, 13.14 and 13.15).

Petechial haemorrhages of the ring and ball type are typically seen in Wernicke's encephalo-pathy (Fig. 13.10), most commonly in the mamillary bodies, but the haemorrhages may occur throughout the periventricular grey matter of the hypothalamus. The pathogenesis of these haemorrhages is obscure. Fat emboli may be found in the hypothalamus in cases of fracture of long bones (Sevitt, personal communication).

Traumatic lesions of the hypothalamus

Few descriptions of traumatic hypothalamic changes are available (Vonderahe 1940; Henzi 1952; Goldman and Jacobs 1960; Orthner and Meyer 1967; Treip 1970). In such cases there is always injury elsewhere in the brain, often severe. Certain lesions are found in the hypothalamus with some regularity. The supraoptic nucleus is the most vulnerable region and damage may be associated with an obvious external lesion such as tearing of the optic tract (Fig. 13.11). Such tearing results in disruption of and haemorrhage into the supraoptic nucleus, and is commonly found in patients dying soon after head injury. Sometimes a haemorrhage into the supraoptic nucleus may be converted into a collection of haemosiderin-laden macrophages occupying most of the nucleus. The vulnerability of the supra-optic nucleus to damage may perhaps be explained anatomically by the tethering of the optic nerve at the optic foramen. When the brain moves suddenly in cerebral trauma a shearing strain is imposed on the angle in which the supraoptic nucleus lies, between the lamina terminalis and the optic nerve, and this results in injury to the nucleus (Fig. 13.12). The paraventricular nucleus often contains petechial haemorrhages and some-times shows striking oedema, which may be circumscribed. The vessels in and around the nuclei may show hyaline necrosis of their walls, possibly the result of spasm at the time of injury followed by increased capillary permeability. The predisposition to haemorrhage in both supraoptic and paraventricular nuclei may be related to the richness of their capillary blood supply, which is greater than anywhere else in the central nervous system.

The commonest traumatic lesion in the infundi-bulum is an acute infarct, which is usually found in the midline, in the tuber cinereum or upper infundibular stem (Fig. 13.13), while bilateral infarction of the ventromedial nucleus may occur (Fig. 13.14). Infarction of the hypothalamus may be widespread (Fig. 13.15). Sometimes a glial scar is seen in the infundibulum. The mechanism of infundibular infarction may be explained by the tethering of the pituitary within the sella turcica by the diaphragma sellae. When the brain moves, the pituitary stalk is stretched and with it the branches of the superior hypophysial

animals there is loss of nerve cells in the supra-optic and paraventricular nuclei and in the remaining cells and their axons there is an excess of neurosecretory material, while in the median eminence and upper part of the hypothalamo-neurohypophysial tract considerable numbers of Herring bodies and many beaded (neurosecretory) nerve fibres are present. The infundibular process on the other hand shows a decrease in stainable

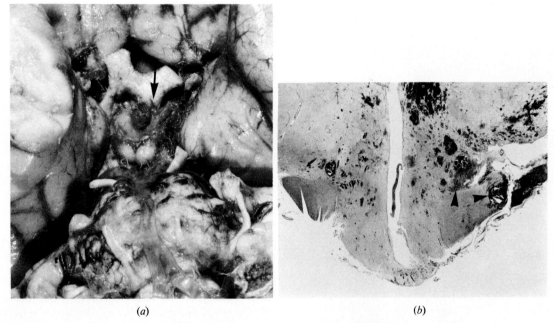

(a)   (b)

Fig. 13.11 A case of head injury. (a) Base of brain showing tearing of left optic tract (arrow), and distortion of the optic chiasma. The stump of the pituitary stalk, below and to the left of the arrow, which had been transected at the time of the accident, is haemorrhagic. (b) Coronal section through the hypothalamus, showing recent haemorrhages in the left optic tract and left supraoptic nucleus (arrows). Haemorrhages are also present in the periventricular region and the right supraoptic nucleus. Luxol fast blue/cresyl violet. × 3·5.

artery supplying the basal hypothalamus. These vessels may go into spasm or rupture with a consequent infarction of their territory of supply (Fig. 13.12). Widespread fibrosis of the hypo-thalamus has occasionally been seen in a patient surviving for many months after head injury (Goldman and Jacobs 1960).

Degenerative and metabolic diseases affecting the hypothalamus

In certain cases of scrapie (a degenerative disease of the brain of sheep) the animals develop some degree of diabetes insipidus. In these

neurosecretory material and an increased density of cells (Beck, Daniel and Parry 1964).

In kuru (see p. 317), a chronic neurological disease seen only in the Fore people of New Guinea, some excess of neurosecretory material may be seen in the tuber cinereum and upper infundibular stem, though obvious loss of cells from the paraventricular and supraoptic nuclei has not been observed (Beck, Daniel, Alpers, Gajdusek and Gibbs 1969). In some cases of Creutzfeldt–Jakob disease there is a similar, but more marked, excess of neurosecretory material (Beck, Daniel, Matthews, Stevens, Alpers, Asher, Gajdusek and Gibbs 1969) (see p. 827).

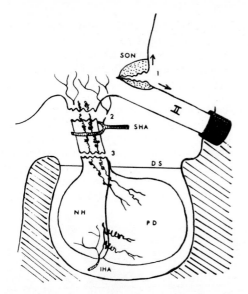

Fig. 13.12 Diagram to illustrate possible mechanisms of hypothalamic and pituitary damage in cases of head injury. (1) Tethering of the optic nerve to the dura at the optic foramen leads to tearing of the supraoptic nuclei as a result of sudden movements of the brain. (2) High transection of the pituitary stalk results in rupture of the branches of the arterial ring which go upwards to the hypothalamus but leaves intact the branches to the stalk which supply the primary capillary bed of the portal vessels. (3) Low stalk transection results in rupture of the long portal vessels supplying most of pars distalis. II = optic nerve. DS = diaphragma sellae. IHA = inferior hypophysial artery. NH = infundibular process. PD = pars distalis. SHA = superior hypophysial artery. SON = supraoptic nucleus.

Acute intermittent porphyria

Disturbances of electrolyte balance found in cases of acute intermittent porphyria have in recent years been linked with the syndrome of 'inappropriate secretion of antidiuretic hormone' (Perlroth, Tschudy, Marver, Costan, Zeigel, Rechcigl and Collins 1966). We have examined the hypothalamus of a case of acute intermittent porphyria with sustained hyponatraemia over a period of two years. Neurosecretory neurons were well preserved and showed an abnormal, excessive amount of intracellular neurosecretory material associated with increased cellularity of the neurohypophysis. This phenomenon appears to be distinct from the cerebral demyelinating lesions most commonly found in acute porphyria (Gibson and Goldberg 1956).

Neurolipidoses

In a case of amaurotic familial idiocy (juvenile type) the cells of the supraoptic nucleus (Fig. 13.16), and to a lesser degree those of the paraventricular nucleus, were found to contain PAS-positive granules, presumably ganglioside, similar to the material found in the cortical neurons.

Changes in the hypothalamus after hypophysectomy and pituitary stalk section

When a hypophysectomy is performed, or if the pituitary stalk is cut, the axons of the hypothalamic cells forming the hypothalamo-neurohypophysial tract are severed. The bulk of the cells from which

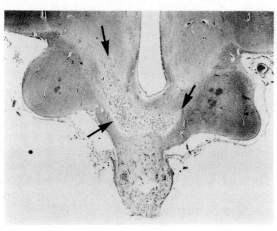

13.13

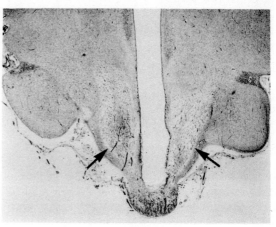

13.14

Fig. 13.13 Coronal section through the hypothalamus in a case of head injury with acute infarction immediately above the pituitary stalk (arrows). Haematoxylin and eosin. × 4·25.

Fig. 13.14 Same case as in Fig. 13.13 showing bilateral acute infarction of the ventromedial nucleus (arrows). Haematoxylin and eosin. × 4·25.

these axons originate are clearly situated in the supraoptic and paraventricular nuclei. Within two months of the operation many cells in the supraoptic nucleus disappear (Fig. 13.17a, b). The cells of the paraventricular nucleus are less severely affected and those cells which disappear seem to be mainly the large neurons. The surviving cells in both nuclei show some increase of neurosecretory material. In long-standing cases there may be very few cells left in the supraoptic nucleus (Daniel and Prichard 1972, 1975). The

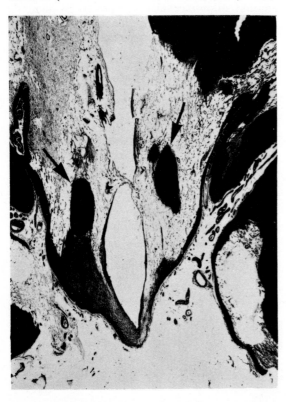

Fig. 13.15 Coronal section through the hypothalamus in a case of long survival after head injury. Extensive old infarcts (pale) of most of the hypothalamus, including the wall of the 3rd ventricle, but sparing the fornices (arrows). Survival 110 days; persistent hypothermia. Loyez. × 5·5.

sites of the nuclei may be indicated by the fibrous gliosis which often develops (Fig. 13.18). Shortly after the pituitary stalk is cut there is a great increase in the quantity of neurosecretory material in the tuber cinereum and upper part of the stalk (Beck, Daniel and Prichard 1969). This suggests that the neurosecretory material has passed down the axons of the hypothalamo-neurohypophysial tract and is dammed up above the level of

transection (Muller 1955). In some animals there is a striking regeneration of the nerve fibres of the hypothalamo-neurohypophysial tract (Daniel and Prichard 1970, 1975; Adams, Daniel and Prichard 1971), but not in man.

Hypothalamic changes after irradiation
The hypothalamus may be damaged when ablation of the pituitary gland is attempted by implantation of such substances as yttrium-90. Accidental damage may also result from displacement of radioactive implants into the 3rd ventricle (Fig. 13.19). The lesions in the hypothalamus

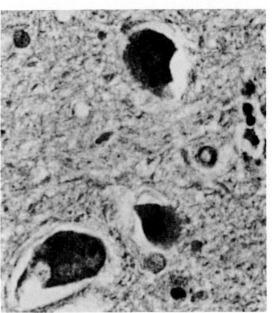

Fig. 13.16 Cells of the supraoptic nucleus from a case of amaurotic familial idiocy (juvenile type). The cells contain large numbers of PAS-positive granules. Periodic-acid-Schiff. × 650.

range from some loss of nerve cells (including cells of the supraoptic nucleus) and occasional glial stars, with slight round cell cuffing of some of the small vessels, to severe necrosis of considerable areas in which the vessels show acute fibrinoid necrosis. In the surviving tissue round the necrotic areas there is astrocytic hypertrophy (see also Crompton and Layton 1961).

Invasive tumours
Diffuse astrocytomas may infiltrate the whole of the hypothalamus (Fig. 13.20) without, in some cases, any appreciable disturbances of endocrine function. A pilocytic astrocytoma of the optic

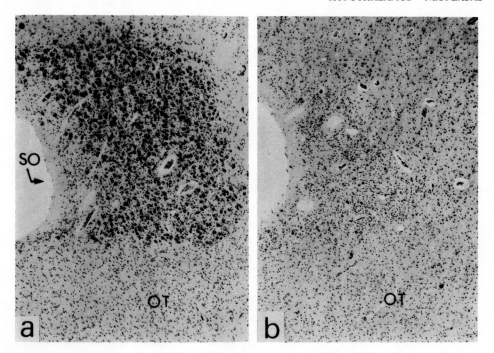

Fig. 13.17   Coronal sections through: (*a*) Normal supraoptic nucleus, SO.   Nissl.   ×40.   (*b*) Supraoptic nucleus 4 months after hypophysectomy.   Note almost total loss of nerve cells and shrinkage of the nucleus.   In both cases the optic tract, OT, lies below the nucleus.   Nissl.   ×40.

nerve or chiasma may spread caudally to replace the hypothalamus in part or in whole.   Such tumours (Fig. 13.21) may, in infants, lead to the development of a 'diencephalic syndrome' (Russell 1951; Braun and Forney 1959).

Seedlings from *medulloblastoma* may be found

invading either the ependyma of the third ventricle (Fig. 13.22) or the outer surface of the hypothalamus and causing varying degrees of destruction.   *Leukaemic deposits* may invade the hypothalamus in the same way.   Occasionally hypothalamic invasion by *microglioma* can give

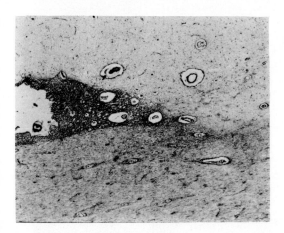

Fig. 13.18   Gliosis (dark triangular area) throughout the entire territory of the supraoptic nucleus 10 months after hypophysectomy.   There was great loss of nerve cells in this nucleus.   Optic tract below.   Holzer.   ×30.

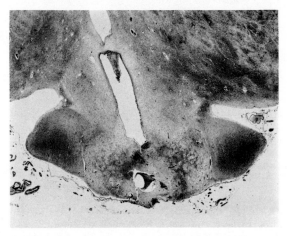

Fig. 13.19   Necrosis and gliosis of walls of 3rd ventricle, caused by the presence of a needle of yttrium-90 in the ventricular cavity.   Haematoxylin and eosin.   ×4.

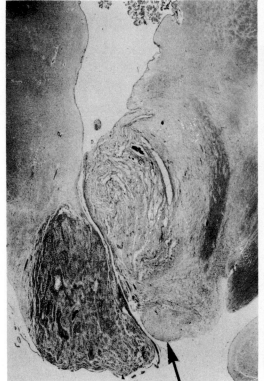

13.20

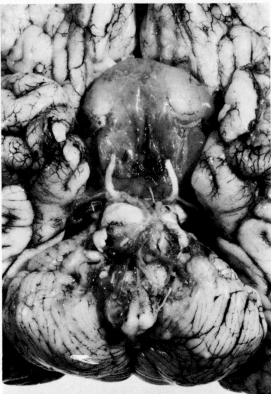

13.21

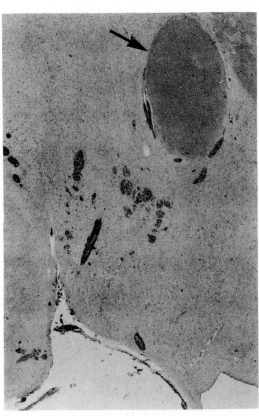

13.22

Fig. 13.20 Coronal section through posterior part of hypothalamus. An astrocytoma has replaced much of this region. Part of the mamillary body (arrow) is seen on the right, though on the left it has been completely replaced by tumour. Haematoxylin and eosin. ×4·5.

Fig. 13.21 Base of brain showing large astrocytoma replacing all the structures of the hypothalamic region. The patient had developed the 'diencephalic syndrome'.

Fig. 13.22 Mid-sagittal section of brain. A medulloblastoma, seen as a haemorrhagic mass replacing much of the cerebellum, has seeded to the 3rd ventricle where a secondary mass (arrow) is destroying the hypothalamus.

Fig. 13.23 Case of 'carcinomatous encephalitis'. Sagittal section through the lateral wall of the hypothalamus. Many of the small vessels show cuffing by carcinoma cells around and below the anterior commissure (arrow). Haematoxylin and eosin. ×9.

13.23

rise to the clinical picture of hypopituitarism (Duchen and Treip 1969).

Secondary carcinoma, as well as forming a single large deposit in the hypothalamus, may spread along the hypothalamic vessels in the form of a 'carcinomatous encephalitis' (Fig. 13.23) or may produce multiple deposits of microscopic size (Fig. 13.24). A special example of metastatic deposit is that not infrequently seen in the pituitary stalk and infundibular process. The circulating tumour cells are presumably trapped in the primary capillary bed of the median

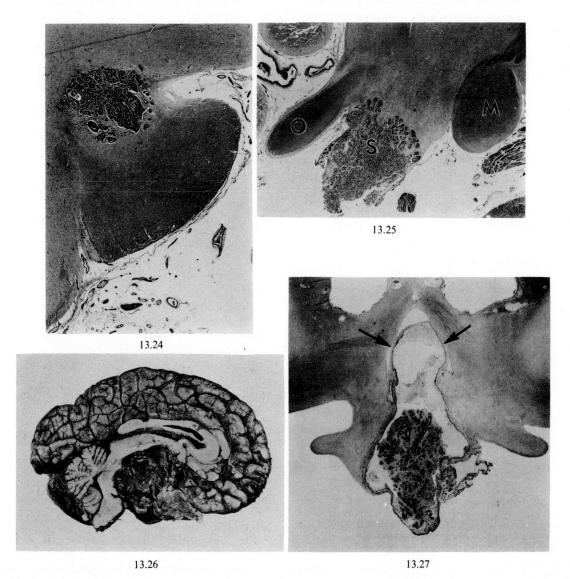

13.25

13.24

13.26

13.27

Fig. 13.24 Secondary deposit from carcinoma of the breast destroying most of one supraoptic nucleus (optic tract below and to the right).   Haematoxylin and eosin.   × 9.

Fig. 13.25 A secondary deposit from a carcinoma of the breast which had destroyed the pituitary stalk.   O, optic chiasma; M, mamillary body; S, stalk expanded by tumour.   Haematoxylin and eosin.   × 4.

Fig. 13.26 Mid-sagittal section to show a chromophobe adenoma of the pituitary which had compressed and distorted the hypothalamic region.   The patient, a man aged 22, was grossly obese and was impotent.

Fig. 13.27 Partly solid and partly cystic craniopharyngioma.   This has grown up into the cavity of the 3rd ventricle, which is expanded and distorted.   Arrows show wall of cyst.   Nissl.   × 2.5.

eminence and infundibular stem (Fig. 13.25). The greater part of the infundibular process and stalk may be destroyed (Duchen 1966, Fig. 15). Diabetes insipidus, usually associated with atrophy of the neurosecretory neurons of the supraoptic and paraventricular nuclei, is a common complication of this lesion. Carcinoma of the breast, bronchus and stomach are the commonest neoplasms to metastasize in this way.

Tumours compressing the hypothalamus

A large *pituitary adenoma* (usually chromophobe) often extends upwards and in addition to compressing the optic chiasma may press upon and distort the hypothalamus. In the case illustrated in Fig. 13.26 there was blindness and gross obesity in a young man. More commonly *craniopharyngiomas* extend upwards, indenting and often destroying a considerable part of the hypothalamus. A craniopharyngioma may fill the

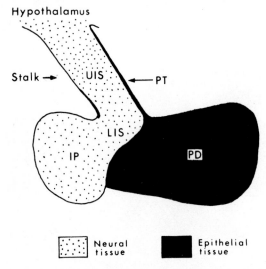

Fig. 13.28 Diagram of the pituitary gland to show the anatomical subdivisions. Black area: epithelial tissue; stippled area: neural tissue (neurohypophysis). UIS: upper infundibular stem; LIS: lower infundibular stem; IP: infundibular process (posterior or neural lobe); PD: anterior lobe or pars distalis; PT: pars tuberalis.

3rd ventricle, producing hypothermia and obesity (Fig. 13.27). A *subependymoma* arising in the wall of the 3rd ventricle may destroy part of the hypothalamus by pressure. Large *colloid cysts* of the 3rd ventricle may compress the hypothalamus. *Pineal teratomas* may sometimes be found within the 3rd ventricle, either ectopically or as a result of anterior displacement of the

neoplasm. The relation of this tumour to precocious puberty may be explained more readily by pressure on hypothalamic structures (Lange-Cosack 1952; Russell and Rubinstein 1971) than by hormonal production by the tumour itself, since evidence of the hormonal role of the pineal is inconclusive (Critchlow and Bar-Sala 1967).

Anatomy of the pituitary gland

The nomenclature used is that of Rioch, Wislocki and O'Leary (1940). The neural downgrowth from the brain forms, from above down, the median eminence, the upper infundibular stem, the lower infundibular stem (Xuereb, Prichard and Daniel 1954*a*) and the infundibular process (the neural or posterior lobe), these elements together forming the neurohypophysis. The epithelial upgrowth from the pharynx gives rise, from its rostral wall, to pars distalis (the anterior lobe). The caudal wall gives rise to pars intermedia in lower animals; this is not seen in man. A diagram of the general arrangements of the human gland is shown in Fig. 13.28 (see also Daniel and Prichard 1975).

Cytology of pars distalis

Pars distalis is composed of epithelial cells, which are supported by a reticulin network and are permeated by sinusoids. Three principal types of glandular cell are found; acidophil, basophil and chromophobe (Romeis 1940). The acidophil cell is typically a large cell with a considerable amount of cytoplasm and contains coarse intracytoplasmic granules which take up acid stains. These cells are concentrated in the posterolateral part of the lobe. The basophil cells contain intracytoplasmic granules staining with basic dyes, and lie largely in the anteromedial region of the lobe, but are also scattered elsewhere. The cytoplasm of chromophobe cells, which are distributed diffusely throughout the lobe, does not have any special tinctorial affinity.

The classification of the granulated cells of the human pars distalis is fraught with difficulty. Nomenclatures of varying complexity have been devised, but since much of the work has been done on animals, and the correlation between man and animal does not appear to be good, no completely satisfying system is available. The various classifications represent attempts to identify individual cell types, stained by various histological or histochemical methods, with the secretion of individual hormones (Romeis 1940; Ezrin and Murray 1963; Purves 1966).

The granules of the acidophil cells appear to be composed of simple proteins, while those of the basophils are composed of glycoprotein as shown by their reaction with the periodic-acid-Schiff (PAS) stain. This seems to be a fundamental difference between the two series of cells. The chromophobe cells are regarded by many as degranulated acidophils or basophils. The Crooke–Russell cell (Crooke and Russell 1935) is a degranulated basophil cell, perhaps an intermediate form.

The precise identification of the nine types of cell in the human pars distalis described by Conklin (1966, 1968), who based his study on Ezrin's classification, depends on the acquisition of material within 3 to 4 hours of death. With such material a tentative classification of cytological type according to hormonal production may be made.

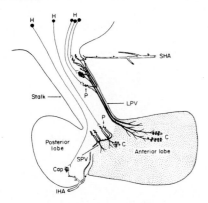

Fig. 13.29 Diagram of the pituitary gland to show sites of the primary capillary beds (P) at which it is believed that releasing factors are transferred from the axons of hypothalamic cells (H) into the blood stream of long (LPV) and short (SPV) portal vessels to be carried to the epithelial cells (C) of pars distalis, which they stimulate to secrete. SHA, superior hypophysial artery; IHA, inferior hypophysial artery.

It is probable, as Conklin (1966) points out, that too much has been made of the importance of identifying a specific cell type with a specific hormonal function. In practice the material normally available to the pathologist is rarely fixed soon enough after death to make an attempt at identification possible. Moreover, any functional interpretation of pituitary histology demands serial sections through pars distalis and differential cell counting to obtain a reliable result.

Vascular connections of the pituitary gland

Pars distalis of the pituitary in man, as in most animals, is supplied solely by portal venous blood (Xuereb *et al.* 1954*a*, *b*; Daniel and Prichard 1975). This is brought mainly by the long portal vessels, originating in the coiled capillaries (gomitoli) of the tuber cinereum and upper infundibular stem and ending distally in the sinusoids of pars distalis. The region of pars distalis adjacent to the lower infundibular stem is supplied by the short portal vessels originating from the primary capillary bed of simple coiled vessels in the lower infundibular stem (Fig. 13.29). The infundibular process itself has a direct arterial supply from the inferior hypophysial artery, supplemented by the artery of the trabecula, derived from the superior hypophysial artery. References to the control of pars distalis will be found in Porter, Mical, Ben-Jonathan and Ondo (1973).

Disorders of the pituitary gland

Agenesis in anencephaly

In most cases of anencephaly the pituitary gland is present (Willis 1962), but abnormal. One-half of the normal amount of pars distalis tissue may be present. The neural tissue of the pituitary is usually lacking. The hypothalamus cannot be identified histologically in these cases. It seems probable that the abnormality of the pituitary is secondary to the failure of the hypothalamus to develop. Target organs of the pituitary such as the thyroid and adrenals may also be deficient in this condition (Potter 1961).

Infective and inflammatory conditions

A metastatic *abscess* of pars distalis may be seen, though it is rare. It must be distinguished from the collections of pus on the diaphragma sellae and around the stalk which are commonly found in purulent meningitis. *Tuberculous infiltration* of the pituitary is uncommon, though we have seen an example.

The pituitary may be involved in *generalized toxoplasmosis* as a metastatic phenomenon or there may be invasive spread of the infection from the brain. *Sarcoidosis* usually involves the meninges (Fig. 13.9) but can involve both the hypothalamus and the pituitary stalk (Fig. 13.8). Such cases not infrequently show clinical signs of pituitary insufficiency, including diabetes insipidus.

Non-specific and giant cell granuloma

Non-specific chronic inflammatory infiltration of the pituitary stalk and infundibular process giving rise to intractable diabetes insipidus may occasionally be seen (Fig. 13.6). In some cases the infiltration may be an extension from the hypothalamus, although granulomatous lesions may not be found elsewhere in the body. These chronic inflammatory conditions of the *neurohypophysis* are to be distinguished from the giant cell granuloma (Rickards and Harvey 1954) in which only *pars distalis* is involved and in which changes may be found in other organs, such as the adrenal. In both conditions the aetiology is obscure.

Effects of pressure on or invasion of the pituitary gland

In cases of *internal hydrocephalus* raised intracranial pressure causes bulging of the tuber cinereum downwards into the sella turcica, compressing the pituitary gland, which assumes a flattened or scaphoid appearance. After a time

internal carotid artery (Fig. 13.30) within the cavernous sinus may also cause hypopituitarism by compression (Orthner 1961).

Primary or secondary neoplasms of the pituitary not only compress but may also replace the gland. Invasive tumours are prone to cause hypopituitarism. Secondary deposits are most commonly seen either in the infundibular process (Fig. 13.31) or in the neural part of the pituitary stalk (Duchen 1966), but may sometimes be found in pars distalis. Hypopituitarism resulting from the commonest pituitary neoplasm, chromophobe adenoma, is usually a late phenomenon, associated with a large tumour (Fig. 13.26).

Traumatic lesions

The pituitary gland may be damaged in head injuries, either directly when a fracture passes through the pituitary fossa, or, much more commonly, by interference with its blood supply (Daniel and Treip 1966a; Ceballos 1966; Orthner and Meyer 1967). In both types of injury the neural tissue of the infundibular process is most

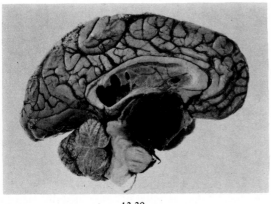
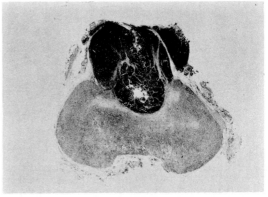

13.30   13.31

Fig. 13.30 Sagittal section showing large, unruptured carotid aneurysm which had damaged the hypothalamus and pituitary by pressure and distortion.

Fig. 13.31 Horizontal section through the pituitary gland. The infundibular process (neural lobe) is wholly replaced by a deposit from a secondary carcinoma (black). Haematoxylin and eosin. × 5.

the sella turcica becomes widened. Clinical hypopituitarism rarely develops. Any mass within or adjacent to the sella turcica may compress and eventually destroy the pituitary, causing hypopituitarism. Simple compression may be exerted by primary or secondary tumours of bone, by meningiomas around the pituitary fossa, by craniopharyngiomas, and by granulomatous infiltration of bone such as occurs in Hand–Schüller–Christian disease. Aneurysms of the

commonly affected, acute haemorrhage being seen in about 45% of cases of fatal head injury. Many of the haemorrhages are small (Fig. 13.32), but occasionally (in from 10 to 15% of cases) they are large. Even in these latter cases, however, diabetes insipidus is uncommon and is scarcely ever permanent. The occurrence of a prolonged or permanent diabetes insipidus is probably dependent on concomitant damage to the infundibulum or to the supraoptic and paraventricular nuclei. Such hypothalamic damage is not uncommon in head injury (see section on the hypothalamus). Necrosis of the infundibular process is rare, being seen only in cases of severe and persistent anoxia such as occurs in prolonged maintenance on artificial respirators (Daniel, Spicer and Treip 1973). If the pituitary stalk is severed by injury (Daniel, Prichard and Treip

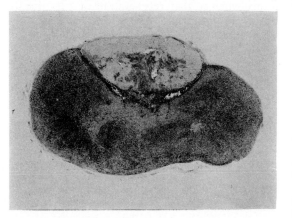

Fig. 13.32 Haemorrhages in the neural tissue of the infundibular process of the pituitary gland in a case of head injury. Haematoxylin and eosin. × 5·7.

1959; Daniel and Treip 1966a) as may sometimes occur, denervation of the infundibular process is soon indicated by an apparent increase in cellularity. Such changes are sometimes associated with the presence of argyrophilic retraction balls (Daniel and Prichard 1966) around the site of transection and pooling of neurosecretory material (Orthner and Meyer 1967). Agonal thrombi may be found in the vessels of the infundibular stem. Atrophy (Lerman and Means 1945; Henzi 1952; Goldman and Jacobs 1960), haemosiderin deposition (Orthner and Meyer 1967) and cystic changes (Marañon 1926) have been recorded, but the number of cases is small.

Acute traumatic haemorrhage in pars distalis is not common (less than 5%) and the foci tend to be small. Small infarcts may occur, usually peripherally and these probably are not of functional importance. Large infarcts, involving up to 90% of pars distalis, are seen in 5 to 10% of fatal head injuries (Daniel and Treip 1966a; Ceballos 1966). The earliest changes in pars distalis may appear within 24 hours of injury. The picture (Fig. 13.33) is the same as that seen after surgical transection of the stalk and is therefore thought to be the result of traumatic

interruption of the portal blood supply of pars distalis. The stalk is not always divided in traumatic injury, and in these cases some other mechanism causing ischaemia, such as stretching of the blood vessels, with consequent spasm, may be inferred. The confinement of the pituitary within the sella turcica by the diaphragma sellae probably makes the stalk particularly vulnerable to the shearing strains imposed by sudden movements of the brain (Kornblum and Fisher 1969). Orthner and Meyer (1967) consider that infarcts occurring in the absence of stalk transection are

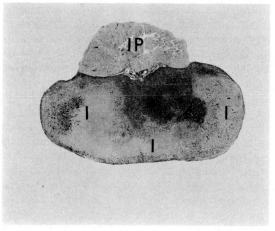

Fig. 13.33 Necrosis of pars distalis caused by traumatic rupture of the pituitary stalk (15 days' survival). Note that a considerable mass of pars distalis cells have survived, adjacent to the infundibular process (IP), nourished by the short portal vessels which retained their blood supply when the stalk was torn across. I, infarct in pars distalis. Haematoxylin and eosin. × 5.

the consequence of hypotensive shock resulting in anoxia, analogous with the postpartum infarcts described by Sheehan (Sheehan 1937; Sheehan and Davis 1968). The distribution of infarction does, however, correspond to the territories supplied by the long portal vessels as described by Xuereb et al. (1954b). The various hypotheses for the mechanism of infarction are reviewed exhaustively by Kovacs (1969) and a further hypotheses was put forward by Daniel, Spicer and Treip (1973). Of special interest are those cases in which pars distalis is not infarcted, though the stalk is transected (Daniel, Prichard and Treip 1959, case 6; Orthner and Meyer 1967, case 3). This apparent anomaly may be explained by high transection of the stalk above the hypophysial arterial ring, which spares the long portal vessels below the ring, but involves the infundibular branches above it, so that in such cases hypothalamic and tuberal, but not anterior pituitary, infarction occurs (Fig. 13.12).

Lesions of pars distalis in chronic hypopituitarism of traumatic origin have rarely been reported. There may be a reduction in size of the gland, haemosiderin deposition and lymphocytic foci (for references, see Daniel and Treip 1966a). Fibrosis appears to be inconstant (Ceballos 1966).

Ischaemic necrosis of pars distalis

In recent years there has been an increasing understanding of ischaemic necrosis of the pituitary partly as a result of a fuller knowledge of its blood supply (Xeureb et al. 1954a, b), partly as a result of experimental work (Daniel and Prichard 1956, 1975; Adams, Daniel and Prichard 1966a) and partly from a study of cases of pituitary stalk section in man (Adams, Daniel and Prichard 1966b). In these latter cases it was found that up to 90% of pars distalis became necrotic. The explanation for this large infarct is that the bulk of the blood supply to the anterior lobe is carried by long hypophysial-portal blood vessels, which run down the stalk (Fig. 13.29), and are transected at operation. Thus the only part of the lobe which survives is that which received its blood supply from the short portal vessels originating in the lower infundibular stem; a rim of tissue, probably nourished by reflux from the venous blood around the pituitary, also commonly survives. Duchen (1966) showed that tumour emboli in the primary capillary bed of the portal vessels caused similar ischaemic necrosis of the anterior lobe. The appearance of an 'empty sella' may be the result of an extensive, clinically silent, infarct. In such cases the sella is not empty, but contains a flattened pituitary remnant, which has maintained normal, or nearly normal, endocrine function.

The pituitary gland after stalk section

The operation of pituitary stalk section is performed in order to inhibit pituitary secretion and thus to decrease hormonal stimulation of various types of carcinoma, most commonly mammary. Not only is up to 90% of the anterior lobe destroyed as a result of the operation, but also those epithelial cells which survive are deprived of the hypothalamic stimuli to secretion normally carried by the short portal vessels. The

infundibular process (neural lobe) is simultaneously denervated since the hypothalamo-neurohypophysial tract is cut in the stalk. The infarct in the anterior lobe shrinks rapidly and after a time only a relatively small scar is found (Adams et al. 1966b). The neural lobe also shrinks and the cells appear to be more densely packed (Adams et al. 1963, 1964, 1966b). There is no evidence that regeneration of pars distalis occurs in man; and there is evidence of only slight regenerative capacity in other mammals such as the sheep (Daniel and Treip 1966b).

Postpartum pituitary necrosis

Simmonds (1914) described a syndrome of chronic pituitary insufficiency and reported finding a severely shrunken fibrotic pituitary in a woman suffering from this condition many years after a complicated delivery. The pituitary gland from

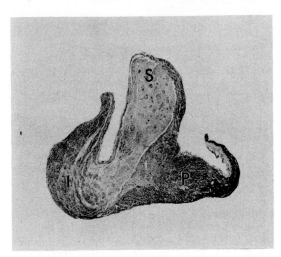

Fig. 13.34 Severely shrunken pituitary gland from a case of Simmonds' disease. There is conspicuous atrophy of pars distalis and the infundibular process. S, stalk; P, pars distalis; I, infundibular process. Haematoxylin and eosin. × 11·5.

a case of long-standing postpartum pituitary necrosis is seen in Fig. 13.34. Sheehan (1937) and Sheehan and Summers (1949) showed that many cases of postpartum haemorrhage and shock were associated with the development of a large infarct in pars distalis of the pituitary. The cause of the pituitary infarct in these cases is still unclear but it seems that infarction must be related to a cessation of blood flow through the long portal vessels, possibly owing to hypotension. Sheehan and Whitehead (1963) have described cases of postpartum anterior pituitary necrosis in which the infundibular process also showed atrophy or scarring.

Other conditions in which anterior pituitary necrosis is found

It has been known for many years that necrosis of pars distalis may be seen in cases of diabetes mellitus (Brennan, Malone and Weaver 1956). In epidemic haemorrhagic fever anterior pituitary necrosis is often found (Hullinghorst and Steer 1953). Small infarcts are often found in cases

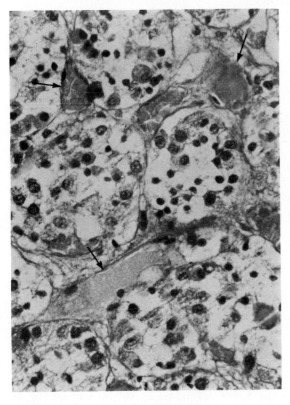

Fig. 13.35 Gargoylism. Pars distalis of the pituitary gland with amorphous material (arrows) lying between acini. The basophil cells show fine vacuolation. Masson's trichrome. × 400.

of raised intracranial pressure (Wolman 1956). There are various reports of pituitary necrosis in shock.

Extensive necrosis of pars distalis may develop in cases that have been kept on an artificial respirator for between 4 and 33 days. The cause for the necrosis is not clear, but Daniel, Spicer and Treip (1973) have suggested that it

may be related to spasm of the superior hypophysial arteries, which is known to occur in some cases of brain swelling. In two of our cases infarction of the infundibular process was also seen, but usually this part of the gland remains intact.

Abnormal depositions in the pituitary

In a number of conditions characterized by widespread deposition of abnormal substances the pituitary gland may be affected; for example in secondary amyloidosis deposits of amyloid material may be seen in the vessels of the capsule and in the trabecula. In gargoylism (Hurler's disease) pars distalis contains many large pale cells with faintly PAS-positive granules and interstitial amorphous material (Fig. 13.35). In a case recently examined there appeared to be a reduction in number of normal basophil cells.

Post-irradiation changes in the pituitary

The pituitary gland has been irradiated as a therapeutic measure in cases of carcinoma of the breast, chromophobe and acidophil adenoma of pars distalis, diabetes mellitus and occasionally exophthalmic ophthalmoplegia. The gland shrinks and may show thickening of its capsule. The epithelial tissue may become necrotic and partly replaced by collagenous scar tissue (Fig. 13.36). Although much of the gland may be destroyed, viable epithelial cells are usually found around the periphery (Oppenheimer 1959).

Changes in the pituitary gland in endocrine disease

Specific changes in the epithelial cells of pars distalis are seen in some endocrine conditions. In myxoedema there is a considerable increase in large cells which are weakly Schiff-positive and are probably thyrotrophic basophils. These cells contain numerous cytoplasmic vesicles within which lipoprotein is found (Thornton 1959). It seems likely that there is a feed-back mechanism activated by lack of thyroid hormone which induces overstimulation of the hypothalamus and hyperplasia of the thyrotrophic cells.

In cases in which the adrenals are severely damaged or are hypoplastic, as in Addison's disease, there is a reduction in the number of normal granulated basophil cells and so-called Crooke–Russell cells appear (Crooke and Russell 1935). These are large cells with basophil cytoplasm which is either hyaline or finely granular in contrast to the normal coarse granules.

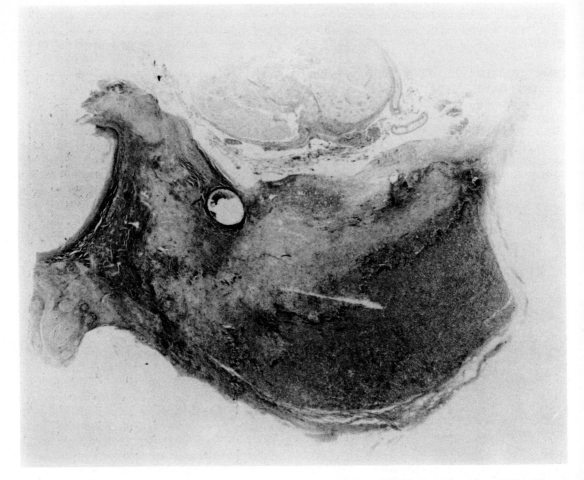

Fig. 13.36 Horizontal section through pituitary gland, to show necrosis caused by implantation of an yttrium-90 seed. The clear ovoid space is the site of the seed. About half of the surrounding pars distalis is necrotic and clearly demarcated from the surviving tissue (infundibular process above). Haematoxylin and van Gieson. × 10.

Clusters of large, basophilic cells, of Crooke–Russell type with finely granular or almost hyaline cytoplasm have been noted in patients who have received massive doses of steroids.

Diabetes insipidus

Modern ideas on diabetes insipidus date from the work of Fisher, Ingram and Ranson (1938), who showed that the control of water metabolism was dependent on the integrity of the hypothalamo-neurohypophysial tract. As the neurosecretory system controlling water metabolism is extensive and diffuse (except in the final common path of the lower infundibular stem), damage to the system has to be widespread to cause symptoms. Hereditary and idiopathic cases of diabetes insipidus are described (Green, Buchan, Alvord and Swanson 1967).

References

Abrahams, V. C., Hilton, S. M. & Zbrozyna, A. W.   (1964) The role of active muscle vasodilatation in the alerting stage of the defence reaction. *Journal of Physiology*, **171**, 189-202.

Adams, J. H., Daniel, P. M. & Prichard, M. M. L.   (1963) The effect of stalk section on the volume of the pituitary gland of the sheep. *Acta Endocrinologica*, **43**, Suppl. 81.

Adams, J. H., Daniel, P. M. & Pritchard, M. M. L. (1964) Transection of the pituitary stalk in the goat and its effect on the volume of the pituitary gland. *Journal of Pathology and Bacteriology*, **87**, 1-14.

Adams, J. H., Daniel, P. M. & Prichard, M. M. L. (1966a) Observations on the portal circulation of the pituitary gland. *Neuroendocrinology*, **1**, 193-213.

Adams, J. H., Daniel, P. M. & Prichard, M. M. L. (1966b) Transection of the pituitary stalk in man; anatomical changes in the pituitary glands of 21 patients. *Journal of Neurology, Neurosurgery and Psychiatry*, **29**, 545-555.

Adams, J. H., Daniel, P. M. & Prichard, M. M. L. (1971) Changes in the hypothalamus associated with regeneration of the hypothalamo-neurohypophysial tract after pituitary stalk section in the ferret. *Journal of Comparative Neurology*, **142**, 109-124.

Bargmann, W. (1954) *Das Zwischenhirn-Hypophysensystem*, Springer Verlag, Berlin.

Bauer, H. G. (1954) Endocrine and other manifestations of hypothalamic disease. *Journal of Clinical Endocrinology*, **14**, 13-31.

Beck, E., Daniel, P. M. & Parry, H. B. (1964) Degeneration of the cerebellar and hypothalamo-neurohypophysial systems in sheep with scrapie and its relationship to human system degenerations. *Brain*, **87**, 153-176.

Beck, E., Daniel, P. M., Alpers, M., Gajdusek, D. C. & Gibbs, C. J. Jr. (1969) Neuropathological comparisons of experimental kuru in chimpanzees with human kuru in Pathogenesis and Etiology of Demyelinating Diseases. Locarno Symposium. Add. ad *International Archives of Allergy*, **36**, 553-562.

Beck, E., Daniel, P. M., Matthews, W. B., Stevens, D. L., Alpers, M. P., Asher, D. M., Gajdusek, D. C. & Gibbs, C. J. Jr. (1969) Creutzfeldt–Jakob disease: the neuropathology of a transmission experiment. *Brain*, **92**, 699-716.

Beck, E., Daniel, P. M. & Prichard, M. M. L. (1969) Regeneration of hypothalamic nerve fibres in the goat. *Neuroendocrinology*, **5**, 161-182.

Besser, G. M. (1974) Hypothalamus as an endocrine organ. *British Medical Journal*, **2**, 560-564; 613-615.

Blackwell, R. E. & Guillemin, R. (1973) Hypothalamic control of adenohypophysial secretions in *Annual Review of Physiology* (Eds. Comroe, J. H., Edelman, I. S. & Sonnenschein, R. R.), Vol. 35, pp. 357-390, Annual Reviews Inc., Palo Alto, California.

Braun, F. C. & Forney, W. R. (1959) Diencephalic syndrome of early infancy associated with brain tumor. *Pediatrics*, **24**, 609-615.

Brennan, C. F., Malone, R. G. S. & Weaver, J. A. (1956) Pituitary necrosis in diabetes mellitus. *Lancet*, **2**, 12-16.

Brobeck, J. R. (1960) Food and temperature. *Recent Progress in Hormone Research*, **16**, 439-466.

Ceballos, R. (1966) Pituitary changes in head trauma (analysis of 102 consecutive cases of head injury). *Alabama Journal of Medical Sciences*, **3**, 185-198.

Christ, J. F. (1966) Nerve supply, blood supply and cytology of the neurohypophysis in *The Pituitary Gland* (Eds. Harris, G. W. & Donovan, B. T.), Vol. 3, Chapter 6, pp. 62-130, Butterworth, London.

Clark, W. E. Le Gros (1938) Morphological aspects of the hypothalamus in *The Hypothalamus* (Eds. Clark, W. E. Le Gros, Beattie, J., Riddoch, G. & Dott, N. M.), pp. 1-68, Oliver and Boyd, Edinburgh.

Clark, W. E. Le Gros (1948) The connexions of the frontal lobes of the brain. *Lancet*, **1**, 353-356.

Conklin, J. L. (1966) The identification of acidophilic cells in the human pars distalis. *Anatomical Record*, **156**, 347-360.

Conklin, J. L. (1968) A histochemical study of mucoid cells in the pars distalis of the human hypophysis. *Anatomical Record*, **160**, 59-78.

Critchlow, V. & Bar-Sala, M. E. (1967) Control of the onset of puberty in *Neuroendocrinology* (Eds. Martini, L. & Ganong, W. F.), Vol. 2, pp. 101-162, Academic Press, New York and London.

Crompton, M. R. (1963) Hypothalamic lesions following the rupture of cerebral berry aneurysms. *Brain*, **86**, 301-314.

Crompton, M. R. & Layton, D. D. (1961) Delayed radionecrosis of the brain following therapeutic X-irradiation of the pituitary. *Brain*, **84**, 85-101.

Crooke, A. C. & Russell, D. S. (1935) The pituitary gland in Addison's disease. *Journal of Pathology and Bacteriology*, **40**, 255-283.

Daniel, P. M. (1966a) The anatomy of the hypothalamus and pituitary gland in *Neuroendocrinology* (Eds. Martini, L. & Ganong, W. F.), Vol. 1, pp. 15-80, Academic Press, New York and London.

Daniel, P. M. (1966b) The blood supply of the hypothalamus and pituitary gland. *British Medical Bulletin*, **22**, 202-208.

Daniel, P. M. & Prichard, M. M. L. (1956) Anterior pituitary necrosis. Infarction of the pars distalis produced experimentally in the rat. *Quarterly Journal of Experimental Physiology*, **41**, 215-229.

Daniel, P. M. & Prichard, M. M. L. (1966) Distal retraction balls in the neurohypophysis after transection of the pituitary stalk. *Journal of Comparative Neurology*, **127**, 321-333.

Daniel, P. M. & Prichard, M. M. L.   (1970) Regeneration of hypothalamic nerve fibres after hypophysectomy in the goat.   *Acta Endocrinologica*, **64**, 696-704.

Daniel, P. M. & Prichard, M. M. L.   (1972) The human hypothalamus and pituitary stalk after hypophysectomy or pituitary stalk section.   *Brain*, **95**, 813-824.

Daniel, P. M. & Prichard, M. M. L.   (1975) Studies of the hypothalamus and the pituitary gland: with special reference to the effects of transection of the pituitary stalk.   *Acta endocrinologica*, **80**, Suppl. 201, 1-216.

Daniel, P. M., Prichard, M. M. L. & Treip, C. S.   (1959) Traumatic infarction of the anterior lobe of the pituitary gland.   *Lancet*, **2**, 927-931.

Daniel, P. M. & Treip, C. S.   (1966a) Lesions of the pituitary gland associated with head injuries in *The Pituitary Gland* (Eds. Harris, G. W. & Donovan, B. T.), Vol. 2, Chap. 18, pp. 535-544, Butterworth, London.

Daniel, P. M. & Treip, C. S.   (1966b) The regenerative capacity of pars distalis of the pituitary gland in *The Pituitary Gland* (Eds. Harris, G. W. & Donovan, B. T.), Vol. 2, Chap. 17, pp. 519-534, Butterworth, London.

Daniel, P. M., Spicer, E. J. F. & Treip, C. S.   (1973) Pituitary necrosis in patients maintained on mechanical respirators.   *Journal of Pathology*, **111**, 135-138.

Dawson, B. H.   (1958) The blood vessels of the human optic chiasma and their relation to those of the hypophysis and hypothalamus.   *Brain*, **81**, 207-217.

Donovan, B. T. & Van der Werff ten Bosch, J. J.   (1965) *Physiology of Puberty*, Arnold, London.

Downey, J. A., Mottram, R. F. & Pickering, G. W.   (1964) The location by regional cooling of central temperature receptors in the conscious rabbit.   *Journal of Physiology*, **170**, 415-441.

Driggs, M. & Spatz, H.   (1940) Pubertas praecox bei einer hyperplastischen Missbildung des Tuber cinereum.   *Virchows Archiv für pathologische Anatomie*, **305**, 567-592.

Duchen, L. W.   (1966) Metastatic carcinoma in the pituitary gland and hypothalamus.   *Journal of Pathology and Bacteriology*, **91**, 347-355.

Duchen, L. W. & Treip, C. S.   (1969) Microgliomatosis presenting with dementia and hypopituitarism.   *Journal of Pathology*, **98**, 143-146.

Duvernoy, H.   (1972) The vascular architecture of the median eminence in *Brain-endocrine Interaction. Median Eminence: Structure and Function* (Eds. Knigge, K. M., Scott, D. E. & Weindl A.), pp. 79-108, Karger, Basel.

Ezrin, C. & Murray, S.   (1963) The cells of the human adenohypophysis in pregnancy, thyroid disease and adrenal cortical disorders in *Cytologie de l'adénohypophyse* (Eds. Benoit, J. & Da Lage, C.), pp. 183-199, CNRS, Paris.

Feldberg, W. & Myers, R. D.   (1965) Changes in temperature produced by micro-injections of amines into the anterior hypothalamus of cats.   *Journal of Physiology*, **177**, 239-245.

Finley, K. H.   (1940) Angio-architecture of the hypothalamus and its peculiarities.   *Research Publications, Association for research in Nervous and Mental Disease*, **20**, 286-309.

Fisher, C., Ingram, W. R. & Ranson, S. W.   (1938) *Diabetes Insipidus and the Neuro-hormonal Control of Water Balance*, Edwards, Ann Arbor, Michigan.

Fitzsimons, J. T.   (1966) The hypothalamus and drinking in *Recent Studies on the Hypothalamus*. *British Medical Bulletin*, **22**, 232-237.

Fitzsimons, J. T.   (1972) Thirst.   *Physiological Reviews*, **52**, 468-561.

Gagel, O.   (1941) Eine Granulationgeschwulst im Gebiete des Hypothalamus.   *Zeitschrift für die gesamte Neurologie und Psychiatrie*, **172**, 710-722.

Gibson, J. B. & Goldberg, A.   (1956) The neuropathology of acute porphyria.   *Journal of Pathology and Bacteriology*, **71**, 495-509.

Goldman, K. P. & Jacobs, A.   (1960) Anterior and posterior pituitary failure after head injury.   *British Medical Journal*, **2**, 1924-1926.

Green, J. D.   (1951) The comparative anatomy of the hypophysis, with special reference to its blood supply and innervation.   *American Journal of Anatomy*, **88**, 225-311.

Green, J. R., Buchan, G. C., Alvord, E. C. & Swanson, A. G.   (1967) Hereditary and idiopathic types of diabetes insipidus.   *Brain*, **90**, 707-714.

Hardy, J. D., Hellon, R. F. & Sutherland, K.   (1964) Temperature-sensitive neurones in the dog's hypothalamus.   *Journal of Physiology*, **175**, 242-253.

Harris, G. W.   (1955) *Neural Control of the Pituitary Gland*, Arnold, London.

Harris, G. W.   (1960) Central control of pituitary secretion in *American Physiological Society Handbook of Neurophysiology*, Section 1, Neurophysiology, Vol. 2, p. 1007-1038, Washington, D.C.

Harris, G. W. & Jacobsohn, D.   (1952) Functional grafts of the anterior pituitary gland.   *Proceedings of the Royal Society, Series B*, **139**, 263-276.

Henzi, H. (1952) Zur pathologischen Anatomie des Diabetes insipidus. *Monatschrift für Psychiatrie und Neurologie*, **123**, 292-316.

Herzog, E. (1955) Histopathologie des vegetativen Nervensystems in *Handbuch der speziellen pathologischen Anatomie und Histologie* (Eds. Lubarsch, O., Henke, F. & Rössle, R.), Vol. 13, Part 5, pp. 361-375, Springer Verlag, Berlin.

Hewer, T. F. & Heller, H. (1949) Non-lipid reticulo-endotheliosis with diabetes insipidus: report of a case with estimation of posterior pituitary hormones. *Journal of Pathology and Bacteriology*, **61**, 499-505.

Hilton, S. M. (1966) Hypothalamic regulation of the cardiovascular system in *Recent Studies on the Hypothalamus. British Medical Bulletin*, **22**, 243-248.

Hinsey, J. C. (1937) The relation of the nervous system to ovulation and other phenomena of the female reproductive tract. *Cold Spring Harbor Symposia on Quantitative Biology*, **5**, 269-279.

Hullinghorst, R. L. & Steer, A. (1953) Pathology of epidemic hemorrhagic fever. *Annals of Internal Medicine*, **38**, 77-101.

Jewell, P. A. & Verney, E. B. (1957) An experimental attempt to determine the site of the neurohypophysial osmoreceptors in the dog. *Philosophical Transactions of the Royal Society Series B*, **240**, 197-324.

Kennedy, G. C. (1966) Food intake, energy balance and growth in *Recent Studies on the Hypothalamus. British Medical Bulletin*, **22**, 216-220.

Kepes, J. J. & Kepes, M. (1969) Predominantly cerebral forms of histiocytosis-X. *Acta Neuropathologica (Berlin)*, **14**, 77-98.

Kornblum, R. N. & Fisher, R. S. (1969) Pituitary lesions in craniocerebral injuries. *Archives of Pathology*, **88**, 242-248.

Kovacs, K. (1969) Necrosis of anterior pituitary in humans. *Neuroendocrinology*, **4**, 170-199; 201-241.

Krabbe, K. H. (1922) La sclérose tubéreuse du cerveau. *Encéphale*, **17**, 281-289.

Kraemer, W. & Paarmann, H. F. (1956) Beitrag zur cerebralen Form der Besnier-Boeck-Schaumannschen Krankheit. Unter Berücksichtigung hypothalamischen Regulationsstörungen. *Nervenarzt*, **27**, 160-165.

Lange-Cosack, H. (1951) Verschiedene Gruppen der hypothalamischen Pubertas praecox (1). *Deutsche Zeitschrift für Nervenheilkunde*, **166**, 499-545.

Lange-Cosack, H. (1952) Verschiedene Gruppen der hypothalamischen Pubertas praecox (2). *Deutsche Zeitschrift für Nervenheilkunde*, **168**, 237-266.

Le Marquand, H. S. & Russell, D. S. (1934-35) A case of pubertas praecox (macrogenitosomia praecox) in a boy associated with a tumour in the floor of the third ventricle. *Royal Berkshire Hospital Reports*, **3**, 31-61.

Lerman, J. & Means, J. H. (1945) Hypopituitarism associated with epilepsy following head injury. *Journal of Clinical Endocrinology*, **5**, 119-131.

Locke, W. & Schally, A. V. (1972) *The Hypothalamus and Pituitary in Health and Disease*, Thomas, Springfield, Ill.

Maccubbin, D. A. & Van Buren, J. M. (1963) A quantitative evaluation of hypothalamic degeneration and its relation to diabetes insipidus following interruption of the human hypophyseal stalk. *Brain*, **86**, 443-464.

Marañon, G. (1926) Über die hypophysäre Fettsucht. *Deutsches Archiv für klinische Medizin*, **151**, 129-153.

McCann, S. M. & Porter, J. C. (1969) Hypothalamic pituitary stimulating and inhibiting hormones. *Physiological Reviews*, **49**, 240-284.

Meyer, A., Beck, E. & McLardy, T. (1947) Prefrontal leucotomy: a neuroanatomical report. *Brain*, **70**, 18-49.

Morton, A. (1970) The time course of retrograde neuron loss in the hypothalamic magnocellular nuclei of man. *Brain*, **93**, 329-336.

Muller, A. (1955) Neurosekretstauung im Tractus supraopticohypophysens des Menschen durch einen raumbeengenden Prozess. *Zeitschrift für Zellforschung*, **42**, 439-442.

Nauta, W. J. H. & Haymaker, W. (1969) Hypothalamic nuclei and fiber connections in *The Hypothalamus* (Eds. Haymaker, W., Anderson, E. & Nauta, W. J. H.), pp. 136-209, Thomas, Springfield, Ill.

Northfield, D. W. C. & Russell, D. S. (1967) Pubertas praecox due to hypothalamic hamartoma: report of two cases surviving surgical removal of the tumour. *Journal of Neurology, Neurosurgery and Psychiatry*, **30**, 166-173.

Oppenheimer, D. R. (1959) Some pathological findings in cases with radioactive pituitary implants. *Journal of Laryngology and Otology*, **73**, 670-678.

Orthner, H. (1955) Pathologische Anatomie und Physiologie der hypophysär-hypothalamischen Krankheiten in *Handbuch der speziellen pathologischen Anatomie und Histologie* (Eds. Lubarsch, O., Henke, F. & Rössle, R.), Vol. 13, part 5, pp. 543-939, Springer Verlag, Berlin.

Orthner, H. (1961) Tumorose Veränderungen im Sellabereich. *Beiträge zur modernen Therapie*, **3**, 313-372.

Orthner, H. & Meyer, Eu. (1967) Der posttraumatische Diabetes insipidus. *Acta neurovegetativa*. **30**, 216-250.

Perlroth, M. G., Tschudy, D. P., Marver, H. S., Costan, W. B., Zeigel, R. F., Rechcigl, M. & Collins, A. (1966) Acute intermittent porphyria. *American Journal of Medicine*, **41**, 149-162.

Porter, J. C., Mical, R. S., Ben-Jonathan, N. & Ondo, J. G. (1973) Neurovascular regulation of the anterior hypophysis in *Recent Progress in Hormone Research* (Ed. Greep, R. O.), Vol. 29, pp. 161-198, Academic Press, New York and London.

Potter, E. L. (1961) *Pathology of the Fetus and the Newborn*, 2nd Edition, Yearbook Publishers, Chicago.

Purves, H. D. (1966) Cytology of the adenohypophysis in *The Pituitary Gland* (Eds. Harris, G. W. & Donovan, B. T.), Vol. 1, Chap. 4, pp. 147-232, Butterworth, London.

Raisman, G. (1966) Neural connexions of the hypothalamus. *British Medical Bulletin*, **22**, 197-201.

Raisman, G. (1970) Some aspects of the neural connections of the hypothalamus in *The Hypothalamus* (Eds. Martini, L., Motta, M. & Fraschini, F.), pp. 1-15, Academic Press, New York and London.

Rasmussen, A. T. (1938) Innervation of the hypophysis. *Endocrinology*, **23**, 263-278.

Rickards, A. G. & Harvey, P. W. (1954) 'Giant-cell granuloma' and the other pituitary granulomata. *Quarterly Journal of Medicine*, **23**, 425-439.

Rinne, U. K. (1960) Neurosecretory material around the hypophysial portal vessels in the median eminence of the rat. *Acta endocrinologica*, Suppl. 57.

Rioch, D. McK., Wislocki, G. B. & O'Leary, J. L. (1940) A précis of preoptic, hypothalamic and hypophysial terminology with atlas. *Research Publications, Association for Research in Nervous and Mental Diseases*, **20**, 3-30.

Romeis, B. (1940) Hypophyse in *Handbuch der mikroskopischen Anatomie des Menschen* (Ed. von Möllendorff, W.), Vol. 6, Part 3, pp. 1-625, Springer Verlag, Berlin.

Russell, A. (1951) A diencephalic syndrome of emaciation in infancy and childhood. *Archives of Disease in Childhood*, **26**, 274.

Russell, D. S. & Rubinstein, L. J. (1971) *Pathology of Tumours of the Nervous System*, 3rd edition, Arnold, London.

Scadding, J. G. (1967) *Sarcoidosis*, Eyre and Spottiswoode, London.

Scharrer, E. & Scharrer, B. (1954) Hormones produced by neurosecretory cells in *Recent Progress in Hormone Research*, **10**, 183-240.

Schmidt, E., Hallervorden, J. & Spatz, H. (1958) Die Entstehung der Hamartom am Hypothalamus mit und

Sheehan, H. L. (1937) Post-partum necrosis of the anterior pituitary. *Journal of Pathology and Bacteriology*, **45**, 189-214.

Sheehan, H. L. (1968) Neurohypophysis and hypothalamus in *Endocrine Pathology* (Ed. Bloodworth, J. M. B. Jr.), pp. 12-74, Williams and Wilkins Co., Baltimore.

Sheehan, H. L. & Davis, J. C. (1968) Pituitary necrosis. *British Medical Bulletin*, **24**, 59-70

Sheehan, H. L. & Summers, V. K. (1949) The syndrome of hypopituitarism. *Quarterly Journal of Medicine*, **18**, 319-378.

Sheehan, H. L. & Whitehead, R. (1963) The neurohypophysis in post-partum hypopituitarism. *Journal of Pathology and Bacteriology*, **85**, 145-169.

Shute, C. C. D. & Lewis, P. R. (1966) Cholinergic and monoaminergic pathways in the hypothalamus in *Recent Studies on the Hypothalamus*. *British Medical Bulletin*, **22**, 221-226.

Simmonds, M. (1914) Ueber Hypophysisschwund mit tödlichem Ausgang. *Deutsche medizinische Wochenschrift*, **40**, 322-323.

Sloper, J. C. (1966) Hypothalamic neurosecretion. *British Medical Bulletin*, **22**, 209-215.

Smith, H. V. & Daniel, P. M. (1947) Some clinical and pathological aspects of tuberculosis of the central nervous system. *Tubercle*, **28**, 64-80.

Smythies, J. R. (1970) *Brain Mechanisms and Behaviour*, 2nd edition, p. 80, Blackwell Scientific Publications, Oxford.

Szentágothai, J., Flerkó, B., Mess, B. & Halász, B. (1968) *Hypothalamic Control of the Anterior Pituitary*, Akadémiai Kiado, Budapest.

Teitelbaum, P. & Epstein, A. N. (1962) The lateral hypothalamic syndrome: recovery of feeding and drinking after lateral hypothalamic lesions. *Psychological Reviews*, **69**, 74-90.

Thornton, K. R. (1959) The cytology of the pituitary gland in myxoedema. *Journal of Pathology and Bacteriology*, **77**, 249-255.

Treip, C. S. (1970) Hypothalamic and pituitary injury in *The Pathology of Trauma*. *Journal of Clinical Pathology*, **23**, Suppl. (*Royal College of Pathologists*), **4**, 178-186.

Vogt, M.   (1954) The concentration of sympathin in different parts of the central nervous system under normal conditions and after the administration of drugs. *Journal of Physiology*, **123**, 451-481.

Vonderahe, A. R.   (1940) Changes in the hypothalamus in organic disease. *Research Publications, Association for Research in Nervous and Mental Disease*, **20**, 689-712.

Weinberger, L. M. & Grant, F. C.   (1941) Precocious puberty and tumors of the hypothalamus. *Archives of Internal Medicine*, **67**, 762-792.

Wilke, G.   (1956) Die granulomatöse Encephalitis mit Bezug auf bekannte oder unbekannte Ätiologie. *Nervenarzt*, **27**, 244-251.

Willis, R. A.   (1962) *The Borderland of Embryology and Pathology*, 2nd edition, Butterworth, London.

Wolman, L.   (1956) Pituitary necrosis in raised intracranial pressure. *Journal of Pathology and Bacteriology*, **72**, 575-586.

Wolman, L. & Balmforth, G. V.   (1963) Precocious puberty due to a hypothalamic hamartoma in a patient surviving to late middle age. *Journal of Neurology, Neurosurgery and Psychiatry*, **26**, 275-280.

Xuereb, G. P., Prichard, M. M. L. & Daniel, P. M.   (1954a) The arterial supply and venous drainage of the human hypophysis cerebri. *Quarterly Journal of Experimental Physiology*, **39**, 199-217.

Xuereb, G. P., Prichard, M. M. L. & Daniel, P. M.   (1954b) The hypophysial portal system of vessels in man. *Quarterly Journal of Experimental Physiology*, **39**, 219-230.

14

Diseases of the Basal Ganglia, Cerebellum and Motor Neurons

Revised by D. R. Oppenheimer

Most of the conditions discussed in this chapter are classified as *primary neuronal degenerations*; that is, diseases in which, for unknown reasons, nerve cells of a particular type or in a particular region successively shrivel and die. Excluded by this definition are diseases due to infections or poisons, or to the 'pathoclitic' effects of hypoxia or epilepsy, or to metabolic deficiencies or avitaminoses; also conditions ascribed to the remote effects of malignant disease elsewhere in the body.

The common characters of the degenerative diseases are: (1) they are selective, affecting one or more 'systems' of neurons in a more or less symmetrical pattern, (2) they are steadily progressive, though not necessarily fatal, and (3) they are variable in their clinical and pathological features and often appear to overlap with one another, making accurate classification difficult if not impossible. Some have a clear genetic basis, others not; in certain diseases with dominant inheritance—for instance, in Huntington's chorea —the disease tends to run a similar course in all the affected members of a family, whereas in other families, such as the one described by Schut and Haymaker (1951), it seems that a single dominant gene may produce a bewildering variety of lesions and syndromes in different individuals. Where a large number of nervous structures is at risk, as in multiple system atrophy of the pontocerebellar type, different combinations of lesions can give rise to a wide variety of clinical pictures, whereas a disease normally affecting one system only, such as Werdnig–Hoffman disease, has a fairly uniform clinical manifestation. Table 14.1 shows the structures at risk in a few of the commoner degenerative diseases.

For the most part, the histology of the lesions reveals no more than focal or systematic loss of neurons, with reactive gliosis. In many instances there is evidence of a 'dying-back' process, in which neuronal atrophy begins at the distal end of the axis cylinder, and proceeds centripetally towards the cell body. This is seen most convincingly in the pyramidal tracts in motor neuron disease, and in the middle cerebellar peduncles in pontocerebellar atrophy. In other cases one may find that the distal parts of long tracts have degenerated, without evidence of progressive degeneration of the proximal parts—for instance, in the long tracts of the spinal cord in Strümpell's familial spastic paraplegia, or the pyramidal tracts in Friedreich's ataxia. Here the impression is that the parent cell body does not die, but is incapable of maintaining the vitality of a long axon.

In many degenerative conditions there is an appearance of 'linked' or 'chain' (i.e. transneuronal) degeneration. Examples are the 'linked' degeneration of the pallidum and subthalamic nucleus in progressive supranuclear palsy; of striatum and substantia nigra, and of pontine nuclei and Purkinje cells, in multiple system atrophy; and of motor neurons and pyramidal tracts in motor neuron disease. Almost nothing is known of the mechanisms involved in such transneuronal degenerations—not even whether it occurs in a prograde or retrograde direction, or both. In any case, 'linked' degeneration does not account for all the combinations of lesions which are found in practice. For instance, in Friedrich's ataxia there is degeneration of the spinocerebellar tracts and of the dentate nuclei, but not of the Purkinje cells which presumably constitute the 'link' between these two.

A few degenerative diseases have peculiar

Table 14.1 *The main sites of neuronal degeneration in various diseases*

	PA	MSA	FA	PSP	MND
Cerebral cortex	(+)	(+)	−	−	(+)
Striatum	(+)	+	−	(+)	−
Pallidum	(+)	−	+	+ +	−
Subthalamic nuclei	(+)	−	+	+ +	−
Pigmented nuclei	+ +	+	−	+ +	−
Pontine nuclei	−	+	−	(+)	−
Inferior olives	−	+	−	(+)	−
Purkinje cells	−	+	−	(+)	−
Dentate nuclei	−	−	+ +	+ +	−
Motor nuclei	−	(+)	−	+	+ +
Thoracic nuclei	−	(+)	+ +	−	(+)
Intermediolateral columns	(+)	+	−	(+)	−
Sensory ganglia	−	−	+ +	−	−
Sympathetic ganglia	+	−	?	?	−
Optic nerves	−	−	+	−	−
Pyramidal tracts	−	+	+ +	(+)	+

PA = Paralysis agitans (Parkinson's disease).   MSA = Multiple system atrophy (pontocerebellar or striatonigral type).   FA = Friedreich's ataxia. PSP = Progressive supranuclear palsy.   MND = Motor neuron disease (amyotrophic lateral sclerosis).

+ + Always or nearly always affected
+ Commonly affected
(+) Occasionally affected
− Seldom if ever affected

histological features, other than simple neuronal loss and gliosis. Examples are the cytoplasmic inclusion bodies described by Lewy (1913) in Parkinson's disease, and the neurofibrillary tangles found in Alzheimer's disease, in progressive supranuclear palsy, and in the Parkinson-dementia complex of Guam. Whether these special features indicate a different type of pathological process from that in the 'simple' neuronal degenerations is still not known. On the other hand there are diseases, of which Jakob–Creutzfeldt disease is an instance, having the histological features of a simple neuronal degeneration, in which it has recently been discovered that material from the diseased brain can be used to transmit a similar, progressive disorder to experimental animals (Beck, Daniel, Matthews, Stevens, Alpers, Asher, Gajdusek and Gibbs 1969). On the assumption that such conditions are acquired by infection, it is now usual to remove them from the category of primary degenerations into that of 'slow virus diseases'. These are discussed in Chapters 8 and 18. It

may well happen that other diseases, at present regarded as primary degenerations, may be found to belong to this group.

There is a much debated question, of medico-legal importance, whether a progressive neuronal degeneration can be caused, or its onset precipitated, by bodily or mental trauma. Evidence on this is mainly of an anecdotal kind, and generally unconvincing, except perhaps in the case of post-traumatic Parkinsonian syndromes, which are discussed below.

In practice, it is often difficult to determine the extent of a neuronal degeneration affecting more than one group of cells. Undoubtedly, lesions are often missed through incomplete examination of the brain and spinal cord; on the other hand, the literature is cluttered with reports of 'slight cell loss' in this nucleus or that, where the reader is left uncertain whether this represents a genuine atrophy, or a senile change, or a subjective impression on the part of the author. The examination of Nissl stained sections is often insufficient, unless it is combined with laborious and carefully controlled cell counts. Where a nucleus has a well-defined efferent tract —for instance, the dentate nucleus—myelin stained sections of this tract may be more informative than the Nissl preparation of the nucleus itself. In the striatum, where the nerve cells are frequently shrivelled and distorted by agonal ischaemic changes, the appearance of the myelinated bundles and of the myelin within the globus pallidus is often more revealing than that of the cell bodies. Positive evidence of disease, in the form of reactive gliosis or of fatty degenera-tion products, may be necessary as confirmation of the negative features of neuronal loss seen in Nissl and myelin preparations.

No attempt will be made here to classify the primary neuronal degenerations. They will be discussed, in this and other chapters, according to the topography of the principal lesions. Alzheimer's and Pick's diseases, in which the main lesions are in the cerebral cortex, are dealt with in Chapter 18: also Huntington's chorea, in which striatal and cortical lesions are com-bined.

Diseases of basal ganglia and brainstem

There is no agreed definition of the term 'basal ganglia'. For present purposes the term is used to cover the *striatum* (i.e. caudate nucleus and putamen), *pallidum* (globus pallidus), *claustrum*, *amygdala*, *substantia innominata*, *subthalamic nucleus* (corpus Luysii), *red nucleus*, and *substantia nigra* (functionally closely related to the preceding structures, but usually classified as a midbrain nucleus). The *thalamus*, though not usually included among the basal ganglia, is included in this section for convenience.

Although much is already known about the anatomical connections of the basal ganglia (Mettler 1968; Kemp and Powell 1971) their functions are still poorly understood. Attempts to reproduce familiar clinical syndromes by means of stimulation or ablation in experimental animals have seldom been successful; and al-though it has been known for many years that various disturbances of movement and posture are associated with lesions in one or other of the basal ganglia, it is still not possible to account for individual symptoms, such as tremor, rigidity or athetosis, in terms of normal or abnormal functioning of a particular nucleus. In other words, one cannot speak confidently of striatal, or pallidal, or nigral syndromes. One reason for this may be that there are lesions of a biochemical kind, which are not shown by routine neurohistological methods. In Parkin-son's disease, for example, routine methods show cell loss in the substantia nigra but not in the striatum. Poirier and Sourkes (1965) showed that destruction of the substantia nigra on one side gave rise, after a delay, to depletion of dopamine in the striatum of the same side, with-out apparent loss of striatal nerve cells. The dramatic effects of L-dopa in alleviating the Parkinsonian disorder are probably exerted through the striatum and other structures, rather than through the remaining cells of the substantia nigra. In general, it is no longer justifiable to explain disorders of function in simple terms of neuronal circuits, with excitatory and inhibitory synapses, and loss of component neurons. If the substantia nigra is regarded merely as part of a neuronal circuit, it is hard to explain why an attack of encephalitis lethargica, with destruc-tion of the substantia nigra, commonly gave rise to a delayed, ingravescent Parkinsonian syndrome rather than to an immediate full-blown Parkin-sonism.

Accounts of the clinical features of diseases of the basal ganglia include those of Denny-Brown (1962, 1968) and Martin (1967). Jellinger (1968a) has reviewed the pathology of a wide variety of degenerative, toxic, metabolic and vascular diseases affecting the striatum and pallidum. These include Wilson's disease and Hallervorden–Spatz disease, which are discussed in Chapter 4 of this book.

Parkinson's disease
(Paralysis agitans)

In his *Essay on the Shaking Palsy* Parkinson (1817) defined the disease which bears his name in these words: 'Involuntary tremulous motion, with lessened muscular power, in parts not in action and even when supported; with a propensity

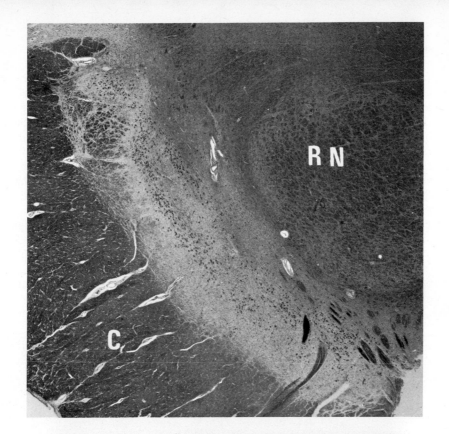

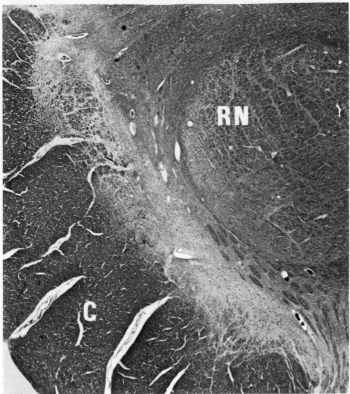

Fig. 14.1 Parkinson's disease. The upper picture shows a normal population of pigmented cells in the substantia nigra, in a 68-year-old man. The lower picture shows depletion of these cells in a 69-year-old woman with Parkinson's disease. RN, red nucleus. C, crus cerebri. Klüver–Barrera stain, 20 μm sections. × 10.

to bend the trunk forwards, and to pass from a walking to a running pace: the senses and intellects being uninjured'. Subsequent clinical descriptions have amplified this picture and emphasized the muscular stiffness, the immobile face, and the mumbling speech of the sufferer.

The disease affects both sexes, and is slowly progressive, with onset most commonly in later middle age. No causative agent is known, and although some families show an undue incidence of the disease, there is no evidence of simple genetic transmission.

Pathology. Trétiakoff (1919), writing a century after Parkinson, appears to have been the first to observe the characteristic lesions of the substantia nigra (Figs. 14.1 and 14.2). Earlier

bear his name (Fig. 14.3). These bodies, which can be seen in melanin-containing cells of the brainstem in almost every case of Parkinson's disease, were observed by Lewy in the nucleus of the substantia innominata. Following Trétiakoff, Foix (1921) studied seven cases of Parkinson's disease and one of the newly observed post-encephalitic Parkinsonism. In the latter, he found gross destructive lesions of the substantia nigra, with residual inflammatory changes. In the other seven, he found loss of pigmented cells from the substantia nigra in all cases; lesions of the striatum, pallidum and hypothalamus were present in some, absent in others.

Hassler (1938) in a study of nine cases of Parkinson's disease found lesions of the substantia nigra and locus ceruleus in every case.

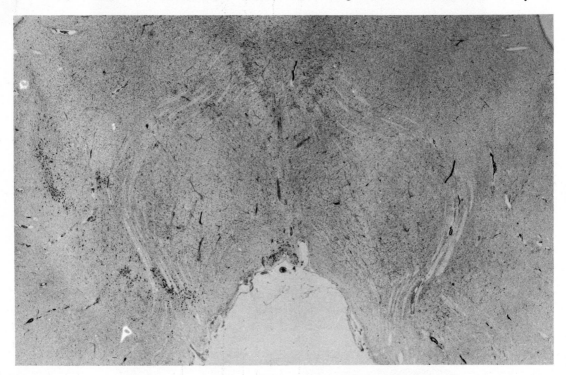

Fig. 14.2 Case of 'hemi-Parkinsonism'. Male, aged 74. On the left of the picture there is mild loss of pigmented cells in the middle zone of the substantia nigra; on the right, the loss is almost complete. Other basal ganglia appeared normal, and symmetrical. Nissl, 20 μm section. × 7·5.

pathologists had described various changes in the basal ganglia, which have since frequently been found in the brains of old people not suffering from Parkinsonism, but had failed to observe lesions in the brainstem. Among these was Lewy (1913), who first described the concentric hyaline cytoplasmic inclusions which

The most severe lesions were in the central part of the zona compacta, where some groups of pigmented cells had almost disappeared. The medial and lateral cell groups were less affected. Cell loss was also seen in the substantia innominata. Lesions of the striatum and pallidum were present in some cases, not in others. Klaue

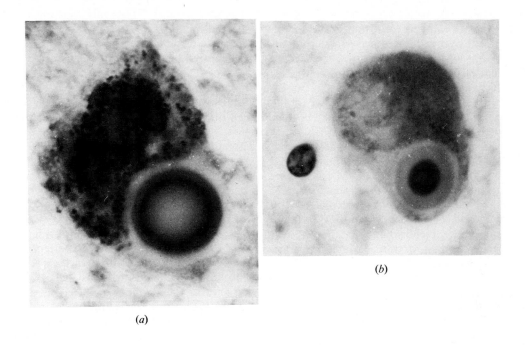

(a)

(b)

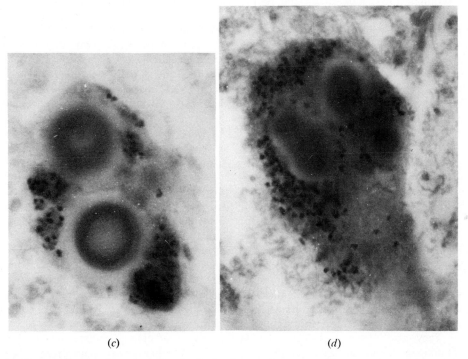

(c)   (d)

Fig. 14.3 Parkinson's disease.   Lewy inclusion bodies in pigmented neurons of locus ceruleus.   (a) and (b) Lendrum's phloxine-tartrazine.   (c) and (d) H & E.   All × 1700.

(1940) in a study of 32 cases of Parkinson's disease, with 22 controls from non-Parkinsonian patients aged over 50, confirmed Hassler's findings. All 32 cases had nigral lesions, which were not present in the controls, the lesions consisting of cell loss, degenerative cell changes, inclusion bodies of Lewy type, and gliosis. Variable lesions of the striatum and pallidum were present in the subjects and in the controls.

Subsequent studies have largely confirmed these findings. In Greenfield and Bosanquet's (1953) study, nigral cell loss and Lewy bodies were constant findings in Parkinson's disease, whereas striatal and pallidal lesions corresponded with those found in brains from non-Parkinsonian elderly subjects. Greenfield and Bosanquet listed a number of staining reactions, which differentiated the Lewy bodies from other types of cell change and of cytoplasmic inclusions. This work was followed up by Bethlem and Jager (1960), who concluded that the central core of the bodies was composed of proteins containing aromatic alpha amino acids, but did not contain any lipids, mucopolysaccharides or nucleic acids. Electron-microscopy (Duffy and Tennyson 1965; Roy and Wolman 1969) has shown the bodies to consist of filaments, loosely packed in the outer zone, densely packed and mixed with granular material in the central core.

It is generally agreed that Lewy bodies are to be found in all, or nearly all, cases of Parkinson's disease, to the extent that it would be difficult to make this histological diagnosis without finding them; on the other hand, they have also been seen in a few cases of well documented postencephalitic Parkinsonism, and occasionally in 'control' material. Lipkin (1959) observed them in 5% of 206 'control' brains, and Forno (1966) in 4% of 400 controls. Whether such brains should be regarded as showing preclinical or subclinical Parkinson's disease is a matter of opinion. Regarding their distribution, they are not confined to the pigmented cells of the substantia nigra, locus ceruleus and dorsal vagal nucleus. Apart from the substantia innominata, which is not pigmented, Jager and Bethlem (1960) found them in numerous brainstem nuclei and in the lateral grey horns of the thoracic cord segments. They also observed bodies, having the same staining reactions but somewhat different shapes, in the cytoplasm and dendrites of nerve cells in sympathetic ganglia. These were not present in control material, and were not found in sensory ganglia. The only other histological report of lesions in the peripheral nervous system appears to be that of Byrnes (1926), who described degenerative changes in muscle spindles in 13 cases of Parkinson's disease, which were not present in controls, or in a case of postencephalitic Parkinsonism. This observation seems to have been neither confirmed nor refuted by subsequent work. The association of Parkinson's disease with autonomic failure discussed on p. 626.

Postencephalitic Parkinsonism

The pathology of the acute phase of *encephalitis lethargica* has been described on p. 311. Selective damage to the substantia nigra had been observed by various authors before Hallervorden (1933, 1935), in a study of 35 cases of postencephalitic Parkinsonism, drew attention to the presence of neurofibrillary changes in nerve cells (Fig. 14.4), not only in the pigmented nuclei but scattered through the cortex, basal ganglia, thalamus, hypothalamus, tegmentum and dentate nuclei. These changes were present in all cases. Subsequent studies (Klaue 1940; Beheim–Schwarzbach 1952; Greenfield and Bosanquet 1953; Forno 1966; Earle 1968) comparing the findings in this condition with those in Parkinson's disease have confirmed that there is at least a statistical difference between the two; that is, Lewy bodies are always or nearly always present in Parkinson's disease, and are rare in controls and in postencephalitic cases, whereas neurofibrillary tangles are nearly always found in postencephalitic cases and are rare in controls and in Parkinson's disease. In a few cases, both changes have been observed; in a few others, neither. Other points of difference are that in postencephalitic cases the destruction in the substantia nigra tends to be more severe and uniformly distributed, and there may be widespread small glial scars, presumably dating from the acute stage of the disease. At present, most neuropathologists regard these two conditions as separate entities, with a small area of unexplained overlap, and would be prepared to make a diagnosis of 'idiopathic' or of postencephalitic Parkinsonism on the basis of the histological findings. When the lesions are those of the postencephalitic disease, in the absence of a history of epidemic encephalitis, the question arises whether other neurotropic viruses may occasionally attack the substantia nigra. The development of immunofluorescent techniques may help to resolve this problem. Gamboa and colleagues have recently (1974) announced the findings of influenza A antigen in the brains of six well documented cases of postencephalitic Parkinsonism. The antigen was not found in five patients with the 'idiopathic' disease, or in two controls.

Striato-nigral degeneration

In 1961 and 1964 Adams, van Bogaert and Vander Eecken drew attention to a group of cases in which the clinical picture was indistinguishable from that of Parkinson's disease. The lesions in the brain consisted of severe cell loss and gliosis

occurring diseases; and it would appear reasonable under the circumstances to use a wider term, such as *multiple system atrophy*, to cover cases showing combinations of degenerative lesions in the striatum, pigmented nuclei, pontine nuclei, cerebellar cortex and inferior olives, including cases displaying the Shy–Drager syndrome (p. 625).

Parkinsonism-dementia complex of Guam

Hirano, Kurland, Krooth and Lessell (1961) described the clinical features of an endemic disease confined to the Chamorro population of Guam, one of the Mariana Islands. It appeared

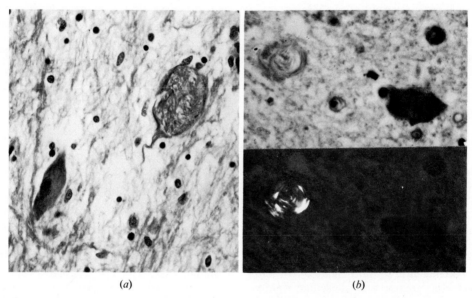

(a)   (b)

Fig. 14.4 Postencephalitic Parkinsonism. Neurofibrillary changes in midbrain. (*a*) Haematoxylin and van Gieson. (*b*) Congo red (the lower half is the same field viewed through crossed Nicol prisms).

in the striatum (especially the putamen) and substantia nigra. Lewy inclusion bodies were not present. There have been further reports of such cases, which have been reviewed by Jellinger and Danielczyk (1968), Adams (1968), Takei and Mirra (1973) and Borit, Rubinstein and Urich (1975). The disease is regarded by some authors as a distinct entity; but it must be pointed out that many recorded patients with pontocerebellar atrophy (see p. 625) have shown clinical Parkinsonism, with lesions in the striatum and pigmented nuclei similar to those described by Adams *et al.*, and that in one of their cases the final diagnosis was of 'striato-nigral degeneration *and* olivo-ponto-cerebellar atrophy'. Presumably the authors did not regard these two as independently

to have a genetic basis, and in many families was associated with the locally prevalent amyotrophic lateral sclerosis described by Kurland and Mulder (1954). In some patients, the two conditions are combined, and they are reasonably regarded as variants of a single disease. The onset is insidious, usually in the fifth and sixth decades, and progresses to death in about four years. About three males are affected to one female. The main clinical features are progressive dementia and Parkinsonism, often with signs of upper motor neuron involvement. The pathological findings in 17 cases were described by Hirano, Malamud and Kurland (1961). To the naked eye there was cortical atrophy, particularly of the frontal and temporal lobes, and loss of pigment from the substantia nigra and locus ceruleus. The microscopic changes consisted in widespread loss of neurons and gliosis, especially in the hippocampus, cerebral cortex, amygdala, hypothalamus, globus pallidus, thalamus, substantia nigra and tegmentum; in the same areas there were numerous intraneuronal neurofibrillary tangles, resembling those seen in Alzheimer's disease, but not associated with 'senile' plaques.

Comparing this with other known diseases, the closest clinical resemblance is with some forms of Jakob–Creutzfeldt disease; these, however, usually run a much more rapid course. The histology of the condition is closer to that of progressive supranuclear palsy (see below).

Other causes of Parkinsonism

At the present time the commonest cause of non-idiopathic Parkinsonism is probably the use of drugs, especially those of the phenothiazine series. The subject is dealt with in Chapter 4, and is discussed in detail, along with other toxic causes (in particular, manganese and carbon monoxide poisoning), by Schwab and England (1968).

Most of the current textbooks of neurology lay stress on arteriosclerosis as a cause of Parkinsonism, and the clinical diagnosis of 'arteriosclerotic Parkinsonism' is commonly made. While it may be the case that the scattered softenings and rarefactions which are so frequently seen in the basal ganglia and thalamus of elderly arteriosclerotic patients are causally related to states of bradykinesia, tremor and muscular rigidity, there is a striking dearth of neuropathological evidence that a full-blown Parkinsonian syndrome can be caused by such lesions. On this subject Schwab and England (1968) conclude that 'arteriosclerosis is not a cause of the disease but exists with it, and greatly adds to the burdens of the patient'.

The same authors discuss at great length the question whether trauma or other forms of stress can cause or precipitate a progressive Parkinsonian disorder, and refer to a previous review of the subject by Grimberg (1934). Apart from the very rare instances in which Parkinsonism was attributable to midbrain trauma, the published evidence is hard to interpret. The authors argue that since various kinds of stress may temporarily exacerbate the symptoms of Parkinsonism, it is reasonable to suppose that stress may unmask symptoms in a case of incipient, subclinical disease. As an argument against trauma actually causing the disease, they note that trauma is not known to precipitate Parkinsonism in young people. Counter to this, the writer once examined the brain of a previously healthy man who had fallen into a dry dock at the age of 21, suffering concussion and minor injuries. During his slow recovery in hospital he developed generalized muscular rigidity, weakness, and later a marked Parkinsonian tremor, mask-like facies, and mumbling dysarthria. All these slowly progressed; the patient became chair-fast, and died at the age of 38. The findings were of severe striatonigral degeneration. There were no Lewy bodies or neurofibrillary tangles, and no traces of brain trauma. Since the usual age of onset in striatonigral degeneration is in the fifth to seventh decades (Adams 1968), it is difficult not to conclude that in this instance the disease had been caused, or its onset prematurely 'triggered', by trauma.

Juvenile paralysis agitans

Ramsey Hunt (1917) described four patients in whom progressive symptoms typical of Parkinson's disease developed before the age of 30. In one case, with onset at age 15 and death at 40, he found a severe loss of large nerve cells from the caudate nucleus, putamen, globus pallidus and substantia innominata. No other lesions were observed. No mention was made of the substantia nigra. In 1930 van Bogaert described a similar case, with onset at age 7 and death at 30. There was degeneration and loss of large cells in the striatum and pallidum, with minor changes in the subthalamic nucleus and substantia nigra. Van Bogaert later (1946) described a series of cases of progressive pallidal and pallidoluysian degeneration, some of which were familial, and which differed clinically from the juvenile Parkinsonism described by Hunt. The relationship between these conditions, which appear to be very rare, is discussed by van Bogaert (1946) and by Jellinger (1968a, b). The relationship with other conditions, such as Friedreich's ataxia and progressive supranuclear palsy, in which there is selective degeneration of the pallidum and subthalamic nucleus, remains obscure.

Progressive supranuclear palsy

In 1964 Steele, Richardson and Olszewski gave an account of nine patients (all male) with a syndrome of progressive paralysis of vertical eye movements, dysarthria, and muscular rigidity, most marked in the muscles of the neck. The disease started in the fifth to seventh decades, and usually led to death in five to seven years. In four of these cases, detailed examination showed widespread symmetrical neuronal loss with gliosis, affecting most conspicuously the globus pallidus, subthalamic nucleus, red nucleus,

have conformed very closely with the findings of Steele *et al.* (1964). Nothing is yet known of the aetiology. Electron-microscopic studies (Tellez-Nagel and Wiśniewski 1973; Powell, London and Lampert 1974; Roy, Datta, Hirano, Ghatak and Zimmerman 1974) have shown a consistent difference in the ultrastructure of the neurofibrillary tangles found in this disease and that of the tangles occurring in Alzheimer's

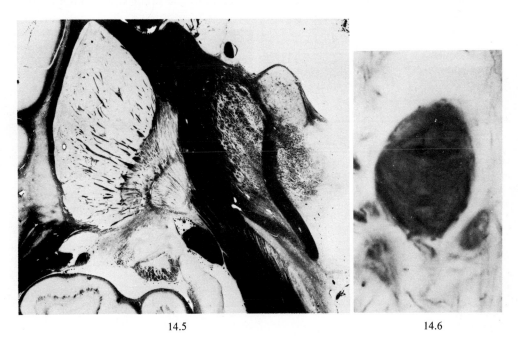

14.5   14.6

Fig. 14.5 Progressive supranuclear palsy. Woman, dying at age 71 after three years' illness. Myelin stain, showing atrophy and loss of myelin in globus pallidus and subthalamic nucleus. × 3.
Fig. 14.6 Progressive supranuclear palsy. Case as in Fig. 14.5. Neurofibrillary tangle in globus pallidus. Hortega double impregnation. × 1700.

substantia nigra, tectum and periaqueductal grey matter, and dentate nucleus (Fig. 14.5). In the same structures, and in many parts of the brain-stem where cell loss was not appreciable, many of the nerve cells showed Alzheimer's neuro-fibrillary change (Fig. 14.6). The cerebral cortex appeared unaffected, and the 'senile plaques' characteristic of Alzheimer's disease were not present.

Subsequent clinical reports on over 40 cases have shown that the disease is rather uniform in its manifestations. Males are affected more than twice as often as females. No familial cases are recorded. Pathological examinations (David, Mackey and Smith 1968; Behrman, Carroll, Janota and Matthews 1969; and others)

disease, Down's syndrome, the Parkinsonism-dementia of Guam, and postencephalitic Parkinsonism, which resemble each other very closely.

Calcification of the basal ganglia

A mild degree of calcification in and around blood vessels in the lentiform nucleus (less frequently in the hippocampus) is a common incidental finding, without associated symptoms, in elderly brains. Calcification of far greater intensity and wider distribution, visible in X-rays of the skull, is an uncommon but very striking post-mortem finding (Fig. 14.7). The condition has been recognized since the middle of the nineteenth century (for references see Löwenthal and Bruyn 1968). Over half of the patients with this condition suffer from a deficiency of parathyroid hormone, either idiopathic or in consequence of radical thyroid surgery. Of the remainder, some have one or other form of Albright's hereditary osteodystrophy; others, including a number of familial cases, have no demonstrable endocrine or metabolic disorder. Clinical disturbances attributed to the lesions in the brain include epilepsy, dementia, abnormal movements, Parkinsonism and ataxia. These

on gross inspection, and may be found in other basal and brainstem nuclei. Calcification occurs in two forms (Fig. 14.11). The first is seen as rows of tiny calcospherites lying along capillary vessels; in the second, calcium salts form tubular deposits in the medial walls of small or medium-sized arteries and veins. Lesions of the first type are seen mainly in grey matter, including the cerebral and cerebellar cortex. The larger concretions, or brain stones, appear to develop

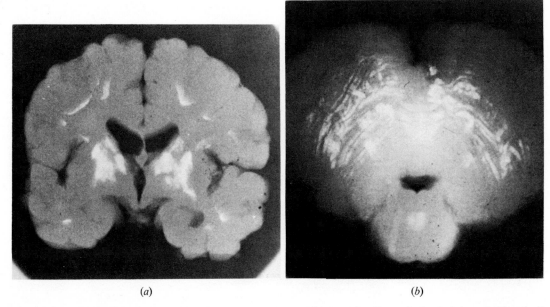

(a)   (b)

Fig. 14.7 Cerebral calcification in a case of hypoparathyroidism. (a) X-ray of a slice at the level of the mamillary bodies. (b) X-ray of pons and superior part of cerebellum. Note the small crescentic shadows cast by cortical calcifications.

symptoms are variable, may be slight or severe, and progress very slowly.

Whatever the underlying disease may be, the distribution of the lesions is rather stereotyped. The heaviest calcifications are found in the globus pallidus, putamen, caudate nucleus, internal capsule, the lateral parts of the thalamus and the dentate nuclei of the cerebellum (Figs. 14.8 and 14.9). Smaller concretions, which may however be visible in X-ray pictures, are present at the junction of cortex and white matter at the bases of cerebral sulci, and in parts of the cerebellar cortex (Fig. 14.10). On slicing the brain, the smaller lesions are felt as a gritty resistance to the knife, whereas the larger concretions ('brain stones') are dislodged, and appear as solid lumps, with an irregular rough surface. Microscopically, the lesions are more widespread than appears

by coalescence of these pericapillary deposits. Calcification of the media of larger vessels is seen mainly in the cerebral and cerebellar white matter. As the lesions enlarge, nervous tissue is destroyed, but healthy looking nerve cells are seen immediately alongside the deposits, and there is no inflammatory, and very little glial, reaction. Involvement of the internal capsules may lead to Wallerian degeneration of the pyramidal tracts. No abnormal calcification is seen in the meninges or choroid plexus.

Chemical analysis of brain stones has shown variable amounts of proteins, polysaccharides and metallic ions—in particular calcium, iron, magnesium and aluminium (Löwenthal and Bruyn 1968). The nature of the biochemical disturbances responsible for calcification is not known. Cerebral calcification associated with

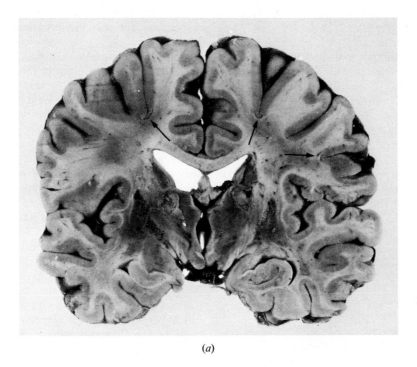

(a)

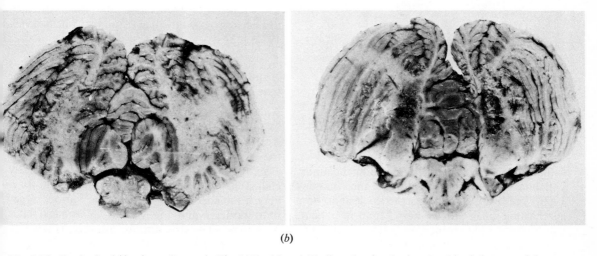

(b)

Fig. 14.8 Cerebral calcification.   Case as in Fig. 14.7.   (a) and (b) slices showing 'brain stones' in thalamus and dentate nuclei, with more diffuse calcification in the lentiform nuclei, cerebellar cortex and white matter, and at the bases of cerebral sulci (arrows).

micrencephaly and other congenital diseases is discussed in Chapter 10.

Effects of focal thalamic and subthalamic lesions

Associations of well-defined clinical disturbances with focal lesions in one or other of the basal ganglia are uncommon. Exceptions are the association of *hemiballism* with lesions of the contralateral subthalamic nucleus, and the '*thalamic syndrome*' described by Déjerine and Roussy in 1906. In both cases the association is strong, but not absolute. Most cases of hemiballism show the expected lesion in the opposite subthalamic nucleus, but some do not; some have

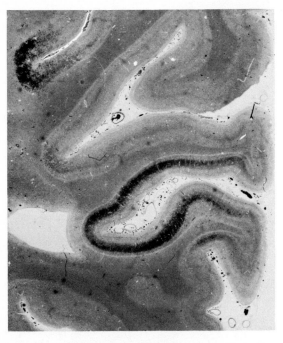

Fig. 14.9 Cerebral calcification. Case as in Fig. 14.7. Calcification of cortex in striate area. H & E. × 3.

solitary lesions in other nuclei, including thalamus, pallidum and striatum (Schwarz and Barrows 1960; Smith 1971) and destructive lesions of a subthalamic nucleus have been found in patients who did not suffer from hemiballism during life. Reviews, with discussion of pathophysiology, include those of Whittier (1947) and Meyers (1968).

The main feature of the thalamic syndrome is a sensory disturbance affecting one side of the body, in which sensory thresholds are raised, but stimulation of the affected side evokes a delayed 'hyperpathic' response, referred to a large area

of the body, and subsiding slowly. The lesion responsible for this is commonly an infarct or haemorrhage involving the posterior ventral nucleus of the opposite thalamus. In the original case descriptions, hemiplegia formed part of the 'syndrome'; but subsequent reports on cases with small lesions and no hemiplegia make it probable that hemiplegia occurs only when the lesions spread into the relevant part of the internal capsule. In a case examined by the writer, a lesion a few millimetres in diameter, involving only the medial part of the posterior ventral nucleus, was associated with hyperpathia affecting only the face on the opposite side. As with hemiballism, lesions in other sites, including the brainstem and parietal cortex and white matter, have been described as responsible for a sensory disorder indistinguishable from that of the thalamic syndrome (see Cassinari and Pagni 1969), and lesions of the posterior ventral nucleus may be associated with sensory loss without hyperpathia. Small vascular lesions in other parts of the thalamus are a common finding in the brains of elderly subjects, and are generally not associated with a recognized clinical disturbance. It is also common to find cell loss and gliosis in the principal thalamic nuclei, associated with destructive lesions of areas of cerebral cortex to which they project. The participation of individual thalamic nuclei in a wide range of degenerative and other diseases has been reviewed in great detail by Martin (1969, 1970).

Neuropathology of various disturbances of muscular tone and movement

Although there is a rough correspondence between disorders of movement and demonstrable lesions in the basal ganglia, and although the clinically described disturbances—chorea, athetosis, myoclonus and so forth—are generally characteristic of particular diseases, there is a very poor correlation between the various types of dyskinesia and the various anatomical sites of lesions. The striatum, for instance, is severely affected in Huntington's disease, in Wilson's disease and in many cases of Jakob–Creutzfeldt disease; but the disorders of movement in these three are different. Chorea occurs in Huntington's disease and in rheumatic fever, but the lesions are different. The same applies to disorders of muscular tone. Zeman and Whitlock

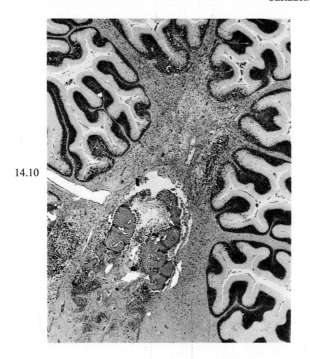

14.10

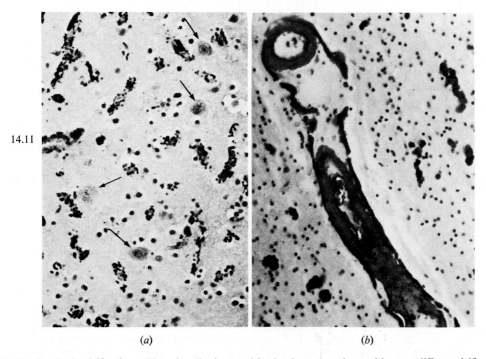

14.11

(a)   (b)

Fig. 14.10 Cerebral calcification. There is a 'brain stone' in the dentate nucleus, with more diffuse calcification in the cerebellar white matter and cortex. H & E. ×5·6.
Fig. 14.11 Cerebral calcification. (a) layer 5 of cerebral cortex, showing pericapillary calcospherites. Note good preservation of nerve cells (arrows). PAS. ×230. (b) vessel in cerebellar white matter, showing medial calcification. H & E. ×230.

(1968) review a number of diseases of widely differing pathology giving rise to 'symptomatic' dystonia. These include various forms of perinatal brain damage, Wilson's and Huntington's diseases, Hallervorden–Spatz disease and other conditions in which lesions of the basal ganglia are consistently present. On the other hand, in *dystonia musculorum deformans*, which appears to be a specific disorder with autosomal dominant inheritance, Zeman and Dyken (1968) maintain

that no characteristic lesions have hitherto been demonstrated—reports to the contrary being attributed to over-enthusiasm leading to self-deception on the part of the investigator, or to the fact that the subjects investigated were suffering from some other disease. Controversies of this kind serve to emphasize the backwardness of present-day central neurophysiology and the inadequacy of conventional neuropathological methods.

Diseases of the cerebellum and its connections

Attempts to classify the cerebellar system degenerations have been unsatisfactory, for several reasons. Clinical classifications are of little use, as indistinguishable states of 'cerebellar ataxia' may result from a variety of different lesions. Even when the disease has a genetic basis, as in the family described by Schut and Haymaker (1951), there may be extreme variation in the clinical and in the pathological expression of the offending gene. The problems of classification and nomenclature are discussed, with refreshing cynicism, by Netsky (1968). General reviews of the subject are those of Greenfield (1954) and Ule (1957). The genetic aspects are discussed by Pratt (1967), and there is a detailed account by Bell and Carmichael (1939) of 242 families, with over 400 cases of hereditary ataxia.

In what follows, three well-known types of cerebellar system degeneration are described: first, cerebellar cortical atrophy, which is almost confined to the Purkinje cells and the inferior olives; second, pontocerebellar atrophy, a multi-system degeneration affecting a selection of cerebellar and other structures; and third, Friedreich's ataxia, in which many structures, including the heart and peripheral nerves, are involved. Brief reference will be made to cases which appear to fall somewhere between these three. Other conditions in which the cerebellum or its afferents degenerate, but in which the aetiology appears to be different, will be dealt with in other chapters of this book. These include carcinomatous cerebellar degeneration (Chapter 5), toxic and metabolic disorders, affecting mainly the Purkinje cells (Chapter 4), and forms of Jakob–Creutzfeldt disease in which the cerebellar cortex or dentate nuclei are particularly involved (Chapter 18).

Atrophy of the granular layer of the cerebellum is described, with other congenital diseases, in Chapter 10.

Cerebellar cortical degeneration
(*Cerebello-olivary degeneration*)

Gordon Holmes (1907) reported a family in which three brothers and one sister became ataxic between the ages of 35 and 40. Four siblings remained well. Gait was first affected, then the finer hand movements. Dysarthria and tremor of the head and limbs appeared later. There was little alteration of deep or superficial reflexes. A post-mortem examination on one patient who reached the age of 70 showed considerable atrophy of the cerebellum, greatest in the superior parts of the vermis and hemispheres (see Fig. 14.12). Histologically there was almost complete disappearance of Purkinje cells from the most affected areas, with proliferation of Bergmann nuclei and fibrous gliosis of the molecular layer. The granule cells were less damaged. There was some loss of myelinated fibres from the folia proportionate to the loss of Purkinje cells, but no degeneration of the pontine or dentate nuclei or of the superior or middle cerebellar peduncles. The inferior and accessory olives had also undergone atrophy, associated with loss of olivocerebellar fibres. This spared to some extent the medial half of the ventral layer and the caudal end of the medial accessory olive. The latter parts of the olivary nucleus were found (Stewart and Holmes 1908) to project to the less affected parts of the cerebellum, whereas the dorsal folia projected to the superior surface. Holmes therefore considered that the olivary degeneration was secondary to atrophy of the cerebellar cortex.

A number of similar, isolated cases were collected by Marie, Foix and Alajouanine (1922) under the name *Late cortical cerebellar atrophy*. In these the onset of the disease was usually later, with an average age of 57 years. In some the cerebellar atrophy was less widespread than in Holmes's case. When the distribution of atrophy in the inferior olives was reported it usually corresponded to that found in Holmes's case in being greater in the dorsal laminae.

Since this report there have been about 20 pathological descriptions of similar cases, and in approximately half of these the disease has been familial (Weber and Greenfield 1942). Hall, Noad and Latham (1941, 1945) reported on a

in a case examined by Blackwood (1952), in which cerebellar cortical degeneration was associated with hereditary sensory radicular neuropathy (Denny-Brown 1951), and the case of Devos (1957), where there was an associated degeneration of the oculomotor nuclei, causing ophthalmoplegia. Here there was a sex-linked dominant inheritance.

Pontocerebellar atrophy
(*Olivopontocerebellar atrophy*)

Menzel (1891) described a form of generalized ataxia affecting three generations of a family. In one patient in the second generation, with three affected siblings, the disease began at the age of 28 and death occurred at 46. Post-mortem

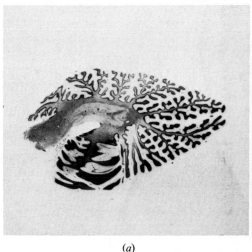 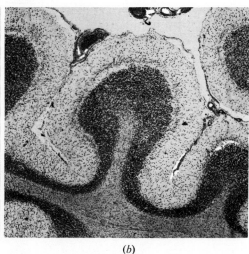

(a)   (b)

Fig. 14.12 Familial cerebellar cortical degeneration (case of Weber and Greenfield 1942). (*a*) Parasagittal section of cerebellum showing atrophy greatest in the superior folia. (*b*) Higher power view of less atrophied folia, showing disappearance of Purkinje cells. Haematoxylin/van Gieson.

large family in which nine members in two generations were known to have been affected. Post-mortem examinations in two members of the older generation, who died aged 80 and 82, showed the atrophy to be limited to the cerebellar cortex and inferior olives. The condition does not generally or appreciably shorten life, but in a family recorded by Akelaitis (1938) the course of the disease was rapid and accompanied by mental confusion, and led to death in less than two years.

Degeneration of Purkinje cells and inferior olives forms part of the pathology of pontocerebellar atrophy, described in the next section. It may also be combined with other lesions, as

examination showed degeneration of the pyramidal and posterior spinocerebellar tracts, thoracic nuclei (Clarke's columns), and the posterior columns of the cord. In the brainstem, there was loss of nerve cells from the gracile, cuneate, hypoglossal, facial and trigeminal nuclei. There was also atrophy of the inferior olives, pontine nuclei and cerebellar cortex, with rarefaction of granule cells and great loss of Purkinje cells, and poverty of myelin in the white matter.

The name *olivopontocerebellar atrophy* was given to a similar, isolated, case by Déjerine and Thomas (1900). This name has persisted; but since the inferior olives normally react to lesions

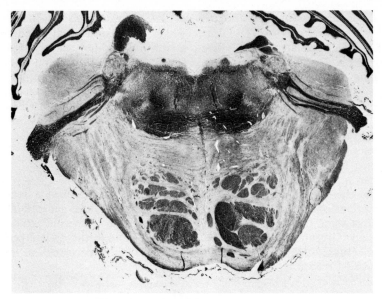

14.13

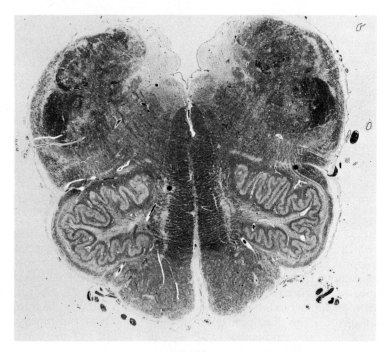

14.14

Fig. 14.13 Pontocerebellar atrophy. Case 4 of Bannister and Oppenheimer 1972. Section of pons, stained for myelin, showing degeneration of transverse fibres and middle cerebellar peduncles, with preservation of tegmentum, trigeminal fibres and pyramidal tracts.

Fig. 14.14 Pontocerebellar atrophy. Case 1 of Bannister and Oppenheimer 1972. Atrophy of inferior olives, loss of olivocerebellar fibres, and pallor of pyramidal and solitary tracts. Myelin stain. (Figures reproduced by courtesy the Editor, *Journal of Neurology, Neurosurgery and Psychiatry.*)

of the cerebellar cortex with retrograde cell loss, and since atrophy of the pons is usually the most striking pathological feature of this condition, it is reasonable to abbreviate the name to *pontocerebellar atrophy*. Since 1900 many cases, both isolated and familial, have been described; and the subject has been reviewed at length by Scherer (1933), Welte (1939) and Rosenhagen (1943).

In a typical case, the most striking naked-eye feature is a gross shrinkage of the ventral part of the pons, which on section may appear wedge-shaped, and of the middle cerebellar peduncles. The cerebellar cortex and the inferior olives may also appear shrunken. In sections stained for myelin, the tegmentum of the pons appears normal or almost so, but there is pallor, which may amount to complete loss of staining, of the transverse fibres in the ventral half, among which the pyramidal tract fibres stand out by their normal staining (Fig. 14.13). In the medulla, there is shrinkage and loss of neurons in the inferior olives, with loss of olivocerebellar fibres (Fig. 14.14). The cerebellar cortex shows a variable—rarely complete—loss of Purkinje cells, the gaps being marked, in silver impregnations, by empty basket formations. The vermis and flocculus tend to be spared, in contrast with the distribution of cell loss in cerebellar cortical atrophy. Granule cells are less affected. The dentate nuclei are gliotic, owing to loss of incoming Purkinje axons, but their cells, and the superior cerebellar peduncles, are well preserved. The cerebellar white matter is grossly deficient in myelinated fibres. It has been observed by several authors that the loss of fibres from the middle peduncles appears disproportionately great in relation to the loss of cells in the pontine nuclei, indicating a 'dying-back' process.

The lesions are not confined to the cerebellar system. There is commonly some degeneration, though not of the severity seen in Friedreich's ataxia, in the long tracts of the spinal cord, and sometimes a loss of motor cells from the anterior horns. In the brain, the commonest associated lesions are loss of cells, with fibrous gliosis, from the striatum (especially the putamen) and the substantia nigra (Fig. 14.15). These features may may make it possible to distinguish clinically between pontocerebellar atrophy and other degenerations of the cerebellar system. In cerebellar cortical degeneration, for instance, pyramidal signs and Parkinsonian disturbances do not

occur, whereas they are sometimes prominent in pontocerebellar atrophy.

The distribution and relative severity of the lesions in this condition vary considerably, even within a single family, such as the one described by Schut and Haymaker in 1951; for instance, there may be only minor changes in the pons, with severe cell loss from the putamen and substantia nigra. Rather than labelling such cases

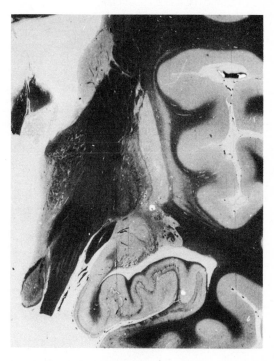

Fig. 14.15 Pontocerebellar atrophy. Case 1 of Bannister and Oppenheimer 1972. Shrinkage and myelin loss in putamen. The pigmented nuclei and intermedio-lateral cell columns were also degenerate. Myelin stain. (Courtesy of the Editor, *Journal of Neurology, Neurosurgery and Psychiatry*.)

'striatonigral degeneration', it is reasonable to include them, along with 'classical' cases of pontocerebellar atrophy, under the general heading of *multiple system atrophy* (p. 615).

Autonomic failure in system degenerations

Shy and Drager (1960) drew attention to a clinical syndrome in which the prominent features are postural (orthostatic) hypotension, urinary incontinence, inability to sweat, muscular rigidity and tremor, and sexual impotence. Cases showing this syndrome are usually sporadic, but an affected family has been described by Lewis (1964). Shy and Drager carried out the first adequate examination of a case of this type, and found widespread symmetrical neuronal degeneration affecting in particular the caudate nucleus, substantia nigra, locus ceruleus pontis, inferior olives, dorsal vagal nuclei, the Purkinje cells of the cerebellum, and in the spinal cord the cells of the ventral and lateral horns and of the thoracic (Clarke's) nuclei. Johnson, Lee, Oppenheimer and Spalding (1966), reported on

autonomic cells. In the first, the only associated lesions have been such as are seen in Parkinson's disease: inclusion bodies of Lewy type in pigmented cells, with or without obvious cell loss from the pigmented nuclei. In the second, larger, group the associated lesions are of a multiple system atrophy of the pontocerebellar or striato-nigral type. Out of 11 such cases, only 6 have had characteristic lesions in the pontine nuclei; but all of them have shown degeneration in the striatum and in the pigmented nuclei, and all

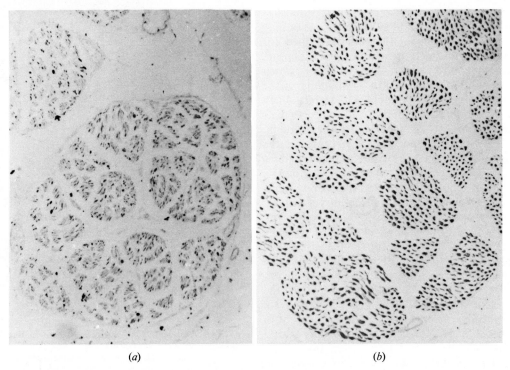

(a)   (b)

Fig. 14.16 Friedreich's ataxia. Onset age 6, death age 10. Lumbar roots, (a) posterior (b) anterior. There is gross loss, especially of thick fibres, in the posterior roots. Holmes silver stain. × 110.

two cases of progressive autonomic failure, attributed the disturbances of sympathetic function to loss of preganglionic cells in the lateral horns (intermediolateral nuclei). In seven such cases which have been examined histologically, controlled counts have been carired out on the intermediolateral cell columns, with the finding of a loss of between 65 and 80% of these cells (Bannister and Oppenheimer 1972). Cell loss and gliosis have repeatedly been observed in the dorsal vagal nuclei, but information on other parasympathetic centres is lacking.

Two groups of patients have been described as showing this form of primary degeneration of

but one showed loss of cells from the Purkinje layer and in the inferior olives. From present evidence one may conclude that so-called idiopathic orthostatic hypotension is not a distinct disease, but an occasional concomitant of two well recognized conditions—Parkinson's disease and multiple system atrophy—resulting from involvement of central autonomic neurons in a primary degenerative process.

Friedreich's ataxia

Friedreich, of Heidelberg, in 1863 and 1876 described a familial form of ataxia with onset

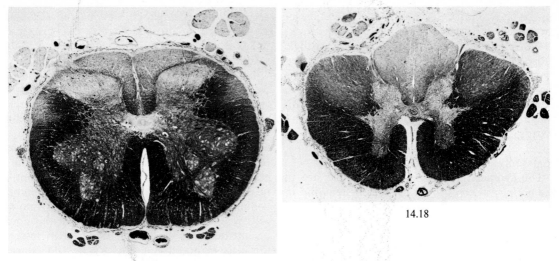

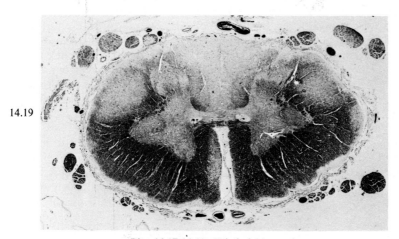

14.17

14.18

14.19

Figs 14.17-14.19 Friedreich's ataxia

Fig. 14.17 Death age 32. Sacral cord. Myelin stain, showing loss of myelin in posterior roots, posterior columns and pyramidal tracts.
Fig. 14.18 Death age 23. Thoracic cord. Myelin stain, showing pallor and shrinkage of posterior columns, and pallor of pyramidal and spinocerebellar tracts.
Fig. 14.19 Death age 31. Cervical cord, showing pallor of posterior roots, posterior columns (gracile more than cuneate), crossed and uncrossed pyramidal tracts, and anterior and posterior spinocerebellar tracts.

under the age of 20. For many years there was reluctance to distinguish between this condition and tabes dorsalis, but the disease is now recognized as one of the commoner hereditary diseases of the nervous system. The proportion of familial cases to 'sporadic' ones is such as would be expected from an autosomal recessive heredity.

The usual presenting symptom is ataxia of gait. This progresses at a variable rate, but by the time of death most patients are unable to walk, even with help. Sensory disturbances, when looked for, are nearly always found, at least in the lower part of the body (Saunders 1913-14). In particular there is loss of joint position sense, vibration sense and two-point discrimination. Other neurological disturbances, in descending order of frequency, include dysarthria, visual deterioration leading to blindness and usually associated with optic atrophy, deafness, dementia or other mental disorders, and epilepsy.

Skeletal deformities, in particular pes cavus

and kyphoscoliosis, develop at an early stage of the disease. In over half of the cases the heart is clinically abnormal, and the commonest single cause of death is heart failure, often complicated by diabetes mellitus, of which the incidence is high in Friedreich's ataxia (Hewer 1968).

The peak age of onset is about 10 years, with roughly equal numbers during the first and second decades. The duration of the disease ranges from under 5 to over 50 years; death occurs most commonly in the third and fourth decades.

The characteristic *pathological changes* are in the peripheral and central nervous system and in the heart.

Peripheral nervous system

The somatic motor fibres, and their cells of origin are usually intact; but degeneration of sensory fibres, posterior roots and ganglion cells is a constant finding (Fig. 14.16). In a series of 18 necropsied and 4 biopsied cases, Hughes, Brownell and Hewer (1968) found severe loss (estimated at about 95%) of thick myelinated fibres, with preservation of large numbers of fine unmyelinated axons, and increase in interstitial fibrous tissue. In the ganglia there was widespread loss of ganglion cells, with proliferation of capsule cells (*Residualknötchen*), and abnormalities of intra-ganglionic nerve fibres. Loss of myelinated fibres from the posterior spinal roots corresponded with that in the peripheral nerves. Comparable data on the state of the trigeminal ganglia and nerves are not at present available.

Central nervous system

The most conspicuous lesions are in the spinal cord (Figs. 14.17, 14.18 and 14.19). The posterior columns are shrunken and degenerate, as is to be expected from the loss of incoming sensory fibres. Fibre loss from the gracile fasciculi is often almost complete, the cuneate fasciculi being affected later and less intensely. Whether there is a 'dying-back' of posterior column fibres towards their cells of origin in sensory ganglia is not known; but 'dying-back' is apparent in the pyramidal tracts, which are often relatively or completely intact at the level of the brainstem, and show progressive loss as they descend through the cord. Degeneration of the thoracic nuclei (Clarke's columns) and the posterior spinocerebellar tracts is constant, and sometimes almost complete. Anterior spinocerebellar tract degeneration is usual, but less marked. The degenerate tracts

are shrunken and gliotic, and overall shrinkage of the cord in cross-section is easily seen by naked eye. In severe cases, there is also visible atrophy of the brainstem.

Lesions in the brain are more variable, and less well documented (Fig. 14.20). Out of 15 personally examined cases of 'classical' Friedreich's ataxia, myelin loss was seen in the descending trigeminal tracts in 11; in the solitary tracts, which consist mainly of primary sensory fibres of the vagus and glossopharyngeal nerves, in 7 cases; in the medullary pyramids in 13; but in no case could degeneration be seen in the cerebral peduncles. In the motor cortex, giant pyramidal cells were absent, or hard to find; but this could be attributed to shrinkage, rather than loss, of the cells in question. The gracile and cuneate nuclei were always densely gliotic, owing to loss of incoming fibres. In addition, there was a variable cell loss in these nuclei, and shrinkage of the ventral (gracile) portion of the medial lemniscus was seen in 12 cases.

Of the cerebellar afferents, the most constantly affected were the accessory cuneate nuclei (the cephalic homologue of the thoracic nuclei), which showed cell loss and cell shrinkage in all 15 cases. Only 5 showed cell loss from the inferior olives, and in these cases there was reason to attribute the loss to circulatory disturbances. The pontine nuclei and middle cerebellar peduncles were never affected. The cerebellar cortex was normal apart from vascular lesions, which were not uncommon. The cerebellar white matter was always gliotic (presumably from degeneration of afferent fibres) but not obviously shrunken. The dentate nuclei showed cell loss, often severe, in 13 cases. This was reflected in a degeneration of the superior cerebellar peduncles, usually more marked in their ventral parts. Cell loss and gliosis were also seen in the vestibular system (especially the medial vestibular nuclei) and in the auditory system (cochlear nuclei and superior olive) in over half the cases. The medial longitudinal bundles were not affected.

Loss of nerve fibres from the optic tracts was seen in about half the cases, and when severe was accompanied by cell loss from the lateral geniculate bodies (regarding the retinal changes occurring in Friedreich's ataxia, and their clinical manifestations, see André-van Leeuwen and van Bogaert 1949). In the basal nuclei, there was cell loss in the external segment of the globus pallidus and subthalamic nucleus in about half the cases.

The cerebral cortex, striatum, thalamus and substantia nigra were unaffected, apart from vascular lesions (Brownell, Hughes and Oppenheimer, unpublished data).

It is clear from this account that several lesions contribute to the dominant clinical feature of the disease—ataxia. They include lesions of sensory nerves, of various cerebellar afferents, and of the cerebellar outflow from the dentate nuclei. The most disabling of these is probably the first, which gives rise to the clinical resemblance, already mentioned, between Friedreich's ataxia and tabes dorsalis.

Heart

In most cases the heart is enlarged, and there are some pericardial adhesions. Microscopical examinations by a number of observers from

due to emboli from mural thrombi within the heart.

Other forms of progressive ataxia

There have been numerous accounts of cases, both sporadic and familial, of progressive ataxia in which the most conspicuous lesions are in the long tracts of the spinal cord. Many of these give the impression of being incomplete manifestations of Friedreich's ataxia (see Fig. 14.21). In these the disease tends to be milder, and the onset is at a later age than in Friedreich's ataxia, especially in cases with dominant inheritance (Bell and Carmichael 1939). In several families (Biemond 1928; Spillane 1940), some siblings show the signs of Friedreich's ataxia and others those of peroneal atrophy. In other families,

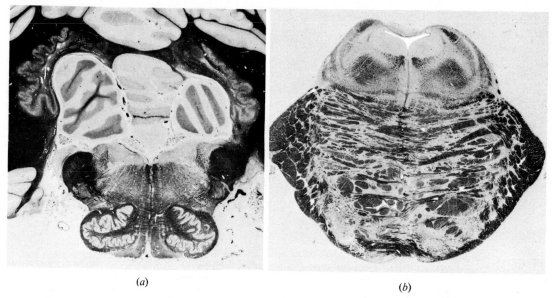

(a)   (b)

Fig. 14.20 Friedreich's ataxia. (*a*) Myelin stain, showing pallor of pyramids, solitary tracts, and hila of dentate nuclei. There is shrinkage of the pyramids and medial lemnisci. (*b*) Myelin stain, showing degeneration of the superior cerebellar peduncles in the upper pons.

Friedreich to Russell (1946) and Hewer (1969) have shown interstitial myocarditis with necrosis or granular degeneration of some fibres and hypertrophy of others. This may be associated with diffuse or focal cellular infiltrations. Valvular lesions of congenital or acquired type are much less common. Intracardial thrombosis has repeatedly been observed at necropsy. Cerebral complications of the heart disease are not uncommon, and take the form either of diffuse hypoxic damage, or of focal infarcts, presumably

pes cavus, ataxia of gait and absence of knee and ankle jerks are combined in some members with atrophy of muscles below the knee and in the hands and forearms. This syndrome was described by Roussy and Lévy in 1926. A long list of similar 'unclassified' diseases could be compiled from published case reports. In the present state of knowledge it would be idle to invent a new name for each of these. Schut (1950) and others have pointed out the great variability, both clinical and anatomical, of these conditions

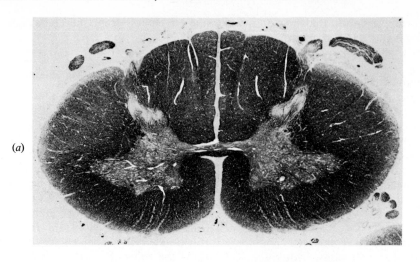

(a)

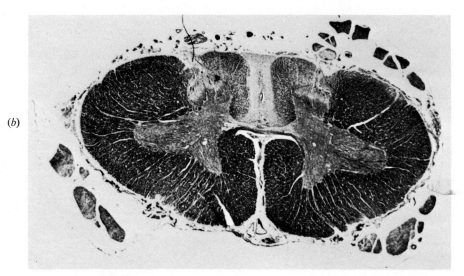

(b)

Fig. 14.21 (a) Cervical cord from a case of familial progressive ataxia, with dominant inheritance. Onset in early middle life, and slow progression. Degeneration of thoracic and accessory cuneate nuclei and spinocerebellar tracts. Mild pyramidal and posterior column degeneration. Similar findings in two other members of the family. Myelin stain. (b) Cervical cord from a sporadic case of progressive ataxia, onset at age 14, death at age 40. Wassermann negative. Severe degeneration of posterior roots and posterior columns. Cerebellum, and its connections, unaffected. Myelin stain.

within a single family, where presumably a single aberrant gene is responsible.

Involvement of the optic, cochlear and vestibular pathways in various types of hereditary ataxia is discussed by van Bogaert and Martin (1974).

Ataxia-telangiectasia (*Louis–Bar syndrome*)

This familial disease of children, characterized by a progressive cerebellar ataxia, with sym-

metrical telangiectases of skin and conjunctiva, was described by Syllaba and Henner in 1926 and by Louis-Bar in 1941. Boder and Sedgwick (1958) described eight cases, one with necropsy, and named the condition *ataxia-telangiectasia*. Since that time many cases have been recorded and much has been discovered about the clinical pathology of the condition. Sedgwick and Boder (1972) list 445 case reports up to that date, including 40 with necropsy. The condition is sometimes classified, along with von Reckling-

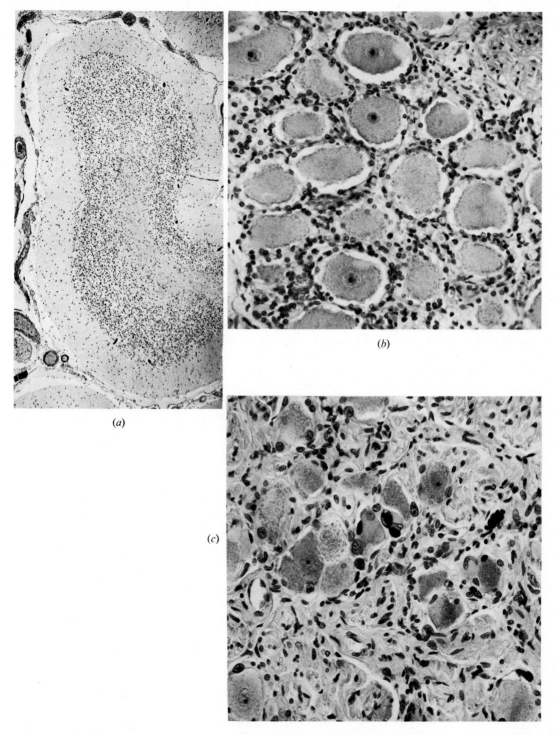

Fig. 14.22 Ataxia-telangiectasia. (*a*) Cerebellar cortex, showing severe loss of both Purkinje and granule cells. H & E. ×42. (Case 1 of Strich 1966.) (*b*) Normal posterior root ganglion with satellite cells. H & E. ×200. (*c*) Posterior root ganglion from case 1 of Strich (1966), showing reduction of satellite cells and abnormal nuclei. H & E. ×200. (By courtesy of the Editor, *Journal of Neurology, Neurosurgery and Psychiatry*.)

hausen's disease, Bournville's disease and the von Hippel–Lindau syndrome, as a *phakomatosis*.

Clinical features. The incidence of the condition is suggestive of autosomal recessive inheritance (Sedgwick and Boder 1972; Koch 1972). In a typical case, the child appears normal at birth. The first signs of ataxia appear in infancy and progress steadily; the child learns to walk and talk, but by the second decade of life is chairfast and grossly dysarthric. Ataxia is often combined with involuntary movements of choreic or athetotic type. Most cases also show progressive abnormalities of eye movements. The appearance of telangiectases, in the conjunctivae and elsewhere, follows the onset of ataxia by a few years. From the beginning, there is a liability to develop respiratory infections, which constitute the commonest immediate cause of death. Bodily growth and sexual development are retarded. The skin and hair show premature ageing. Mental deterioration sometimes occurs in the later stages of the disease. There is a strong tendency to develop malignant disease—most frequently a malignant lymphoma—this being the second commonest cause of death. Few patients survive into the third decade.

Laboratory investigations reveal abnormalities which serve to distinguish this disease from other causes of progressive ataxia, such as Friedreich's ataxia. Immunological studies, originally prompted by the patients' proneness to respiratory infections, led to the discovery that in ataxia-telangiectasia there is a consistent deficiency of IgA in serum and other body fluids, a defect of delayed hypersensitivity responses, aplasia or hypoplasia of the thymus and decreased blast cell transformation of lymphocytes cultured *in vitro* with phytohaemagglutinin (Peterson, Kelly and Good 1964; Leikin, Bazelon and Park 1966).

Pathological changes. The *thymus* is absent, or rudimentary, without Hassall's corpuscles. *Lymphoid* tissue is reduced, with loss of lymphoid follicles, in tonsils, adenoids, lymph nodes and spleen; along with this, there is an apparent hyperplasia of reticulum cells. *Gonads* (particularly the ovaries) are hypoplastic. Other viscera are not abnormal, apart from the presence of scattered large cells with bizarre nuclei. Such cells have repeatedly been observed in the anterior lobe of the *pituitary*. The cutaneous and conjunctival *telangiectases* take the form of dilated, tortuous venules. The *lungs* show the expected changes due to chronic and recurrent infections.

In the *central nervous system*, the constant feature is atrophy of the cerebellar cortex, with extensive loss of Purkinje and granule cells (Fig. 14.22). Remaining Purkinje cells may show irregular dendritic expansions and eosinophilic cytoplasmic inclusion bodies have been observed (Strich 1966). In many cases (especially those of longer duration) there is degeneration in the posterior columns of the spinal cord, affecting the gracile more than the cuneate fasciculi. Apart from these features, there are no striking changes in the brain or cord. Abnormally dilated meningeal veins have been noted in a few cases, but as a rule the vasculature appears normal.

Changes in the peripheral nervous system are less well documented. Strich (1966) observed changes in posterior root ganglia in all of her three cases. These showed a paucity of satellite cells, and the ganglion cells appeared smaller than normal. Among the interstitial cells there were abnormal large cells with bizarre nuclei. In some cases, neurogenic muscle atrophy has been observed.

The condition has been exhaustively reviewed by Sedgwick and Boder (1972). These authors consider that the disease is underdiagnosed and is probably commoner than Friedreich's ataxia. Its prevalence has probably been much increased by the use of antibiotics in controlling the recurrent respiratory infections.

Diseases of motor neurons and pyramidal tracts

Selective destruction of lower motor neurons occurs in a variety of inflammatory and degenerative conditions. The best known of these are *acute anterior poliomyelitis*, which is described in Chapter 8, the various forms of *motor neuron disease*, and *Werdnig–Hoffmann disease*. Motor cells may also be lost in a number of multisystem degenerations, such as *pontocerebellar atrophy*;

in *peroneal muscular atrophy* (see Chapter 16), which is generally regarded as a primary neuropathy, with 'dying back' of motor root fibres; and in chronic (especially syphilitic) radiculopathies, which are discussed in Chapter 6.

It is doubtful whether a pure degeneration of the pyramidal tracts (the 'primary lateral sclerosis' of some authors) ever occurs. Severe pyramidal tract degeneration, without motor cell loss, is characteristic of *Friedreich's ataxia*. Concomitant pyramidal and motor cell lesions are typical of *motor neuron disease*, and of the amyotrophic form of *Jakob–Creutzfeldt disease*, in which the histology of the spinal cord may be indistinguishable from that of classical motor neuron disease.

Motor neuron disease
(*Progressive muscular atrophy: progressive bulbar palsy: amyotrophic lateral sclerosis*)

The term *progressive muscular atrophy* was introduced by Aran (1850) and his teacher Duchenne (1853), who described a series of cases of progressive muscular weakness and wasting in middle-aged patients. They did not suspect damage to the nervous system. In 1860 Duchenne also described the syndrome which later became known as *progressive bulbar palsy*. In his paper of 1853 Duchenne mentioned the observation, made by Cruveilhier on one of his patients, of relative atrophy of the anterior spinal roots, but the

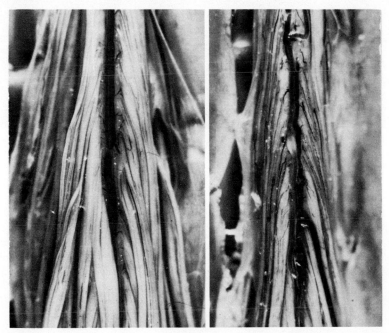

Fig. 14.23 Motor neuron disease. Atrophy of anterior roots in lumbosacral region. Normal subject on left.

The simultaneous involvement of upper and lower motor neurons in these conditions strongly suggest a 'linked' degeneration; but the process can hardly be one of simple trans-synaptic degeneration, either prograde or retrograde. Motor cells are not known to disappear in cases of long-standing cord transection, hemiplegia, or Friedreich's ataxia; nor do the pyramidal tracts atrophy following an attack of poliomyelitis.

In this section we are concerned only with changes observed in the central nervous system. The changes in muscle resulting from denervation are described in Chapter 19.

involvement of the central nervous system in progressive muscular atrophy was first demonstrated in 1869 by Charcot and Joffroy, and in progressive bulbar palsy by Charcot (1870). The discovery of pyramidal tract lesions in cases of progressive muscular atrophy led Charcot (1874) to introduce the term '*amyotrophic lateral sclerosis*'.

During the next 30 years there were numerous neuropathological studies on such cases. Kojewnikow (1885) was able to trace pyramidal tract degeneration upwards through the brainstem and internal capsules to the cerebral cortex, and

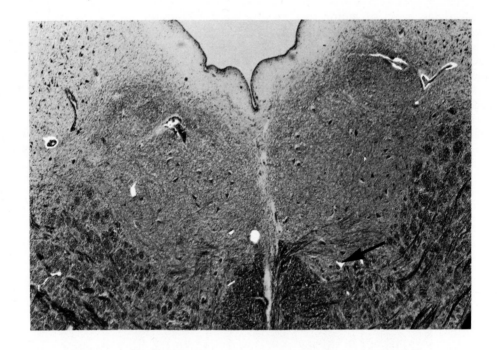

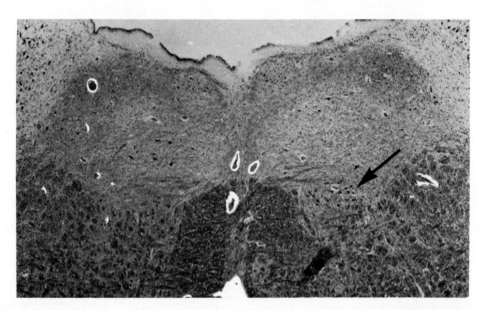

Fig. 14.24(a)   Motor neuron disease.   Loss of motor cells in hypoglossal nuclei.   × 30.   The nucleus of Roller (arrows) is unaffected.   Normal subject is shown in upper illustration.

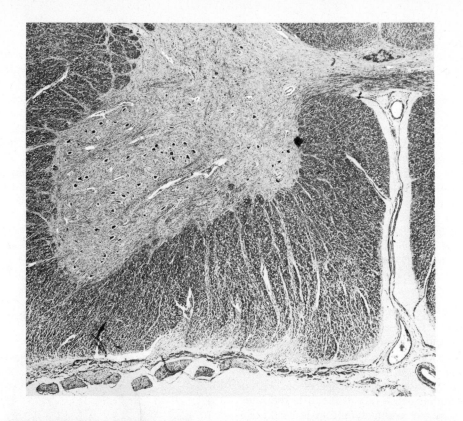

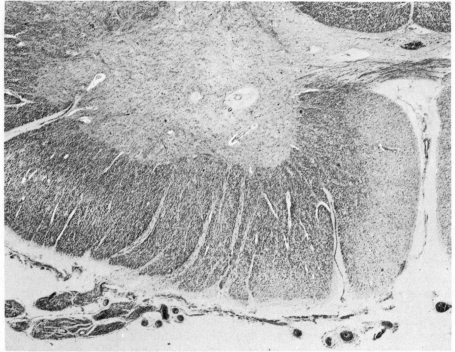

Fig. 14.24(*b*) Motor neuron disease. Loss of motor cells in anterior horn of sixth cervical segment. × 25. Normal subject is shown in upper illustration.

Probst (1898, 1903), using the Marchi technique, demonstrated a widespread but systematic fibre degeneration in the cerebral hemispheres, including parts of the corpus callosum. Déjerine (1883) put forward the view—hotly debated for many years, but now generally accepted by both clinicians and pathologists—that progressive muscular atrophy, progressive bulbar palsy and amyotrophic lateral sclerosis are one and the same condition, with variations in the local distribution and relative severity of the lesions in grey matter and white. The nomenclature of this condition varies in different parts of the world; in the British Isles, the term *motor neuron disease* is commonly used to cover all its variants. For a detailed review of the subject, see Colmant (1958*a*, *c*).

Clinical features. The disease occurs in all parts of the world. In general, it is not familial. In most series males are affected about 1·7 times as often as females (Kurland, Nung Won Choi and Sayre 1969). It is a disease of middle-aged and elderly people, rare before the age of 35, with a rapidly rising incidence rate in the fifth and later decades. The presenting symptom is weakness, often accompanied by pain, in one or two limbs, or in the bulbar musculature. The weakness progresses, involving more and more of the body, and though in the early stages it may be one-sided, it tends to become symmetrical. The external ocular muscles are not affected. Sensation is intact, and there is no sign of involvement of the cerebellar system. Physical signs include muscular wasting and fasciculation, with a very variable admixture of upper motor neuron signs. The cerebrospinal fluid is usually normal. The average duration from the first symptom till death is two or three years, but cases with a duration of five or more years are not uncommon and a benign, very chronic form has been described by Pearce and Harriman (1966). The cause of death in most cases is respiratory failure, often with a terminal aspiration pneumonia.

Pathological changes. To the naked eye, the most striking changes are in the affected muscles, which are pale and shrunken, and in the anterior spinal nerve roots (Fig. 14.23). In some cases there is selective atrophy of the precentral gyri (see Colmant 1958*c*), which becomes more apparent after stripping off the leptomeninges.

The essential histological change is a loss of large motor cells, with resulting gliosis (Fig.

14.24). This is most easily observed in the anterior horns of the lumbar and cervical enlargements and in the hypoglossal nuclei. Remaining motor neurons are commonly shrunken and pyknotic; but this change may be hard to distinguish from post-mortem shrinkage. Large, pale 'ghost' cells may be present, but typical central chromatolysis is rarely seen. Figures of neuronophagia are often present, especially in cases running a rapid course (Fig. 14.25). In the motor nuclei of the facial and trigeminal

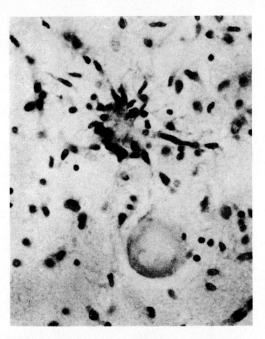

Fig. 14.25 Motor neuron disease. Neuronophagia and 'ghost' cell in anterior horn. Nissl. × 345. (Case 2 of Brownell *et al.* 1970.

nerves, and in the nuclei ambigui, it is often easier to find such changes than to demonstrate an actual loss of cells. The nuclei of the oculomotor, trochlear and abducent nerves are rarely if ever affected.

Changes in the white matter of the spinal cord are variable. The commonest is a degeneration (sometimes asymmetrical) of the pyramidal tracts. When this is severe it can be traced upwards into the white matter of the cerebral hemispheres (Fig. 14.26). In other cases it may be undetectable above the medulla, or even the cervical cord (Davison 1941). In a series of 45 necropsied cases Brownell, Oppenheimer and Hughes (1970) found degeneration extending into the hemi-

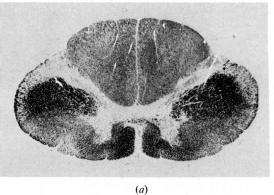

(a)

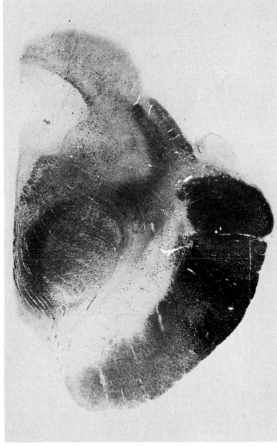

(b)

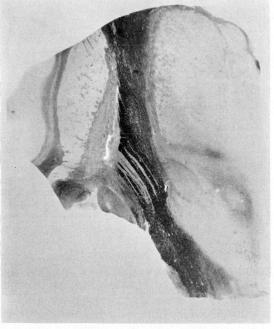

(c)

Fig. 14.26 Motor neuron disease. Marchi preparations, showing pyramidal tract degeneration in (a) cervical cord, (b) midbrain, and (c) internal capsule. (Courtesy of Dr Marion Smith.)

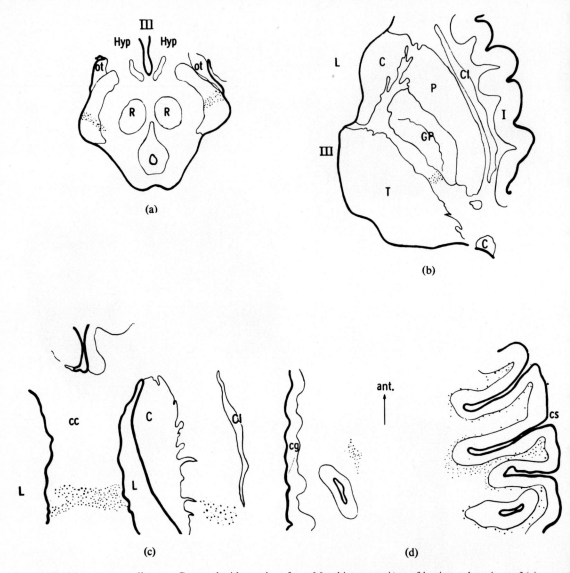

Fig. 14.27 Motor neuron disease. Camera lucida tracings from Marchi preparations of horizontal sections of (*a*) upper midbrain, (*b*) basal nuclei, (*c*) centrum ovale and corpus callosum, and (*d*) superior fronto-parietal region. The stippled areas indicate positive Marchi degeneration. Abbreviations: C = caudate nucleus; cc = corpus callosum; cg = cingulate gyrus; Cl = claustrum; cs = central sulcus; GP = globus pallidus; Hyp = hypothalamus; I = insula; L = Lateral ventricle; ot = optic tract; P = putamen; R = red nucleus; T = thalamus; III = third ventricle. (Case 18 of Brownell *et al.* 1970.)

spheres in under half; and in 10 cases they were unable to observe pyramidal degeneration at any level (it is worth remarking that these 10 cases, clinically and pathologically diagnosed as suffering from motor neuron disease, would be excluded by definition from the diagnosis of amyotrophic lateral sclerosis).

At higher levels, the degenerate tracts occupy the middle thirds of the crura of the cerebral peduncles. Above that, they form discrete bundles in the posterior part of the posterior limbs of the internal capsules (Bertrand and van Bogaert 1925; Smith 1960; Brownell *et al.* 1970) —i.e. well behind the position usually assigned to the pyramidal tracts in textbooks of anatomy. Above this they fan out widely towards their origins in the precentral and postcentral gyri and beyond. There is also a discrete bundle of degenerate fibres running across the middle of the corpus callosum (see Fig. 14.27). Loss of pyramidal cells from the pre- and postcentral gyri may be severe enough to be obvious without formal cell counts. Loss of the giant pyramidal cells of Betz from the precentral gyrus is often apparent, but may be due to shrinkage, rather than to disappearance, of these cells. Cell loss and astrocytic gliosis have been reported in other parts of the brain, in particular the basal ganglia and thalamus; as with Parkinson's disease, however, the significance of these changes in the brains of elderly subjects is doubtful.

In the spinal white matter, in addition to degeneration of the crossed and uncrossed pyramidal tracts, there is often a diffuse loss of

neuron disease has so far yielded nothing substantial. Cases in which some degree of dementia is present, or in which status spongiosus is observed in parts of the cerebral cortex, have suggested a relationship with Jakob–Creutzfeldt disease (Meyer 1929; Brownell et al. 1970); but repeated attempts to transmit the disease to experimental animals have been unsuccessful. Instances in which there is reason to suspect that a progressive atrophy of motor cells is caused by a virus, 'slow', latent, or otherwise, are discussed below. The epidemiology of the disease is discussed by Kurland et al. (1969) and Kurtzke (1969).

Motor neuron disease, if it is a single entity, is a very variable one. In the series of Brownell

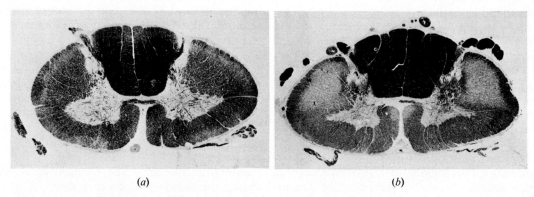

(a)   (b)

Fig. 14.28 Motor neuron disease. Sections from the cervical enlargement. Myelin stain (a) From a case with 9 month's history of bulbar palsy. No abnormal physical signs in the arms or legs. (b) From a typical case with wasting of the small hand muscles and spastic paraplegia.

stainable myelin in the anterior and lateral columns, with intact posterior columns (Fig. 14.28). Whether this is due to demyelination or to degeneration of axons is not known. In Marchi preparations, where the pyramidal tracts are clearly marked by degeneration products, these are rarely seen in the remainder of the anterior and lateral columns, and loss of axons is not detectable in silver impregnations. Degeneration of the dorsal spinocerebellar tracts, with loss of cells from the thoracic nuclei, has been described, but appears to be rare (Brownell et al. 1970). Loss of myelin in a narrow subpial zone is a common finding in elderly subjects, and should not be mistaken for specific tract degeneration.

Problems of classification. The search for genetic, metabolic and environmental causes for motor

et al., there were two cases in which muscular wasting progressed over 10 years. Post-mortem examination showed an almost total loss of motor cells from the anterior horns and hypoglossal nuclei; the pyramidal tracts were intact, and there were no other lesions in the central nervous system. In contrast, there were three cases of progressive spastic paraparesis, with death after 16, 22 and 30 months of illness. In these, motor cell loss was slight, but there was very heavy pyramidal tract degeneration, and intense gliosis in thalamus and basal ganglia. In the present state of knowledge it is impossible to decide whether these represent the extreme ends of a spectrum, or two different diseases.

Familial forms of motor neuron disease
There have been numerous reports (see Colmant 1958c) of motor neuron disease occurring in

several members of a family, with an apparently autosomal dominant inheritance. According to Kurland and Mulder (1954) such cases probably account for 5 to 10% of all cases dying of motor neuron disease in the United States. Clinically, and in most instances pathologically, these cases are indistinguishable from the more usual sporadic cases. In 1959, however, Engel, Kurland and Klatzo described two families in which clinically typical motor neuron disease occurred as an autosomal dominant; in three cases with necropsy they found, in addition to motor cell loss and pyramidal degeneration, symmetrical patches of myelin loss in the posterior columns and degeneration in the spinocerebellar tracts, with loss of cells from the thoracic nuclei. In 1967 Hirano, Kurland and Sayre reported on five familial cases (three from the families described by Engel *et al.*). In four of these they observed similar lesions of motor neurons, pyramidal tracts, spinocerebellar tracts and posterior columns; in addition they found swollen motor cells, containing concentric hyaline cytoplasmic inclusions, in the anterior horns and hypoglossal nuclei. Whether this constitutes a distinct disease, and whether it occurs sporadically, is at present uncertain.

Motor neuron disease in Guam

Following earlier reports of a high incidence of motor neuron disease in the island of Guam, Kurland and Mulder (1954) made a detailed epidemiological survey, which showed that among the Chamorro population (but not among other inhabitants of the island) the disease was at least 50 times commoner than in most parts of the world, and accounted for 8 to 10% of adult deaths. Males were affected nearly twice as often as females. Dominant inheritance was suspected, but it is still uncertain whether genetic or environmental and cultural factors are the main cause. The pathology in 22 of these cases was described by Malamud, Hirano and Kurland in 1961. The consistent findings were loss of motor cells from the cervical and lumbar enlargements and hypoglossal nuclei, degeneration, usually severe, of the pyramidal tracts, and neurofibrillary tangles, widely distributed in the brain, and occasionally in motor cells of the spinal cord. The appearance of these tangles, and their distribution, corresponded closely with the same authors' findings in the Parkinsonian-dementia complex of Guam (p. 615); and they concluded that the two conditions were different

expressions of the same disease. An indication that the disease is not confined to the Chamorros is the report by Shiraki (1969) of similar pathological findings in patients from the Kii peninsula, in Japan, where the incidence of motor neuron disease is abnormally high.

Infantile spinal muscular atrophy of Werdnig and Hoffmann

Various conditions, some of which are still poorly understood, may give rise to congenital amyotonia (the 'floppy baby' syndrome). Of these the best known, the most rapidly lethal, and probably the commonest, is the disease described by Werdnig (1891, 1894) and Hoffmann (1893, 1900). Clinically, a progressive muscular weakness, sparing only the diaphragm and the muscles supplied by the upper brainstem, usually leads to death in a matter of months from respiratory failure, often hastened by aspiration pneumonia. The floppiness is often detectable at birth, and the mother may have noticed feebleness of fetal movements. In general, the earlier the onset, the more rapid the course. The disease is transmitted by simple autosomal recessive inheritance. For a detailed discussion, see the monograph by Brandt (1950).

Pathological changes. The changes in skeletal muscle are those of progressive denervation, as described in Chapter 19. They are widespread and severe, but there is marked sparing of the diaphragm, the 'strap' muscles of the neck, the external ocular and masticator muscles. Those supplied by the lower cranial nerves are not spared (Byers and Banker 1961).

On naked-eye examination there is atrophy of the anterior spinal roots. Microscopically, there is loss of motor cells from most levels of the spinal cord, from the nuclei ambigui and from the hypoglossal and facial nuclei (Fig. 14.29). Among the remaining motor cells, there are frequent figures of neuronophagia, and pale, swollen cells, resembling the 'ghost' cells seen in motor neuron disease. These are commonly described as showing central chromatolysis, but it may be doubted whether the change is a true axonal reaction. Long tracts in the brainstem and spinal cord appear intact. Gruner and Bargeton (1952) reported, as a constant finding in nine otherwise typical cases, a symmetrical loss of nerve cells, with 'ghost' cells and neuronophagia, from the posteroventral nucleus of the thalamus—a finding confirmed in other reported cases in which the thalamus has been carefully examined (Fig. 14.30). Lesions elsewhere in the brain tend to be of a non-specific kind, attributable to cerebral hypoxia.

There have been several reports on cases diagnosed as Werdnig–Hoffmann disease, with lesions additional to the 'classical' ones listed above. Radermecker (1951) observed lesions in parts of the cerebellar system and in optic nerves. In some reports, one cannot but wonder whether the case was truly one of Werdnig–Hoffmann disease, and if so whether a second disease was present. Such is the case reported by Ajuriaguerra, Heuyer and Lebovici (1950) of a mentally defective 16-year-old girl showing, in addition to motor cell loss and amyotrophy, a severe loss of spinal ganglion cells, with degeneration of the posterior columns; and the case reported by Norman (1961) of a 6-month-old child with

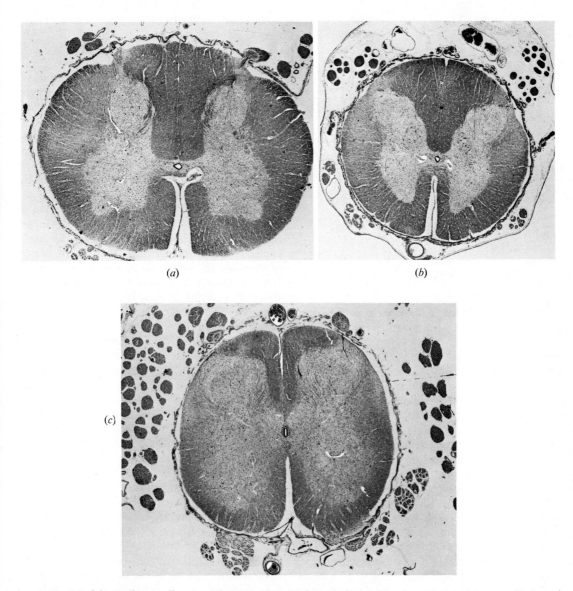

(a)

(b)

(c)

Fig. 14.29 Werdnig–Hoffmann disease. Three-month-old infant. Spinal cord, (a) cervical enlargement, (b) thoracic (note well-preserved cells in thoracic nuclei) and (c) sacral (note relative atrophy of anterior roots). There is a severe loss of motor cells at all levels. Klüver–Barrera. × 18.

cerebellar hypoplasia and severe degenerative changes in the thalamus, globus pallidus and subthalamic nucleus.

There appears to be no distinct upper age limit for this disease. Late infantile, juvenile and adolescent forms of spinal amyotrophy, with autosomal recessive inheritance, have been described by Wohlfart, Fex and Eliasson (1955), Kugelberg and Welander (1956), Smith and Patel

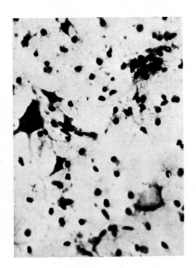

Fig. 14.30 Werdnig–Hoffmann disease. Thalamus, showing a degenerate nerve cell and a figure of neuronophagia. Carbol azure.

(1965), Gardner-Medwin, Hudgson and Walton (1967), and others. In general, the later the onset the slower the progression and the more favourable the prognosis. In the juvenile and adolescent forms the proximal limb muscles are often affected, bulbar muscles are spared, and the disease may be mistaken for a muscular dystrophy. The diagnosis of neurogenic atrophy depends on electromyography and muscle biopsy. Because of the benign course of the disease, there is a dearth of anatomical reports on the central nervous system in these cases. The same is true of the neurogenic muscular atrophies with dominant inheritance (discussed by Gardner-Medwin *et al.* 1967, and by Fenichel 1969), in which the clinical course is even slower.

The condition of *arthrogryposis multiplex congenita* (deformed and rigid joints, associated with muscular wasting) results, according to Drachman (1969) from paralysis of, or interference with, muscular activity in the fetus. The causes of this are various, and include primary muscle

disorders (Banker, Victor and Adams 1957); most commonly, there is a primary disease of the central nervous system, which may be a gross malformation (such as meningomyelocele), or merely a deficit of anterior horn cells. Drachman (1969) lists 21 necropsy reports, in 14 of which loss of motor cells was observed. In all but three of these, which showed some pyramidal tract degeneration, this was the only lesion in the central nervous system. On this basis, it is thought that Werdnig–Hoffmann disease, with early onset, constitutes a major cause of congenital arthrogryposis.

Other conditions affecting motor neurons

The separation of a degenerative motor neuropathy, with 'dying-back' of axons, from a primary degeneration of motor cells is somewhat artificial. In the case of *peroneal muscular atrophy* (Charcot–Marie–Tooth disease: see Chapter 16) the pathological changes in the motor cells of the spinal cord are indistinguishable from those in various conditions described above (Hughes and Brownell 1972), and the concomitant degeneration of sensory ganglion cells and their processes resembles that found in Friedreich's ataxia (Hughes, Brownell and Hewer 1968). The distinction appears even more unreal in view of reports of families in which some members show the clinical features of Friedreich's ataxia and others those of peroneal atrophy (p. 629).

In the degenerative conditions hitherto mentioned, other than progressive supranuclear palsy, there is a striking, and unexplained, tendency for the external ocular muscles to be spared. In rare cases, however, there appears to be a selective denervation of these muscles. The clinical condition of *progressive external ophthalmoplegia* occurs sometimes in apparent isolation, sometimes associated with a generalized myopathy, and sometimes with evidence of disease of the peripheral or central nervous system. Muscle biopsies have been suggestive of myopathy in some cases, of denervation in others. Few such cases have had full neuropathological studies, and in these the interpretation of the findings has been difficult. The subject has been reviewed by Colmant (1958b), Drachman (1968), and Rosenberg, Schotland, Lovelace and Rowland (1968).

In addition to the acute destruction of motor cells in poliomyelitis, it has often been suspected that these cells may be progressively attacked by a 'slow' or latent infection. Zilkha (1962) presented figures showing a very high incidence of a past history of acute poliomyelitis in patients with motor neuron disease. Greenfield and Matthews (1954) and others have described cases of postencephalitic Parkinsonism, later developing a progressive amyotrophy, with loss of motor cells. A number of recent authors (Brain, Croft and Wilkinson 1965; Norris and Engel 1965; Norris, McMenemey and Barnard 1969) maintain that there is an association, beyond what would be expected by chance, between a form of motor neuron disease and malignant disease. Here, too,

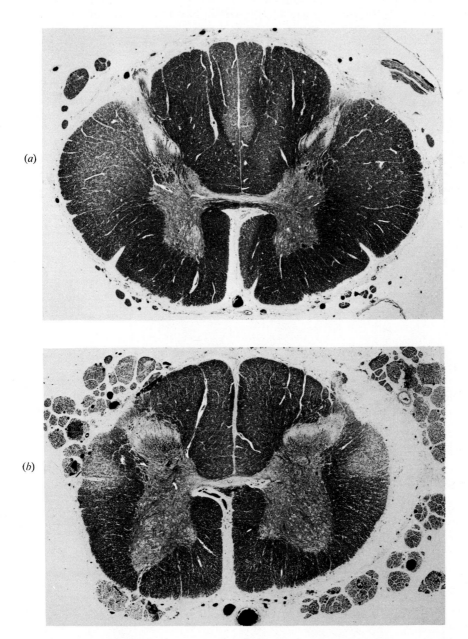

Fig. 14.31 Familial spastic paraplegia. Dominant inheritance. Early onset, death age 74. (*a*) Fourth cervical level. (*b*) Lower lumbar level. The posterior columns are more affected at the higher level, and the pyramidal tracts at the lower one. Myelin stain.

the suggestion has been made of an 'opportunistic' virus infection. The evidence for the association of malignancy and motor cell disease in humans is hard to assess; but an experimental approach to the subject has been made by Klüver and Weil (1948), who, having observed loss and vacuolation of motor cells in a monkey with a carcinoma of the tongue, implanted carcinoma cells into the tongue of another monkey; the tumour grew apace, and the recipient subsequently showed a disease of the motor cells similar to that of the donor.

A possible association between motor neuron disease and pancreatic malfunction is discussed by Quick (1969). Various toxic and metabolic conditions affecting motor cells and long tracts

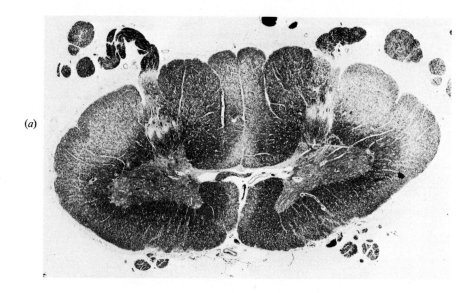

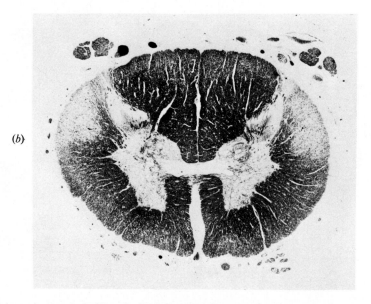

Fig. 14.32 Familial spastic paraplegia (Case 2 of Behan and Maia). Dominant inheritance. Onset age 55, death age 66. (*a*) Cervical level. (*b*) Upper lumbar level. Tract degeneration as in Fig. 14.31 but more severe. Myelin stain. (Courtesy of the Editor, *Journal of Neurology, Neurosurgery and Psychiatry*.)

are dealt with in Chapter 4. Spontaneous diseases of motor neurons in other mammals are reviewed by Andrews and Maxwell (1969).

Familial spastic paraplegia

Strümpell (1880) described two brothers in whom spastic paraplegia, with very little involvement of the arms or face, developed in middle life. On post-mortem examination of the younger patient (1886) he found degeneration of the pyramidal tracts, beginning below their decussation and most definite in the lower thoracic and lumbar segments. Degeneration of the posterior columns was slight at the lumbar level but became more evident in the upper thoracic and cervical segments, in which the fasciculus gracilis was extensively, and the fasciculus cuneatus slightly, involved. Degeneration of the spinocerebellar tracts was also evident at these levels. In 1904 Strümpell described another familial case, with onset at 35, slow progression, and death at 69. The lesions in the cord were almost identical with those in the first case.

Since that time there have been many clinical, and a few pathological, reports on families affected with spastic weakness of the lower limbs. As in the case of familial ataxias, these families show a great variety of clinical syndromes, with various combinations of degenerative lesions; it is at present unprofitable to attempt to classify and name separate conditions. Within single families, there are wide variations in age of onset, severity of symptoms, and associated disabilities. In some cases, spasticity and weakness are followed by loss of motor neurons and amyotrophy. In others (Bickerstaff 1950; van Bogaert 1952a) there is optic neuropathy, leading to blindness; and in a number of cases lesions of long motor tracts are combined with degeneration of parts of the cerebellar system. The subject has been reviewed by Schwarz (1952) and Schwarz and Liu (1956), and the genetic aspects are discussed by van Bogaert (1952b). According to Schwarz (1952) the published reports constitute 'a hodgepodge of varied disorders of the nervous system, with paraparesis or paraplegia simply one of the occurrences in the illness, not the main or only factor'. Cases closely resembling those of Strümpell, with late onset, slow progression, and degeneration practically confined to the long cord tracts, include the case of Schwarz and Liu (1956) and two cases reported by Behan and Maia (1974) (see Figs. 14.31 and 14.32). Fig. 14.31 is from an unpublished case of this type.

Degeneration of the distal portions of long axons, without appreciable loss of parent cell bodies, is characteristic of these cases. It is uncertain whether or not this represents a retarded 'dying-back' process, of the kind seen in other degenerative conditions, where the parent cell body eventually disappears. An alternative explanation would be in terms of a generalized failure of nerve cells to maintain the vitality of the distal parts of long axons. It is also uncertain to what extent the spasticity and weakness in this condition are due to involvement of motor pathways other than the pyramidal tracts. It is noteworthy that, although posterior columns are involved, sensory loss is never severe and is often undetected.

References

Adams, R. D. (1968) The striatonigral degenerations in *Handbook of Clinical Neurology* (Eds. Vinken, P. J. & Bruyn, G. W.), Vol. 6, Chapter 26, pp. 694-702, North Holland Publishing Co., Amsterdam.

Adams, R. D., Bogaert, L. van & Vander Eecken, H. (1961) Dégénérescences nigro-striées et cérébello-nigro-striées. *Psychiatria et Neurologia*, **142**, 219.

Adams, R. D., Bogaert, L. van & Vander Eecken, H. (1964) Striato-nigral degeneration. *Journal of Neuropathology and Experimental Neurology*, **23**, 584-608.

Ajuriaguerra, J. de, Heuyer, G. & Lebovici, S. (1950) Maladie de Werdnig–Hoffmann. Examen anatomo-clinique. *Revue Neurologique*, **83**, 312-314.

Akelaitis, A. J. (1938) Hereditary form of primary parenchymatous atrophy of the cerebellar cortex associated with mental deterioration. *American Journal of Psychiatry*, **94**, 1115-1140.

André-van Leeuwen, M. & Bogaert, L. van (1949) Hereditary ataxia with optic atrophy of the retrobulbar neuritis type, and latent pallido-luysian degeneration. *Brain*, **72**, 340-363.

Andrews, J. M. & Maxwell, D. S. (1969) Motor neuron diseases in animals in *Motor Neuron Diseases* (Eds. Norris, F. H. & Kurland, L. T.), Chapter 35, Grune and Stratton, New York.

Aran, F. A. (1850) Recherches sur une maladie non encore décrite du système musculaire (atrophie musculaire progressive). *Archives Générales de Médecine*, **24**, 5-35, 172-214.

Banker, B. Q., Victor, M. & Adams, R. D.   (1957) Arthrogryposis multiplex due to congenital muscular dystrophy. *Brain*, **80**, 319-334.

Bannister, R. & Oppenheimer, D. R.   (1972) Degenerative diseases of the nervous system associated with autonomic failure. *Brain*, **95**, 457-474.

Beck, E., Daniel, P. M., Matthews, W. B., Stevens, D. L., Alpers, M. P., Asher, D. M., Gajdusek, D. C. & Gibbs, C. J.   (1969) Creutzfeldt–Jakob disease: the neuropathology of a transmission experiment. *Brain*, **92**, 699-716.

Behan, W. M. H. & Maia, M.   (1974) Strümpell's familial spastic paraplegia: genetics and neuropathology. *Journal of Neurology, Neurosurgery and Psychiatry*, **37**, 8-20.

Beheim-Schwarzbach, D.   (1952) Über Zelleibveränderungen im Nucleus coeruleus bei Parkinsonsymptomen. *Journal of Nervous and Mental Disease*, **116**, 619-632.

Behrman, S., Carroll, J. D., Janota, I. & Matthews, W. B.   (1969) Progressive supranuclear palsy: clinico-pathological study of four cases. *Brain*, **92**, 663-677.

Bell, J. & Carmichael, E. A.   (1939) On hereditary ataxia and spastic paraplegia in *The Treasury of Human Inheritance* (Ed. Fisher, R. A.), Vol. 4, Part 3, Cambridge University Press, London.

Bertrand, I. & Bogaert, L. van   (1925) Rapport sur la sclérose latérale amyotrophique (anatomie pathologique). *Revue Neurologique*, **1**, 779-806.

Bethlem, J. & Jager, W. A. den H.   (1960) The incidence and characteristics of Lewy bodies in idiopathic paralysis.agitans. *Journal of Neurology, Neurosurgery and Psychiatry*, **23**, 74-80.

Bickerstaff, E. R.   (1950) Hereditary spastic paraplegia. *Journal of Neurology, Neurosurgery and Psychiatry*, **13**, 134-145.

Biemond, A.   (1928) Neurotische Muskelatrophie und Friedreichsche Tabes in derselben Familie. *Deutsche Zeitschrift für Nervenheilkunde*, **104**, 113-145.

Blackwood, W.   (1952) Biopsy technique in the diagnosis of peripheral neuropathies. *Proceedings of the 1st International Congress of Neuropathology* (*Rome*), Vol. 3, pp. 415-424, Rosenberg & Sellier, Torino.

Boder, E. & Sedgwick, R. P.   (1958) Ataxia-telangiectasia: a familial syndrome of progressive cerebellar ataxia, oculocutaneous telangiectasia and frequent pulmonary infection. *Pediatrics*, **21**, 526-554.

Bogaert, L. van   (1930) Contribution clinique et anatomique à l'étude de la paralysie agitante juvénile primitive. *Revue Neurologique*, **37**, 315-326.

Bogaert, L. van   (1946) Aspects cliniques et pathologiques des atrophies pallidales et pallido-luysiennes pro-gressives. *Journal of Neurology, Neurosurgery and Psychiatry*, **9**, 125-157.

Bogaert, L. van   (1952*a*) Etudes sur la paraplégie spasmodique familiale. V: forme classique pure avec atrophie optique massive. *Acta neurologica et psychiatrica belgica*, **52**, 795-807.

Bogaert, L. van   (1952*b*) Etude génétique sur les paraplégies spasmodiques familiales. *Journal de Génétique Humaine*, **1**, 6-23.

Bogaert, L. van & Martin, L.   (1974) Optic and cochleovestibular degenerations in the hereditary ataxias. *Brain*, **97**, 15-40.

Borit, A., Rubinstein, L. J. & Urich, H.   (1975) The striatonigral degenerations: putaminal pigments and noso-logy. *Brain*, **98**, 101-112.

Brain, Lord, Croft, P. B. & Wilkinson, M.   (1965) Motor neurone disease as a manifestation of neoplasm. *Brain*, **88**, 479-500.

Brandt, S.   (1950) *Werdnig–Hoffmann's Infantile Progressive Muscular Atrophy*, Munksgaard, Copenhagen.

Brownell, B., Oppenheimer, D. R. & Hughes, J. T.   (1970) The central nervous system in motor neurone disease. *Journal of Neurology, Neurosurgery and Psychiatry*, **33**, 338-357.

Byers, R. K. & Banker, B. Q.   (1961) Infantile muscular atrophy. *Archives of Neurology* (*Chicago*), **5**, 140-164.

Byrnes, C. M.   (1926) A contribution to the pathology of paralysis agitans. *Archives of Neurology and Psychiatry* (*Chicago*), **15**, 407-443.

Cassinari, V. & Pagni, C. A.   (1969) *Central Pain: a Neurosurgical Survey*, Harvard University Press, Cam-bridge, Mass.

Charcot, J.-M.   (1870) Note sur un cas de paralysie glosso-laryngée suivi d'autopsie. *Archives de Physiologie*, **3**, 247-260.

Charcot, J.-M.   (1874) De la sclérose latérale amyotrophique. *Progrès Médicale*, **2**, 325-327, 341-342, 453-455.

Charcot, J.-M. & Joffroy, A.   (1869) Deux cas d'atrophie musculaire progressive avec lésions de la substance grise et des faisceaux antérolatéraux de la moëlle épinière. *Archives de Physiologie* (*Paris*), **2**, 354-367, 629-649, 744-760.

Colmant, H.-J.   (1958*a*) Die chronisch-progressive Bulbärparalyse in *Handbuch der speziellen pathologischen Anatomie und Histologie* (Eds. Lubarsch, O., Henke, F. & Rössle, R.), Vol. 13/2B, pp. 2571-2584, Springer Verlag, Berlin.

Colmant, H.-J.   (1958b) Die chronisch-progressive exteriore Ophthalmoplegie in *Handbuch der speziellen pathologischen Anatomie und Histologie* (Eds. Lubarsch, O., Henke, F. & Rössle, R.), Vol. 13/2B, pp. 2585-2623, Springer Verlag, Berlin.

Colmant, H.-J.   (1958c) Die myatrophische Lateralsklerose in *Handbuch der speziellen pathologischen Anatomie und Histologie* (Eds. Lubarsch, O., Henke, F. & Rössle, R.), Vol. 13/2B, pp. 2624-2692, Springer Verlag, Berlin.

David, N. J., Mackey, E. A. & Smith, J. L.   (1968) Further observations in progressive supranuclear palsy *Neurology (Minneapolis)*, **18**, 349-356.

Davison, C.   (1941) Amyotrophic lateral sclerosis.   Origin and extent of the upper motor neuron lesion. *Archives of Neurology and Psychiatry (Chicago)*, **46**, 1039-1056.

Déjerine, J.   (1883) Etude anatomique et clinique sur la paralysie labio-glosso-laryngée.   *Archives de Physiologie Normale et Pathologique, Série 3*, **2**, 180-227.

Déjerine, J. & Roussy, G.   (1906) La syndrome thalamique.   *Revue Neurologique*, **12**, 521-532.

Déjerine, J. & Thomas, A.   (1900) L'atrophie olivo-ponto-cérébelleuse.   *Nouvelle Iconographie de la Salpêtrière*, **13**, 330-370.

Denny-Brown, D.   (1951) Hereditary sensory radicular neuropathy.   *Journal of Neurology, Neurosurgery and Psychiatry*, **14**, 237-252.

Denny-Brown, D.   (1962) *The Basal Ganglia and their Relation to Disorders of Movement*, Oxford Neurological Monographs, Oxford University Press, London.

Denny-Brown, D.   (1968) Clinical symptomatology of diseases of the basal ganglia in *Handbook of Clinical Neurology* (Eds. Vinken, P. J. & Bruyn, G. W.), Vol. 6, Chapter 5, pp. 133-172, North Holland Publishing Co., Amsterdam.

Devos, J.   (1957) Atrophie cérébelleuse tardive, à hérédité dominante avec paralysies oculaires.   *Psychiatria et Neurologia*, **133**, 46-62.

Drachman, D. A.   (1968) Ophthalmoplegia plus: the neurodegenerative disorders associated with progressive external ophthalmoplegia.   *Archives of Neurology (Chicago)*, **18**, 654-674.

Drachman, D. B.   (1969) Congenital deformities produced by neuromuscular disorders of the developing embryo in *Motor Neuron Diseases* (Eds. Norris, F. H. & Kurland, L. T.), Chapter 10, Grune and Stratton, New York.

Duchenne, G. B. A.   (1853) Etude comparée des lésions anatomiques dans l'atrophie musculaire progressive et dans la paralysie générale.   *Union Médicale*, **7**, 246-247.

Duchenne, G. B. A.   (1860) Paralysie musculaire progressive de la langue, du voile du palais et des lèvres. *Archives générales de Médicine*, **16**, 283-296, 431-445.

Duffy, P. E. & Tennyson, V. M.   (1965) Phase and electron microscopic observations of Lewy bodies and melanin granules in the substantia nigra and locus ceruleus in Parkinson's disease. *Journal of Neuropathology and Experimental Neurology*, **24**, 398-414.

Earle, K. M.   (1968) Studies on Parkinson's disease, including X-ray fluorescent spectroscopy of formalin-fixed brain tissue. *Journal of Neuropathology and Experimental Neurology*, **27**, 1-14.

Engel, W. K., Kurland, L. T. & Klatzo, I.   (1959) An inherited disease similar to amyotrophic lateral sclerosis with a pattern of posterior column involvement. *Brain*, **82**, 203-220.

Fenichel, G. M.   (1969) The spinal muscular atrophies in *Motor Neuron Diseases* (Eds. Norris, F. H. & Kurland, L. T.), Chapter 11, Grune and Stratton, New York.

Foix, M. C.   (1921) Les lésions anatomiques de la maladie de Parkinson.   *Revue Neurologique*, **28**, 593-600.

Forno, L. S.   (1966) Pathology of Parkinsonism: a preliminary report of 24 cases.   *Journal of Neurosurgery*, **24**, 266-271.

Friedreich, N.   (1863) Ueber degenerative Atrophie der spinalen Hinterstränge.   *Virchows Archiv für pathologische Anatomie*, **26**, 391-419, 433-459; **27**, 1-26.

Friedreich, N.   (1876) Ueber Ataxie mit besonderer Berücksichtigung der hereditären Formen.   *Virchows Archiv für pathologische Anatomie*, **68**, 145-245.

Gamboa, E. T., Wolf, A., Yahr, M. D., Harter, D. H., Duffy, P. E., Barden, H. & Hsu, K. C.   (1974) Influenza virus antigen in postencephalitic Parkinsonism brain.   *Archives of Neurology (Chicago)*, **31**, 228-232.

Gardner-Medwin, D., Hudgson, P. & Walton, J. N.   (1967) Benign spinal muscular atrophy arising in childhood and adolescence. *Journal of the Neurological Sciences*, **5**, 121-158.

Greenfield, J. G.   (1954) *The Spino-cerebellar Degenerations*, Blackwell, Oxford.

Greenfield, J. G. & Bosanquet, F. D.   (1953) The brain-stem lesions in Parkinsonism.   *Journal of Neurology, Neurosurgery and Psychiatry*, **16**, 213-226.

Greenfield, J. G. & Matthews, W. B.   (1954) Post-encephalitic Parkinsonism with amyotrophy.   *Journal of Neurology, Neurosurgery and Psychiatry*, **17**, 50-56.

Grimberg, L. (1934) Paralysis agitans and trauma. *Journal of Nervous and Mental Diseases*, **79**, 14-42.

Gruner, J.-E. & Bargeton, E. (1952) Lésions thalamiques dans la myatonie du nourisson. *Revue Neurologique*, **86**, 236-242.

Hall, B., Noad, K. B. & Latham, O. (1941) Familial cortical cerebellar atrophy. *Brain*, **64**, 178-194.

Hall, B., Noad, K. B. & Latham, O. (1945) Familial cortical cerebellar atrophy: a contribution to the study of heredo-familial cerebellar disease in Australia. *Medical Journal of Australia*, **1**, 101-108.

Hallervorden, J. (1933) Zur Pathogenese des postencephalitischen Parkinsonismus. *Klinische Wochenschrift*, **12**, 692-694.

Hallervorden, J. (1935) Anatomische Untersuchungen zur Pathogenese des postencephalitischen Parkinsonismus. *Deutsche Zeitschrift für Nervenheilkunde*, **136**, 68-77.

Hassler, R. (1938) Zur Pathologie der Paralysis agitans und des postenzephalitischen Parkinsonismus. *Journal für Psychologie und Neurologie (Leipzig)*, **48**, 387.

Hewer, R. L. (1968) Study of fatal cases of Friedreich's ataxia. *British Medical Journal*, **3**, 649-652.

Hewer, R. L. (1969) The heart in Friedreich's ataxia. *British Heart Journal*, **31**, 5-14.

Hirano, A., Kurland, L. T., Krooth, R. S. & Lessell, S. (1961) Parkinsonism-dementia complex, an endemic disease on the island of Guam. I. Clinical features. *Brain*, **84**, 642-661.

Hirano, A., Kurland, L. T. & Sayre, G. P. (1967) Familial amyotrophic lateral sclerosis. *Archives of Neurology (Chicago)*, **16**, 232-243.

Hirano, A., Malamud, N. & Kurland, L. T. (1961) Parkinsonism-dementia complex, an endemic disease on the island of Guam. II. Pathological features. *Brain*, **84**, 662-679.

Hoffmann, J. (1893) Ueber chronische spinale Muskelatrophie im Kindesalter auf familiäre Basis. *Deutsche Zeitschrift für Nervenheilkunde*, **3**, 427-470.

Hoffmann, J. (1900) Ueber die hereditäre progressive spinale Muskelatrophie im Kindesalter. *Münchener medizinische Wochenschrift*, **47**, 1649-1651.

Holmes, G. (1907) A form of familial degeneration of the cerebellum. *Brain*, **30**, 466-489.

Hughes, J. T. & Brownell, B. (1972) Pathology of peroneal muscular atrophy. *Journal of Neurology, Neurosurgery and Psychiatry*, **35**, 648-657.

Hughes, J. T., Brownell, B. & Hewer, R. L. (1968) The peripheral sensory pathway in Friedreich's ataxia. *Brain*, **91**, 803-818.

Hunt, J. R. (1917) Progressive atrophy of the globus pallidus. *Brain*, **40**, 58-148.

Jager, W. A. den H. & Bethlem, J. (1960) The distribution of Lewy bodies in the central and autonomic nervous systems in idiopathic paralysis agitans. *Journal of Neurology, Neurosurgery and Psychiatry*, **23**, 283-290.

Jellinger, K. (1968a) Degenerations and exogenous lesions of the pallidum and striatum in *Handbook of Clinical Neurology* (Eds. Vinken, P. J. & Bruyn, G. W.), Vol. 6, Chapter 25, pp. 632-693, North Holland Publishing Co., Amsterdam.

Jellinger, K. (1968b) Progressive Pallidum-atrophie. *Journal of the Neurological Sciences*, **6**, 19-44.

Jellinger, K. & Danielczyk, W. (1968) Striato-nigrale Degeneration. *Acta Neuropathologica (Berlin)*, **10**, 242-257.

Johnson, R. H., Lee, G. de J., Oppenheimer, D. R. & Spalding, J. M. K. (1966) Autonomic failure with orthostatic hypotension due to intermediolateral column degeneration. *Quarterly Journal of Medicine*, **35**, 276-292.

Kemp, J. M. & Powell, T. P. S. (1971) The connections of the striatum and globus pallidus: synthesis and speculation. *Philosophical Transactions of the Royal Society, London, Series B*, **262**, 441-457.

Klaue, R. (1940) Parkinsonsche Krankheit (Paralysis agitans) und postencephalitischer Parkinsonismus. *Archiv für Psychiatrie und Nervenkrankheiten*, **111**, 251-321.

Klüver, H. & Weil, A. (1948) Carcinomas of the tongue in monkeys and pathologic changes in the central nervous system. *Journal of Neuropathology and Experimental Neurology*, **7**, 144-153.

Koch, G. (1972) Genetic aspects of the phakomatoses in *Handbook of Clinical Neurology* (Eds. Vinken, P. J. & Bruyn, G. W.), Vol. 14, Chapter 20, pp. 515-517, North Holland Publishing Co., Amsterdam.

Kojewnikow, A. (1885) Ein Fall von lateraler amyotrophischer Sclerose. *Zentralblatt für Nervenheilkunde*, **8**, 409-414.

Kugelberg, E. & Welander, L. (1956) Heredofamilial juvenile muscular atrophy simulating muscular dystrophy. *Archives of Neurology and Psychiatry (Chicago)*, **75**, 500-509.

Kurland, L. T. & Mulder, D. W. (1954) Epidemiologic investigations of amyotrophic lateral sclerosis, I. *Neurology (Minneapolis)*, **4**, 355-378, 438-448.

Kurland, L. T., Nung Won Choi & Sayre, G. P. (1969) Implications of incidence and geographic patterns on the classification of amyotrophic lateral sclerosis in *Motor Neuron Diseases* (Eds. Norris, F. H. & Kurland, L. T.), Chapter 4, Grune and Stratton, New York.

Kurtzke, J. F. (1969) Comments on the epidemiology of amyotrophic lateral sclerosis in *Motor Neuron Diseases* (Eds. Norris, F. H. & Kurland, L. T.), Chapter 8, Grune and Stratton, New York.

Leikin, S. L., Bazelon, M. & Park, K. H. (1966) In vitro lymphocyte transformation in ataxia-telangiectasia. *Journal of Pediatrics*, **68**, 477-479.

Lewis, P. (1964) Familial orthostatic hypotension. *Brain*, **87**, 719-728.

Lewy, F. H. (1913) Zur pathologischen Anatomie der Paralysis agitans. *Deutsche Zeitschrift für Nervenheilkunde*, **50**, 50-55.

Lipkin, L. E. (1959) Cytoplasmic inclusions in ganglion cells associated with Parkinsonian states. *American Journal of Pathology*, **35**, 1117-1133.

Louis-Bar, D. (1941) Sur un syndrome progressif comprenant des télangiectasies capillaires cutanées et conjonctivales symétriques, à disposition naevoïde, et des troubles cérébelleux. *Confinia neurologica (Basel)*, **4**, 32-42.

Löwenthal, A. & Bruyn, G. W. (1968) Calcification of the striopallidodentate system in *Handbook of Clinical Neurology* (Eds. Vinken, P. J. & Bruyn, G. W.), Vol. 6, Chapter 27, pp. 703-725, North Holland Publishing Co., Amsterdam.

Malamud, N., Hirano, A. & Kurland, L. T. (1961) Pathoanatomic changes in amyotrophic lateral sclerosis on Guam. *Archives of Neurology (Chicago)*, **5**, 401-415.

Marie, P., Foix, C. & Alajouanine, T. (1922) De l'atrophie cérébelleuse tardive à prédominance corticale. *Revue Neurologique*, **29**, 849-885, 1082-1111.

Martin, J. J. (1969) Thalamic syndromes in *Handbook of Clinical Neurology* (Eds. Vinken, P. J. & Bruyn, G. W.), Vol. 2, Chapter 17, pp. 469-496, North Holland Publishing Co., Amsterdam.

Martin, J. J. (1970) Contribution à l'étude de l'anatomie du thalamus et de sa pathologie au cours des maladies dégénératives dites abiotrophiques. *Acta neurologica belgica*, **70**, 5-212.

Martin, J. P. (1967) *The Basal Ganglia and Posture*, Pitman Medical, London.

Menzel, P. (1891) Beitrag zur Kenntnis der hereditären Ataxie und Kleinhirnatrophie. *Archiv für Psychiatrie*, **22**, 160-190.

Mettler, F. A. (1968) Anatomy of the basal ganglia in *Handbook of Clinical Neurology* (Eds. Vinken, P. J. & Bruyn, G. W.), Vol. 6, Chapter 1, pp. 1-55, North Holland Publishing Co., Amsterdam.

Meyer, A. (1929) Ueber eine der amyotrophischen Lateralsklerose nahestehende Erkrankung mit psychischen Störungen. *Zeitschrift für die gesamte Neurologie und Psychiatrie*, **121**, 107-138.

Meyers, R. (1968) Ballismus in *Handbook of Clinical Neurology* (Eds. Vinken, P. J. & Bruyn, G. W.), Vol. 6, Chapter 19, pp. 476-490, North Holland Publishing Co., Amsterdam.

Netsky, M. G. (1968) Degenerations of the cerebellum and its pathways in *Pathology of the Nervous System* (Ed. Minckler, J.), Vol. I, Chapter 87, McGraw-Hill, New York.

Norman, R. M. (1961) Cerebellar hypoplasia in Werdnig–Hoffmann disease. *Archives of Disease in Childhood*, **36**, 96-101.

Norris, F. H. & Engel, W. K. (1965) Carcinomatous amyotrophic lateral sclerosis in *The Remote Effects of Cancer on the Nervous System* (Eds. Brain, Lord & Norris, F. H.), Chapter 4, Grune and Stratton, New York.

Norris, F. H., McMenemey, W. H. & Barnard, R. O. (1969) Anterior horn pathology in carcinomatous neuromyopathy compared with other forms of motor neuron disease in *Motor Neuron Diseases* (Eds. Norris, F. H. & Kurland, L. T.), Chapter 9, Grune and Stratton, New York.

Parkinson, J. (1817) *An Essay on the Shaking Palsy*, London. Reproduced in *James Parkinson* (Ed. Critchley, M.) (1955), Macmillan, London.

Pearce, J. & Harriman, D. G. F. (1966) Chronic spinal muscular atrophy. *Journal of Neurology, Neurosurgery and Psychiatry*, **29**, 509-520.

Peterson, R. D. A., Kelly, W. D. & Good, R. A. (1964) Ataxia-telangiectasia: its association with a defective thymus, immunological deficiency disease and malignancy. *Lancet*, **1**, 1189-1193.

Poirier, L. J. & Sourkes, T. L. (1965) Influence of the substantia nigra on the catecholamine content of the striatum. *Brain*, **88**, 181-192.

Powell, H. C., London, G. W. & Lampert, P. W. (1974) Neurofibrillary tangles in progressive supranuclear palsy: electron microscopic observations. *Journal of Neuropathology and Experimental Neurology*, **33**, 98-106.

Pratt, R. T. C. (1967) *The Genetics of Neurological Disorders*, Oxford University Press, London.

Probst, M. (1898) Zu der fortschreitenden Erkrankungen der motorischen Leitungsbahnen. *Archiv für Psychiatrie und Nervenkrankheiten*, **30**, 766-844.

Probst, M. (1903) Zur Kenntnis der amyotrophischen Lateralsklerose. *Sitzungsberichte der Akademie der Wissenschaften in Wien*, **112**, Abt. 3, 683-824.

Quick, D. T. (1969) Pancreatic dysfunction in amyotrophic lateral sclerosis in *Motor Neuron Diseases* (Eds. Norris, F. H. & Kurland, L. T.), Chapter 20, Grune and Stratton, New York.

Radermecker, J. (1951) L'amyotrophie spinale de l'enfance (Werdnig–Hoffmann) comme hérédo-dégénérescence. *Revue Neurologique*, **84**, 14-31.

Rosenberg, R. N., Schotland, D. L., Lovelace, R. E. & Rowland, L. P. (1968) Progressive ophthalmoplegia. *Archives of Neurology (Chicago)*, **19**, 362-376.

Rosenhagen, H. (1943) Die primäre Atrophie des Brückenfusses und der unteren Oliven. *Archiv für Psychiatrie*, **116**, 163-228.

Roussy, G. & Lévy, G. (1926) Sept cas d'une maladie familiale particulière. *Revue Neurologique*, **33**, 427-450.

Roy, S., Datta, C. K., Hirano, A., Ghatak, N. R. & Zimmerman, H. M. (1974) Electron microscopic study of neurofibrillary tangles in Steele–Richardson–Olszewski syndrome. *Acta Neuropathologica (Berlin)*, **29**, 175-179.

Roy, S. & Wolman, L. (1969) Ultrastructural observations in Parkinsonism. *Journal of Pathology*, **99**, 39-44.

Russell, D. S. (1946) Myocarditis in Friedreich's ataxia. *Journal of Pathology and Bacteriology*, **58**, 739-748.

Saunders, P. W. (1913-14) Sensory changes in Friedreich's ataxia. *Brain*, **36**, 166-192.

Scherer, H.-J. (1933) Extrapyramidale Störungen bei der olivopontocerebellaren Atrophie. *Zeitschrift für die gesamte Neurologie und Psychiatrie*, **145**, 406-419.

Schut, J. W. (1950) Hereditary ataxia: clinical study through six generations. *Archives of Neurology and Psychiatry (Chicago)*, **63**, 535-568.

Schut, J. W. & Haymaker, W. (1951) Hereditary ataxia: a pathologic study of five cases of common ancestry. *Journal of Neuropathology and Clinical Neurology*, **1**, 183-213.

Schwab, R. S. & England, A. C. (1968) Parkinson syndromes due to various specific causes in *Handbook of Clinical Neurology* (Eds. Vinken, P. J. & Bruyn, G. W.), Vol. 6, Chapter 9, þp. 227-247, North Holland Publishing Co., Amsterdam.

Schwarz, G. A. (1952) Hereditary (familial) spastic paraplegia. *Archives of Neurology and Psychiatry (Chicago)*, **68**, 655-682.

Schwarz, G. A. & Barrows, L. J. (1960) Hemiballism without involvement of Luys' body. *Archives of Neurology (Chicago)*, **2**, 420-434.

Schwarz, G. A. & Liu, C.-N. (1956) Hereditary (familial) spastic paraplegia. *Archives of Neurology and Psychiatry (Chicago)*, **75**, 144-162.

Sedgwick, R. P. & Boder, E. (1972) Ataxia-telangiectasia in *Handbook of Clinical Neurology* (Eds. Vinken, P. J. & Bruyn, G. W.), Vol. 14, Chapter 10, pp. 267-339, North Holland Publishing Co., Amsterdam.

Shiraki, H. (1969) The neuropathology of amyotrophic lateral sclerosis in the Kii peninsula and other areas of Japan in *Motor Neuron Diseases* (Eds. Norris, F. H. & Kurland, L. T.), Chapter 7, Grune and Stratton, New York.

Shy, G. M. & Drager, G. A. (1960) A neurological syndrome associated with orthostatic hypotension. *Archives of Neurology (Chicago)*, **2**, 511-527.

Smith, J. B. & Patel, A. (1965) The Wohlfart–Kugelberg–Welander disease: review of the literature and report of a case. *Neurology (Minneapolis)*, **15**, 469-473.

Smith, M. C. (1960) Nerve fibre degeneration in the brain in amyotrophic lateral sclerosis. *Journal of Neurology, Neurosurgery and Psychiatry*, **23**, 269-282.

Smith, M. C. (1971) Pathology of unilateral Parkinsonism and of hemiballismus in *Symposium Bel-Air IV (Geneva)* (Ed. Ajuriaguerra, J. de), pp. 263-267, Georg, Geneva.

Spillane, J. D. (1940) Familial pes cavus and absent tendon jerks: its relationship with Friedreich's disease and peroneal muscular atrophy. *Brain*, **63**, 275-290.

Steele, J. C., Richardson, J. C. & Olszewski, J. (1964) Progressive supranuclear palsy. *Archives of Neurology (Chicago)*, **10**, 333-359.

Stewart, T. G. & Holmes, G. (1908) On the connection of the inferior olives with the cerebellum in man. *Brain*, **31**, 125-137.

Strich, S. J. (1966) Pathological findings in three cases of ataxia-telangiectasia. *Journal of Neurology, Neurosurgery and Psychiatry*, **29**, 489-499.

Strümpell, A. (1880) Beiträge zur Pathologie des Rückenmarks. *Archiv für Psychiatrie*, **10**, 676-717.

Strümpell, A. (1886) Ueber eine bestimmte Form der primären combinierten Systemerkrankung des Rückenmarks. *Archiv für Psychiatrie*, **17**, 217-238.

Strümpell, A. (1904) Die primäre Seitenstrangsklerose (spastische Spinalparalyse). *Deutsche Zeitschrift für Nervenheilkunde*, **27**, 291-339.

Syllaba, L. & Henner, K.   (1926) Contribution à l'indépendance de l'athétose double idiopathique et congénitale.   Atteinte familiale, syndrome dystrophique, signe du réseau vasculaire conjonctival, intégrité psychique.   *Revue Neurologique*, **1**, 541-562.

Takei, Y. & Mirra, S. S.   (1973) Striatonigral degeneration: a form of multiple system atrophy with clinical Parkinsonism.   *Progress in Neuropathology*, **2**, 217-251.

Tellez-Nagel, I. & Wiśniewski, H. M.   (1973) Ultrastructure of neurofibrillary tangles in Steele–Richardson–Olszewski syndrome.   *Archives of Neurology (Chicago)*, **29**, 324-327.

Trétiakoff, C.   (1919) Contribution à l'étude de l'anatomie pathologique du locus niger.   Thesis, University of Paris.

Ule, G.   (1957) Die systematischen Atrophien des Kleinhirns in *Handbuch der speziellen pathologischen Anatomie und Histologie* (Eds. Lubarsch, O., Henke, F. & Rössle, R.), Vol. XIII/1A, pp. 934-988, Springer Verlag, Berlin.

Weber, F. P. & Greenfield, J. G.   (1942) Cerebello-olivary degeneration: an example of heredo-familial incidence.   *Brain*, **65**, 220-231.

Welte, E.   (1939) Die Atrophie des Systems des Brückenfusses und der unteren Oliven.   *Archiv für Psychiatrie*, **109**, 649-698.

Werdnig, G.   (1891) Zwei frühinfantile hereditäre Fälle von progressiver Muskelatrophie.   *Archiv für Psychiatrie*, **22**, 437-480.

Werdnig, G.   (1894) Die frühinfantile progressive spinale Amyotrophie.   *Archiv für Psychiatrie*, **26**, 706-744.

Whittier, J. R.   (1947) Ballism and the subthalamic nucleus.   *Archives of Neurology and Psychiatry (Chicago)*, **58**, 672-692.

Wohlfart, G., Fex, J. & Eliasson, S.   (1955) Hereditary spinal muscular atrophy.   *Acta psychiatrica et neurologica scandinavica*, **30**, 395-406.

Zeman, W. & Dyken, P.   (1968) Dystonia musculorum deformans in *Handbook of Clinical Neurology* (Eds. Vinken, P. J. & Bruyn, G. W.), Vol. 6, Chapter 21, pp. 517-543, North Holland Publishing Co., Amsterdam.

Zeman, W. & Whitlock C. C.   (1968) Symptomatic dystonias in *Handbook of Clinical Neurology* (Eds. Vinken, P. J. & Bruyn, G. W.), Vol. 6, Chapter 22, pp. 544-566, North Holland Publishing Co., Amsterdam.

Zilkha, K. J.   (1962) Discussion on motor neurone disease.   *Proceedings of the Royal Society of Medicine*, **55**, 1028-1029.

15

Diseases of the Spine and Spinal Cord

Revised by J. T. Hughes

Although the skull and vertebral column normally protect the brain and spinal cord, disease or malformation of these bony envelopes may cause local or more widespread pressure either on the nervous parenchyma or on the blood vessels which supply it, with effects which resemble those of tumours arising in these bones. But in some the pressure is more widely spread, in others is more sharply localized and in most cases is more chronic. The pathogenesis of these lesions has been somewhat neglected although many are common and some are severely disabling. Very few studies of the effects of diffuse, long-continued pressure on the brain have been made and even the simpler pathology of spinal cord compression is imperfectly understood. In many acute early cases the loss of function is greater than can easily be explained by the lesions found, but the reverse may be true in long-standing cases in which the lower limbs retain useful function in spite of very severe lesions in the cord. In some cases the pathogenesis of the functional disability may be suggested by the character of the minor lesions which are found, but in other cases it remains uncertain. Mechanical pressure would seem to be more likely to compress blood vessels than solid tissue, and veins more than arteries. Many of the effects of pressure have therefore been attributed to venous stasis and oedema and others to compression or spasm of small arteries. Myelin seems to be more vulnerable both to mechanical pressure and to minor degrees of anoxia than nerve cells and axons. Certainly in the spinal cord the effects of pressure are usually greatest in the myelin of the white columns. Movement of the cord or lower medulla over bony prominences on the dorsal surface of the vertebral bodies may have a specially deleterious effect on nervous tissue. This effect may be secondary to ischaemic or vascular stasis, but McAlhany and Netsky (1955) found that the greatest demyelination often lay either immediately under a tumour or on the opposite side of the cord and attributed this to the direct effects of pressure.

The type of lesion which is found in the spinal cord under conditions of acute or more chronic compression is well established. The earliest lesion is usually a rounded or wedge-shaped area of vacuolar degeneration in the posterior part of the lateral columns. This may be unilateral or bilateral and consists of distended myelin sheaths many of which contain swollen axons. In more advanced cases these lesions become more extensive and similar areas often appear in the deeper parts of the dorsal columns. The ventral third of the white matter usually remains intact. Areas of more frank necrosis in which the neuroglial scaffolding also suffers may appear in the centre of the older areas and there may also be areas of softening in the grey matter, most often near the base of the ventral horns. Cavitation often appears in the deeper parts of the dorsal columns or in the region of the grey commissure. In chronic cases the myelin loss is replaced by overgrowth of neuroglial and connective tissue fibres, among which many axons still persist. There is usually shrinkage of the ventral horns associated with atrophy and loss of nerve cells, and hyaline thickening of the small intramedullary vessels.

Although this progressive type of degeneration is very common in cases of subacute or chronic compression of the cord, many cases of sudden paraplegia due to pressure are associated in their early stages with frankly necrotic changes in the cord which may involve all its transverse section or be confined to some part of this. In such cases a vascular causation is most probable but thrombosis of vessels is rarely found. It seems likely that they are due to compression of an important radicular vessel in or close to the intervertebral foramen.

The effects of compression of the brain have been less studied, but definite changes have been found in the cerebellar cortex by Scharenberg (1953) and others. These consist of atrophy, degeneration and loss of nerve cells, affecting first the Purkinje cells, and gliosis of the granular and molecular layers. These effects are greatest near the surface of the parts subjected to most direct pressure. In cases with tonsillar herniation, atrophy and gliosis is often severe in the herniated parts.

Osteitis deformans
(*Paget's disease of bone*)

The skull and spinal columns are common sites of osteitis deformans, and this may produce lesions in the central nervous system or in the cranial or spinal nerve roots. The rarefaction of the bony trabeculae, which constitutes the early stage of the disease, makes the bone less able to resist the effects of gravity in spite of its increased thickness, so that, as it thickens, it becomes moulded to a new shape. The vault of the skull becomes wider, slightly longer in its antero-posterior diameter and reduced in height. But as there is no great change in its capacity the brain is not compressed. A similar change at the base of the skull, especially round the foramen magnum, is one of the causes of platybasia and basilar invagination (Bull, Nixon, Pratt and Robinson 1959). In such cases the inferior surface of the cerebellum may be compressed by flattening of the base of the posterior fossa.

In some cases optic atrophy results from narrowing of the optic foramina. Loss of hearing and nystagmus may be due either to changes in the bones of the cochlea and labyrinth or to narrowing of the internal auditory meatus. Involvement of other cranial nerves is rare.

In osteitis deformans of the spine there is usually some degree of kyphosis, and in some cases this may be a rather sharp curvature. But the paraplegia, which sometimes results, appears to be more often due to the general reduction in the lumen of the canal, or to more local pressure by bony prominences which may form on the dorsal surfaces of the vertebral bodies. In two cases reported by Wyllie (1923) laminectomy showed a loss of the space which normally exists between the cord and the bone, and absence of pulsation in the cord. In the more serious case, on which Greenfield performed a necropsy, bony projections from the dorsal surfaces of the 6th and 8th thoracic vertebral bodies compressed the cord at these levels. The dura mater was everywhere in contact with the walls of the spinal canal and was abnormally adherent to them. The changes in the spinal cord are those already described as resulting from compression.

Bony abnormalities in the region of the foramen magnum

Abnormalities in the floor of the posterior fossa, or in the articulation of the skull with the atlas or of the atlas with the axis may be the cause of serious neurological symptoms. The most common of these are (1) *occipitalization or assimilation of the atlas*, that is partial or more complete bony fusion of the atlas with the ring of the foramen magnum, (2) *basilar invagination* or *impression* and (3) *anomalies* either in the *odontoid process* itself or in its relation to the atlas. In over 100 patients with bony abnormalities in the region of the foramen magnum McRae (1953) found 28 instances of the first type, 21 of the second and 17 of the third, and others with combinations of these. Since in most cases these are congenital abnormalities, symptoms often begin in childhood or early adult life. In some cases they appear to follow an injury to the head or neck.

(1) Assimilation or fusion of the atlas with the margin of the foramen magnum does not of itself cause compression or abnormal angulation of the medulla but it may be combined with other abnormalities, such as an odontoid process which is abnormally long, angulated backwards or placed unusually high or a reduction in size of the foramen magnum. In McRae's series neurological signs were always present if the antero-posterior diameter of the spinal canal behind the odontoid process was less than 20 mm. The lack of movement between the skull and atlas may also throw an abnormal strain on the atlanto-axial joint and produce abnormally free movement of the odontoid process in relation to the arch of the atlas or actual dislocation at this joint. This strain may be increased by fusion

of the 2nd and 3rd cervical vertebrae as in List's case 3 (1941). Assimilation of the atlas may also be associated with platybasia or basilar invagination.

(2) Basilar invagination has been defined in relation to lateral radiographs of the skull as an abnormal protrusion of the tip of the odontoid process above Chamberlain's line, that is a line drawn from the back of the hard palate to the posterior margin of the foramen magnum. There is some uncertainty as to the limits of the normal in this respect. The tip of the dens not infrequently lies 5 mm above Chamberlain's line in normal individuals and occasionally 1 or 2 mm higher (Saunders 1943), but in basilar invagination it is often more than 10 mm above this line. The condition has also been defined in anteroposterior views by the relation of the tip of the odontoid process to a line joining the tips of the mastoid processes. This line normally passes through the occipito-atlantal joints which lie at about the same level as the dens.

Basilar invagination is often associated with platybasia, that is flattening of the angle between the orbital plates and the clivus of the sphenoid. This angle, which normally is 135° or less, becomes 145° or more in platybasia. These malformations are usually developmental and Bull et al. (1959) have found evidence of hereditary transmission. In rare cases they result from softening of the base of the skull by osteitis deformans, rickets, osteomalacia or osteogenesis imperfecta. In most cases the atlas is tilted in relation to the skull, so that its anterior arch, carrying the odontoid process with it, may lie at a higher level than the spinous processes. Basilar invagination is not uncommonly associated with fusion of two or more cervical vertebrae. It may produce abnormal angulation of the lowest part of the medulla, or the first cervical segment over the prominence formed by the odontoid process and transverse ligament. This angulation and pressure vary with the position of the head and some patients relate their symptoms to head movements. Thickening of the transverse ligament of the atlas and of the dural sheath are often present and increase the constriction of the cord and medulla. The effect on these structures is usually gradual but eventually there is degeneration of white matter and reduction in the size of the cord, especially in its anteroposterior diameter. In some cases the cord has been described as a fibrous ribbon and in one of Greenfield's cases, associated with extensive fusion of cervical vertebrae (Klippel–Feil malformation, Fig. 15.4), it measured only 2 mm in its anteroposterior diameter.

(3) Separation of the odontoid process from the axis may result either from fracture across the base of the odontoid or from tearing of a persistent cartilaginous union at this level. Fusion of the dens with the body of the axis normally occurs during the 3rd to 4th year, but in many normal subjects some hyaline cartilage persists here throughout life. In most cases this is no more than a central disc, but in some it is larger and may cover most of the plane of junction. Greenfield (1953) examined a case in which the lower surface of the separated odontoid process was covered by cartilage. Separations which result from slight strains or injuries may be explained most easily on these lines. In these cases the inferior surface of the separated odontoid usually has a smooth horizontal line. Other congenital anomalies may be associated. In two of McRae's cases the tip of the odontoid was fused to the anterior lip of the foramen magnum. The separated odontoid process, which is often shorter and smaller than normal, retains its relation to the anterior arch of atlas, but the separation allows abnormal anteroposterior movement of the atlas on the axis and in many cases there is permanent forward dislocation of the head and atlas at this level. In some such cases the appearance of nervous symptoms and signs may be delayed for weeks (Wallace and Bruce 1910) or even years (Bachs, Barraquer-Bordas, Barraquer-Ferre, Canadell and Modolell 1955); three of McRae's cases were asymptomatic. But in most cases there is a gradual or more rapid onset of signs of compression of the spinal cord.

In atlanto-axial dislocation the atlas is displaced forward in relation to the axis and lower cervical spine and the odontoid process is separated from the anterior arch of the atlas. In these cases McRae found little or no gliding of the atlas on the axis and little anteroposterior movement of the skull on the atlas; flexion and extension movements occurred chiefly at lower levels of the cervical spine. In his cases the dens lay from 5 to 17 mm behind the arch of the atlas and the anteroposterior diameter of the spinal canal at this level was correspondingly reduced, but in spite of this four of his six cases showed no signs of spinal compression.

The relationship of malformations in the region of the foramen magnum to syringomyelia is not altogether clear. McRae and others have found these anomalies common in cases with clinical evidence of syringomyelia, and it might be considered that obstruction to the venous drainage of the cord by bony pressure or dural constriction may produce oedema and eventual cavitation of the cervical cord. On the other hand List (1941) found the Arnold–Chiari or Chiari's Type I malformation in three, and hydromyelia in another, of his seven cases of bony malformations at this level. He concluded that these had no causal relationship to one another but were all equally the results of a developmental disturbance at about the third week of intrauterine life. The relationship of the Arnold–Chiari malformation to syringomyelia has already been referred to and List's theory appears all the more probable since cavitation of the cervical cord does not commonly occur in cases of acquired compression either by bony lesions or tumours at this level. It is, however, important to distinguish the Arnold–Chiari malformation from the tonsillar herniation, sometimes combined with transverse grooving on the dorsal surface of the medulla, which may result from reduction in size of the posterior fossa of the skull by acquired basilar invagination.

Degenerations and protrusions of intervertebral discs

Protrusion of intervertebral discs appears to have been first recognized by Luschka (1858), who also described the small neurocentral joints of the cervical vertebrae which play an important part in the pathology of cervical discs. Cases of spinal compression due to this cause were described by Middleton and Teacher (1911) and by Goldthwait (1911).

Anatomical considerations. The anatomy of intervertebral discs was studied by Luschka (1858), Schmorl and Junghans (1959), Andrae (1929) and Beadle (1931). The central part of the disc consists of soft cellular fibrocartilage, with very fine collagenous fibres, the *nucleus pulposus*. This is surrounded by a ring of much firmer fibrocartilage, the *annulus fibrosus*, which is attached directly to the margin of the vertebral bodies. Between the nucleus pulposus and the spongiosa of the bone there is a thin layer of hyaline cartilage. These three forms of cartilage merge into one another without any abrupt transition. In the central part of the nucleus pulposus, in addition to numerous cartilage cells, there may be a few myxomatous or physaliphorous cells which are vestigial remains of the notochord. The ring of the annulus fibrosus is thicker anteriorly than posteriorly, so that the nucleus pulposus lies eccentrically. This may explain why herniations seldom take place in a forward direction. In the child the nucleus pulposus constitutes by far the greater part of the disc, but as age advances it becomes gradually encroached on by the annulus fibrosus, and after middle age becomes considerably dehydrated and shrinks in its vertical diameter. In children and young adults it is under considerable tension, so that on sawing through the vertebral bodies in a sagittal plane the nuclei bulge out from the surface. When bearing the weight of the body, this tension must be even greater. The normal disc has been compared to a fully inflated tyre; it allows rocking and, to a minor degree, torsion movements between the vertebral bodies, while at the same time it absorbs jars in the longitudinal direction. At the thoracic level the ribs and intercostal muscles limit the forward and backward flexion of the spine and very little rotation is possible. The thoracic intervertebral discs are thus protected from many of the stresses and strains to which those at higher and lower levels are subject and protrusions at this level are relatively rare.

Pathology. Three types of lesions of intervertebral discs may cause neurological symptoms: (1) Horizontal tearing. (2) Herniation of the nucleus pulposus. (3) Degeneration leading to osteophytosis. These are often combined.

(1) *Tearing* may occur at the lower thoracic and lumbar levels in severe lesions associated with dislocation. Spondylolisthesis at the lumbosacral or lower lumbar level is also probably associated with horizontal tearing of the disc and tearing or more gradual stretching of the anterior and posterior longitudinal ligaments. At the cervical level tearing, usually of a single disc, is found in the sudden traumatic subluxations which will be described on p.665. Such tears, without herniation of the nucleus, are most often seen in middle-aged or elderly subjects in whom the nucleus is less tense.

(2) *Herniation of the nucleus pulposus* occurs almost always in a backward direction, since the annulus fibrosus is thinner posteriorly. The nucleus may herniate through a weakened or torn part of the annulus, or between annulus and bone or, in rare cases, through the spongy bone to its posterior or posterolateral surface

(Beadle). The herniations through the hyaline cartilage into the spongy tissue of the vertebral body, which may be seen near the centre of the disc in about 38% of normal subjects (Schmorl), are of themselves of little importance, but by reducing tension in the nucleus pulposus they may lead to bulging of the annulus fibrosus and to osteophytosis. Their effects are therefore similar to those of degeneration of the nucleus pulposus. Herniation of the nucleus pulposus is most common in young adults in whom the nucleus is more tense and the annulus thinner than in older subjects. They may be caused either by trauma or by sudden or severe muscular strain. Posterior or posterolateral herniations may burst through the annulus into the spinal canal either as a single mass or in several fragments, but more commonly they are checked by the outer fibres of the annulus and the posterior longitudinal ligament and so form a localized bulge into the spinal canal or intervertebral foramen. Owing to the firm central strands of the posterior longitudinal ligament in the lumbar region herniations here are usually posterolateral rather than posteromedian. They may be unilateral or bilateral.

(3) Degeneration of intervertebral discs is so common as to be almost physiological after the age of 50. As has been seen the nucleus pulposus loses water during life so that the percentage in its composition falls from 88% at birth to 70% at the age of 70. This desiccation of the nucleus is associated with shrinkage and increase in its fibrous tissue so that the transition from nucleus to annulus fibrosus becomes more gradual. There is also loss of tension which allows of some bulging of the annulus fibrosus in all directions when any pressure is put on the disc. The condition then resembles that of a partially deflated tyre. This is commonly followed by bony outgrowths from the margins of the upper and lower surfaces of the vertebral bodies, forming the *lipping* which is very commonly seen after middle age especially on the ventral surface of the lower thoracic and lumbar vertebral bodies. Schmorl found this condition in 10% of young adults in the third decade, in 35% in the fourth decade, in 70% in the fifth decade and in 90% of men over 50 and women over 60 years of age (Collins 1950). In most cases it remains slight at the cervical and upper thoracic levels where the pressure on the discs in the erect posture is less. But if for any reason, such as Schmorl's intra-osseous herniations, there is con-

siderable loss of nuclear substance in a disc, lipping tends to occur above and below it. At the cervical level some loss of disc space associated with ventral lipping is recognized by radiologists as an early sign of degeneration of a disc. Schmorl recognized this process to be degenerative and distinguished it from rheumatic and inflammatory conditions by the term *spondylosis deformans*. Collins (1950) prefers the term *osteophytosis*, but it is probable that formation of osteophytes is secondary to the bulging of the annulus fibrosus which is itself secondary to loss of disc substance, and that bone formation follows the curve which the annulus assumes when pressure is applied to the disc. Anterior lipping causes no neurological symptoms and many cases with minor degrees of posterior lipping are also asymptomatic. But in a minority of cases bony transverse ridges on the dorsal surface of the cervical vertebrae associated with protrusions of disc substance are the cause of paraplegia or tetraplegia. Osteophytes in relation to the neurocentral joints of the lower cervical vertebrae also may cause signs of pressure on the roots of the brachial plexus. Degeneration of discs and osteophytosis is thus a common cause of neurological symptoms at the cervical level whereas herniation of nuclear substance is the usual cause of symptoms at the lumbar level. Since the causes and effects of protrusions of intervertebral discs differ in this and other ways according to the level at which they are situated, those at the cervical, thoracic and lumbar levels will be considered separately.

Cervical discs

Anatomical considerations. The lower five cervical vertebrae differ from all the others in the shape of their bodies. These are considerably wider in the transverse than in the anteroposterior direction and are saddle-shaped. When viewed from the front the lateral margins of the upper surface are seen to be curved sharply upwards, and the upper edges of these 'uncinate processes' come into contact through fibrocartilage with recesses on the outer margins of the inferior surface of the body of the upper vertebra, and thus form a joint in which there is usually a cavity (Frykholm 1951; Bull 1948). These *neurocentral joints* prevent lateral displacement of the vertebral bodies and also ensure that in flexion and extension movements of the neck the vertebral bodies rock on a pivot near their centre. The superior surfaces of the vertebral bodies are slightly convex in the

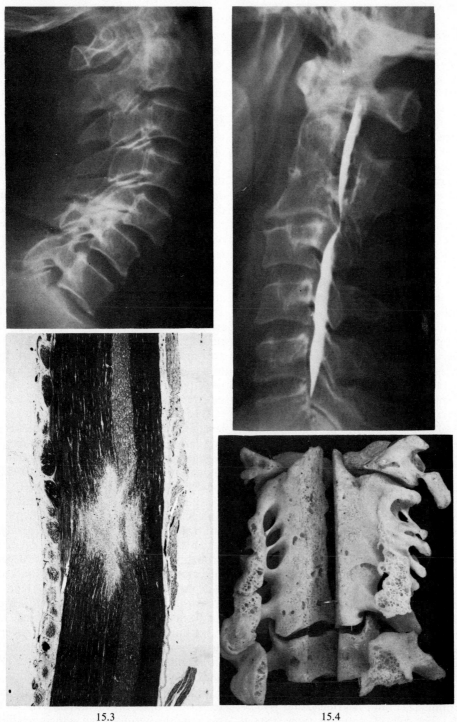

15.1

15.2

15.3

15.4

Fig. 15.1 X-ray photograph. Degeneration of the disc between C5 and C6 is made more evident by hyperextension of the neck.

Fig. 15.2 Myelogram of cervical spine, showing narrowing of the disc space and backward protrusion of the disc between C3 and C4. Note the congenital fusion of C2 and C3. (Case 1 of Mair and Druckman 1953.)

Fig. 15.3 Longitudinal section of the cervical cord from a case with 18 years' history of slight paraplegia due to degeneration of the disc between C7 and Th1. Myelin stain. (Case 4 of Mair and Druckman 1953.)

Fig. 15.4 Klippel–Feil deformity. Congenital fusion of vertebrae from C2 to C6. This was associated with basilar impression. Severe paraplegia resulted from angulation of the cord over the protruding odontoid process.

anteroposterior direction, and the inferior surfaces correspondingly concave, with their anterior lips slightly overhanging the body of the subjacent bone. The shortness of the spinous processes at the cervical level allows more backward movement (extension) than at the thoracic level where the spines are imbricated. Forward flexion also is more free. Lateral flexion and rotation are limited by the neurocentral joints and articular processes, but the joint between the latter is rather lax and allows some movement. These movements are associated with moulding of the intervertebral discs. Owing to the position of the neurocentral joints there is little difference between the tensions produced within the discs by full flexion and full (backward) extension of the neck.

Pathology. A few cases in which sudden flexion of the neck by external force has caused tearing of the annulus fibrosus and backward herniation of a large mass of nucleus pulposus have been verified by operation or postmortem examination. These have usually been in young adults. The spinal cord is compressed by the herniated tissue and when this has been removed by operation there has sometimes been considerable or even apparently complete restoration of its function. Small central or posterolateral protrusions which encroach on the canal or the intervertebral foramina are more common. Many of these cases are caused by trauma such as blows by which the head is suddenly jerked backwards or forwards. When sudden pain in the arm, shoulder or trunk has been felt at the time of the injury it is probable that there has been a herniation of the nucleus pulposus through a torn or stretched part of the annulus. Operation or postmortem-examination shows a posteromedian or postero-lateral protrusion of disc material which in the early stages may be fairly soft, but later becomes firmer and often fibrous or partly calcified or may be covered with a thin layer of bone. In the cervical region the posterior longitudinal ligament is rather weaker at its centre than more laterally and therefore herniations are likely to be either median or in close relation to the inter-vertebral foramina (Brain, Northfield and Wilkinson 1952). The age of onset in such cases is usually below 40.

In cases of degeneration of discs, symptoms come on more gradually. There may be no history of injury, or trauma, often of minor degree, may have occurred several months or

years previously. X-ray examination in these cases may show loss of disc space at one or more levels, often associated with anterior and posterior osteophytosis and this may also be seen by oblique views in the intervertebral canals. In some cases paraplegia may come on suddenly after a degree of flexion or extension of the neck which is not very abnormal; for example, cases of paraplegia after tooth extraction and after tonsillectomy have occurred. In such cases also there is often radiological evidence of previous degeneration of one or more discs. It is in fact doubtful whether paraplegia can follow such minor strains unless there is already degeneration of a disc. In patients over middle life the backward protrusion of the annulus fibrosus, which is the chief cause of pressure on the cord, may be visualized by myelography, but may not be visible at operation with the head in the normal position and the muscles relaxed. Surgeons therefore tend to stress the importance of the transverse bony ridges with which the bulging is associated. On post-mortem examination also no protrusion may be visible, but on flexion and extension of the neck there is abnormal mobility at one or more intervertebral joints.

Whereas nuclear herniations at the cervical level are most often found either between the 5th and 6th, or the 6th and 7th bodies, chronic degenerations are equally common in the two discs next above these (Brain *et al.* 1952). Their incidence at these levels may be partly explained by their tendency to occur immediately below congenitally fused vertebrae, usually the 2nd and 3rd or the 2nd, 3rd and 4th. The strong leverage which the fused segments exert on this disc is probably the cause of its premature degeneration. In cases of severe degeneration limited to one disc the vertebrae above it may tend to move forward out of line with those below it especially on flexion or extension of the neck. In other cases bony ridges may be seen at several levels, or in myelograms the column of myodil is seen to be indented opposite several discs (Figs. 15.1 and 15.2).

Protrusions of intervertebral discs, whether due to herniation or degeneration, give rise to hyper-plasia of the fibrous tissue in their neighbourhood. The dura mater becomes thickened and adherent to the posterior longitudinal ligament and there is also thickening and fibrosis of the pia arachnoid especially round the roots. Narrowing of one or more intervertebral canals by cartilaginous protrusion and osteophytosis, along with thickening of the fibrous tissue of the dural sleeve (Frykholm 1951), may cause degeneration of the nerve roots that pass through them. This is most common between the 5th and 6th and 6th and 7th vertebrae and is usually bilateral but may be greater on one side. Although in most cases both ventral and dorsal components of the root are damaged, in some cases the position of the protrusion is such that it presses chiefly on the ventral root.

The effects of disc protrusion on the spinal

fresh neurites from the axons proximal to the level of damage and these may form a stump neuroma at the entrance to the intervertebral foramen or, more commonly, leashes of myelinated fibres which run in the meninges or pass along the walls of blood vessels into the tissues of the cord. Such regenerative phenomena are very common in chronic cases of lesion of cervical discs.

(2) Posteromesial or posterolateral protrusions may press on the ventral surface of the cord,

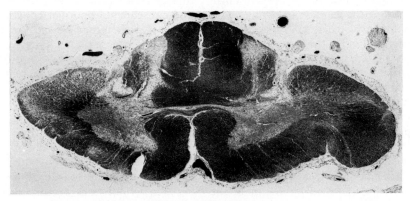

15.5

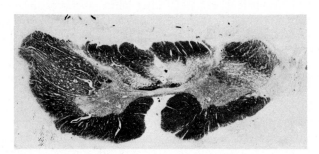

15.6

Fig. 15.5 Cervical disc protrusion. Section of the cord at the level of C4-C5 from a case with multiple disc protrusions involving chiefly the intervertebral foramina at the lower cervical level. The cord is flattened anteroposteriorly as a result of pressure and tension on the ligamentum denticulatum and shows degeneration in the dorsal columns due to lesions of the lower cervical nerve roots. Myelin stain.

Fig. 15.6 Section of the cord at the level of a disc protrusion (C6-C7) showing degeneration in the region of attachment of the ligamentum denticulatum on one side and degeneration in the ventral part of the dorsal columns chiefly on the same side. Myelin stain.

cord vary in different cases according to variations in the causative factors.

(1) *Lesions of roots* in the intervertebral foramina show themselves by wedge-shaped areas of degeneration in the dorsal columns which pass medially and become narrower in successively higher segments (Fig. 15.5). When a ventral root is severely damaged there is an outgrowth of

and encroach on the restricted space of the spinal canal. Normally the anteroposterior diameter of the spinal canal from C3 to C7, with the neck in the neutral position, as measured by radiographs, is 17 mm (Wolf, Khilnani and Malis 1956) but in cases of cervical spondylosis with myelopathy this measurement averages 14 mm (Payne and Spillane 1957). When the neck is extended this distance, from the spur on the postero-inferior aspect of one vertebra to the base of the spinous process of the vertebra below, may be reduced by 2 mm and if there is any posterior movement of one vertebra upon the other, as may occur (Penning 1962), the distance is even further reduced. Posteriorly, in hyper-extension, the ligamentum flavum may be infolded and press upon the cord (Nugent 1959). The effects of pressure by the firm boss of cartilage on the anterior spinal artery are probably even more important than pressure on the substance of the cord, since at the cervical level this vessel supplies not only the ventrolateral white columns and grey matter but also the ventral third or quarter of the dorsal columns (Bolton 1939). The tension of the ligamentum denticulatum aids this pressure since by its attachment to the dura mater, which is itself anchored by the root sleeves, it prevents the cord from moving back-wards. Allen (1952) observed that flexion of the neck during operations might produce blanch-ing of the cord at the level of disc protrusion, and it is possible that the mechanical effects of compression are supplemented by spasm of the artery. To these effects may be added in some cases those of compression of the nutrient branches in their course through the intervertebral foramina. These branches are very variable both in position and importance, but a common arrangement is for a fairly large branch, which may be unilateral or bilateral, to enter along with the root of C6 or C7. The flow in the anterior spinal artery is caudad and, as Bolton (1939) showed, a valvular arrangement at the junction of branches with the main vessel prevents them from supplying the cord above the level at which they join it. These factors explain the ischaemic changes in the ventral horns which are frequently seen in one or two segments below the level of com-pression. For example, loss of nerve cells and ischaemic changes in those that remain may be found in the 1st thoracic segment when the cord has been compressed by protrusion of the disc between the 5th and 6th cervical vertebrae (7th cervical segment) (Mair and Druckman 1953).

The greatest changes are seen in the spinal cord at the level of compression (Wilkinson 1960; Höök, Lidvall and Åström 1960). Here the cord is flatter than normal from compression in its anteroposterior diameter. Not infrequently there is some demyelination of the white matter at the point of attachment of the thickened liga-mentum denticulatum in a line passing inwards from this towards the base of the ventral horns, suggesting the lines of tension to which the cord has been subjected. Ill-defined areas of demye-lination are also commonly found in the ventral parts of the dorsal columns either in the midline or at one or both sides (Fig. 15.6). These are not so easily explained. They may be due to ischaemia in the area of terminal supply of the anterior spinal artery or to venous stasis.

(3) In cases of severe disc lesions there is the further factor of abnormal mobility of the spine and consequent abnormal bending of the spinal cord. This is most likely to occur in cases with fusion of vertebrae. In all these cases the lesions of the nervous parenchyma are often associated with hyaline changes in the walls of the intra-medullary vessels.

Thoracic discs

Protrusions of intervertebral discs at the thoracic level are, for the reasons stated, comparatively rare. Some are due to trauma, but in a few cases the spinal injury has been masked by fractures of the legs or has only begun to cause paraplegia after some weeks or months. On the available evidence the great majority of protrusions at this level begin as herniations of nuclear tissue which later becomes more fibrous and may undergo calcification or bone formation. The normal slight kyphosis at the thoracic level brings the spinal cord into constant contact with these firm or hard projections and in its slight upward and downward movements it is rubbed against them. This may cause necrosis and loss of tissue on the ventral surface of the cord, resulting in a cavity in which the nodule is embedded. In other respects the lesions in the cord are a com-bination of the effects of pressure, tension and ischaemia similar to that seen at the cervical level.

Logue (1952), from a review of the literature and his own experience, considered that pro-trusions at this level constituted only about 2 to 3% of all disc protrusions. Most occurred in patients of middle or later age and few appeared to be related to trauma. They were only found in the lower 9 discs and seldom above the level of the 6th. In his cases the damage to the cord appeared to be disproportionate to the degree of protrusion, suggesting that it was due more to ischaemia than to pressure.

Lumbar discs

Although the lumbar spine is robust and well supported by muscles it has to withstand very heavy compressive strains, especially in athletic young adults. Lesions of lumbar discs are therefore very common under the age of forty. They may be caused by external violence, such as a fall on the sacrum, but many cases can be attributed to severe muscular strain, especially lifting heavy weights in a stooping position. As the majority of protrusions at this level occur between the lower lumbar vertebrae or between the lowest of these (4th, 5th or 6th) and the sacrum, they do not damage the spinal cord and their effects are those of compression or attrition of the roots of the cauda equina. Almost all are due to herniation of the nucleus pulposus, but spondylolisthesis due to tearing of the disc may occur between the lowest lumbar vertebra and the sacrum or between the two lowest lumbar vertebrae. Herniations are usually posterolateral. When they project chiefly into the intervertebral foramen they compress only the corresponding root, usually the 4th or 5th lumbar. They are usually associated with thickening of the connective tissue around the articular joints and this may contribute to the narrowing of the intervertebral foramina. When they project into the canal the roots which pass over them to a lower level are affected. Usually only a few roots are involved, but in a few cases there is severe damage to most of the lower roots of the cauda equina. In these cases flaccid paralysis and anaesthesia of the ankles and feet, and loss of sphincter control, may come on suddenly or progressively over a few days. In 17 cases of this kind Jennett (1956) found large herniations of nucleus pulposus which almost filled the spinal canal. In a further 8 cases the herniation was not so large but the nerve roots were bound together by thickened arachnoid.

Degeneration of lumbar discs with osteophytosis is also very common at the lumbar level, but prominent bony ridges on the dorsal surface of the vertebral bodies are proportionately rarer than at the cervical level. In severe cases osteophytes may occlude the intervertebral canal which contains the important *arteria radicis anterior magna* or other important vessel going to the lumbosacral segments of the cord. These vessels are usually unpaired and their occlusion may lead to partial or even complete necrosis of the tissues of the cord at this level. Suh and

Alexander (1939) found that the arteria radicis magna most often entered along with the 2nd lumbar root, but in different subjects it ranged from the 8th thoracic to the 4th lumbar root. A fairly large posterior spinal artery usually enters the spinal canal along a different root.

Spillane (1952) drew attention to the frequency of severe protrusions at the lumbar level in achondroplasics, and related it to the dorsolumbar kyphosis which is common in these dwarfs.

Lumbar puncture and radiography

In cases of cervical disc protrusion there is very seldom any increase in the cell count in the cerebrospinal fluid but some excess of protein is found in about one-third of the cases and partial or complete spinal block in a similar proportion. When no block can be demonstrated by the usual technique Clarke and Robinson (1956) recommend 'postural manometry', i.e. compressing the jugular veins with the neck fully flexed or fully extended. By using the latter position they could demonstrate spinal block in 10 cases in which none was found in the normal position.

When the site of the protruded disc is at the thoracic level protein increase and spinal block become more common. Protrusions in the lumbar region are most often below the usual level of puncture, through the third interspace, so that no spinal block is found unless there are considerable arachnoidal adhesions. But there is often a considerable rise in protein in the cerebrospinal fluid. In severe lesions of the cauda equina Jennett (1956) constantly found a complete spinal block and considerable excess of protein when the puncture was made below the level of the protrusion; in two of his cases the fluid was yellow and clotted spontaneously.

The diagnosis rests chiefly on radiography both by direct views and by myelograms with opaque media. At the cervical level anteroposterior views are of little value owing to the shape of the vertebral bodies but oblique views outlining the intervertebral foramina are useful especially in cases with root symptoms. As some degree of degeneration of cervical discs is very common in middle-aged patients, slight indentation of the opaque medium, usually at several levels, may be seen in many normal cervical spines, especially when the myelogram is taken with the neck fully extended. This appearance may usually be discounted. Deeper indentations, especially if associated with posterior lipping, are more important.   Protrusions at a single level are less common and are more often the result of trauma. Some, especially those between C3 and 4, may be secondary to fusion of vertebrae.

Pott's paraplegia
(Paraplegia associated with spinal caries)

The name *Pott's disease* should be reserved for the association of paraplegia with spinal curvature

the spinal disease until a later publication in 1782.

Pott's paraplegia occurs in from 5 to 20% of all cases of spinal caries involving the cervical and thoracic vertebrae.   As is well known, spinal caries is most common in the thoracic vertebrae and paraplegia is therefore most often due to lesions at this level, but caries of cervical vertebrae carry an equal risk of paraplegia (Butler 1935).   This may precede obvious disease of the spine, especially in adults, but usually follows either very soon after its appearance or at a shorter

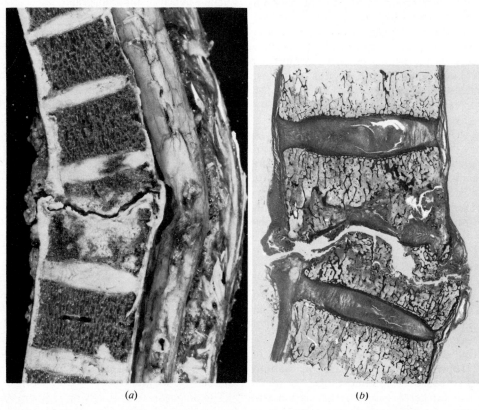

(a)   (b)

Fig. 15.7 Pott's paraplegia.   (a) Right half of a sagittally sawn specimen of thoracic cord.   There is collapse of T7 and T8 vertebral bodies due to a tuberculous osteitis which has spread into the T7-8 intervertebral disc.   The anterior aspect of the spinal cord is compressed by the kyphosis.   (b) Decalcified section of spine seen in previous figure.   (Taken with permission from *Pathology of the Spinal Cord*, 2nd ed., Lloyd-Luke, London.)

due to tuberculous caries, since Percival Pott in 1779 was the first to draw attention to this association in English literature.   But as the name is often used for the spinal disease alone (although this was described by Galen) the term *Pott's paraplegia* is here used to avoid ambiguity.   A fuller account of the condition was published in France in the same year by David and indeed Pott did not recognize the tuberculous nature of

or longer interval.   In cases with angular kyphosis due to caries of one or more vertebral bodies three factors may combine to damage the spinal cord: (1) The presence of granulation tissue or a cold abscess in the epidural space, (2) bending of the cord, and (3) compression or disease of its nutrient vessels.   The first of these factors is probably the most important and has received most attention, but either or both of the latter may contribute to cause the more severe and permanent forms of paraplegia.

(1) Whether the primary disease is in the vertebral bodies or, as rarely occurs, in the laminae, granulation tissue tends to reach the epidural space, where it spreads both up and down the canal and around the cord. It soon fills the space between cord and bone and becomes adherent to the dura mater; but this usually resists invasion and becomes thickened by the formation of new fibrous tissue on its outer surface. The granulation tissue compresses the cord and probably produces oedema in it by impeding the venous drainage. The formation of a cold abscess in the epidural space will probably have the same effect. This compression of the cord is the most probable cause of the minor degrees of paraplegia which improve after treatment. In some such cases improvement coincides with, and appears to be due to, the tracking of a cold abscess into the soft paravertebral tissues.

The most useful lesion in early cases is a vacuolar type of myelin degeneration in the lateral or anterolateral columns. This is often more diffuse than that which is seen in ischaemic lesions and may be due to oedema secondary to venous obstruction. The myelin is often more damaged than the axons. In three cases of Pott's paraplegia, associated with a sharp kyphosis and epidural granulation tissue, Holmes (1906) could find no evidence of Wallerian degeneration of long tracts above or below the lesion in spite of considerable damage to myelin at this level But in some cases there are more severe degenerative or necrotic lesions of the white or grey matter.

(2) Prolonged angulation of the cord over a sharp kyphosis usually results in thinning of the cord at that level, especially in its anteroposterior diameter (Fig. 15.7a and b). This may not be associated with much damage to the white columns of the cord, but there is evident loss of tissue, and in many cases, definite demyelination at this level. More acute and severe lesions of the cord may be produced in cases of rapid collapse of a vertebral body, or when the cord is bent over a relatively intact intervertebral disc between two diseased vertebrae, or is compressed by a sequestrum which is pushed backwards into

the spinal canal by the angulation (Seddon 1935). Dislocation of the spine is also liable to produce severe damage to the cord.

(3) In all these cases an important radicular artery may be compressed in the intervertebral foramen or may be the seat of tuberculous arteritis before it enters the dural sheath. This may account for some cases of severe paraplegia of rapid onset in cases in which the vertebral and epidural disease is not unusually severe.

Compression of the spinal cord in other inflammatory diseases of the spine

A number of other microorganisms may cause osteomyelitis of the vertebral bodies or laminae with spread of inflammatory granulation tissue into the epidural space. Of these the most common is *Staphylococcus pyogenes*, which may produce an epidural abscess which tracks down the spinal canal, or a more localized mass of granulomatous tissue which compresses the cord. Subacute cases of this kind may occur after one or more attacks of staphylococcal infection in other parts of the body. Sometimes, in the writer's experience, they contain little or no pus and their aetiology has only been proved by bacteriological examination. But more frankly purulent abscesses also may compress the spinal cord. In most cases the effects on the cord are reversible so that function returns after pressure is relieved.

Typhoid spine is another form of osteomyelitis or periostitis in which compression of the cord may occur. In such cases paraplegia may be the first, or an early symptom, but it is usually preceded by pain in the back, or round the body. The interval, sometimes of months or years, between the initial infection and the spinal disease may confuse the diagnosis in these cases.

Cerebrospinal fluid

In Pott's paraplegia, and other forms of epidural granuloma, a complete spinal block is almost always found. The protein is raised, often to very high levels, but there is rarely any increase in the cell count. In cases of *typhoid spine* the fluid usually contains a relatively high titre of antibodies to the causative organism.

Traumatic lesions of the spinal cord

The spinal cord is protected from injury by its bony casing and, except in the cervical region, a considerable degree of violence is needed to damage this to such an extent as to injure the spinal cord. Fracture dislocation of the lower thoracic or lumbar spine is, however, a well-recognized lesion in mining accidents due to falls of the roof, and may be caused in many other ways. The cervical spine is much more vulnerable and, as in the lower animals, fracture at this level is a common cause of death. On the other hand direct injuries to the spinal cord by stab wounds, bullets or fragments of shell or bomb casing are as common at the thoracic as at the cervical level. Wounds of the spine and spinal cord by high-velocity bullets have special pathological features due to the severity of the jar to the spinal column. Traumatic lesions of the spinal cord may be classified as (1) *Direct* due to injury of the cord by stab wounds or missiles which penetrate the cord. (2) *Indirect* due to fracture dislocations, or subluxations of the spine or to acute jars to the bone which are transmitted to the spinal cord. (3) *A combination of direct and indirect violence* as in wounds with high-velocity bullets, or in cases of fracture dislocation where the cord is lacerated or pierced by a spicule of bone.

Direct injuries to the spinal cord

The spinal cord may be directly injured without obvious or serious injury to the spine by stab wounds or by bullets or fragments of explosive which pass between the vertebral laminae. *Stab wounds* are of special interest to clinicians owing to the close correlation which may be traced between the lesions and the symptoms they cause. Three of the cases showing his syndrome, in the series which Brown–Séquard published in 1868, were of this kind. Their chief interest to the pathologist is the opportunity they may give for the study of the course and termination of the longer spinal nerve tracts and the phenomena of Wallerian degeneration.

As the imbrication of the spines of the thoracic vertebrae protect the spinal canal on its dorsal surface, stab wounds must enter it dorsolaterally. The severance of nerve tracts in the spinal cord is therefore greater on one side than the other and the dorsal columns are usually more severely damaged than the ventrolateral. But in some cases the cord is more or less completely severed. There is usually little bleeding except from the epidural veins and comparatively slight bruising of the tissues of the cord. The lesion is therefore quite local and, unless complicated by sepsis or injury to the anterior spinal artery, is limited to the level of the wound and a few millimetres on either side of this where the nervous tissue is bruised and softened. Within a few hours swellings appear on the severed axons at the ends which remain in continuity with the cell body, and the softened nervous tissue becomes gradually broken up and engulfed by phagocytes. Unless the spinal cord has been completely divided the wound is eventually closed by a glio-conjunctival scar through which neurites arising from the severed axons run irregularly, chiefly along connective tissue trabeculae.

The effects of direct injuries to the spinal cord by bullets or shell fragments have been well described by Roussy and Lhermitte (1918). The degree of damage to the cord in such cases bears a relation both to the size and to the velocity of the missile. When pierced by high-velocity missiles, as a bullet fired at close range, the nervous tissue may be disintegrated over one or more segments above and below the level of entry. Shell fragments usually cause more local lesions, but may produce softening or pulping and destruction of the whole thickness of the cord. The hole in the dura mater appears small in relation to the extent of damage to the cord; it may be a longitudinal slit or a ragged tear, the edges of which tend to rejoin. It is very rare for the dura mater to be completely torn across, so that in the more severe injuries the ends of the cord are held in approximation, if not in apposition, by the dural sheath. Intramedullary haemorrhage is usually slight but there may be considerable bleeding in the epi- and subdural spaces where the blood is mixed with cerebrospinal fluid. Some subarachnoid haemorrhage is also present. When examined at an interval of weeks after the injury the dura mater is found to adhere both to the bony wall of the canal and more firmly and extensively to the pia arachnoid, which is thickened and united with the glio-conjunctival scar tissue within the cord. The latter is shrunken and yellowish and may contain one or more cysts where tissue has been lost. Many of the nerve fibres that remain are demyelinated so that stains for myelin give an appearance of more complete destruction of nerve fibres than has actually taken place. The amount of secondary degeneration is therefore often considerably less than might be expected from the appearances at the level of the lesion.

Indirect injuries of the spinal cord

Subluxation and fracture dislocation of the spine

In civil life these are the most common form of traumatic lesion of the spinal cord. They may be caused by flying or road accidents, by diving into shallow water, by falls from horseback and by accidents in other sports and games as well as by industrial accidents. In some cases head injuries due to blows on the back of the head are complicated by fracture or subluxation of the cervical spine. Indeed, when the slenderness of the cervical spine is considered in relation to the weight of the head and the stresses to which it is commonly subjected, it is surprising that it is not more often the site of fracture dislocations or of subluxations. Sudden hyperflexion of the cervical spine in a forward direction may tear the interspinous and dorsal common ligaments of the vertebrae as well as the annulus fibrosis of one or more intervertebral discs without causing any fracture of bone. Lateral and backward hyperflexions are more likely to be associated with bony fracture but this may be limited to a pedicle or lamina or to severance of an articular process. After these slighter degrees of injury the spine returns to its normal alignment, and the fracture may not be easily visible in radiographs. Whether or not there is fracture dislocation the injury to the spinal cord is caused chiefly at the time of the accident by the sudden mechanical stresses to which the nervous tissue is subjected. But when there is dislocation with pressure on the cord, or continuous stretching of the cord over a bony or cartilaginous protrusion, the ischaemia caused in this way produces additional lesions or, at least, hinders recovery.

In some cases herniation and protrusion of the nucleus pulposus, causing serious compression of the spinal cord, results immediately from an injury to the cervical spine (Schneider 1951) but in most cases injuries to cervical intervertebral discs produce symptoms of a more chronic and progressive character which differ little from those seen in cases of cervical spondylosis in which no history of trauma is obtained. There appears, however, to be no doubt that in patients with existing degeneration of cervical discs paraplegia may be brought on by comparatively minor accidents, or even by voluntary flexion of the neck. In these cases the cord is subjected to abnormal stresses by being stretched over a cartilaginous or bony protrusion at the level of the degenerated disc.

Thus, whether or not there is fracture of the vertebrae, sudden flexion of the neck may damage the spinal cord either (1) by immediate mechanical stresses, or (2) by compression. These effects are often combined.

Subluxation

In many cases in which paraplegia results immediately from an accident involving sudden flexion of the neck, operation or post-mortem examination shows no gross abnormality in the spine or spinal canal. The spine may, however, be unduly mobile at one intervertebral joint, or there may be fracture of a pedicle or lamina. Sometimes bleeding under the posterior common ligament of the vertebrae or the separation of a small exostosis from the upper or lower margin of a vertebral body is the only or most obvious evidence of damage to the spine. In such cases the injury to the spinal cord may be severe or slight and largely recoverable. In the early stages the cord is usually swollen over one or two segments at the level at which the greatest flexion occurred. Later it becomes shrunken at this level, but this may only be obvious when the finger is passed gently in an upward or downward direction over the cord.

On section, in early cases, the damaged area may be grossly softened. More often it is diffusely swollen and shows small haemorrhagic points in the grey columns. It is seldom very haemorrhagic. The demarcation of grey from white matter is often blurred and the tissue may appear abnormally pale. Occasionally cylindrical cores of softened tissue can be seen passing upwards and downwards from the most softened area. The usual position of these cores is the base of the dorsal horns or the ventral part of the dorsal columns. They are greyish or brownish, sometimes creamy, less often frankly haemorrhagic. The name *traumatic haematomyelia* is often given to cases of this kind, but the name is almost always a misnomer since red blood corpuscles rarely form more than a minor part of the contents of the core. These consist of softened débris of myelin and axons, sometimes contained in phagocytic cells, along with serous fluid. Cores of this kind are most commonly found when there is gross softening of the cord at one level, without tearing of the pia arachnoid. The swelling of the tissues and outpouring of serum associated with softening is restrained by the firm pia mater and thus the softened tissue tends to track in an upward and downward direction along the grey columns or in the line of the nerve fibres. While there is no doubt, both from human and experimental observations, that these cores may exist before death, it is probable that some may be formed, or at least enlarged, by careless removal of the spinal cord at the post-mortem examination.

Microscopically in mild cases transverse sections may show only swelling of axons and myelin sheaths in the damaged segment of the cord. This may be diffuse and slight, but is usually more severe in one area which may, however, be very limited both in its transverse and longitudinal extent. The characteristic appearances are most easily recognized in longitudinal sections stained for axons which may be diffusely swollen or show beaded swellings on their course or end bulbs where they are torn across. These appearances may persist for some weeks. The myelin sheaths show distensions conforming to those of the axons which they contain. There are also, in most cases, some changes in the nerve cells, although these may be slight and limited to a minor degree of central chromatolysis. Ghost cells are sometimes seen, and later some loss of nerve cells may be found by comparative counts. The experiments of Groat, Windle and Magoun (1945) indicate that the small internuncial neurones, both in the dorsal and ventral grey columns, suffer more than the large motor cells. Both they and Roussy and Lhermitte described agglutination of Nissl granules as a characteristic minor change in cases of this kind.

Whether or not the swelling of the spinal cord in the early stages is due to oedema is not easily determined although the spread of paralysis in an upward direction in some cases makes this probable. Although no serous transudate can be seen between the nerve fibres, it is possible that they are separated more than normally by thin unstainable fluid, as in the minor grades of cerebral oedema. On the other hand the swelling of the cord may possibly be explained by the swelling of axons and distension of myelin sheaths.

At a later stage the only obvious abnormality may be small cysts, or loss of nerve fibres in some parts of the white matter. In cases due to sudden forward flexion of the neck, loss of fibres is commonly limited to the dorsal columns and this may be compatible with a remarkable degree of clinical recovery. It would appear that the damage to nerve fibres in these cases is due to longitudinal stretching or angulation or to a combination of these two processes. These mechanical stresses probably affect a large proportion of the nerve fibres of the cord in a minor degree, which in the great majority of the fibres is recoverable. This would account for the transient nature of the paraplegia in some cases and for the remarkable degree of recovery in others.

'Blast injuries' of the spinal cord

Both in the first and second World Wars cases were reported in which paraplegia resulted from close exposure to the blast of an explosion (Claude and Lhermitte 1915; Davison 1945). It was at first thought that the lesions in the spinal cord were caused by sudden changes in air pressure, but when a full history could be obtained it was shown that the patient had been forcibly thrown to the ground or bruised by earth, so that subluxation of the spine, especially at the cervical level, could never be excluded and in some cases this was definitely proved. This theory of causation was confirmed by British experience during 1939–45 which showed that blast by itself had little effect on the brain or spinal cord and that lesions in either organ following bomb explosions were due to other factors, especially CO poisoning in the case of the brain and subluxation of the spine in the case of the spinal cord. Both in animals and humans exposed to blast, death was commonly caused by the effects of sudden changes in air pressure on the lungs, but paraplegia due to this cause alone was not observed.

Fracture dislocations of the cervical spine

These are most common at the level of the 5th to 6th vertebrae. In them the cord is stretched over a bony or cartilaginous prominence and the effects of pressure ischaemia are added to the immediate mechanical trauma. Occasionally the cord may be pierced by spicules of bone, but in most cases it is protected by the dural sheath. One or more nerve roots are also commonly compressed by the dislocation, and this may contribute to the amyotrophy caused by the destruction of motor nerve cells in the cord.

Fracture dislocations of the thoracic and lumbar spine

These are most common at the lower thoracic level. They are more often caused by crushing, as by an excessive weight on the shoulders in falls of the roof of mines, or by extreme forward or backward flexion of the spine in falls or road accidents. They are often therefore less sudden than fracture dislocations of the neck and the effects on the cord are due more to compression and less to the sudden jar of the accident. The degree of damage to the spinal cord varies greatly. As the space between it and the bony canal is rather greater at the thoracic than at the cervical level the cord is less constantly damaged, and its injury is often incomplete and compatible with considerable recovery of function. In severe cases, however, there may be complete or almost complete destruction of nervous tissue at the level of the lesion. Lesions of the lumbar spine may damage the conus terminalis, with permanent effects, or may compress the less vulnerable roots of the cauda equina. In the latter case considerable recovery of function is possible.

When the spine is examined weeks or months after the injury, the canal at the level of the fracture dislocation contains dense fibrous scar tissue formed by the fusion and thickening of periosteum and dura mater. The leptomeninges are often adherent to this scar but a subarachnoid space may still exist either all round the cord or, more often, on one side only. The cord itself is thinned and sclerotic. In severe cases it may be represented by an ochreous fibrous band. In less severe cases it is partially or more completely demyelinated with fibrous gliosis in the degenerated areas or throughout. Sclerosis by collagenous tissue also may be present in the more severe cases.

Indirect spinal injuries from high-velocity bullets

High-velocity bullets which pass through the vertebral bodies or spines can cause severe jars to the spinal column. Even when they do not touch either the dura mater or cord they may cause complete or incomplete softening of the nervous tissue at the level of impact and minor lesions for a distance of several segments above and below this. Holmes (1915) describes small disseminated haemorrhages spread through two or more segments on either side of the wound especially in the cervical region, and moniliform or beaded swelling of axons especially near the surface of the cord. Both he and Roussy and Lhermitte also found superficial areas of necrosis in the white columns at some distance from the main lesion. These resembled the effects of thrombosis of small meningeal arteries, but although the vessels were engorged they were not thrombosed. In some the glial trabeculae were preserved and traversed the necrotic area, or the astrocytes also might be degenerated or necrotic. Holmes found these areas especially in the dorsal and ventral columns. In Roussy and Lhermitte's cases they were most common in the marginal zone of the lateral columns and the middle root zone of the dorsal columns. More rarely they were seen in the ventral horns. Lesions of nerve cells at some distance from the chief lesions were also seen by Holmes. These lesions appear to be caused by the sudden shock to the spinal column, as similar lesions have been found in experimental animals in which the spine has been struck (Schmaus 1890; Jakob 1919). In Schmaus' experiments he struck a wooden board placed against the animal's back, and the effects of the blow therefore were probably distributed over many vertebrae. It has been suggested that the shock of the blow, in these and other experiments, is transmitted by a wave of cerebrospinal fluid but this appears to be no better substantiated than Duret's similar hypothesis of the mechanics of head injury.

Late pathological changes

The preceding description refers to the pathological changes seen when the interval between the spinal injury and the necropsy is relatively short. Gradually the macroscopical and histological appearances change and when the survival period exceeds five years the pathological picture is totally different.

There is now a traumatic scar composed mainly of acellular collagenous connective tissue uniting all the layers of the meninges to the spinal canal and to the spinal cord. Within this connective tissue scar the anatomical planes of the spinal cord and of its meninges are quite indistinct. The histological features are best demonstrated in a connective tissue stain which will show that the grossly damaged part of the spinal cord has now been replaced by connective tissue and that the site of the earlier blood clot and destroyed spinal cord now consists of scar tissue. The less damaged parts of the spinal cord and invariably the region which was situated immediately above and immediately below the main site of damage now present as a region of intense astrocytic fibrous gliosis. The area of partial cord damage is filled with spongy glia and sometimes a syrinx has formed. Wallerian degeneration is present in the long tracts of the white columns of the spinal cord.

A constant feature in spinal cord injury after about five years is the presence of regenerating nerve fibres growing within the connective tissue scar situated in the damaged region of the spinal cord. There is evidence which is discussed elsewhere (Hughes 1974) that these fibres originate by the regeneration of the central processes of the neuron cell bodies in the posterior spinal root ganglia. These processes, possessing a Schwann cell sheath, have the same capacity to regenerate after trauma as have the axons within the peripheral nerve trunks. In severe spinal cord trauma, it frequently happens that some of the spinal ganglia are not damaged and their central processes regrow often into the connective tissue scar replacing the spinal cord. These fibres have a Schwann cell sheath and grow within the connective tissue but not within the glia areas. This regrowth phenomenon should not be confused with regeneration occur-ring within the spinal cord. There is no evidence that fibres arising and terminating within the spinal cord (e.g. the cells concerned in the spino-cerebellar tracts) are regenerated after trauma.

Post-traumatic syringomyelia

A common phenomenon seen at necropsy in a case of spinal injury is a longitudinal cavity in the spinal cord. These post-traumatic syringes were noted long ago, among others, by Holmes (1915). The syrinx replaces part or all of the spindle-shaped zone of haemorrhagic necrosis present in the acute stage of the injury. The lining of this cavity is of glia and connective tissue and these may form a thick wall.

The interest in this common, but relatively unknown, feature of spinal cord trauma is the occasional development of progressive post-traumatic syringomyelia (Hughes 1974). Many months and sometimes years after the original injury, and when the traumatic neurological deficit has been stable for some time, further symptoms and signs develop. These take the form clinically of an upward extension of the signs of the spinal cord lesion which may ascend to the medulla. Dissociated anaesthesia in the arms may be found.

At necropsy the appearances are similar to those of idiopathic syringomyelia except that the cavity extends upwards from a traumatic scar. Downward cavitation can occur but is clinically silent because of the existing spinal cord lesion above. I have seen in one case a combination of syringomyelia both above and below the region of trauma. The exact mechanism of these post-traumatic syringes has never been demonstrated but in some there is a suspicion that a communication exists between the syrinx and the subarachnoid space laterally near the posterior root entry zone.

Syringomyelia and syringobulbia

The name *syringomyelia* (syrinx = a tube) is used for a disease in which there is tubular cavitation of the spinal cord extending over many segments. Cavities which involve only two or three segments are not usually considered syringomyelic, although they may be of essentially similar nature. When the cavitation is merely a distension of the central canal of the cord the condition is called *hydromyelia* and the actual cavity a *hydromyelus*. It is not always possible even at necropsy to distinguish syringomyelia from hydromyelia, but the distinction is important as will appear when the aetiology of the two conditions is considered. The name *syringobulbia* is used for a similar condition in which the cavities are situated in the medulla and these syringes are often associated with syringomyelia. The name is rather less appropriate because the cavities are more slit-like than tubular. Rarely the cavitation extends into the pons and in exceptional cases it may reach the midbrain and even the internal capsule (Spiller 1906). Clinically the disease usually begins during the second and third decade and is slowly progressive, or the symptoms may increase at first rapidly and then more slowly. They may cease to progress at any time. Unless associated with bulbar symptoms, the disease rarely causes death directly but considerable disability is produced by the weakness of limbs and trunk and by the almost invariable spinal deformity.

Pathological changes in syringomyelia

When exposed at operation or autopsy the spinal cord appears swollen and tense in the cervical region and may fill the spinal canal. During life

numerous transverse sections but clearly a thorough examination at every segmental level is a very time-consuming task. A complete examination throughout the cord would require many thousands of sections and is scarcely feasible. In cases carefully examined at necropsy the following features recur. The cavity is usually found to be largest in the cervical region but is often absent from the first cervical segment. In the consideration of some of the theories of aetiology of syringomyelia this complete absence of any trace of the syrinx at this high cervical level is important. The syrinx commonly extends through the upper thoracic segments for a varying distance and usually terminates at a lower thoracic level. The lumbosacral enlargement is rarely involved. In typical cases the cavity in the cervical enlargement extends transversely across the cord, involving the more posterior parts of the ventral horns and passing across the midline behind the central canal. It often extends also into the posterior horns (Fig. 15.8a). When very large it occupies most of the cross-sectional area of the cord; the more anterior groups of motor nerve cells lie in front of it but

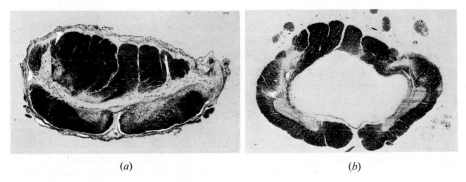

(a)   (b)

Fig. 15.8 Syringomyelia. (a) Cavity extends into both dorsal horns. (b) Cavity merges with the central canal.

this enlargement can be demonstrated radiologically by myelography, an important diagnostic procedure in the disease. Externally, apart from the swelling, the spinal cord appears normal and there is no leptomeningeal thickening. The syrinx is filled with a clear fluid, which in many cases (Gardner 1973) proves to have a similar composition to that of cerebrospinal fluid. The syrinx fluid may however be yellow with a high protein content. When at necropsy the fluid within the syrinx is allowed to escape, the cord becomes flattened, most often in its anteroposterior diameter. The syrinx may best be examined by

otherwise little grey matter remains, and the lateral and posterior white columns are reduced by compression to a narrow zone of fibres (Fig. 15.8b). Extensions in the midline, or more laterally into the posterior columns, are common and the anterior white commissure is often destroyed either by pressure or by a midline anterior extension of the cavity. A transverse cavity with midline posterior and anterior extensions, such as is sometimes seen at this level, closely resembles the cruciform shape of the central canal during the stage of fetal development before the altar and basal laminae fuse with one another. That this is more than a chance resemblance is shown by the most usual position of the cavity in the medulla which also lies between the nuclei arising respectively from the alar and the basal laminae. In the thoracic cord the cavity commonly lies in the posterior horns and is often unilateral. When bilateral the cavities may be separate or may be joined in the region of the grey commissure and so form a single U-shaped cavity. Serial sections show that cavities which are double at one level usually join into a single cavity at some point above, and it is usual for the cavity on one side to end at a higher level than the other. More rarely two cavities join in the lower thoracic region. Although the grey matter is the common site of cavitation, extensions into the posterior or lateral columns or across the white commissure are not unusual, and the cavity may reach the pial surface at the tips of the dorsal horns at any level. It is possible, though usually difficult to prove, that in some cases the syrinx may communicate here with the subarachnoid space.

The walls of the cavity vary greatly in character, especially from case to case but also in different parts of the same cavity. Greenfield believed that these variations depended on the age of the cavity and the degree of tension within it. Where there is recent extension the wall is irregular and consists of degenerated neuroglial and neural elements. Myelinated nerve fibres enclosed by sheaths of Schwann cells are commonly found in the wall of syrinx and have been thought (Hughes and Brownell 1963) to arise by regeneration from damaged posterior nerve roots. The myelin around the syrinx stains poorly, as it does in oedematous white matter, and the appearances suggest tearing of the tissues and transudation of serous fluid into them. When the cavity has been established for a longer time there is neuroglial hyperplasia around it with large fibre-forming astrocytes lying chiefly in a tangential direction. These finally form a dense concentric wall of neuroglial sclerosis which may be 1 or 2 mm in thickness. It is common to find a thin layer of collagen covering some part of the wall. Thicker strands of collagen, or blood vessels with hyalinized walls, may be seen passing across the cavity from one wall to another. Where the cavity communicates with the central canal, as it not uncommonly does especially in the cervical region, part of the central wall of the cavity is lined with ependymal cells, but in most places these take no part in the formation of the wall. This is an obvious but sometimes overlooked feature distinguishing syringomyelia from hydromyelia. When in syringomyelia there is a lining of ependyma the layer of neuroglial tissue which is deep to the ependymal layer is usually thinner than that surrounding the rest of the cavity.

Syringobulbia

Slit-like cavities in the medulla usually lie in one of three positions (Jonesco-Sisesti 1932). (1) The most common is a slit running out in an anterolateral direction from the floor of the 4th ventricle external to the hypoglossal nucleus. It may communicate with the cavity of the ventricle but sometimes begins anterior to this. It passes outwards and forwards for a variable distance towards the descending root of the trigeminal nerve, usually destroying the fasciculus solitarius and the fibres which pass dorsally from the nucleus ambiguus to join those arising in the dorsal vagal nucleus (Fig. 15.9c). A cavity in this position is most commonly limited to the lower half or two-thirds of the medulla where it interrupts the fibres passing from the nuclei gracilis and cuneatus to form the decussation of the medial lemniscus. It may also descend low enough to interrupt many of the decussating pyramidal fibres. At this level it extends transversely from the grey matter lateral to the central canal to a position anterior to the substantia gelatinosa and descending root of the trigeminal nerve. Cavities in this position usually have thin walls of neuroglial tissue. Occasionally the slit is replaced by a neuroglial scar which interrupts the fibre system as completely as a slit or cavity. Such appearances are not uncommon at the upper and lower ends of a cavity and may arise from secondary fusion of its walls. These cavities are usually unilateral but may be bilateral and roughly symmetrical (Fig. 15.9b). In such a case one cavity extends to a higher or lower level than the other. (2) Almost equally common is an extension of the 4th ventricle along the median raphe for a shorter or longer distance. This is usually lined by ependyma, but occasionally is replaced by a neuroglial scar containing ependymal cells or small ependyma lined tubules, like those seen in forking of the aqueduct (Fig. 15.9b). By interrupting the decussation of fibres passing from the descending vestibular nucleus to the median longitudinal fasciculus these slits may cause nystagmus, but are otherwise asymptomatic. When this median extension is small and is not associated with other cavitation in the medulla it scarcely merits the name of syringobulbia. (3) A rarer position for a cavity is where they may destroy the fibres of the 6th or 7th cranial nerves, or the central tegmental tract. They may pass down posterior to the olive for a short distance. Extensions of the cavity to a higher level are extremely rare. In Spiller's case the cavity in one pyramid passed up among the

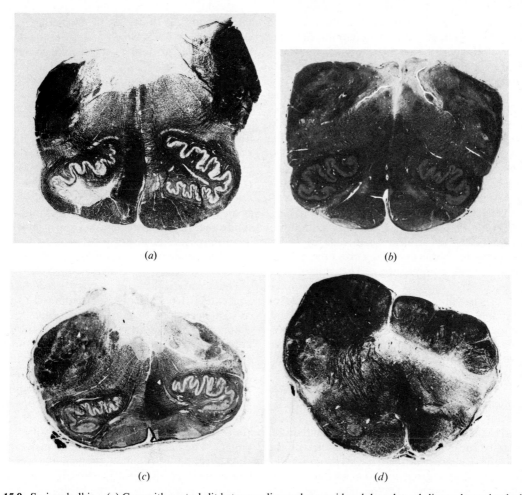

(a)

(b)

(c)

(d)

Fig. 15.9 Syringobulbia. (a) Case with ventral slit between olive and pyramid and dorsolateral slit at a lower level which has produced degeneration of the contralateral medial lemniscus. (b) Case with bilateral dorsolateral and dorsomedial slits. (c) Case with dorsolateral slit producing degeneration of the medial lemniscus. (d) Section at the level of the pyramidal decussation. The lateral extension of the cavity has destroyed the crossed pyramidal fibres.

between the pyramid and the inferior olive where it interrupts the emerging fibres of the hypoglossal nerve (Fig. 15.9a). These cavities are usually unilateral; in Spiller's case they were bilateral, although only one was large enough to cause atrophic palsy of the tongue. A cavity in this situation may also damage the anteromedian part of the olive or the posterior part of the pyramid.

Cavities in the pons usually lie in the tegmentum

corticospinal fibres, destroying also the substantia nigra and ended in the internal capsule and caudate and lenticular nuclei.

Secondary degenerations

Secondary degenerations follow destruction of tracts and fibre systems both in syringomyelia and syringobulbia. The pyramidal tracts may be pressed on by an anterior cavity between the pyramid and medullary olive or a slit at a lower level may interrupt pyramidal fibres during their decussation. In the latter case there is commonly some retrograde degeneration of the pyramidal fibres in the medulla. Alternatively a large cavity in the cervical region may destroy much of the pyramidal tract by compression. The *spinocerebellar tracts* may degenerate owing to destruction of their cells of origin in the grey matter of the cord or of the fibres leaving these. The fibres passing in the posterior columns may be compressed or destroyed by extensions of the cavity in the cord. In cases of syringobulbia the fibres relayed to the thalamus from the nuclei gracilis and cuneatus are commonly destroyed as they pass towards the decussation of the medial lemniscus so that there is more or less complete absence of the medial lemniscus on the side opposite to the lesion (Figs. 15.9a and c); retrograde degeneration occurs in the nerve cells of the nuclei gracilis et cuneatus. Fibres passing to the spinothalamic tracts are very commonly involved either at or near their cells of origin in the posterior horns or as they cross the midline in the central commissure. The dorsolateral cavities in the medulla commonly interrupted some of the fibres passing inwards from the descending trigeminal nucleus to the medial lemniscus. The destruction of the motor fibres arising in the nucleus ambiguus and hypoglossal nuclei and destruction of the tractus solitarius have already been mentioned.

Symptomatology

The symptomatology of syringomyelia is closely related to the extent of the destruction of individual cells and fibres. Wasting of the muscles of the hands and forearms is related to lesions of the posterolateral cell groups in the anterior horns of the cervical cord. Dissociated anaesthesia results from damage to spinothalamic fibres and autonomic symptoms to destruction of the cells of the intermediolateral tract in the upper thoracic segments. Anaesthesia to all forms of sensibility is usually attributable to a combination of a spinothalamic lesion either with a lesion in the posterior columns or more often with a cavity in the medulla which interrupts the decussating fibres going to the medial lemniscus. Loss of appreciation of position and vibration may also result from a lesion of this system of fibres. The position of the medullary cavities explains the paralyses of the lower cranial nerves and the

facial and corneal analgesia. Rarely extensions into the pons may cause paralysis of one abducens nerve or of conjugate deviation to one side, or by destruction of the central tegmental tract may lead to the syndrome of palatolaryngeal nystagmus. Nystagmus, or lateral deviation of the eyes, which is very common in cases with dorsolateral slits, is most easily explained by the destruction of fibres which pass from the descending vestibular nucleus to the medial longitudinal fasciculus.

Hydromyelia

The name *hydromyelus* is given to a congenital dilatation of the central canal of the cord and the condition is called *hydromyelia*. Although minor degrees of hydromyelia may be found in routine necropsies there is an important association with spina bifida occulta, spina bifida cystica (meningomyelocele), the Arnold–Chiari syndrome, and diastematomyelia. Thus there is an important correlation between hydromyelia and developmental malformations of the neural tube.

The hydromyelic cavities vary greatly in size and extent, from narrow slits confined to a few cervical segments, to fairly large tubular cavities running through most of the length of the spinal cord. The smaller cavities are either transverse slits or are triangular on cross-section with their base lying transversely in the grey commissure and their apex in relation to the dorsomedian septum (Figs. 15.10a and b). Anteroposterior slits are less common. Larger cavities are sometimes cruciform recalling the shape of the fetal canal. The wall is lined by ependymal cells but this covering is often incomplete, especially in the corners of the cavity. Where ependyma is absent it is replaced by thickening of the subependymal neuroglia which may project as granulations into the lumen of the cavity. In some cases, especially when hydromyelia is associated with the Arnold–Chiari malformation in the adult, only the ventral wall of the cavity may be covered by ependyma and the remainder by a thick firm layer of neuroglial fibres.

Secondary syringomyelia

This term should be reserved for longitudinal cysts secondary to clearly evident causes. Tumours, trauma, adhesive arachnoiditis, haematomyelia and vascular softenings account for most cases. Most of the cysts are small but in tumours the associated cystic lesion may be extensive and progressive.

Poser (1956) reviewed 254 necropsied cases of syringomyelia and found that 40 (16·4%) had an associated intramedullary tumour. Out of 209 cases of intramedullary tumours there was an incidence of 31% of syringomyelia. Extrinsic tumours can cause syringomyelia as in the case reported by Kosary, Braham, Shaked and Tadmor (1969) who found an occipital meningioma.

one or two segments above and below the tumour. Such cavities may arise as a result of transudation from the tumour. In other cases the cavities may be very extensive and may involve most of the spinal cord above and below the tumour. Such cavities are most often associated either with tumours of ependymal character or with haemangioblastomas. In the former case it is possible that the cavitation was a true syringomyelia and preceded the growth of the tumour. In two cases examined at the National Hospital, Queen Square, an ependymal tumour

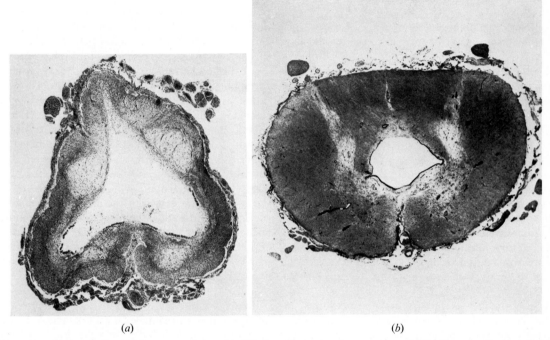

(a)

(b)

Fig. 15.10 Hydromyelia. (*a*) In a case of Arnold–Chiari malformation in a newborn child with early gliosis replacing lines of ependyma in the dorsal extension. (*b*) In a man of 25 who died of poliomyelitis. Both hydromyelia and Chiari's Type I deformity were clinically silent.

Post-traumatic syringomyelia is dealt with on p. 668. Syringomyelia has occasionally been described following adhesive arachnoiditis (Schwartz 1897) and a more recent case was described by Appleby, Bradley, Foster, Hankinson and Hudgson (1969) following tuberculous meningitis. Carroll (1967) described syringomyelia following an attack of acute anterior poliomyelitis and reviewed other case reports of this association.

The cavitation associated with spinal tumours presents a more difficult problem. In some cases there is only a small cavity which extends for

at the midthoracic level was associated with cavitation which extended from the 2nd cervical segment to the conus terminalis. This had all the characters of a syringomyelic cavity but had not caused any anaesthesia or other symptoms above the level of the tumour. The cavitation associated with haemangioblastomas of the spinal cord may, like the cerebellar cysts, be caused by transudation from the tumour acting over many years. Such cavities also are often very extensive. Brain, Greenfield and Northfield (1943) reported a case with a tumour at the 9th thoracic level, and cavitation extending from the medulla to the conus terminalis, and in the cases of Craig, Wagener and Kernohan (1941) the cavity was almost equally extensive. It would appear that cavities associated with tumours extend into the lumbosacral enlargement more often than those of simple syringomyelia. The venous congestion which is often found below the level of a spinal tumour may be a contributory factor to this lumbosacral extension. The linkage of syringomyelia to cerebral tumours on which Langhans based his theory of pathogenesis is probably a chance association since asymptomatic cavitation of the cervical cord is not rare.

Aetiology and pathogenesis
The inclusion of syringomyelia in the large group covered by the name *craniorachischisis* appears justified at first sight on anatomical grounds, but this may not be correct and in any case brings us little nearer to an understanding of its cause. One difficulty is the distinction of syringomyelia from hydromyelia. In hydromyelia there is an undoubted association with neural tube malformations. It is also possible in some cases to trace the development of a syringomyelic cavity from hydromyelia, for example in cases of the Arnold–Chiari malformation in the adult. But this is only true for a minority of cases. Syringomyelia is rarely familial. The so-called 'hereditary lumbosacral syringomyelia' has been shown to be affection of the dorsal root ganglia and primary sensory neurons (Denny-Brown 1951).

Several different factors may be combined in the pathogenesis of cavitation in syringomyelia: (1) instability in the lines of junction of the alar and basal laminae with each other; (2) the constant movements of flexion and torsion to which the cervical cord and lower medulla are exposed; (3) the tendency for cysts within nervous tissue to undergo alterations of tension and so to enlarge.

(1) As has been seen the cavitation, both in the spinal cord and especially in the medulla, tends to occur along lines of fusion which take place comparatively late in fetal life. The ventral

cavity in the medulla may thus be related to the migration of the olivary cells from the rhomboid lip across the median raphe to their final position behind the pyramids. Many of the older writers have described the cells in the walls of a syringomyelic cavity as of embryonal character (Gowers and Taylor 1899). There is little evidence of this in many cases which have been expertly examined. Ependymal cells are often seen in the tissue in front of the cavity; in those that result from a hydromyelia they may also be found under its lateral walls; but these cells do not differ from those seen in the grey commissure in normal cords. The theory that cavitation takes place by the breakdown of abnormal neuroglial tissue appears to have no firm histological basis since this is a feature of no other pathological conditions either in the medulla or the spinal cord.

(2) The reason why syringomyelic cavities tend to begin in the cervical region of the cord, and attain their greatest size there, may well be related to the great mobility of the cervical spine. Bending of the neck in all directions and torsion when the head is turned (Schaltenbrandt 1951) must impose stresses and strains on the cervical cord to which it is less subject at lower levels, and which may well cause small tears of the tissue in the centre of the cord. Movements of the head on the atlanto-occipital joint must affect the lower medulla in a similar way.

(3) Once cavitation in the spinal cord has begun it may be enlarged by transudation of fluid into it under pressure. This expansion is more likely to occur in the grey matter than in the firmer columns of white matter and owing to the restricting investment of pia mater must take place chiefly upwards and downwards. It is favoured by anything which increases venous congestion in the body cavity, such as muscular effort, since there are no valves on the veins draining the spinal cord, but it may also depend to some extent on the electrolyte content of the blood. In this relation the fact that a syringomyelic cavity usually ceases at the 2nd cervical level and has no communications with the 4th ventricle may be of considerable importance (see also Barnett *et al.* 1973).

Vascular disorders of the spinal cord

Anatomy

Adamkiewicz (1881, 1882), then professor at the Institute of Experimental Pathology at Krakow, and his pupil Kadyi (1889) laid the foundations of our modern understanding of the blood supply of the human spinal cord. To this has been added the findings of injection studies (Bolton 1939; Suh and Alexander 1939; Herren and Alexander 1939) and of experimental work on the spinal cord of the monkey (Sahs 1942; Yoss 1950). Monographs on the vasculature of the human spinal cord have been written by Corbin (1961) and by Jellinger (1966).

Embryology

In the embryo the arterial supply of the spinal cord accurately follows the segmental arrangement of vertebrate development. The aorta, which first appears as a capillary ventral to the neural tube, gives off branches to each spinal cord segment and these arteries are among the first in the body to develop and for a time are the largest and the most important vessels. At this stage each spinal cord segment is supplied by a pair of anterior and a pair of posterior radicular arteries. Each radicular artery gives off an ascending and a descending branch which anastomose with the corresponding branches belonging to adjacent segments. With the passage of time many of these radicular arteries become rudimentary or disappear, but the anastomotic channels increase in calibre and importance, resulting in one large anterior anastomotic channel, or anterior spinal artery, and two smaller posterior anastomotic channels, or posterior spinal arteries. The adult arterial vasculature is based on these three vessels of which the first described is by far the most important.

Arteries

The anterior spinal artery begins by the union of the anterior spinal branches of each vertebral artery which usually takes place at the level of the foramen magnum but in about 10% of cases is delayed as far down as the lower cervical region. Very rarely the anterior spinal artery is duplicated throughout most of its length but small parts of the artery are commonly double. In position the anterior spinal artery lies in approximate relation to the anterior median sulcus but pursues a zig-zag course determined by the entry of the radicular tributaries. The calibre of the artery is widest in the lumbosacral region and narrowest in the thoracic region but also varies at various segments, being wider just caudal to the entry of a large tributary artery. From this observation, from the results of injection experiments and from some radiological evidence it is thought that during life the blood flow in the human anterior spinal artery is in the caudal direction. The artery throughout the length of the spinal cord is maintained by the contributions of the radicular arteries which enter the anterior spinal artery in a caudal direction and supply the spinal cord below the point of their entry.

The two posterior spinal arteries arise from the vertebral arteries or more rarely from the posterior inferior cerebellar arteries. The channel of a posterior spinal artery is much less distinct than that of the anterior spinal artery and the posterior spinal artery usually appears as a vascular network rather than a single vessel. When the artery can be recognized as a single structure it is very tortuous and often moves medially or laterally away from its usual position at the region of entry of the posterior nerve roots. Frequently the arteries are discontinuous and sometimes one artery moves across to supply the other side. It is rare for the posterior radicular tributaries to be seen easily as they frequently end in a plexus of small arteries. The blood flow of the posterior spinal arteries is probably caudal in the cervical and thoracic regions and in an upward direction in the lumbosacral region. There is a good anastomosis around the cauda equina between the anterior spinal artery and the posterior spinal arteries.

Of the radicular tributary arteries, those accompanying the anterior spinal nerve roots (the anterior radicular arteries) are of considerable importance. Anterior radicular tributaries accompany nearly every anterior spinal nerve root but some of these provide a blood supply only for the root itself. A small and variable number are large and supply the anterior spinal artery. The larger tributaries usually number from three to nine. The largest anterior tributary is usually a substantial vessel and has been called the artery of Adamkiewicz. In 12 out of 40 human cords (Hughes 1967) this artery accompanied the left T10 anterior nerve root. In the remainder of the cases this major artery usually accompanied one of the anterior roots from T9 to L1. These radicular tributaries may be subdivided into two groups, the first being those derived from the subclavian artery and the second those arising more directly from the aorta. It follows that somewhere in the region of the second thoracic spinal cord segment there is a change of arterial supply from a subclavian supply to a direct aortic supply and this anatomical feature is sometimes of clinical importance.

The sulcal arteries arise from the anterior spinal artery and pass backwards in the anterior median sulcus. They enter the grey commissure and by turning either left or right supply the grey matter and central white matter of one side. These vessels and their branches form what is termed the centrifugal arterial system. The centripetal arterial system, of lesser importance, is formed by radial arteries proceeding inwardly as branches from the coronal arterial plexus surrounding the spinal cord.

It is a remarkable fact that certain kinds of vascular disease affect the vessels of the spinal cord much less than those of the brain. Atherosclerosis is very rare and hypertensive arterial and arteriolar changes are much less severe in the spinal cord than in the brain of the same patient.

Veins

The spinal venous system is prominent on the posterior aspect of the spinal cord, particularly in the lumbosacral region. The venous network is irregular and there is considerable anastomosis between the large venous trunks. There is, however, with regularity a single large median posterior vein, applied to the posterior aspect of the spinal cord in the region of the posterior median septum, and this vessel appears to have no arterial counterpart. It receives draining veins from the posterior columns and parts of the posterior horns. The anterior spinal vein accompanies the anterior spinal artery and receives small sulcal veins in a corresponding manner to the origin of the sulcal

arteries from the anterior spinal artery. Both the anterior spinal veins and the median posterior vein are themselves drained by radicular veins, which accompany the anterior or posterior spinal nerve roots. These radicular veins are commoner than the corresponding radicular arteries and like them some are especially large. These large veins can be termed major radicular draining veins and sometimes accompany major radicular arterial tributaries but often are independent. The radicular veins drain into the paravertebral and intervertebral plexuses, which in turn communicate with the pelvic venous plexuses.

Pathological changes

Occlusion of the anterior spinal artery

The anterior spinal artery, which arises by the union of a spinal branch from each vertebral artery, supplies the anterior and median portion of the lower medulla, in which the following structures are present: the pyramids and pyramidal decussations, the medial lemnisci, the medial longitudinal fasciculi, the caudal portions of the hypoglossal and dorsal vagal nuclei, the nucleus and tractus solitarius on each side (at the level of the decussation), the lateral spinothalamic and ventral spinocerebellar tracts (Gower's tracts), the olivocerebellar fibres as they cross the midline, part of the inferior olivary nuclei and the internal and ventral external arcuate fibres and nuclei. In the spinal cord this artery supplies about two-thirds of the cross-sectional area of the cord and this includes all the cord except the posterior parts of the posterior white columns and the posterior grey columns. Obstruction of the beginning of this artery in the medulla is uncommon. Davison (1937, 1944) described five cases with occlusion of the medullary portion of the artery (in two cases both branches of origin). The structures which were damaged were the pyramids, the medial lemnisci, the medial longitudinal fasciculi and the ventral part of the inferior olivary nuclei (three cases). The hypoglossal nuclei and nerves were not affected. In association with this infarct the patient shows contralateral or bilateral pyramidal tract involvement, sensory disturbance referable to the posterior columns, and sometimes urinary and faecal incontinence.

The occlusion of the spinal part of the anterior spinal artery, commonly by thrombosis of the upper part of the vessel, causes a well-recognized clinical syndrome. The onset is sudden with pain in the back and in the neck and with paraesthesiae experienced in the upper limbs. In a few hours the condition progresses to a flaccid paralysis of both arms with loss of pain and temperature sensation below a sensory level. Touch, joint and position sense are preserved. The lower limbs may develop a spastic paraplegia and paralysis of bowel and bladder are common. The prognosis is reasonably good with considerable improvement in the neurological deficit except for the lower motor neuron paralysis in the arm which is usually permanent.

Published accounts of this syndrome with confirmation of the pathology by necropsy are surprisingly few.

The account of Margulis (1930) refers to three cases (cases 1, 2 and 7) in which syphilitic arteritis caused anterior spinal artery thrombosis and these cases are similar to several described earlier in this century. Syphilis is no longer the common predisposing cause of the condition. In the case of Schott (1915) the thrombosis was attributed to minor trauma and this was also the cause in the report of Grinker and Guy (1927). In their case, a 15-year-old boy developed thrombosis of the upper part of the anterior spinal artery, apparently caused by subluxation of the cervical spine. Similar minor trauma was postulated in the case of Hughes and Brownell (1964) in which cervical spondylosis was present. That part of the anterior spinal artery affected by thrombosis was compressed by a large spondylotic protrusion. This case, in which cervical spondylosis was complicated by anterior spinal artery thrombosis, is relevant to the problem of chronic myelopathy due to spondylosis. In these cases, Mair and Druckman (1953) considered that the changes which occur in the spinal cord, in association with protrusion of cervical intervertebral discs, are secondary to compression of the anterior spinal artery and its branches.

Proved cases of occlusion of the caudal portion of the anterior spinal artery are also few. They were reviewed by Zeitlin and Lichtenstein (1936). All were due to syphilis. Their own case was unusual in that the extent of the lesion was in the middle segment of the cord from C5 to T10, being maximal at T7. This case was also exceptional in that the thrombosis occurred in an anterior spinal artery which was affected by atheroma. Atheroma has very rarely been reported in the anterior spinal artery and most authors comment on its rarity.

Occlusion of the posterior spinal artery

The syndrome of anterior spinal artery occlusion is well known, but that of obstruction of the posterior spinal arteries is scarcely recognized. Hughes (1970), in describing a case with necropsy confirmation of the diagnosis, could only find seven previous case reports. Clinically the onset begins with pain or dysaesthesia but paresis or paralysis of the lower limbs and trunk rapidly supervene. The bladder and bowel are also paralysed. This description refers to the period immediately following the onset of the neurological syndrome when, because of swelling and oedema, there is a temporary disability of the spinal cord amounting to a cord transection. If the patient survives this acute phase, considerable neurological improvement may occur, and recovery may be almost complete. The lower limb and trunk paresis may disappear, normal control of bladder and bowel are regained, and only a moderate sensory deficit may persist, demonstrable only on neurological examination and causing no symptoms. This would be the expected loss of function from destruction of the spinal cord in the territories of the posterior spinal arteries. The predisposing cause of the occlusion of the posterior spinal artery is usually apparent in the case history, and in the case of Hughes (1970) the thrombosis was caused by an intrathecal phenol injection. Thrombosis is generally present and in the earlier reports was caused by syphilitic arteritis. In the case of Stone and Roback (1937) the onset of the neurological syndrome followed minor indirect trauma. Two cases were described by Perier, Demanet, Henneaux and Nunès-Vincente (1960) and the second of these was exceptional in that the posterior spinal arteries were obstructed by embolic atheromatous material.

Neurological complications of the adult type of coarctation of the aorta

Coarctation of the aorta, first described by Morgagni in 1761, is a congenital stenosis of the isthmus of the aorta, which is that part of the aorta between the origin of the left subclavian artery and the ductus arteriosus. It has been customary to divide cases into two types: 'infantile' with extensive obliteration of the aortic isthmus, and 'adult' type in which there is a small segment of narrowing which may be before, at, or (the usual situation) beyond the origin of the left subclavian artery. In the adult type the ductus arterosus closes and there is an extensive anastomotic circulation between the arteries supplying the upper trunk and limbs and those arising beyond the aortic constrictions which supply the lower trunk and lower limbs. These 'adult' type cases alone concern us in a consideration of neurological complications. An important factor is the arterial hypertension in the upper parts of the body which contrasts with the hypotension in the lower parts of the body.

In the combined figures of Abbott (1928) and Reifenstein, Levine and Gross (1947) which cover 304 cases of the adult type of coarctation, death was considered on clinical grounds to be due to an intracranial haemorrhage in 36 cases and this diagnosis was confirmed *post mortem* in 29 of them. In 10 cases a ruptured saccular aneurysm of the Circle of Willis was found and this mechanism is probably a common cause of intracranial haemorrhage complicating coarctation of the aorta.

Neurological complications affecting the spinal cord are fewer and are of two types:

1. *Those due to a reduced blood supply to the more caudal part of the spinal cord.* These complications formed the majority of the case reports recorded by Tyler and Clark (1958). The symptoms and signs of paresis, sensory and sphincteric disturbance were attributed by these authors to ischaemia and hypotension of that part of the spinal cord supplied by arteries derived from the aorta distal to the constriction.

2. *Complications due to the hypertension present in the body in arteries arising proximal to the aortic constriction.* The anastomotic circulation we have mentioned includes the anterior spinal artery. The blood passes from the heart to the subclavian arteries, then via the vertebral arteries into the upper part of the anterior spinal artery, and via the ascending cervical branches of the thyreocervical trunks into the upper radicular tributaries of the anterior spinal artery. The blood by-passes the aortic obstruction by flowing down the anterior spinal artery to reach the spinal branches of the aortic intercostals below the obstruction. In such cases the anterior spinal artery becomes enlarged and tortuous (Fig. 15.11).

This change in the anterior spinal artery usually causes no clinical ill effects. However, Haberer (1903) found, in a woman aged 47 who died 4 months after the sudden onset of a transverse

myelitis, that the spinal cord at Th2 was compressed and necrotic. This he considered to be a compression myelopathy secondary to pronounced dilatation and tortuosity of the anterior spinal artery at this level. Greenfield had a case in which there was a saccular false aneurysm of the anterior spinal artery at Th1 (Fig. 15.11). In each of these cases the anterior spinal artery became markedly dilated and tortuous immediately inferior to the point of entry of an enlarged lower cervical radicular artery, of which indeed the anterior spinal artery appeared to be the continuation. A similar case was described by Christian and Noder (1954).

Neurological complications of dissecting aneurysm of the aorta

In dissecting aneurysm of the aorta there is an extensive haemorrhage into the tunica media of the aorta and within this plane the aortic wall is forced apart into two layers. The dissection by this haemorrhage may extend along the tunica media to involve the innominate, carotid or femoral arteries, narrowing the lumen and impairing the blood flow. It may surround, stretch, or even tear apart the intercostal and lumbar arteries and obliterate their lumen. Thrombosis may occur in these narrowed arteries. There are several accounts of the pathology of the condition and some more recent reports are listed by Braunstein (1963). In its commonest form the condition is associated with arteriosclerosis in which systemic hypertension and aortic dilatation probably predispose to the dissection. The commonest finding at necropsy is severe atherosclerosis and a tear through the intima of the aorta which is sited on an atheromatous plaque. More rarely dissecting aneurysm of the aorta is seen in Marfan's syndrome and there is also an uncommon association with pregnancy, aortic stenosis and myxoedema. Syphilitic aortitis does not seem to be linked to dissection of the aorta.

Neurological complications are common in dissecting aneurysm of the aorta. Shennan (1934) found neurological complications in 45 out of 317 cases and Lindsay and Hurst (1967) 26 out of 62. Weisman and Adams (1944) divided the neurological complications into three groups:

(1) *Ischaemic necrosis of peripheral nerves.* This is the commonest neurological complication and is usually associated with extension of the haemor-

rhage into the subclavian or iliac arteries thus causing impairment of blood supply to the nerves of the limbs.

(2) *Ischaemic necrosis of the brain.* This is the least common complication. It is usually associated with extension of the dissection into the innominate or carotid arteries. The effects are

reports as in the case of Kalischer (1914) and the first case of Lange-Cosack and Köhn (1962) it is probable that death supervened before the changes in the spinal cord became evident. This explanation will not suffice for all these instances and, for example, in the case of Moersch and Sayre (1950), despite a sufficient interval to death, no changes were found. Several cases have had a

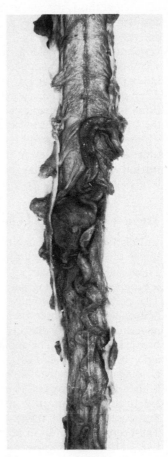

Fig. 15.11 Coarctation of the aorta. Ventral aspect of the spinal cord of a girl who, when aged 14, had transient headache and twitching of the legs followed 5 days later by weakness of the right leg. Gradual complete recovery. Aged 16 onset of progressive motor and sensory loss to level of the nipple line. Aged 18 died after negative exploratory laminectomy. At necropsy, left-sided cardiac hypertrophy and coarctation of aorta. The cranial portion of the anterior spinal artery was slightly larger than normal. At C5, on the left, a dilated and thick-walled radicular artery joined the anterior spinal artery. At Th1 there was a rounded thick-walled aneurysmal sac lying partly within and partly anterior to the thin orange-coloured substance of the spinal cord. This sac lay posterolateral to the tortuous dilated anterior spinal artery, with which it communicated through a small aperture in the wall of the artery. It appeared that the aneurysm was a false aneurysm, which had formed as the result of haemorrhage from the tortuous anterior spinal artery. At Th3 the anterior spinal artery divided into two, one branch passing laterally as an anterior radicular artery on the left side and the other branch continuing onwards for a few more segments until it too joined a radicular artery.

similar to occlusion of the carotid artery, which has already been considered.

(3) *Ischaemic necrosis of the spinal cord.* The involvement of the spinal cord in cases of dissecting aneurysm of the aorta requires more detailed comment.

Reviewing the literature of this association and considering only the accounts with necropsy, about 11 case reports are readily accessible. It is evident from these reports that the dissection of the aorta causes more extensive spinal damage in some cases than in others. In some case

complete necrosis of the whole cross-sectional area of the spinal cord and affecting several consecutive spinal cord segments. To this belong the cases of Schwartz, Shorey and Anderson (1950), Ballentine (1952), and Hill and Vasquez (1962).

The striking differences in the extent of spinal cord involvement can be explained by the pattern of blood supply to the spinal cord. The obstructive effect of the dissecting aneurysm, which may involve a variable extent of the aortic media, may occlude one or several of the intercostal and lumbar arteries. The degree of interference with the blood flow in these spinal branches accounts for the variations in the extent of the spinal cord infarction. The other complicating factor is the importance to the spinal cord of these spinal branches and in particular whether a large tributary or small insignificant tributaries are affected.

In general, the portion of the spinal cord which is severely damaged is the mid- and lower-thoracic region and this is the region supplied by the inter-costal arteries. The upper part of the cord, which derives its blood supply from branches of the vertebral arteries, is seldom involved. The lumbo-sacral cord, which is supplied by the lumbar, ilio-lumbar and lateral sacral arteries, is sometimes damaged when the aneurysmal dissection has been extensive. The ischaemic necrosis always involves the grey matter and the adjacent white matter. The white matter at the periphery of the cord is some-times spared but, in severe cases, the whole cross-section of the cord may be necrotic at certain levels.

Arteriovenous aneurysm of the spinal cord

In 1926 Foix and Alajouanine described two cases under the title 'La myélite nécrotique subaigue'. These male patients aged 19 and 27 had developed a progressive ascending paralysis and anasthesia. The paralysis was initially of the upper motor neuron type but later became flaccid, and the anaesthesia, initially dissociated in character, later became complete. The spinal fluid was remark-able in that a massive protein increase was accompanied by only a slight lymphocytosis. In both cases the progressive course of the illness led to a fatal issue in 2 years 9 months in the first case and in 11 months in the second case. The necropsy findings in both cases were distinc-tive. The lower thoracic, lumbar and sacral parts of the spinal cord were affected by large areas of necrosis. The grey matter was completely destroyed but the white matter damage, although extensive, was incomplete. The histological picture in the severely affected spinal cord seg-ments was remarkable not only for the necrosis and numerous lipid phagocytes but also because of the striking vascular changes. In both cases the authors observed enlargement and thickening of the extramedullary and of the intramedullary vessels of the spinal cord, the veins being chiefly affected. These vascular changes were termed 'endomesovascularitis' and were attributed to some toxic or infective agent which had also caused the parenchymal destruction in the spinal cord.

This paper, containing the two case reports described above, directed attention to a condition which is sometimes called Foix–Alajouanine disease and was renamed *Angiodysgenetische nekrotisierende Myelopathie* by Scholtz and Manuelidis (1951). The underlying pathology in many of these cases is now considered (Antoni 1962) to be a spinal arteriovenous aneurysm or fistula. The numerous case reports of the con-dition are reviewed in the following monographs: Wyburn-Mason (1943), Corbin (1961), Jellinger (1966), Neumayer (1967).

Spinal cord angiography

The great advance in our understanding of these cases has come from the development of angio-graphic procedures directed at the spinal cord. Formerly angiomatous malformations were recog-nized by myelography but this technique added little to our knowledge of the type of malfor-mation present. In 1962 Djindjian and his co-workers (Djindjian 1970) reported their first angiographic investigation of an intraspinal arteriovenous aneurysm and in 1966 this group (Djindjian, Fauré and Hurth 1966) published 12 cases of intraspinal arteriovenous aneurysms ex-amined by this technique. An important part of the technique depends on removing the opacity of overlying bone structure by cancelling the image components common to the preliminary and subsequent (contrast filled) radiographs. These radiographic studies, now widely employed (Di Chiro and Wener 1973), have shown that the commonest type of spinal angioma is an arterio-venous communication in which one or more of the spinal arteries forms a cluster of vessels which allow flow into one or more of the draining veins without the blood passing in the normal way through the capillary bed of the spinal cord. The feeding artery or arteries to one of these angio-matous malformations has a normal origin and direction but is enormously enlarged. If this arterial pedicle can be identified and ligated then the progressive enlargement of the malformation can be arrested. These angiographic observations, which have so elegantly demonstrated the haemo-dynamics of these spinal angiomas, now direct attention to the pathological findings which are consistent with the presence of an abnormal arteriovenous communication in the spinal vessels.

Morbid anatomy

The macroscopical appearances at necropsy are remarkably uniform in these cases. However, the complexity of the various components of the spinal cord vasculature makes a complete assessment difficult even for the expert and very confusing to the inexperienced pathologist.

The anterior spinal artery is normal or slightly enlarged. The posterior spinal arteries are normal. The spinal venous system is normal in its fundamental anatomy but abnormal in the hypertrophy and distension of most of the spinal veins. The anterior spinal vein, for example, is always normally situated. A constant finding is a very abnormal large thick-walled tortuous vessel pursuing an irregular course longitudinally on the posterior aspect of the spinal cord. At necropsy (and by some surgeons during life) this tortuous convoluted vessel can be dissected away from the spinal cord as a single continuous vascular channel greatly exceeding in length that of the whole spinal cord. This abnormal vessel is now known from the angiographic studies during life to be part of an abnormal vascular communication between the arterial and venous systems of the spinal cord. It is difficult at necropsy, but easy during life with the angiographic techniques mentioned, to determine the artery or arteries feeding into this large complex vessel and the veins which drain it (Fig. 15.12).

Histological findings (Figs. 15.13, 15.14, 15.15)

The microscopical findings are so unusual that, in many of the published reports, attention has been directed away from the more informative macroscopical appearances. Furthermore, the anatomy of the malformation described above becomes difficult to elucidate after the spinal cord is sliced transversely and tissue blocks are taken.

The histological changes are more advanced in the caudal part of the spinal cord, being very evident in the lumbosacral enlargement. There are many capillaries and other small thick-walled channels the size and position of which suggests that they are altered capillaries and veins. These vessels have thick hyaline walls which are sometimes calcified. Recent thrombosis may be seen within these intramedullary vessels and others show changes indicative of the organization of earlier thrombus. Thrombosis may also be seen in the large extramedullary vessels. The examination by elastic stains of the tunica media of the

large abnormal vessels shows them to have the structure of arterialized veins.

The substance of the spinal cord is affected by an unusual form of incomplete necrosis which

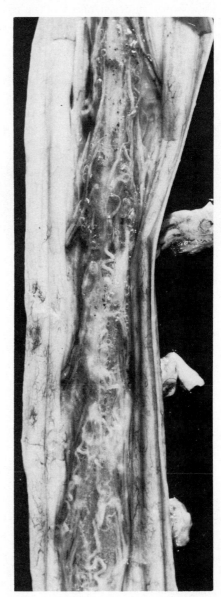

Fig. 15.12 Arteriovenous aneurysm of the spinal cord. Posterior aspect of the spinal cord after the dura has been opened and reflected. Note the coiled vessels in the subarachnoid space. (Taken with permission from *Pathology of the Spinal Cord*, 2nd ed., Lloyd-Luke, London.)

involves grey and white matter but particularly the central parts of the cord. The majority of the neuron cell bodies are lost but some, although apparently dead, are encrusted with material that stains for iron and calcium. Lipid phagocytes are common but acute inflammatory cells are usually absent. The upper parts of the spinal cord show Wallerian degeneration of the upward directed long tracts.

Spinal thrombophlebitis

Proved cases of a syndrome caused by spinal thrombophlebitis are extremely rare. In the

in some of the abnormal vessels. This condition has been described above. Here we are only considering acute thrombophlebitis.

One of the earliest cases of this type of venous infarction of the spinal cord was that reported by Wyss (1898) under the name 'acute haemorrhagic myelitis'. In this report an extensive haemorrhagic infarction of the spinal cord was associated with thrombosis of the veins of the spinal cord and those of the spinal meninges. The cause of the venous thrombosis was a tumour

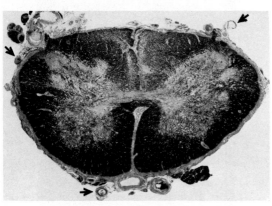

15.13

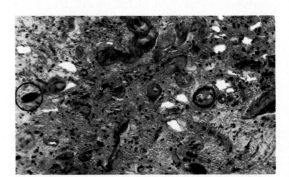

15.14

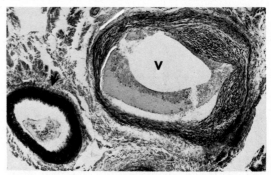

15.15

Fig. 15.13 Arteriovenous aneurysm. Second lumbar segment, myelin preparation. Note the enlarged and thickened veins. The arteries (arrows) appear healthy. There is extensive degeneration of the white matter. Weigert Pal.
Fig. 15.14 Part of the anterior grey horn, same case as Fig. 15.11 showing marked hyaline fibrous thickening of the small vessels. The parenchyma is damaged but some nerve cells (circle) are still present. Celloidin, haematoxylin van Gieson.
Fig. 15.15 Anterior spinal vessels, same case as Fig. 15.11, different level, showing healthy artery (arrow) and enlarged vein (v) with internal fibrous thickening. Celloidin, haematoxylin van Gieson.

reported cases, the occlusion of the spinal veins has led to an acute haemorrhagic venous infarction of the spinal cord which has caused the rapid development of an acute syndrome of spinal cord destruction. The name spinal thrombophlebitis has also been applied to cases which now would be recognized as an angiomatous malformation of the spinal cord with thrombosis

of the spinal cord which was said to be a gliosarcoma. In the same year, Petren (1898) described spinal cord infarction due to venous thrombosis associated with extensive generalized septicaemia. There are now at least seven case reports (Hughes 1971) in which necropsy has shown venous infarction of the spinal cord caused by acute thrombophlebitis. In these reviewed case reports the clinical features and the pathological findings are remarkably constant.

Clinical features. The onset of the condition is rapid and invariably with pain which is felt either in the back, legs or abdomen. After one or two days, weakness and loss of sensation in the legs and trunk develop and these symptoms are usually combined with paralysis of the bladder and bowel. The spinal fluid shows an elevation of cells and of protein but these changes may be slight or absent. If myelography is performed it gives findings indicative of moderate swelling of the spinal cord with the appearances of a partial hold-up of the myodil column rather than a complete obstruction. In all cases the illness has been rapidly progressive and the outcome has been death in the first or second week of the neurological illness. In these reviewed cases the poor prognosis has been due to the gravity of the associated illness which causes the venous infarction of the spinal cord. The actual prognosis of the condition may be less grave because only cases verified by necropsy have been diagnosed. It is possible that a milder form of the condition exists but is not recognized clinically.

Pathological findings. In nearly all the cases there is an obvious causative disease to explain the extensive venous thrombosis found. The commonest causative condition has been generalized sepsis but other causes have been a spinal cord tumour and a generalized thrombotic syndrome.

The spinal veins are always greatly distended and are usually extensively thrombosed. The venous obstruction may however be sited in the plexus of veins in the spinal canal or in the veins in the pelvis and abdomen. The spinal cord itself is disrupted by a severe haemorrhagic necrosis in which small haematomas are conspicuous. The worst affected parts of the spinal cord are the central areas and the infarction is much more haemorrhagic than arterial. The extent of the infarction both longitudinally and in its cross-sectional area is greater even than an extensive thrombosis of the anterior spinal artery.

Subacute and chronic spinal thrombophlebitis

The above description refers to acute infarction caused by an acute thrombophlebitis. Whether a subacute or chronic spinal cord syndrome can be produced by a more gradual venous thrombotic occlusion is a matter for debate. Many, but certainly not all, of these cases have been examples of spinal vascular malformations. The findings of thrombosed veins either around the spinal cord or in the abdomen and pelvis is not conclusive. These obscure myelopathies invariably suffer from a paraplegic syndrome in which pressure sores and urinary tract infection in a recumbent patient commonly lead to venous thrombosis. In many of these cases the venous thrombosis demonstrated at necropsy is likely to have been caused by the paraplegia rather than to be itself the primary condition.

Haematomyelia

The expression haematomyelia should be used only for a large intramedullary haemorrhage extending over several segments of the spinal cord. These haemorrhages occur predominantly in the grey matter, which may be largely destroyed, but extension is possible into and along the white columns in which there is separation rather than destruction of the nerve fibres. The most frequent cause of haematomyelia is bleeding from an angiomatous malformation (Richardson 1938), and the next most common cause is bleeding associated with a haemorrhagic diathesis. In venous infarction of the spinal cord (Hughes 1971) there is often considerable intramedullary bleeding, and haematomyelia has also been reported in association with arteriosclerosis, meningovascular syphilis, spinal tumour and syringomyelia.

It is very doubtful whether mechanical trauma ever produces haematomyelia. It is true that, after a severe fracture-dislocation or bullet wound of the spine (Holmes 1915), the naked-eye appearances will often be those of haemorrhagic pulping of the cord at the level of the injury, together with a thin pencil of blood-stained material which runs upwards and downwards from this site for several segments. Microscopical examination, however, shows that the material is composed principally of disintegrating nervous tissue, which has been produced at the site of the lesion by pulping and haemorrhagic infarction, and has been forced upwards and downwards. It is not haemorrhage and the condition is not haematomyelia.

References

Abbott, M. E. (1928) Coarctation of aorta of adult type; statistical study and historical retrospect of 200 recorded cases with autopsy, of stenosis or obliteration of descending arch in subjects above age of 2 years. *American Heart Journal*, **3**, 574-618.

Adamkiewicz, A. (1881) Die Blutgefässe des menschlichen Rückenmarkes. 1 Theil. Die Gefässe der Rückenmarkssubstanz. *Sitzungsberichte der Akademie der Wissenschaften in Wien. Mathematisch-naturwissenschaftliche Klasse*, **84**, 469-502.

Adamkiewicz, A. (1882) Die Blutgefässe des menschlichen Rückenmarkes. II Theil. Die Gefässe der Rückenmarksoberfläche. *Sitzungsberichte der Akademie der Wissenschaften in Wien. Mathematisch-naturwissenschaftliche Klasse*, **85**, 101-130.

Allen, K. L. (1952) Neuropathies caused by bony spurs in the cervical spine with special reference to surgical treatment. *Journal of Neurology, Neurosurgery and Psychiatry*, **15**, 20-36.

Andrae, R. (1929) Ueber Knorpelknötchen am hinteren Ende der Wirbelbandscheiben im Bereich des Spinalkanals. *Beiträge zur pathologischen Anatomie und zur allgemeinen Pathologie*, **82**, 464-474.

Antoni, N. (1962) Spinal vascular malformation (angiomas) and myelomalacia. *Neurology (Minneapolis)*, **12**, 795-804.

Appleby, A., Bradley, W. G., Foster, J. B., Hankinson, J. & Hudgson, P. (1969) Syringomyelia due to chronic arachnoiditis at the foramen magnum. *Journal of the Neurological Sciences*, **8**, 451-464.

Bachs, A., Barraquer-Bordas, L., Barraquer-Ferre, L., Canadell, J. M. & Modolell, A. (1955) Delayed myelopathy following atlanto-axial dislocation by separated odontoid process. *Brain*, **78**, 537-553.

Ballentine, H. T. (1952) Case records of the Massachusetts General Hospital. *New England Journal of Medicine*, **247**, 326-329.

Barnett, H. J. M., Foster, J. B. & Hudgson, P. (1973) *Syringomyelia*, Saunders, London.

Beadle, O. C. ·(1931) *M.R.C. Special Report Series* **161**, H. M. Stationery Office, London.

Bolton, B. (1939) Blood supply of the human spinal cord. *Journal of Neurology and Psychiatry*, **2**, 137-148.

Brain, W. R., Greenfield, J. G. & Northfield, D. W. C. (1943) A case of atypical Lindau's disease. *Journal of Neurology and Psychiatry*, **6**, 32-37.

Brain, W. R., Northfield, D. & Wilkinson, M. (1952) The neurological manifestations of cervical spondylosis. *Brain*, **75**, 187-225.

Braunstein, H. (1963) Pathogenesis of dissecting aneurysm. *Circulation*, **28**, 1071-1080.

Bull, J. W. D. (1948) Discussion on rupture of the intervertebral disc in the cervical region. *Proceedings of the Royal Society of Medicine*, **41**, 513-516.

Bull, J. W. D., Nixon, W. L. B., Pratt, R. T. C. & Robinson, P. K. (1959) Paget's disease of the skull and secondary basilar impression. *Brain*, **82**, 10-22.

Butler, R. W. (1935) Paraplegia in Pott's disease with special reference to pathology and etiology. *British Journal of Surgery*, **22**, 738-768.

Carroll, J. D. (1967) Syringomyelia as a possible complication of poliomyelitis. *Neurology (Minneapolis)*, **17**, 213-215.

Christian, P. & Noder, N. (1954) Akute Rückenmarkssyndrome bei Isthmusstenose der Aorta als Folge eines pathologischen Kollateralkreislaufs über die *A. spinalis* anterior. *Zeitschrift für Kreislaufforschung*, **43**, 125-131.

Clarke, E. & Robinson, P. K. (1956) Cervical myelopathy: a complication of cervical spondylosis. *Brain*, **79**, 483-510.

Claude, H. & Lhermitte, J. (1951) Étude clinique et anatome-pathologique de la commotion médullaire directe per projectiles de guerre. *Annales de Médecine*, **2**, 479-506.

Collins, D. H. (1950) *The Pathology of Articular and Spinal Diseases*, Arnold, London.

Corbin, J. L. (1961) *Anatomie et pathologie artérielles de la moelle*, Masson, Paris.

Craig, W. M., Wagener, H. P. & Kernohan, J. W. (1941) Lindau-von Hippel disease. *Archives of Neurology and Psychiatry (Chicago)*, **46**, 36-58.

Davison, C. (1937) Syndrome of anterior spinal artery of medulla oblongata. *Archives of Neurology and Psychiatry (Chicago)*, **37**, 91-107.

Davison, C. (1944) Syndrome of the anterior spinal artery of the medulla oblongata. *Journal of Neuropathology and Experimental Neurology*, **3**, 73-80.

Davison, C. (1945) *In Trauma of the Central Nervous System. Research Proceedings, Association for Research in Nervous and Mental Disease*, **24**, 151-187.

Denny-Brown, D. (1951) Hereditary sensory radicular neuropathy. *Journal of Neurology, Neurosurgery and Psychiatry*, **14**, 237-252.

Di Chiro, G. & Wener, L. (1973) Angiography of the spinal cord. *Journal of Neurosurgery*, **39**, 1-29.

Djindjian, R. (1970) *Angiography of the Spinal Cord*, University Park Press, Baltimore.

Djindjian, R., Fauré, C. & Hurth, M. (1966) Explorations artériographiques des anéurismes artério-veineux de la moelle épinière. *Annales de Radiologie, Monograph* No. 1.

Frykholm, R. (1951) Lower cervical vertebrae and intervertebral discs. Surgical anatomy and pathology. *Acta chirurgica scandinavica*, **101**, 345-359.

Gardner, W. J. (1973) *The Dysraphic States*, Excerpta Medica, Amsterdam.

Goldthwait, J. E. (1911) The lumbo-sacral articulation; an explanation of many cases of 'lumbago', sciatica and paraplegia. *Boston Medical and Surgical Journal*, **164**, 365-372.

Gowers, W. R. & Taylor, J. (1899) *A Manual of Diseases of the Nervous System*, 3rd Edn., Churchill, London.

Greenfield, J. G. (1953) Malformations et dégénérescences des disques intervertébraux de la région cervicale. *Revue Médicale de la Suisse Romande*, **73**, 227-250.

Grinker, R. & Guy, C. (1927) Sprain of cervical spine causing thrombosis of the anterior spinal artery. *Journal of the American Medical Association*, **88**, 1140-1142.

Groat, R. A., Windle, W. F. & Magoun, H. W. (1945) Functional and structural changes in monkey's brain during and after concussion. *Journal of Neurosurgery*, **2**, 26-35.

Haberer, H. (1903) Ein Fall seltenes Collateralkreislauf bei geborener Obliteration der Aorta und dessen Folgen. *Zeitschrift für Heilkunde*, **24**, 26-38.

Herren, R. Y. & Alexander, I. (1939) Sulcal and intrinsic blood vessels of human spinal cord. *Archives of Neurology and Psychiatry (Chicago)*, **41**, 678-687.

Hills, S. & Vasquez, J. M. (1962) Massive infarction of spinal cord and vertebral bodies as a complication of dissecting aneurysm of the aorta. *Circulation*, **25**, 997-1000.

Holmes, G. (1906) On the relation between loss of function and structural change in focal lesions of the central nervous system, with special reference to secondary degeneration. *Brain*, **29**, 514-523.

Holmes, G. (1915) The Goulstonian lectures on spinal injuries of warfare. *British Medical Journal*, **2**, 769-774.

Höök, O., Lidvall, H. & Åström, K.-E. (1960) Cervical disk protrusions with compression of the spinal cord. *Neurology (Minneapolis)*, **10**, 834-841.

Hughes, J. T. (1967) The blood supply and vascular disorders of the human spinal cord. D.Phil. thesis, University of Oxford.

Hughes, J. T. (1970) Thrombosis of the posterior spinal arteries. A complication of an intrathecal injection of phenol. *Neurology (Minneapolis)*, **20**, 659-664.

Hughes, J. T. (1971) Venous infarction of the spinal cord. *Neurology (Minneapolis)*, **21**, 794-800.

Hughes, J. T. (1974) Pathology of spinal cord damage in spinal injuries in *Brock's Injuries of the Brain and Spinal Cord* (Ed. Feiring, E. H.), 5th Edn., Chapter 21, Springer Pub. Co. Inc., New York.

Hughes, J. T. & Brownell, B. (1963) Aberrant nerve fibres within the spinal cord. *Journal of Neurology, Neurosurgery and Psychiatry*, **26**, 528-534.

Hughes, J. T. & Brownell, B. (1964) Cervical spondylosis complicated by anterior spinal artery thrombosis. *Neurology (Minneapolis)*, **14**, 1073-1077.

Jakob, A. (1919) Zur Pathologie der Rückenmarkerschütterung. *Zeitschrift für die gesamte Neurologie und Psychiatrie*, **51**, 247-258.

Jellinger, K. (1966) *Zur Orthologie und Pathologie der Rückenmarksdurchblutung*, Springer Verlag, Berlin.

Jennett, W. B. (1956) A study of 25 cases of compression of the cauda equina by prolapsed intervertebral discs. *Journal of Neurology, Neurosurgery and Psychiatry*, **19**, 109-116.

Jonesco-Sisesti, N. (1932) *La Syringobulbie*, Masson, Paris.

Kadyi, H. (1889) *Ueber die Blutgefässe des menschlichen Rückenmarkes*, Gubrynowicz and Schmidt, Lemberg.

Kalischer, O. (1914) Demonstration eines Präparates (Aneurysma dissecans der Aorta mit Paraplegie). *Berliner Klinische Wochenschrift*, **51**, 1286-1288.

Kosary, I. Z., Braham, J., Shaked, I. & Tadmor, R. (1969) Cervical syringomyelia associated with occipital meningioma. *Neurology (Minneapolis)*, **19**, 1127-1130.

Lange-Cosack, H. & Köhn, K. (1962) Ischämische Rückenmarkschädigung bei Aneurysm dissecans der Aorta. *Münchener medizische Wochenschrift*, **104**, 410-413.

Lindsay, J. & Hurst, J. W. (1967) Clinical features and prognosis in dissecting aneurysm of the aorta. *Circulation*, **35**, 880-888.

List, C. F. (1941) Neurologic syndromes accompanying developmental anomalies of occipital bone, atlas and axis. *Archives of Neurology and Psychiatry*, **45**, 577-616.

Logue, V. (1952) Thoracic intervertebral disc prolapse with spinal cord compression. *Journal of Neurology, Neurosurgery and Psychiatry*, **15**, 227-241.

Luschka, H. von   (1858) *Die Halbgelenke des menschlichen Körpers*, Reiner, Berlin.

McAlhany, H. J. & Netsky, M. G.   (1955) Compression of spinal cord by extrameduallary neoplasms; clinical and pathologic study. *Journal of Neuropathology and Experimental Neurology*, **14**, 276-287.

McRae, D. L.   (1953) Bony abnormalities in region of foramen magnum: correlation of anatomic and neurologic findings. *Acta radiologica*, **40**, 335-355.

Mair, W. G. P. & Druckman, R.   (1953) The pathology of spinal cord lesions and their relation to clinical features in protrusions of cervical intervertebral discs. *Brain*, **76**, 70-91.

Margulis, M. W.   (1930) Pathologische Anatomie und Klinik der akuten thrombotischen Erweichungen bei spinaler Lues. *Deutsche Zeitschrift für Nervenheilkunde*, **113**, 113-145.

Middleton, G. S. & Teacher, J. H.   (1911) Injury of the spinal cord due to rupture of an intervertebral disc during muscular effort. *Glasgow Medical Journal*, **76**, 1-6.

Moersch, F. P. & Sayre, G.   (1950) Neurologic manifestations associated with dissecting aneurysm of the aorta. *Journal of the American Medical Association*, **144**, 1141-1148.

Neumayer, E.   (1967) *Die vasculäre Myelopathie*, Springer Verlag, Berlin.

Nugent, G. R.   (1959) Clinicopathologic correlations in cervical spondylosis. *Neurology (Minneapolis)*, **9**, 273-281.

Payne, E. E. & Spillane, J. D.   (1957) The cervical spine. An anatomico-pathological study of 70 specimens (using a special technique) with particular reference to the problem of cervical spondylosis. *Brain*, **80**, 571-596.

Penning, L.   (1962) Some aspects of plain radiography of the cervical spine in chronic myelopathy. *Neurology (Minneapolis)*, **12**, 513-519.

Perier, O., Demanet, J. C., Henneaux, J. & Nunès-Vincente, A.   (1960) Existe-t-il un syndrome des artères spinales posterieures? *Revue Neurologique*, **113**, 396-409.

Petren, K.   (1898) Ein Fall von akuter Infektionskrankeit mit Thrombosen in den pialen Gefässen des Rückenmarks. *Nordiskt medicinskt arkiv*, **7**, 1-48.

Poser, C. M.   (1956) *The Relationship between Syringomyelia and Neoplasm*, Thomas, Springfield, Ill.

Reifenstein, G. H., Levine, S. A. & Gross, R. E.   (1947) Coarctation of aorta: review of 104 autopsied cases of 'adult type', 2 years of age or older. *American Heart Journal*, **33**, 146-168.

Richardson, J. C.   (1938) Spontaneous haematomyelia: short review and report of cases illustrating intramedullary angioma and syphilis of spinal cord as possible causes. *Brain*, **61**, 17-36.

Roussy, J. & Lhermitte, J.   (1918) *Blessures de la moelle et de la queue de cheval*, Masson, Paris.

Sahs, A. L.   (1942) The vascular supply of the spinal cord in monkeys. *Journal of Comparative Neurology*, **76**, 403-415.

Saunders, W. W.   (1943) Basilar impression; position of normal odontoid. *Radiology*, **41**, 589-590.

Schaltenbrandt, G.   (1951) *Die Nervenkrankheiten*, Thieme, Stuttgart.

Scharenberg, K.   (1953) Atrophy of cerebellum following pressure; study with silver carbonate. *Journal of Neuropathology and Experimental Neurology*, **12**, 11-23.

Schmaus, H.   (1890) Beiträge zur pathologischen Anatomie der Rückenmarkerschülterung. *Virchows Archiv für pathologische Anatomie*, **122**, 326-356.

Schmorl, G. & Junghans, H.   (1959) *The Human Spine in Health and Disease*, 1st American edn. (Trans. and Ed. Wilk, S. P.), Grune and Stratton, New York.

Schneider, R. C.   (1951) Syndrome in acute cervical spine injuries for which early operation is indicated. *Journal of Neurosurgery*, **8**, 360-367.

Scholtz, W. & Manuelidis, E. F.   (1951) Angiodysgenetische nekrotisierende Myelopathie. *Deutsche Zeitschrift für Nervenheilkunde*, **165**, 56-71.

Schott, E.   (1915) Schwere Rückenmarksläsion nach leichtem Trauma. *Medizinische Klinik*, **9**, 43-45.

Schwartz, E.   (1897) Präparate von einem Falle syphilitischer Meningomyelitis mit Höhlenbildung im Rückenmarke und besonderen degenerativen Veränderungen der Neuroglia. *Wiener klinische Wochenschrift*, **110**, 177.

Schwartz, G. A., Shorey, W. K. & Anderson, N. S.   (1950) Myelomalacia secondary to dissecting aneurysm of the aorta. *Archives of Neurology and Psychiatry (Chicago)*, **64**, 401-416.

Seddon, H. J.   (1935) Pott's paraplegia, prognosis and treatment. *British Journal of Surgery*, **22**, 769-799.

Shennan, T.   (1934) *Special Report Series Medical Research Council, London* No. 193, H.M. Stationery Office, London.

Spillane, J. D.   (1952) Three cases of achondroplasia with neurological complications. *Journal of Neurology, Neurosurgery and Psychiatry*, **15**, 246-252.

Spiller, W. G.   (1906) Syringomyelia, extending from the sacral region of the spinal cord through the medulla oblongata, right side of the pons and right cerebral peduncle to the upper part of the right internal capsule (syringobulbia). *British Medical Journal*, **2**, 1017-1021.

Stone, L. & Roback, H. N. (1937) Myelomalacia without thrombosis following indirect trauma (strain). *Journal of the American Medical Association*, **108**, 1698-1701.

Suh, T. H. & Alexander, L. (1939) Vascular system of the human spinal cord. *Archives of Neurology and Psychiatry (Chicago)*, **41**, 659-677.

Tyler, H. R. & Clark, O. B. (1958) Neurological complications in patients with coarction of aorta. *Neurology (Minneapolis)*, **8**, 712-718.

Wallace, D. & Bruce, A. (1910) Case of dislocation between the atlas and the axis vertebrae, with probable fracture of the odontoid process, reduction, recovery. *Review of Neurology and Psychiatry (Edinburgh)*, **8**, 1-7.

Weisman, A. D. & Adams, R. A. (1944) The neurological complications of dissecting aortic aneurysm. *Brain*, **67**, 69-92.

Wilkinson, M. (1960) The morbid anatomy of cervical spondylosis and myelopathy. *Brain*, **83**, 589-617.

Wolf, B. S., Khilnani, M. & Malis, L. I. (1956) Sagittal diameter of bony cervical canal and its significance in cervical spondylosis. *Journal of Mt. Sinai Hospital (New York)*, **23**, 283-292.

Wyburn-Mason, R. (1943) *The Vascular Abnormalities and Tumours of the Spinal Cord and its Membranes*, Kimpton, London.

Wyllie, W. G. (1923) The occurrence in osteitis deformans of lesions of the central nervous system with a report of four cases. *Brain*, **46**, 336-351.

Wyss, O. (1898) Über acute hämorrhagische Myelitis. *Deutsche medizinische Wochenschrift*, **24**, 81V.

Yoss, R. E. (1950) Vascular supply of the spinal cord: the production of vascular syndromes. *Univ. Michigan Medical Bulletin (Ann Arbor)*, **16**, 333-345.

Zeitlin, H. & Lichtenstein, B. W. (1936) Occlusion of the anterior spinal artery. *Archives of Neurology and Psychiatry (Chicago)*, **36**, 96-111.

16

Diseases of Peripheral Nerves

H. Urich

General pathology of the peripheral nervous system

The peripheral nervous system differs from the central in the nature of its supporting cell, the cell of Schwann taking the place of neuroglial cells (Schwann 1839). It extends from the glio-Schwannian junction in the cranial nerves and spinal roots to the termination of the nerve fibres in their end-organs and includes the posterior root ganglia as well as those of the autonomic nervous system.

The fundamental disease processes were studied in the last decades of the nineteenth century, largely on preparations of teased individual fibres. Subsequently teased preparations were superseded by stained sections, which yielded more information about the general structure of the nerves than on changes within the conductive elements. Even modern methods of simultaneous visualization of axons and myelin sheaths allow only tentative conclusions on the nature of the processes affecting nerve fibres.

The recent revival of interest may be ascribed on one hand to clinical progress, based on advances of applied neurophysiology and on the development of nerve and muscle biopsy, and on the other to a technical revolution which consists of a reinstatement of ancient techniques and development of new ones, particularly electron-microscopy. The latter has contributed an immense amount of information in the 25 years since the pioneering studies of Sjöstrand (1950) and Fernandez-Morán (1950). Up-to-date accounts of the ultrastructure of peripheral nerves may be found in reviews by Bischoff (1970), Peters, Palay and Webster (1970) and Wechsler (1970).

The study of teased preparations of individual fibres is now supported by quantitative measure-ments (Fullerton, Gilliatt, Lascelles and Morgan-Hughes 1965) and electron-microscopy (Spencer and Thomas 1970). Other quantitative studies are still in their infancy (Thomas 1970). Limited but important studies on normal human material have already been carried out by light (Swallow 1966; O'Sullivan and Swallow 1968) and electron-microscopy (Ochoa and Mair 1969a, b).

Observations on human material have been vastly extended by studies on experimental animals. All basic pathological processes have been adequately reproduced experimentally. Satis-factory models for some human diseases may either occur naturally or be induced artificially.

The composite picture derived from all these sources and techniques underlies our present con-ception of disease processes in the peripheral nervous system.

The components of peripheral nerves and their reactions in disease

The nerve fibre
The anatomical terminology of the peripheral nervous system is confused. The concept of a nerve fibre usually embraces the axon and its myelin sheath. As the latter is now known to be part of the cell of Schwann this cell must be included in the concept. Furthermore, the Schwann cells are surrounded by a basement membrane (probably identical with the sheath of Plenk and Laidlaw), which runs continuously over the cells supporting an individual axon, thus con-taining the whole fibre in a single unit. The term 'neurilemma' is best avoided as it has been used by various authors to denote different structures.

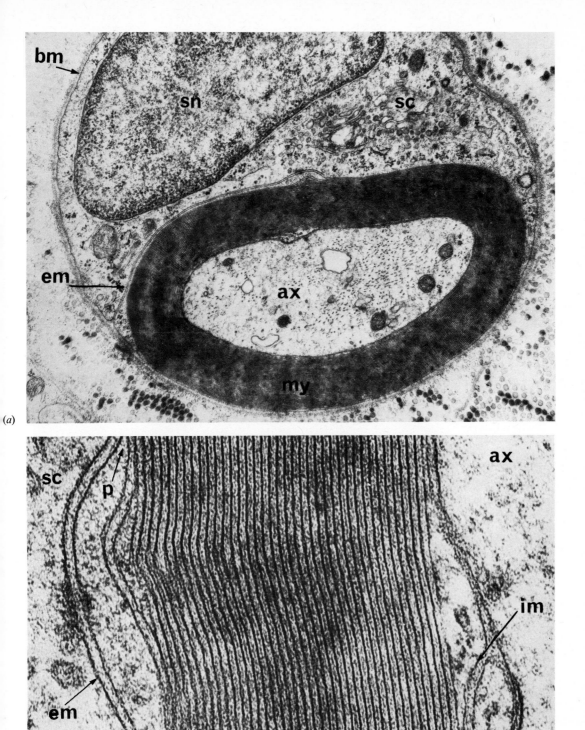

(a)

(b)

Fig. 16.1 (a) Transverse section of a human myelinated nerve fibre at the level of the Schwann cell nucleus (ax = axon, bm = basement membrane, em = external mesaxon, my = myelin sheath, sc = Schwann cell cytoplasm, sn = Schwann cell nucleus). ×26,600. (b) Higher magnification of part of the same myelin sheath showing period and intraperiod lines (ax = axon, em = external mesaxon, im = internal mesaxon, p = origin of period line, sc = Schwann cell cytoplasm). ×190,000. (By courtesy of Dr R. O. Weller and the Editor, *Journal of Neurology, Neurosurgery and Psychiatry*.)

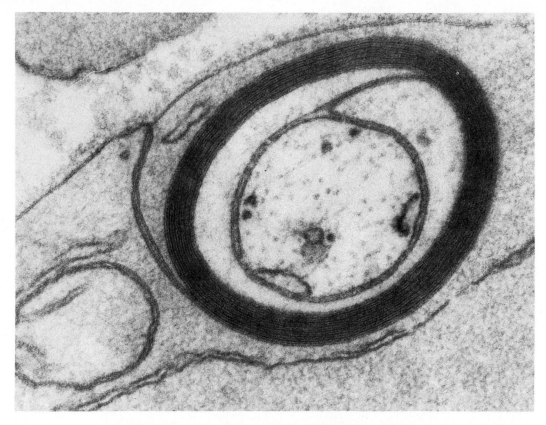

Fig. 16.2 Schwann cell of the giant nerve of the crayfish with a myelinated axon embedded in it. The laminated structure of the myelin, and both the outer and inner mesaxons are clearly demonstrated. × 24,000. (By courtesy of Professor J. D. Robertson, and the Editor, *Annals of the New York Academy of Sciences* (1961, **94**, 350, Fig. 9).)

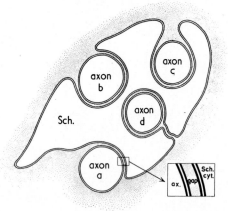

Fig. 16.3 Diagram showing a Schwann cell with four associated axons in different stages of envelopment. Only axon *d* is sufficiently deeply embedded to have a complete mesaxon formed by the enveloping double Schwann cell membranes. Robertson's 'Unit' (shown also enlarged) consists of the double membranes of both axon and cell. (Reproduced from *Electronmicroscopy in Anatomy*, London 1961, by courtesy of Professor J. D. Robertson.)

The axis cylinder

Strictly speaking, only the efferent, centrifugal fibres are axons, while the afferent, centripetal ones are dendrites. The long dendrites of the sensory peripheral nerves are, however, structurally indistinguishable from axons and it has become conventional to refer to both types of fibres by this term. The axons are roughly cylindrical in shape, but taper slightly towards the periphery. In their course they show several minor irregularities, such as constriction at the nodes of Ranvier with expansion in the paranodal regions, indentation in the region of the Schwann cell nucleus and slight narrowing at the Schmidt–Lantermann incisures.

Ultrastructurally the normal axon contains numerous neurofilaments and microtubules, a sparse smooth endoplasmic reticulum, vesicular bodies, and scanty mitochondria.

The basic pathological response of the axon is by localized swelling. These swellings, single or multiple, fusiform or ovoid, are due to excessive accumulation of fluid in the axoplasm and throw little light on the nature of the pathological process. Electron-microscopy reveals that different changes in cell organelles occur in various degenerative and regenerative processes. The various patterns described by Lampert (1967) in central axons are probably applicable to peripheral fibres as well.

Occasionally, intra-axonal inclusions, resembling corpora amylacea in structure and staining properties may be seen, particularly in peripheral ramifications. These are probably identical with the spherical expansions seen in supravitally stained preparations of intramuscular nerve endings. They apparently constitute an ageing phenomenon.

The peculiar axonal swellings found in the central nervous system in infantile neuro-axonal dystrophy also occur in the peripheral (Bérard-Badier, Gambarelli, Pinsard, Hassoun and Toga 1971) and autonomic nervous systems (Bérard-Badier, Toga, Gambarelli, Hassoun, Pellissier, Pinsard and Bernard 1974).

An unusual type of expansion has been described by Asbury, Gale, Cox, Baringer and Berg (1972) in which large fusiform or ovoid axonal swellings were filled with tangled neurofilaments. This was found in a case of a slowly progressive polyneuropathy in childhood ('giant axonal neuropathy').

The Schwann cell and the myelin sheath

The supporting cells of the peripheral nervous system are intimately associated with the axons throughout their course. It is now known that every axon is invaginated into the cytoplasm of a Schwann cell, carrying the plasma membrane of that cell with it. The membrane surrounds the axon and is connected with the surface by a mesaxon (Gasser 1955) which represents the infolded surfaces of the membrane in close apposition. Several unmyelinated axons may share a single Schwann cell, but myelinated fibres are invariably single. The cells carrying unmyelinated axons are sometimes called Remak cells.

The myelin sheath is part of the cell of Schwann and consists of the reduplicated cell membrane wound spirally around the axon. In transverse electronmicrographs it forms a laminated structure in which the lighter lines represent the layer of the plasma membrane separated by darker lines of fusion (Fig. 16.1). Of the latter, the less dense line (the intraperiod line) is in continuity with the line of fusion of the mesaxon, while the dense line (the period line) represents the line of fusion of the cytoplasmic surfaces. The periodicity of peripheral myelin differs slightly from that of central myelin, the lamellae being thicker. The distance between the centres of adjacent dense lines is 11·9 nm in sections (Karlsson 1966) and 18·5 nm in freeze-etched preparations (Bischoff and Moor 1967). Two parts of the mesaxon remain separate from the fused myelin sheath: that joining the myelin sheath to the surface of the Schwann cell (the external mesaxon) and that joining it to the axon (the internal mexason) (Fig. 16.2). The structure of the sheath has been largely elucidated by studies of myelination in animal embryos (Geren 1945; Robertson 1955) (Fig. 16.3). The developing unmyelinated axons invaginate the cytoplasm of the Schwann cells forming several mesaxons (Fig. 16.4). Prior to myelination, the Schwann cell divides, leaving one axon per cell. A rotation of the mesaxon now begins, with apposition of layer upon layer of the reduplicated cell membrane around the axon. To begin with, layers are separated by Schwann cell cytoplasm, which subsequently disappears during the process of condensation, leaving only a thin layer of cytoplasm on the surface of the sheath, and larger accumulations in the nuclear region, at the nodes of Ranvier and in the clefts of Schmidt–Lantermann. This process has now been confirmed in human embryos (Dunn 1970).

Longitudinally, the myelin sheaths form segments co-extensive with the length of the cell of Schwann. These segments vary in length with the size of the fibre and the thickness of the myelin sheath: the larger the fibre the longer the segments (Key and Retzius 1876; Vizoso and Young 1948). Between two adjacent segments, there is a gap known as the node of Ranvier (Ranvier 1878) (Fig. 16.5). This is now known to be filled by the cytoplasm of the two adjacent Schwann cells interlocked by nodal processes. In the paranodal regions the reduplicated layers of the myelin form closed loops, ensuring the continuity of the invaginated and convoluted cell membrane.

In the longitudinal course of each myelin segment there are several oblique or spiral gaps, known as the clefts or incisures of Schmidt–Lantermann (Schmidt 1874; Lantermann 1877). Ultrastructurally they do not represent breaches in continuity of the lamellae, but areas where the lamellae are separated by persistent Schwann cell

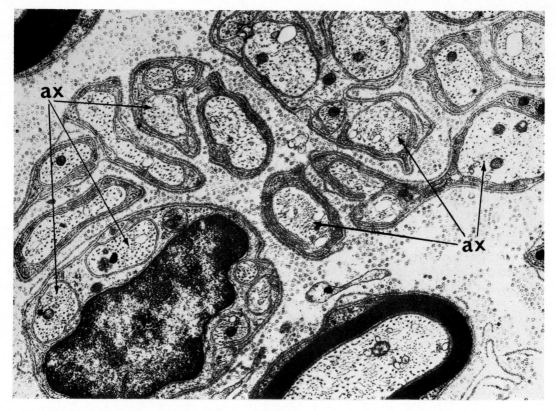

Fig. 16.4 Transverse section through nerve of human infant, showing predominance of unmyelinated axons, several of which share the same Schwann cell (ax = axon). ×13,500. (By courtesy of Dr R. O. Weller and the Editor, *Journal of Neurology, Neurosurgery and Psychiatry.*)

cytoplasm (Robertson 1958). Their significance is conjectural; according to Dunn (1970) they represent growth zones in the progressive elongation of the Schwann cells and myelin segments.

The Schwann cell is remarkably stable. Once the association of axon and Schwann cell has been established, it remains constant throughout life except in pathological conditions. The Schwann cell grows in length with the growing axon and apparently does not multiply after the onset of myelination.

The situation changes in pathological conditions, whether in primary diseases of the Schwann cell or of the axon. Once the Schwann cell has lost its fixed relationship to the axon it may become mobile (the migratory phase of Young 1942 and of Lubinska 1961a). It becomes capable of mitotic division and in all regenerative conditions replaces the lost long internodes by several short ones. Some demyelination and remyelination may also occur with advancing age (Lascelles and Thomas 1966; Arnold and Harriman 1970).

The cell of Schwann appears to have phagocytic properties. It is capable of autophagy, or destruction of its own components, viz. the myelin sheath. It also engulfs fragments of the degenerated axon and breaks it down into smaller components. Whether it is capable of chemical as well as mechanical degradation of the products of breakdown is debatable. The prevailing view favours the macrophages as the site of chemical change in the structure of lipids.

Another controversial issue is the formation of collagen fibres by the Schwann cell. Some authorities (Causey 1960; Barton 1962) maintain that this cell has fibroblastic properties. Others (Thomas 1963) believe that all collagen fibres in the nerve bundles are produced by endoneurial fibroblasts. Gamble and Eames (1964) observed pockets of collagen invaginated into the cytoplasm of Schwann cells. As these are separated from the plasma membrane by an intact basement membrane it seems unlikely that the collagen fibres should be a product of the Schwann cells.

The connective tissues of the nerve

The nerve fibres are joined together into fascicles or funiculi. These are not constant throughout the course of the nerve but join together to form larger bundles and separate again into smaller fascicles, forming complicated plexiform arrangements. The connective tissues which bind the fibres together follow the course of the funiculi.

The *endoneurium* consists of predominantly longitudinally orientated collagen fibres condensed around each nerve fibre (the sheath of Key and Retzius) and more loosely arranged between nerve fibres. A few larger septa, containing blood vessels of arteriolar or venular calibre, separate each fascicle into several compartments. The cellular composition of the endoneurium is still

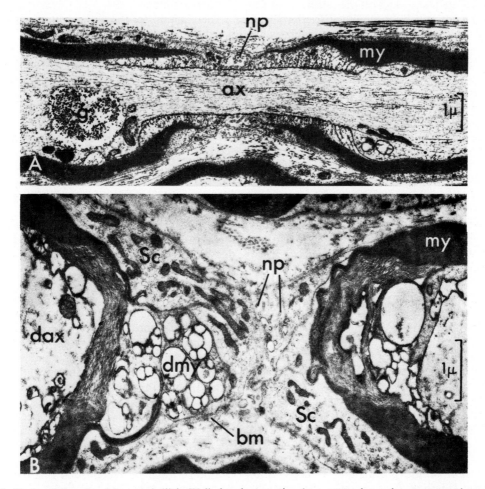

Fig. 16.5 Nodes of Ranvier: (*a*) normal, (*b*) in Wallerian degeneration (ax = axon, bm = basement membrane, dax = degenerating axon, dmy = degenerating myelin, g = glycogen, my = myelin, np = Schwann cell nodal processes, sc = Schwann cell cytoplasm). (*a*) ×10,000, (*b*) ×16,000. (By courtesy of Professor P. K. Thomas.)

Their terminology is confused and it is desirable to keep their classification as simple as possible by dividing them into three compartments (Key and Retzius 1873): the endoneurium which represents all connective tissue structures within the funiculi, the perineurium which forms a specialized sheath around each fascicle and the epineurium which is the extrafascicular connective tissue.

controversial. Estimates of the population of endoneurial fibroblasts range from 5% (Causey 1960) to 30 to 40% (Thomas 1963).

The spaces between the collagenous sheaths and septa contain fluid. This is separated from the blood stream by a 'blood nerve barrier', depending largely on tight junctions between endothelial cells, and from the epineurial lymphatics by the perineurium (Olsson and Reese 1971). Both a centrifugal (Weiss, Wang, Taylor and Edds 1945) and centripetal (Brierley and Field 1949) flow of endoneurial fluid have been demonstrated. Its connections with the subarachnoid (Brierley and Field 1948) or subdural space (Dorang and Matzke 1960) are still controversial. The communication is not entirely free, as there seems to be a block for particulate matter and cellular elements at the level of the posterior root ganglion (Brierley 1950). Accumulation of watery endoneurial fluid, which does not take up stains, is seen in pathological conditions. The significance of this endoneurial oedema is not clear. Krücke (1941-42) considers it a primary lesion, due to increased capillary permeability and leading to fibrosis of the endo-neurium by organization. Weiss (1943) ascribes it to obstruction of the endoneurial flow by scarring due to other causes. Occasionally the oedema fluid contains basophilic material, with the staining properties of an acid mucopolysaccharide ('mucoid degeneration', Krücke 1939).

Fibrosis is the typical response of the endoneurium to damage. It is particularly conspicuous in the terminal stages of Wallerian degeneration (see p. 696) and is often a useful indication of axonal loss in degenerative processes.

Small nodules of hyalinized collagen (bodies of Rénaut 1881) are often found in the endoneurium of major nerves, particularly in areas where the nerves are subject to pressure. They are devoid of pathological significance.

Mast cells are present in the normal endoneurium in small numbers (Torp 1961; Gamble and Goldby 1961). They undergo marked proliferation in a variety of pathological conditions (Enerbäck, Olsson and Sourander 1965; Olsson 1968; Olsson and Sjöstrand 1969).

The *perineurium* begins at the level of the radicular nerve, the nerve roots being invested by an extension of the pia mater. It consists of concentric layers of fusiform cells separated by collagen fibres and elastic laminae. The origin of the cells is controversial, both a mesenchymal and neuroectodermal derivation being postulated. Ultrastructurally they resemble Schwann cells, but differ from them by the presence of pinocytotic vesicles.

The thickness of the perineurium varies considerably within the same nerve, generally smaller bundles having a thinner perineurium than the larger ones. The function of the perineurium is that of a diffusion barrier separating the endo-

neurial fluid from epineurial lymph (Feng and Liu 1949; Olsson 1966). This diffusion barrier is maintained by tight junctions between perineurial cells (Olsson and Reese 1971; Kristensson and Olsson 1971) and may be damaged in pathological conditions such as trauma (Olsson and Kristensson 1973). The elastic component of the perineurium may also provide tensile strength to the nerve bundles.

The reactions of the perineurium in disease are poorly understood. Hyperplasia of the perineurium may be more apparent than real and due to collapse and shrinkage of a large fascicle. Fibrosis of the perineurium usually follows fibrosis of the endoneurium, so that in the end-stage of Wallerian degeneration they may fuse together to form solid fibrous cords.

A selective fibrosis of the perineurium, consequent upon inflammatory infiltration, and affecting random branches of cutaneous nerves, has been described by Asbury, Picard and Baringer (1972) under the name 'sensory perineuritis'.

The *epineurium* consists of loose areolar tissue separating the fascicles and surrounded by a denser fibrous sheath. It contains the vasa nervorum, the detailed anatomy of which was described by Adams (1941-42). It also contains lymphatics which drain into the regional lymph nodes. Small amounts of adipose tissue are a normal constituent of the interfascicular epineurium.

The epineurium is particularly subject to processes affecting the nerves from outside, such as trauma, pressure and inflammatory processes extending from the neighbourhood. It responds by fibrosis, the loose areolar connective tissue being replaced by dense collagenous scars.

The posterior root ganglia

Our knowledge of the normal anatomy of the sensory ganglia (reviewed by de Castro 1932a and by Stöhr 1928) is still far from complete. The ganglion cells are predominantly spherical in shape and can be subdivided into three groups according to size: large (50 to 100 mμ diameter), medium-sized (30 to 50 mμ) and small (15 to 30 mμ). The composition of individual ganglia varies, most of the large cells being found in the cervical and lumbar regions. The nucleus of a ganglion cell shows a typical neuronal structure. Nissl bodies are generally small and aggregated round the periphery. Melanin pig-

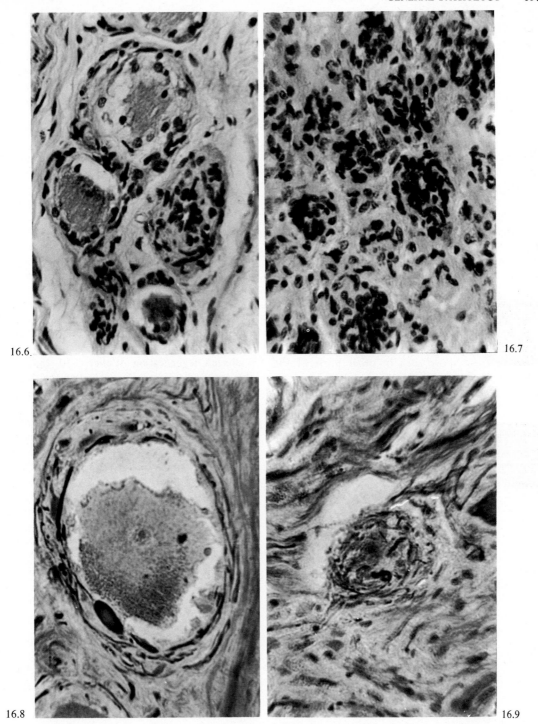

Fig. 16.6 Group of degenerating neurons in posterior root ganglion: vacuolation of cytoplasm and proliferation of capsule cells. H & E.   ×450.
Fig. 16.7 Group of residual nodules of Nageotte. H & E.   ×450.
Fig. 16.8 Degenerating neuron surrounded by argyrophilic 'basket' fibres. Glees-Marsland and Luxol fast blue.   ×540.
Fig. 16.9 Tangle of argyrophilic fibres persisting in nodule of Nageotte. Glees-Marsland and Luxol fast blue.   ×540.

ment is present in most of the medium-sized cells. Lipofuscin appears in the cytoplasm relatively early in life and increases with age.

Most of the ganglion cells are unipolar, a single process emerging from the axon hillock and, after a variable course, dividing into a usually larger peripheral dendrite and a more slender centrally directed axon. The proximal part of the process tends to form loops, which take a particularly complicated form in medium-sized cells. Numerous fine afferent fibres terminate on the surface of the ganglion cell.

Each neuron is surrounded by a layer of small cells, the capsule or satellite cells. They are of neuroectodermal origin and may be considered to be modified Schwann cells. These are not evenly distributed around the neuronal body, there being usually an aggregation of capsule cells near the axon hillock, this being particularly abundant when the axon forms an elaborate loop which is completely ensheathed by capsule cells.

In addition the ganglion is traversed by bundles of myelinated nerve fibres which do not differ in structure from those seen in other parts of the peripheral nervous system.

The pathology of the posterior root ganglia has been reviewed by de Castro (1932a) and more recently by Döring (1955). While various types of degeneration of the ganglion cells have been described, their common feature is fenestration with peripheral vacuoles appearing in the cytoplasm. This may proceed to complete disintegration of the cell. Degeneration of the ganglion cell is accompanied by two additional phenomena: proliferation of the capsule cells and hypertrophy of the circumferential afferent nerve terminals (Fig. 16.6).

The capsule cells undergo hyperplasia and invade the disintegrating nerve cells, displaying phagocytic properties. When the remnants of the neuron are completely removed, the capsule cells become pyknotic and form tightly packed cellular nodules, *the residual nodules of Nageotte* (1907) (Fig. 16.7). The subsequent fate of these nodules is not clear. Presumably they also disappear in time, as their number in totally destroyed ganglia is far smaller than the original population of ganglion cells.

The hypertrophy of the fine fibres which terminate on the cell body is a more erratic phenomenon. Around some degenerating neurons these fibres become very conspicuous and form argyrophilic baskets (Fig. 16.8). These may

persist to the stage of formation of nodules of Nageotte, while other nodules are devoid of nerve fibres (Fig. 16.9). The significance of these formations is unknown, but their presence provides additional evidence of a degenerative process.

In evaluating the lesions in posterior root ganglia three factors should be taken into consideration: post-mortem artefacts, the patient's age and his drug history. Artefacts are common and tend to mimic degenerative changes in neurons, which should be dismissed in the absence of vital reactions. Loss of ganglion cells occurs with advancing age, and occasional nodules of Nageotte in the elderly are of no significance. Finally, the ganglia are sensitive to the action of neurotoxic drugs as they are not protected by a blood–nerve barrier. It is therefore essential to obtain a full drug history before attempting an interpretation of the findings.

Degenerative and regenerative processes in the peripheral nervous system

Wallerian degeneration (Waller 1850, 1852)

This term was originally applied to the degeneration of the distal portion of a mechanically transected fibre of a peripheral nerve. It has been legitimately extended to include degeneration of any severed axon, irrespective of the nature of the process which has separated it from its cell body and it is probably correct to use the term in this context both in the central and in the peripheral nervous systems. The concept does not include degenerative processes in an axon which remains in continuity with the cell body and should not be applied either to retrograde changes in the proximal stump or to the 'dying-back' phenomenon. If structural changes reminiscent of Wallerian degeneration are found in these circumstances they may be called Wallerian-type degeneration.

The sequence of structural changes, as seen under the light microscope, has been extensively studied and repeatedly described. Excellent accounts of the classical findings are those of Ramón y Cajal (1928) and Nageotte (1932). The lesions, as observed in an experimental animal (rabbit), may be summarized as follows. The changes in axons, as demonstrated by silver impregnation, start as irregular swellings which give an axon a moniliform or varicose appearance. This occurs within hours of transection and is well seen in many axons after 12 hours. The second phase is that of granular disintegration of the neurofibrils, which begins after 24 hours and is widespread at the end of 4 days. The third stage consists of fragmentation of the axon and longitudinal retraction of the fragments, which become irregularly convoluted into spiral or helicoidal forms. This process occurs at different speeds in different axons, some beginning to break up about the second day, others keeping their continuity until the latter part of the first week. The final stage is that of resorption, which

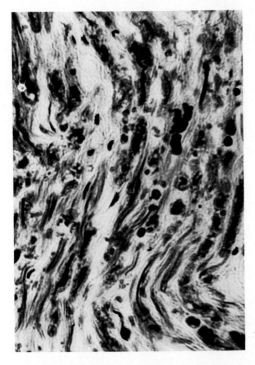

Fig. 16.10 Fragmentation of axons and myelin sheaths in Wallerian degeneration. Glees-Marsland and Luxol fast blue. × 500.

begins at the end of the first week and is complete after 3 weeks.

Pari passu with changes in the axons, structural alterations occur in the myelin sheath. The first changes can be observed in some sheaths after 14 or 16 hours. They consist of retraction of myelin from the nodes of Ranvier, with widening of the nodal gaps. The clefts of Schmidt–Lantermann also become wider and more prominent. Subsequently the myelin tubes split in the line of the clefts and subsidiary clefts appear, which leads to further splitting of the sheath into short cylinders. The speed of the

process varies in different fibres, but the fragmentation is complete by the fourth day. The fragments of myelin enclose the broken-up pieces of axon, forming ovoids or 'digestion chambers' (Fig. 16.10). Apart from axonal remnants, these ovoids contain a certain amount of unstainable fluid. During the subsequent days the large ellipsoids break up into smaller fragments. At this stage a chemical change with increasing sudanophilia also takes place. From the tenth day onwards the fragments have become largely converted into fatty droplets, which are gradually removed. All fatty remnants disappear by the end of 3 months.

During this process of myelin disintegration the Schwann cell undergoes reactive changes. The cytoplasm of the perinuclear region becomes more abundant, fills the cleft between the myelin fragments and reaches the axon by the second day. After the fourth day, the cytoplasm of the Schwann cells forms a continuous cylinder containing engulfed myelin debris. At the same time, mitotic division begins in the Schwann nuclei and this process reaches its height between the sixth and ninth days, gradually declining during the third week. The end-result is the filling of the endoneurial sheaths by columns of short Schwann cells, known as the *cell-bands of Büngner* (1891).

The subsequent fate of the affected fibres depends on the presence or absence of regeneration. If this is inhibited, the Schwann cells undergo gradual atrophy with simultaneous multiplication of the endoneurial collagen fibres, until ultimately the tube is converted into a solid fibrous cord.

This sequence of events is common to all species, the only significant variation being in the speed of reaction. Very little is known of the time-table of Wallerian degeneration in man; it is, however, highly probable that the evolution of the process is far slower than that observed in small laboratory animals.

Electron-microscopy of Wallerian degeneration has been the subject of several studies (Vial 1958; Glimstedt and Wohlfart 1960; Barton 1962; Webster 1962; Wechsler and Hager 1962; Nathaniel and Pease 1963; O'Daly and Imaeda 1967). In summary, the findings indicate that changes in the axons precede those seen in the myelin sheath. They consist of disintegration of the neurofilaments, swelling of the mitochondria and vesicular bodies and the appearance of dense

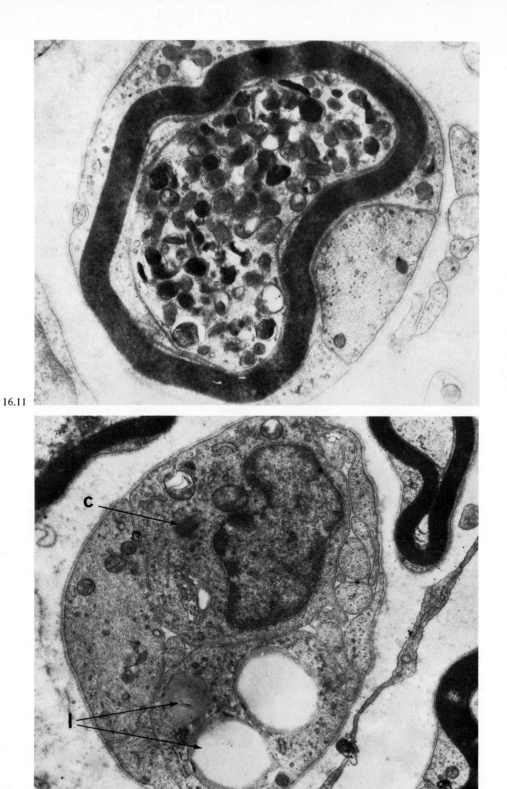

16.11

16.12

Fig. 16.11 Dense membranous bodies in axon undergoing early Wallerian degeneration. ×21,000. (By courtesy of Dr R. O. Weller.)

Fig. 16.12 Cluster of Schwann cells devoid of axons in late stage of Wallerian degeneration: cell band of Bungner (c = centriole, 1 = lipid droplets). ×12,500. (By courtesy of Dr R. O. Weller.)

membranous bodies (Fig. 16.11). These may represent degenerate mitochondria (Webster 1962) or lysosomes (Holtzman and Novikoff 1965) or both (Ballin and Thomas 1969*a*). Progressive degenerative changes in the organelles are associated with fragmentation of the axoplasm. Changes in the myelin sheath begin at the nodes of Ranvier where the myelin loops retract from the nodes, while the cytoplasm of the Schwann cell remains in continuity (Ballin and Thomas 1969*a*). Separation of the myelin lamellae also occurs at the clefts of Schmidt–Lantermann, the free edges of the short segments of myelin coming together to form ovoids, which encircle the axonal fragments while retaining their normal laminated structure. The ovoids and their contents remain within the cytoplasm of the Schwann cells, where they undergo a gradual disintegration into smaller fragments. Finally the fragments are extruded into the cytoplasm of macrophages, which appear in large numbers first in the endoneurium and then penetrate the basement membrane of the nerve fibre. The Schwann cells undergo both hypertrophy and hyperplasia and arrange themselves into clusters which represent the cell-bands of Büngner (Fig. 16.12). Simultaneously new collagen fibres appear around them, mainly within the original inner endoneurial sheaths, (Thomas 1964). As these become more abundant the cell-bands become thinner and their nuclei sparse.

Degeneration and regeneration of unmyelinated fibres has been studied by Dyck and Hopkins (1972). The changes in the axon resemble those seen in Wallerian degeneration in myelinated fibres, but are not accompanied by appropriate changes in the Schwann cells. Both degeneration and regeneration proceed more rapidly in unmyelinated than in myelinated fibres.

Changes in the proximal segment: axonal reaction
Alteration in structure at the proximal stump of the transected segment starts within a few hours of transection (Cajal 1928). Apart from the degeneration and disintegration of mechanically damaged portions, every nerve fibre breaks up, up to the level of the first node of Ranvier above the level of section. In its details this process resembles that seen in Wallerian degeneration. When the viable portion of the fibre is reached, the first change is swelling of the axon, which develops a club-like terminal expansion (Fig. 16.13), which may vary considerably in shape and size: most are oval, some are imperfectly formed, conical or spindle shaped, and giant forms are occasionally observed. The latter are thought to be degenerating and not to give rise to sprouts of regenerating fibres; the term 'retraction bulbs' may be legitimately applied to them. All terminal expansions show a great affinity for silver, thought to be due to multiplication of neurofibrils. Electron-microscopy (Lampert 1967)

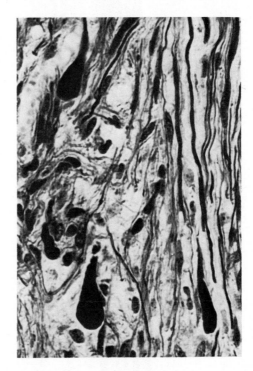

Fig. 16.13 Club-like expansions of end of proximal portions of severed axons. Glees-Marsland. ×650. (By permission of the Editor, *Brain*.)

confirms this proliferation of microtubules and neurofilaments and also shows the presence of large and prominent mitochondria; dense bodies on the other hand are scanty.

The proximal fibre remains myelinated, but teased preparations show widening of the nodes of Ranvier, extending over up to three terminal segments (Lubinska 1961*b*). Some division of the Schwann cells also occurs.

The changes of axonal reaction in the parent cell body are described in Chapter 1.

Regeneration of nerve fibres
The formation of terminal expansions is a preliminary to the formation of axoplasmic sprouts,

which thus become growth bulbs analogous to embryonic growth cones. Terminal sprouting begins in the experimental animal about 24 hours

fibres in which the terminal bulb has been imperfectly formed, the new axonal sprouts may arise collaterally from a more proximal part of

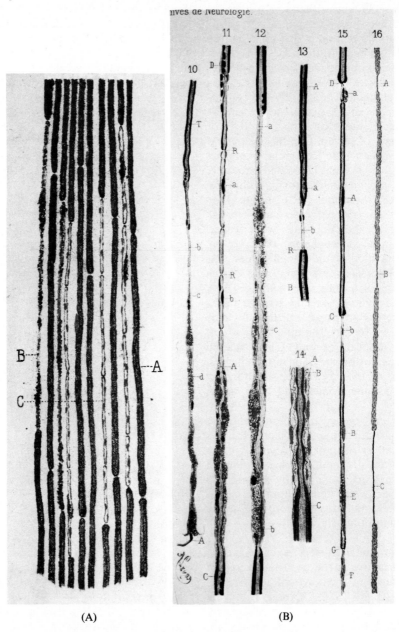

(A)   (B)

Fig. 16.14 Lead neuropathy. Segmental demyelination. Illustrations from Gombault's article on experimental lead neuropathy. Osmic acid and picrocarmine.

after the transection. Several fine fibres originate from every growth bulb, most of which grow in parallel bundles in the direction of the original axon, but some retrograde fibres also appear. In

the axon. These often arrange themselves spirally and form tangled skeins around the remnant of the original axons. These formations are known as the *spirals of Perroncito* (1907). The subsequent growth and organization of the axonal sprouts depends largely on the conditions at the site of transection: these will be considered in connection with traumatic lesions of peripheral nerves.

All axonal sprouts behave like unmyelinated fibres and initially several of them share the cytoplasm of the same Schwann cell. Their subsequent separation, during the process of myelination, resembles normal embryonic development.

Collateral sprouting

Whenever an axon is destroyed, neighbouring nerve fibres react by collateral sprouting (Edds 1949). Fine axonal branches, originating from the nodes of Ranvier, grow in the direction of the denervated end-organ, leading to its partial re-innervation. This mechanism is best observed on preterminal intramuscular fibres stained intravitally. It is probably responsible for the functional recovery of partially denervated muscle in situations where regeneration is impossible (e.g. after acute poliomyelitis). The end-result is the formation of giant motor units, in which a far larger number of muscle fibres is stimulated by a single anterior horn cell than in the normal situation.

The 'dying-back' phenomenon

The term 'dying-back' was first used by Greenfield (1954) to describe the peripheral accentuation of loss of nerve fibres in systemic degenerations of the central nervous system. It was applied to the peripheral nervous system by Cavanagh (1964) to denote processes in which damage to the neuron manifests itself first in the most distal parts of the cell processes. It may then progress until the cell body is ultimately destroyed, or may become arrested and be followed by regeneration of the destroyed peripheral parts. If this view of a diseased cell unable to maintain the metabolic demands of the periphery is correct, lesions should be observed both in the centrifugal and centripetal fibres of the affected cells. This has indeed been demonstrated (Prineas 1969a, b) in the sensory fibres which enter the posterior columns, where the first degenerative changes are found in the *boutons terminaux* of the gracile and cuneate nuclei. The pattern of breakdown of the degenerating axons and the associated changes in the Schwann cells resemble closely those seen in Wallerian degeneration. In addition, some changes may occur in Schwann cells surrounding

the still viable axon; breakdown of myelin may occur at the nodes of Ranvier with widening of the nodal gap (Hopkins 1968).

Ultrastructural studies (Prineas 1969a, b) have demonstrated considerable differences in the pattern of axonal degeneration in various 'dying-back' conditions. It appears that different noxious agents may damage different cell organelles, leading to diverse electron-microscopic appearances of the dystrophic axon.

Segmental demyelination

This process occurs in primary diseases of the Schwann cell in which the axon remains substantially unaffected. It was first described by Gombault (1880-81) in experimental lead poisoning in the guinea pig (Fig. 16.14), and subsequently studied in greater detail by Stransky

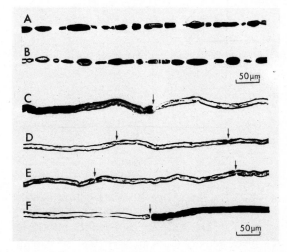

Fig. 16.15 Teased single fibre preparations contrasting segmental demyelination (C-F) with Wallerian degeneration (A-B). The demyelinated internode shows early remyelination in five short segments. Osmium tetroxide. × 130. (By courtesy of Professor P. K. Thomas.)

(1902-03). Meyer (1881) first reported it in human nerves in diphtheritic neuropathy. The basic lesion consists of degeneration of individual Schwann cells with loss of myelin in the appropriate internodes (Fig. 16.15). The destroyed Schwann cell is then replaced by several new cells, usually four to five, in heavily myelinated fibres. Remyelination gradually takes place, the new myelin sheaths slowly increasing in thickness until the original segment is replaced by several short, but otherwise normal, internodes (Fig. 16.16).

The exact nature of the process was largely elucidated by electron-microscopy. This was carried out on experimental diphtheritic neuropathy by Webster, Spiro, Waksman and Adams (1961) and Weller (1965), on lead poisoning in rats by Lampert and Schochet (1968) and on experimental allergic neuritis by Lampert (1969) and by Schröder and Krücke (1970). The findings, in summary, indicate that the first change is a swelling in the Schwann cell cytoplasm. In small fibres this is associated with increased lysosomal activity, which leads to a breakdown of myelin along the entire length of an internode (Weller and Mellick 1966). In large fibres, this

lamellae ultimately reconstitutes the myelin sheath (Fig. 16.18). Throughout this process the basement membrane of the nerve fibre remains intact and all multiplication and migration of Schwann cells occurs within it. Electron-microscopic studies of remyelination include those of Allt (1969, 1972) Ballin and Thomas (1969b) and Prineas (1971).

In human pathology, the process of segmental demyelination has been shown to occur in diphtheria (Fisher and Adams 1956), in acute infective polyneuritis (Asbury, Arnason and Adams 1969), in diabetes (Thomas and Lascelles 1966), in metachromatic leucodystrophy (Webster 1962;

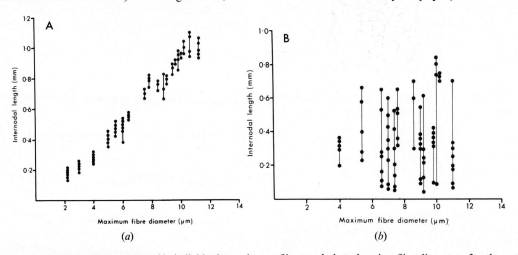

Fig. 16.16 Internodal lengths measured in individual teased nerve fibres and plotted against fibre diameter, after the method of Fullerton *et al.*, in (A) normal nerve and (B) segmental demyelination and remyelination. Note large number of abnormally short internodes in (B). (By courtesy of Professor P. K. Thomas.)

lysosomal activity is not apparent and the damage starts at the nodes of Ranvier (Weller and Nester 1972). This is followed by splitting of the myelin lamellae, both along the dense and the less dense lines. Concurrently with these degenerative phenomena, proliferation of Schwann cells takes place and cytoplasmic processes of several new cells insert themselves between and around the myelin fragments, establishing contact with the denuded axon (Fig. 16.17). These cells engulf the debris of the old myelin, which undergoes further disintegration though probably without chemical degradation. The latter takes place within macrophages, to which the myelin debris is transmitted. When the new Schwann cells establish contact with the axon, remyelination begins by the formation of a mesaxon and its spiralling round the axon. The fusion of the

Dayan 1967), in hypertrophic neuropathy (Thomas and Lascelles 1967) and probably in some other conditions.

Hypertrophic interstitial neuropathy

For a long time this was thought to be a specific lesion characteristic of the familial hypertrophic neuropathy of Déjerine and Sottas. The typical appearances of this condition consist of swelling of the nerves, in which widely separated and poorly myelinated axons are surrounded by concentric 'onion-bulb' structures consisting of Schwann cells and collagen fibres (Fig. 16.19). The Schwannian nature of these structures, first suggested by Bertrand (Marie and Bertrand 1918; Souques and Bertrand 1921), has been confirmed by electron-microscopy (Garcin, Lapresle, Fardeau and Recondo 1966; Weller 1967; Webster,

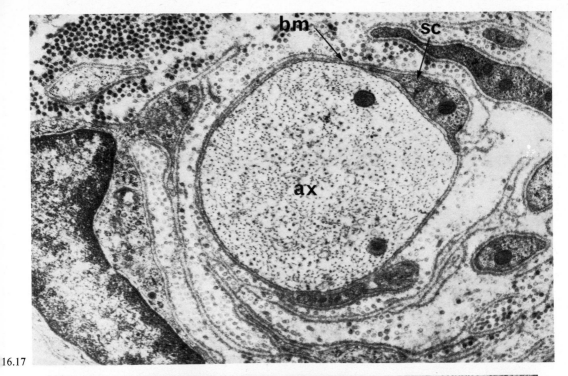

16.17

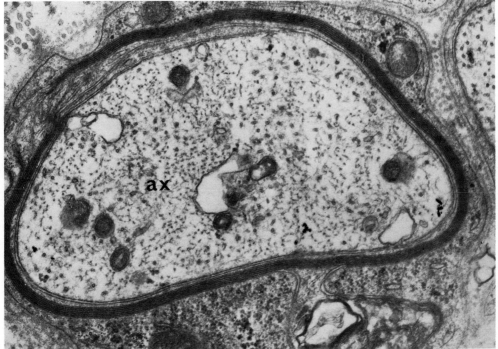

16.18

Fig. 16.17 Completely demyelinated large axon adjacent to Schwann cell cytoplasm (ax = axon, bm = basement membrane, sc = Schwann cell cytoplasm). ×17,500. (By courtesy of Dr R. O. Weller and the Editor, *Journal of Neurology, Neurosurgery and Psychiatry*.)

Fig. 16.18 Remyelinating axon surrounded by a thin, incompletely fused myelin sheath (ax = axon). ×29,700. (By courtesy of Dr R. O. Weller and the Editor, *Journal of Neurology, Neurosurgery and Psychiatry*.)

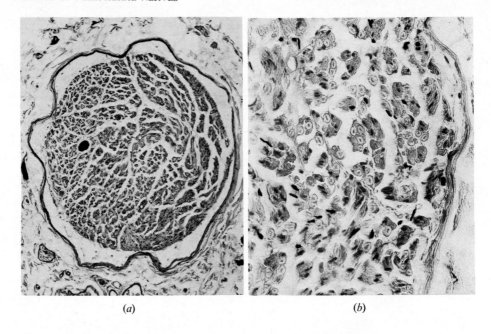

(a)   (b)

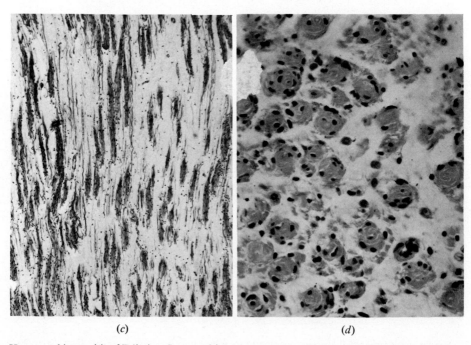

(c)   (d)

Fig. 16.19 Hypertrophic neuritis of Déjerine–Sottas. (a) Low-power view of a nerve bundle to show the loose, wrinkled perineurium and the space under it. ×75. (b) Transverse section of nerve. Many axons are still seen surrounded by myelin (unstained). Haematoxylin van Gieson. (c) Longitudinal section of nerve showing great separation of fibres. (By courtesy of Dr Bosanquet.) (d) Transverse section of a nerve with considerable collagenous thickening round the individual fibres.

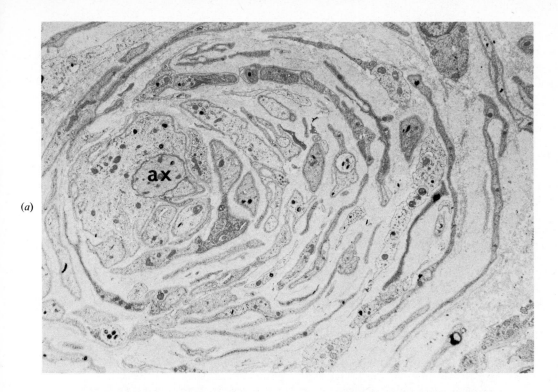

(a)

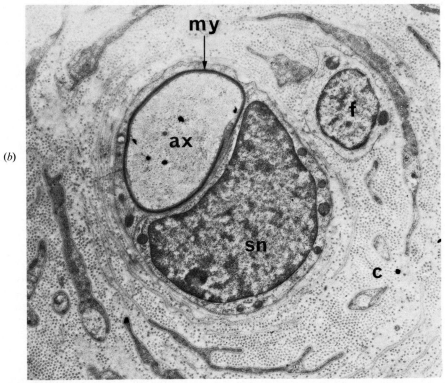

(b)

Fig. 16.20 (*a*) Low-power electronmicrograph of 'onion-bulb' formation in hypertrophic neuropathy showing concentric arrangement of Schwann cell processes (ax = axon). ×2880. (*b*) Higher power view of 'onion-bulb' with remyelinating axon in centre, surrounded by concentric Schwann cell processes separated by collagen fibres (ax = axon, c = collagen, f = fibroblast, my = myelin, sn = Schwann cell nucleus). ×6000. (By courtesy of Dr R. O. Weller and the Editor, *Journal of Neurology, Neurosurgery and Psychiatry*.)

Schröder, Asbury and Adams 1967). They consist of concentric layers of Schwann cell processes, separated by sparse collagen fibres (Fig. 16.20). They are apparently the result of repeated, or continuous, hyperplasia of Schwann cells in the course of a chronic demyelinating process. This lesion may occur, albeit on a limited scale, in any disease associated with segmental demyelination (Thomas and Lascelles 1967) and can be reproduced experimentally (Weller and Das Gupta 1968; Dyck 1969).

Intercalated segments

Not infrequently short internodes are found between two apparently normal segments (Rénaut 1881). These were called 'intercalated internodes' by Lubinska (1958). They occur in any condition in which a widening of the node of Ranvier has led to the formation of a nodal gap which cannot be bridged by extension of the neighbouring Schwann cells and is filled by a new one (Allt 1969). Considering the large variety of processes which may lead to widening of the nodal gaps, such as incomplete segmental demyelination, axonal reaction, the dying-back process etc., intercalated segments must be considered the end-result of a non-specific reparative process which throws no light on the nature of the original disease.

Pathophysiological correlations

Owing to the development of clinical electrophysiology, it is now possible to correlate abnormalities of function with structural alterations (Gilliatt 1969). The Schwann cell appears to play an important part in conductivity and, in human disease, severe slowing of conduction is associated with segmental demyelination. Conduction remains normal or slightly impaired in primary disease of the axon, at least as long as some large, fast-conducting axons are preserved, there being a positive correlation between conduction velocity and thickness of the myelin sheath (Sanders and Whitteridge 1946).

It is more difficult to establish a correlation between conduction velocity and effective function. In the early stages of massive demyelination, there is a total conduction block leading to abolition of function. Function, however, tends to recover rapidly, and this recovery may precede histological evidence of remyelination and the return of conduction velocity to normal figures

(Morgan-Hughes 1965). Mere slowing of conduction velocity appears to affect only those functions which depend on a strict synchronicity of discharges, such as tendon reflexes and perception of vibration.

An additional question arises, whether the enveloping Schwann cell is essential not only for the normal function but also for the maintenance of the integrity of the axon. It is well established that for most of its metabolic needs, particularly protein and enzyme synthesis, the axon depends on its parent cell body, and the continuous axoplasmic flow maintains the uniformity of its internal composition (Lubinska 1964). Nevertheless, there is evidence that, for some of its metabolic needs, the axon may depend on the Schwann cell (Schmidt 1958). Transport of labelled amino acids through the Schwann cell to the axon has been demonstrated by Singer and Salpeter (1966). The evidence is far from conclusive, yet on the answer to this question depends the interpretation of many phenomena in the pathology of peripheral nerves.

Conversely, it may be asked to what extent the Schwann cell depends on the axon. It obviously can survive and proliferate in the absence of an axon, as in Wallerian degeneration, but changes in the myelin sheaths, widening of the nodal gaps and the appearance of intercalated segments occur in primary diseases of the axon and suggest repercussions on the Schwann cell of processes taking place in the axons. Until the nature of the axon–Schwann cell relationship is fully clarified, our understanding of diseases of peripheral nerves is bound to be incomplete and the interpretation of findings largely arbitrary.

Classification of diseases of the peripheral nervous system

There is at present no satisfactory classification of diseases involving the peripheral nervous system. In the absence of sufficient aetiological data, a classification based on pathogenetic mechanisms is the best available. The subdivision of diseases into those which affect primarily the Schwann cell and those which attack the neuron, or part of it, is theoretically attractive, yet leads to considerable difficulties in practice.

In the first place, not all conditions have been fully examined by modern methods. Furthermore, many diseases show evidence both of axonal and Schwannian damage. The interpretation of these depends largely on the author's views on the axon–Schwann cell relationship. Finally, strict enforcement of this classification would often lead to separation of closely related conditions. To avoid such absurdities, some difficulties and inconsistencies have to be overlooked.

The well-established demyelinating neuropathies, as outlined by Gilliatt (1966), form a definite group. To these may be added others in which evidence is accumulating that Schwann cell disease plays an important part.

The conditions in which damage to the neuronal elements is the important, though sometimes doubtfully primary, feature may be subdivided into three groups. One consists of focal axonal lesions, single or multiple, and includes all vascular and traumatic disorders. The second group includes diffuse axonal lesions, most of them based on the dying-back phenomenon. The third forms a heterogeneous group of conditions, in which the lesions in peripheral nerves are secondary to destruction of their parent cell bodies. Only those affecting the posterior root ganglia, or ganglioradicular neuropathies, are diseases of the peripheral nervous system in the strict sense. Their motor equivalents are due to lesions in the anterior horn cells of the spinal cord and are described elsewhere.

The demyelinating neuropathies

Diphtheria

Diphtheritic neuropathy is now a condition of largely historical interest. It was first noted in the eighteenth century, and adequately described by Trousseau and Lassègue in 1851. According to Rolleston (1904), significant neurological involvement occurred in about 20% of cases of diphtheria.

Clinically, a slowly evolving paralysis appears after a latent period during which the original faucial infection may have cleared up. Palatal paralysis appears first, between the fifth and twelfth day of the disease. Soon afterwards other cranial nerve palsies may develop; of these ciliary paralysis with loss of accommodation and blurring of vision is the most characteristic. These signs usually clear up within 3 weeks of onset. In a minority of cases the paralysis spreads to the trunk and limbs, usually between the fifth and eighth weeks. It ranges in severity from mild weakness and sensory disturbances to severe paralysis leading to fatal respiratory failure. Survivors recover completely within weeks or months. The neurological illness is afebrile. The cerebrospinal fluid shows raised protein values, but otherwise remains normal.

In cutaneous diphtheria, resulting from infected war-wounds, palatal paralysis does not occur and paralysis of accommodation is less common. In some cases the onset of paralysis is at a site anatomically related to the infective focus, but the final polyneuritic pattern is remarkably constant irrespective of the site of infection (Walshe 1918-1919). In a similar series examined in the second World War, Gaskill and Korb (1946) failed to find any correlation between the focus of infection and the initial site of the paralysis.

The first pathological observations were those of Charcot and Vulpian (1862) who found evidence of myelin breakdown in a nerve of the soft palate. In a detailed post-mortem examination, Meyer (1881) found lesions of segmental demyelination with sparing of axis cylinders in all nerves of the body, although to a variable degree. These observations have been confirmed by several authors, more recently by Veith (1949), by Scheid and Peters (1952) and by Fisher and Adams (1956). The latter observers emphasized the striking tendency for the demyelinating process to be localized within the sensory ganglia and the paraganglionic regions of the nerve roots and spinal nerves. Wallerian degeneration is uncommon (Preisz 1895; Hechst 1934). Contrary to some earlier observations, inflammatory infiltration has not been found by recent observers.

Experimental work has largely confirmed and extended the observations on human material. The early work culminated in the monograph of Dreyer (1900), who studied diphtheritic neuropathy induced by injection of toxin–antitoxin mixtures in several species, particularly the guinea pig. Ransom (1900) demonstrated that diphtheria toxin acted locally if injected in the neighbourhood of a peripheral nerve. Recent work includes that of Waksman, Adams and Mansmann (1957) in the rabbit and guinea pig, McDonald (1963) in the cat and of Cavanagh and Jacobs (1964) in the chicken. These experiments have formed the material for electron-microscopic studies by Webster, Spiro, Waksman and Adams (1961) and by Weller (1965). This work has confirmed that diphtheria toxin is directly responsible for the lesions, which consist almost exclusively of segmental demyelination without significant damage to the axons and without inflammatory infiltration.

The pathogenesis of human diphtheritic neuropathy resembles that observed in experimental animals. That toxin alone is responsible was demonstrated by the accidental injection of pure unmodified toxin into 14 children, four of whom developed a typical polyneuropathy within a month (Jakovleva 1927). The mode of action of the toxin on the Schwann cell is not clearly understood, nor is the long latency and slow progression of the disease.

Idiopathic polyneuritis

In 1916 Guillain, Barré and Strohl described two cases of an acute illness in young, previously healthy adults, characterized by motor weakness, abolition of tendon reflexes, paraesthesiae, muscular tenderness and elevation of the protein level in the cerebrospinal fluid with a normal cell count. There is now little doubt that the condition was identical with that previously described by Landry (1859) as acute ascending paralysis, and by numerous other authors under a bewildering variety of names (Roseman and Aring 1941). As little is known of its aetiology, a non-committal term such as idiopathic polyneuritis (Asbury, Arnason and Adams 1969) appears most satisfactory at present.

It is a relatively common condition, frequently encountered in clinical practice. The classical clinical picture (Marshall 1963; Wiederholt, Mulder and Lambert 1964) is that of predominantly motor paralysis affecting both the spinal and the cranial nerves, frequently associated with subjective sensory disturbances, less commonly with objective sensory loss, sometimes accompanied by disturbances of sphincter control and by evidence of autonomic dysfunction. The onset is usually acute with rapid spread of the motor weakness, either ascending or descending.

Cranial nerves, particularly the facial and glossopharyngeal are frequently involved; in some cases the disease is confined to the cranial territory (Munsat and Barnes 1965). The condition is self-limiting and leads to spontaneous recovery, unless death occurs from respiratory paralysis. Mortality rates differ widely in various reported series, ranging from nil (Guillain 1936) to 42% (Forster, Brown and Merritt 1941).

Atypical recurrent or chronic cases have also been recorded (Austin 1958; Thomas, Lascelles, Hallpike and Hewer 1969; Prineas 1970; Currie and Knowles 1971). These form a heterogeneous group, part of which is probably related to the classical syndrome.

The disease is often preceded by a vague febrile illness which usually takes the form of an upper respiratory infection. In isolated instances acute polyneuritis has been recorded as a complication of specific virus infections such as mumps (Collens and Rabinowitz 1928), measles (Urquhart 1934), vaccinia (Spillane and Wells 1964) or herpes zoster (Dayan, Ogul and Graveson 1972). Polyneuritis occurs in the course of infectious mononucleosis (Gautier-Smith 1965), after surgical operations (Arnason and Asbury 1968), after fever therapy (Garvey, Jones and Warren 1940) and after prophylactic vaccination against rabies (Marinesco and Draganesco 1938).

Changes in the cerebrospinal fluid, consisting of a high protein and a normal cell count, were included by Guillain, Barré and Strohl in the definition of the syndrome. However, these findings are not constant. The level of protein may be variable, being low in the early stages of the disease and rising gradually, or falling rapidly from an initially high level. Pleocytosis has been recorded in several cases reviewed by Haymaker and Kernohan (1949). Furthermore, the 'albumino-cytological dissociation' occurs in other neuropathies, particularly of the demyelinating type. The cause of this rise in protein is not known. It is generally ascribed to involvement of the nerve roots, but other theories involving the exchange of fluid between the subarachnoid and endoneurial spaces have also been put forward (Greenfield and Carmichael 1925).

Electrophysiological studies have shown conduction block in the affected nerves during the early acute stage of the disease, followed by marked slowing of conduction velocities (Bannister and Sears 1962).

Accounts of the pathology of idiopathic polyneuritis differ considerably. There is no general agreement on the site of the lesions. Involvement of nerve roots was emphasized by Casamajor (1919) and by Margulis (1927). Haymaker and Kernohan (1949) placed the main lesions at the point where the anterior and posterior roots unite to form the spinal nerve, but admit that little peripheral material was available for examination. The widespread distribution of the lesions was repeatedly pointed out by Pette and Környey (1936), Krücke (1955), Matsuyama and Haymaker (1967) and Asbury, Arnason and Adams (1969). In fact, lesions may occur in any part of the peripheral nervous system, and vary in their detailed distribution from case to case, reflecting the clinical pattern of the disease.

The predominant lesion in all affected nerves is segmental demyelination, and that is accompanied to a greater or lesser extent by Wallerian degeneration (Asbury, Arnason and Adams). Inflammatory infiltration is a common, possibly constant, feature. It has always figured predominantly in accounts given in the German and French literature, but until recently has been played down by English-speaking writers. Thus Gilpin, Moersch and Kernohan (1936) and Scheinker (1947) found no evidence of an inflammatory process, while Bradford, Bashford and Wilson (1918-19) and Haymaker and Kernohan (1949) ascribed to it a secondary significance. Asbury, Arnason and Adams (1969) found that lymphocytic infiltration was a constant feature of the disease in all its stages and considered it to be of primary pathogenetic significance. They found perivascular aggregations of lymphocytes at all sites where demyelination was prominent. Many of the lymphocytes are 'transformed' and apparently in a stage of immunological activity: these cells have abundant cytoplasm and pale, oval or irregular nuclei. However, the inflammatory reaction may be modified by treatment with steroids and it is not uncommon to find it suppressed in autopsy material from treated cases.

Despite occasional reports to the contrary, the central nervous system is probably not primarily affected in this condition, but secondary lesions may occur when Wallerian degeneration is widespread.

Animal models. There are two possibly relevant conditions which bear sufficient similarity to the human disease to form useful experimental models. One is a naturally occurring disease in dogs, which develop polyneuritis 7 to 14 days after raccoon bites ('coonhound paralysis', Cummings and Haas 1967). The disease closely resembles human polyneuritis both in its clinical course and its pathology, the only difference being the absence of changes in the cerebrospinal fluid.

The other condition is experimental allergic neuritis (EAN) (Waksman and Adams 1955). This is induced by sensitizing rabbits to foreign peripheral nerve tissue with the addition of Freund's adjuvant. Two weeks after immunization the animals develop paralysis, which increases over the next few days. Some animals die, others recover fully after a few weeks. The lesions are those of segmental demyelination associated with perivascular lymphocytic infiltration. Segmental demyelination was confirmed by Cragg and Thomas (1964a, b) in experimental neuritis in the guinea pig by study of conduction-velocities and examination of individual teased fibres.

The early lesions of EAN were examined by phase contrast and electron-microscopy by Åström, Webster and Arnason (1968), who demonstrated that the first changes consist of attachment of activated lymphocytes to the endothelial cells of venules in peripheral nerves. They penetrate the endothelial cells, and migrate to the nervous parenchyma where they insinuate themselves between the nerve fibres. During migration the lymphocytes enlarge and transform. In further electron-microscopic studies on rats, Lampert (1969) demonstrated that the mononuclear cells traversed the basement membrane of the Schwann cells, penetrated the outer mesaxon, then surrounded and destroyed the myelin sheath. Schröder and Krücke (1970) confirmed the penetration of the Schwann cell by infiltrating mononuclear cells, but also observed breakdown of myelin remote from inflammatory cells.

The invasion of the myelin sheath by large mononuclear cells, both macrophages and non-phagocytic cells, presumably transformed lymphocytes, has now been confirmed on biopsies from human cases of polyneuritis (Wisniewski, Terry, Whitaker, Cook and Dowling 1969; Prineas 1971).

Immunological research has confirmed the important part which the lymphocyte plays both in EAN and in idiopathic polyneuritis. EAN can be passively transferred by transplantation of lymphocytes (Åström and Waksman 1962). Lymphocytes, both from animal and human cases, destroy myelin in tissue culture of posterior root ganglia (Winkler 1965; Arnason, Winkler and Hadler 1969). There is increased DNA synthesis in circulating lymphocytes in idiopathic polyneuritis, particularly in the active stage of the disease (Cook and Dowling 1968; Cook, Dowling and Whitaker 1970). Lymphocytes respond by transformation to antigenic stimulation by a basic protein obtained from sciatic nerve (Currie and Knowles 1971). The active fraction of this protein has now been isolated and characterized (Brostoff, Burnet, Lampert and Eylar 1972).

Humoral factors may also play some part in the process. Melnick (1963) was the first to describe circulating antibodies to peripheral nerve tissue in idiopathic polyneuritis. The myelinolytic action of serum on tissue cultures has been demonstrated both in EAN (Yonezawa, Ishihara and Matsuyama 1968) and in human polyneuritis (Murray, Cook and Dowling 1970; Cook, Dowling, Murray and Whitaker 1971).

The case in favour of an allergic pathogenesis of idiopathic polyneuritis thus seems very strong. A note of caution has, however, been struck by Drachman, Paterson, Berlin and Roguska (1970), who reported the occurrence of a typical acute polyneuritis in a totally immunosuppressed patient.

Leprosy

Leprosy is a disease which involves the skin, superficial mucous membranes, peripheral nerves and organs of the reticuloendothelial system. It is a condition of great complexity, which can be only briefly summarized here; for a detailed account the reader is referred to specialized textbooks (e.g. Cochrane and Davey 1964).

Little is known of the early stages of the infection by *Mycobacterium leprae* in man. It appears to be a disease of low infectivity, contagion occurring only after prolonged exposure. The disease becomes overt after a long latent period and usually manifests itself in the form of cutaneous lesions, less commonly in involvement of major peripheral nerves.

The modern classification of the disease is based on the host-parasite relationship which may be extraordinarily varied. At one end of the scale the patient may exhibit a total lack of cellular immunity, in which case the organisms multiply freely in the infected cells in the absence of an inflammatory reaction. At the other end

of the spectrum a patient with high immunity will show an intense inflammatory reaction, and the growth of organisms will be suppressed. The Madrid (1953) classification subdivides leprosy into two clear-cut types, lepromatous and tuberculoid and two additional groups, indeterminate and borderline (dimorphous). The *lepromatous* type is associated with low immunity. It tends to be progressive and presents with infiltrated skin lesions. The basic lesion consists of aggregations of macrophages containing numerous ingested acid-fast bacilli. In older lesions these cells become foamy or coarsely vacuolated (lepra cells). The lepromin skin test is negative. The *tuberculoid* type occurs in patients with high immunity. It tends to run a benign, non-progressive course. The basic lesion is an inflammatory granuloma, consisting of epithelioid cells, multinucleated giant cells and abundant lymphocytes in the periphery. The lesions have a tendency to central necrosis. Acid-fast bacilli are not found in the lesions. The lepromin test is strongly positive. The *indeterminate* group consists of early cases which do not show any characteristic features of either polar type. They may evolve towards the lepromatous or the tuberculoid type. The *borderline* (dimorphous) group includes all cases which show intermediate features between the two polar types and vary in their inflammatory response, bacterial content and lepromin reaction. It forms a continuous spectrum between the polar types, some cases being nearer the lepromatous, others nearer the tuberculoid end. It has been subdivided into three subgroups: the borderline-lepromatous, borderline-intermediate and borderline-tuberculoid (Ridley and Jopling 1966). Changes in the immunological state of the patient may occur, with corresponding transformation of the clinico-pathological picture. The indeterminate and borderline cases tend to be more unstable than the polar types. The immunological aspects of the various types of leprosy have been studied by Turk (1969) and Turk and Waters (1971).

Clinically, involvement of the major peripheral nerve occurs in all forms of leprosy, with the possible exception of the indeterminate. In tuberculoid leprosy the nerve trunks get involved relatively early in the disease. The disease attacks individual nerves asymmetrically, usually one or at most two at a time (Jopling and Morgan Hughes 1965). The major nerves in the limbs, particularly the ulnar, median and lateral popliteal

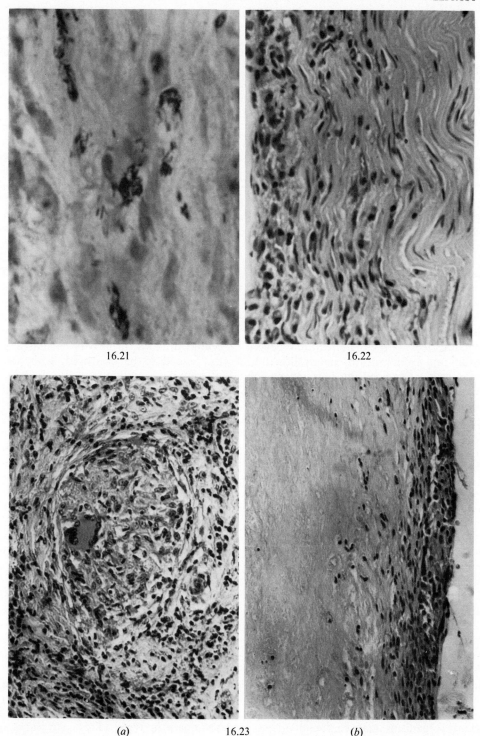

16.21   16.22

(a)   16.23   (b)

Fig. 16.21 Lepromatous leprosy: clusters of acid fast bacilli in nerve biopsy. Ziehl-Neelsen.   × 1500.
Fig. 16.22 Lepromatous leprosy: fibrosis and hyalinization of nerve; the presence of a few inflammatory cells puts the case into the borderline-lepromatous group. H & E.   × 500.
Fig. 16.23 Tuberculoid leprosy. (a) Epithelioid and giant cell granuloma. H & E.   × 270. (b) Massive necrosis of fascicle ('nerve abscess') with thin rim of granulation tissue. H & E.   × 270.

nerves are commonly affected. Of the cranial nerves only the trigeminal and the facial may be damaged. Cutaneous sensory nerves may also be involved and palpably and visibly swollen, usually irregularly. Some less common manifestations have been reviewed by Browne (1965).

In lepromatous leprosy clinical involvement occurs late in the disease. It is usually symmetrical and polyneuritic. The nerves are slightly and uniformly thickened to begin with and gradually transformed into thin, fibrous cords.

There are remarkably few electrophysiological studies on peripheral nerves in leprosy. Dash (1967) measured conduction velocities and found them considerably reduced in all types of leprosy. Similar findings in single cases were reported by Jopling and Morgan Hughes (1965) and by Rosenberg and Lovelace (1968).

The *pathology* of peripheral nerves was first described by Virchow (1864). Recent accounts include those of Fite (1943), Dastur (1955, 1967), Khanolkar (1964) and Job and Desikan (1968). In lepromatous leprosy the main feature is severe loss of axons and myelin sheaths and proliferation of Schwann cells. The Schwann cells are swollen and contain numerous acid-fast bacilli in their cytoplasm (Fig. 16.21). Some macrophages containing bacteria may also be present. The endoneurium may show oedema in the early stages, and that is followed by progressive fibrosis of a singularly dense and hyaline character (Fig. 16.22). In pure lepromatous lesions there are no inflammatory cells, but in borderline-lepromatous cases some lymphocytic infiltration may be present and there is a tendency towards epithelioid transformation of macrophages.

In tuberculoid leprosy the main feature is the formation of epithelioid cell granulomata, irregularly distributed along the course of the nerve (Fig. 16.23). There is intense lymphocytic infiltration, particularly at the periphery of the lesions. Central necrosis of a colliquative type occurs in the granulomata leading to the formation of so-called 'nerve abscesses'. In the affected areas both the axons and the Schwann cells are completely destroyed; the fibres distal to the lesions show Wallerian degeneration. Acid-fast bacilli are not seen, other than in borderline-tuberculoid lesions where scanty organisms may be found on prolonged search.

The early *electron-microscopic* studies (Nishiura 1960; Imaeda and Convit 1963) have largely confirmed the appearances found on light microscopy.

More recently Job (1970), in his study of lepromatous leprosy, found both intact and degenerating mycobacteria, the latter surrounded by electron-transparent zones which may enlarge to form vesicular spaces. Organisms were seen in Schwann cells, macrophages, capillary endothelial cells and occasionally in perineurial cells. When present in axons they were separated from the axoplasm by double membranes, thus suggesting invagination of a tongue of Schwann cell cytoplasm. Several infected Schwann cells contained normal fully myelinated axons. Demyelinated and degenerating axons were also present. Similar observations were made by Dastur, Ramamohan and Shah (1972a) on four cases of lepromatous leprosy. There was depletion of large myelinated fibres with proliferation of Schwann cells. *M. leprae* almost constantly parasitized Schwann cells, endothelial and perineurial cells. Bacilli were not seen in myelin sheaths or axons. *M. leprae* had a greater predilection for the Schwann cells of unmyelinated fibres. Both myelinated and unmyelinated axons, in heavily bacillated Schwann cells, tended to be destroyed, with consequent Wallerian degeneration.

In their ultrastructural studies on nerve biopsies from eight early cases of tuberculoid leprosy, Dastur, Ramamohan and Shah (1972b) observed the following features. There was loss of large myelinated fibres; in the remaining fibres the Schmidt–Lantermann clefts were prominent, indicating early Wallerian degeneration. Advanced stages of such degeneration were also present. There was evidence of regeneration both of myelinated and unmyelinated fibres. Some irregular proliferation of Schwann cells was seen, as well as an excessive increase of endoneurial collagen. The perineurium showed initially proliferative, later degenerative changes with fibrosis. Inflammatory cells, including epithelioid and plasma cells, were seen in significant numbers only in two cases. Bacilli were present in one case only.

Animal experiments have developed rapidly in recent years. Human leprosy has been successfully transferred to the footpads of the mouse (Shepard 1960; Rees 1964) and other rodents. The lesions remained largely localized and indeterminate in type. The main value of these experiments was the reproduction of early lesions, particularly the clear demonstration of early involvement of Schwann cells in cutaneous nerves. Further progress was made by the use of thymectomized and irradiated mice (Rees 1966), in which the disease becomes generalized and closely resembles human lepromatous leprosy. The present state of experimental research has been reviewed by Rees and Waters (1972). In brief, it has been shown that the generalized disease develops in a stereotyped pattern, irrespective of the strain of *M. leprae* and of the portal of entry. In peripheral nerves the organisms multiply in Schwann cells, perineurial cells and macrophages. In the early stages of the disease, bacillary multiplication also occurs in striated muscle, a finding since confirmed in human leprosy (Job, Karat, Karat and Mathan 1969; Pearson, Rees and Weddell 1970).

These experimental data, together with electron-microscopic appearances and recent studies on teased nerve fibres (Dayan and Sanbank 1970; Dastur and Razzak 1971; Swift 1974), leave no doubt about the correctness of the Schwannian theory of spread of neural leprosy, already convincingly presented by Lumsden in 1964. The axonal theory (Khanolkar 1951; Terada 1953) must now be considered obsolete.

Diabetes mellitus

Marchal de Calvi's (1853) observation on the association of diabetes mellitus with a paraplegia which improved on dietary treatment is generally accepted as the beginning of the history of diabetic neuropathy. In fact, cases of diabetes with neuritic symptoms had been described before (Rollo 1798) and many single case reports followed. More recently large clinical surveys have appeared (Jordan 1936; Rundles 1945; Martin 1953). It is a common disorder, yet its prevalence has been difficult to assess. Published figures range from 5% to over 90%, depending on the degree of refinement of diagnostic methods.

The clinical manifestations include pain, muscle weakness, sensory loss, penetrating ulcers, ataxia, autonomic disorders and isolated cranial and spinal nerve palsies. It is possible to subdivide the condition into two main types, one of rapid onset, associated with pain and motor weakness and wasting (the 'diabetic amyotrophy' of Garland 1955), the other insidious, predominantly sensory, associated with penetrating ulcers of the feet and with ataxia of a sensory type. Perhaps this classification is an over-simplification, as there is much overlap between the clinical pictures and this disease may be considered to form a con-tinuous spectrum covering various manifestations (Greenbaum 1964). Reduced conduction velocities have been found in motor nerves in both types of neuropathy but not in isolated nerve palsies where the functional impairment was local (Gilliatt and Willison 1964).

Observations on the pathology of diabetic neuropathy have yielded a number of contradictory data. Some authors placed the lesion in the peripheral nerves (Woltman and Wilder 1929; Goodman, Baumoel, Frankel, Marcus and Wasserman 1953; Dolman 1963; Thomas and Lascelles 1965, 1966), others described lesions involving the entire lower motor or primary sensory neuron (Kraus 1922; Alderman 1938; Bosanquet and Henson 1957; Greenbaum Richardson, Salmon and Urich 1964).

Studies of teased preparations and measurements of internodal lengths have confirmed that the fundamental lesion in diabetic neuropathy is segmental demyelination (Thomas and Lascelles 1965, 1966; Chopra and Fannin 1971). This is fully in accordance with electrophysiological findings. These changes, however, are also found in diabetics in the absence of overt clinical neuropathy (Chopra and Hurwitz 1969; Chopra, Hurwitz and Montgomery 1969). In cases of florid neuropathy, Wallerian degeneration of some nerve fibres is almost constantly observed and manifests itself in denervation atrophy of skeletal muscles (Greenbaum *et al.* 1964; Reske-Nielson and Lundbaek 1968). Whether this is secondary to severe Schwann cell disease or caused independently is debatable. Minor changes in anterior horn cells and posterior root ganglia may be retrograde in nature, but severe selective loss of anterior horn cells (Alderman 1938), or almost total devastation of posterior root ganglia (Bosanquet and Henson 1957), are difficult to explain (Fig. 16.24).

Ultrastructurally (Bischoff 1970), degenerative changes with lipid inclusions are present in Schwann cells, with or without demyelination. Evidence of axonal breakdown and Wallerian degeneration is common. A characteristic feature is the thickening and reduplication of basement membranes, both around Schwann cells and capillaries.

The relative importance of vascular and metabolic factors in the pathogenesis of diabetic neuropathy remains controversial. Woltman and Wilder (1929) believed that the neuropathy was ischaemic in origin and due to atheroma of the

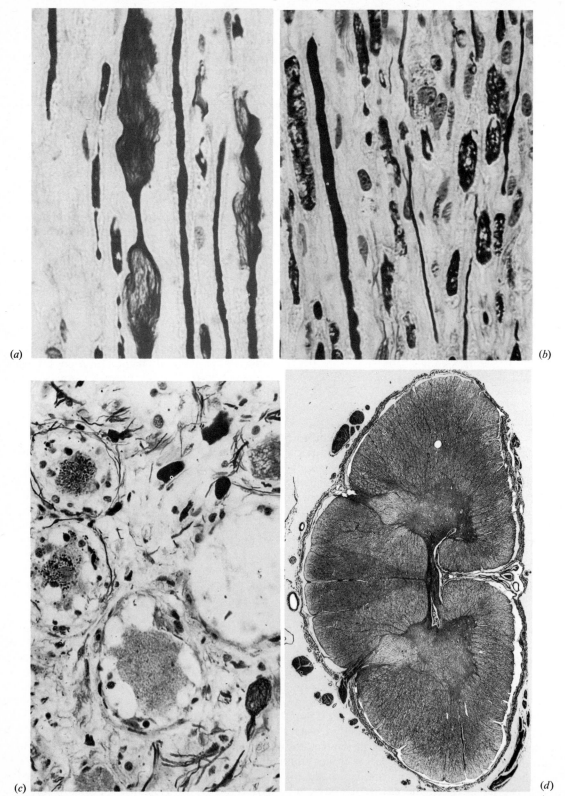

Fig. 16.24 Diabetes mellitus (*a*) Early Wallerian-type degeneration in anterior root. Glees-Marsland. ×500. (*b*) More advanced stage of Wallerian type degeneration in posterior root. Glees-Marsland. ×500. (*c*) Degenerative changes in posterior root ganglion. Glees-Marsland. ×470. (*d*) Cervical cord: gliosis of anterior horns and fasciculus gracilis. Holzer. ×9. (By permission of the Editor, *Brain*.)

vasa nervorum. Most of their material, however, consisted of limbs amputated for occlusive arterial disease. Fagerberg (1959) ascribed the neuropathy to a diabetic microangiopathy, in which the intrafascicular arterioles are thickened and narrowed due to accumulation of PAS-positive material in their walls. There is, however, no obvious correlation between these lesions and changes in nerve fibres. Probably some neurological manifestations of diabetes, such as single nerve palsies, are due to vascular factors (Dreyfus, Hakim and Adams 1957; Raff, Sangalang and Asbury 1968; Asbury, Aldridge, Hershberg and Fisher 1970).

Experimental models do not completely reproduce the human situation yet have the advantage of relative simplicity. Alloxan diabetes in rats produces a subclinical demyelinating neuropathy demonstrated by slowing of conduction-velocities (Eliasson 1964, 1969; Preston 1967). This was thought to be completely uncomplicated by vascular factors and therefore particularly suitable for the study of metabolic disturbances. Of these the abnormalities in the sorbitol pathway have attracted particular attention (Gabbay and O'Sullivan 1968). In rats rendered diabetic with alloxan there is an accumulation of sorbitol and fructose in the sciatic nerves. There is also a diminution of aldose reductase, an enzyme localized in the Schwann cell and essential for the series of reactions which maintain the normal sorbitol pathway. Similar high levels of sorbitol have been demonstrated in human material (Ward 1971). On the other hand Seneviratne (1972) emphasized the importance of vascular factors in experimental diabetic neuropathy. He demonstrated increased capillary permeability and breakdown of the blood nerve barrier and suggested that leakage of protein into the endoneurial fluid was responsible for damage to Schwann cells and segmental demyelination.

Haemochromatosis

Finch and Finch (1955) found evidence of peripheral neuropathy in 14% of their cases of primary haemochromatosis. The main clinical features are pains in the extremities, cutaneous hyperaesthesiae, muscle tenderness and cramps. Muscular weakness and wasting, with diminished tendon reflexes, may also be found. Most sufferers from haemochromatosis are also diabetic and in some cases at least the neuropathy is indistinguishable from the diabetic (Jarrett and Barter 1964). In addition, alcoholism appears to be an important aggravating factor (McDonald and Mallory 1960) and this may account for involvement of the peripheral nervous system in some cases.

Published reports of pathological findings in peripheral nerves are rare. Mallory, Parker and Nye (1920-21) found deposits of haemosiderin and haemofuscin in peripheral nerves. Melnick and Whitfield (1962) found iron deposition in the axons of intramuscular nerves in a patient with haemochromatosis who apparently developed a coincidental idiopathic polyneuritis.

Hypoglycaemia

See Chapter 2.

Uraemia

The association of peripheral neuropathy with chronic renal failure was known to Osler (1892), but interest in the condition has been revived only recently with the advent of intermittent haemodialysis. The occurrence of severe neuropathy in patients undergoing this form of treatment was reported by Hegstrom, Murray, Pendras, Burnell and Scribner (1961, 1962). At the same time, Marin and Tyler (1961) described two cases of neuropathy associated with hereditary interstitial nephritis but did not ascribe it to uraemia. The association of neuropathy with uraemia, irrespective of the nature of the underlying renal disease, was firmly established by Asbury, Victor and Adams (1963).

The clinical findings are initially those of a sensory neuropathy, presenting with pain, tingling, numbness and burning paraesthesiae, affecting the lower limbs more severely than the upper. Loss of vibration sense is an early sign. Peripheral muscular weakness and wasting supervene in untreated cases. The correlation with the severity of renal failure is variable; while all affected patients have raised levels of blood urea and low creatinine clearances (Konotey-Ahulu, Baillod, Comty, Heron, Shaldon and Thomas 1965) many sufferers from severe and prolonged uraemia never develop neurological symptoms. Males are more liable to develop uraemic neuropathy (Tyler 1968) and older patients are more frequently affected (Tenckhoff, Boen, Hebsen and Spiegler 1965). The condition tends to improve on haemodialysis and symptoms do not develop after adequate treatment has begun (Konotey-Ahulu *et al.* 1965). In some cases, however, either the onset or deterioration of the neuropathy could be dated to the earlier stages of haemodialysis (Hegstrom *et al.* 1961; Tenckhoff *et al.* 1965). Improvement invariably occurs after successful renal transplantation (Tenckhoff *et al.* 1965; Funck-Brentano, Chaurmont, Vantelon and Zingraff

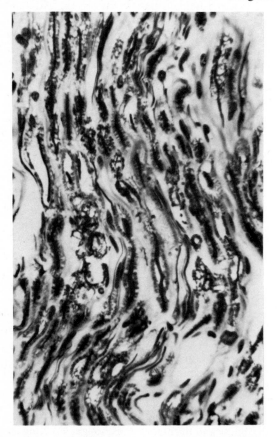

Fig. 16.25 Uraemic neuropathy: Wallerian-type degeneration of axons and myelin sheaths. Glees-Marsland and Luxol fast blue. × 460.

1968). The sensory symptoms improve first, followed by a slow recovery of the motor disability.

The pathology of the neuropathy of chronic renal failure is predominantly that of a Wallerian-type degeneration of axons (Fig. 16.25), most prominent in the distal parts of the limbs (Asbury *et al.* 1963; Dayan, Gardner-Thorpe, Down and Gleadle 1970; Thomas, Hollinrake, Lascelles, O'Sullivan, Baillod, Moorhead and Mackenzie 1971). Segmental demyelination, if present, is usually inconspicuous. Dyck, Johnson, Lambert

and O'Brien (1971) consider it a phenomenon secondary to axonal damage.

On the other hand, in acute renal failure the lesions are exclusively demyelinating in type (Dayan *et al.* 1970). Temporary conduction block has been observed by Buchthal (1970).

Subclinical involvement of peripheral nerves, which manifests itself only in slowing of conduction-velocities and is associated with segmental demyelination, may occur both in acute and in chronic renal failure (Prestwick and Jeremy 1964; Dinn and Crane 1970; Appenseller, Kornfeld, Albuquerque and McGee 1971).

The relationship of the two types of uraemic neuropathy remains obscure. The causative mechanisms are unknown and various metabolic and vascular factors have been postulated. These are fully discussed by Thomas *et al.* (1971).

Hepatic failure

See Chapter 4.

The neuropathies of malignant disease

Reports of neurological disorders in which autopsy failed to reveal involvement of the nervous system by the primary malignant tumour or its metastases have appeared sporadically since the end of the last century. The historical aspects of these paraneoplastic disorders of the nervous system have been fully reviewed by Appicciutoli and Bignami (1962).

The modern approach to the problem began with the description of the sensory neuropathy associated with carcinoma of the bronchus (Denny-Brown 1948), followed by the report on the association of peripheral neuropathy with bronchial carcinoma (Lennox and Pritchard 1950), the identification of cerebellar syndromes (Brain, Daniel and Greenfield 1951) and the review of the clinical and pathological aspects of the whole field by Henson, Russell and Wilkinson (1954).

The central and peripheral nervous systems, as well as skeletal muscles, may be involved in a large variety of clinical patterns. As little is known about the pathogenetic mechanisms which cause the individual lesions, the only acceptable classification at present is purely anatomical, based on the level of the nervous system involved (Brain and Adams 1965).

The incidence of these paraneoplastic disorders is difficult to assess and figures given by different

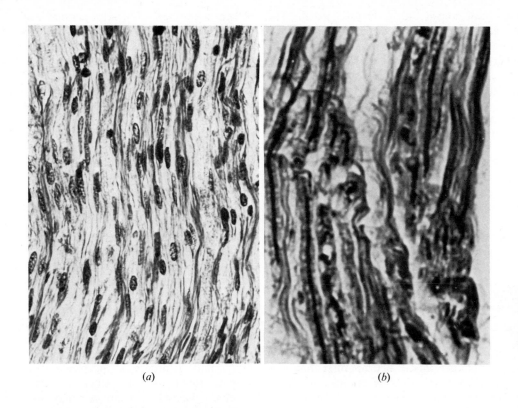

(a)

(b)

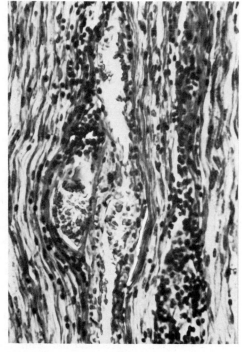

Fig. 16.26 Peripheral neuropathy associated with malignant disease. (*a*) Increased cellularity of nerve due to Schwann cell proliferation. van Gieson. × 500. (*b*) Wallerian-type degeneration of some nerve fibres. Sarnaker's silver impregnation and Luxol fast blue. × 500. (*c*) Sparse perivascular lymphocytic infiltration in peripheral nerve. van Gieson. × 300. (By permission of the Editor, *Brain*.)

(c)

authors have ranged widely (Henson 1970). The high figures obtained by the London Hospital research team (Croft and Wilkinson 1963, 1965) are due on one hand to inclusion of minimal lesions apparent only in a systematic survey and on the other to a high referral rate to a specialized centre. If only clinically significant syndromes were included, a realistic assessment would probably not exceed 4% in bronchial carcinoma and 1% in other cancers.

Carcinoma of the bronchus undoubtedly accounts for the majority of non-metastatic neurological complications (Croft and Wilkinson 1965, 1969). Of the various histological types, oat-cell carcinoma accounts for the majority of cases of encephalomyelitis and ganglioradiculitis and for a little more than one half of other types of neuropathy (Dayan, Croft and Wilkinson 1965).

Tumours other than carcinoma are rarely associated with remote effects on the nervous system, with the exception of neoplasms of the lymphoreticular system (Hutchinson, Leonard, Maudsley and Yates 1958; Currie, Henson, Morgan and Poole 1970). Of these myeloma shows a high incidence of peripheral neuropathies but this tumour presents a variety of specific problems. Peripheral neuropathies also occur in lymphomas, particularly Hodgkin's disease, in the leukaemias and in polycythaemia.

The affections of the peripheral nervous system fall into two well-defined groups: the peripheral mixed polyneuropathies and the sensory ganglioradicular neuropathies. Whether a purely motor peripheral neuropathy exists is open to doubt: it is, however, possible that some of the cases of 'motor neuron disease' associated with carcinoma (Brain, Croft and Wilkinson 1965) have a peripheral component.

The clinical picture of the *polyneuropathies* is that of a mixed peripheral neuropathy affecting both the motor and the sensory systems (Croft, Urich and Wilkinson 1967). The course may be acute or subacute, continuous or relapsing. The onset may precede or follow other manifestations of carcinoma. In a substantial group of cases a mild neuropathy develops only terminally. The lower limbs are generally more severely affected than the upper. Cranial nerves are rarely involved. In severe cases the cerebrospinal fluid protein is raised, with an abnormal Lange curve, but without pleocytosis. Electrophysiological studies show evidence of denervation, sometimes with reduction of conduction velocities.

The pathology of carcinomatous polyneuropathies shows the features both of segmental demyelination and of axonal degeneration, one or the other feature predominating (Fig. 16.26a, b). The nerves of the lower limbs are usually more severely affected, but the lesions can be widespread and affect the spinal roots as well as the periphery. Posterior root ganglia show secondary degenerative changes in severe cases; they are relatively mild compared with the massive destruction seen in ganglioradiculitis. Evidence of inflammation is usually absent, but in some cases sparse perivascular lymphocytic infiltration has been noted in peripheral nerves (Fig. 16.26c). No ultrastructural data are available at present, nor has the condition been reproduced in experimental animals.

Both the clinical and pathological data suggest that the carcinomatous polyneuropathies form a heterogeneous group in which a variety of pathogenetic mechanisms may play a part. Toxic and metabolic factors were the first to be considered (Brain and Henson 1958). In the search for specific factors, nutritional deficiencies (Victor 1965) and disorders of porphyrin metabolism (Vavra 1965) were investigated with negative results. Allergic mechanisms may well be involved in cases of demyelinating neuropathies with an inflammatory component, resembling the subacute or relapsing forms of idiopathic polyneuritis. Demyelinating antibodies (Murray *et al.* 1970) and increased DNA synthesis in circulating lymphocytes (Cook and Dowling 1968) have been reported in some cases of carcinomatous neuropathy.

The preponderance of bronchial carcinoma among the causative tumours has led to the suggestion that it is pulmonary disease rather than neoplasia which is responsible for the neuropathy. The occasional occurrence of neuropathy in pulmonary tuberculosis has been known since the work of Oppenheim (1886). Caughey, Farpour and Etemadee (1967) described three cases of neuropathy associated with bronchiectasis. These cases, however, are rare and do not support the contention of Wilner and Brody (1968) that the incidence of neuropathy in bronchial carcinoma is the same as that found in other chronic pulmonary disease.

Sensory neuropathy is a less common though better defined paraneoplastic complication. Several single case reports preceded the definition of the syndrome by Denny-Brown (1948), the first being

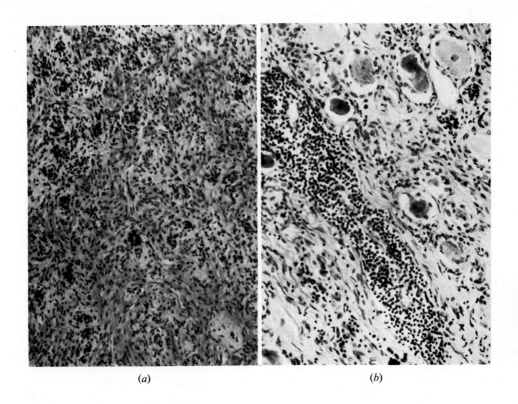

(a)   (b)

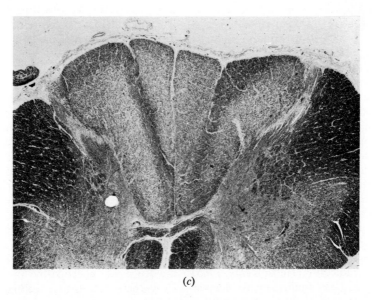

(c)

Fig. 16.27 Sensory neuropathy with carcinoma. (a) Almost total loss of neurons in posterior root ganglion and replacement by nodules of Nageotte. H & E.   ×130. (b) Perivascular lymphocytic infiltration in posterior root ganglion. H & E.   ×170. (c) Degeneration of posterior columns. Klüver-Barrera.   ×12. (By permission of the Editor, *Brain*.)

that reported by Williamson (1908). Most cases are associated with bronchial carcinoma, almost exclusively of the oat-cell type. In many instances the primary tumour is small and its spread may be limited to the regional lymph nodes, leading to diagnostic difficulties. Exceptionally the condition has been reported with squamous cell (Gray, Woolf and Wright 1955) or with undifferentiated carcinoma of the bronchus (Henson et al. 1954) as well as with cancers of the oesophagus (Dodgson and Hoffman 1953), thyroid (Beardwell 1961) and uterus (Henson, Hoffman and Urich 1965).

The clinical picture is that of a sensory neuropathy affecting all modalities (Croft, Henson, Urich and Wilkinson 1965). Paraesthesiae and ataxia constitute the main symptoms. Loss of positional sense may be severe enough to lead to pseudo-athetosis. The disability may affect the upper or lower limbs predominantly and may be asymmetrical. The onset may be insidious or sudden. After the sensory loss has reached its peak it remains stationary. Signs of associated involvement of the spinal cord, brainstem or cerebral cortex are common. The cerebrospinal fluid may be normal or show an excess of protein; pleocytosis is rare.

The *pathology* is that of a ganglioradiculitis with extensive destruction of neurons in the posterior root ganglia, proliferation of capsule cells and formation of residual nodules of Nageotte (Fig. 16.27a). Perivascular lymphocytic infiltration is almost invariably found in some, if not all, affected ganglia (Fig. 16.27b). Wallerian degeneration follows in the posterior columns and the sensory components of peripheral nerves (Fig. 16.27c). The cervical and lumbar ganglia are usually more severely affected than the thoracic, but a random distribution is not uncommon. It may be asymmetrical, affect only individual ganglia, or single ganglia may escape from otherwise global destruction.

Ganglioradiculitis is commonly associated with limbic encephalitis, bulbar encephalitis or myelitis. Most cases of sensory neuropathy show at least minimal involvement of the neuraxis (Croft et al. 1965) and, conversely, many cases of carcinomatous encephalomyelitis show some, if limited, evidence of ganglioradiculitis (Henson et al. 1965). This association has been confirmed by independent observers (Alemà, Bignami and Appicciutoli 1963; Ulrich, Spiess and Huber 1967). This co-existence of inflammatory lesions at

various levels of the nervous system and their almost specific association with one type of tumour must be taken into account in the formulation of pathogenetic theories. The resemblance of the central lesions to virus encephalitides has led to the infective theory (Henson et al. 1954). Search for causative viruses has remained largely unfruitful, but structures resembling virus particles have been reported by Walton, Tomlinson and Pearce (1968) in a case of subacute myelitis associated with Hodgkin's disease and by Norris, McMenemey and Barnard (1970) in encephalomyelitis with oat-cell carcinoma.

Russell (1961) pointed out that the inflammatory nature of the lesions did not necessarily denote infection, but could be due to an immune reaction. Wilkinson (1964) discovered a circulating anti-brain antibody in the sera of patients suffering from sensory neuropathy. The antibody is organ specific and directed against a cytoplasmic component of neurons (Wilkinson and Zeromski 1965). The search for common antigenic determinants between oat-cell cancers and nervous tissue, which might explain the appearance of such an antibody, has been unsuccessful.

The dysproteinaemias

These conditions form a heterogeneous group of diseases with one common feature, a persistent abnormality in the protein profile of the serum. They include the paraproteinaemias, the immunoglobulin deficiencies and the alipoproteinaemias.

Paraproteinaemias

Paraproteinaemia may be defined as a primary excess of one or more immunoglobulins, produced in the absence of antigenic stimulation. All classes of immunoglobulin may be represented, in multiple myeloma usually IgG or IgA, in macroglobulinaemia IgM. Incomplete immunoglobulins may also be produced. Monoclonal and polyclonal patterns have been recorded. The term 'cryoglobulin' does not refer to any specific class of immunoglobulin, but to the physical property of precipitation on cooling. This may be of some pathological significance as reflected in a 7% incidence of neuropathy in cryoglobulinaemia (Logothetis, Kennedy, Ellington and Williams 1968).

The mechanisms by which paraproteinaemias affect the peripheral nervous system are obscure.

Garcin, Mallarmé and Rondot (1962) suggested three possibilities: cellular infiltration, sludging of red cells and allergic vasculitis. There is remarkably little evidence to support any of these hypotheses.

Peripheral neuropathy occurs in about 8% of cases of *Waldenström's disease* (Logothetis, Silverstein and Coe 1960). Different clinical patterns have been recorded: sensorimotor polyneuritis, mononeuritis, mononeuritis multiplex, sensory polyneuritis and cranial neuritis. The protein in the cerebrospinal fluid may be elevated. A

(1966) interpreted the findings in their case of macrocryoglobulinaemia as those of a demyelinating neuropathy, but their evidence is not conclusive.

In *myeloma* the incidence of peripheral neuropathy is about 3% (Currie *et al*. 1970). It occurs in multiple myelomatosis as well as in association with solitary plasmacytoma. In view of this relatively high incidence it would be tempting to ascribe the damage to peripheral nerves to the paraproteinaemia, yet in fact there is little evidence in favour of this hypothesis. Both clinically and

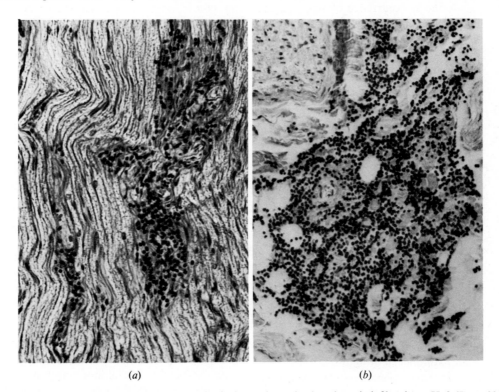

(a)   (b)

Fig. 16.28 Neuropathy with myeloma. (*a*) Intrafascicular perivascular lymphocytic infiltration. H & E.   × 225. (*b*) Lymphocytic infiltration of interfascicular epineurium. H & E.   × 210. (By permission of the Editor, *Journal of the Neurological Sciences*.)

variety of lesions have been described in peripheral nerves. Aarseth, Ofstad and Torvik (1961) noted lymphocytic infiltration as well as degenerative changes in axons and myelin sheaths. Darnley (1962) described deposition of a homogeneous, strongly PAS-positive substance in the perineurium. Intraneural and perivascular amyloid was found by Nick, Contamin, Brion, Guillard and Guiraudon (1963), by Le Bourhis, Fève, Besançon and Leroux (1964) and by Bigner, Olsen and McFarlin (1971). Dayan and Lewis

pathologically the condition closely resembles the polyneuropathies of other malignant neoplasms. It affects both the sensory and the motor nerves, usually symmetrically, but with a predilection for the lower limbs, and runs a variable clinical course. The cerebrospinal fluid protein is usually raised. Both segmental demyelination and loss of axons are found in the affected nerves (Scheinker 1938; Victor, Banker and Adams 1958; Dayan, Urich and Gardner-Thorpe 1970). The lesions are usually purely degenerative, but in some cases lymphocytic infiltration may be present (Fig. 16.28).

It is surprising that amyloidosis plays a very small part in the pathogenesis of myelomatous neuropathy. Small amounts of amyloid may be present in the walls of blood vessels but no lesions have been reported comparable with those seen in primary amyloid neuropathy. On the other hand deposition of amyloid in ligaments and synovial membranes may cause a bilateral carpal tunnel syndrome in myelomatosis (Fig. 16.29).

Another factor of possible importance may be the frequent terminal occurrence of renal failure due to myelomatous nephropathy. However,

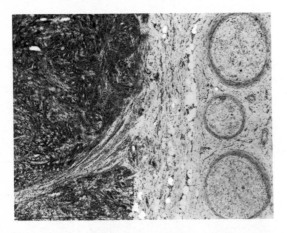

Fig. 16.29 Amyloidosis with myeloma. Median nerve in carpal tunnel compressed by flexor retinaculum infiltrated with amyloid. Congo red. × 33. (By permission of the Editor, *Journal of the Neurological Sciences*.)

none of the recorded cases of myelomatous neuropathy can be ascribed to uraemia, either on clinical or on pathological grounds.

A promising experimental model has been evolved in mice bearing transplanted plasma cell myelomas. Some of these animals develop a mild peripheral neuropathy. This occurs only in association with tumours producing free light chains (Dayan and Stokes 1972).

Immunoglobulin deficiencies: ataxia telangiectasia

See Chapter 14.

Alipoproteinaemias

Alpha-lipoprotein deficiency (Tangier disease)

This rare condition, described by Fredrickson, Altrocchi, Avioli, Goodman and Goodman (1961)

is characterized by an almost complete absence of plasma high density lipoproteins and the storage of cholesterol esters in many tissues of the body (Fredrickson 1966). Clinical features include enlargement and yellowish discoloration of the tonsils, while the pharyngeal and rectal mucosa are orange in colour. Hepatosplenomegaly, lymphadenopathy and corneal infiltration may occur.

Peripheral neuropathy has been described by Kocen, Lloyd, Lascelles, Fosbrooke and Williams (1967), by Engel, Dorman, Levy and Fredrickson (1967) and by Kummer, Laissue, Spiess, Pflugshaupt and Bucher (1968). Pathological data are still scanty and confined to routine examinations of nerve biopsies. Kocen *et al.* found loss of axons and myelin sheaths, endoneurial fibrosis and cells containing sudanophil material in close proximity to nerve fibres. Engel *et al.* found no significant lesions in a nerve biopsy. In a further study Kocen, King, Thomas and Haas (1973) found axonal loss, both of myelinated and unmyelinated fibres, but not segmental demyelination. There was extensive accumulation of cholesterol within Schwann cells and an excess of collagen in the endoneurium.

Beta-lipoprotein deficiency (Bassen–Kornzweig's disease)

This rare disease affects the nervous system, the retina, the gastrointestinal system, the heart and the red blood cells which show acanthocytosis (Bassen and Kornzweig 1950; Kornzweig and Bassen 1957).

Neurological symptoms are mainly central, with cerebellar ataxia, dysarthria, proprioceptive sensory loss and extensor plantar responses. The symptoms appear in childhood and progress into adult life. Peripheral neuropathy may occur and manifests itself in cutaneous sensory loss and abolition of tendon jerks.

Post-mortem findings were recorded by Sobrevilla, Goodman and Kane (1964). In the central nervous system they found degeneration of posterior columns and spinocerebellar tracts, also loss of neurons in the cerebellar cortex and in anterior horns. Sections of peripheral nerves showed 'focal areas of demyelination'. In a sural nerve biopsy Schwartz, Rowland, Eder, Marks, Osserman, Hirschberg and Anderson (1963) reported a severe loss of myelin disproportionate to the slight loss of axons, also a mild increase of sheath cell nuclei and endoneurial connective tissue. Further studies are required to elucidate the nature of the neuropathy, in particular to exclude nutritional factors consequent upon the malabsorption syndrome which is a common feature of the disease.

A somewhat similar neurological syndrome associated with acanthocytosis has also been described in the absence of abeta-lipoproteinaemia (Estes, Morley, Levine and Emerson 1967; Critchley, Clark and Wikler 1968; Aminoff 1972).

Inborn errors of lipid metabolism

See Chapter 12.

The hypertrophic neuropathies

The hypertrophic neuropathies form a heterogeneous group of conditions which share the common feature of clinically detectable enlargement of nerves due to hyperplasia of Schwann cells in response to chronic or recurrent demyelination (see p. 702). This is associated with considerable slowing of conduction velocities (Gilliatt and Sears 1958; Andermann, Lloyd-Smith, Mavor and Mathieson 1962; Ulrich, Esslen, Regli and Bischoff 1965; Thomas and Lascelles 1967). The protein in the cerebrospinal fluid is usually raised, except possibly in some of the most slowly progressive cases (Dyck and Lambert 1968a, b). An abnormal protein, between the beta- and gamma-globulin fraction, was present in the cerebrospinal fluid, serum and urine in a family described by Gibberd and Gavrilescu (1966).

The principal feature of the pathology of the affected nerves is hyperplasia of Schwann cells with 'onion bulb' formation. Teased single fibre preparations show evidence of demyelination and remyelination. The axis cylinders are almost invariably affected and both degenerating and regenerating axons may be seen. It is not uncommon to find 'onion bulbs' devoid of axons. The cords of hyperplastic Schwann cells may be widely separated by oedematous endoneurium which occasionally contains mucoid material. This oedema is, however, an inconstant feature. Changes in the posterior root ganglia are probably secondary to axonal degeneration, as are tract degenerations in the posterior columns.

The distribution of the lesions varies considerably, ranging from involvement of single nerves (Imaginario, Coelho, Tomé and Luis 1964; Simpson and Fowler 1966) to a generalized neuropathy. The spinal nerve roots are frequently involved. In some cases their enlargement may cause compression of the spinal cord and myelographic block (Symonds and Blackwood 1962).

The subject has been fully reviewed by Austin (1956), Dyck and Lambert (1968), Gathier and Bruyn (1970) and by Thomas, Lascelles and Stewart (1973). As a result of these studies it is now possible to subdivide hypertrophic neuropathy into genetic and sporadic types. Both recessive and dominant modes of inheritance have been recorded. The former include the condition originally described by Déjerine and Sottas, and also Refsum's disease. The dominant group includes the majority of reported familial cases. Those associated with von Recklinghausen's disease form a separate subgroup. The sporadic cases may be subdivided into those running a steadily progressive course and into remitting and relapsing ones.

Déjerine–Sottas disease

Déjerine and Sottas (1893) described two siblings with a progressive neurological disorder starting in childhood with bilateral foot deformity and difficulty in walking. There was wasting in the distal muscles of all four limbs, starting in the lower limbs with weakness of the affected muscles. Distal sensory loss was symmetrical and the patients complained of lightning pains. Eye signs included nystagmus, miosis and sluggish reaction of pupils to light. Thickening of peripheral nerves was a striking feature.

The post-mortem findings on one sibling were reported in the original article, on the other in a subsequent communication by Déjerine and Thomas (1906). The authors acknowledged the similarity of their findings to those of Gombault and Mallet (1889) in a case reported as tabes dorsalis. The findings were those outlined above.

Other clinical variants have been reported subsequently. Marie (1906) and Boveri (1910) described cases in which pupillary abnormalities were absent, and the prominent features were ataxia and intention tremor. It is indeed far from clear whether all cases conforming to the definition of Déjerine–Sottas disease, i.e. inherited as an autosomal recessive, starting in infancy and running a steadily progressive course, represent a single entity. This would require elucidation of the underlying metabolic error. Dyck, Ellefson, Lais, Smith, Taylor and Van Dyck (1970) noted an abnormality in the metabolism of ceramide hexosides and hexoside sulphates in one case.

Refsum's disease

In 1946 Refsum described a new familial clinical syndrome to which he gave the name 'heredopathia ataxica polyneuritiformis'. The outstanding features were atypical retinitis pigmentosa, night-blindness, peripheral neuropathy and increased cerebrospinal fluid protein content. A previous similar case was reported by Thiébault, Lemoyne and Guillaumat (1939) and subsequently identified by the same authors (1961) as a case of Refsum's disease. Several further cases have been recorded and the condition has been reviewed by Refsum (1960), by Veltema and Verjaal (1961) and by Kolodny, Hass, Lane and Drucker (1965).

The disease affects both sexes equally and is probably inherited as an autosomal recessive. Symptoms begin in childhood with night-blindness, hearing defects, ichthyosis, weakness of the limbs or ataxia. The disease runs a variable course, rapidly or slowly progressive, sometimes with long periods of arrest, in other instances with exacerbations or remissions. Death may be due to respiratory failure or to cardiomyopathy which is a common concomitant of the disease.

Peripheral neuropathy occurs in all cases, although the symptoms may not appear for some years after the onset of visual and auditory disorders. The neuropathy is usually symmetrical and starts in the lower limbs, gradually involving the upper limbs and trunk. Muscular wasting may be severe, and palpable thickening of peripheral nerves may be detected in advanced cases. The ataxia is predominantly cerebellar in type. The cerebrospinal fluid protein is almost constantly raised and may reach values of 600 mg per 100 ml.

Pathological descriptions include those of Cammermeyer (1956), Edström, Gröntoft and Sandring (1959), Alexander (1966) and of van Bogaert, van Mechelen, Martin and Guazzi (1967). The changes in the peripheral nerves are those of a hypertrophic neuropathy similar to the lesions seen in Déjerine–Sottas disease. Most writers emphasize the presence of abundant mucoid material in the endoneurial spaces. Alexander (1966) found an eosinophilic exudate, weakly PAS-positive and containing droplets of sudanophilic lipid. Cammermeyer also noted an abundance of mast cells.

Electron-microscopy confirmed the typical Schwannian hyperplasia of hypertrophic neuropathy (Dereux 1963; Dereux and Gruner 1963). In addition, Fardeau and Engel (1969) found osmiophilic droplets in the cytoplasm of Schwann cells and crystalline-like inclusions in their mitochondria.

In the central nervous system, axonal reaction in the anterior horn cells and degeneration of posterior columns are secondary to the peripheral lesions. Additional lesions include tract degenerations in the medial lemniscus and in cerebellar connections, particularly the olivocerebellar fibres. Droplets of sudanophilic lipid have been found in the leptomeninges, the choroid plexus, the ependyma, the glial cells of the globus pallidus and the red zone of the substantia nigra, but only in one instance (Cammermeyer) in neurons. Granular ependymitis was seen in several cases. Cerebellar lesions are inconspicuous, only one group of authors mentioning degenerative changes in Purkinje cells (Edström et al.).

Skeletal muscles show denervation atrophy. The heart may show a cardiomyopathy with focal scarring, resembling the lesions found in Friedreich's ataxia (Alexander 1966). The liver and kidney show fatty infiltration.

These findings suggested to Refsum that the condition was an inborn error of lipid metabolism. The problem has been clarified by the discovery of the presence of 3,7,11,15-tetramethyl-hexadecanoic (phytanic) acid in the fat of various tissues (Klenk and Kahlke 1963; Kahlke and Richterich 1965). Phytanic acid appears to be of dietary origin, being found in butter and other animal fats, but most of it is probably derived from phytol, present in green vegetables. The metabolic error involves an inability to degrade phytanic acid, which accumulates in the tissues (Steinberg, Mize, Avigan, Fales, Eldjarn, Try, Stokke and Refsum 1966). The pathogenetic mechanism by which phytanic acid affects various cells, and in particular the Schwann cells, remains obscure.

Polyneuropathy with optico-acoustic degeneration

Rosenberg and Chutorian (1967) reported a family, consisting of two brothers and a nephew, with a syndrome consisting of optic atrophy, nerve deafness and a polyneuropathy resembling peroneal muscular atrophy. Nerve conduction velocities were slow. A similar condition, affecting a brother and sister, was reported by Iwashita, Inoue and Kuroiwa (1969). A sural nerve biopsy carried out on the brother showed typical hypertrophic changes with onion-bulb formation on electron-microscopy (Ohta 1970). If this condition is indeed a single entity its mode of inheritance remains obscure. The American cases suggest a sex-linked, the Japanese an autosomal recessive mode.

The dominant variant of hypertrophic neuropathy
The eponym of Déjerine–Sottas disease has often been extended to include cases of later onset, lesser severity and slower progression, inherited as a dominant trait with a variable degree of penetrance. Detailed family studies include those of Russell and Garland (1930) subsequently reviewed by Croft and Wadia (1957) and those of Sears (1931), of Cooper (1936) and of Bedford and James (1956). Clinically this condition closely resembles peroneal muscular atrophy. In analysing a large clinical material of peroneal muscular atrophy, Dyck and Lambert (1968a) separated from it a group of cases characterized by marked reduction of motor conduction velocities. The pathology of the affected nerves is that of segmental demyelination and remyelination, revealed by teased fibre preparations of sural nerve biopsies (Gutrecht and Dyck 1966). The marked hyperplasia of Schwann cells leads to 'onion bulb' formation, best demonstrated by electron-microscopy. On reviewing the literature Dyck and Lambert concluded that the 'dominant form of Déjerine–Sottas disease' and the 'demyelinating variety of Charcot–Marie–Tooth's disease' probably represented the same entity. The use of both eponyms is probably incorrect and the condition is best defined as the dominant form of familial hypertrophic neuropathy.

Hypertrophic neuropathy associated with neurofibromatosis
The pathology of von Recklinghausen's disease is outside the scope of this book, but it may be noted that tissue reactions of hypertrophic neuritis have been observed in neurofibromatosis (Bielschowsky 1922; Bailey and Hermann 1938; Austin 1956). Borderline cases which may be interpreted either as atypical cases of hypertrophic neuropathy or of neurofibromatosis have also been recorded (Krücke 1942–43; Bruns 1951; Reisner and Spiel 1952).

Sporadic cases
Roussy and Cornil (1919) drew attention to the occurrence of sporadic cases of hypertrophic neuropathy starting in middle life and running a steadily progressive course. Previous reports include those of Long (1906) and Dide and Courjon (1918). Other cases have been reported in which the disease ran a relapsing and remitting course (Harris and Newcombe 1929). The pathological features of these cases are indistinguishable from those described in the genetic variants. The 'Roussy–Cornil syndrome' probably represents a mixed group of chronic demyelinating neuropathies of obscure aetiology. Some may be examples of chronic or recurrent idiopathic polyneuritis which ultimately develop a hypertrophic pattern (Cazzato 1965).

Infantile polyneuropathy
The syndrome of the 'floppy infant' (Walton 1969) may be due to a variety of causes. While the central and muscular lesions are well documented, those due to abnormalities in peripheral nerves are poorly understood. Chambers and MacDermot (1957), Byers and Taft (1957) and Tasker and Chutorian (1969) all reported series of cases of chronic polyneuropathy with hypotonia starting in infancy or early childhood. If cases of metachromatic leucodystrophy and obvious hypertrophic neuropathy are excluded, the residue consists of a variety of obscure polyneuropathies, some progressive, some relapsing, others self-limiting or responding to treatment with steroids. Light-microscopic examination of biopsies usually showed loss of myelin, some loss of axons, excess of collagen and patchy neurogenic atrophy of muscles.

Electron-microscopic studies, in a few similar cases, revealed lesions of hypertrophic neuropathy, even when they were not apparent under the light microscope (Dyck 1966; Webster et al. 1967; Weller 1967; Joosten, Gabreëls, Gabreëls-Festen, Vrensen, Korten and Notermans 1974).

A few cases which fall outside this range have been recorded. Lyon (1969) reported the case of a girl, hypotonic from early infancy, unable to walk without support at $2\frac{1}{2}$ years, with moderate distal muscle wasting and absent tendon jerks. A sural nerve biopsy showed almost total disappearance of myelin sheaths, apparent preservation of axons and increase in endoneurial collagen. Electron microscopy revealed concentric structures resembling the 'onion-bulbs' of hypertrophic neuropathy, but consisting almost entirely of reduplicated basement membranes with scanty Schwann cell processes. The axons were either totally demyelinated or possessed very thin, often irregular sheaths. Other Schwann cell abnormalities were also noted.

Similar findings were described by Kennedy, Sung, Berry and Mastri (1971) in a 5½-year-old girl, hypotonic, scoliotic and areflexic, whose sister had died of a similar condition at the age of 10 months. A sural nerve biopsy, examined by light- and electron-microscopy, showed some reduction in the number of large axons, most of which were unmyelinated. In the rare myelinated fibres the thickness of the sheath was greatly reduced. Onion-bulb formations consisted mainly of double lamellae of basement membranes, frequently without intervening Schwann cell processes. Collagen fibres were abundant. The authors interpreted the findings as evidence of primary hypomyelination in which the Schwann cells were unable to manufacture or maintain a significant amount of myelin.

Another case is that of a boy, floppy since early life with progressive muscular weakness, diagnosed clinically as Werdnig–Hoffmann's disease. Death from respiratory failure occurred at the age of 8 months. At autopsy no lesions were found in the central nervous system, but there was apparently total loss of myelin in cranial nerves, dorsal and ventral spinal nerve roots and samples of peripheral nerves (Karch and Urich 1975).

The disparity of materials and methods make these cases difficult to compare. Their nosology and, in particular, their relationship to hypertrophic neuropathies remains obscure. Joosten et al. (1974) consider Lyon's case a variant of hypertrophic neuropathy on the strength of finding similar lesions side by side with typical onion-bulbs in their familial case.

Globular neuropathy

Dayan, Graveson, Robinson and Woodhouse (1968) described four cases of a progressive peripheral sensorimotor neuropathy affecting members of three generations of one family and one member of another, unrelated one. The study of sural nerve biopsies from two cases revealed evidence of axonal degeneration and regeneration as well as of segmental demyelination and remyelination. In addition bizarre globules of lipid, with ultrastructural properties of a complex phospholipid, were found incorporated into the myelin sheaths. The nosological position of this disorder remains obscure. Its relationship to the 'sausage-body' neuropathy (Behse, Buchthal, Carlsen and Knappes 1972) has been discussed by Madrid and Bradley (1975).

Focal lesions

The vascular neuropathies

Occlusions of major vessels

The involvement of peripheral nerves in ischaemia due to chronic occlusive arterial disease was first described by Joffroy and Achard (1889). Similar changes may be produced by arterial embolism (Blackwood 1944) and by arterial injury (Tinel 1917). The abundant literature on the subject has been reviewed by Richards (1951).

The incidence of significant clinical involvement of peripheral nerves in vascular occlusion is difficult to assess, the figures differing according to the criteria adopted. Hutchinson and Liversedge (1956) found neurological abnormalities in 58·8% of their patients and Mufson (1952) in 53%. Eames and Lange (1967) found evidence of sensory neuropathy in 87·5% of 32 patients studied, but their series included those in whom

loss of vibration sense was the only abnormality present. Symptoms of ischaemic neuropathy include lightning pains, painful paraesthesiae and pain at rest. Objective loss of one or more sensory modalities is commonly present. Vibration sense is most frequently lost, but impairment of sense of position and patchy loss of superficial sensation may also be found. Motor symptoms, including weakness and wasting, occur less frequently than sensory manifestations.

The older literature emphasized the common occurrence of Wallerian degeneration but gave little indication of the nature of the process. A detailed modern study by Eames and Lange (1967), which included examination of teased individual fibres and electron microscopy, revealed widespread demyelination and remyelination of large and, to a lesser extent, medium-sized fibres. Some regenerated fibres with uniformly short internodes were also found. Axonal damage was probably more severe than the small numbers of regenerating fibres would suggest. There was an appreciable diminution in the total number of axons and a marked increase in the amount of endoneurial collagen. The authors also emphasized the changes found in the vasa nervorum, which frequently showed endothelial proliferation, occlusion by fibrin thrombi and marked

Polyarteritis nodosa

Peripheral neuropathy figured prominently in Kussmaul and Maier's (1866) original description of polyarteritis ('periarteritis') nodosa. The older literature has been fully reviewed by Wohlwill (1923) and by Baló (1926), the more recent work has been briefly summarized by Bignami (1961).

The incidence of neurological complications has been reported as ranging from 12 to 60% of cases.

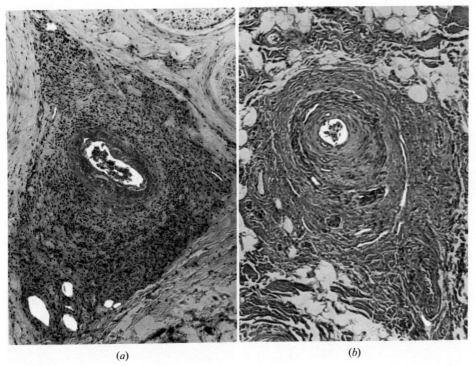

(a)   (b)

Fig. 16.30 Polyarteritis nodosa. (a) Acute lesion with fibrinoid necrosis of arterial wall and inflammatory infiltration of adventitia. H & E. × 120. (b) Healed lesion with fibrosis of all coats of arterial wall and total loss of internal elastica. Elastic van Gieson. × 120.

thickening and reduplication of endothelial basement membranes. They thought that these secondary occlusive phenomena in the vasa nervorum might play an important part in determining focal nerve damage.

The occurrence of segmental demyelination and remyelination in ischaemic nerves was confirmed on sural nerve biopsies by Chopra and Hurwitz (1967), who suggested that segmental demyelination may be the initial pathological response to ischaemia.

Lovshin and Kernohan (1948) found clinical evidence of peripheral neuropathy in 52% of their series of 25 patients.

The classical clinical picture is that of progressive involvement of several peripheral nerves in succession, a sequence of events to which Kernohan and Woltman (1938) gave the name of 'mononeuritis multiplex'. Both the motor and sensory functions are commonly affected. The onset may be abrupt or gradual, the spread into successive nerves rapid or in well spaced out episodes. The final distribution may be symmetrical or asymmetrical; if all four limbs are affected more or less simultaneously the picture resembles that of an acute polyneuropathy. The most common initial symptom is pain; this is frequently accompanied by paraesthesiae and motor weakness. The natural course of the disease is usually steadily progressive, but spontaneous regressions occur and many cases respond favourably to treatment with corticosteroids.

The lesions are those of a necrotizing arteritis involving the vasa nervorum (Fig. 16.30). They resemble those seen in other parts of the body

degeneration, which may affect isolated funiculi or parts thereof. Through a summation effect these lesions are more prominent in the distal than in the proximal parts of the nerves.

Wegener's granulomatosis

The triad of granulomata of the respiratory tract, arteritis and nephritis, known as Wegener's granulomatosis, involves peripheral nerves in a similar way to polyarteritis nodosa, yet has received little attention. There is no mention of peripheral neuropathy in Wegener's (1939)

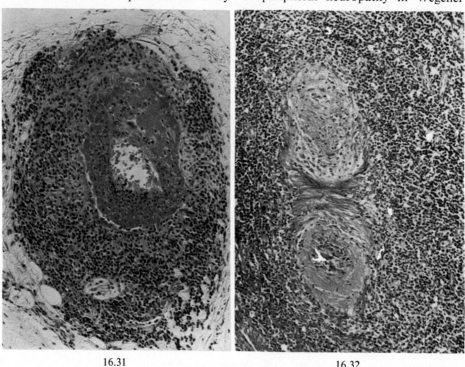

16.31   16.32

Fig. 16.31 Wegener's granulomatosis. Acute necrotizing arteritis indistinguishable from polyarteritis nodosa. H & E. × 120.

Fig. 16.32 Lymphomatoid granulomatosis. Necrotizing arterial lesion surrounded by massive lymphocytic infiltrate. Elastic van Gieson. × 120.

and may go through various stages of evolution (Arkin 1930). The effects of these vascular lesions on the nerves are variable. The anastomotic circulation in the vasa nervorum is exceptionally rich (Sunderland 1945a, b) and multiple occlusions are necessary to produce ischaemic lesions. Lovshin and Kernohan (1948) refer to nerve 'infarcts' without describing them in detail. Foci of demyelination without loss of axons have been described (Holtermann 1924; Bignami 1961). The most prominent lesion is, however, Wallerian

account, but subsequent reviews (Walton 1958; Drachman 1963) have revealed a high incidence of neurological complications.

Drachman (1963) divided them into three groups. The first consists of contiguous invasion of nervous structures by nasal and paranasal granulomata, which may cause external ocular palsies and involvement of branches of the trigeminal nerve. The rare second group includes random lesions in single peripheral nerves involved in granulomata remote from the respiratory tract.

The third and largest group presents as a 'mononeuritis multiplex'. This is due to a widespread arteritis indistinguishable from polyarteritis nodosa (Stern, Hoffbrand and Urich 1965) (Fig. 16.31).

Lymphomatoid granulomatosis

Liebow, Carrington and Friedman (1972) isolated a group of cases of a granulomatous condition affecting the lungs and many other organs, characterized by a necrotizing arteritis, extensive necrosis and infiltration predominantly by atypical lymphocytes and plasmacytoid cells. The relationship of the condition to Wegener's granulomatosis on one hand and to the lymphomas on the other remains obscure.

Both the central and the peripheral nervous systems may be involved. The lesions in peripheral nerves are those of a 'mononeuritis multiplex' due to necrotizing arteritis of the vasa nervorum. The condition may be distinguished from classical polyarteritis nodosa by the nature of the perivascular cellular infiltrate (Fig. 16.32).

Rheumatoid neuropathy

The occurrence of a peripheral neuropathy in the course of rheumatoid arthritis was first reported by Pitres and Vaillard (1887) and infrequent accounts of this complication have appeared in subsequent literature. The advent of corticosteroid therapy and its controversial effects on various aspects of rheumatoid disease have led to a revival of interest in the neurological complications (Hart, Golding and Mackenzie 1957; Mason and Steinberg 1957–58).

In their review of 30 cases of rheumatoid arthritis with peripheral neuropathy, Pallis and Scott (1965) classified the clinical manifestations into five patterns: (I) Upper limb : single nerve lesions; (II) Upper limb : digital neuropathy; (III) Lower limb : single nerve lesions; (IV) Lower limb : distal sensory neuropathy; (V) All four limbs : mixed sensorimotor neuropathy.

Types I and III are entrapment neuropathies occurring in the neighbourhood of affected joints. Type II is a patchy ischaemic neuropathy secondary to digital arteritis, a common feature of rheumatoid disease (Scott, Hourihane, Doyle, Steiner, Laws, Dixon and Bywaters 1961). Types IV and V represent the mild and severe forms of rheumatoid polyneuropathy respectively. The latter usually follows the pattern of 'mononeuritis multiplex' and carries a serious prognosis

most patients dying within a year from occlusive vascular disease elsewhere. Predominantly it affects male patients.

In the pathology of the condition many points still require elucidation. The earlier accounts (Freund, Steiner, Leichtentritt and Price 1942; Morrison, Short, Ludwig and Schwab 1947) are not entirely satisfactory. They described inflammatory nodules in the perineurium (meaning epineurium) which they equated with the subcutaneous rheumatoid nodules. Their illustrations suggest that they were describing vascular lesions.

Recent post-mortem studies are largely confined to the severe polyneuropathies (Hart *et al.* 1957; Mason and Steinberg 1957–58; Hart and Golding 1960; Pallis and Scott 1965). With the exception of two mild cases of Hart and Golding, which did not fall into Type V, all the reported cases showed evidence of obliterative arteritis of the vasa nervorum. The nature and severity of the arteritic lesions vary considerably (Schmid, Cooper, Ziff and McEwen 1961).

The common type is represented by a bland intimal proliferation leading to total or subtotal occlusion of the lumen with preservation of the internal elastica (Bywaters 1957) (Fig. 16.33*a*). Mild inflammatory infiltration and some deposition of fibrinoid material may be found in some vessels (Fig. 16.33*b* and *c*). At the other end of the scale there are acute necrotising lesions indistinguishable from polyarteritis nodosa. The superimposition of these on a pre-existing Bywaters' arteritis may lead to difficulties in interpretation (Fig. 16.33*d*).

Far less is known about the benign forms. Weller, Bruckner and Chamberlain (1970) carried out clinical and electrophysiological studies on five cases of rheumatoid neuropathy, supported by histological examination of sural nerve biopsies. Two cases were of the severe sensorimotor variety, one of which showed the expected vascular lesions. The remaining three were mild distal sensory neuropathies which electromyographically also showed evidence of motor denervation. Sural nerve biopsies showed evidence of obliterative arteritis in one case, severe loss of large myelinated axons likely to be caused by more proximal ischaemia in another, and no significant lesions in the third. The authors support the view that even the mild forms are secondary to vascular involvement.

Haslock, Wright and Harriman (1970) studied

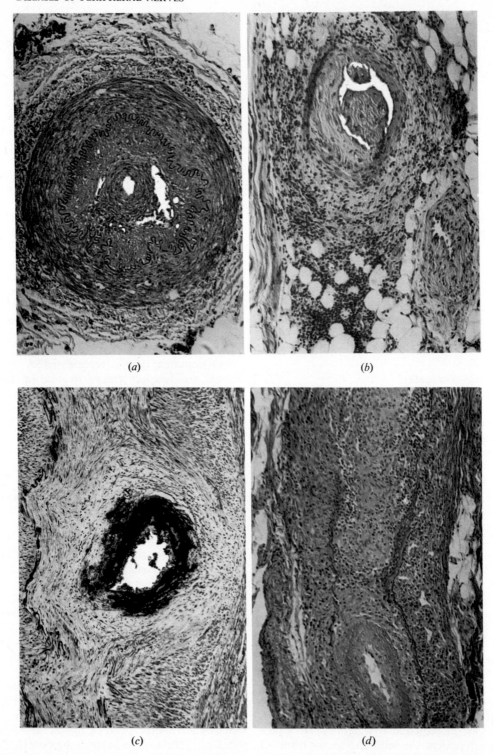

Fig. 16.33 Rheumatoid neuropathy. (*a*) Bywaters' arteritis with intimal fibrosis but otherwise intact vessel wall. H & E. × 120. (*b*) Lymphocytic infiltration in Bywaters' arteritis. H & E.   × 120. (*c*) Deposition of fibrinoid in Bywaters' arteritis. Mallory's PTAH.   × 120. (*d*) Polyarteritis nodosa superimposed on Bywaters' arteritis: the process is largely confined to the thickened intima and the elastica is partially preserved. Elastic van Gieson.   × 120.

nerve and muscle biopsies from nine cases of rheumatoid neuropathy, one of which subsequently came to autopsy. They reached the conclusion that while all severe neuropathies were caused by vascular lesions, only some of the milder cases were due to bland endarteritis, while others showed segmental demyelination. Beckett and Dinn (1972) examined sural nerve biopsies from cases of rheumatoid arthritis with or without neuropathy. Segmental demyelination with complete remyelination was found in patients without clinical neurological manifestations. Overt neuropathy was associated with vascular lesions and Wallerian degeneration. In an intermediate group vascular lesions were present, as well as segmental demyelination with partial remyelination. There is thus substantial evidence for the occurrence of segmental demyelination independent of vascular lesions, but its significance requires further investigation.

Systemic lupus erythematosus
The peripheral nervous system is less commonly involved in systemic lupus than in rheumatoid arthritis (Bennett, Hughes, Bywaters and Holt 1972). In a consecutive study of 100 patients only three were found to have evidence of neuropathy (Clark and Bailey 1954). It may take the form of a symmetrical distal sensorimotor neuropathy or of a mononeuritis multiplex. Pathological observations are scanty. Most of them revealed vascular lesions, either in the form of an acute necrotizing arteritis or of a bland endarteritis with preserved elastica (Sedgwick and Van Hagen 1948; Heptinstall and Sowry 1952; Bailey, Sayre and Clark 1956; Anderson 1965). In two cases the lesions were thought to be purely degenerative (Schienberg 1956; Goldberg and Chitanondh 1959). Haematoxyphil bodies were found in peripheral nerves only in Schienberg's case.

Amyloid neuropathy
Deposition of amyloid occurs in peripheral nerves in cases of primary amyloidosis. It is confined to the type of amyloid which deposits on collagen fibres (the pericollagen type of Heller, Missmahl, Sohar and Gafni 1964). The condition was first described by De Bruyn and Stern (1929) but misinterpreted as an example of hypertrophic neuropathy. Other sporadic cases were reported by de Navasquez and Treble (1938), Götze and Krücke (1941), Kernohan and Woltman (1942),

and Munsat and Poussaint (1962). Andrade (1952) drew attention to the familial occurrence of the disease in Portuguese fishermen of the Oporto region and many other affected families have been recorded in various parts of the world (Kantarjian and Dejong 1953; Rukavina, Block, Jackson, Falls, Carey and Curtis 1956; Schlesinger, Duggins and Masucci 1962; Castaigne, Cambier and Augustin 1965; Araki, Mawatari, Ohta, Nakajima and Kuroiwa 1968; Zalin, Darby, Vaughan and Raftery 1974). The mode of inheritance in familial cases affects predominantly males, as also does the sporadic form. The age of onset is earlier in the familial form, usually between 20 and 40 years, while the sporadic form tends to present in later middle age. The florid type of amyloid neuropathy rarely, if ever, occurs in myelomatosis, despite the pericollagen distribution of amyloid in this disease. Small amounts of perivascular amyloid may, however, be found on histological examination of the nerves.

The clinical picture is that of a sensorimotor neuropathy of insidious onset and slowly progressive course. Sensory symptoms are usually prominent, and commonly begin in the lower limbs. They consist of pains, sometimes of lightning type, dysaesthesiae of various types, hyperaesthesia of the skin and muscular tenderness. Dissociated anaesthesia with distal loss of appreciation of pain and temperature may occur at an early stage. As the disease progresses, all sensory modalities become affected and signs of lower motor neuron involvement become apparent. Involvement of the cranial nerves may also occur and can be the predominant feature as in the familial Finnish cases reported by Meretoja (1969). Ultimately the patient becomes totally disabled, and the disease ends fatally after a course of 1 to 10 years.

The neurological manifestations are accompanied by signs of involvement of other systems, most commonly the gastrointestinal tract and the heart. Renal involvement leading to death in uraemia was a prominent feature of the familial cases described by Van Allen, Frohlich and Davis (1969).

The pathological findings are similar in sporadic (de Navasquez and Treble 1938; Götze and Krücke 1941) and in familial cases (Andrade 1952). The lesions consist of deposits of amyloid mainly in the endoneurium and to a lesser extent in the interfunicular epineurium. These deposits are irregular, but roughly globular in shape and variable in size. Many of them are demonstrably related to blood vessels, where amyloid is deposited both in the media and in the adventitia (Fig. 16.34). The gradual thickening of the vessel wall leads to progressive reduction and, finally, obliteration of the lumen. The adventitial deposits are often eccentric, crescentic in shape and extend deeply into the parenchyma of the nerve.

The distribution of lesions within the nerves is random, but tends to be more abundant in distal parts. Amyloid deposits may be found in the posterior root ganglia, leading to their visible enlargement (de Navasquez and Treble 1938). In

to amyloid nodules. In their study of the Portuguese familial cases Coimbra and Andrade (1971b) failed to confirm this selective predilection for small unmyelinated fibres. Large myelinated fibres were equally affected, and their degeneration did not follow a strictly Wallerian pattern in that disintegration of the myelin sheath preceded changes in the axon.

The pathogenesis of these lesions is obscure. In Kernohan and Woltman's (1942) view the damage is due entirely to obliteration of the vasa nervorum; they included amyloidosis of peripheral nerves among ischaemic neuropathies.

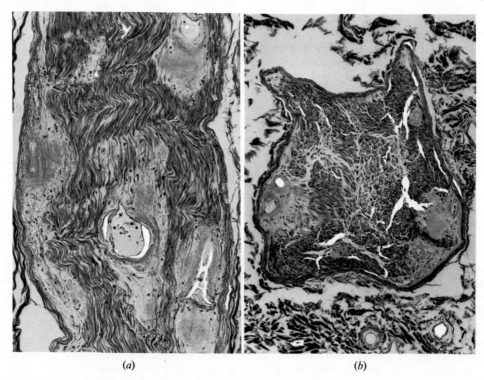

(a)   *(b)*

Fig. 16.34 Amyloid neuropathy. (*a*) Longitudinal and (*b*) transverse sections of nerve showing perivascular distribution of amyloid. Lendrum's method for amyloid. × 135.

Krücke's (1959*a*, *b*) opinion the ganglia are the sites of the most severe lesions, but that is not necessarily so. The posterior roots may be severely affected; the anterior roots usually escape.

Dyck and Lambert (1969) examined biopsies of sural nerves of two patients suffering from the familial form of the disease. Electron-microscopy revealed selective loss of unmyelinated axons and, to a lesser extent, of small myelinated fibres. Preparations of teased fibres showed predominantly Wallerian degeneration, while demyelination and remyelination was seen only in fibres adjacent

While ischaemia may play a part in amyloid neuropathy it is open to doubt whether this is the main pathogenetic mechanism. Coimbra and Andrade (1971*a*, *b*) believe that degeneration of nerve fibres is independent of deposition of amyloid. This view is based on observations in early cases where amyloid was scanty and fibre degeneration already advanced. The non-Wallerian pattern of degeneration militates against interruption of axons proximal to the site of biopsy.

A localized form of amyloidosis, apparently

confined to the Gasserian ganglion, has been found in two patients in whom these ganglia were surgically removed for the treatment of trigeminal neuralgia (Daly, Love and Dockerty 1957; Borghi and Tagliabue 1961). At the time of operation these patients showed no evidence of systemic amyloidosis or of neuropathy, and their trigeminal symptoms were unilateral. In the absence of adequate follow-up studies, the nosological position of localized Gasserian amyloidosis remains uncertain.

An unusual form of trigeminal amyloidosis was found in a case of trigeminal neuropathy described by Spillane and Wells (1959, case 15). This patient showed degeneration of the entire sensory root of the 5th nerve, with deposition of a substance showing all staining reactions of amyloid at the glio-schwannian junction and of an atypical substance, sharing some staining reactions with amyloid, along the course of the degenerated fibres. Similar deposits were found in the walls of the blood vessels of the spinal tract of the trigeminal nerve and in degenerated long tracts in the spinal cord (Spillane and Urich 1976).

Peripheral nerves may be involved indirectly in amyloidosis of connective tissue structures which may cause entrapment of individual nerves. Bilateral carpal tunnel syndromes have been repeatedly described in myelomatosis (Grokoest and Demartini 1954; Kyle and Bayrd 1961; Hamilton and Bywaters 1961; Dayan, Urich and Gardner-Thorpe 1970). In these cases the flexor retinaculum is grossly thickened and heavily infiltrated with amyloid.

Sarcoidosis of the peripheral nervous system

See Chapter 6.

Xanthomatous neuropathy

A sensory neuropathy may occur in the course of primary biliary cirrhosis associated with hypercholesterolaemia and xanthomatosis (Thomas and Walker 1965). The clinical features include unpleasant paraesthesiae, hyperaesthesia, pain and distal sensory loss. Nerve biopsies showed small yellowish swellings visible to the naked eye. These were due to infiltration of the perineurium, and to a lesser extent the endoneurium, by lipid-laden foam cells. A secondary overgrowth of con-

nective tissue would follow, leading ultimately to complete disorganization of the architecture of the nerve.

Idiopathic hyperlipaemia

Fulton (1952) described a patient with hyperlipaemia, gout, a sensory neuropathy of glove-and-stocking distribution and myocardial changes. In a somewhat similar case Sandbank, Bechar and Bornstein (1971) carried out a nerve biopsy and found changes suggestive of segmental demyelination on light-microscopy. Electron-microscopy showed axons surrounded by accumulations of myelin figures ('disorganized hypermyelination'), invagination of Schwann cell cytoplasm into axons and multiplication of basement membranes.

Fabry's disease

Angiokeratoma corporis diffusum (Fabry 1898) is a genetically determined disorder of lipid metabolism transmitted as a sex-linked recessive. The abnormality consists of a deficiency of the enzyme ceramide trihexosidase, which results in the accumulation of ceramid trihexose in the tissues (Brady, Gall, Bradley, Martensson, Warshaw and Laster 1967). The tissues affected are blood vessels, skin, eyes, kidneys, heart and the nervous system.

In the nervous system some lesions are secondary to vascular involvement, others to lipid storage in neurons of various parts of the brain and in the ganglia of the autonomic nervous system (Rahman and Lindenberg 1963).

Peripheral manifestations are confined to attacks of severe pain in the limbs, the cause of which remains obscure. Lesions in peripheral nerves have been described on biopsy material by Bischoff, Fierz, Regli and Ulrich (1968) and by Kocen and Thomas (1970). The latter found granules of sudanophil, PAS-positive lipid in the perineurium, as well as some loss of myelinated axons, particularly in the smaller fibre range. Electron-microscopy revealed lamellated inclusions in the cytoplasm of perineurial cells with a periodicity of ± 4 nm. Bischoff et al. reported similar findings but state the periodicity of the lamellae to be 5-6 nm. In addition, they found degenerative changes in unmyelinated axons. Neither group of authors found any evidence of demyelination.

Traumatic lesions of peripheral nerves

Acute injuries

Seddon (1942, 1943, 1972) classified injuries of peripheral nerves into three categories: neurapraxia, axonotmesis and neurotmesis.

Neurapraxia implies a degree of injury to the axons in which their function is temporarily abolished without anatomical disruption. Wallerian degeneration does not occur and function is usually completely restored. This type of injury is commonly caused by pressure or blows.

Axonotmesis described lesions in which there is disruption of continuity of the nerve fibres due to destruction of axons at the site of injury. The connective tissue sheaths are, however, preserved. Wallerian degeneration occurs in the severed axons, but regeneration along pre-existing endoneurial tubes proceeds unimpeded as there is no neuroma formation. Axonotmesis commonly occurs in areas of severe bruising, as in fractures involving peripheral nerves.

In *neurotmesis* there is disruption of the connective tissue sheaths as well as of the nerve fibres. A neuroma forms at the site of the lesion and recovery is delayed. Injuries of this type may be caused by cuts, gun-shot wounds or severe traction.

Sunderland (1968), in his monograph which deals exhaustively with all aspects of the subject, divides nerve injuries into five degrees. A first-degree injury involves interruption of conduction with preservation of the continuity of axons. In the second degree there is loss of continuity of axons without breaches in the endoneurium. The third degree comprises injuries with intrafunicular rupture of the endoneurium, but preservation of the perineurium. Rupture of the perineurium with loss of continuity of entire funiculi constitutes the fourth degree, while severance of the entire nerve trunk occurs in the fifth. The first and second degrees correspond to Seddon's neurapraxia and axonotmesis respectively, while the higher degrees are subdivisions of the category of neurotmesis, their main importance being in the size and position of the ensuing neuroma.

Very little is known of the pathology of neurapraxia in man and most of our data are derived from experimental work. Denny-Brown and Brenner (1944a) studied the effects of percussion on the nerves and of various forms of pressure (1944b). Denny-Brown and Doherty (1945) examined the effects of stretching on peripheral nerves.

The effects of percussion varied depending on severity. Severe blows led to extensive local necrosis of axons and myelin sheaths with Wallerian degeneration of the distal portion of the injured fibres. Milder percussion led to a transient paralysis in which the lesions consisted of localized interstitial oedema ('pseudoneuroma') and local demyelination affecting mainly the large fibres. This local demyelination outlasted the transient paralysis. The compression lesions appear to act on the nerves largely through ischaemia and their effects are therefore similar to those produced by transient or prolonged impairment of blood supply. Recently, however, Ochoa, Danta, Fowler and Gilliatt (1971) produced evidence of direct damage to myelin sheaths by pressure. Application of a sphygmomanometer to the limb of a baboon and inflation to 1000 mm Hg caused dislocation and invagination of paranodal myelin with subsequent localized demyelination. The nodal displacement is maximal under the edges of the cuff, with relative or complete sparing under its centre, the direction of displacement always being away from the cuff towards uncompressed tissue, suggesting that the pressure gradient within the nerve, between its compressed and its uncompressed parts, is the factor responsible for the movement (Ochoa, Fowler and Gilliatt 1972).

Slow, progressive compression leads to local segmental demyelination most conspicuous in the superficial fibres of the compressed nerve (Aguayo, Nair and Midgley 1971).

Stretching experiments revealed a remarkable resistance to this type of injury. Nerves could be stretched to nearly double their length without damage to their perineurium or blood vessels with only transient paralysis. When stretching is carried to the point of rupture of blood vessels, ischaemic lesions ensue. There is, however, no general agreement on the tensile strength of nerves as outlined by Denny-Brown and Doherty. Figures obtained by various authors on different species range from 10 to 100% of elongation before mechanical failure. Sunderland and Bradley (1961) investigated the problem on fresh human post-mortem material and obtained results ranging from 7 to 32%. Tensile strength depends essentially on the perineurium, and varies in individual nerves according to their funicular structure, nerves being stronger when they are composed of numerous small funiculi. Nerve roots, being devoid of perineurium, are more vulnerable than nerve trunks. Another important factor is that of time, slow stretching over long periods being far less damaging than rapid stretching (Sunderland 1968).

The lesions of axonotmesis have been studied in experimental animals by Gutmann and Sanders (1943). The fundamental processes of Wallerian degeneration and regeneration have already been outlined in the general section. In the absence of neuroma formation, the regenerative process remains unimpeded and the regenerating fibres follow the intact endoneurial tubes. The end-result is restoration of the nerves almost to their original condition, with the exception of considerable shortening of internodal lengths.

In neurotmesis the regenerative phenomena are modified and delayed by the absence of a continuous pathway for the regenerating axons. The gap between the cut ends is filled with blood and plasma, which after a few days becomes organized by invading fibroblasts. Some of these follow the orientation of the nerve, others are arranged obliquely. As the axonal sprouts leave the endoneurial tubules of the proximal segments they come into contact with these fibroblasts and tend to run along them, the fibroblasts forming collagenous tubules around the new axons, several of which may be contained within one tubule (Denny-Brown 1946). With the varying orientation of the fibroblasts the axons tend to grow in haphazard directions, mostly obliquely to the line of the nerve and a neuroma is formed. The size and shape of the neuroma depends on the nature and degree of the injury. If the perineurium remains intact the neuroma remains intrafunicular (spindle neuroma). Where the perineurium is breached but not severed, fibroblastic proliferation occurs through the gap and a lateral neuroma is formed. When the perineurium is severed but the ends have not retracted, a small neuroma will rapidly bridge the gap. With wide retraction of the cut ends, such as occurs in total severance of a nerve (fifth-degree injury), swellings develop at both cut ends, known as the proximal and distal bulbs. Both bulbs consist of fibroblastic and Schwannian elements, the proximal bulb also containing regenerating axons. If the gap is small, the proximal unites with the distal by fibroblastic granulation tissue which is gradually invaded by axons and Schwann cells. If the gap is too large to be bridged, a stump, or terminal neuroma forms at the proximal end. Even in this situation a few axons may find

their way through the intervening scar tissue to the endoneurial tubes of the distal segment (Sunderland 1953) (Fig. 16.35).

It remains controversial whether proliferation of columns of Schwann cells precedes (Nageotte 1932) or follows (Denny-Brown 1946) the growth of regenerating axons. Electron-microscopic studies (Spencer 1971) have revealed the immense complexity of processes affecting the various cellular components of neuromas, but have left many problems unsolved.

Both terminal and collateral axonal sprouting occurs and tends to be more profuse in neuroma formation than after simple crush injuries (Shawe 1955). A single regenerating axon may give rise to as many as 50 sprouts. Several of these may grow into a single endoneurial tube of the distal end, but usually only a few acquire a myelin sheath. Ultimately one tends to dominate the growth pattern and the others fail to survive (Weddell 1942). On the other hand a single axon may innervate several endoneurial tubes by branching. A confusion of growth occurs and fibres may be misdirected to a functionally different end-organ.

Remyelination proceeds *pari passu* with regeneration. Holmes and Young (1942) observed myelination immediately below the suture line 15 days after surgical repair and concluded that the process began as soon as the axon came into contact with Schwann cytoplasm.

The rate of growth of the regenerating axons has been the subject of several studies, both in experimental animals and, indirectly, in man. The original delay depends on the degree of neuroma formation and may extend to several months. Once the axons reach the endoneurial tubes of the distal end growth proceeds unimpeded. It was held until recently that the rate of growth was constant throughout the length of the nerve. In fact, the rate of advance of the axon tip gradually diminishes over the whole period of recovery and is slower at the distal than at the proximal end of the nerve (Sunderland 1947). In rabbits the mean growth is approximately 3 mm per day (Gutman, Guttmann, Medawar and Young 1942). In man Seddon, Medawar and Smith (1943) estimated the average rate to be approximately 1·5 mm per day. Sunderland (1947) found rates of 3 mm per day in the arm and thigh, 0·5 mm per day at the wrist and ankle.

The ultimate pattern of the regenerated nerve depends on several factors, among others the

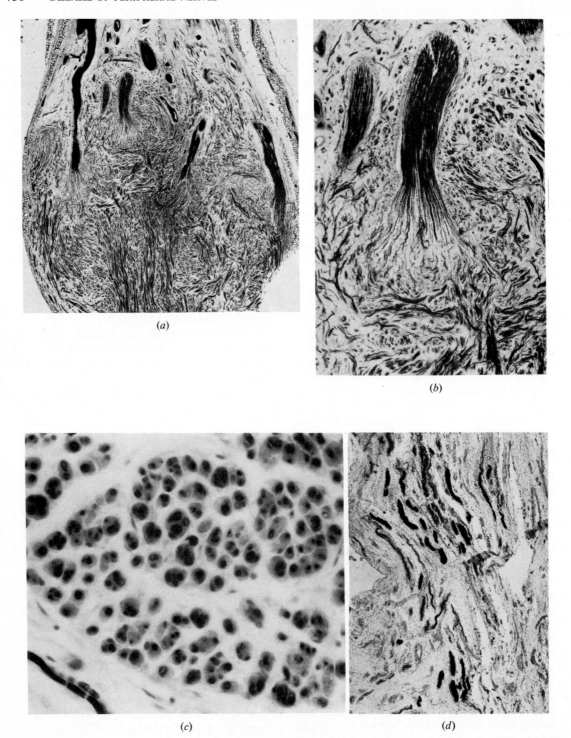

Fig. 16.35 Trauma of peripheral nerves. (*a*) and (*b*) Low and higher power view of traumatic neuroma. Myelin. Towards the lower end the fibres are again becoming longitudinally orientated. (*c*) Transverse sections of sprouting nerve fibres near their origin from old nerve fibres. Note that several small fibres arise from one old fibre. Myelin. (*d*) New nerve fibres running in scar tissue joining proximal and distal cut ends of a nerve.

size of the endoneurial tubes which the new axons occupy. In simple crush injuries, where axons are guided back into their original tubes, they regain their original diameter and thickness of myelin sheath (Gutmann and Sanders 1943). Constriction of endoneurial tubes by fibrosis, more likely to occur after a long period of delay, may however prevent the axon from reaching its full size. Similarly, the entry of a sprout of a large axon into a tube previously occupied by a small one will affect its expansion (Sanders and Young 1944, 1946). Another factor affecting the size of the regenerating nerve fibres is the establishment of abnormal functional relationships. Axons which are misdirected to a functionally unrelated end-organ fail to regain their original diameter or degree of myelination (Weiss, Edds and Cavanaugh 1945). Nevertheless a good functional recovery may be obtained.

Even in cases of satisfactory functional recovery some electrophysiological disturbances may remain. Sanders and Whitteridge (1946) described full recovery of conduction velocity in fibres below a simple crush injury and emphasized the close correlation between conduction velocity and myelin thickness independent of internodal distance. Other authors, however, found considerably reduced velocities in regenerated nerves. Cragg and Thomas (1964b) found velocities reduced by 24% below normal 16 months after crushing a nerve and were not satisfied that the residual reduction in fibre diameter accounted for the conduction defect. Perhaps that is due to disordered reconstruction of myelin sheaths; small regenerated nerve fibres tend to have relatively thick myelin sheaths, while large axons may acquire relatively thin sheaths (Schröder 1970).

Avulsion injuries

Violent traction on the arm may induce lesions commonly ascribed to the brachial plexus. In fact, most of them are due to intradural avulsion of cervical roots, first described by Flaubert (1827). Various mechanisms may operate to produce this type of injury. Upward traction on the arm, as occurs when the arm is caught by moving machinery, will lead to damage of the lower roots, particularly T1, C8 and C7. Forcible separation of head and shoulder, which may happen in falls, tends to put the stress on the upper roots, particularly C5, C6 and C7. Similar mechanisms operate in birth palsies of the upper

limb, associated with the name of Erb (1874) and Klumpke (1885).

The anterior roots are far more vulnerable than the posterior. As a result of this, the clinical picture of avulsion injuries tends to be purely motor and in lesions involving T1 is associated with Horner's syndrome. There is no regeneration and the paralysis remains permanent.

There are relatively few pathological studies on avulsion injuries. The early literature includes the cases of Flaubert (1827), Apert (1898) and Déjerine-Klumpke (1908). The recent revival of interest in the condition has produced several reports of cases confirmed at autopsy, operation or by myelography. The subject is fully reviewed by Taylor (1962).

Avulsion usually occurs at the junction of the anterior roots with the spinal cord, in some cases causing superficial tears in the cord itself. Cicatrization between the cord and meninges frequently occurs, with fibrous thickening of the arachnoid and adhesions to the dura. The severed root undergoes complete atrophy and the distal segment of the nerve irreversible Wallerian degeneration. Retrograde degeneration leads to loss of anterior horn cells. In cases where tears occur in the substance of the spinal cord, long tract degeneration may ensue (Boyer 1912).

Pressure palsies

Prolonged or repeated pressure on a nerve may cause localized lesions in peripheral nerves. The effects of pressure are a combination of the direct effect on axons as in acute blows and the compression of blood vessels with ensuing ischaemia. Paralysis and sensory impairment appear 15 to 45 minutes after a limb is compressed or rendered ischaemic (Lewis, Pickering and Rothschild 1931; Merrington and Nathan 1949). Function is restored within seconds after compression lasting up to 30 minutes. After 40 minutes' ischaemia the nerve takes several hours to recover, more prolonged injuries may lead to protracted disabilities.

The lesions vary according to the severity and duration of ischaemia. The early changes have only been studied experimentally (Denny-Brown and Brenner 1944c). Swelling of myelin sheaths and axons occurs, even in nerves in which recovery is almost immediate. More severe lesions result in focal demyelination, often associated with damage to a few axons.

Interference with the venous circulation leads to congestion and oedema of the compressed nerve. This, if prolonged, may stimulate fibro-blastic proliferation, with subsequent dense fibrosis of the endoneurium and perineurium which interferes with regenerative processes. In severe persisting compression the affected segment of nerve may ultimately become converted into a strand or ribbon of ischaemic fibrous tissue.

The common sites of pressure palsies are dictated by anatomical considerations. The radial nerve may be compressed in the axilla ('crutch palsy') or against the shaft of the humerus in the spiral canal ('Saturday night palsy'). In the lower limb the lateral popliteal nerve may be compressed against the neck of the fibula. Tourniquet palsies occur more frequently in the upper limb than in the lower. The radial nerve is most commonly affected, but the median and ulnar may be involved in addition to the radial. Ill-fitting plaster casts may damage the lateral popliteal nerve. Pressure palsies, both in the upper and lower limbs, may occur during operations due to malposition of the anaesthetized patient on the operating table. Occupational palsies include the tailor's crossed-leg palsy with damage to the lateral popliteal nerve, the ulnar palsy of glass-blowers due to leaning on the forearm against a hard surface, and lesions to the distal branches of the ulnar and median nerves caused by pressure of tools on the palm of the hand.

Other traumatic pressure palsies may occur as a result of fractures or dislocations of bones. The nerves of the upper limb are more commonly affected than those of the lower. The radial nerve is again the most vulnerable, but the axillary nerve may be compressed by the dislocated head of the humerus, the ulnar nerve may be involved in fractures or dislocation of the lower end of the humerus and the median nerve in injuries to the wrist.

Nerves may be subject to pressure by haematomas. This is particularly common in haemophilia (Silverstein 1964). The femoral nerve is most commonly affected, but the median, ulnar, sciatic, peroneal and radial nerves can also be involved. Similar accidents have been reported in patients receiving anticoagulant therapy (De Bolt and Jordan 1966; Gallois, Dhers and Badaron 1967).

Hereditary neuropathy with liability to pressure palsies

Some individuals are prone to recurrent pressure palsies. This tendency runs in families and is inherited as an autosomal dominant (de Jong 1947; Earl, Fullerton, Wakefield and Schutta 1964). Examination of sural nerve biopsies in patients suffering from this pressure-sensitive neuropathy revealed striking changes in myelin sheaths (Behse et al. 1972). Apart from evidence of demyelination and remyelination, the sheaths showed localized sausage-like swellings resembling those found in globular neuropathy (p. 726). However, the 'sausages' were much larger than the 'globules' (40 μm diameter as opposed to 8 to 12 μm). They occurred in fully myelinated segments and consisted of an increased number of myelin lamellae (up to 560), while globules are formed by apparently unabsorbed products of myelin breakdown incorporated into the myelin sheath.

Madrid and Bradley (1975) studied four cases of this 'sausage-body' or 'tomaculous' neuropathy. Clinically two of them were examples of recurrent familial brachial neuropathy and one of chronic distal sensorimotor neuropathy. Electron-microscopy of sural nerve biopsies revealed six types of lesions responsible for the formation of 'sausages': (1) Hyper-myelination with an excessive number of lamellae for the axonal circumference, similar to the observations of Behse et al. (1972); (2) Redundant loop formation with the surplus loop wrapping round the original myelin sheath; (3) Branching and duplication of the mesaxon; (4) Transnodal myelination with spread of the sheath of one internode into the region of the next, as described by Dinn (1970); (5) Participation of two or more Schwann cells in the formation of one myelin sheath; (6) Degeneration of myelin with retention of products of breakdown between an outer intact layer of myelin and the axon, as described by Dayan et al. (1968) in globular neuropathy. Redundant loop formation was the commonest lesion.

Not all cases of acute brachial palsy, or 'neuralgic amyotrophy' (Parsonage and Turner 1948) display this abnormality. This syndrome forms a heterogeneous group, some cases being familial, others sporadic, with or without tendency to recurrence, painful or painless (Bradley, Madrid, Thrush and Campbell 1975). Only the familial recurrent cases in their material showed evidence of tomaculous neuropathy.

Entrapment neuropathies

These are defined as localized injuries in a peripheral nerve, caused by mechanical irritation from an infringing anatomical neighbour. They may occur at a point at which a nerve goes through a fibrous or fibro-osseous tunnel or at which the nerve changes its course over a fibrous or muscular band (Koppell and Thompson 1963). Although not necessarily or obviously traumatic in origin, these lesions are best considered in conjunction with pressure palsies of which they form a variant.

Entrapment of nerve roots may occur in disorders of the vertebral column, both traumatic and degenerative (see Chapter 15). In the periphery numerous sites have been described, of which only a few are common (Koppell and Thompson 1963; Sunderland 1968; Seddon 1972).

The main clinical feature of the entrapment neuropathies is pain, which may be acute and correspond in distribution to the areas innervated by the affected nerve, or may be an ill-defined, deep-seated ache with muscular tenderness, or may take the form of painful paraesthesiae. Objective sensory loss is less common. Motor weakness and muscular wasting occur in severe cases. Autonomic dysfunction in the affected area may also be present.

The commonest peripheral entrapment neuropathy in the upper limb is the *carpal tunnel syndrome*. Compression of the median nerve under the flexor retinaculum, first described by Marie and Foix (1913), has been the subject of a large literature (Brain, Wright and Wilkinson 1947; Watson-Jones 1949; Heathfield 1957 and many others). The position of the nerve between the flexor tendons, in a tunnel formed by the bones of the wrist and the transverse ligament, renders it particularly vulnerable to compression. Apart from fracture and dislocation of carpal bones, the size of the tunnel may be reduced by arthritis of the wrist joint or by thickening of the flexor retinaculum, either due to repeated trauma or to amyloidosis (p. 733). The contents of the tunnel may be increased in tumours, ganglia and inflammatory lesions of the tendon sheaths. An increase in connective tissue leading to median nerve compression has been described in acromegaly (Schiller and Kolb 1954) and in myxoedema (Murray and Simpson 1958). There remains an 'idiopathic' group, common with advancing age, in which there is clear evidence of involvement of the median nerve at the level of the carpal tunnel and in which other aetiological factors have been excluded.

The pathology of the median nerve is similar to that seen in other chronic pressure palsies. The nerve, as seen during surgical decompression, appears swollen and greyish pink. This is due partly to oedema and partly to fibrosis, mainly epineurial. The nerve fibres usually show extensive local demyelination and a variable loss of axons. The changes in fibre size have been investigated by Thomas and Fullerton (1963). More recently Neary, Ochoa and Gilliatt (1975) adduced evidence that mechanical rather than ischaemic factors played a major part in the production of lesions in the carpal tunnel syndrome. The lesions are similar to those observed in the guinea pig. In this species, animals develop a compressive lesion of the median and ulnar nerves at the wrist as they grow older. There is local demyelination at the site of compression, followed by Wallerian degeneration in severe cases (Fullerton and Gilliatt 1967; Anderson, Fullerton, Gilliatt and Hern 1970). The earliest lesion is a distortion of the internodes of the myelinated fibres which become asymmetrical, with tapering at one end and bulbous swelling at the other. The swollen end is always that more distant from the site of compression. Demyelination begins at the tapering end. The appearances suggest a gradual slipping of myelin lamellae, due to repeated pressure waves arising at the site of entrapment (Ochoa and Marotte 1973).

The *thoracic inlet syndrome*, reviewed by Walshe (1951), has lately been the subject of severe criticism. There is no doubt that many nerve compressions in the upper limb were wrongly ascribed to involvement of the brachial plexus, while in fact the lesion was either more proximal (cervical spondylosis) or more distal (carpal tunnel syndrome). However, a group of cases remains in which cervical ribs, fully developed or rudimentary, may cause repeated trauma to the adjacent trunks of the brachial plexus and the subclavian artery.

In the lower limbs the majority of entrapment neuropathies affect the sciatic nerve. By far the greatest number of cases of *sciatica* are due to involvement of roots by prolapsed intervertebral discs or by narrowing of the intervertebral foramina in chronic lumbar spondylosis (p. 661). Rare cases of compression of the sciatic nerve in the pelvis and in the buttock also occur.

A specific instance of an entrapment neuropathy in the foot is *Morton's metatarsalgia* (Morton 1876). It is due to compression of a digital nerve between the heads of two adjacent metatarsal bones, usually the third and fourth. The lesion is a localized fusiform swelling, usually less than 1 cm in diameter, circumscribed, but not encapsulated, and adherent to neighbouring structures. Microscopically there is marked fibrosis of the epineurium, perineurium and endoneurium, with increase in mucoid material in the endoneurial spaces. Intrafascicular, rounded, concentric nodules of hyalinized, acellular collagen form a prominent feature of some cases. There is severe loss of myelin sheaths and a variable loss of axons (Harkin and Reed 1969). Apart from changes in the nerve, lesions may be found in plantar digital arteries, in fat lobules and fibrous septa and in the lining of synovial cavities (Meachim and Abberton 1971).

Effect of cold on peripheral nerves

Blackwood (1944) reported the findings in cases of immersion foot in seamen. In all cases there was degeneration of axons and myelin sheaths in the nerves of the foot, but in the cases in which immersion was of shorter duration this did not involve all fibres. Evidence of regeneration was present in long-standing cases.

The effects of cold have been extensively studied experimentally and the results largely agree with the findings in man. Blackwood and Russell (1943) kept the tails of rats in water at a temperature of 4 to 5° for 3 to 4 days, producing degenerative changes in the intramuscular branches of nerves. Immediately after exposure there was irregularity in the outline of myelin sheaths in a large proportion of fibres. Three days after immersion had been discontinued, these changes progressed to disintegration of axons and myelin sheaths. In later stages denervation atrophy appeared in muscles. Denny-Brown, Adams, Brenner and Doherty (1945) studied the sciatic nerve of rabbits after freezing with CO_2 or enclosing them for 2 hours in chambers filled with brine at the temperature of $-4°$. Lesions of different severity were produced according to the temperature and duration of the exposure. Freezing for 5 minutes caused total necrosis of all structures within the perineurium, with the exception of capillary endothelia. This was followed by an intense inflammatory reaction and by Wallerian degeneration of the distal segment. Complete regeneration occurred within 3 months. After shorter freezing, or after chilling for 1 to 2 hours, there was no massive necrosis, but only destruction of large and medium-sized fibres. Slighter degrees of chilling produced only transient paralysis with local swelling of axons and myelin sheaths, without Wallerian degeneration. Injection of indian ink into the vasa nervorum failed to reach the necrotic parts of the nerves, but there were no significant changes in the vessels in minor degrees of cold injury. The authors concluded that the more severe lesion may have been caused by ischaemia, while the milder lesions were probably a direct effect of cold on the lipoproteins of the myelin sheath.

More recently Denny-Brown's experiments were repeated under strictly controlled conditions by Schaumberg, Byck, Herman and Rosengart (1967). They support the view that degeneration of axons and myelin sheaths was independent of ischaemia, but failed to confirm any differential vulnerability of large axons.

Chemical injury

Chemical injury to peripheral nerves is usually due to accidental injection of therapeutic agents into a nerve. This occurs most commonly in the buttock, and on the outer aspect of the upper arm, leading to damage of the sciatic or radial nerves. The extent and severity of the damage are influenced by the internal structure of the nerve, the amount of material injected and its sclerosing and toxic properties. A wide range of therapeutic substances has been implicated (Woodhall, Mahaley, Boone and Hunneycutt 1962).

Intrathecal injections of phenol were used for the relief of chronic severe pain, on the assumption that phenol affected predominantly fine nerve fibres, the large and medium-sized fibres being protected by their myelin sheaths. Pathological studies do not support this view and reveal indiscriminate degeneration of both large and small fibres (Berry and Olszewski 1963; Smith 1964).

Exposure to radiation

Peripheral nerves are remarkably resistant to ionizing radiation. Very little is known about radiation damage to peripheral nerves in man. Experimental work has been mainly neurophysiological, and pathological observations are scanty. Janzen and Warren (1942) failed to produce either histological or physiological changes in peripheral nerves of the rat exposed to X-rays in doses up to 10,000 rads. However, exposure up to 1200 to 1600 millicurie hours of gamma radiation caused complete degeneration of nerve fibres. Bergström (1962) subjected rat sciatic nerves to doses of proton radiation from 20 to 40 kilorads and followed the pathological changes in serial studies over a period of 4 months. The changes ranged from hyperaemia and oedema, through inflammatory infiltration and fibroblastic proliferation in the epineurium, to fragmentation of myelin sheaths and degeneration of axons. Focal areas of necrosis associated with lesions in blood vessels appeared after 15 to 16 days. Surprisingly, proliferation of Schwann cells was prominent, and evidence of regeneration, both functional and structural, was present at the end of 4 months.

The studies on the effect of implanted radium needles on peripheral nerves have given conflicting results. The best controlled studies (Dobrovolskaia-Zavadskaia 1924, Goulston 1930) again confirmed the radioresistance of nerves which retained their anatomical continuity even where they traversed areas of tissue necrosis. Large doses of radiation damaged some nerve fibres, the sensory ones before the motor. There was a latent period of 20 to 30 days before histological changes were observed and myelin fragmentation appeared to precede the degeneration of axons. There was marked fibrosis and little regeneration in the damaged nerves.

Damage to peripheral nerves may also be indirect and due to secondary strangulation by the surrounding scar tissue (Holtzmann and Howes 1940).

The parenchymatous neuropathies

Peroneal muscular atrophy

The disease commonly associated with the names of Charcot and Marie (1886) and of Tooth (1886), but previously described by several German writers (reviewed by Schultze 1930), is a slowly progressive condition leading to muscular weakness and wasting involving first the feet and legs and later the hands and forearms. The symptoms are predominantly motor, but sensory signs may be present (Hoffmann 1893; England and Denny-Brown 1952).

The disease is genetically determined and the mode of inheritance is dominant in most cases. In this context the family reported by Eichhorst (1873) in which members of six generations were affected is of interest. Other modes of inheritance, such as autosomal or sex-linked recessive, have also been recorded, as well as sporadic cases (Bell 1935). Genetic links have been suggested with other system degenerations, such as Friedreich's ataxia (Greenfield 1954) and the Roussy-Lévy syndrome (Yudell, Dyck and Lambert 1965).

The early accounts of the pathology of the condition (Virchow 1855; Friedreich 1873; Marinesco 1894; Biemond 1928) emphasized a variety of lesions such as loss of anterior horn cells, loss of myelinated fibres in peripheral nerves, increase in the amount of connective tissue in the nerves, and degeneration of posterior columns. Recent studies have cast doubt on whether the clinical syndrome represents a single pathological entity. Dyck and Lambert (1968a, b) suggested that it included at least three groups of diseases, a neuronal atrophy, a peripheral demyelinating process and possibly a distal myopathy. The demyelinating variety is probably identical with the dominant form of hypertrophic neuropathy (p. 725).

The neuronal group (Dyck and Lambert 1968b) consists of all those cases in which motor nerve conduction velocities are not significantly reduced and in which nerve biopsies reveal only loss of fibres without evidence of segmental demyelination or remyelination. This group may include cases with primary destruction of anterior horn cells or posterior root ganglia, and those in which a 'dying-back' mechanism affects the distal parts of the axons. Dyck and Lambert divide their cases into four sub-groups: the neuronal type of Charcot-Marie-Tooth's disease with dominant inheritance, sporadic cases of spinal muscular atrophy with peroneal presentation, cases associated with Friedreich's ataxia, either sporadic or recessive, and cases associated with dominantly inherited familial spastic paraplegia.

In their detailed post-mortem study of four typical cases of Charcot-Marie-Tooth's disease, Hughes and Brownell (1972) demonstrated severe atrophy of peripheral nerves, both motor and sensory, with degenerative changes and loss of neurons in the anterior horns and posterior root ganglia and corresponding degeneration of the posterior columns. Those findings agree with those reported in the older literature.

Porphyria

Neurological complications occur in two types of porphyria: acute intermittent porphyria, the Swedish type (Waldenström and Haeger-Aronsen 1962) and porphyria variegata, the South African type (Dean 1963). The two conditions are similar yet appear to be genetically and biochemically distinct. In both conditions porphobilinogen and delta-aminolaevulinic acid are excreted in the urine during acute attacks. In the Swedish type smaller quantities of these compounds are also excreted during remission. In the South African type the urine is normal during latent periods, but the faeces always contain increased amount of protoporphyrin and coproporphyrin.

The clinical picture (Berman 1961; Ridley 1969) consists of acute attacks heralded by abdominal pain, constipation, nausea and vomiting, followed by neurological and psychiatric symptoms. Skin manifestations, mainly due to photosensitivity, are common in the South African type, but are said to be absent in the Swedish form. Acute attacks may be precipitated by a variety of drugs, of which barbiturates are the most important.

The peripheral neuropathy is predominantly motor. The patient commonly complains of pains in the proximal parts of the limbs followed by severe and extensive flaccid paralysis with depression or abolition of the tendon reflexes. The nerves of the trunk and the cranial nerves may also be involved, leading to respiratory difficulties. The mortality is high (up to 15%); other patients make a slow, but usually complete recovery. The cerebrospinal fluid remains normal throughout the course of the disease.

The pathology of the neurological complications of porphyria has been studied by several authors (Erbslöh 1903; Baker and Watson 1945; Denny-Brown and Sciarra 1945; Gibson and Goldberg 1956; Hierons 1957; Cavanagh and Mellick 1965). The common feature in all reports are the breakdown and loss of axons in peripheral nerves, frequently accompanied by central chromatolysis in anterior horn cells. Hierons (1957) in addition found some degeneration of posterior columns. The earlier writers emphasized the disproportionate loss of myelin compared with destruction of axons, and interpreted the condition as a demyelinating neuropathy. Some were impressed by the patchy character of the lesions, which suggested a possible vascular mechanism (Denny-Brown and Sciarra 1945). Cavanagh and Mellick (1965) studied teased preparations of nerve fibres and failed to find any evidence of segmental demyelination. The only lesion observed was a Wallerian-type degeneration, affecting the motor and, to a lesser extent, the sensory fibres. The process was most pronounced in the terminal ramifications of the motor nerves, but in advanced cases was also present in proximal parts of the nerve trunks, when it was associated with central chromatolysis in anterior horn cells and corresponding changes in posterior root ganglia. These findings suggest a 'dying-back' mechanism. The presence of unmyelinated or thinly unmyelinated fibres could be ascribed to regeneration.

The nature of the biochemical disturbance causing neuronal damage is unknown. It has been suggested that a deficiency of pyridoxal phosphate, induced by excessive consumption of this co-enzyme by abnormally large amounts of delta-amino-laevulic acid synthetase during an acute attack, may be an important aetiological factor (Cavanagh and Ridley 1967).

Deficiency diseases

See Chapter 5.

Toxic neuropathies

See Chapter 4.

The ganglioradicular neuropathies

Herpes zoster

See Chapter 8.

Hereditary sensory radicular neuropathy

In 1852 Nélaton briefly described a case of a man who developed recurrent trophic ulcers of his feet and sequestration of his metatarsal bones. Two of his five brothers were similarly affected. Bruns (1903), in reporting a similar family, tentatively ascribed the condition to lumbosacral syringomyelia. This concept of 'familial lumbosacral syringomyelia' remained unchallenged for many years despite the lack of pathological confirmation. Many families were described in various countries, among others that of Hicks (1922) in which 11 members out of 36 were affected in four generations, and that of Jackson (1949) which included 26 affected members in four generations. Pathological evidence that syringomyelia was not the cause of the syndrome was produced by Jughenn, Krücke and Wadulla (1949) but they offered no alternative explanation owing to inadequate material available for examination. Denny-Brown (1951) examined a member of the family originally described by Hicks, demonstrated conclusively a degenerative process in the posterior root ganglia and coined the term 'hereditary sensory radicular neuropathy'. Subsequent post-mortem reports (Blackwood 1952; van Bogaert 1953; Heller and Robb 1955; Vignon, Mégard and Martin 1956) confirmed Denny-Brown's findings.

The *clinical picture*, reviewed by Thévenard (1942, 1953), is dominated by sensory loss, affecting predominantly, sometimes exclusively, the lower limbs, and accompanied by trophic changes. The onset of the disease is insidious, in the third or fourth decade in some families, earlier in others. Subjective sensory disturbances are uncommon; shooting pains featured prominently only in the family described by Hicks. Objective sensory loss may affect all modalities, present as dissociated anaesthesia affecting pain and temperature only, or may be total distally

and dissociated proximally. The lower limbs are affected earlier and more severely than the upper. Trophic changes leading to penetrating ulcers are frequently the first manifestation. Necrosis and sequestration of bones often follows, but in some cases (e.g. van Bogaert's) osteolytic changes preceded the appearance of skin lesions. In the upper limbs ulceration of the fingers is not uncommon, but bony changes are rarely observed. The tendon reflexes, particularly the ankle jerks, are often lost early in the disease but may persist for a long time. The cerebrospinal fluid is normal as a rule, but a slight rise in protein has been reported in some cases.

Other neurological symptoms and signs include deafness (Hicks, Blackwood), external ocular palsies, nystagmus, choreiform movements and intellectual impairment.

Pathology. The prominent lesion in all cases was degeneration and disappearance of nerve cells in posterior root ganglia, mainly in the lumbosacral and to a lesser extent in the lower cervical regions. This was accompanied by proliferation of capsule cells, formation of nodules of Nageotte and hypertrophy of 'basket' fibres. The corresponding posterior roots were atrophic, the degeneration extending into the posterior columns (Fig. 16.36). Peripheral nerves also showed some atrophy. Hyaline bodies, mainly related to blood vessels, were found in the affected ganglia by Denny-Brown (1951) and by van Bogaert (1953). In the former case the hyaline material stained with Congo red.

There was extensive loss of Purkinje cells in the cerebellum and some loss of neurons in the inferior olives in Blackwood's case. Hallpike (1967) reporting on the temporal bones of this case, described slight degeneration of the cells and nerve fibres of the spiral ganglion with very severe degeneration of the cochlear end organs and stria vascularis. Moderate degeneration was also present of the cells and nerve fibres of Scarpa's ganglion with very severe disorganization of the maculae of the saccule and utricle and of the cristae of the semicircular canals. In a recent examination of the temporal bones of Denny-Brown's case Hallpike and Scott (unpublished) found degenerative changes in the sensory neural apparatus of the cochlea and vestibule which

they found extensive vacuolation of fibroblasts which they considered unique at the time. Subsequent studies revealed that this phenomenon occurred in other chronic scarring conditions of

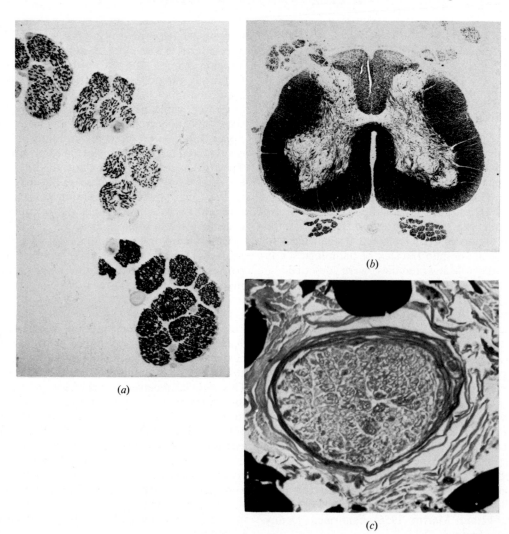

Fig. 16.36 Hereditary sensory radicular neuropathy. (a) Dorsal and ventral roots. (b) Lumbar cord. The degeneration is greatest in Lissauer's area, and slightly less in the posterior root zone. The middle root zone is relatively intact. (c) Fascicle of sensory nerve (medial terminal branch of deep peroneal) showing total absence of myelinated fibres. Osmium tetroxide. × 300. (Courtesy of Prof. W. Blackwood.)

in degree and character resembled very closely those described by Hallpike (1967) in Blackwood's case.

Ultrastructural studies on sural nerve biopsies were carried out on two cases by Schoene, Asbury, Åström and Masters (1970). In addition to the expected loss of myelinated fibres, proliferation of columns of Schwann cells and marked fibrosis,

peripheral nerves (Asbury, Cox and Baringer 1971).

As to the *nosological position* of the disease, it is best classified among the familial system degenerations. Its occasional associations with peroneal muscular atrophy (England and Denny-Brown 1952; Barraquer-Ferré and Barraquer-Bordas 1953; Campbell and Hoffman 1964; Dyck,

Kennel, Magal and Kraybill 1965) and with spino-cerebellar degenerations (van Bogaert 1957) strongly support this view. It may be added that the lesions of the peripheral sensory pathway found in classical cases of Friedreich's ataxia (Hughes, Brownell and Hewer 1968) and of Charcot–Marie–Tooth's disease (Hughes and Brownell 1972) are similar in nature if not in severity.

Sensory neuropathy associated with carcinoma

See p. 718.

The autonomic nervous system

Our knowledge of the pathology of the autonomic nervous system is still rudimentary. Abundant pathophysiological data are available but little is known about structural changes.

The sympathetic system

The preganglionic fibres of the sympathetic system originate in the intermediolateral cell group of the spinal cord and form the rami communicantes which reach the sympathetic chain. The postganglionic fibres have their cells of origin in the ganglia of the sympathetic chain and in the coeliac ganglion. The normal anatomy of the ganglia was fully described by de Castro (1932*b*). The nerve cells can be classified into three groups: large (35 to 55 μm), intermediate (25 to 32 μm) and small (15 to 22 μm). The intermediate group accounts for the largest number of cells. Most cells have one vesicular nucleus with a prominent nucleolus. Binucleate and multinucleate forms occur, but their significance is debatable and may be pathological. Nissl bodies vary in size and are irregularly distributed. Melanin pigment is present in many cells, particularly the small ones. Cell processes vary in number and in length; some dendrites show elaborate ramifications. The capsule cells resemble those of the posterior root ganglia.

Infections

Acute inflammatory changes in sympathetic ganglia were found in *typhus fever* (Lubimoff 1874; Herzog 1935) in herpes zoster (Bielschowsky 1914) and in rabies (Chachina 1926). Lesions resembling those seen in other peripheral nerves were found in the sympathetic chain and sensory ganglia of the vagus in *leprosy* (Takino and Miyake 1935).

The Guillain–Barré syndrome

The clinical manifestations of involvement of the autonomic nervous system in acute idiopathic polyneuritis include abolition of vascular reflexes and of sweating, disorders of heart rate and of blood pressure, particularly postural hypotension. Lesions in the myelinated fibres of the sympathetic chain were described by Matsuyama and Haymaker (1967). These consisted of patchy demyelination with preservation of axons, proliferation of Schwann cells and focal perivascular infiltration by a variety of mononuclear cells. Similar findings were recorded by Asbury, Arnason and Adams (1969).

Diabetes

Autonomic disturbances are common in diabetic neuropathy (Martin 1953; Colby 1965). They include absence of circulatory reflexes, such as vasoconstriction on cooling or vasodilatation on heating, altered sudomotor activity, orthostatic hypotension, impotence, disturbance of bladder function and disorders of gastrointestinal motility. Among the latter may be noted gastric dilatation, impaired motility of the oesophagus and small intestine, intractable constipation or diarrhoea, particularly nocturnal in pattern. Little is known about the site or nature of the lesions. Dolman (1963) examined the lumbar sympathetic chain in 20 out of her 36 diabetic cases and found no significant lesions. Berge, Sprague and Bennett (1956) reported chromatolysis, vacuolation of cytoplasm and pyknosis of neurons in the plexuses of Auerbach and Meissner with intact nerve fibres; the findings are of doubtful significance.

Parkinson's disease

See Chapter 14.

Raynaud's disease

Most of the studies on the pathology of this condition were carried out on surgically removed sympathetic ganglia. Post-mortem studies are scanty and include that of Gagel and Watts (1932) who failed to find significant abnormalities in sympathetic ganglia, but described central chromatolysis in the neurons of the intermediolateral cell group in the spinal cord. Craig and Kernohan (1933) and Kuntz (1934) studied ganglia removed surgically and found only non-specific degenerative change in neurons. On the other hand Hagen (1934-35, 1948-50) demonstrated a bizarre hypertrophy of dendrites in surgically removed ganglia. As similar changes were also found in other vascular diseases and in bronchial asthma their specific nature remains open to doubt.

Familial dysautonomia

This syndrome, described by Riley, Day, Greeley and Langford (1949) and subsequently reviewed by Riley (1957), by Riley and Moore (1966) and by Brunt and McKusick (1970), affects predominantly Jewish children and is inherited as an autosomal recessive. Essential clinical features include feeding difficulties from birth, defective lacrimation, absent corneal reflexes and tendon jerks, postural hypotension, emotional lability, indifference to pain, absent fungiform papillae in tongue and abnormal responses to intradermal histamine. Pathological observations are scanty and inconsistent. Some authors emphasize degenerative lesions in the reticular substance of the brainstem (Cohen and Solomon 1955; Brown, Beauchemin and Linde 1964), while others found lesions in sympathetic ganglia and the myenteric plexus (Brown et al. 1964; Solitare and Cohen 1965). Yatsu and Zussman (1964) failed to find any abnormality in the central, peripheral or autonomic systems. In a sural nerve biopsy Aguayo, Nair and Bray (1971) found a severe selective loss of unmyelinated nerve fibres.

Search for an underlying biochemical defect revealed consistent abnormalities in catecholamine metabolism. The urinary excretion of vanillyl-mandelic acid (VMA) is very low, implying reduced noradrenaline turnover, while the excretion of homovanillic acid (HVA) is high, implying increased dopamine turnover (Smith, Taylor and Wortis 1963). Similarly the levels of HVA in the cerebrospinal fluid are excessively high (Andersson, Hange and Roos 1973). These findings suggest a deficiency in dopamine-β-

hydroxylase, an enzyme which converts dopamine into noradrenaline, and indeed absence of this enzyme has been found in about 25% of cases (Weinshilboum and Axelrod 1971). The deficiency of noradrenaline manifests itself in an exaggerated response to an infusion of this substance (Smith and Dancis 1964). However, a similarly exaggerated response to cholinergic agents (methacholine) suggest other transmitter substance deficiencies (Smith, Hirsch and Dancis 1965). Finally, the observation of greatly increased plasma renin activity in the supine position, falling after 4 hours in the upright position, remains completely unexplained (Rabinowitz, Landau, Rosler, Moses, Rotem and Freier 1974).

The parasympathetic system

The preganglionic fibres of the parasympathetic system originate in the brainstem and the sacral cord. The postganglionic fibres originate in the peripheral parasympathetic ganglia, situated in close proximity to their end-organs.

The normal anatomy of the autonomic innervation of the gut was first described by Remak (1847). A detailed description of the myenteric plexus by Auerbach followed in 1864. Its structure, as summarized by Smith (1970, 1972), is that of a geometrical network of nerve fibres with neurons at the angles. There are two types of myenteric neurons, distinguished by their affinity for silver. The argyrophil cells constitute between 5 and 20% of the total number. They are multipolar and frequently multiaxonal, their processes terminating around other neurons in the same ganglion or neighbouring ones. Their axons do not leave the plexus and do not reach muscle fibres. The argyrophobe cells, which are strongly cholinergic, supply the muscle fibres. They produce acetylcholine, which fires the muscle fibres, while the argyrophils act as co-ordinators of peristalsis, intercalated between vagal fibres and the cholinergic cells. Functionally the loss of argyrophil cells has the same denervating effect as total loss of myenteric neurons.

The effect of damage to the myenteric plexus is loss of co-ordinated muscle action which propels the contents of the gut towards the anus. The denervated segment remains stationary and the peristaltic wave does not cross it, as demonstrated experimentally by Hukuhara, Kotani and Sato (1961). As it is refilled from above it dilates and undergoes segmentation, which is a response of the muscle to stretching, independent of innervation. The muscle coat undergoes gross hypertrophy. This may be partially work hypertrophy, partially a direct response to denervation, as there is some evidence that denervated smooth muscle hypertrophies in contrast to skeletal muscle (Alvarez 1949). The hypertrophy, which is much greater than that seen behind an organic obstruction, may exacerbate the functional obstruction by adding an organic element to it.

Chagas' disease

The infection with *Trypanosoma cruzi* (Chagas 1909), endemic in Brazil, runs in two stages. The first or acute septicaemic phase usually occurs in childhood and subsides spontaneously. The chronic stage or, more accurately, the stage of sequelae is the result of destruction of ganglion cells in the peripheral autonomic system which has occurred in the acute phase. The destruction of neurons is due to liberation of a neurotoxin from parasites dying in the neighbourhood of ruptured pseudocysts (Köberle 1956). The parasympathetic plexuses are severely affected, while the ganglia of the sympathetic chain escape.

The main effects are on the heart and on the gut. Chagas' cardiomegaly consists of severe loss of ganglion cells in the heart followed by sympathetic overstimulation (Köberle 1957). This leads, through a mechanism not clearly understood, to dilatation, followed by hypertrophy and finally by foci of necrosis and scarring. The condition has been reproduced experimentally by Alcantara (1959).

The common gut lesions (Köberle 1963) are megaoesophagus and megacolon, which develop after a variable time lag largely dependent on the degree of denervation. The lesions in the myenteric plexus of the colon were described by Smith (1967a). Less common sites of functional obstruction and dilatation include the stomach, duodenum and jejunum, and also the bronchi, ureters and bladder.

Achalasia of the cardia

This is due to a destructive lesion of the myenteric plexus in the oesophagus and the gastro-oesophageal segment (Rake 1927). The loss of neurons is often extensive and may be total. In some cases, however, neurons have been seen in biopsy specimens (Adams, Marples and Trounce 1960). These appear to be exclusively argyrophobes. The denervation of the gastro-oesophageal segment leads to loss of peristalsis and gross hyperplasia of the sphincter. Vagal lesions in achalasia were described by Cassella, Ellis and Brown (1965). If confirmed they would suggest a system degeneration involving the primary and secondary neurons. On the other hand inflammatory infiltration of the plexus (Misiewicz, Waller, Anthony and Gummer 1969) raises the possibility of a virus infection or an auto-immune reaction.

Infantile hypertrophic pyloric stenosis

This condition develops during the first few weeks of life (Wallgren 1946). It appears to be due to failure of the pyloric pump (Edwards 1961). The fundamental lesion is a complete absence of argyrophil cells (Rintoul and Kirkman 1961), presumably due to a localized maturation defect in which the innervation of the pyloric canal remains inadequate. The denervated pylorus remains patent, until the development of muscular hypertrophy leads to narrowing of the canal and obstruction. In infants who survive without surgical treatment the symptoms disappear, but the radiological abnormalities and pyloric 'tumour' may persist (Armitage and Rhind 1951). Some cases may remain asymptomatic in infancy and present in adult life (Lumsden and Truelove 1958).

Myenteric denervation in the small intestine

This may be congenital or acquired. Congenital absence of neurons usually occurs in the duodenum. The acquired form usually presents as a subacute intestinal obstruction (Dyer, Dawson, Smith and Todd 1969). Occasionally it may cause a malabsorption syndrome of the 'blind-loop' variety, due to bacterial infection of the stagnant segment of bowel (Naish, Capper and Brown 1960). The myenteric plexus in these cases shows loss of argyrophil cells with degenerative changes in survivors.

Hirschsprung's disease

Congenital megacolon (Hirschsprung 1888) is the commonest lesion of the myenteric plexus. Its clinical manifestations range from intestinal obstruction in the newborn, through the pot-bellied child, to intractable constipation in the adult. The factor which decides the mode of presentation is the length of the contracted aganglionic segment. The absence of ganglion cells was first demonstrated by Dalla Valle (1920). This was confirmed in a detailed study by Whitehouse and Kernohan (1948) who also demonstrated the presence of abnormal bundles of unmyelinated fibres. Further observations include those of Bodian, Stephens and Ward (1949) and of Bodian, Carter and Ward (1951). The complete pattern of the lesion was revealed in thick sections by Smith (1967b). The plexus in the contracted segment shows no neurons and is replaced by a network of fine unmyelinated fibre trunks, different in morphology from the normal ones. In addition, a network of single argyrophil fibres is present in the muscle coat in areas where normally no axons are seen. These fibres are probably adrenergic (Bennett, Garrett and Howard 1968). The proximal dilated segment contains neurons of abnormal morphology, often devoid of processes. The unmyelinated nerve trunks are still present and show fragmentation or thickening of axons. Where axons of a mature parasympathetic type are present they are often uneven in calibre and have abnormal anatomical connections. The muscle coat both in the contracted and in the dilated segments is extremely thick (see also Meier-Ruge 1974).

Drug lesions of the parasympathetic plexuses

The most important of these is the cathartic colon (Smith 1968) caused by abuse of anthraquinone purgatives, which in small doses stimulate the myenteric plexus and damage it when given in large amounts. The lesions consist of a partial loss of argyrophil cells and their axons. The remaining neurons show degenerative changes which vary with the length of the history. In young patients, they are pale and enlarged with thick and irregular processes. In patients who have taken purgatives for 30 to 40 years the neurons are dark, shrunken and their processes clubbed. The lesions are always more severe on the right side of the colon.

Other drugs may affect the myenteric plexus and cause constipation as a side-effect. These include the anticholinergics, particularly the tranquillizers, the vinca alkaloids and many of the antimitotic drugs. Smith (1967c) induced lesions in the plexus experimentally in mice, using vinblastine, mepacrine and isoniazid.

Selective damage to parasympathetic neurons in the heart may be caused by rubidomycin (Smith 1969).

References

Aarseth, S., Ofstad, E. & Torvik, A. (1961) Macroglobulinaemia Waldenström: A case with haemolytic anaemia and involvement of the nervous system. *Acta medica scandinavica*, **169**, 691-699.

Adams, C. W. M., Marples, E. A. & Trounce, J. R. (1960) Achalasia of the cardia and Hirschsprung's disease. The amount and distribution of cholinesterases. *Clinical Science*, **19**, 473-481.

Adams, W. E. (1941-42) The blood supply of nerves I: Historical review. *Journal of Anatomy*, **76**, 323-341.

Aguayo, A. J., Nair, C. P. V. & Bray, G. M. (1971) Peripheral nerve abnormalities in the Riley–Day syndrome. *Archives of Neurology* (*Chicago*), **24**, 106-116.

Aguayo, A., Nair, C. P. V. & Midgley, R. (1971) Experimental progressive compression neuropathy in the rabbit: histologic and electrophysiologic studies. *Archives of Neurology* (*Chicago*), **24**, 358-364.

Alcantara, F. G. de (1959) Experimentelle Chagas-Kardiopathie. *Zeitschrift für Tropenmedizin und Parasitologie*, **10**, 296-303.

Alderman, J. E. (1938) Diabetic anterior neuropathy. Clinical and pathological observations. *Journal of Mt. Sinai Hospital*, **5**, 396-402.

Alemà, G., Bignami, A. & Appicciutoli, L. (1963) La neuropatia carcinomatosa: studio clinico e anatomico di uno caso con sindrome sensoriale. *Rivista di neurobiologia*, **9**, 237-256.

Alexander, W. S. (1966) Phytanic acid in Refsum's syndrome. *Journal of Neurology, Neurosurgery and Psychiatry*, **29**, 412-416.

Allt, G. (1969) Repair of segmental demyelination in peripheral nerves: An electron microscope study. *Brain*, **92**, 639-646.

Allt, G. (1972) An ultrastructural analysis of remyelination following segmental demyelination. *Acta Neuropathologica* (*Berlin*), **22**, 333-344.

Alvarez, W. C. (1949) A simple explanation for cardiospasm and Hirschsprung's disease. *Gastroenterology*, **13**, 422-429.

Aminoff, M. J. (1972) Acanthocytosis and neurological disease. *Brain*, **95**, 749-760.

Andermann, F., Lloyd-Smith, D. L., Mavor, H. & Mathieson, G. (1962) Observations on hypertrophic neuropathy of Déjerine and Sottas. *Neurology* (*Minneapolis*), **12**, 712-724.

Anderson, I. F. (1965) Peripheral neuritis in systemic lupus erythematosus. *Medical Proceedings*, **11**, 31-33.

Anderson, M. H., Fullerton, P. M., Gilliatt, R. W. & Hern, J. E. C. (1970) Changes in the forearm associated with median nerve compression at the wrist in the guinea-pig. *Journal of Neurology, Neurosurgery and Psychiatry*, 30, 393-402.

Andersson, H., Hagne, I. & Roos, B. E. (1973) Homovanillic acid and 5-hydroxyindolacetic acid in cerebro-spinal fluid of a child with familial dysautonomia. *Acta paediatrica scandinavica*, 62, 46-48.

Andrade, C. (1952) A peculiar form of peripheral neuropathy: familial atypical generalized amyloidosis with special involvement of the peripheral nerves. *Brain*, 75, 408-427.

Apert, E. (1898) Paralysie traumatique radiculaire inférieure du plexus brachial. Autopsie trente-trois ans après l'accident. *Bulletin et mémoires de la Société médicale des hôpitaux de Paris*, 15, 613-619.

Appenseller, O., Kornfeld, M., Albuquerque, N. M. & McGee, J. (1971) Neuropathy in chronic renal disease. A microscopic, ultrastructural and biochemical study of sural nerve biopsies. *Archives of Neurology (Chicago)*, 24, 449-461.

Appicciutoli, L. & Bignami, A. (1962) La neuropatia carcinomatosa. *Recenti Progressi in Medicina (Rome)*, 32, 406-417.

Araki, S., Mawatari, S., Ohta, M., Nakajima, A. & Kuroiwa, Y. (1968) Polyneuritic amyloidosis in a Japanese family. *Archives of Neurology (Chicago)*, 18, 593-602.

Arkin, A. (1930) A clinical and pathological study of periarteritis nodosa: a report of five cases, one histologically healed. *American Journal of Pathology*, 6, 401-426.

Armitage, G. & Rhind, J. A. (1951) The fate of the tumour in infantile hypertrophic pyloric stenosis. *British Journal of Surgery*, 39, 39-43.

Arnason, B. G., & Asbury, A. K. (1968) Idiopathic polyneuritis after surgery. *Archives of Neurology (Chicago)*, 18, 500-507.

Arnason, B. G., Winkler, G. F. & Hadler, N. M. (1969) Cell-mediated demyelination of peripheral nerve in tissue culture. *Laboratory Investigation*, 21, 1-10.

Arnold, N. & Harriman, D. G. F. (1970) The incidence of abnormality in control human peripheral nerves studied by single axon dissection. *Journal of Neurology, Neurosurgery and Psychiatry*, 33, 55-61.

Asbury, A. K., Aldridge, H., Hershberg, R. & Fisher, C. M. (1970) Oculomotor palsy in diabetes mellitus: A clinico-pathological study. *Brain*, 93, 555-566.

Asbury, A. K., Arnason, B. G. & Adams, R. D. (1969) The inflammatory lesion in idiopathic polyneuritis: its role in pathogenesis. *Medicine (Baltimore)*, 48, 173-215.

Asbury, A. K., Cox, S. C. & Baringer, J. R. (1971) The significance of giant vacuolation of endoneurial fibroblasts. *Acta Neuropathologica (Berlin)*, 18, 123-131.

Asbury, A. K., Gale, M. K., Cox, S. C., Baringer, J. R. & Berg, B. O. (1972) Giant axonal neuropathy—a unique case with segmental neurofilamentous masses. *Acta Neuropathologica (Berlin)*, 20, 237-247.

Asbury, A. K., Picard, E. H. & Baringer, J. R. (1972) Sensory perineuritis. *Archives of Neurology (Chicago)*, 26, 302-312.

Asbury, A. K., Victor, M. & Adams, R. D. (1963) Uremic polyneuropathy. *Archives of Neurology (Chicago)*, 8, 413-428.

Åström, K. E. & Waksman, B. H. (1962) The passive transfer of experimental allergic encephalomyelitis and neuritis with living lymphoid cells. *Journal of Pathology and Bacteriology*, 83, 89-106.

Åström, K. E., Webster, H. de F. & Arnason, B. G. (1968) The initial lesion in experimental allergic neuritis. A phase and electron microscope study. *Journal of Experimental Medicine*, 128, 469-495.

Auerbach, L. (1864) Fernere vorläufige Mitteilung über den Nervenapparat des Darmes. *Virchows Archiv für pathologische Anatomie*, 30, 457-460.

Austin, J. H. (1956) Observations on the syndrome of hypertrophic neuritis (the hypertrophic interstitial radiculo-neuropathies). *Medicine (Baltimore)*, 35, 187-237.

Austin, J. H. (1958) Recurrent polyneuropathies and their cortico-steroid treatment. *Brain*, 81, 157-192.

Bailey, A. A., Sayre, G. P. & Clark, E. C. (1956) Neuritis associated with systemic lupus erythematosus. *Archives of Neurology and Psychiatry*, 45, 250-259.

Bailey, P. & Hermann, J. (1938) The role of the cells of Schwann in the formation of tumors of the peripheral nerves. *American Journal of Pathology*, 14, 1-38.

Baker, A. B. & Watson, C. J. (1945) The central nervous system in porphyria. *Journal of Neuropathology and Experimental Neurology*, 4, 68-76.

Ballin, R. H. M. & Thomas, P. K. (1969a) Changes at the nodes of Ranvier during Wallerian degeneration: an electron microscope study. *Acta Neuropathologica (Berlin)*, 14, 237-249.

Ballin, R. H. M. & Thomas, P. K. (1969b) Electron microscopic observations on demyelination and remyelination in experimental allergic neuritis II. Remyelination. *Journal of the Neurological Sciences*, 8, 225-237.

Baló, J.   (1926) Ueber eine Häufung von Periarteritis-nodosa-Fällen, nebst Beiträgen zur Polyneuritis infolge von Periarteritis nodosa.   *Virchows Archiv für pathologische Anatomie*, **259**, 773-794.

Bannister, R. G. & Sears, T. A.   (1962) The changes in nerve conduction in acute idiopathic polyneuritis.   *Journal of Neurology, Neurosurgery and Psychiatry*, **25**, 321-328.

Barraquer-Ferré, L. & Barraquer-Bordas, L.   (1953) De la sémiologie ganglio-radiculaire postérieure dans l'amyotrophie de Charcot–Marie–Tooth: troubles trophiques, douleurs fulgurantes, troubles sensitifs.   *Acta neurologica et psychiatrica belgica*, **53**, 55-70.

Barton, A. A.   (1962) An electron microscope study of degeneration and regeneration of nerve.   *Brain*, **85**, 799-808.

Bassen, F. A. & Kornzweig, A. L.   (1950) Malformation of erythrocytes in a case of atypical retinitis pigmentosa.   *Blood*, **5**, 381-387.

Beardwell, A.   (1961) Peripheral neuropathy in association with carcinoma of the thyroid.   *British Medical Journal*, **1**, 1012-1013.

Beckett, V. L. & Dinn, J. J.   (1972) Segmental demyelination in rheumatoid arthritis.   *Quarterly Journal of Medicine*, **41**, 71-80.

Bedford, P. D. & James, F. E.   (1956) A family with the progressive hypertrophic polyneuritis of Déjerine and Sottas.   *Journal of Neurology, Neurosurgery and Psychiatry*, **19**, 46-51.

Behse, F., Buchthal, F., Carlsen, F. & Knappes, G. G.   (1972) Hereditary neuropathy with liability to pressure palsies.   *Brain*, **95**, 777-794.

Bell, J.   (1935) On the peroneal type of progressive muscular atrophy in *Treasury of Human Inheritance: Nervous Disease and Muscular Dystrophies* (Ed. Fisher, R. A.), Vol. 4, pp. 69-139, Cambridge University Press, London.

Bennett, A., Garrett, J. R. & Howard, E. R.   (1968) Adrenergic myenteric nerves in Hirschsprung's disease.   *British Medical Journal*, **1**, 487-489.

Bennett, R., Hughes, G. V. R., Bywaters, E. G. L. & Holt, P. J. L.   (1972) Neuropsychiatric problems in systemic lupus erythematosus.   *British Medical Journal*, **4**, 342-345.

Bérard-Badier, M., Gambarelli, D., Pinsard, N., Hassoun, J. & Toga, M.   (1971) Infantile neuroaxonal dystrophy or Seitelberger's disease.   II: Peripheral nerve involvement: electron microscopic study in one case.   *Acta Neuropathologica (Berlin) Suppl. V*, 30-39.

Bérard-Badier, M., Toga, M., Gambarelli, D., Hassoun, J., Pellissier, J. F., Pinsard, N. & Bernard, R.   (1974) Infantile neuroaxonal dystrophy or Seitelberger's disease.   IV. Autonomic nervous system involvement.   Electron microscopic study in two siblings.   *Acta Neuropatholigica (Berlin)*, **28**, 261-267.

Berge, K. G., Sprague, R. G. & Bennett, W. A.   (1956) The intestinal tract in diabetic diarrhoea: a pathologic study.   *Diabetes*, **5**, 289-294.

Bergström, R.   (1962) Changes in peripheral nerve tissue after irradiation with high energy protons.   *Acta radiologica*, **58**, 301.

Berman, S.   (1961) Neurologic disorders in porphyria.   A brief clinical study of 81 cases in *Proceedings of the 7th International Congress of Neurology (Rome)*, pp. 33-38.

Berry, K. & Olszewski, J.   (1963) Pathology of intrathecal phenol injection in man.   *Neurology (Minneapolis)*, **13**, 152-154.

Bielschowsky, M.   (1914) Herpes zoster in *Handbuch der Neurologie* (Ed. Lewandowsky), Vol. 5, pp. 316-341, Springer Verlag, Berlin.

Bielschowsky, M.   (1922) Familiäre hypertrophische Neuritis und Neurofibromatose.   *Journal für Psychologie und Neurologie*, **29**, 182.

Biemond, A.   (1928) Neurotische Muskelatrophie und Friedreichsche Tabes in derselben Familie.   *Deutsche Zeitschrift für Nervenheilkunde*, **104**, 113-145.

Bignami, A.   (1961) Le neuriti nella periarterite nodosa.   *Il Policlinico*, **68**, 577-595.

Bigner, D. D., Olson, W. H. & McFarlin, D. E.   (1971) Peripheral polyneuropathy, high and low molecular weight IgM and amyloidosis.   *Archives of Neurology (Chicago)*, **24**, 365-373.

Bischoff, A.   (1970) in *Ultrastructure of the Peripheral Nervous System and sense Organs* (Ed. Bischoff, A.), Thieme, Stuttgart; Churchill, London.

Bischoff, A., Fierz, U., Regli, F. & Ulrich, J.   (1968) Peripherneurologische Störungen bei der Fabryschen Krankheit (Angiokeratoma corporis diffusum universale).   Klinische-elektronenmikroskopische Befunde bei einem Fall.   *Klinische Wochenschrift*, **46**, 666-671.

Bischoff, A. & Moor, H.   (1967) The ultrastructure of the 'difference factor' in the myelin.   *Zeitschrift für Zellforschung und mikroskopische Anatomie*, **81**, 571-580.

Blackwood, W.   (1944) A pathologist looks at ischaemia.   *Edinburgh Medical Journal*, **51**, 131-143.

Blackwood, W.   (1944) Studies in the pathology of human 'immersion foot'.   *British Journal of Surgery*, **31**, 329-350.

Blackwood, W.   (1952) Biopsy technique in the diagnosis of peripheral neuropathies (especially hereditary and sensory neuropathy) in *Proceedings of the 1st International Congress of Neuropathology (Rome)*, Vol. 3, pp. 415-424, Rosenberg and Sellier, Turin.

Blackwood, W. & Russell, H.   (1943) Experiments on the study of immersion foot.   *Edinburgh Medical Journal*, **50**, 385-398.

Bodian, M., Carter, C. O. & Ward, B. C. H.   (1951) Hirschsprung's disease.   *Lancet*, **1**, 302-309.

Bodian, M., Stephens, F. D. & Ward, B. C. H.   (1949) Hirschsprung's disease and idiopathic megacolon.   *Lancet*, **1**, 6-11.

Bogaert, L. van   (1953) Étude histopathologique d'une observation d'arthropathie mutilante symétrique familiale.   Sa non-appartenance à la syringomyélie.   Ses rapports aves la neuropathie radiculaire sensorielle héréditaire (Hicks et Denny-Brown).   *Acta neurologica et psychiatrica belgica*, **53**, 37-54.

Bogaert, L. van   (1957) Familial ulcers, mutilating lesions of the extremities and acro-osteolysis.   *British Medical Journal*, **2**, 367-371.

Bogaert, L. van, Mechelen, P. van, Martin, J. J. & Guazzi, G. C.   (1967) Sur la neuropathologie de la maladie de Refsum-Thiébault (Protocole de l'observation de Richterich, Kahlke, van Mechelen et Rossi, 1963).   *Revue Neurologique*, **116**, 229-240.

Borghi, G. & Tagliabue, G.   (1961) Primary amyloidosis in the Gasserian ganglion.   *Acta neurologica et psychiatrica scandinavica*, **37**, 105-110.

Bosanquet, F. D. and Henson, R. A.   (1957) Sensory neuropathy in diabetes mellitus.   *Folia psychiatrica, neurologica et neurochirurgica neerlandica*, **60**, 107-117.

Boveri, P.   (1910) De la névrite hypertrophique familiale (type Pierre Marie).   *La Semaine Médicale*, **30**, 145-150.

Boyer, G. F.   (1912) The complete histopathological examination of the nervous system of an unusual case of obstetrical paralysis forty-one years after birth and a review of the pathology.   *Proceedings of the Royal Society of Medicine*, **5**, *(Neurology)*, 31-58.

Bradford, J. R., Bashford, E. F. & Wilson, J. A.   (1918-19) Acute infective polyneuritis.   *Quarterly Journal of Medicine*, **12**, 88-126.

Bradley, W. G., Madrid, R., Thrush, D. C. & Campbell, M. J.   (1975) The syndromes of brachial plexus neuropathy.   *Brain* (in press).

Brady, R. O., Gall, A. G., Bradley, R. M., Martensson, E., Warshaw, A. L. & Laster, L.   (1967) Enzymatic defect in Fabry's disease: ceramide trihexosidase deficiency.   *New England Journal of Medicine*, **276**, 1163-1168.

Brain, Lord & Adams, R. D.   (1965) A guide to the classification and investigation of neurological disorders associated with neoplasms in *Remote Effects of Cancer on the Nervous System* (Eds. Brain, Lord & Norris, F. H.), pp. 216-221, Grune and Stratton, New York.

Brain, Lord, Croft, P. B. & Wilkinson, M.   (1965) Motor neurone disease as a manifestation of neoplasm.   *Brain*, **88**, 479-500.

Brain, W. R., Daniel, P. M. & Greenfield, J. G.   (1951) Subacute cortical cerebellar degeneration and its relation to carcinoma.   *Journal of Neurology, Neurosurgery and Psychiatry*, **14**, 59-75.

Brain, W. R. & Henson, R. A.   (1958) Neurological syndromes associated with carcinoma: the carcinomatous neuromyopathies.   *Lancet*, **2**, 971-974.

Brain, W. R., Wright, A. D. & Wilkinson, M.   (1947) Spontaneous compression of both median nerves in the carpal tunnel.   Six cases treated surgically.   *Lancet*, **1**, 277-282.

Brierley, J. B.   (1950) The penetration of particulate matter from the cerebrospinal fluid into the spinal ganglia, peripheral nerves and the perivascular spaces of the posterior root ganglia.   *Journal of Neurology, Neurosurgery and Psychiatry*, **13**, 203-215.

Brierley, J. B. & Field, E. J.   (1948) The connexion of the spinal subarachnoid space with the lymphatic system.   *Journal of Anatomy*, **82**, 153-166.

Brierley, J. B. & Field, E. J.   (1949) The fate of an intraneural injection as demonstrated by the use of radioactive phosphorus.   *Journal of Neurology, Neurosurgery and Psychiatry*, **12**, 86-99.

Brostoff, S., Burnet, P., Lampert, P. & Eylar, E. H.   (1972) Isolation and characterization of a protein from Sciatic Nerve Myelin responsible for Experimental Allergic Neuritis.   *Nature New Biology*, **235**, 210-212.

Browne, S. G.   (1965) Some less common neurological findings in leprosy.   *International Journal of Leprosy*, **33**, 881-891.

Brown, W. J., Beauchemin, J. A. & Linde, L. M.   (1964) A neuropathological study of familial dysautonomia (Riley–Day Syndrome) in siblings.   *Journal of Neurology, Neurosurgery and Psychiatry*, **27**, 131-139.

Bruns, G.   (1951) Zur Kenntnis der hypertrophischen Neuritis (Roussy-Cornil).   *Beiträge zur pathologischen Anatomie*, **3**, 407-418.

Bruns, O.   (1903) Familiale symetrische Gangrän und Arthropathie an den Füssen, möglicherweise beruhend auf familiärer Syringomyelie im Lumbosacralmark.   *Neurologisches Zentralblatt*, **22**, 599-600.

Brunt, P. W. & McKusick, V. A.   (1970) Familial dysautonomia. A report of genetic and clinical studies with a review of the literature.   *Medicine (Baltimore)*, **49**, 343-374.

Buchthal, F.   (1970) Electrophysiological abnormalities in metabolic myopathies and neuropathies.   *Acta neurologica scandinavica Suppl.* **43**, 129-176.

Büngner, O.   (1891) Über die Degenerations—und Regenerationsvorgänge am Nerven nach Verletzungen.   *Beiträge zur pathologischen Anatomie*, **10**, 321-393.

Byers, R. K. & Taft, L. T.   (1957) Chronic multiple peripheral neuropathy in childhood.   *Pediatrics*, **20**, 517-537.

Bywaters, E. G. L.   (1957) Peripheral vascular obstruction in rheumatoid arthritis and its relationship to other vascular lesions.   *Annals of the Rheumatic Diseases*, **16**, 84-103.

Cajal, S. Ramón y   (1928) *Degeneration and Regeneration of the Nervous System* (Translated May, R. M.), Vol. 1, Oxford University Press, London.

Cammermeyer, J.   (1956) Neuropathological changes in hereditary neuropathies: manifestation of the syndrome heredopathia atactica polyneuritiformis in the presence of interstitial hypertrophic neuropathy.   *Journal of Neuropathology and Experimental Neurology*, **15**, 340-361.

Campbell, A. M. G. & Hoffman, H. L.   (1964) Sensory radicular neuropathy associated with muscle wasting in two cases.   *Brain*, **87**, 67-79.

Casamajor, L.   (1919) Acute ascending paralysis among troops, pathologic findings.   *Archives of Neurology and Psychiatry*, **2**, 605-620.

Cassella, R. R., Ellis, F. H. & Brown, A. L.   (1965) Fine structure changes in achalasia of esophagus I. Vagus nerves.   *American Journal of Pathology*, **46**, 279-288.

Castaigne, P., Cambier, J. and Augustin, P.   (1965) La neuropathie amyloïde.   *Presse Médicale*, **73**, 1171-1176.

Castro, F. de   (1932a) Sensory ganglia of the cranial and spinal nerves, normal and pathological in *Cytology and Cellular Pathology of the Nervous System* (Ed. Penfield, W.), Vol. 1, pp. 91-143, Hoeber, New York.

Castro, F. de   (1932b) Sympathetic ganglia, normal and pathological in *Cytology and Cellular Pathology of the Nervous System* (Ed. Penfield, W., Vol. 1, pp. 317-379, Hoeber, New York.

Caughey, J. E., Farpour, A. & Etemadee, A. A.   (1967) Peripheral neuropathy with bronchiectasis.   *New Zealand Medical Journal*, **66**, 1-6.

Causey, G.   (1960) *The Cell of Schwann*, Livingstone, Edinburgh and London.

Cavanagh, J. B.   (1964) The significance of the 'dying-back' process in experimental and human neurological disease.   *International Review of Experimental Pathology*, **7**, 219-267.

Cavanagh, J. B. & Jacobs, J. M.   (1964) Some quantitative aspects of diphtheritic neuropathy.   *British Journal of Experimental Pathology*, **45**, 309-322.

Cavanagh, J. B. & Mellick, R. S.   (1965) On the nature of the peripheral nerve lesions associated with acute intermittent porphyria.   *Journal of Neurology, Neurosurgery and Psychiatry*, **28**, 320-327.

Cavanagh, J. B. & Ridley, A.   (1967) The nature of the neuropathy complicating acute intermittent porphyria.   *Lancet*, **2**, 1023-1024.

Cazzato, G.   (1965) Rapporti fra 'poliradiculonevriti recidivanti' e 'nevrite interstiziale ipertrofica sporadica dell' adulto'.   *Rivista di Patologia nervosa e mentale*, **86**, 325-354.

Chachina, S.   (1926) Veränderungen der sympathischen Ganglien bei Tollwut.   *Virchows Archiv für pathologische Anatomie*, **261**, 795-801.

Chagas, C.   (1909) Nova tripanozomiaze humana.   *Memorias do Instituto Oswaldo Cruz*, **1**, 159-218.

Chambers, R. & MacDermot, V.   (1957) Polyneuritis as a cause of 'amyotonia congenita'.   *Lancet*, **1**, 397-401.

Charcot, J. M. & Marie, P.   (1886) Sur une forme particulière d'atrophie musculaire progressive souvent familiale débutant par les pieds et les jambes et atteignant plus tard les mains.   *Revue de Médecine (Paris)*, **6**, 97-138.

Charcot, J. M. & Vulpian, E. F. A.   (1862) Note sur l'état des muscles et des nerfs du voile du palais dans un cas d'angine diphthéritique.   *Comptes rendus des Séances de la Société de Biologie et de ses Filiales*, **14**, 173-176.

Chopra, J. S. & Fannin, T.   (1971) Pathology of diabetic neuropathy.   *Journal of Pathology*, **104**, 175-184.

Chopra, J. S. & Hurwitz, L. J.   (1967) Internodal length of sural nerve fibres in chronic occlusive vascular disease.   *Journal of Neurology, Neurosurgery and Psychiatry*, **30**, 207-214.

Chopra, J. S. & Hurwitz, L. J.   (1969) A comparative study of peripheral nerve conduction in diabetes and non-diabetic chronic occlusive peripheral vascular disease.   *Brain*, **92**, 83-96.

Chopra, J. S., Hurwitz, L. J. & Montgomery, D. A. D. (1969) The pathogenesis of sural nerve changes in diabetes mellitus. *Brain*, **92**, 391-418.

Clark, E. C. & Bailey, A. A. (1954) Neurologic and psychiatric findings in lupus erythematosus. *Transactions of the American Neurological Association*, **79**, 15-18.

Cochrane, R. G. & Davey, T. F. (1964) *Leprosy in Theory and Practice*, 2nd Edn., J. Wright & Sons, Bristol.

Cohen, P. & Solomon, N. H. (1955) Familial dysautonomia: case report with autopsy. *Journal of Pediatrics*, **46**, 663.

Coimbra, A. & Andrade, C. (1971a) Familial amyloid polyneuropathy: an electron microscope study of the peripheral nerve in five cases I. Interstitial changes. *Brain*, **94**, 199-206.

Coimbra, A. & Andrade, C. (1971b) Familial amyloid polyneuropathy: an electron microscope study of the peripheral nerve in five cases II. Nerve fibre changes. *Brain*, **94**, 207-212.

Colby, A. O. (1965) Neurologic disorders of diabetes mellitus. *Diabetes*, **14**, 424-429, 516-525.

Collens, W. S. & Rabinowitz, M. A. (1928) Mumps polyneuritis quadriplegia with bilateral facial paralysis. *Archives of Internal Medicine*, **41**, 61-65.

Cook, S. D. & Dowling, P. C. (1968) Neurologic disorders associated with increased DNA synthesis in peripheral blood. *Archives of Neurology (Chicago)*, **19**, 583-590.

Cook, S. D., Dowling, P. C., Murray, M. R. & Whitaker, J. N. (1971) Circulating demyelinating factors in acute idiopathic polyneuropathy. *Archives of Neurology (Chicago)*, **24**, 136-144.

Cook, S. D., Dowling, P. C. & Whitaker, J. N. (1970) The Guillain–Barré Syndrome: relationship of circulating immunocytes to disease activity. *Archives of Neurology (Chicago)*, **22**, 470-474.

Cooper, E. L. (1936) Progressive familial hypertrophic neuritis (Déjerine–Sottas). *British Medical Journal*, **1**, 793-794.

Cragg, B. G. & Thomas, P. K. (1964a) Changes in nerve conduction in experimental allergic neuritis. *Journal of Neurology, Neurosurgery and Psychiatry*, **27**, 106-115.

Cragg, B. G. & Thomas, P. K. (1964b) The conduction velocity of regenerated nerve fibres. *Journal of Physiology (London)*, **171**, 164-175.

Craig, W. McK. & Kernohan, J. W. (1933) The surgical removal and histological studies of sympathetic ganglia in Raynaud's disease, thrombo-angiitis obliterans, chronic infectious arthritis, and scleroderma. *Surgery, Gynaecology and Obstetrics*, **56**, 767-778.

Critchley, E. M. R., Clark, D. B. & Wikler, A. (1968) Acanthocytosis and neurological disorder without abetalipoproteinemia. *Archives of Neurology (Chicago)*, **18**, 134-140.

Croft, P. B., Henson, R. A., Urich, H. & Wilkinson, P. C. (1965) Sensory neuropathy with bronchial carcinoma: a study of four cases showing serological abnormalities. *Brain*, **88**, 501-514.

Croft, P. B., Urich, H. & Wilkinson, M. (1967) Peripheral neuropathy of sensorimotor type associated with malignant disease. *Brain*, **90**, 31-66.

Croft, P. B. & Wadia, N. H. (1957) Familial hypertrophic polyneuritis; review of a previously reported family. *Neurology (Minneapolis)*, **7**, 356-366.

Croft, P. B. & Wilkinson, M. (1963) Carcinomatous neuromyopathy: its incidence in patients with carcinoma of the lung and carcinoma of the breast. *Lancet*, **1**, 184-188.

Croft, P. B. & Wilkinson, M. (1965) The incidence of carcinomatous neuromyopathy in patients with various types of carcinoma. *Brain*, **88**, 427-448.

Croft, P. B. & Wilkinson, M. (1969) The course and prognosis in some types of carcinomatous neuromyopathy. *Brain*, **92**, 1-8.

Cummings, J. F. & Haas, D. C. (1967) Coonhound paralysis: an acute idiopathic polyradiculoneuritis in dogs resembling the Landry–Guillain–Barré Syndrome. *Journal of the Neurological Sciences*, **4**, 51-81.

Currie, S., Henson, R. A., Morgan, H. G. & Poole, A. J. (1970) The incidence of the non-metastatic neurological syndromes of obscure origin in the reticuloses. *Brain*, **93**, 629-640.

Currie, S. & Knowles, M. (1971) Lymphocyte transformation in the Guillain–Barré syndrome. *Brain*, **94**, 109-116.

Dalla Valle, A: (1920) Ricerche istologiche su un caso di megacolon congenito. *Pediatria (Napoli)*, **28**, 740-752.

Daly, D. D., Love, J. G. & Dockerty, M. B. (1957) Amyloid tumour of Gasserian ganglion. *Journal of Neurosurgery*, **14**, 347-352.

Darnley, J. D. (1962) Polyneuropathy in Waldenström's macroglobulinaemia. Case report and discussion. *Neurology (Minneapolis)*, **12**, 617-623.

Dash, M. S. (1967) Studies in conduction velocity of the sensory fibres of the ulnar nerve in leprosy. *International Journal of Leprosy*, **35**, 460-469.

Dastur, D. K.   (1955) Cutaneous nerves in leprosy: relationship between histopathology and cutaneous sensibility. *Brain*, **78**, 615-633.

Dastur, D. K.   (1967) The peripheral neuropathology of leprosy in *Symposium on Leprosy* (Eds. Antia, N. H. & Dastur, D. K., pp. 57-71, Bombay University Press.

Dastur, D. K., Ramamohan, Y. & Shah, J. S.   (1972*a*) Ultrastructure of lepromatous nerves.   Neural pathogenesis in leprosy. *International Journal of Leprosy*, **41**, 47-80.

Dastur, D. K., Ramamohan, Y. & Shah, J. S.   (1972*b*) Ultrastructure of nerves in tuberculoid leprosy. *Neurology (India)*, **20** (*Suppl. 1*), 89-99.

Dastur, D. K. & Razzak, Z. A.   (1971) Degeneration and regeneration in teased nerve fibres I.   Leprous neuritis. *Acta Neuropathologica (Berlin)*, **18**, 286-298.

Dayan, A. D.   (1967) Peripheral neuropathy of metachromatic leucodystrophy: observations on segmental demyelination and remyelination and the intracellular distribution of sulphatide. *Journal of Neurology, Neurosurgery and Psychiatry*, **30**, 311-318.

Dayan, A. D., Croft, P. B. & Wilkinson, M.   (1965) Association of carcinomatous neuromyopathy with different histological types of carcinoma of the lung. *Brain*, **88**, 435-448.

Dayan, A. D., Gardner-Thorpe, C., Down, P. F. & Gleadle, R. I.   (1970) Peripheral neuropathy in uremia. *Neurology, (Minneapolis)*, **20**, 649-658.

Dayan, A. D., Graveson, C. S., Robinson, P. K. & Woodhouse, M. A.   (1968) Globular neuropathy: a disorder of axons and Schwann cells. *Journal of Neurology, Neurosurgery and Psychiatry*, **31**, 552-560.

Dayan, A. D. & Lewis, P. D.   (1966) Demyelinating neuropathy in macrocryoglobulinomia. *Neurology (Minneapolis)*, **16**, 1141-1144.

Dayan, A. D., Ogul, R. & Graveson, G. S.   (1972) Polyneuritis and herpes zoster. *Journal of Neurology, Neurosurgery and Psychiatry*, **35**, 170-175.

Dayan, A. D. & Sanbank, U.   (1970) Pathology of the peripheral nerves in leprosy: report of a case. *Journal of Neurology, Neurosurgery and Psychiatry*, **33**, 586-591.

Dayan, A. D. & Stokes, M. I.   (1972) Peripheral neuropathy and experimental myeloma in the mouse. *Nature New Biology*, **236**, 117-118.

Dayan, A. D., Urich, H. & Gardner-Thorpe, C.   (1970) Peripheral neuropathy and myeloma. *Journal of the Neurological Sciences*, **14**, 21-35.

Dean, G.   (1963) The prevalence of the porphyrias. *South African Journal of Laboratory and Clinical Medicine*, **9**, 145-151.

De Bolt, W. L. & Jordan, J. C.   (1966) Femoral neuropathy from heparin haematoma. *Bulletin of the Los Angeles Neurological Society*, **31**, 45-50.

De Bruyn, R. S. & Stern, R. O.   (1929) Case of progressive hypertrophic polyneuritis of Déjerine and Sottas, with pathological examination. *Brain*, **52**, 84-107.

Déjerine-Klumpke, A.   (1908) Paralyse radiculaire totale du plexus brachial avec phénomenes oculo-pupillaires autopsiée trente-six jours après l'accident. *Revue Neurologique*, **16**, 637-645.

Déjerine, J. & Sottas, J.   (1893) Sur la névrite interstitielle hypertrophique et progressive de l'enfance. *Comptes Rendus des Séances de la Société de Biologie et de ses filiales*, **45**, 63-96.

Déjerine, J. & Thomas, A.   (1906) Sur la névrite interstitielle hypertrophique progressive de l'enfance. *Nouvelle Iconographie de la Salpêtrière*, **19**, 477-509.

De Jong, J. G. Y.   (1947) Over families met hereditaire dispositie tot het optreten van neuritiden, gecorreleerd met migraine. *Psychiatrische en Neurologische bladen (Amst.)*, **50**, 60-76.

Denny-Brown, D.   (1946) Importance of neural fibroblasts in the regeneration of nerve. *Archives of Neurology and Psychiatry*, **55**, 171-215.

Denny-Brown, D.   (1948) Primary sensory neuropathy with muscular changes associated with carcinoma. *Journal of Neurology, Neurosurgery and Psychiatry*, **11**, 73-87.

Denny-Brown, D.   (1951) Hereditary sensory radicular neuropathy. *Journal of Neurology, Neurosurgery and Psychiatry*, **14**, 237-252.

Denny-Brown, D., Adams, R. D., Brenner, C. & Doherty, M. M.   (1945) The pathology of injury to nerve induced by cold. *Journal of Neuropathology and Experimental Neurology*, **4**, 305-325.

Denny-Brown, D. & Brenner, C.   (1944*a*) The effect of percussion of nerve. *Journal of Neurology, Neurosurgery and Psychiatry*, **7**, 76-95.

Denny-Brown, D. & Brenner, C.   (1944*b*) Paralysis of nerve induced by direct pressure and by tourniquet. *Archives of Neurology and Psychiatry*, **51**, 1-26.

Denny-Brown, D. & Brenner, C.   (1944*c*) Lesions in peripheral nerve resulting from compression by spring clip. *Archives of Neurology and Psychiatry*, **52**, 1-19.

Denny-Brown, D. & Doherty, M. M. (1945) Effects of transient stretching on peripheral nerve. *Archives of Neurology and Psychiatry*, **54**, 116-129.

Denny-Brown, D. & Sciarra, D. (1945) Changes in the nervous system in acute porphyria. *Brain*, **68**, 1-16.

Dereux, J. (1963) La maladie de Refsum. *Revue Neurologique*, **109**, 599-608.

Dereux, J. & Gruner, J. E. (1963) La maladie de Refsum: étude d'une biopsie nerveuse au microscope électronique. *Revue Neurologique*, **109**, 564.

Dide, M. & Courjon, R. (1918) Un cas de névrite hypertrophique de l'adulte. *Nouvelle Iconographie de la Salpêtrière*, **28**, 377-383.

Dinn, J. J. (1970) Transnodal remyelination. *Journal of Pathology*, **102**, 51-53.

Dinn, J. J. & Crane, D. L. (1970) Schwann cell dysfunction in uraemia. *Journal of Neurology, Neurosurgery and Psychiatry*, **33**, 605-608.

Dobrovolskaia-Zavadskaia, N. (1924) Action des rayonnements du radium sur les nerfs périphériques. *Comptes rendus des Séances de la Société de Biologie et de ses Filiales*, **91**, 1322-1324.

Dodgson, M. C. H. & Hoffman, H. L. (1953) Sensory neuropathy associated with carcinoma of the esophagus: report of a case. *Annals of Internal Medicine*, **38**, 130-135.

Dolman, C. L. (1963) The morbid anatomy of diabetic neuropathy. *Neurology (Minneapolis)*, **13**, 135-142.

Dorang, L. & Matzke, H. A. (1960) The fate of a radio-opaque medium injected into the sciatic nerve. *Journal of Neuropathology and Experimental Neurology*, **19**, 25-32.

Döring, G. (1955) Pathologische Anatomie der Spinal- und Hirnnervenganglion, einschliesslich der Wurzelnerven in *Handbuch der speziellen pathologischen Anatomie und Histologie* (Eds. Lubarsch, O., Henke, I. & Rössle, R.,) Vol. 13, pt. 5, pp. 249-356, Springer Verlag, Berlin.

Drachman, D. A. (1963) Neurological complications of Wegener's granulomatosis. *Archives of Neurology (Chicago)*, **8**, 145-155.

Drachman, D. A., Paterson, P. Y., Berlin, B. S. & Roguska, J. (1970) Immunosuppression and the Guillain–Barré syndrome. *Archives of Neurology*, **23**, 385-393.

Dreyer, G. (1900) *Experimentelle undersøgelser over differigiftens toxoner*, Copenhagen.

Dreyfus, P. M., Hakim, S. & Adams, R. D. (1957) Diabetic ophthalmoplegia. *Archives of Neurology and Psychiatry*, **77**, 337-349.

Dunn, J. S. (1970) Developing myelin in human peripheral nerve. *Scottish Medical Journal*, **15**, 108-117.

Dyck, P. J. (1966) Histologic measurements and fine structure of biopsied sural nerve: normal and in peroneal muscular atrophy, hypertrophic neuropathy and congenital sensory neuropathy. *Proceedings of the Staff Meetings of the Mayo Clinic*, **41**, 742-774.

Dyck, P. J. (1969) Experimental hypertrophic neuropathy. Pathogenesis of onion-bulb formations produced by repeated tourniquet applications. *Archives of Neurology (Chicago)*, **21**, 73-95.

Dyck, P. J., Ellefson, R. D., Lais, A. C., Smith, R. C., Taylor, W. F. & van Dyck, R. A. (1970) Histologic and lipid studies of sural nerves in inherited hypertrophic neuropathy: preliminary report of a lipid abnormality in nerve and liver in Déjerine–Sottas disease. *Mayo Clinic Proceedings*, **45**, 286-327.

Dyck, P. J. & Hopkins, A. P. (1972) Electron microscopic observations on degeneration and regeneration of unmyelinated fibres. *Brain*, **95**, 223-234.

Dyck, P. J., Johnson, W. J., Lambert, E. H. & O'Brien, P. C. (1971). Segmental demyelination secondary to axonal degeneration in uremic neuropathy. *Mayo Clinic Proceedings*, **46**, 400-431.

Dyck, P. J., Kennel, A. J., Magal, I. V. & Kraybill, E. N. (1965) A Virginia kinship with hereditary sensory neuropathy, peroneal muscular atrophy and pes cavus. *Proceedings of the staff Meetings of the Mayo Clinic*, **40**, 685-694.

Dyck, P. J. & Lambert, E. H. (1968a) Lower motor and primary sensory neuron diseases with peroneal muscular atrophy I. Neurologic, genetic and electrophysiologic findings in hereditary polyneuropathies. *Archives of Neurology*, **18**, 603-618.

Dyck, P. J. & Lambert, E. H. (1968b) Lower motor and primary sensory neuron diseases with peroneal muscular atrophy II. Neurologic genetic and electrophysiologic findings in various neuronal degenerations. *Archives of Neurology (Chicago)*, **18**, 619-625.

Dyck, P. J. & Lambert, E. H. (1969) Dissociated sensation in amyloidosis. *Archives of Neurology (Chicago)*, **20**, 490-507.

Dyer, N. H., Dawson, A. M., Smith, B. F. & Todd, I. P. (1969) Obstruction of bowel due to lesion in the myenteric plexus. *British Medical Journal*, **1**, 686-689.

Eames, R. A. & Lange, L. S. (1967) Clinical and pathological study of ischaemic neuropathy. *Journal of Neurology, Neurosurgery and Psychiatry*, **30**, 215-226.

Earl, C. J., Fullerton, P. M., Wakefield, G. S. & Schutta, H. S. (1964) Hereditary neuropathy with liability to pressure palsies. *Quarterly Journal of Medicine*, **33**, 481-498.

Edds, MacV. (1949) Experiments on partially deneurotized nerves: II. Hypertrophy of residual fibres. *Journal of Experimental Zoology*, **112**, 29-47.

Edström, R., Gröntoft, O. & Sandring, H. (1959) Refsum's disease: three siblings, one autopsy. *Acta psychiatrica scandinavica*, **34**, 40-50.

Edwards, D. A. W. (1961) Physiological concepts of the pylorus. *Proceedings of the Royal Society of Medicine*, **54**, 930-933.

Eichhorst, H. (1873) Über Heredität der progressiven Muskelatrophie. *Klinische Wochenschrift*, **10**, 497-499, 511-514.

Eliasson, S. G. (1964) Nerve conduction changes in experimental diabetes. *Journal of Clinical Investigation*, **43**, 2353-2358.

Eliasson, S. G. (1969) Properties of isolated nerve fibres from alloxanised rats. *Journal of Neurology, Neurosurgery and Psychiatry*, **32**, 525-529.

Enerbäck, L., Olsson, Y. & Sourander, P. (1965) Mast cells in normal and sectioned peripheral nerves. *Zeitschrift für Zellforschung*, **66**, 596-608.

Engel, W. K., Dorman, J. D., Levy, R. I. & Fredrickson, D. S. (1967) Neuropathy in Tangier disease. *Archives of Neurology (Chicago)*, **17**, 1-9.

England, A. C. & Denny-Brown, D. (1952) Severe sensory changes, and trophic disorder, in peroneal muscular atrophy (Charcot–Marie–Tooth type). *Archives of Neurology and Psychiatry*, **67**, 1-22.

Erb, W. (1874) *Über eine eigenthümliche Lokalisation von Lähmungen im Plexus brachialis*, Heidelberg.

Erbslöh, W. (1903) Zur Pathologie und pathologischen Anatomie der toxischen Polyneuritis nach Sulfonalgebrauch. *Deutsche Zeitschrift für Nervenheilkunde*, **23**, 197-204.

Estes, J. W., Morley, T. J., Levine, I. M. & Emerson, C. P. (1967) A new hereditary acanthocytosis syndrome. *American Journal of Medicine*, **42**, 868-881.

Fabry, J. (1898) Ein Beitrag zur Purpura haemorrhagica nodularis (Purpura papulosa haemorrhagica Hebrae). *Archiv für Dermatologie und Syphilis, Suppl.* **43**, 187-200.

Fagerberg, S. E. (1959) Diabetic neuropathy: a clinical and histological study on the significance of vascular affections. *Acta medica scandinavica, Suppl.* 345.

Fardeau, M. & Engel, W. K. (1969) Ultrastructural study of peripheral nerve biopsy in Refsum's disease. *Journal of Neuropathology and Experimental Neurology*, **28**, 278-294.

Feng, T. P. & Liu, Y. M. (1949) The connective tissue sheath of the nerve as effective diffusion barrier. *Journal of Cellular and Comparative Physiology*, **34**, 1-16.

Fernandez-Morán, H. (1950) *a.* Electron microscope observations on the structure of the myelinated nerve fibre sheath. *Experimental Cell Research*, **1**, 143-149. *b.* Sheath and axon structures in the internode portion of vertebrate myelinated nerve fibres. *Experimental Cell Research*, **1**, 309-340.

Finch, S. C. & Finch, C. A. (1955) Idiopathic hemochromatosis, an iron storage disease. *Medicine (Baltimore)*, **34**, 381-430.

Fisher, C. M. & Adams, R. D. (1956) Diphtheritic polyneuritis—a pathological study. *Journal of Neuropathology and Experimental Neurology*, **15**, 243-268.

Fite, G. L. (1943) Leprosy from the histologic point of view. *Archives of Pathology*, **35**, 611-644.

Flaubert, M. (1827) Mémoire sur plusieurs cas de luxation. *Réport général d'Anatomie, de Physiologie, de Pathologie, de clinique et de Chirurgie*, **3**, 55-69.

Forster, F. M., Brown, M. & Merritt, H. M. (1941) Polyneuritis with facial diplegia: a clinical study. *New England Journal of Medicine*, **225**, 51-56.

Fredrickson, D. S. (1966) Familial high-density lipoprotein deficiency: Tangier disease in *The metabolic basis of inherited disease* (Eds. Stanbury, J. B., Wyngaarden, J. B. & Fredrickson, D. S.), 2nd Edn., pp. 486-508, McGraw-Hill, New York.

Fredrickson, D. S., Altrocchi, P. H., Avioli, L. V., Goodman, W. S. & Goodman, H. C. (1961) Tangier disease. *Annals of Internal Medicine*, **55**, 1016-1033.

Freund, H. A., Steiner, C., Leichtentritt, B. & Price, A. E. (1942) Peripheral nerves in chronic atrophic arthritis. *American Journal of Pathology*, **18**, 865-885.

Friedreich, N. (1873) *Über progressive Muskelatrophie, über wahre und falsche Muskelhypertrophie*, A. Hirschwald, Berlin.

Fullerton, P. M. & Gilliatt, R. W. (1967) Median and ulnar neuropathy in the guinea-pig. *Journal of Neurology, Neurosurgery and Psychiatry*, **30**, 393-402.

Fullerton, P. M., Gilliatt, R. W., Lascelles, R. G. & Morgan-Hughes, J. A. (1965) The relation between fibre diameter and internodal length in chronic neuropathy. *Journal of Physiology*, **178**, 26P-28P.

Fulton, J. K. (1952) Essential lipemia, acute gout, peripheral neuritis and myocardial disease in a negro. Response to corticotrophin. *Archives of Internal Medicine*, **89**, 303-308.

Funck-Brentano, U. L., Chaumont, P., Vantelon, J. & Zingraff, J.   (1968) Polynévrite au cours de l'urémie chronique.   Evolution après transplantation renale (10 observations personelles).   *Nephron*, **5**, 31-42.

Gabbay, K. H. & O'Sullivan, J. B.   (1968) The sorbitol pathway: enzyme localization and content in normal and diabetic nerve and cord.   *Diabetes*, **17**, 239-243.

Gagel, O. & Watts, J. W.   (1932) Zur Pathogenese der Raynaudschen Gangräne.   *Zeitschrift für klinische Medizin*, **122**, 110-117.

Gallois, P., Dhers, A. & Badaron, G.   (1967) Deux cas de paralysie nerveuse périphérique par hématome spontané au cours de traitement anticoagulant.   *Lyon Médical*, **218**, 401-406.

Gamble, H. J. & Eames, R. A.   (1964) An electron microscopic study of the connective tissues of human peripheral nerve.   *Journal of Anatomy (London)*, **98**, 655-663.

Gamble, H. J. & Goldby, S.   (1961) Mast cells in peripheral nerve trunks.   *Nature (London)*, **189**, 766-767.

Garcin, R., Mallarmé, J. & Rondot, P.   (1962) Névrites dysglobulinémiques.   *Presse Médicale*, **70**, 111-114.

Garcin, R., Lapresle, J., Fardeau, M. & Recondo, J. de (1966) Étude au microscope électronique du nerf périphérique prélevé par biopsie dans quatre cas de névrite hypertrophique se Déjerine–Sottas.   *Revue Neurologique*, **115**, 917-932.

Garland, H.   (1955) Diabetic amyotrophy.   *British Medical Journal*, **2**, 1287-1290.

Garvey, P. H., Jones, N. & Warren, S. L.   (1940) Polyradiculoneuritis (Guillain–Barré syndrome) following the use of sulfanilamide and fever therapy.   *Journal of the American Medical Association*, **115**, 1955-1959.

Gaskill, H. S. & Korb, M.   (1946) Occurrence of multiple neuritis in cases of cutaneous diphtheria.   *Archives of Neurology and Psychiatry*, **55**, 559-572.

Gasser, H. S.   (1955) Properties of the dorsal root unmedullated fibres on the two sides of the ganglion.   *Journal of General Physiology*, **38**, 709-728.

Gathier, J. C. & Bruyn, C. W.   (1970) Hypertrophic interstitial neuropathy (Déjerine–Sottas) in *Handbook of Clinical Neurology* (Eds. Vinken, P. J. & Bruyn, C. W.), Vol. 8, pp. 169-179, North-Holland Publishing Co., Amsterdam.

Gautier-Smith, P. C.   (1965) Neurological complications of glandular fever (infectious mononucleosis).   *Brain*, **88**, 323-334.

Geren, B. B.   (1945) The formation from the Schwann cell surface of myelin in the peripheral nerves of chick embryos.   *Experimental Cell Research*, **7**, 558-562.

Gibberd, F. B. & Gavrilescu, K.   (1966) A familial neuropathy associated with a paraprotein in the serum, cerebro-spinal fluid and urine.   *Neurology (Minneapolis)*, **16**, 130-134.

Gibson, J. B. & Goldberg, A.   (1956) The neuropathy of acute porphyria.   *Journal of Pathology and Bacteriology*, **71**, 495-510.

Gilliatt, R. W.   (1966) Nerve conduction in human and experimental neuropathies.   *Proceedings of the Royal Society of Medicine*, **59**, 989-993.

Gilliatt, R. W.   (1969) Experimental peripheral neuropathy in *The Scientific Basis of Medicine Annual Reviews*, pp. 202-219, Athlone Press, London.

Gilliatt, R. W. & Sears, T. A.   (1958) Sensory nerve action potentials in patients with peripheral nerve lesions.   *Journal of Neurology, Neurosurgery and Psychiatry*, **21**, 109-118.

Gilliatt, R. W. & Willison, R. G.   (1964) Peripheral nerve conduction in diabetic neuropathy.   *Journal of Neurology, Neurosurgery and Psychiatry*, **25**, 11-18.

Gilpin, S. F., Moersch, F. P. & Kernohan, J. W.   (1936) Polyneuritis, a clinical and pathologic study of a special group of cases frequently referred to as instances of neuronitis.   *Archives of Neurology and Psychiatry*, **35**, 937-963.

Glimstedt, G. & Wohlfart, G.   (1960) Electron microscope observations on Wallerian degeneration in peripheral nerves.   *Acta morphologica neerlando-scandinavica*, **3**, 135-146.

Goldberg, M. & Chitanondh, H. (1959) Polyneuritis with albuminocytologic dissociation in the spinal fluid in systemic lupus erythematosus.   *American Journal of Medicine*, **27**, 342-350.

Gombault, A.   (1880-81) Contribution à l'étude anatomique de la névrite parenchymateuse subaigüe et chronique: névrite segmentaire périaxile.   *Archives de Neurologie (Paris)*, **1**, 11-38, 177-190.

Gombault, A. & Mallet,   (1889) Un cas de tabès ayant débuté dans l'enfance.   *Archives de Médecine Expérimentale*, **1**, 385-415.

Goodman, J. I., Baumoel, S., Frankel, L., Marcus, J. L. & Wassermann, S.   (1953) *The Diabetic Neuropathies*, Thomas, Springfield, Ill.

Götze, W. & Krücke, W.   (1941) Über Paramyloidose mit besonderer Beteiligung der peripheren Nerven.   *Archiv für Psychiatrie und Nervenkrankheiten*, **114**, 183-213.

Goulston, D. L.   (1930) The action of radiation from radium needles on nerves.   *Medical Journal of Australia*, **2**, 651-660.

Gray, K. W., Woolf, A. L. & Wright, E. A. (1955) Two cases of primary sensory neuropathy associated with carcinoma. *Guy's Hospital Reports*, **104**, 157-176.

Greenbaum, D. (1964) Observations on the homogeneous nature·and pathogenesis of diabetic neuropathy. *Brain*, **87**, 215-232.

Greenbaum, D., Richardson, P. C., Salmon, M. V. & Urich, H. (1964) Pathological observations on six cases of diabetic neuropathy. *Brain*, **87**, 201-214.

Greenfield, J. G. (1954) *The Spino-cerebellar Degenerations*, p. 31, Blackwell Scientific, Oxford.

Greenfield, J. G. & Carmichael, A. E. (1925) *The Cerebrospinal Fluid in Clinical Diagnosis*, pp. 160-161, Macmillan, London.

Grokoest, A. W. & Demartini, F. E. (1954) Systemic disease and the carpal tunnel syndrome. *Journal of the American Medical Association*, **155**, 635-637.

Guillain, G. (1936) Radiculoneuritis with acellular hyperalbuminosis of the cerebrospinal fluid. *Archives of Neurology and Psychiatry*, **36**, 975-990.

Guillain, G., Barré, J. A. & Strohl, A. (1916) Sur un syndrome de radiculo-névrite avec hyperalbuminose du liquide céphalo-rachidien sans réaction cellulaire: Remarques sur les caractères cliniques et graphiques des réflexes tendineuses. *Bulletin de la Societé Médicale de l'Hôpital de Paris*, **40**, 1462-1470.

Gutmann, E., Guttmann, L., Medawar, P. B. & Young, J. Z. (1942) The rate of regeneration of nerve. *Journal of Experimental Biology*, **19**, 14-44.

Gutmann, E. & Sanders, F. K. (1943) Recovery of fibre numbers and diameters in the regeneration of peripheral nerves. *Journal of Physiology (London)*, **101**, 489-518.

Gutrecht, J. A. & Dyck, P. J. (1966) Segmental demyelinization in peroneal muscular atrophy: nerve fibres teased from sural nerve biopsy specimens. *Mayo Clinic Proceedings*, **41**, 775-777.

Hagen, E. (1943-45) Beitrag zur Histopathologie des Halsgrenzstranges bei der Raynaudschen Erkrankung. *Zeitschrift für Zellforschung und mikroskopische Anatomie*, **33**, 68-85.

Hagen, E. (1948-50) Beobachtungen zur pathologischen Histologie des vegetativen Nervensystems bei verschiedenen Erkrankungen des Gefässapparates. *Zeitschrift für Anatomie und Entwicklungsgeschichte*, **114**, 420-437.

Hallpike, C. S. (1967) Observations on the structural basis of two rare varieties of hereditary deafness. *Ciba Foundation Symposium on Myotatic, Kinaesthetic and Vestibular Mechanisms* (Ed. de Reuck, A. V. S. and Knight, Julie), pp. 285-289, Churchill, London.

Hamilton, E. B. & Bywaters, E. G. L. (1961) Joint symptoms in myelomatosis and similar conditions. *Annals of the Rheumatic Diseases*, **20**, 353-362.

Harkin, J. C. & Reed, R. J. (1969) Tumors of the Peripheral Nerves, *A.F.I.P. Atlas of Tumor Pathology*, 2nd Series, Fascicle 3, pp. 24-27, Armed Forces Institute of Pathology, Washington.

Harris, W. & Newcombe, W. D. (1929) A case of relapsing interstitial hypertrophic polyneuritis. *Brain*, **52**, 84-107.

Hart, F. D. & Golding, J. R. (1960) Rheumatoid neuropathy. *British Medical Journal*, **1**, 1594-1600.

Hart, F. D., Golding, J. R. & Mackenzie, D. H. (1957) Neuropathy in rheumatoid disease. *Annals of the Rheumatic Diseases*, **16**, 471-480.

Haslock, D. I., Wright, V. & Harriman, D. G. F. (1970) Neuromuscular disorders in rheumatoid arthritis: a motor-point muscle biopsy study. *Quarterly Journal of Medicine*, **39**, 335-358.

Haymaker, W. & Kernohan, J. W. (1949) Landry–Guillain–Barré syndrome: 50 fatal cases and a critique of the literature. *Medicine (Baltimore)*, **28**, 59-141.

Heathfield, K. W. G. (1957) Acroparaesthesiae and the carpal tunnel syndrome. *Lancet*, **2**, 663-666.

Hechst, B. (1933-34) Über pathologisch-anatomische Veränderungen im Nervensystem bei postdiphtherischen Nervenerkrankungen. *Archiv für Psychiatrie und Nervenkrankheiten*, **101**, 1-18.

Hegstrom, R. M., Murray, J. S., Pendras, J. P., Burnell, J. M. & Scribner, B. H. (1961) Hemodialysis in the treatment of chronic uremia. *Transactions of the American Society for Artificial Internal Organs*, **7**, 136-152.

Hegstrom, R. M., Murray, J. S., Pendras, J. P., Burnell, J. M. & Scribner, B. H. (1962) Two years' experience with periodic hemodialysis in the treatment of chronic uremia. *Transactions of the American Society for Artificial Internal Organs*, **8**, 266-275.

Heller, H., Missmahl, H. P., Sohar, E. & Gafni, J. (1964) Amyloidosis, its differentiation into perireticulin and pericollagen types. *Journal of Pathology and Bacteriology*, **88**, 15-34.

Heller, I. H. & Robb, P. (1955) Hereditary sensory neuropathy. *Neurology (Minneapolis)*, **5**, 15-29..

Henson, R. A. (1970) Non-metastatic neurological manifestations of malignant disease in *Modern Trends in Neurology* (Ed. Williams, D.), Vol. 5, pp. 209-225, Butterworth, London.

Henson, R. A., Hoffman, H. L. & Urich, H. (1965) Encephalomyelitis with carcinoma. *Brain*, **88**, 449-464.

Henson, R. A., Russell, D. S. & Wilkinson, M. I. P. (1954) Carcinomatous neuropathy, a clinical and pathological study. *Brain*, **77**, 82-121.

Heptinstall, R. H. & Sowry, G. S. C. (1952) Peripheral neuritis in systemic lupus erythematosus. *British Medical Journal*, **2**, 525-527.

Herzog, E. (1935) Histopathologische Veränderungen des Vagus und Sympathicus beim Fleckfieber. *Virchows Archiv für pathologische Anatomie*, **296**, 403-415.

Hicks, E. P. (1922) Hereditary perforating ulcer of the foot. *Lancet*, **1**, 319-321.

Hierons, R. (1957) Changes in the nervous system in acute porphyria. *Brain*, **80**, 176-192.

Hirschsprung, H. (1888) Stuhlträgheit Neugeborener in Folge von Dilatation und Hypertrophie des Colons. *Jahrbuch für Kinderheilkunde und physische Erziehung*, **27**, 1-7.

Hoffmann, J. (1893) Über chronische spinale Muskelatrophie im Kindesalter, auf familiärer Basis. *Deutsche Zeitschrift für Nervenheilkunde*, **3**, 427-470.

Holmes, W. & Young, J. Z. (1942) Nerve regeneration after immediate and delayed suture. *Journal of Anatomy (London)*, **77**, 63-96.

Holtermann, C. (1924) Ein Beitrag zur pathologischen Anatomie der Periarteritis nodosa. *Beiträge zur pathologischen Anatomie*, **72**, 344-348.

Holtzman, E. & Novikoff, A. B. (1965) Lysosomes in the rat sciatic nerve following crush. *Journal of Cell Biology*, **27**, 651-669.

Holtzmann, I. N. & Howes, W. E. (1940) Peripheral nerve destruction: an unusual sequel to radium therapy. *American Journal of Roentgenology*, **43**, 426-427.

Hopkins, A. P. (1968) Experimental neuropathy in the Baboon. M.D. Thesis, London.

Hughes, J. T. & Brownell, B. (1972) Pathology of peroneal muscular atrophy (Charcot–Marie–Tooth disease) *Journal of Neurology, Neurosurgery and Psychiatry*, **35**, 648-657.

Hughes, J. T., Brownell, B. & Hewer, R. L. (1968) The peripheral sensory pathway in Friedreich's ataxia. *Brain*, **91**, 803-818.

Hukuhara, T., Kotani, S. & Sato, G. (1961) Effects of destruction of intramural ganglion cells on colon motility: possible genesis of congenital megacolon. *Japanese Journal of Physiology*, **11**, 635-640.

Hutchinson, E. C., Leonard, B. J., Maudsley, C. & Yates, P. O. (1958) Neurological complications of the reticuloses. *Brain*, **81**, 75-92.

Hutchinson, E. C. & Liversedge, L. A. (1956) Neuropathy in peripheral vascular disease. *Quarterly Journal of Medicine*, **25** (N.S.), 267-274.

Imaeda, T. & Convit, J. (1963) Electron-microscopic study of cutaneous nerves in leprosy. *International Journal of Leprosy*, **31**, 188-210.

Imaginario, J. da G., Coelho, B., Tomé, F. & Luis, M. L. S. (1964) Névrite interstitielle hypertrophique monosymptomatique. *Journal of the Neurological Sciences*, **1**, 340-347.

Iwashita, H., Inoue, N. & Kuroiwa, Y. (1969) Familial optic and acoustic nerve degeneration with distal amyotrophy. *Lancet*, **2**, 219-220.

Jackson, M. (1949) Familial lumbo-sacral syringomyelia and the significance of developmental errors of the spinal cord and column. *Medical Journal of Australia*, **1**, 433-439.

Jakovleva, J. (1927) Diphtherie polyneuritis nach (versehentlicher). Einspritzung von Diphtherietoxin (Abstr.). *Zentralblatt für die gesamte Neurologie und Psychiatrie*, **47**, 203.

Janzen, A. H. & Warren, S. (1942) Effect of Roentgen-rays on the peripheral nerve of the rat. *Radiology*, **38**, 333-337.

Jarrett, E. & Barter, A. (1964) Polyneuritis in haemochromatosis. *Postgraduate Medical Journal*, **40**, 95.

Job, C. K. (1970) Mycobacterium leprae in nerve lesions in lepromatous leprosy: an electron-microscopic study. *Archives of Pathology*, **89**, 195-207.

Job, C. K. & Desikan, K. V. (1968) Pathologic changes and their distribution in peripheral nerves in lepromatous leprosy. *International Journal of Leprosy*, **36**, 257-270.

Job, C. K., Karat, A. B. A., Karat, S. & Mathan, M. (1969) Leprous myositis—a histopathological and electron-microscopic study. *Leprosy Review*, **40**, 9-16.

Joffroy, A. & Achard, C. (1889) Névrite périphérique d'origine vasculaire. *Archives de Médecine Expérimentale*, **1**, 229-240.

Joosten, E., Gabreëls, F., Gabreëls-Festen, A., Vrensen, G., Korten, J. & Notermans, S. (1974) Electron microscopic heterogeneity of onion-bulb neuropathies of the Déjerine–Sottas type. Two patients in one family with the variant described by Lyon. *Acta Neuropathologica (Berlin)*, **27**, 105-118.

Jopling, W. H. & Morgan-Hughes, J. A. (1965) Pure neural tuberculoid leprosy. *British Medical Journal*, **2**, 799-800.

Jordan, W. R. (1936) Neuritic manifestations in diabetes mellitus. *Archives of Internal Medicine*, **57**, 307-366.

Jughenn, H., Krücke, W. & Wadulla, H.   (1949) Zur Frage der familiären Syringomyelie (Klinisch-anatomische Untersuchungen über 'familiäre neurovasculäre Dystrophie der Extremitäten') *Archiv für Psychiatrie und Nervenkrankheiten*, **182**, 153-176.

Kahlke, W. & Richterich, R.   (1965) Refsum's disease (heredopathia atactica polyneuritiformis): an inborn error of lipid metabolism with storage of 3,7,11,15-tetramethyl-hexadecanoic acid.   II. Isolation and identification of the storage product. *American Journal of Medicine*, **39**, 237-242.

Kantarjian, A. D. & Dejong, R. N.   (1953) Familial primary amyloidosis with nervous system involvement. *Neurology (Minneapolis)*, **3**, 399-409.

Karch, S. B. & Urich, H.   (1975) Infantile polyneuropathy with defective myelination: an autopsy study. *Developmental Medicine and Child Neurology*, **17**, 504-511.

Karlsson, U.   (1966) Comparison of the myelin period of peripheral and central origin by electron microscopy. *Journal of Ultrastructure Research*, **15**, 451-468.

Kennedy, W. R., Sung, J. H., Berry, J. F. & Mastri, A.   (1971) Hypertrophic neuropathy with primary failure of peripheral myelination. *Transactions of the American Neurological Association*, **96**, 75-79.

Kernohan, J. W. & Woltman, H. W.   (1938) Periarteritis nodosa: a clinico-pathologic study with special reference to the nervous system. *Archives of Neurology and Psychiatry*, **39**, 655-686.

Kernohan, J. W. & Woltman, H. W.   (1942) Amyloid neuritis. *Archives of Neurology and Psychiatry*, **47**, 132-140.

Key, A. & Retzius, G.   (1873) Studien in der Anatomie des Nervensystems. *Archiv für mikroskopische Anatomie*, **9**, 308-386.

Key, A. & Retzius, G.   (1876) *Studien in der Anatomie des Nervensystems und des Bindegewebes*, Samson and Wallin, Stockholm.

Khanolkar, V. R.   (1951) *Studies in the Histology of Early Lesions in Leprosy*, Indian Council for Medical Research, Special Report Series No. 19.

Khanolkar, V. R.   (1964) Pathology of leprosy in *Leprosy in theory and practice* (Eds. Cochrane, R. G. & Davey, T. F.), pp. 125-151, Wright, Bristol.

Klenk, E. & Kahlke, W.   (1963) Über das Vorkommen der 3,7,11,15-tetramethyl-Hexadecansäure in den Cholesterinestern und anderen Lipoidfraktionen der Organe bei einem Krankheitsfall unbekannter Genese (Verdacht auf Heredopathia atactica polyneuritiformis—Refsum-Syndrom). *Hoppe-Seyler's Zeitschrift für physiologische Chemie*, **333**, 133-139.

Klumpke, A.   (1885) Contributions à l'étude des paralysies radiculaires du plexus brachial. *Revue Medicale*, **5**, 591-616, 739-790.

Köberle, F.   (1956) Über das Neurotoxin des Trypanosoma cruzi. *Zeitschrift für allgemeine Pathologie und pathologische Anatomie*, **95**, 468-475.

Köberle, F.   (1957) Die chronische Chagaskardiopathie. *Virchows Archiv für pathologische Anatomie*, **330**, 267-295.

Köberle, F.   (1963) Enteromegaly and cardiomegaly in Chagas disease. *Gut*, **4**, 399-405.

Kocen, R. S., King, R. H. M., Thomas, P. K. & Haas, L. F.   (1973) Nerve biopsy findings in two cases of Tangier disease. *Acta Neuropathologica (Berlin)* **26**, 317-327.

Kocen, R. S., Lloyd, J. K., Lascelles, P. T., Fosbrooke, A. S. & Williams, D.   (1967) Familial α-lipoprotein deficiency (Tangier disease) with neurological abnormalities. *Lancet*, **1**, 1341-1345.

Kocen, R. S. & Thomas, P. K.   (1970) Peripheral nerve involvement in Fabry's disease. *Archives of Neurology (Chicago)* **22**, 81-88.

Kolodny, E. H., Hass, W. K., Lane, B. & Drucker, W. D.   (1965) Refsum's syndrome.   Report of a case including electron-microscopic studies of the liver. *Archives of Neurology (Chicago)*, **12**, 583-596.

Konotey-Ahulu, F. I. D., Baillod, R., Comty, C. M., Heron, J. R., Shaldon, S. & Thomas, P. K.   (1965) Effect of periodic dialysis on the peripheral neuropathy of end-stage renal failure. *British Medical Journal*, **2**, 1212-1215.

Koppel, H. P. & Thompson, W. A. L.   (1963) *Peripheral Entrapment Neuropathies*, William and Wilkins, Baltimore.

Kornzweig, A. L. & Bassen, F. A.   (1957) Retinitis pigmentosa, acanthocytosis and heredodegenerative neuro-muscular disease. *Archives of Ophthalmology*, **58**, 183-187.

Kraus, W. M.   (1922) Involvement of the peripheral neurons in diabetes mellitus. *Archives of Neurology and Psychiatry*, **7**, 202-209.

Kristensson, K. & Olsson, Y.   (1971) The perineurium as a diffusion barrier to protein tracers.   Differences between mature and immature animals. *Acta Neuropathologica (Berlin)*, **17**, 127-138.

Krücke, W.   (1939) Die mucoide Degeneration der peripheren Nerven. *Virchows Archiv für pathologische Anatomie*, **304**, 442-463.

Krücke, W.   (1941-42) Ödem und seröse Entzündung im peripheren Nerven. *Virchows Archiv für pathologische Anatomie*, **308**, 1-13.

Krücke, W.   (1942-43) Zur Histopathologie der neuralen Muskelatrophie, der hypertrophischen Neuritis und Neurofibromatose. *Archiv für Psychiatrie und Nervenkrankheiten*, **115**, 180-236.

Krücke, W.   (1955) Die primär-entzündliche Polyneuritis unbekannter Ursache in *Handbuch der speziellen Pathologischen Anatomie und Histologie* (Eds. Lubarsch, O., Henke, F. and Rössle, G.), Vol. 13/5, pp. 164-182, Springer Verlag, Berlin.

Krücke, W.   (1959a) Die Paramyloidose. *Ergebnisse der inneren Medizin und Kinderheilkunde*, **11**, 299-378.

Krücke, W.   (1959b) Histopathologie der Polyneuritis und Polyneuropathie. *Deutsche Zeitschrift für Nervenheilkunde*, **180**, 1-39.

Kummer, H., Laissue, J., Spiess, H., Pflugshaupt, R. & Bucher, U.   (1968) Familiäre Analphalipoproteinämie (Tangier-Krankheit). *Schweizerische medizinische Wochenschrift*, **98**, 406-412.

Kuntz, A.   (1934) Sympathetic ganglions removed surgically: a histopathologic study. *Archives of Surgery*, **28**, 920-935.

Kussmaul, A. & Maier, R.   (1866) Über eine bisher nicht beschriebene eigenthümliche Arterienerkrankung (Periarteritis nodosa) die mit Morbus Brightii und rapid fortschreitender allgemeiner Muskellähmung einhergeht. *Deutsches Archiv für klinische Medizin*, **1**, 484-518.

Kyle, R. A. & Bayrd, E. D.   (1961) Primary systemic amyloidosis and myeloma. *Archives of Internal Medicine*, **107**, 344-353.

Lampert, P.   (1967) A comparative electron-microscopic study of reactive, degenerating, regenerating and dystrophic axons. *Journal of Neuropathology and Experimental Neurology*, **26**, 345-368.

Lampert, P.   (1969) Mechanism of demyelination in experimental allergic neuritis. *Laboratory Investigation*, **20**, 127-138.

Lampert, P. W. & Schochet, S. S. jr.   (1968) Demyelination and remyelination in lead neuropathy-electron microscopic studies. *Journal of Neuropathology and Experimental Neurology*, **27**, 527-545.

Landry, O.   (1859) Note sur la paralysie ascendante aiguë. *Gazette Hebdomadaire de Médecine*, **6**, 472-474, 486-488.

Lantermann, A. J.   (1877) Über den feineren Bau der markhaltigen Nervenfasern. *Archiv für mikroskopische Anatomie*, **13**, 1-8.

Lascelles, R. G. & Thomas, P. K.   (1966) Changes due to age in internodal length in the sural nerve in man. *Journal of Neurology, Neurosurgery and Psychiatry*, **29**, 40-44.

Le Bourhis, J., Fève, J. R., Besançon, C. & Leroux, M. J.   (1964) Neuropathie périphérique avec infiltration amyloide des nerfs au cours d'une macroglobulinémie de Waldenström. *Revue Neurologique*, **111**, 474-478.

Lennox, B. & Prichard, S.   (1950) Association of bronchial carcinoma and peripheral neuritis. *Quarterly Journal of Medicine*, (N.S.), **19**, 97-109.

Lewis, T., Pickering, G. W. & Rothschild, P.   (1931) Centripetal paralysis arising out of arrested blood flow to the limb including notes on a form of tingling. *Heart*, **16**, 1-32.

Liebow, A. A., Carrington, C. R. B. & Friedman, P. J.   (1972) Lymphomatoid granulomatosis. *Human Pathology*, **3**, 457-558.

Logothetis, J., Kennedy, W. R., Ellington, A. & Williams, R. C.   (1968) Cryoglobulinemic neuropathy: incidence and clinical characteristics. *Archives of Neurology* (*Chicago*), **19**, 389-397.

Logothetis, J., Silverstein, P. & Coe, J.   (1960) Neurological aspects of Waldenström's macroglobulinemia: report of cases. *Archives of Neurology* (*Chicago*), **3**, 564-573.

Long, E.   (1906) Atrophie musculaire progressive, type Aran-Duchenne, de nature névritique (névrite interstitielle hypertrophique). *Revue Neurologique* **14**, 1198-1199.

Lovshin, L. L. & Kernohan, J. W.   (1948) Peripheral neuritis in periarteritis nodosa: a clinicopathologic study. *Archives of Internal Medicine*, **82**, 321-338.

Lubimoff, A.   (1874) Beiträge zur Histologie und pathologischen Anatomie des sympathischen Nervensystem. *Virchows Archiv für pathologische Anatomie*, **61**, 145-207.

Lubinska, L.   (1958) 'Intercalated' internodes in nerve fibres. *Nature* (*London*), **181**, 957-958.

Lubinska, L.   (1961a) Sedentary and migratory states of Schwann cells. *Experimental Cell Research*, **8**, 74-90.

Lubinska, L.   (1961b) Demyelination and remyelination in the proximal parts of regenerating nerve fibres. *Journal of Comparative Neurology*, **117**, 275-289.

Lubinska, L.   (1964) Axoplasmic streaming in regenerating and in normal nerve fibres in *Progress in Brain Research, Mechanisms of Neural Regeneration* (Eds. Singer, M. & Schade, J. P.), Vol. 13, pp. 1-71, Elsevier, Amsterdam.

Lumsden, C. E.   (1964) Leprosy and the Schwann cell in vivo and in vitro in *Leprosy in theory and practice* (Eds. Cochrane and Davey), pp. 221-250, Wright, Bristol.

Lumsden, K. & Truelove, S. C.   (1958) Primary hypertrophic pyloric stenosis in the adult.   *British Journal of Radiology*, **31**, 261-266.

Lyon, G.   (1969) Ultrastructural study of a nerve biopsy from a case of early infantile chronic neuropathy. *Acta Neuropathologica (Berlin)*, **13**, 131-142.

Macdonald, R. A. & Mallory, C. K.   (1960) Hemochromatosis and hemosiderosis.   Study of 211 autopsied cases.   *Archives of Internal Medicine*, **105**, 686-700.

McDonald, W. I.   (1963) The effects of experimental demyelination on conduction in peripheral nerve: a histological and electrophysiological study.   I. Clinical and histological observations.   *Brain*, **86**, 481-524.

Madrid, R. & Bradley, W. G.   (1975) The pathology of neuropathies with focal thickening of the myelin sheath (tomaculous neuropathy): studies on the formation of the abnormal myelin sheath.   *Journal of the Neurological Sciences*, **25**, 415-448.

Madrid Classification   (1953) Technical resolutions.   *International Journal of Leprosy*, **21**, 504-516.

Mallory, F. B., Parker, F. & Nye, R. N.   (1920-21) Experimental pigment cirrhosis due to copper and its relation to haemochromatosis.   *Journal of Medical Research*, **42**, 461-490.

Marchal de Calvi, J.   (1853) Note pour servir à l'histoire du diabète.   *Compte rendu hebdomadaire des séances de l'Academie des sciences Paris*, **37**, 346-348.

Margulis; M. S.   (1927) Pathologie und Pathogenese der akuten primären infektiösen Polyneuritiden.   *Deutsche Zeitschrift für Nervenheilkunde*, **99**, 165-192.

Marie, P.   (1906) Forme spéciale de névrite interstitielle hypertrophique de l'enfance.   *Revue Neurologique*, **14**, 557-560.

Marie, P. & Bertrand, I.   (1918) Contribution à l'anatomie pathologique de la névrite hypertrophique familiale. *Annales de Médecine*, **5**, 209-258.

Marie, P. & Foix, C.   (1913) Atrophie isolée de l'éminence thénar d'origine névritique, rôle du ligament annulaire du carpe dans la pathogénie de la lésion.   *Revue Neurologique*, **26**, 647-649.

Marin, O. S. M. & Tyler, H. R.   (1961) Hereditary interstitial nephritis associated with polyneuropathy. *Neurology (Minneapolis)*, **11**, 999-1005.

Marinesco, G.   (1894) Contribution à l'étude de l'amyotrophie Charcot-Marie.   *Archives de Médecine Expérimentale*, **6**, 921-965.

Marinesco, G. & Draganesco, S.   (1938) Contribution à l'étude des accidents post-vaccino-rabiques (à l'occasion d'un cas avec examen anatomo-clinique).   *Annales de l'Institut Pasteur*, **60**, 477-498.

Marshall, J.   (1963) The Landry–Guillain–Barré syndrome.   *Brain*, **86**, 55-66.

Martin, M. M.   (1953) Diabetic neuropathy: a clinical study of 150 cases.   *Brain*, **76**, 594-624.

Mason, R. M. & Steinberg, V. L.   (1957-58) Rheumatoid arthritis.   *Annals of Physical Medicine*, **4**, 265-273.

Matsuyama, H. & Haymaker, W.   (1967) Distribution of lesions in the Landry–Guillain–Barré syndrome, with emphasis on the involvement of the sympathetic system.   *Acta Neuropathologica (Berlin)*, **8**, 230-241.

Meachim, G. & Abberton, M. J. (1971)   Histological findings in Morton's metatarsalgia.   *Journal of Pathology*, **103**, 209-217.

Meier-Ruge, W.   (1974) Hirschsprung's disease: aetiology, pathogenesis and differential diagnosis.   *Current Topics in Pathology*, **59**, 131-179.

Melnick, S. C.   (1963) Thirty-eight cases of the Guillain–Barré syndrome: an immunological study.   *British Medical Journal*, **1**, 368-373.

Melnick, S. C. & Whitfield, A. G.   (1962) Polyneuritis in haemochromatosis.   *Postgraduate Medical Journal*, **38**, 580-583.

Meretoja, J.   (1969) Familial systemic paramyloidosis with lattice dystrophy of the cornea, progressive cranial neuropathy, skin changes and various internal symptoms.   *Annals of Clinical Research*, **1**, 314-324.

Merrington, W. R. & Nathan, P. W.   (1949) A study of post-ischaemic paraesthesiae.   *Journal of Neurology, Neurosurgery and Psychiatry*, **12**, 1-18.

Meyer, P.   (1881) Anatomische Untersuchungen über diphtheritische Lähmung.   *Virchows Archiv für pathologische Anatomie*, **85**, 181-226.

Misiewicz, J. J., Waller, S. L., Anthony, P. P. & Gummer, J. W. P.   (1969) Achalasia of the cardia: pharmacology and histopathology of isolated cardiac sphincteric muscle from patients with or without achalasia. *Quarterly Journal of Medicine*, **38**, 17-30.

Morgan-Hughes, J. A.   (1965) Changes in motor nerve conduction velocity in diphtheritic polyneuritis. *Rivista di Patologia nervosa e mentale*, **86**, 253-260.

Morrison, L. R., Short, C. L., Ludwig, A. O. & Schwab, R. S.   (1947) The neuromuscular system in rheumatoid arthritis.   *American Journal of Medical Science*, **214**, 33-49.

Morton, T. G.   (1876) A peculiar and painful affection of the fourth metatarso-phalangeal articulation. *American Journal of Medical Science*, **71**, 37-45.

Mufson, I.   (1952) Diagnosis and treatment of neural complications of peripheral arterial obliterative disease. *Angiology*, **3**, 392-396.

Munsat, T. L. & Barnes, J. E.   (1965) Relation of multiple cranial nerve dysfunction to the Guillain–Barré syndrome. *Journal of Neurology, Neurosurgery and Psychiatry*, **28**, 115-120.

Munsat, T. L. & Poussaint, A. F.   (1962) Clinical manifestations and diagnosis of amyloid polyneuropathy. Report of three cases. *Neurology (Minneapolis)*, **12**, 413-422.

Murray, I. P. C. & Simpson, J. A.   (1958) Acroparaesthesia in myxoedema a clinical and electromyographic study. *Lancet*, **1**, 1360-1363.

Murray, M. R., Cook, S. D. & Dowling, P. C.   (1970) Myelinotoxic activity of Guillain–Barré serum on cultures of peripheral nerve tissue in *Proceedings of the VI International Congress of Neuropathology (Paris)*, pp. 611-627.

Nageotte, J.   (1907) Neurophagie dans les greffes de ganglions rachidiens. *Revue Neurologique*, **15**, 933-944.

Nageotte, J.   (1932) Sheaths of the peripheral nerves, nerve degeneration and regeneration in *Cytology and Cellular Pathology of the Nervous System* (Ed. Penfield, W.), Vol. 1, pp. 189-239, Hoeber, New York.

Naish, J. M., Capper, W. M. & Brown, N. J.   (1960) Intestinal pseudo-obstruction with steatorrhoea. *Gut*, **1**, 62-66.

Nathaniel, E. J. H. & Pease, D. C.   (1963) Degenerative changes in rat dorsal roots during Wallerian degeneration. *Journal of Ultrastructure Research*, **9**, 511-532.

Navasquez, S. de & Treble, H. A.   (1938) A case of primary generalized amyloidosis with involvement of the nerves. *Brain*, **61**, 116-128.

Neary, D., Ochoa, J. & Gilliatt, R. W.   (1975) Subclinical entrapment neuropathy in man. *Journal of the Neurological Sciences*, **24**, 283-298.

Nélaton, A.   (1852) Affection singulière des os du pied. *Gazette des hôpitaux civils et militaires Paris*, **25**, 13.

Nick, J., Contamin, F., Brion, S., Guillard, A. & Guiraudon, Mme   (1963) Macroglobulinémie du Waldenström avec neuropathie amyloïde. Observation anatomo-clinique. *Revue Neurologique*, **109**, 21-30.

Nishiura, M.   (1960) The electron microscopic basis of the pathology of leprosy. *International Journal of Leprosy*, **28**, 357-400.

Norris, F. H., McMenemey, W. H. & Barnard, R. O.   (1970) Unusual particles in a case of carcinomatous neuronal disease. *Acta Neuropathologica (Berlin)*, **14**, 350-353.

Ochoa, J., Danta, G., Fowler, T. J. & Gilliatt, R. W.   (1971) Nature of the nerve lesion caused by a pneumatic tourniquet. *Nature (London)*, **233**, 265-266.

Ochoa, J., Fowler, T. J. & Gilliatt, R. W.   (1972) Anatomical changes in peripheral nerves compressed by a pneumatic tourniquet. *Journal of Anatomy*, **113**, 433-455.

Ochoa, J. & Mair, W. C. P.   (1969a) The normal sural nerve in man, Part 1: Ultrastructure and numbers of fibres and cells. *Acta Neuropathologica (Berlin)*, **13**, 197-216.

Ochoa, J. & Mair, W. C. P.   (1969b) The normal sural nerve in man Part 2: Changes in the axons and Schwann cells due to ageing. *Acta Neuropathologica (Berlin)*, **13**, 217-239.

Ochoa, J. & Marotte, L.   (1973) The nature of the nerve lesion caused by chronic entrapment in the guinea-pig. *Journal of the Neurological Sciences*, **19**, 491-495.

O'Daly, J. A. & Imaeda, T.   (1967) Electron microscopic study of Wallerian degeneration in cutaneous nerves caused by mechanical injury. *Laboratory Investigation*, **17**, 744-766.

Ohta, M.   (1970) Electron microscopic observations of sural nerve in familial opticoacoustic nerve degeneration with polyneuropathy. *Acta Neuropathologica (Berlin)*, **15**, 114-127.

Olsson, Y.   (1966) Studies on vascular permeability in peripheral nerves: I.   Distribution of circulating fluorescent serum albumin in normal, crushed and sectioned rat sciatic nerve. *Acta Neuropathologica (Berlin)*, **7**, 1-15.

Olsson, Y.   (1968) Mast cells in the nervous system. *International Review of Cytology*, **24**, 27-70.

Olsson, Y. & Kristensson, K.   (1973) The perineurium as a diffusion barrier to protein tracers following trauma to nerves. *Acta Neuropathologica (Berlin)*, **23**, 105-111.

Olsson, Y. & Reese, T. S.   (1971) Permeability of vasa nervorum and perineurium in mouse sciatic nerve studied by fluorescence and electron microscopy. *Journal of Neuropathology and Experimental Neurology*, **30**, 105-119.

Olsson, Y. & Sjöstrand, J.   (1969) Proliferation of mast cells in peripheral nerves during Wallerian degeneration. A radioautographic study. *Acta Neuropathologica (Berlin)*, **13**, 111-121.

Oppenheim, H.   (1886) Beiträge zur Pathologie der 'multiplen Neuritis' und Alkohol-Lähmung. *Zeitschrift für klinische Medizin*, **11**, 232-262.

Osler, W.   (1892) *The Principles and Practice of Medicine*, New York.

O'Sullivan, D. J. & Swallow, M.   (1968) The fibre size and content of the radial and sural nerves.   *Journal of Neurology, Neurosurgery and Psychiatry*, **31**, 464-470.

Pallis, C. A. & Scott, J. T.   (1965) Peripheral neuropathy in rheumatoid arthritis.   *British Medical Journal*, **1**, 1141-1147.

Parsonage, M. J. & Turner, J. W. A.   (1948) Neuralgic amyotrophy.   *Lancet*, **1**, 973-978.

Pearson, J. M. H., Rees, R. J. W. & Weddell, A. G. M.   (1970) Mycobacterium leprae in the striated muscle of patients with leprosy.   *Leprosy Review*, **41**, 155-166.

Perroncito, A.   (1907) Die Regeneration des Nerven.   *Beiträge zur pathologischen Anatomie*, **42**, 354-446.

Peters, A., Palay, S. L. & Webster, H. de F.   (1970) *The Fine Structure of the Nervous System*, Hoeber, New York.

Pette, H. & Környey, S.   (1930) Zur Histologie und Pathogenese der akutentzündlichen Formen der Landryschen Paralyse.   *Zeitschrift für die gesamte Neurologie und Psychiatrie*, **128**, 390-412.

Pitres, A. & Vaillard, L.   (1887) Névrites périphériques dans le rhumatisme chronique.   *Revue Médicale (Paris)*, **7**, 456-468.

Preisz, H.   (1895) Beiträge zur Anatomie der diphtheritischen Lähmungen.   *Deutsche Zeitschrift für Nervenheilkunde*, **6**, 95-114.

Preston, G. M.   (1967) Peripheral neuropathy in the alloxan diabetic rat.   *Journal of Physiology*, **189**, 49-50.

Preswick, G. & Jeremy, D.   (1964) Subclinical polyneuropathy in renal insufficiency.   *Lancet*, **2**, 731-732.

Prineas, J. W.   (1969a) The pathogenesis of dying-back polyneuropathies Part I.   An ultrastructural study of experimental tri-ortho-cresyl phosphate intoxication in the cat.   *Journal of Neuropathology and Experimental Neurology*, **28**, 571-597.

Prineas, J. W.   (1969b) The pathogenesis of dying-back polyneuropathies Part II.   An ultrastructural study of experimental acrylamide intoxication in the cat.   *Journal of Neuropathology and Experimental Neurology*, **28**, 598-621.

Prineas, J. W.   (1970) Polyneuropathies of undetermined cause.   *Acta neurologica scandinavica*, **44**, *Suppl. 46*, 1-72.

Prineas, J. W.   (1971) Demyelination and remyelination in recurrent idiopathic polyneuropathy.   An electron microscope study.   *Acta Neuropathologica (Berlin)*, **18**, 34-57.

Rabinowitz, D., Landau, H., Rosler, A., Moses, S. W., Rotem, Y. & Freier, S.   (1974) Plasma renin activity and aldosterone in familial dysautonomia.   *Metabolism*, **23**, 1-5.

Raff, M. C., Sangalang, V. & Asbury, A. K.   (1968) Ischemic mononeuropathy multiplex associated with diabetes mellitus.   *Archives of Neurology*, **18**, 487-499.

Rahman, A. N. & Lindenberg, R.   (1963) The neuropathology of hereditary dystopic lipidosis.   *Archives of Neurology (Chicago)*, **9**, 373-385.

Rake, G. W.   (1927) On the pathology of achalasia of the cardia.   *Guy's Hospital Reports*, **77**, 141-150.

Ransom, F.   (1900) Diphtheritic paralysis and antitoxine.   *Journal of Pathology and Bacteriology*, **6**, 397-414.

Ranvier, M. L.   (1878) *Leçons sur l'histologie du système nerveux*, F. Savy, Paris.

Rees, R. J. W.   (1964) Limited multiplication of acid-fast bacilli in the foot-pads of mice inoculated with mycobacterium leprae.   *British Journal of Experimental Pathology*, **45**, 207-218.

Rees, R. J. W.   (1966) Enhanced susceptibility of thymectomized and irradiated mice to infection with mycobacterium leprae.   *Nature (London)*, **211**, 657-658.

Rees, R. H. W. & Waters, M. F. R.   (1972) Recent trends in leprosy research.   *British Medical Bulletin*, **28**, 16-21.

Refsum, S.   (1946) Heredopathia atactica polyneuritiformis: familial syndrome not hitherto described.   A contribution to the clinical study of hereditary diseases of the nervous system.   *Acta psychiatrica scandinavica, Suppl.* **38**.

Refsum, S.   (1960) Heredopathia atactica polyneuritiformis: a reconsideration.   *World Neurology*, **1**, 334-347.

Reisner, H. & Spiel, W.   (1952) Zur Frage der Polyneuritis hypertrophicans.   *Wiener Zeitschrift für Nervenheilkunde*, **5**, 388-403.

Remak, R.   (1847) *Über ein selbständiges Darmnervensystem*, Berlin.

Rénaut, J.   (1881) Recherches sur quelques points particuliers de l'histologie des nerfs.   *Archives de Physiologie Normale et de Pathologie*, **13**, 161-190.

Reske-Nielsen, E. & Lundbaek, K.   (1968) Pathological changes in the central and peripheral nervous system of young long-term diabetics II: The spinal cord and peripheral nerves.   *Diabetologia*, **4**, 34-43.

Richards, R. L.   (1951) Ischaemic lesions of peripheral nerves: a review.   *Journal of Neurology, Neurosurgery and Psychiatry*, **14**, 76-87.

Ridley, A.   (1969) The neuropathy of acute intermittent porphyria.   *Quarterly Journal of Medicine*, **38**, 307-333.

Ridley, D. S. & Jopling, W. H. (1966) Classification of leprosy according to immunity. *International Journal of Leprosy*, **34**, 255-273.

Riley, C. M. (1957) Familial dysautonomia. *Advances in Pediatrics*, **9**, 157-190.

Riley, C. M., Day, R. L., Greeley, D. M. & Langford, W. S. (1949) Central autonomic dysfunction with defective lacrimation. Report of 5 cases. *Pediatrics*, **3**, 468-478.

Riley, C. M. & Moore, R. H. (1966) Familial dysautonomia differentiated from related disorders. Case reports and discussion of current concepts. *Pediatrics*, **37**, 435-446.

Rintoul, J. R. & Kirkman, N. F. (1961) The myenteric plexus in infantile hypertrophic pyloric stenosis. *Archives of Disease in Childhood*, **36**, 474-480.

Robertson, J. D. (1955) The ultrastructure of adult vertebrate peripheral myelinated nerve fibres in relation to myelinogenesis. *Journal of Biophysical and Biochemical Cytology*, **1**, 271-278.

Robertson, J. D. (1958) The ultrastructure of Schmidt-Lantermann clefts and related shearing defects of the myelin sheath. *Journal of Biophysical and Biochemical Cytology*, **4**, 39-46.

Rolleston, J. D. (1904) Clinical observations on diphtheritic paralysis. *Practitioner*, **73**, 597-623.

Rollo, J. (1798) *Cases of the Diabetes Mellitus*, C. Dilly, London.

Roseman, E. & Aring, C. D. (1941) Infectious polyneuritis. *Medicine* (*Baltimore*), **20**, 463-494.

Rosenberg, R. N. & Chutorian, A. (1967) Familial opticoacoustic nerve degeneration and polyneuropathy. *Neurology* (*Minneapolis*), **17**, 827-832.

Rosenberg, R. N. & Lovelace, R. E. (1968) Mononeuritis multiplex in lepromatous leprosy. *Archives of Neurology*, **19**, 310-314.

Roussy, G. & Cornil, L. (1919) Névrite hypertrophique progressive non-familiale de l'adulte. *Revue Neurologique* **34**, 590-592.

Rukavina, J. G., Block, W. D., Jackson, C. E., Falls, H. F., Carey, J. H. & Curtis, A. C. (1956) Primary systemic amyloidosis: a review and an experimental genetic and clinical study of 29 cases with particular emphasis on the familial form. *Medicine* (*Baltimore*), **35**, 239-334.

Rundles, R. W. (1945) Diabetic neuropathy: general review with report of 125 cases. *Medicine* (*Baltimore*), **24**, 111-160.

Russell, D. S. (1961) Encephalomyelitis and 'carcinomatous neuropathy' in *Encephalitides* (Eds. van Bogaert, L., Radermecker, J., Hozay, J. & Lowenthal, A., pp. 131-135, Elsevier, Amsterdam.

Russell, W. R. & Garland, H. G. (1930) Progressive hypertrophic polyneuritis, with case reports. *Brain*, **53**, 376-384.

Sandbank, U., Bechar, M. & Bornstein, B. (1971) Hyperlipemic polyneuropathy. Case report: histological and electron-microscopical study. *Acta Neuropathologica* (*Berlin*), **19**, 290-300.

Sanders, F. K. & Whitteridge, D. (1946) Conduction velocity and myelin thickness in regenerating nerve fibres. *Journal of Physiology* (*London*), **105**, 152-174.

Sanders, F. K. & Young, J. Z. (1944) The role of the peripheral stump in the control of fibre diameter in regenerating nerves. *Journal of Physiology* (*London*), **103**, 119-136.

Sanders, F. K. & Young, J. Z. (1946) The influence of peripheral connexion on the diameter of regenerating nerve fibres. *Journal of Experimental Biology*, **22**, 203-212.

Schaumberg, H., Byck, R., Herman, R. & Rosengart, C. (1967) Peripheral nerve damage by cold. *Archives of Neurology* (*Chicago*), **16**, 103-109.

Scheid, W. & Peters, G. (1952) Über die tödlich verlaufenden Diphtherielähmungen unter besonderer Berücksichtigung der anatomischen Befunde. *Deutsche Zeitschrift für Nervenheilkunde*, **167**, 355-390.

Scheinker, I. (1938) Myelom und Nervensystem: über eine bisher nicht beschriebene mit eigentümlichen Hautveränderungen einhergehende Polyneuritis bei einem plasmazellulären Myelom des Sternums. *Deutsche Zeitschrift für Nervenheilkunde*, **147**, 247-273.

Scheinker, M. (1947) Pathology and pathogenesis of infectious polyneuritis. *Transactions of the American Neurological Association*, **72**, 141-143.

Schienberg, L. (1956) Polyneuritis in systemic lupus erythematosus: review of the literature and report of a case. *New England Journal of Medicine*, **255**, 416-421.

Schiller, F. & Kolb, F. O. (1954) Carpal tunnel syndrome in acromegaly. *Neurology* (*Minneapolis*), **4**, 271-282.

Schlesinger, A. S., Duggins, V. A. & Masucci, E. F. (1962) Peripheral neuropathy in familial primary amyloidosis. *Brain*, **85**, 357-370.

Schmid, F. R., Cooper, B. S., Ziff, M. & McEwen, C. (1961) Arteritis in rheumatoid arthritis. *American Journal of Medicine*, **30**, 56-83.

Schmidt, F. O. (1958) Axon-satellite cell relationship in peripheral nerve fibres. *Experimental Cell Research*, *Suppl.*, **5**, 33-57.

Schmidt, H. D. (1874) On the construction of the dark or double-bordered nerve fibre. *Monthly Microscopical Journal*, **11**, 200-221.

Schoene, W. C., Asbury, A. K., Åström, K. E. & Masters, R. (1970) Hereditary sensory neuropathy: a clinical and ultrastructural study. *Journal of the Neurological Sciences*, **11**, 463-487.

Schröder, J. M. (1970) Zur Feinstruktur und quantitativen Auswertung regenerierter peripherer Nervenfasern. *Proceedings of the 6th International Congress of Neuropathology (Paris)*, pp. 628-646.

Schröder, J. M. & Krücke, W. (1970) Zur Feinstruktur der experimentellallergischen Neuritis beim Kaninchen. *Acta Neuropathologica (Berlin)*, **14**, 261-283.

Schultze, F. (1930) Über die vererbbare neurale oder neurospinale Muskelatrophie. *Deutsche Zeitschrift für Nervenheilkunde*, **112**, 1-19.

Schwann, T. (1839) Mikroskopische Untersuchungen über die Übereinstimmung in der Struktur und dem Wachsthum der Thiere und Pflanzen, Berlin.

Schwartz, J. F., Rowland, L. P., Eder, H., Marks, P. A., Osserman, E. F., Hirschberg, E. & Anderson, H. (1963) Bassen–Kornzweig syndrome. *Archives of Neurology (Chicago)*, **8**, 438-454.

Scott, J. T., Hourihane, D. O'B., Doyle, F. H., Steiner, R. E., Laws, J. W., Dixon, A. St. J. & Bywaters, E. G. L. (1961) Digital arteritis in rheumatoid disease. *Annals of the Rheumatic Diseases*, **20**, 324-334.

Sears, W. G. (1931) Progressive hypertrophic polyneuritis. *Journal of Neurology and Psychopathology*, **12**, 137-147.

Seddon, H. J. (1942) A classification of nerve injuries. *British Medical Journal*, **2**, 237-239.

Seddon, H. J. (1943) Three types of nerve injury. *Brain*, **66**, 237-288.

Seddon, H. J. (Sir Herbert) (1972) *Surgical Disorders of the Peripheral Nerves*, Churchill Livingstone, Edinburgh and London.

Seddon, H. J., Medawar, P. B. & Smith, H. (1943) Rate of regeneration of peripheral nerve in man. *Journal of Physiology (London)*, **102**, 191-215.

Sedgwick, R. P. & Van Hagen, K. O. (1948) The neurological manifestations of lupus erythematosus and periarteritis nodosa: report of ten cases. *Bulletin of the Los Angeles Neurological Society*, **13**, 129-142.

Seneviratne, K. N. (1972) Permeability of blood nerve barriers in the diabetic rat. *Journal of Neurology, Neurosurgery and Psychiatry*, **35**, 156-162.

Shawe, G. D. H. (1955) On the number of branches formed by regenerating nerve fibres. *British Journal of Surgery*, **42**, 474-488.

Shepard, C. C. (1960) The experimental disease that follows the injection of human leprosy bacilli into footpads of mice. *Journal of Experimental Medicine*, **112**, 445-454.

Silverstein, A. (1964) Neuropathy in hemophilia. *Journal of the American Medical Association*, **190**, 554-555.

Simpson, D. A. & Fowler, M. (1966) Two cases of localized hypertrophic neurofibrosis. *Journal of Neurology, Neurosurgery and Psychiatry*, **29**, 80-84.

Singer, M. & Salpeter, M. M. (1966) Transport of tritium-labelled l-histidine through the Schwann and myelin sheaths into the axon of peripheral nerves. *Nature (London)*, **210**, 1225-1227.

Sjöstrand, F. S. (1950) Electron-microscopic demonstration of a membrane structure isolated from nerve tissue. *Nature (London)*, **165**, 482-483.

Smith, A. A. & Dancis, J. (1964) Exaggerated response to infused norepinephrine in familial dysautonomia. *New England Journal of Medicine*, **270**, 704-707.

Smith, A. A., Hirsch, J. I. & Dancis, J. (1965) Responses to infused methacholine in familial dysautonomia. *Pediatrics*, **36**, 225-230.

Smith, A. A., Taylor, T. & Wortis, S. B. (1963) Abnormal catecholamine metabolism in familial dysautonomia. *New England Journal of Medicine*, **268**, 705-707.

Smith, B. (1967a) The myenteric plexus in Chagas' disease. *Journal of Pathology and Bacteriology*, **94**, 462-463.

Smith, B. (1967b) Myenteric plexus in Hirschsprung's disease. *Gut*, **8**, 308-312.

Smith, B. (1967c) The myenteric plexus in drug-induced neuropathy. *Journal of Neurology, Neurosurgery and Psychiatry*, **30**, 506-510.

Smith, B. (1968) Effect of irritant purgatives on the myenteric plexus in man and the mouse. *Gut*, **9**, 139-143.

Smith, B. (1969) Damage to the intrinsic cardiac neurones by rubidomycin (daunorubicin). *British Heart Journal*, **31**, 607-609.

Smith, B. (1970) Disorders of the myenteric plexus. *Gut*, **11**, 271-274.

Smith, B. (1972) *The Neuropathology of the Alimentary Tract*, Arnold, London.

Smith, M. C. (1964) Histological findings following intrathecal injection of phenol solutions for the relief of pain. *British Journal of Anaesthesia*, **36**, 387-406.

Sobrevilla, L. A., Goodman, M. L. & Kane, C. A. (1964) Demyelinating central nervous disease, macular atrophy and acanthocytosis (Bassen–Kornzweig syndrome). *American Journal of Medicine*, **37**, 821-832.

Solitare, G. B. & Cohen, G. S. (1965) Peripheral autonomic nervous system lesions in congenital or familial dysautonomia (Riley–Day syndrome). *Neurology (Minneapolis)*, **15**, 321-327.

Souques, A. & Bertrand, I. (1921) Contribution à l'étude anatomo-pathologique de la névrite hypertrophique familiale. *Annales de Médecine*, **9**, 305-329.

Spencer, P. S. (1971) Light and electron microscopic observations on localised peripheral nerve injuries. Ph.D. Thesis, University of London.

Spencer, P. S. & Thomas, P. K. (1970) The examination of isolated nerve fibres by light and electron microscopy with observations on demyelination proximal to neuromas. *Acta Neuropathologica (Berlin)*, **16**, 177-186.

Spillane, J. D. & Urich, H. (1976) Trigeminal neuropathy with nasal ulceration: report of two cases and one autopsy. *Journal of Neurology, Neurosurgery and Psychiatry* (in press).

Spillane, J. D. & Wells, C. E. C. (1959) Isolated trigeminal neuropathy. A report of 16 cases. *Brain*, **82**, 391-416.

Spillane, J. D. & Wells, C. E. C. (1964) The neurology of Jennerian vaccination. *Brain*, **87**, 1-44.

Steinberg, D., Mize, C., Avigan, J., Fales, H. M., Eldjarn, L., Try, K., Stokke, O. & Refsum, S. (1966) On the metabolic error in Refsum's disease. *Transactions of the American Neurological Association*, **91**, 168-172.

Stern, G. M., Hoffbrand, A. V. & Urich, H. (1965) The peripheral nerves and skeletal muscles in Wegener's granulomatosis: a clinico-pathological study of four cases. *Brain*, **88**, 151-164.

Stöhr, P. (1928) Die Anteile des cerebrospinalen Nervensystems. I. Die Ganglien in *Handbuch der mikroskopischen Anatomie des Menschen* (Ed. Möllendorf, W. V., Vol. 4, part 1, pp. 202-213.

Stransky, E. (1902-03) Über discontinuierliche Zerfallsprozesse an der peripheren Nervenfaser. *Journal für Psychologie und Neurologie*, **1**, 169-199.

Sunderland, S. (1945a) Blood supply of the nerves of the upper limb in man. *Archives of Neurology and Psychiatry*, **53**, 91-115.

Sunderland, S. (1945b) Blood supply of the sciatic nerve and its popliteal divisions in man. *Archives of Neurology and Psychiatry*, **54**, 283-289.

Sunderland, S. (1947) Rate of regeneration in human peripheral nerves. *Archives of Neurology and Psychiatry*, **58**, 251-295.

Sunderland, S. (1953) The capacity of regenerating axons to bridge long gaps in nerves. *Journal of Comparative Neurology*, **99**, 481-488.

Sunderland, S. (1968) *Nerves and Nerve Injuries*, Livingstone, Edinburgh and London.

Sunderland, S. & Bradley, K. C. (1961) Stress-strain phenomena in human peripheral nerve trunks. *Brain*, **84**, 120-124.

Swallow, M. (1966) Fibre size and content of the anterior tibial nerve in the foot. *Journal of Neurology, Neurosurgery and Psychiatry*, **29**, 205-213.

Swift, T. R. (1974) Peripheral nerve involvement in leprosy. Quantitative histologic aspects. *Acta Neuropathologica (Berlin)*, **29**, 1-8.

Symonds, C. P. & Blackwood, W. (1962) Spinal cord compression in hypertrophic neuritis. *Brain*, **85**, 251-259.

Takino, M. & Miyake, S. (1935) Die Veränderungen der vegetativen Nerven bei der Lepra, besonders bei der infiltrativen Form. *Acta Scholae medicinalis Universitatis in Kioto*, **18**, 85-115.

Tasker, W. & Chutorian, A. M. (1969) Chronic polyneuritis of childhood. *Journal of Pediatrics*, **74**, 699-708.

Taylor, P. E. (1962) Traumatic intradural avulsion of the nerve roots in the brachial plexus. *Brain*, **85**, 579-602.

Tenckhoff, H. A., Boen, F. S. T., Hebsen, R. H. & Spiegler, J. H. (1965) Polyneuropathy in chronic renal insufficiency. *Journal of the American Medical Association*, **192**, 1121-1124.

Terada, M. (1953) Electron-microscopic studies on leprosy bacilli. *Journal of Electronmicroscopy*, **1**, 51-53.

Thévenard, A. (1942) L'acropathie ulcéro-mutilante familiale. *Revue Neurologique*, **74**, 193-212.

Thévenard, A. (1953) L'acropathie ulcéro-mutilante familiale. *Acta neurologica et psychiatrica belgica*, **53**, 1-23.

Thiébault, F., Lemoyne, J. & Guillaumat, L. (1939) Deux syndromes oto-neuro-oculistiques d'origine congénitale. Leurs rapports avec les phacomatoses et van der Hoeve et autres dysplasies neuro-ectodermiques. *Revue Neurologique*, **72**, 71-75.

Thiébault, F., Lemoyne, J. & Guillaumat, L. (1961) Maladie de Refsum. *Revue Neurologique*, **104**, 152-154.

Thomas, P. K. (1963) The connective tissue of peripheral nerves. *Journal of Anatomy (London)*, **97**, 35-44.

Thomas, P. K. (1964) Changes in the endoneurial sheaths of peripheral myelinated nerve fibres during Wallerian degeneration. *Journal of Anatomy (London)*, **98**, 175-182.

Thomas, P. K. (1970) The quantitation of nerve biopsy findings. *Journal of the Neurological Sciences*, **11**, 285-295.

Thomas, P. K. & Fullerton, P. M. (1963) Nerve fibre size in the carpal tunnel syndrome. *Journal of Neurology, Neurosurgery and Psychiatry*, **26**, 520-527.

Thomas, P. K., Hollinrake, K., Lascelles, R. G., O'Sullivan, D. J., Baillod, R. A., Moorhead, J. F. & Mackenzie, J. C. (1970) The polyneuropathy of chronic renal failure. *Brain*, **94**, 761-780.

Thomas, P. K. & Lascelles, R. G. (1965) Schwann cell abnormalities in diabetic neuropathy. *Lancet*, **1**, 1355-1357.

Thomas, P. K. & Lascelles, R. G. (1966) Pathology of diabetic neuropathy. *Quarterly Journal of Medicine*, **35**, (N.S.) 489-509.

Thomas, P. K. & Lascelles, R. G. (1967) Hypertrophic neuropathy. *Quarterly Journal of Medicine*, **36** (N.S.), 223-238.

Thomas, P. K., Lascelles, R. G., Hallpike, J. F. & Hewer, R. L. (1969) Recurrent and chronic relapsing Guillain–Barré polyneuritis. *Brain*, **92**, 589-606.

Thomas, P. K., Lascelles, R. G. & Stewart, G. (1975) Hypertrophic neuropathy in *Handbook of Clinical Neurology* (Eds. Vinken, P. J. & Bruyn, C. W.), Vol. 21, Part I, Chap. 8, pp. 145-170, North Holland Publishing Co., Amsterdam.

Thomas, P. K. and Walker, J. G. (1965) Xanthomatous neuropathy in primary biliary cirrhosis. *Brain*, **88**, 1079-1088.

Tinel, J. (1917) *Nerve Wounds* (Trans. Rothwell, F., Ed. Joll, G.), Baillière, Tindall & Cox, London.

Tooth, H. H. (1886) *The Peroneal Type of Progressive Muscular Atrophy*, H. K. Lewis & Co., London.

Torp, A. (1961) Histamine and mast cells in nerve. *Medicina experimentalis*, **4**, 180-182.

Trousseau, A. & Lassègue, C. (1851) Du raisonnement de la paralysie du voile du palais. *L'Union médicale*, **5**, 471.

Turk, J. L. (1969) Cell-mediated immunological processes in leprosy. *Bulletin of the World Health Organisation*, **41**, 779-792.

Turk, J. L. & Waters, M. F. R. (1971) Immunological significance of changes in lymph nodes across the leprosy spectrum. *Clinical and Experimental Immunology*, **8**, 363-376.

Tyler, H. R. (1968) Neurologic disorders in renal failure. *American Journal of Medicine*, **44**, 734-748.

Ulrich, J., Esslen, E., Regli, F. & Bischoff, A. (1965) Die Beziehungen der Nervenleitgeschwindigkeit zum histologischen Befund am peripheren Nerven. *Deutsche Zeitschrift für Nervenheilkunde*, **187**, 770-786.

Ulrich, J., Spiess, H. & Huber, R. (1967) Neurologische Syndrome als Fernwirkung maligner Tumoren (Ammonshornsklerose bei Bronchuskarzinom). *Schweizerisches Archiv für Neurologie, Neurochirurgie und Psychiatrie*, **99**, 83-100.

Urquhart, D. A. (1934) Multiple peripheral neuritis as a complication of measles. *British Medical Journal*, **2**, 115-116.

Van Allen, M. W., Frohlich, J. A. and Davis, J. R. (1969) Inherited predisposition to generalized amyloidosis. Clinical and pathological study of a family with neuropathy, nephropathy and peptic ulcer. *Neurology (Minneapolis)*, **19**, 10-25.

Vavra, J. (1965) Porphyria and neoplasms in *The Remote Effects of Cancer on the Nervous System* (Ed. Brain, W. R. & Norris, F.), pp. 172-184, Grune and Stratton, New York.

Veith, G. (1949) Untersuchungen über die Histologie der Polyneuritis diphtheritica. *Beiträge zur pathologischen Anatomie*, **110**, 567-606.

Veltema, A. N. & Verjaal, A. (1961) Sur un cas d'hérédopathie ataxique polyneuritique. *Revue Neurologique*, **104**, 15-23.

Vial, J. D. (1958) The early changes in the axoplasm during Wallerian degeneration. *Journal of Biophysical and Biochemical Cytology*, **4**, 551-556.

Victor, M. (1965) The effects of nutritional deficiency on the nervous system. A comparison with the effects of carcinoma in *The Remote Effects of Cancer on The Nervous System* (Eds. Brain, W. R. & Norris, F.), pp. 134-161, Grune and Stratton, New York.

Victor, M., Banker, B. Q. & Adams, R. D. (1958) The neuropathy of multiple myeloma. *Journal of Neurology, Neurosurgery and Psychiatry*, **21**, 73-78.

Vignon, G., Megard, M. & Martin, A. (1956) Une observation anatomo-clinique d'acropathie ulcéro-mutilante *Presse médicale*, **64**, 1954-1956.

Virchow, R. (1855) Ein Fall von progressiver Muskelatrophie. *Virchows Archiv für pathologische Anatomie*, **8**, 537-540.

Virchow, R. (1864) *Die krankhaften Geschwülste*, Vol. 2, pp. 494-531, A. Hirschwald, Berlin.

Vizoso, A. D. & Young, J. Z. (1948) Internode length and fibre diameter in developing and regenerating nerve. *Journal of Anatomy (London)*, **82**, 110-134.

Waksman, B. H. & Adams, R. D.   (1955) Allergic neuritis: an experimental disease of rabbits induced by the injection of peripheral nervous tissue and adjuvants. *Journal of Experimental Medicine*, **102**, 213-235.

Waksman, B. H., Adams, R. D. & Mansmann, H. C. Jr.   (1957) Experimental study of diphtheritic polyneuritis in the rabbit and guinea pig: I. Immunologic and histopathologic observations. *Journal of Experimental Medicine*, **105**, 591-614.

Waldenström, J. & Haeger-Aronsen, B.   (1962) Different patterns of human porphyria. *British Medical Journal*, **2**, 272-276.

Waller, A.   (1850) Experiments on the section of the glossopharyngeal and hypoglossal nerves of the frog, and observations of the alterations produced thereby in the structure of their primitive fibres. *Philosophical Transactions of the Royal Society London, Series B*, **140**, 423-429.

Waller, A.   (1852) Sur la reproduction des nerfs et sur la structure et les fonctions des ganglions spineaux. *Müllers Archiv für Anatomie and Physiologie*, 392-401.

Wallgren, A.   (1946) Preclinical stage of infantile hypertrophic pyloric stenosis. *American Journal of Diseases of Children*, **72**, 371-376.

Walshe, F. M. R.   (1918-19) On the pathogenesis of diphtheritic paralysis: Part II. Clinical observations on the paralysis of faucial and extrafaucial diphtheria with an analysis of 30 cases following skin and wound infections. *Quarterly Journal of Medicine*, **13**, 14-37.

Walshe, F. M. R.   (1951) Nervous and vascular pressure syndromes of the thoracic inlet and cervico-axillary canal in *Modern Trends in Neurology* (Ed. Feiling, A.), pp. 542-566, Butterworth, London.

Walton, E. W.   (1958) Giant-cell granuloma of the respiratory tract (Wegener's granulomatosis). *British Medical Journal*, **2**, 265-270.

Walton, J. N.   (1969) The floppy infant syndrome in *Brain's Diseases of the Nervous System* (Eds. Brain, Lord & Walton, J. N.), 7th Edn, pp. 878-881, Oxford University Press, London.

Walton, J. N., Tomlinson, B. E. & Pearce, G. W.   (1968) Subacute "poliomyelitis" and Hodgkin's disease. *Journal of the Neurological Sciences*, **6**, 435-445.

Ward, J. D.   (1971) Functional and metabolic studies in diabetic peripheral nerve. M.D. Thesis, University of London, p. 124.

Watson-Jones, R.   (1949) Léri's pleonosteosis, carpal tunnel compression of the medial nerves and Morton's metatarsalgia. *Journal of Bone and Joint Surgery*, **31B**, 560-571.

Webster, H. de F.   (1962) Schwann cell alterations in metachromatic leucodystrophy: preliminary phase and electron microscopic observations. *Journal of Neuropathology and Experimental Neurology*, **21**, 534-541.

Webster, H. de F.   (1962) Transient focal accumulation of axonal mitochondria during the early stages of Wallerian degeneration. *Journal of Cell Biology*, **12**, 361-383.

Webster, H. de F., Schröder, J. M., Asbury, A. K. & Adams, R. D.   (1967) The role of Schwann cells in the formation of 'onion bulbs' found in chronic neuropathies. *Journal of Neuropathology and Experimental Neurology*, **26**, 276-299.

Webster, H. de F., Spiro, D., Waksman, B. & Adams, R. D.   (1961) Phase and electron microscopic studies of experimental demyelination. Part 2: Schwann cell changes in guinea pig sciatic nerves during experimental diphtheritic neuritis. *Journal of Neuropathology and Experimental Neurology*, **20**, 5-34.

Wechsler, W.   (1970) The development and structure of peripheral nerves in vertebrates in *Handbook of Clinical Neurology* (Eds. Vinken, P. J. & Bruyn, G. W.), Vol. 7/1, pp. 1-39, Elsevier, Amsterdam.

Wechsler, W. & Hager, H.   (1962) Elektronmikroskopische Untersuchung der Wallerschen Degeneration des peripheren Säugetiernerven. *Beiträge zur pathologischen Anatomie*, **126**, 352-380.

Weddell, G.   (1942) Axonal regeneration in cutaneous nerve plexuses. *Journal of Anatomy (London)*, **77**, 49-62.

Wegener, F.   (1939) Über eine eigenartige rhinogene Granulomatose mit besonderer Beteiligung des Arteriensystems und der Nieren. *Beiträge zur pathologischen Anatomie*, **102**, 36-68.

Weinshilboum, R. M. & Axelrod, J.   (1971) Reduced plasma dopamine-β-hydroxylase activity in familial dysautonomia. *New England Journal of Medicine*, **285**, 938-942.

Weiss, P.   (1943) Endoneurial edema in constricted nerves. *Anatomical Record*, **86**, 491-522.

Weiss, P., Edds, McV. & Cavanaugh, M.   (1945) The effect of terminal connections on caliber of nerve fibres. *Anatomical Record*, **92**, 215-233.

Weiss, P., Wang, H., Taylor, A. C. & Edds, McV.   (1945) Proximo-distal fluid convection in the endoneurial spaces of peripheral nerves, demonstrated by colored and radioactive (isotope) tracers. *American Journal of Physiology*, **143**, 521-540.

Weller, R. O.   (1965) Diphtheritic neuropathy in the chicken: an electron-microscope study. *Journal of Pathology and Bacteriology*, **89**, 591-598.

Weller, R. O.   (1967) An electron microscope study of hypertrophic neuropathy of Déjerine and Sottas. *Journal of Neurology, Neurosurgery and Psychiatry*, **30**, 111-125.

Weller, R. O., Bruckner, F. E. & Chamberlain, M. A.   (1970) Rheumatoid neuropathy: a histological and electrophysiological study. *Journal of Neurology, Neurosurgery and Psychiatry*, **33**, 592-604.

Weller, R. O. & Das Gupta, T. K.   (1968) Experimental hypertrophic neuropathy: an electron microscope study. *Journal of Neurology, Neurosurgery and Psychiatry*, **31**, 34-42.

Weller, R. O. & Mellick, R. S.   (1966) Acid phosphatase and lysosome activity in diphtheritic neuropathy and Wallerian degeneration. *British Journal of Experimental Pathology*, **47**, 425-434.

Weller, R. O. & Nester, B.   (1972) Early changes at the node of Ranvier in segmental demyelination. Histochemical and electron microscopic observations. *Brain*, **95**, 665-674.

Whitehouse, F. R. & Kernohan, J. W.   (1948) Myenteric plexus in congenital megacolon. *Archives of Internal Medicine*, **82**, 75-111.

Wiederholt, W. C., Mulder, D. W. & Lambert, E. H.   (1964) The Landry–Guillain–Barré–Strohl syndrome or polyradiculoneuropathy: historical review, report on 97 patients and present concepts. *Mayo Clinic Proceedings*, **39**, 427-451.

Wilkinson, P. C.   (1964) Serological findings in carcinomatous neuromyopathy. *Lancet*, **1**, 1301-1303.

Wilkinson, P. C. & Zeromski, J.   (1965) Immunofluorescent detection of antibodies against neurones in sensory carcinomatous neuropathy. *Brain*, **88**, 529-538.

Williamson, R. T.   (1908) *Diseases of the Spinal Cord*, p. 377, Hodder and Stoughton, London.

Wilner, E. C. & Brody, J. A.   (1968) An evaluation of the remote effects of cancer on the nervous system. *Neurology (Minneapolis)*, **18**, 1120-1124.

Winkler, G. F.   (1965) In vitro demyelination of peripheral nerve induced with sensitized cells. *Annals of the New York Academy of Sciences*, **122**, 287-296.

Wisniewski, H., Terry, R. D., Whitaker, J. N., Cook, S. D. & Dowling, P. C.   (1969) Landry–Guillain–Barré Syndrome: a primary demyelinating disease. *Archives of Neurology*, **21**, 269-276.

Wohlwill, F.   (1923) Über die nur mikroskopisch erkennbare Form der Periarteritis nodosa. *Virchows Archiv für pathologische Anatomie*, **246**, 377-411.

Woltman, H. W. & Wilder, R. M.   (1929) Diabetes mellitus: pathologic changes in the spinal cord and peripheral nerves. *Archives of Internal Medicine*, **44**, 576-603.

Woodhall, B., Mahaley, S., Boone, S. & Hunneycutt, H.   (1962) The effect of chemotherapeutic agents upon peripheral nerves. *Journal of Surgical Research*, **2**, 373-381.

Yatsu, F. & Zussman, W.   (1964) Familial dysautonomia (Riley–Day Syndrome). Case report with postmortem findings of a patient at age 31. *Archives of Neurology (Chicago)*, **10**, 459-463.

Yonezawa, T., Ishihara, Y. & Matsuyama, H.   (1968) Studies on experimental allergic peripheral neuritis. 1. Demyelinating patterns studied in vitro. *Journal of Neuropathology and Experimental Neurology*, **27**, 453-463.

Young, J. Z.   (1942) The functional repair of nervous tissue. *Physiological Reviews*, **22**, 318-374.

Yudell, A., Dyck, P. J. & Lambert, E. H.   (1965) A kinship with the Roussy–Lévy Syndrome. *Archives of Neurology*, **13**, 432-440.

Zalin, A., Darby, A., Vaughan, S. & Raftery, E. B.   (1974) Primary neuropathic amyloidosis in three brothers. *British Medical Journal*, **1**, 65-66.

17

Epilepsy

Revised by J. A. N. Corsellis and B. S. Meldrum

In an epileptic attack the normal activity of the central nervous system is temporarily disturbed. In some people the initial fault is a toxic or a metabolic illness and the disorder lies outside the central nervous system. More often, clinical evidence will be found of an abnormality within the skull. In either situation the epilepsy will be classified as symptomatic.

However, in many people no adequate explanation of the attacks can be found during life and these form the cryptogenic, or idiopathic, group.

The role of the pathologist, and particularly of the neuropathologist, is to take this diagnostic process a stage further either by studying the patient's nervous system after death or by investigating some fragment of tissue that has been removed surgically during life.

Sometimes, even after an extensive histological search, a significant abnormality cannot be found and the diagnosis of cryptogenic epilepsy is upheld. At other times some kind of structural abnormality is disclosed which may well point to a diagnosis of symptomatic epilepsy; it is then essential to clarify as far as possible the relationship of the abnormality to the attacks. This may not be difficult when a gross fault such as a tumour, a cortical scar or a malformation is present, for it is then reasonable to look on the epileptic attacks as its consequence. Often, however, the position is less straightforward, for a cerebral abnormality that gives rise to fits in one person may not do so in another, while, as will be described later, the effect of the disorganization of brain structure may vary according to the time of life at which the insult occurs. Finally, even if there seems to be conclusive evidence of a direct link between the abnormal state of the brain and the occurrence of epileptic attacks the abnormality may be a consequence of the attacks and not their cause.

These difficulties in interpretation have beset the neuropathological study of epilepsy from the outset and because they proved so intractable it began in the 1920s to look as if little progress would be made. Then in the 1930s the introduction of electroencephalography and developments in the neurosurgical treatment of epilepsy, combined with an experimental approach to the subject, began to produce information which had not been available to the classical workers in the field. During the last 30 or so years, therefore, many of the old problems in the neuropathology of epilepsy have had to be re-investigated, and although there are still many questions left unanswered, the relation between structure and function in epilepsy is perhaps better understood now than at any time in the past.

This increase in knowledge about the nature and the localization of epileptic foci has led to the epileptic attacks in an increasing number of patients being attributed to focal abnormalities of the brain. It follows from this that the cryptogenic group is gradually getting smaller, but even if all the epilepsies proved to be focal in origin it is likely that other factors also, such as the genetic and the environmental, sometimes play an important part in the development of the illness. Familial inheritance is frequently found in those with cryptogenic epilepsy (Metrakos and Metrakos 1974) and it is not absent in the symptomatic and overtly focal forms. Cortical dysrhythmia, identified in the electroencephalogram, was found to be six times more frequent in the relatives of those suffering from cryptogenic epilepsy than in a normal control group (Lennox, Gibbs and Gibbs 1940). The nature of the predisposing factor, however, is not known.

Symptomatic epilepsy

Brain and Walton (1969) list the systemic disorders that may precipitate convulsions. These have been reviewed by Millichap (1974) and Meldrum (1975). They include derangements of body fluids and electrolytes, renal failure, hypoglycaemia, anoxia and other endocrine and metabolic disorders, including exogenous poisonings. Convulsions associated with childhood fever form a separate group and are discussed in the following section.

Almost any disease of the brain may be associated with epilepsy. The more common local causes of symptomatic epilepsy include cerebral tumours, encephalitis, meningitis, cerebral abscess, trauma, vascular accidents, congenital abnormalities and degenerative processes.

It is difficult to be precise about the incidence of the different types of abnormality, since the figures vary not only according to the source but also according to the age range of the patients being studied. Bridge (1949) in his analysis of 742 children attending an epileptic clinic considered that birth and neonatal injuries were the commonest causes since they accounted for nearly 25% of the cases. Vascular accidents and head injury after the neonatal period accounted for 12% and 7% respectively, while acute infection, malformation and cerebral tumour were all considerably lower. In 20% of the cases cerebral injury of uncertain cause was suspected and in nearly one-third no evidence of brain disease was found.

A more recent study (Rose and Lombroso 1970) confined to seizures in the neonatal period (full-term infants, 0 to 21 days old) suggests that metabolic disorders (hypocalcaemia and hypoglycaemia) account for 25% of seizures, and intracranial birth injury (especially subarachnoid haemorrhage) and CNS infection for another 25%. Congenital malformations and perinatal anoxia each appeared to be responsible for less than 10% of seizures.

When fits develop in the adult, *tumour* and *trauma* become the more important of the identifiable factors. Although generalizations are of limited value, almost 50% of patients with intracranial tumours suffer from epileptic attacks at some time during the illness (Ketz 1974). In 60 to 80% of tumour patients with fits the epileptic attacks are the presenting symptom. Tumours are more likely to give rise to an epileptic fit when they are situated in the cerebral hemispheres than when they lie below the tentorial opening. Within the hemispheres the position of the tumour and its nearness to the cortex are important. Lund (1952), for example, in his study of 'epilepsy with intracranial tumour' found that the most sensitive region was the frontal and parietal cortex around the central fissure, either generalized or focal attacks being recorded in 75% of patients with a tumour in this area. The figure for the temporal lobes was 50% and for other regions it was still lower. Patients with slowly growing tumours develop fits more often than those with rapidly invasive tumours. A recent survey by Ketz (1974) of the relationship between the occurrence of epilepsy and the type of tumour gave 71% in cases of oligodendroglioma, 59% in astrocytoma, 37% in meningioma and 29% in glioblastoma, the last named being particularly associated with focal seizures. These figures are not a true indication of the difference in epileptogenicity of the type of tumour, but they do reflect the important role in epileptogenesis of elapsed time following the onset of any pathological change in the brain (Penfield, Erickson and Tarlov 1940).

The reason why some patients with tumours have seizures and others do not is obscure. The patient's genetic predisposition to epilepsy can play a role but is probably critical in only a minority of cases. Kirstein (1942) found that 7% of tumour patients with seizures had a relative with epilepsy, while among those without seizures only 2% had such a relative. Lund (1952) on similar grounds concluded that a hereditary tendency to epilepsy possibly contributed to the occurrence of seizures in 10% of patients with tumours.

The immediate pathogenetic mechanism is often broadly described as 'hypoxia' or 'ischaemia' of the grey matter adjacent to the tumour but this should not be interpreted in any direct sense. Although generalized cerebral hypoxia may trigger off epileptic seizures, there is little reason to believe that a degree of focal cortical hypoxia, which is too slight to result in cellular damage, will have the same effect. It is well established that the occurrence of fits, symptomatic of tumours, is little related to the general physiological state of the patient (Janz 1964) and this would suggest that they are unrelated to acute fluctuations in the oxygen tension around the tumour. The failure of fast-growing and invasive tumours to show any excess of seizures also argues against the acute effects of hypoxia. On the contrary, slowly developing neuronal and glial changes are more likely to be the important factors. Since cellular mechanisms of this kind are, however, common to many forms of epilepsy they are discussed later in a separate section.

Neurosurgical excision of the tumour abolished the seizures in about 50% of cases, but according to Ketz about 10% of patients who had no seizures before operation develop them subsequently.

Epilepsy following *head injury* is more likely to occur in open than in closed wounds. Russell and Whitty (1952) found that attacks had developed in 40% of their patients during the five-year period after a penetrating injury to the skull. As with tumours, the most sensitive region was the cerebral cortex adjacent to the central fissure. There seems to be no evident difference in the incidence of traumatic epilepsy in the two World Wars, in spite of the improved methods of treatment and of combating infection. In closed head injuries the incidence is much lower. Jennett (Jennett and Lewin 1960; Jennett 1965) gave the overall figure as less than 10%, but he emphasized that the risk varied greatly according to the severity of the injury and the nature of the complications. Thus prolonged post-traumatic amnesia when combined with a depressed skull fracture carried a higher risk than on its own. Jennett (1969) later emphasized that 'early fits', or those occurring during the first week after an injury, are commonly of the focal motor variety and it is only after this period that temporal lobe attacks are liable to develop.

The damage responsible for fits during the first few hours after cerebral trauma is likely to be a combination of shearing of nerve cell processes and of capillaries, cerebral oedema and other early consequences of focal ischaemia. The late seizures which may occur ten or more years after the trauma are presumably due to cellular changes, similar to those occurring in relation to tumours and abscesses (see p. 787).

Acute *infections*, especially viral meningoencephalitides are not infrequent causes of focal or generalized seizures. Protozoal infections such as toxoplasmosis or cerebral malaria (in tropical countries) are causes of seizures that may be diagnosed sometimes only after death. Intracranial infections are also liable to give rise to epileptic attacks after the acute episode. Legg, Gupta and Scott (1973) found that in 72% of patients with a history of cerebral abscess, occasional fits occurred which commonly started during the first year although in many there was an interval of three or more years.

In later adult life and in old age, epilepsy may occur in association with various degenerative conditions of the brain (reviewed by Radermecker 1974). Alzheimer's disease, Huntington's chorea and, occasionally, senile dementia are examples. Cerebrovascular disease is also an important cause of seizures in later life. Fits occur in 13% of cerebral haemorrhages or infarcts (Richardson, Dodge and Victor 1954). Venous thrombosis and subdural haematomas may cause seizures at any age but are commonest at the two extremes of life.

At all ages, however, there are some epileptic patients in whom no underlying disturbance is to be found either within the nervous system or outside it. The figures quoted earlier from Bridge strongly substantiate this, for aetiological factors could be identified in only about half the children. Similarly, in a clinical study of late onset epilepsy in adults, Serafetinides and Dominian (1963) found no cause for the fits in as many as three-quarters of the patients. Such cases make up the cryptogenic group. The pathological findings in this group, however, are bound up with the type of brain damage that may occur in association with, or as a result of, convulsions particularly in early life and when status epilepticus develops. The main features of these conditions will therefore be described first.

Febrile convulsions and status epilepticus

Generalized seizures in infants and young children during the course of an acute febrile illness occur in temperate climates in 29 to 72 per 1000 (Lennox-Buchthal 1973). The incidence rate is apparently higher in tropical countries (Lessell, Torres and Kurland 1962; Hall 1964; Egdell and Stanfield 1972). This contrasts with the 5 in 1000 incidence of epilepsy in adults.

'Febrile convulsions', in which the primary infection does not involve the brain, are usually distinguished from seizures secondary to meningitis and encephalitis (Millichap 1968; Lennox-Buchthal 1973). In practice the distinction is not easily made partly because the primary infection in many febrile illnesses is not identified (exanthem subitum is commonly not recognized), and even when a viral agent is identified the degree of direct cerebral involvement is hard to ascertain (Wallace and Zealley 1970).

Febrile convulsions are important because of the risk of status epilepticus and of damage to the brain, particularly if the episode is prolonged. The cerebral consequences may be graded as:

(i) generalized damage, but involving principally those areas vulnerable to any form of cerebral hypoxia (neocortex, cerebellum, thalamus, hippocampus) (Fowler 1957; Zimmerman 1938);

(ii) cerebral hemiatrophy, associated with hemiparesis and sometimes hemiconvulsions (Gastaut, Poirier, Salamon, Toga and Virouroux 1960; Isler 1969; Aicardi and Chevrie 1970; Aicardi and Baraton 1971;

(iii) Ammon's horn sclerosis or other 'ischaemic' pathology of the hippocampus and temporal lobe. This may be a more restricted form of (ii). It is the lesion found in 50% of anterior temporal specimens when the operation is performed for temporal lobe epilepsy (Falconer 1974);

(iv) 'minimal changes'. Approximately one-third of children show EEG abnormalities one week or more after the convulsion, usually asymmetrical slowing in the occipital or temporal regions, which is sometimes replaced by a spike focus (Lennox-Buchthal 1973).

One-third of 208 children followed for up to seven years after febrile convulsions showed behavioural disturbance or educational retardation (Frantzen 1971). The nature of the brain damage underlying this has not been demonstrated, but a similar behavioural disorder has been described prior to the onset of temporal lobe epilepsy (Aird, Venturini and Spielman 1967) in which it has been suggested that the abnormality is similar to, but milder than, that of sclerosis of the medial temporal areas.

Analysis of the neurological and pathological sequelae of febrile convulsions is complicated by two factors. (i) Pre-existing brain damage (commonly arising from perinatal asphyxia or trauma) predisposes to febrile convulsions (Peterman 1950, 1952; Millichap 1968; Wallace 1972; Lennox-Buchthal 1973). (ii) Viral infections (even when

signs of encephalitis are not present) may give rise to neurological sequelae whether or not convulsions occur (Wallace and Zealley 1970).

Although these two factors may introduce a variable bias into collected series, there is a good correlation between seizure duration and incidence and severity of sequelae both within and between reported series. Further, prompt medical care of febrile convulsions leads to fewer severe sequelae, including non-febrile convulsions, although it possibly has less effect on minor sequelae (Frantzen 1971; Lennox-Buchthal 1973).

Status epilepticus may be defined broadly as a convulsive episode lasting over an hour, without an intervening period of consciousness. It has long been recognized as a serious danger to life at any age (Hunter 1959), but it offers a special threat in the early years. Aicardi and Chevrie (1970) found that of a series of children under 15 years with an episode of status, about 40% were young infants in whom mortality was high. In 85% the status occurred before the age of 5 years. Three out of four affected children who survived for more than a year had further epileptic attacks. Aicardi and Chevrie considered that in 50% of their patients the status was due to organic cerebral disease. In more than half of those in whom no cause could be identified, the status had developed following a non-specific febrile episode.

Oxbury and Whitty (1971) made a comparable study of status epilepticus in adults and found it to have been symptomatic in 63% of their series. Tumours, vascular disease, infections and trauma, all involving the brain, were the most common causes and, in so far as any localization was identified, the abnormalities tended to involve the frontal lobes. Whitty (1961) had already observed this association in relation to trauma while Janz (1964) had described status epilepticus as the particular presenting sign of a frontal tumour. Oxbury and Whitty emphasized that status may also affect patients with long-established cryptogenic epilepsy.

The prognosis in an attack of symptomatic status usually depends more on the underlying cerebral disease than on damage resulting from the attack itself. When, therefore, the status has no known cause the immediate outlook is better, but the risk of permanent brain damage or even death is always there.

Since, as already mentioned, the risk is much greater in the earlier years of life, it is not surprising that the neuropathological aspects have been studied most intensively in the brains of young children (Zimmerman 1938; Meyer, Beck and Shepherd 1955). Norman (1964; Ounsted, Lindsay and Norman 1966) in a study of 11 cases found that the brain is usually, but not always, slightly swollen; some congestion is common and occasional petechial haemorrhages may occur.

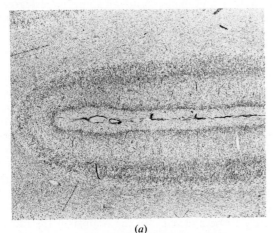

(a)

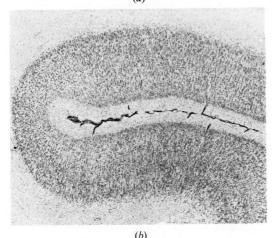

(b)

Fig. 17.1 (a) Cerebral cortex of an infant dying shortly after an episode of status epilepticus. Extensive neuronal necrosis has destroyed the middle layers, and particularly the third. The resulting pallor is seen when compared with the normal cortex in (b). Cresyl violet. × 12.

There is often a striking difference between the relatively normal appearance of the fixed brain and the structural devastation seen under the microscope, or even that seen by the naked eye on the stained slide. In the latter, using a cell stain such as cresyl violet, wide expanses of the cortical ribbon stand out as abnormally pale (Fig. 17.1). Sometimes the outer, or less often the deeper layers are affected. This is due to the extensive neuronal necrosis which tends to follow a pattern. Thus the calcarine cortex and the parahippocampal gyri are usually spared whereas the hippocampus (Fig. 17.3b) and uncus appear blanched. The hippocampus in particular may have a swollen outline in the region of the Sommer sector and the dentate fascia. Other cortical regions are affected to a more variable degree. The deep grey matter, and particularly the thalamus, may be patchily necrotic. In the affected parts the neuronal changes are similar to those commonly seen in severe hypoxia or ischaemia (Chapter 2). The 'ischaemic nerve cell change' of Spielmeyer is common. In this the cell body becomes scarcely visible with a Nissl stain, but is eosinophilic in haematoxylin and eosin preparations. At the same time the cell outline and the cell nucleus both take on a triangular shape while the nucleus becomes small and darkly stained so that the nucleolus can no longer be identified. Many other nerve cells disappear, only small tags of eosinophilic cytoplasm and disintegrating nuclei being visible. In the cerebellum the Purkinje cells are commonly affected in many folia or lobules. The cytoplasm then loses its Nissl substance and becomes eosinophilic, while the nucleus may be dark and shrunken or at times it may stain faintly.

In any of the affected parts of the brain a microglial and astrocytic reaction occurs. The microglia are the more prominent in the early stages and neutral fat may be seen in their processes if survival has been for more than a few days. As the length of survival increases, the astrocytic reaction becomes more noticeable and eventually a dense fibrous gliosis may be laid down. The necrosis is rarely extensive enough to result in the breakdown of tissue or cyst formation. The white matter may show slight diffuse pallor in the more oedematous brains.

The neuronal necrosis and glial reaction following severe serial convulsions or an episode of status are acute and tend to be considerably more extensive than the chronic scarring found when an epileptic patient has died after many years of recurrent epileptic fits, that is to say in an adult patient with cryptogenic epilepsy.

Cryptogenic epilepsy

There are many people, some living in the community and others in long-stay hospitals, who have suffered for much or all of their lives from an epilepsy of which the cause is not known. These belong to the cryptogenic group. The absence of any clear-cut cause for the disease, however, does not mean that all pathological change is absent, and in many cases it is present. There are two main types. The first is superficial erosion and scarring of the orbital, frontal and temporal cortex. Stauder (1935) remarked on this, having observed it in 25% of a series of chronic epileptic brains. He also pointed out that 16 of 77 contused brains investigated by Spatz

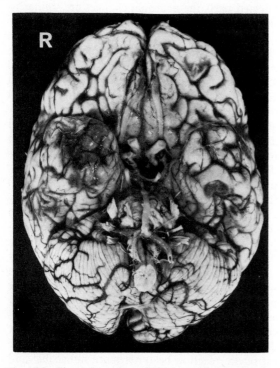

Fig. 17.2 The undersurface of the brain showing contre-coup bruising and scarring in an adult patient with life-long epilepsy. The right temporal lobe has suffered in a recent fall whereas there is older cortical scarring at a more posterior level in both temporal lobes. The left orbital area also shows a shallow cortical 'ulcer' due to past trauma and scarring. × 0.5.

had come from epileptic patients and he rightly emphasized that such damage was considerably commoner in chronic epilepsy than was generally recognized. Sano and Malamud (1953) found the incidence as high as 36% but the figure given by Margerison and Corsellis (1966) was lower at 11%. The impression of the present writers is that this damage has become less common in recent years. It is clearly of the contre-coup type and although it may occasionally be the result

of a closed head injury preceding the onset of the epilepsy, it is much more commonly the result of a fall during a fit. This can at times be obvious when both old and recent damage is seen in the same brain (Fig. 17.2).

The second type of cerebral damage is the commoner, for in at least half the patients with cryptogenic epilepsy, and much less often in those with the symptomatic forms, an appreciable degree of neuronal loss accompanied by a glial reaction can be found. Not all parts of the brain are equally vulnerable, but the best known and also the most often damaged areas are the Ammon's horn followed by the cerebellum. Spielmeyer originally observed that 80% of the 125 epileptic brains that he had examined were damaged in one or both of these regions. Later studies, and particularly those of Scholz (1951) and Peiffer (1963), have extended the range of vulnerability to include the thalamus and the cerebral neo-cortex, while Meyer and Beck (1955) added the amygdaloid nucleus and the grey matter adjacent to it to the list. The striatum and pallidum seem rarely to be affected. In the brainstem the most vulnerable areas are the inferior olives.

The damage, wherever it occurs, looks much the same. The acute stages are found at their most severe in the brains of young children who have died during or shortly after a bout of status epilepticus, and have been described in the previous section. In the great majority of people with long-standing cryptogenic epilepsy, however, the histological abnormality, when present, is one of scarring and appears to be the result of one or more insults well in the past, for acute damage of this kind is rarely seen in such people even if they have died shortly after an attack.

The histological minutiae of the process may be particularly well studied in the hippocampus, or Ammon's horn as it is also known. The final stage of scarring in this region is the lesion known as Ammon's horn or hippocampal sclerosis. The normal structure is illustrated in Fig. 17.3a in which the ribbon of nerve cells has been divided into the simplified areas as proposed by Scholz (1951). The first part is the Sommer sector or the h1 field, and is the commonest site for severe neuronal loss and gliosis (Fig. 17.3c). The end folium, or h3 field, is also highly vulnerable while a remarkably constant and inexplicable feature is the marked tendency for a short run of nerve cells lying between these two fields to be relatively spared—this is the resistant part or h2. The small, dark, densely packed neurons of the dentate fascia are also often more or less erased. In its chronic stage the atrophy is usually obvious to the naked eye (Fig. 17.4). It can, with some exceptions (Bodechtel 1930), be seen running through the full length of the hippocampal formation, although it becomes more patchy anteriorly in the pes and is then less easily identified.

In the cerebellum the Purkinje cells are the most vulnerable and their numbers may be greatly reduced over many folia. Along the line of the

in the occasional folium, often then around its base, and only detectable with the microscope (Fig. 17.7).

The same process of selective neuronal necrosis and gliosis can affect one or both cerebral hemispheres more widely and occasionally an entire hemisphere is smaller than the other leading to a clear cut hemiatrophy (Fig. 17.8). More often the damage is less marked and is patchy, ranging from localized neuronal loss (Fig. 17.9) and gliosis scattered through the cerebral neocortex to more

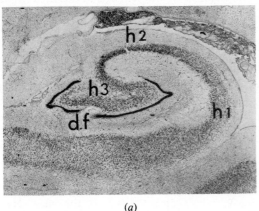

(a)

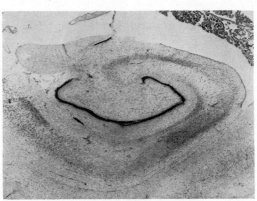

(b)

Fig. 17.3 (a) The normal hippocampus (see text); (b) acute selective necrosis of hippocampus following status epilepticus; (c), the classical Ammon's horn, or hippocampal sclerosis. (a), (b) and (c). Cresyl violet. ×7.

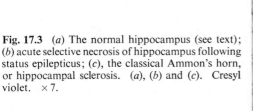

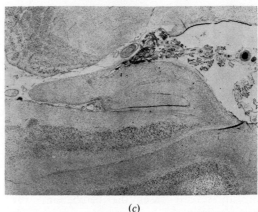

(c)

Purkinje cell loss, the astrocytes (or Bergmann glia) proliferate and spread out into the overlying molecular layer which can become heavily gliosed (Fig. 17.5). Considerable destruction of the granular layer sometimes occurs as well; and dense fibrous gliosis of the deep white matter spreads into the dentate nucleus which may also lose nerve cells. The severity of the cerebellar damage, therefore, ranges from the gross atrophy of many or most folia easily seen with the naked eye (Fig. 17.6) to the restricted loss of nerve cells

extensive damage which runs horizontally, in a laminar way, mainly through the intermediate layers of the cortex. In the deep grey matter of the hemisphere the area most frequently affected is the thalamus and, particularly in the presence of hemiatrophy, a gross inequality between the two thalami may be seen. The neuronal loss in the thalamus is distributed throughout the different nuclei and shows no systematic or anatomical preference (Fig. 17.10). The mamillary body may also be grossly shrunken (Fig. 17.11).

The incidence of damage in the vulnerable areas was studied by Peiffer (1963) and by Margerison and Corsellis (1966). The latter study found that one or both hippocampi were affected in 50% to 60% of cases of chronic cryptogenic epilepsy, and that unilateral damage was far the commoner, a classical Ammon's horn sclerosis being found bilaterally in only 3%. The cerebellum was damaged in 45% of the cases and the thalamus, the amygdaloid nucleus and the cerebral cortex each, not necessarily together, in about 25%. Nearly all cases in which the hippocampus was

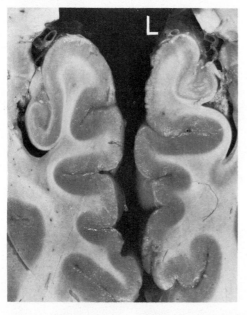

Fig. 17.4 Naked-eye coronal view of the two hippocampi from an epileptic brain with the adjacent gyri placed side by side. The right side is normal, on the left the hippocampus and the parahippocampal gyrus are greatly shrunken and sclerosed. × 1·4.

affected showed some damage elsewhere in the brain. In several cases the cerebellum was affected although the hippocampi were not. It should be emphasized that most, if not all, studies in this field have been based on patients whose epileptic illness had been severe enough to bring them into the long-stay hospitals. Considerably less is therefore known about the incidence and extent of cerebral damage in those less seriously afflicted.

The pathogenesis of 'epileptic' brain damage
The origin of the kind of damage just described has long been discussed and there is still no completely satisfactory solution to the problem. The controversy began in 1825 when Bouchet and Cazauvieilh noticed that one or both Ammon's horns in the brains of some epileptic patients were unusually small and hard. No conclusions were drawn at that time from this macroscopic observation, but in the following years the Ammon's horn came to be looked on by other workers as an important part of the motor and sensory pathways in the brain, and the idea germinated that epileptic attacks could be triggered off by the sclerosis in this area (Sommer 1880). This view was not without its opponents, however, who rightly pointed out that in many patients with epilepsy no demonstrable abnormality could be found in the hippocampus or indeed elsewhere in the brain. Pfleger (1880) added further doubts to this belief in the epileptogenic importance of an abnormal hippocampus by proposing, on the basis of his observations on the brains of patients who had died during an attack, that the neuronal necrosis in the Ammon's horn was recent in origin and was indeed a sequel to the fits.

The same interpretation soon came to be applied to Chaslin's observations on the glia. He had described in 1889 the way in which the delicate network of fine glial fibres covering the surface of the normal cerebral cortex could thicken up in epileptic brains to form a dense subpial 'carpet' spreading down into the deeper cortical layers. Chaslin saw this 'marginal gliosis' as a primary proliferation of fibres that indicated the presence of a pathological process which underlies the epilepsy and could be compared to the formation of glial tumours. Alzheimer (1898), however, considered the gliosis to be a secondary reaction following the loss of nerve cells from the cortex. This controversy, like that about the hippocampus, continued for many years, and as Scholz (1959) emphasized, the hypothesis of a progressive cerebral process as the cause of idiopathic epilepsy was widely accepted until the major contribution from Spielmeyer in 1927. He had analysed both the nature and the pathogenesis of the neuronal and of the glial abnormalities in many epileptic brains and come down firmly on the side of those who saw the changes as secondary to the fits or, more precisely in his view, to the vascular spasm that was believed to occur at the onset of an epileptic attack. Although the precise mechanism proposed by Spielmeyer proved unacceptable, the view that the scarring and atrophy were the con-

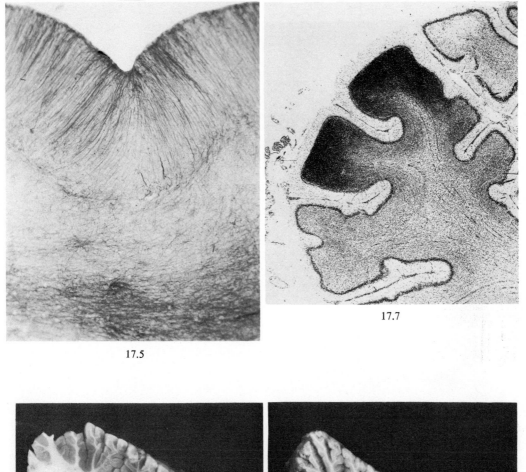

17.7

17.5

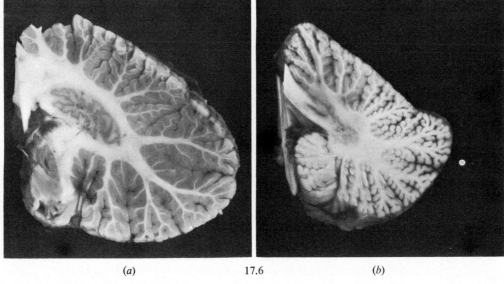

(a)   17.6   (b)

Fig. 17.5 Cerebellar cortex and subadjacent white matter showing an intense fibrous gliosis spreading through the molecular layer, less in the granular layer and more intense in the white matter. Holzer stain. × 110.

Fig. 17.6 (a) the normal cerebellum for comparison with (b), which shows the naked-eye appearance of atrophy that is not infrequently seen in chronic epileptic patients. In this case the folial atrophy is most marked in the posterior and inferior parts of the lateral lobe. (a) and (b) × 1·25.

Fig. 17.7 Cerebellar folia with extensive loss of Purkinje cells and almost complete destruction of the granular layer. A few deeply stained patches of surviving granular cells are seen. Cresyl violet. × 13.

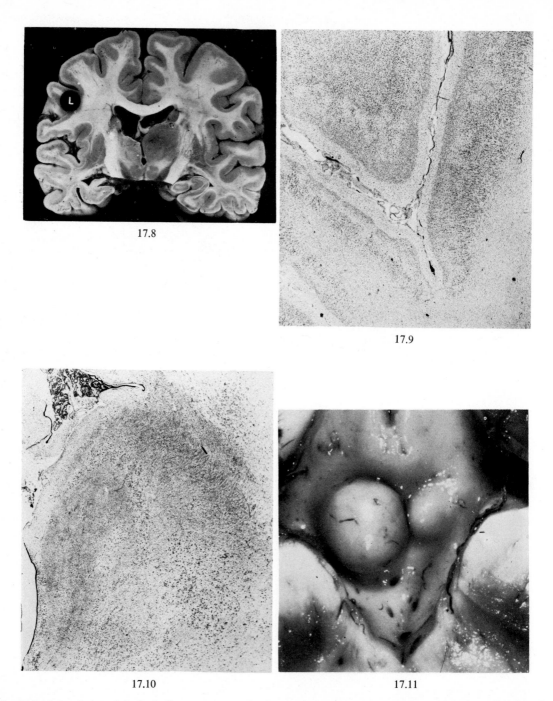

Fig. 17.8 Coronal view of the brain from a patient with long-standing epilepsy. The left hemisphere is smaller than the right, the hippocampus and the thalamus being particularly severely affected.   × 0·5.

Fig. 17.9 Patchy neuronal loss in the cortex of the convexity of the occipital lobe. Cresyl violet.   × 12.

Fig. 17.10 Medial part of the thalamus showing irregular areas of neuronal loss and dense glial proliferation, which has stained darkly. Cresyl violet.   × 15.

Fig. 17.11 Severe atrophy of the left mamillary body in the same specimen as shown in Fig. 17.8.   × 5.

sequence of interference with the blood and oxygen supply to certain parts of the brain persisted and was supported by Scholz (1951), and later by Peiffer (1963). Since the damage was, therefore, described as a result of the fits there was no contradiction in the fact that although this change was present the epilepsy was classified as cryptogenic.

This view of the inertness of the cerebral scarring was accepted for some years and it only began to be questioned, particularly in so far as the hippocampus was concerned, after psychomotor attacks and the electrical abnormalities associated with them had been found to occur in many patients with atrophy of the medial temporal grey matter (which includes the parahippocampal gyrus, the hippocampus, the uncus and the amygdaloid nucleus).

It was then postulated by Penfield and his colleagues that the hypoxia leading to the sclerosis was not the consequence of fits but that the initial damage had occurred during the process of birth, by deformation of the skull and herniation of the medial temporal gyri through the incisura of the tent. According to this view, the distortion of the brain impedes the blood supply via the branches of the posterior cerebral artery to the grey matter in and around the hippocampus, and the resultant scar, or 'incisural sclerosis' as it was called, becomes liable to ripen after months or years into an epileptogenic focus. Penfield, however, did not regard birth as the only time during which this damage could occur and Gastaut and his colleagues (1959) extended the concept to include other pathological events, such as a head injury or cerebral infarction. According to this view, the common factor was the development of cerebral oedema which led to transtentorial herniation with compression of the anterior choroidal and posterior cerebral arteries. This hypothesis was given added weight by Lindenberg (1955), who had concluded that 'a typical vascular sclerosis of the Ammon's horn generally signifies at least one phase of increased supratentorial pressure during the life of the individual'.

Although the hypotheses of Penfield and Gastaut were soon preferred by many to that of the German school there are cogent reasons why they should be questioned. Firstly, Ounsted et al. (1966) pointed out that the distribution of the damage, with the emphasis on the hippocampus and the almost invariable sparing of the calcarine cortex, is radically different from that which usually results from an obstruction of the posterior cerebral artery. Furthermore, the explanation also fails to take into account that damage of a similar nature is often encountered in other parts of the brain, well away from the tentorial opening and not lying in the territory of any vessel manifestly at risk in the same way as the posterior cerebral artery. Although the evidence quoted both for and against such hypotheses is too often drawn from studies of the mature rather than the developing brain, there is little doubt that the so-called hypoxic cerebral changes seen in epileptic children and in adults can develop in the absence of brain swelling: conversely, the changes that usually result from brain swelling are not merely those of hypoxia. Secondly, Veith (1970) found no evidence that herniation of the temporal lobes at birth could be held responsible for the neuronal changes that he had occasionally encountered in a histological study of several hundred infant brains. The reasons just given not only make Penfield's theory of the origin of incisural sclerosis difficult to accept, at least as the common causal mechanism, but also militate against the unqualified acceptance of that proposed by Gastaut.

The important fact in both hypotheses is the emphasis that they lay on the occurrence of some initial catastrophe at birth or in the first few years of life. Insults such as a severe infection or a head injury may well be important factors in some cases, but the most sinister event most commonly found to have occurred in epileptic patients with 'hypoxic' brain damage is the onset of the fits in infancy or in childhood (Falconer, Serafetinides and Corsellis 1964; Veith 1970). If the fits are serial or if status supervenes the outlook is particularly ominous, for there is then a good chance that irretrievable destruction of nerve cells will result and in due course scar tissue will form. A widely held view, which is essentially that taught by Scholz and latterly by Norman, attributes the selective damage in the brain to the hypoxia occurring during the course of these attacks. This remains compatible with the view that the scarring, however caused, is liable to perpetuate the attacks and by its localization to influence their clinical pattern (Margerison and Corsellis 1966).

The need remains, however, to define more precisely the course of the physiological events by which the pathological changes are produced. As McMenemey (1940) put it in another context, the morbid anatomist has only the battlefield to work on after the battle has been lost.

The result of experimental studies in sub-human primates (Meldrum and Horton 1973; Meldrum and Brierley 1973; Meldrum, Vigouroux and Brierley 1973) has been to emphasize other systemic and local cerebral changes, all of which tend to impair cerebral energy metabolism. Measurements of the physiological changes during drug-induced status epilepticus and the incidence and severity of ischaemic cell change in the perfusion-fixed brain a few hours after the episode of status, failed to show any correlation between the early transient systemic hypoxia and brain damage. On the other hand, physiological events occurring after 30 minutes of sustained seizure activity did show a relationship to brain damage. Hyperpyrexia and arterial hypotension appeared to play a critical role in producing cerebellar damage (i.e. ischaemic cell change in Purkinje and basket cells, especially in the boundary zone between the arterial territories of the superior cerebellar artery and the posterior inferior cerebellar artery). The incidence of ischaemic cell change in the neocortex, hippo-campus and thalamus was related to the total duration of seizure activity in the range $1\frac{1}{2}$ to 5 hours. An impaired neuronal energy metabolism results from the combination of excessive neuronal activity and the cumulative effects of secondary changes such as hypoxia, hypoglycaemia, arterial hypotension and hyperpyrexia. If the secondary changes are prevented or markedly diminished by peripheral muscular paralysis, neuronal changes can still occur in the neocortex, thalamus and hippocampus but only after relatively more pro-longed seizures (3 to 8 hours) (Meldrum *et al.* 1973). These experiments in sub-human primates have provided a good model in physiological and pathological terms for studying the lesions in man resulting from status epilepticus.

It is also possible experimentally to produce a pattern of damage that involves predominantly the hippocampus, and more closely resembles the lesions found in chronic epileptic patients and especially those with temporal lobe epilepsy (see below). In experimental primates this has been achieved by using allylglycine (an inhibitor of the cerebral enzyme glutamate decarboxylase (Horton and Meldrum 1973) to produce recurrent brief seizures (Meldrum and Brierley 1972; Meldrum, Horton and Brierley 1974). The generalized physiological changes associated with

a sequence of 26 to 62 brief tonic-clonic seizures in 8 to 13 hours are relatively mild, and the baboons appear neurologically normal 1 to 2 days later. However, examination of the hippo-campus after a 1 to 6 week survival period showed neuronal loss in the Sommer sector (h1) and the endfolium (h3) and an associated pro-liferation of fibrous astrocytes and microglia. As in temporal lobe epileptics the h1 lesions tended to be unilateral whereas the h3 lesions were symmetrical. Systemic factors such as hypoxia and arterial hypotension appeared to be less important than local factors secondary to the local epileptic activity. The appearance of hippo-campal lesions in cats after sustained limbic seizures induced by septal injections of ouabain supports this conclusion (Baldy-Moulinier, Arias and Passouant 1973). Swelling of astrocytic end-feet as a result of seizure activity (De Robertis, Alberici and De Lores Arnaiz 1969) or local increase in cerebral venous pressure could impede local capillary circulation, and thus induce ischaemic neuronal changes.

This newer experimental evidence therefore further supports the view that the physiological changes and the disturbed energy metabolism occurring during prolonged epileptic activity are able to cause irrevocable neuronal damage of the kind and distribution so long recognized in epi-leptic human patients.

Epilepsy and the temporal lobes

During the period in which the interpretation of the various histological abnormalities in the brains of epileptic patients was the subject of so much controversy, Hughlings Jackson and his colleagues (Anderson 1886; Jackson and Beevor 1889) described a complex pattern of epileptic attacks in which auras of smell or taste occurred. Feelings of unreality or familiarity and dream-like illusory experiences were also common. Visual hallucina-tions could display an organized scenic character. In the brains of several people with such symp-toms, focal abnormalities were found lying close to the hippocampus, but centred on the region of the uncus and the amygdaloid nucleus. Other workers confirmed these observations and the existence of a focal form of symptomatic epilepsy became established which was linked to the temporosphenoidal regions, much as the motor attacks of Jacksonian epilepsy had been associated with the frontal, and particularly with the pre-central cortex.

In 1935 Stauder claimed to have made a comparable correlation based on the hippocampus. He carefully analysed the nature of the attacks in 53 patients with long-standing epilepsy and found the Ammon's horn, or hippocampus, to be sclerotic in 36 of them. In all but three of these 36 the clinical picture had pointed to a lesion in the temporal lobes although in some brains there was also frontotemporal scarring of the contrecoup type. None of the 17 patients in whose brains the Ammon's horns were normal had shown signs of a temporal lobe disturbance.

Less attention was paid to Stauder's observations than to the more notable contribution by Hughlings Jackson, but both took on a new importance when the neurosurgical treatment of the focal epilepsies began to be combined with the use of the electroencephalogram. The introduction of this technique led to the identification of abnormal paroxysmal electric discharges in tracings obtained from epileptic patients and one particular type of these was claimed by Gibbs, Gibbs and Lennox in 1937 to be characteristic of what had by then come to be known as 'psychomotor epilepsy'. In 1951 Jasper, Pertuisset and Flanigin introduced the term 'temporal lobe seizures' to embrace the wide spectrum of complex attacks that could range from the dreamy states of Hughlings Jackson to the psychomotor epilepsies.

The common factor in the EEG records of patients suffering from temporal lobe seizures was the occurrence, during the interictal period, of spikes or sharp waves thought to originate in the affected temporal lobe (Jasper and Kershman 1941). This was an observation of great practical as well as theoretical importance since about half the epileptic patients living in long-stay hospitals were found to fall into the category of temporal lobe epilepsy (Liddell 1953; Gastaut 1954), even if the precise incidence depends on the definition of its clinical and electrical criteria (Margerison and Liddell 1961).

The next step was taken by the neurosurgeons, who began to remove the affected temporal lobe from such people and reports on the effects of the operation appeared at the beginning of the 1950s (Penfield and Flanigin 1950; Green, Duisburg and McGrath 1951). According to what was already known from post-mortem studies it was not unreasonable to expect that the resected tissue might be found to contain either the kind of focal abnormalities described by Hughlings Jackson or, conceivably, a sclerotic hippocampus. At first, however, there was little apparent incidence of any kind of lesion. In 1951 Bailey and Gibbs reported that they had failed to find anything abnormal in about half the 25 temporal lobes that they had resected. The figure given by Morris (1956) was of the same order while Haberland (1958) observed histopathological changes in only 19 out of 47 specimens; in 6 of the 19 the lesion was a typical Ammon's horn sclerosis.

Others however had been more successful, for in 1953 Earle, Baldwin and Penfield claimed to have found macroscopical or histological abnormalities in all the temporal lobes removed from 157 epileptic patients. In 57 of these cases a postnatal abnormality was found which was usually tumorous in nature or had occurred as a sequel to trauma or infection. In the remaining 100 cases, however, a variable degree of atrophy was found which could range from the shrinkage of a single convolution to that of the entire temporal lobe. The uncus, amygdaloid nucleus and the parahippocampal gyrus were the areas most often affected but the extent could not be precisely defined. This was partly because no systematic histological investigations had been undertaken and partly because the more medial grey matter, and particularly the hippocampus, was not included in the resected tissue. Nevertheless, the distribution and the nature of the atrophic changes seemed similar to those seen when an Ammon's horn sclerosis was present. Penfield and his colleagues, however, preferred to label the condition 'incisural sclerosis' since its origin, in their view, depended on the medial parts of the temporal lobes being displaced through the incisura during birth. Meyer, Falconer and Beck (1954) followed these positive observations with the statement that they too had found some kind of abnormality in all the 14 specimens they had examined. Crome (1955) was loath to accept that the degree of gliosis described in some of the cases was beyond the range of normal and further suggested that the epileptogenic significance of the sclerotic changes was doubtful. By 1958 Cavanagh, Falconer and Meyer had increased the number of cases to 50. They agreed that in about 30% the glial reaction was relatively slight and as Meyer commented in 1963 'it is certainly justifiable to doubt its value as a substrate of the psychomotor attacks and in not a few cases, it was of doubtful pathological significance altogether'. Other studies have been reported since then by Green and Scheetz (1964), Falconer *et al.* (1964) and Jann-Brown (1973) and the incidence of some kind of clearcut abnormality has settled down to about 75% of the specimens examined.

Although there are exceptions, there is a marked tendency for the abnormalities, irrespective of their nature, to lie deep in the temporal lobe and less often towards the convexity. It is these deeper limbic parts, which include the uncus, the amygdaloid nucleus and the hippocampus, that lie on the edge of most resections and are therefore liable to be sucked away or lost during the operation. At other times their removal may not have been intended. The tissue available for examination can therefore range from the full coronal extent of the temporal lobe with a major part of the amygdala and the hippocampus to no more than some part of the three temporal gyri. Abnormalities will therefore be found less often if only the latter, neocortical, areas are examined. This fact helps to explain the variable incidence that has been reported by different observers. It is also important to emphasize that not all lesions can be seen, or even suspected with the naked eye. A few may therefore be overlooked if the tissue is not sampled histologically at several levels, or occasionally by an interrupted run of serial sections.

The abnormalities may be divided into those which tend to be focal and those which are more diffuse. In the former there is a small number with cortical scarring following trauma (Cavanagh *et al.* 1958; Corsellis 1970), with a patch of old infarction or with evidence of past infection such as an abscess or rarely an encephalitis (Aguilar and Rasmussen 1960). The main focal group comprises abnormalities which range from small discrete masses, obvious to the naked eye, to aggregations of bizarre neurons and glia identifiable only under the microscope. The label of tumour is often inappropriate in this connection, at least without qualification, since the lesions appear to replace rather than to expand and indeed in most series patients suffering primarily from a cerebral tumour have been deliberately excluded. The masses that are found, even in patients with an epileptic history lasting for many years, are small, measuring a few millimetres to about two centimetres across. They may not be

identified at operation; very occasionally they are calcified. The lesions are usually single, but multiple islets of abnormal cells may be found. The histological picture varies greatly; the cellular population is usually mainly glial, appearing as an astrocytoma, an oligodendroglioma or as a mixed glial tumour (Cavanagh 1958) (Fig. 17.12). Not infrequently abnormal neurons are present and the overall picture resembles that of a ganglioglioma; less often the growth is predominantly vascular (Edgar and Baldwin 1960). There is usually little or no evidence of recent growth or of infiltration. Many of the masses seem therefore to be more in the nature of malformation than of neoplasm. The term hamartoma is applicable in many instances, although not invariably, since sometimes the mass appears frankly neoplastic while at others the lesion is clearly that of a malformation or 'hamartia'. Very occasionally patches of typical heterotopic grey matter are seen deep in the white matter. Another, and more common, abnormality is a form of cortical dysplasia in which large, and even giant, malformed neurons are scattered through one or more short runs of cortex and may be accompanied by bizarre glial cells spreading into the subjacent white matter (Fig. 17.13). These can at times be reminiscent histologically of the tuber in tuberous sclerosis, but there are usually many clinical and histological points of difference which make this diagnosis unacceptable (Taylor, Falconer, Bruton and Corsellis 1971). Perot, Weir and Rasmussen (1966) and others have, however, described classical tuber formation in tissue resected from epileptic patients with tuberous sclerosis.

Ammon's horn or hippocampal sclerosis is the diffuse type of abnormality (Fig. 17.14). This has been identified in 50 to 60% of resected temporal lobes and it is therefore the commonest lesion found. Its pathological features and its pathogenesis have been discussed in the previous sections and they will be reconsidered here only in so far as they may throw light on the role in epilepsy of the sclerotic hippocampus, or more correctly sclerosis of the medial temporal areas, since the scarring tends to spread out anteriorly to the amygdaloid nucleus (Fig. 17.15) and uncus as well as laterally into the parahippocampal gyrus and beyond. It is important to emphasize that there are other ways in which the hippocampus may be damaged besides the classical Ammon's horn sclerosis. Thus the hippocampus

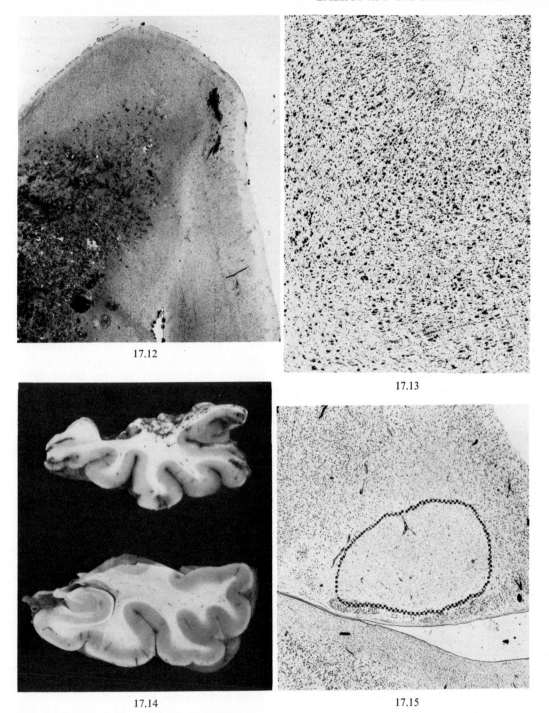

17.12

17.13

17.14

17.15

Fig. 17.12 Atypical glioma in the region of uncus and amygdaloid complex. Haematoxylin and eosin. ×8.

Fig. 17.13 Cortical dysplasia—a population of large anomalous neurons scattered through all but the first cortical layer. The cortical ribbon is widened and the lamination is lost. Cresyl violet. ×30.

Fig. 17.14 The upper view is of a temporal lobectomy specimen which has been cut coronally. A typical hippocampal sclerosis can be seen when compared with normal picture in the lower view.

Fig. 17.15 Part of the amygdaloid nucleus in a lobectomy specimen. A sizeable patch of neuronal loss is outlined. The edge of the resection is seen at the top right hand corner. Cresyl violet. ×20.

may be largely destroyed by atheromatous occlusion of the posterior cerebral artery or less severely by micro-infarcts due to the degeneration of its small vessels. It is also peculiarly liable to disintegrate with the almost total loss of the Sommer sector in senile dementia and in Alzheimer's disease (Morel and Wildi 1956; Corsellis 1957). Haymaker, Pentschew, Margoles and Bingham (1958) found no history of epilepsy in 21 infants with kernicterus in all of whose brains the large hippocampal neurons were destroyed. Similarly, they found that fits were a far from constant feature in a large series of infants with inclusion body encephalitis that had damaged the temporal lobes. In none of these conditions is the sporadic convulsion, let alone any form of long-standing epilepsy, particularly liable to appear. It is only when 'hypoxic' damage occurs, but does not kill during the acute stages, that the classical sclerosis will have time to develop and, as Penfield put it, ripen into a scar. It is in this situation, which is particularly prone to occur in the first few years of life, that the risk of an epilepsy becoming permanently established is greatest, whether or not fits or status epilepticus had occurred as a feature of the initial hypoxic episode. The hippocampal sclerosis may then be seen as part of a post-hypoxic scarring process which preferentially, but not exclusively, affects the medial temporal grey matter and which, like scarring elsewhere in the brain, may sooner or later lead to epileptic attacks which tend to be of a particular kind or constellation because of the pattern and localization. This hypothesis does not require either that temporal lobe seizures should inevitably follow the development of the scarring or that such damage should be the only determining factor. The genetic side is also important since a family history of epilepsy was found in nearly 40% of a group of epileptic patients with sclerosis of the Ammon's horn (Margerison and Corsellis 1966).

The clinicopathological problem is further complicated by the fact that no clear-cut structural abnormality can be found in about every fifth temporal lobe that is fully resected, but there are other possibilities. Sometimes the specimen is incomplete; it is also conceivable that lateralization had been wrong, while both Falconer, Driver and Serafetinides (1962) and Schneider, Crosby and Farhat (1965) have reported instances of temporal lobe epilepsy due to distant, extra-temporal lesions.

The most difficult histological problem, however, is set by findings which lie in the borderlands between normal and abnormal. The commonest of these is an apparent astrocytic proliferation with some degree of fibrous gliosis similar to that described by Chaslin (1889). This is usually seen most clearly in the subpial surface of the cortex and spreading into the deeper cortical layers, but the white matter and the amygdaloid nucleus may also be affected. This kind of glial reaction is most often seen when a typically sclerosed hippocampus is present and there is then no special problem. The difficulty arises when no hippocampal tissue is present, or when this is normal, or at least no more gliotic than the rest of the lobe. Crome (1955) was particularly critical of attributing any special importance to such uncertain changes which can vary from person to person with age and are not specific either to the temporal lobes or to the epileptic brain. It seems wisest therefore only to accept as abnormal a gliosis which is not only unquestionably severe but is also accompanied by neuronal loss. Unfortunately this is also notoriously difficult to estimate both in the neocortex and in the complex architecture of the uncus and the amygdaloid nucleus. In other words, these changes lie along a continuum and the point at which they become abnormal is an arbitrary one.

Finally, it is important that consideration of the temporal lobes should not lead to the exclusion of the rest of the brain. As Williams (1957) pointed out, the anatomical limits of the temporal lobe are artificial and 'the brain involved in the origin and spread of the epileptic events in temporal lobe epilepsy widely transcends the morphological boundaries of the temporal lobe'. The same is certainly true at times of the pathological changes. Nevertheless, even if the relation of structural abnormality to the epilepsy may be questioned in an individual case, it is in the temporal lobe that a lesion is most often found. Several reports, moreover, have pointed out that the abnormalities tend to lie in the limbic parts of the lobe. The same reports have also emphasized that the prognosis is materially better when these deeper areas are included in the resection and when they are found to include a focal lesion or to consist of a sclerosis of the hippocampus and the adjacent temporal grey matter (Falconer et al. 1964; Green 1967; Bengzon, Rasmussen, Gloor, Dussault and Stephens 1970; Jann-Brown 1973).

Cytological changes and epileptogenesis

Cerebral grey matter, when it is the focus of origin of epileptic discharges, shows a variety of cytological changes irrespective of the primary cause of the lesion (e.g. underlying tumour, infection, trauma, febrile convulsion, local ischaemia). Similar cytological changes are found in damaged grey matter that is not the substrate of epileptic activity. There are theoretical and speculative reasons for thinking that some of these changes may be involved in epileptogenesis but in no case is definite proof available.

It is natural to enquire if the reactive or fibrous astrocytes that are so abundant in these lesions could play a role in epileptogenesis. Normal astrocytes are believed to (a) transport glucose and various metabolic precursors from capillaries to neurons, (b) take up and metabolize various amino acid transmitters and (c) participate in the regulation of the ionic composition of the extracellular fluid. A failure in the latter function could be critical, as an increase in the extracellular fluid content of potassium can lead to local epileptiform discharges (Zuckermann and Glaser 1970). However, the resting potential of reactive astrocytes (in a freezing lesion) is very high (Grossman and Rosman 1971), indicating a high intracellular, and low extracellular, potassium concentration. Physiological studies of glial membrane properties in a focus have also provided evidence against the disordered potassium transport hypothesis (Glötzner 1973).

A loss of neurons is also characteristic and, although this is obviously non-selective in the centre of a traumatic lesion or abscess, in some situations there are elements of selectivity, especially when ischaemia is the intermediate agent. This creates the possibility of a partially selective destruction of inhibitory interneurons. Thus there is evidence that the spasticity that follows a period of spinal cord ischaemia results from the preferential destruction of inhibitory interneurons containing glycine (Werman, Davidoff and Aprison 1968). In the cerebellum the two types of cells (Purkinje and basket cells) that are selectively vulnerable to ischaemia (Brierley, Meldrum and Brown 1973) are both inhibitory (Curtis and Johnston 1974). For the neocortex such clear evidence is not yet available, but the third and fifth laminae—in which the smaller neurons tend to be vulnerable to ischaemia —do contain inhibitory interneurons. A loss of local inhibitory feedback could facilitate epileptic discharges.

Traumatic or space-occupying lesions may also partially de-afferent areas of cortex. Experimental undercutting of the cortex prolongs the afterdischarge that can be induced by electrical stimulation (Halpern 1972), suggesting that de-afferentation could be a significant factor in the genesis of a focus.

A loss of dendritic spines, identified in Golgi impregnations, can provide evidence of de-afferentation (Globus and Schiebel 1966). A reduction in dendritic branching and a loss of dendritic spines have been observed in the neurons in an epileptogenic focus induced by alumina cream in the sensorimotor cortex of rhesus monkeys (Westrum, White and Ward 1965; Ward 1969). A similar shrinkage of the apical dendrite system, loss of dendritic spines, and the appearance of terminal nodules have been described in hippocampal pyramidal neurons and dentate granular cells in temporal lobectomy specimens from patients with temporal lobe epilepsy (Scheibel and Scheibel 1973; Scheibel, Crandall and Scheibel 1974). It is possible that such pathologically altered neurons are abnormally excitable. They could be the histological counterpart of the 'epileptic neurons' identified electrophysiologically by Ward (1969).

Myoclonus epilepsy

Brief myoclonic contractions may affect a small group of muscle fibres, an individual muscle or many different muscles. The effect may therefore be too slight for a limb to move or it may throw a person to the ground.

Myoclonic contractions are common in epileptic patients; Muskens (1909) observed them in about two-thirds of all patients suffering from convulsions. Epilepsy and myoclonus, occurring together as a progressive, familial and often hereditary illness, were first reported by Unverricht (1891) and Lundborg (1903). Similar cases have been described by Lafora and Glück (1911), Westphal and Sioli (1921), Ostertag (1925), Hodskins and Yakovlev (1930) and van Bogaert (1949). More recent studies, including detailed chemical and electron-microscopical analyses, have been made by Seitelberger, Jacob, Peiffer and Colmant (1964), Seitelberger (1968), Kraus-Ruppert (1969) and Bergener and Gerhard (1970). The disease is rare; it is commoner in girls and usually begins between the ages of 10 and 16 years. The first sign is the onset of generalized, and often nocturnal, convulsions. Myoclonic jerks develop during the next few years and may gradually render the patient helpless. Dementia supervenes and the patient wastes away, death usually occurring 10 to 15 years after the onset. During the later stages the epilepsy may disappear while the myoclonus persists.

The pathological basis of this syndrome is varied and at times inconclusive. The most striking group of cases, and therefore the most fully documented (Seitelberger 1968), is that in which the brain appears only slightly atrophic and there is some diffuse neuronal loss with a mild fibrous gliosis. The salient feature is the presence of Lafora inclusion bodies. These appear as concentric rounded inclusions of varying size lying in the neuronal cytoplasm. Davison and Keschner (1940) described two types, homo-geneous and concentric. The homogeneous bodies are separated from the other contents of the cell body by a narrow capsule of unstain-able material; some have a central core of cruci-form or stellate shape. The concentric bodies have a deeply stained core with paler rings around this or with dark radial striae in the pale outer zone. Their size ranges from about 1 to 30 micrometres in diameter; there may be several in a single cell. Lafora and Glück (1911) pictured a cell of the vagal nucleus with one large and seven small inclusions, but so many is exceptional. They may be found in dendrites, axons or ap-parently free in the tissue. This last may indicate the loss of the parent cell, although their presence does not necessarily lead to cell degeneration and death, as Nissl granules are often normally present in the surrounding cytoplasm. Harriman and Miller (1955), in a careful histochemical study of these bodies, first showed them to contain an acid mucopolysaccharide. They are readily dis-tinguished from the Lewy inclusions of paralysis agitans in being basophilic with all stains, in giving γ metachromasia with methyl violet and toluidin blue, and in staining with the PAS method for one to two glycol groupings after extraction with solvents for lipid, hyaluronic acid and glycogen. Both the intraneuronal bodies and those found by Harriman and Millar in heart muscle and liver differ from amyloid, as commonly seen in tissue, in being basophilic and in failing to stain with Congo Red or to be aniso-tropic after this stain.

The distribution of Lafora bodies in the brain has varied considerably in the 40 or so cases so far reported (Seitelberger 1968). They occur throughout the cerebral cortex but are usually best seen in the central gyrus and the anterior frontal cortex. The thalamus, globus pallidus, and both zones of the substantia nigra tend to be heavily involved. The number drops lower down the brainstem, only scattered bodies being seen in the superior and inferior olives. The cerebellar cortex contains many and there may also be a patchy loss of Purkinje cells and granule cells with some glial increase. The dentate nucleus is one of the most severely affected regions, both because of the number of large Lafora bodies and the neuronal loss. Few bodies are seen below the medulla.

In some patients, however, the illness runs a similar course to that described but Lafora bodies are not found. Hodskins and Yakovlev (1930) found that they had been present in only 7 of the 19 cases reported up to that time. They were also absent from the example reported in 1949 by van Bogaert in his clinicopathological review of the condition. His case showed, in addition to the myoclonic and epileptic phenomena, an extrapyramidal syndrome reminiscent of paralysis agitans. The histological changes, which con-sisted of neuronal loss and gliosis, were most marked in the inferior olives, the compact zone of the substantia nigra and the centromedian nucleus of the thalamus, with less marked changes in the dentate nucleus and the cerebellar cortex. The cerebral cortex, Ammon's horn and corpus striatum were not involved. Van Bogaert was inclined to attribute the Parkinsonian-like features in his case to the nigral damage and the myoclonic features to the olivary and dentate involvement. More recently, Haltia, Kristensson and Sourander (1969) have recorded three Scandinavian cases in which the pattern of cerebral disease was merely that of widespread non-specific degenerative changes, mainly affecting the cerebellum, the medial thalamus and the peripheral nervous system. Another example was described by Matthews, Howell and Stevens (1969) in which only the cerebellum was affected.

The third group of cases consists of those in which the myoclonus is part of another cerebral disorder. It is, for example, common in subacute sclerosing panencephalitis and is seen in some cases of Creutzfeldt–Jakob disease. It is also encountered occasionally in the lipidoses, the leucodystrophies, in gliotic encephalopathy and in tuberous sclerosis (Crome and Stern 1972).

Myoclonus epilepsy (familial or sporadic) has also been found together with spinocerebellar degeneration. Dentatorubral atrophy, which Greenfield (1954) named 'the Ramsay Hunt syndrome', is an important example. In Hunt's (1921) case the cerebellar cortex was intact, the dentate nucleus was atrophic and the myelin was rarefied in the superior cerebellar peduncle. In a similar case of Louis-Bar and van Bogaert (1947) there was severe neuronal loss in the cerebellar nuclei with some loss of granule cells in the cortex. The superior olives, superior vestibular nuclei and the spinal root of the trigeminal nucleus were also atrophic; the superior cerebellar peduncle stained palely. In an earlier case of Hänel and Bielschowsky, quoted by Greenfield, the cerebellar cortex and the medullary olives were more severely affected than either the dentate nucleus or the superior cerebellar peduncles.

Action or intention myoclonus is sometimes a prominent feature of the 'Ramsay Hunt syndrome'. It is also seen in patients with ischaemic brain damage following cardiac arrest, asphyxia or blunt head injury (Lance and Adams 1963; Boudin, Pepin, Lauras, Masson and Barraine 1963). Correlative clinicopathological studies of myoclonus and hypoxic encephalopathy are lacking. Cerebellar damage is of course common after cerebral hypoxia, and it is found in other myoclonic syndromes. However, conventional neurological signs of cerebellar damage are often lacking. Clinical features such as chorea, athetosis and Parkinsonism, which suggest basal ganglia disease, may be present. The syndrome sometimes responds dramatically to the oral or intravenous administration of 5-hydroxytryptophan, the immediate precursor of serotonin (Lhermitte, Marteau and Degos 1972). This does not necessarily indicate, however, that the primary abnormality lies in the serotoninergic system. Neurons containing serotonin, the cell bodies of which lie in the nuclei of the median raphe, have terminals within the basal ganglia and their influence could be critically modified by pathological changes in either the cerebellum or basal ganglia.

The pathological basis of myoclonus is thus both aetiologically diverse and anatomically varied. Electrophysiological studies in patients (and in animals treated with excitant drugs) have been reviewed by Halliday (1967). Myoclonic activity can be differentiated according to the level showing abnormal responsiveness. In some cases of familial myoclonic epilepsy there is an apparent excessive responsiveness of the cortex which yields exceptionally high voltage responses following peripheral nerve stimulation. Pyramidal tract activity determines the myoclonus. In other patients the abnormality is within the extrapyramidal system, or can be demonstrated at the segmental or spinal level.

Convulsive treatment

The wide employment of convulsive therapy in psychiatry calls for a description of its pathology. In recent years the provocation of convulsions by chemical substances such as cardiazol and related drugs has been almost universally superseded by electroconvulsive treatment.

Fatalities from both chemical and electroconvulsive treatment have been in the main due to complications, particularly independent disease of the cardiovascular system. This emerges clearly in the review by Maclay (1953) and in the reports of Paarmann and Veltin (1955), Madow (1956), Gaitz, Pokorny and Mills (1956) and Stensrud (1958). A rare complication is fat embolism following bone fracture or mobilization of other fat depots (Meyer and Teare 1945; Paarman and Veltin). In electrically induced convulsions death may be due to faulty placing of the electrodes allowing the current to flow through the hind brain (Alexander and Löwenbach 1944). These same authors do not believe that the current, if used in therapeutic strength, is itself strong enough to cause irreversible damage of an appreciable degree. The prior injection of muscle relaxants may in certain circumstances act cumulatively with the anoxia resulting from the convulsions and thus prove dangerous or fatal (Maclay).

Much discussion and experimental work has been directed to the question whether uncomplicated convulsive therapy, particularly electroconvulsive therapy, causes brain damage. The problem has been reviewed by Corsellis and Meyer (1954). Most reviewers, including Alpers (1946) and Will, Rehfeldt and Neumann (1948), consider that irreversible damage in such uncomplicated cases is unlikely. Where experimental conditions approximated to 'therapeutic' dosage histological findings in the brains of animals were either negative or negligible (Cerletti and Bini 1940; Barrera, Lewis, Pacella and Kalinowsky 1942; Winkelman and Moore 1944; Alexander and Löwenbach 1944; Sickert, Williams and Windle 1950), or they were not severe (Neuburger, Whitehead, Rutledge and Ebaugh 1942; Lidbeck 1944; Ferraro and Roizin 1949). The problem has been investigated and comprehensively discussed also by Hartelius (1952), who found significant changes in nerve cells, blood vessels and glia, although by far the greater proportion of these seemed to be reversible. This does not preclude the possibility that occasionally, particularly after a large number of convulsions or after intensive treatment, mild changes of the kind seen after spontaneous convulsions may occur both in human patients and in experimental animals (Ferraro and Roizin 1949; Corsellis and Meyer 1954). Such changes may take the form of a marginal gliosis and astrocytic proliferation within the white matter. In a large material of brains of patients who had previously undergone electric shock treatment and had died from intercurrent disease, Ammon's horn sclerosis and lobular sclerosis of the cerebellum were never seen by Meyer. In the literature only one worker, Zeman (1950), has observed necrosis in Ammon's horn and the cerebellum, but in the few cases he studied the effect of the convulsions was aggravated by serious complications (endocarditis and pneumonia). Corsellis and Meyer concluded that the absence of appreciable neuronal loss in Ammon's horn, cerebellum and cerebral cortex was a further indication of the mildness of the sequelae which rarely may follow electrically induced convulsions. It is possible that the slight memory defect, which not infrequently lasts for some time, may in some cases be associated with these minimal changes.

References

Aguilar, M. J. & Rasmussen, T. (1960) Role of encephalitis in pathogenesis of epilepsy. *Archives of Neurology* (*Chicago*), **2**, 663-676.

Aicardi, J. & Baraton, J. (1971) A pneumonencephalographic demonstration of brain atrophy following status epilepticus. *Developmental Medicine and Child Neurology*, **13**, 660-667.

Aicardi, J. & Chevrie, J. J. (1970) Convulsive status epilepticus in infants and children. A study of 239 cases. *Epilepsia*, **11**, 187-197.

Aird, R. B., Venturini, A. M. & Spielman, P. M. (1967) Antecedents of temporal lobe epilepsy. *Archives of Neurology* (*Chicago*), **16**, 67-73.

Alexander, L. & Löwenbach, H. (1944) Experimental studies on electroshock treatment: the intracerebral vascular reaction as an indicator of the path of the current and the threshold of early changes within the brain tissue. *Journal of Neuropathology and Experimental Neurology*, **3**, 139-171.

Alpers, B. J. (1946) The brain changes associated with electrical shock treatment: a critical review. *Digest of Neurology and Psychiatry*, **14**, 136-137.

Alzheimer, A. (1898) Ein Beitrag zur pathologischen Anatomie der Epilepsie. *Monatschrift für Psychiatrie und Neurologie*, **4**, 345-369.

Anderson, J. (1886) On sensory epilepsy. *Brain*, **9**, 385-395.

Bailey, P. & Gibbs, F. A. (1951) Surgical treatment of psychomotor epilepsy. *Journal of the American Medical Association*, **145**, 365-370.

Baldy-Moulinier, M., Arias, L. P. & Passouant, P. (1973) Hippocampal epilepsy produced by ouabain. *European Neurology*, **9**, 333-348.

Barrera, S. E., Lewis, N. D. C., Pacella, B. L. & Kalinowsky, L. B. (1942) Brain changes associated with electrically induced seizures: Studies in Macacus rhesus. *Transactions of the American Neurological Association*, **68**, 31-35.

Bengzon, A. R. A., Rasmussen, T., Gloor, P., Dussault, J. & Stephens, M. (1968) Prognostic factors in the surgical treatment of temporal lobe epileptics. *Neurology* (*Minneapolis*), **18**, 717-731.

Bergener, M. & Gerhard, L. (1970) Myoklonuskörperkrankheit und progressive Myoklonusepilepsie. *Nervenarzt*, **41**, 166-173.

Bodechtel, G. (1930) Die Topik der Ammonshornschädigung. *Zeitschrift für die gesamte Neurologie und Psychiatrie*, **123**, 485-535.

Bouchet, C., & Cazauvieilh (1825) De l'épilepsie considereé dans ses rapports avec l'aliénatih mentale. *Archives générales de Médecine* (*Paris*), **9**, 510-542.

Boudin, G., Pepin, B., Lauras, A., Masson, S. & Barraine, R. (1963) Myoclonies intentionelles persistantes après réanimation cardiaque. *Revue Neurologique*, **109**, 468-472.

Brain, R. & Walton, J. N. (1969) *Diseases of the Nervous System*, 7th Edn., Oxford University Press, London.

Bridge, E. M. (1949) *Epilepsy and Convulsive Disorders in Childhood*, McGraw Hill, New York.

Brierley, J. B., Meldrum, B. S. & Brown, A. W. (1973) The threshold and neuropathology of cerebral 'anoxic-ischaemic' cell change. *Archives of Neurology (Chicago)*, **29**, 367-374.

Cavanagh, J. B. (1958) On certain small tumours encountered in the temporal lobe. *Brain*, **81**, 389-405.

Cavanagh, J. B., Falconer, M. A. & Meyer, A. (1958) Some pathogenic problems of temporal lobe epilepsy in *Temporal Lobe Epilepsy* (Eds. Baldwin, M. & Bailey, P.), pp. 140-148, Thomas, Springfield, Ill.

Cerletti, U. & Bini, L. (1940) Le alterazioni istopatologiche del sistema nervoso in seguito all E.S. *Rivista sperimentale di freniatria e medicina legale delle alienazioni mentale*, **64**, 311-359.

Chaslin, P. (1889) Note sur l'anatomie pathologique de l'épilepsie dite essentielle—La sclérose nevroglique. *Compte rendu des Séances de la Société de Biologie (Paris)*, **1**, 169-171.

Corsellis, J. A. N. (1957) The incidence of Ammon's horn sclerosis. *Brain*, **80**, 193-208.

Corsellis, J. A. N. (1970) The neuropathology of temporal lobe epilepsy in *Modern Trends in Neurology* (Ed. Williams, D.), pp. 254-270, Butterworth, London.

Corsellis, J. A. N. & Meyer, A. (1954) Histological changes in the brain after uncomplicated ECT. *Journal of Mental Science*, **100**, 375-383.

Crome, L. (1955) A morphological critique of temporal lobectomy. *Lancet*, **1**, 882-884.

Crome, L. & Stern, J. (1972) *Pathology of Mental Retardation*, Churchill Livingstone, Edinburgh and London.

Curtis, D. R. & Johnston, G. A. R. (1974) Amino acid transmitters in the mammalian central nervous system. *Ergebnisse der Physiologie*, **69**, 98-188.

Davison, C. & Keschner, M. (1940) Myoclonus epilepsy. *Archives of Neurology and Psychiatry (Chicago)*, **43**, 524-546.

De Robertis, E., Alberici, M. & De Lores Arnaiz, G. R. (1969) Astroglial swelling and phosphohydrolases in cerebral cortex of metrazol convulsant rats. *Brain Research*, **12**, 461-466.

Earle, K. M., Baldwin, M. & Penfield, W. (1953) Incisural sclerosis and temporal lobe seizures produced by hippocampal herniation at birth. *Archives of Neurology and Psychiatry (Chicago)*, **69**, 27-42.

Edgar, R. & Baldwin, M. (1960) Vascular malformation associated with temporal lobe epilepsy. *Journal of Neurosurgery*, **17**, 638-656.

Egdell, H. P. & Stanfield, J. P. (1972) Pediatric neurology in Africa: A Ugandan report. *British Medical Journal*, **1**, 548-552.

Falconer, M. A. (1974) Mesial temporal (Ammon's horn) sclerosis as a common cause of epilepsy. Aetiology, treatment and prevention. *Lancet*, **2**, 767-770.

Falconer, M. A., Driver, M. V. & Serafetinides, E. A. (1962) Temporal lobe epilepsy due to distant lesions: two cases relieved by operation. *Brain*, **85**, 521-534.

Falconer, M. A., Serafetinides, E. A. & Corsellis, J. A. N. (1964) Etiology and pathogenesis of temporal lobe epilepsy. *Archives of Neurology (Chicago)*, **10**, 233-248.

Ferraro, A. & Roizin, L. (1949) Cerebral morphologic changes in monkeys subjected to a large number of electrically induced convulsions (32-100). *American Journal of Psychiatry*, **106**, 278-284.

Fowler, M. (1957) Brain damage after febrile convulsions. *Archives of Disease in Childhood*, **32**, 67-76.

Frantzen, E. (1971) Round table discussion on febrile convulsions. *Epilepsia*, **12**, 191-194.

Gaitz, C. M., Pokorny, A. D. & Mills, M. (1956) Death following electroconvulsive therapy. *Archives of Neurology and Psychiatry (Chicago)*, **75**, 493-499.

Gastaut, H. (1954) in *Colloque sur les problèmes d'anatomie normale et pathologique posés par les décharges épileptiques*. Editions Acta Medica Belgica, Bruxelles, Belgium.

Gastaut, H., Meyer, A., Naquet, R., Cavanagh, J. B. & Beck, E. (1959) Experimental psychomotor epilepsy in the cat: Electro-clinical and anatomo-pathological correlations. *Journal of Neuropathology and Experimental Neurology*, **18**, 270-293.

Gastaut, H., Poirier, H., Salamon, G., Toga, M. & Vigouroux, M. (1960) H.H.E. syndrome. Hemiconvulsions, hemiplegia, epilepsy. *Epilepsia*, **1**, 418-447.

Gibbs, F. A., Gibbs, E. L. & Lennox, W. G. (1937) Epilepsy: A paroxysmal cerebral dysrhythmia. *Brain*, **60**, 377-388.

Globus, A. & Scheibel, A. B. (1966) Loss of dendritic spines as an index of presynaptic terminal patterns. *Nature*, **212**, 463-465.

Glötzner, F. L. (1973) Membrane properties of neuroglia in epileptogenic gliosis. *Brain Research*, **55**, 159-171.

Green, J. R. (1967) Temporal lobectomy with special reference to selection of epileptic patients. *Journal of Neurosurgery*, **26**, 584-593.

Green, J. R., Duisberg, R. E. H. & McGrath, W. B. (1951) Focal epilepsy of psychomotor type. A preliminary report of observations on effects of surgical therapy. *Journal of Neurosurgery*, **8**, 157-172.

Green, J. R. & Scheetz, D. G.   (1964) Surgery of epileptogenic lesions of the temporal lobe.   *Archives of Neurology (Chicago)*, **10**, 135-148.

Greenfield, J. G.   (1954) *The Spino-Cerebellar Degenerations*, Blackwell Scientific Publications, Oxford.

Grossman, R. G. & Rosman, L. J.   (1971) Intracellular potentials of inexcitable cells in epileptogenic cortex undergoing fibrillary gliosis after a local injury.   *Brain Research*, **28**, 181-201.

Haberland, C.   (1958) Histological studies in temporal lobe epilepsy based on biopsy materials.   *Psychiatria et Neurologia (Basel)*, **135**, 12-29.

Hall, J.   (1964) A pattern of convulsions in childhood.   *West Indian Medical Journal*, **13**, 244-248.

Halliday, A. M.   (1967) The electrophysiological study of myoclonus in man.   *Brain*, **90**, 241-284.

Halpern, L. M.   (1972) *Experimental Models of Epilepsy*.   *Chronic isolated aggregates of mammalian cerebral cortical neurons studied* in situ.   Raven Press, New York.

Haltia, M., Kristensson, K. & Sourander, P.   (1969) Neuropathological studies in three Scandinavian cases of progressive myoclonus epilepsy.   *Acta neurologica scandinavica*, **45**, 63-77.

Harriman, D. G. & Millar, J. H.   (1955) Progressive familial myoclonic epilepsy in three families: Its clinical features and pathological basis.   *Brain*, **78**, 325-349.

Hartelius, U.   (1952) Cerebral changes following electrically induced convulsions.   An experimental study on cats.   *Acta psychiatrica (Copenhagen)*, suppl. 77.

Haymaker, W., Pentschew, A., Margoles, C. & Bingham, W. G.   (1958) Occurrence of lesions in the temporal lobe in the absence of convulsive seizures, in *Temporal Lobe Epilepsy* (Eds. Baldwin, M. & Bailey, P.), Thomas, Springfield, Ill.

Hodskins, M. B. & Yakovlev, P. I.   (1930) Anatomico-clinical observations on myoclonus in epileptics and on related symptom complexes.   *American Journal of Psychiatry*, **9**, 827-848.

Horton, R. W. & Meldrum, B. S.   (1973) Seizures induced by allylglycine, 3-mercaptopropionic acid and 4-deoxypyridoxine in mice and photosensitive baboons, and different modes of inhibition of cerebral glutamic acid decarboxylase.   *British Journal of Pharmacology*, **49**, 52-63.

Hunt, J. R.   (1921) Dyssynergia cerebellaris myoclonica—primary atrophy of the dentate system.   *Brain*, **44**, 490-538.

Hunter, R. A.   (1959) Status epilepticus.   History, incidence and problems.   *Epilepsia (Amsterdam)*, **1**, 162-188.

Isler, W.   (1969) *Akute Hemiplegien und Hemisyndrome im Kindesalter*, Thieme, Stuttgart.

Jackson, H. & Beevor, C. E.   (1889) Case of tumour of the right temporo-sphenoidal lobe bearing on the localisation of the sense of smell and on the interpretation of a particular variety of epilepsy.   *Brain*, **12**, 346-357.

Jann-Brown, W.   (1973) Structural substrates of seizure foci in the human temporal lobe.   *UCLA Forum in Medical Sciences*, **17**, 339-374.

Janz, D.   (1964) Status epilepticus and frontal lobe lesions.   *Journal of the Neurological Sciences*, **1**, 446-457.

Jasper, H. & Kershman, J.   (1941) Electroencephalographic classification of the epilepsies.   *Archives of Neurology and Psychiatry*, **45**, 903-943.

Jasper, H., Pertuisset, B. & Flanigin, H.   (1951) E.E.G. and cortical electrograms in patients with temporal lobe seizures.   *Archives of Neurology and Psychiatry (Chicago)*, **65**, 272-290.

Jennett, W. B.   (1965) Predicting epilepsy after blunt head injury.   *British Medical Journal*, **1**, 1215-1216.

Jennett, W. B.   (1969) Early traumatic epilepsy.   *Lancet*, **1**, 1023-1025.

Jennett, W. B. & Lewin, W.   (1960) Traumatic epilepsy after closed head injury.   *Journal of Neurology, Neurosurgery and Psychiatry*, **23**, 295-301.

Ketz, E.   (1974) Brain tumours and epilepsy in *Handbook of Clinical Neurology*, **16**, (Eds. Vinken, P. J. & Bruyn, G. W.), pp. 254-269.   North Holland Publishing Co., Amsterdam.

Kirstein, L.   (1942) Epilepsie bei intrakraniellen expansiven Processen.   *Acta medica scandinavica*, **110**, 56-68.

Kraus-Ruppert, R.   (1969) Zur Frage der idiopathischen Randzonensiderose (Rosenthal) um Tierversuch.   *Zentralblatt für die allgemeine Pathologie*, **112**, 332-334.

Lafora, G. R. & Glück, B.   (1911) Beitrag zur Kenntnis der Alzheimerschen Krankheit oder Präsenilen Demenz mit Herdsymptomen.   *Zeitschrift für die gesamte Neurologie und Psychiatrie*, **6**, 1-20.

Lance, J. W. & Adams, R. D.   (1963) The syndrome of intention or action myoclonus as a sequel to hypoxic encephalopathy.   *Brain*, **86**, 111-136.

Legg, N. J., Gupta, P. C. & Scott, D. F.   (1973) Epilepsy following cerebral abscess—A clinical and EEG study of 70 patients.   *Brain*, **96**, 259-268.

Lennox-Buchthal, M. A.   (1973) *Febrile Convulsions*, Elsevier, Amsterdam.

Lennox, W. G., Gibbs, F. A. & Gibbs, E. L.   (1940) Inheritance of cerebral dysrhythmia and epilepsy.   *Archives of Neurology and Psychiatry (Chicago)*, **44**, 1155-1183.

Lessell, S., Torres, J. M. & Kurland, L. T.   (1962) Seizure disorders in a Guanamanian village.   *Archives of Neurology (Chicago)*, **7**, 37-44.

Lhermitte, F., Marteau, R. & Degos, C. F.   (1972) Analyse pharmacologique d'un nouveau cas de myoclonies d'intention et d'action post-anoxiques.   *Revue Neurologique*, **126**, 107-114.

Libdeck, W. J.   (1944) Pathological changes in the brain after electric shock.   *Journal of Neuropathology and Experimental Neurology*, **3**, 81-86.

Liddell, D. W.   (1953) Observations on epileptic automatism in a mental hospital population.   *Journal of Mental Science*, **99**, 732-748.

Lindenberg, R.   (1955) Compression of brain arteries as pathogenetic factor for tissue necroses and their areas of predilection.   *Journal of Neuropathology and Experimental Neurology*, **14**, 223-243.

Louis-Bar, D. & van Bogaert, L.   (1947) Sur la dyssynergie cérébelleuse myoclonique (Hunt).   *Monatschrift für die Psychiatrie und Neurologie*, **113**, 215-247.

Lund, M.   (1952) Epilepsy in association with intracranial tumour.   *Acta psychiatrica scandinavica, Suppl.*, 81.

Lundborg, H.   (1903) *Die Progressive Myoklonus-Epilepsie (Unverrichts Myoklonie)*, Almquist and Wiksells, Uppsala.

Maclay, W. S.   (1953) Death due to treatment.   *Proceedings of the Royal Society of Medicine*, **46**, 13-20.

Madow, L.   (1956) Brain changes in electroshock therapy.   *American Journal of Psychiatry*, **113**, 337-347.

Margerison, J. H. & Corsellis, J. A. N.   (1966) Epilepsy and the temporal lobes. A clinical, electroencephalographic and neuropathological study of the brain in epilepsy, with particular reference to the temporal lobes.   *Brain*, **89**, 499-530.

Margerison, J. H. & Liddell, D. W.   (1961) The incidence of temporal lobe epilepsy among a hospital population of long-stay female epileptics.   *Journal of Mental Science*, **107**, 909-920.

Matthews, W. B., Howell, D. A. & Stevens, D. L.   (1969) Progressive myoclonus epilepsy without Lafora bodies.   *Journal of Neurology, Neurosurgery and Psychiatry*, **32**, 116-122.

McMenemey, W. H.   (1940) Alzheimer's disease.   *Journal of Neurology and Psychiatry*, **3**, 211-240.

Meldrum, B. S.   (1975) Pathophysiology in *Textbook of Epilepsy*, Eds. Laidlaw, J. & Richens, A., Churchill-Livingstone, Edinburgh.

Meldrum, B. S. & Brierley, J. B.   (1972) Neuronal loss and gliosis in the hippocampus following repetitive epileptic seizures induced in adolescent baboons by allylglycine.   *Brain Research*, **48**, 361-365.

Meldrum, B. S. & Brierley, J. B.   (1973) Prolonged epileptic seizures in primates: Ischaemic cell change and its relation to ictal physiological events.   *Archives of Neurology (Chicago)*, **28**, 10-17.

Meldrum, B. S. & Horton, R. W.   (1973) Physiology of status epilepticus in primates.   *Archives of Neurology (Chicago)*, **28**, 1-9.

Meldrum, B. S., Horton, R. W. & Brierley, J. B.   (1974) Epileptic brain damage in adolescent baboons following seizures induced by Allylglycine.   *Brain*, **97**, 407-418.

Meldrum, B. S., Vigouroux, R. A. & Brierley, J. B.   (1973) Systemic factors and epileptic brain damage.   *Archives of Neurology (Chicago)*, **29**, 82-87.

Metrakos, K. & Metrakos, J. D.   (1974) Genetics of epilepsy in *Handbook of Clinical Neurology*, **15** (Eds. Vinken, P. J. & Bruyn, G. W.), North Holland Publishing Co., Amsterdam.

Meyer, A.   (1963) Epilepsy in *Greenfield's Neuropathology*, 2nd Edn., Arnold, London.

Meyer, A. & Beck, E.   (1955) Hippocampal formation in temporal lobe epilepsy.   *Proceedings of the Royal Society of Medicine*, **48**, 457-462.

Meyer, A. & Teare, D.   (1945) Cerebral fat embolism after electric convulsion therapy.   *British Medical Journal*, **2**, 42-44.

Meyer, A., Beck, E. & Shepherd, M. (1955) Unusually severe lesions in the brain following status epilepticus.   *Journal of Neurology and Psychiatry*, **18**, 24-33.

Meyer, A., Falconer, M. A. & Beck, E.   (1954) Pathological findings in temporal lobe epilepsy.   *Journal of Neurology and Psychiatry*, **17**, 276-285.

Millichap, J. G.   (1968) *Febrile Convulsions*, MacMillan, New York.

Millichap, J. G.   (1974) Metabolic and endocrine factors in *Handbook of Clinical Neurology*, **15**. (Eds. Vinken, P. J. & Bruyn, G. W.), pp. 311-324, North Holland Publishing Co., Amsterdam.

Morel, F. & Wildi, E.   (1956) Sclérose ammonienne et épilepsies (Étude anatomopathologique et statistique).   *Acta neurologica belgica*, **2**, 61-74.

Morris, A. A.   (1956) Temporal lobectomy with removal of uncus, hippocampus and amygdala.   *Archives of Neurology and Psychiatry (Chicago)*, **76**, 479-496.

Muskens, L. J. J.   (1909) Regional and myclonic convulsions.   *Epilepsia (Amst.)*, **1**, 161-178.

Neuburger, K. T., Whitehead, R. W., Rutledge, E. K. & Ebaugh, F. C.   (1942) Pathologic changes in the brains of dogs given repeated electric shocks.   *American Journal of Medical Science*, **204**, 381-387.

Norman, R. M.   (1964) The neuropathology of status epilepticus.   *Medical Science Law*, **4**, 46-51.

Ostertag, B.   (1925) Zur Histopathologie der Myoklonus epilepsie (Eine weitere Studie über die intragangliocellulären, corpusculären Einlagerungen).   *Archiv für Psychiatrie und Nervenkrankheiten*, **73**, 633-656.

Ounsted, C., Lindsay, J. & Norman, R.   (1966) *Biological factors in temporal lobe epilepsy.   Clinics in Developmental Medicine* 22, Heinemann Medical, London.

Oxbury, J. M. & Whitty, C. W. M.   (1971) Causes and consequences of status epilepticus in adults.   A study of 86 cases.   *Brain*, **94**, 733-744.

Paarmann, H. F., & Veltin, A.   (1955) Zur Frage tödlicher Komplikationen nach Elektroschock (Bericht über 3 Beobachtungen).   *Nervenarzt*, **26**, 106-111.

Peiffer, J.   (1963) *Morphologische Aspekte der Epilepsien*, Springer, Berlin.

Penfield, W., Erickson, T. C. & Tarlov, J.   (1940) Relation of intracranial tumours and symptomatic epilepsy.   *Archives of Neurology and Psychiatry (Chicago)*, **44**, 300-315.

Penfield, W. & Flanigin, H.   (1950) Surgical therapy of temporal lobe seizures.   *Archives of Neurology and Psychiatry (Chicago)*, **64**, 491-500.

Perot, P., Weir, B. & Rasmussen, T.   (1966) Tuberous sclerosis.   *Archives of Neurology (Chicago)*, **15**, 498-506.

Peterman, M. G.   (1950) Febrile convulsions in children.   *Journal of the American Medical Association*, **143**, 728-730.

Peterman, M. G.   (1952) Febrile convulsions.   *Journal of Pediatrics*, **41**, 536-540.

Pfleger, L.   (1880) Beobachtungen über Schrumpfung und Sklerose des Ammonshorns bei Epilepsie.   *Allgemeine Zeitschrift für Psychiatrie*, **36**, 359-365.

Radermecker, J.   (1974) Epilepsy in the degenerative diseases in *Handbook of Clinical Neurology*, (Eds. Vinken, P. J. & Bruyn, G. W.) North Holland Publishing Co., Amsterdam.

Richardson, E. P., Dodge, P. R. & Victor, M.   (1954) Recurrent convulsive seizures as a sequel to cerebral infarction; a clinical and pathological study.   *Brain*, **77**, 610-638.

Rose, A. L. & Lombroso, C. T.   (1970) Neonatal seizure states.   *Pediatrics*, **45**, 404-425.

Russell, W. R. & Whitty, C. W. M.   (1952) Studies in traumatic epilepsy.   I. Factors influencing the incidence of epilepsy after brain wounds.   *Journal of Neurology, Neurosurgery and Psychiatry*, **15**, 93-98.

Sano, K. & Malamud, N.   (1953) Clinical significance of sclerosis of the Cornu Ammonis.   *Archives of Neurology and Psychiatry (Chicago)*, **70**, 40-53.

Scheibel, M. E., Crandall, P. H. & Scheibel, A. B.   (1974) The hippocampal-dentate complex in temporal lobe epilepsy.   *Epilepsia*, **15**, 55-80.

Scheibel, M. E. & Scheibel, A. B.   (1973) Hippocampal pathology in temporal lobe epilepsy.   A Golgi survey.   *UCLA Forum in Medical Sciences*, **17**, 311-337.

Schneider, R. C., Crosby, E. C. & Farhat, S. M.   (1965) Extratemporal lesions triggering the temporal lobe syndrome.   The role of Association Bundles.   *Journal of Neurosurgery*, **22**, 246-263.

Scholz, W.   (1951) *Die Krampfschädigungen des Gehirns*, Springer, Berlin.

Scholz, W.   (1959) The contribution of patho-anatomical research to the problem of epilepsy.   *Epilepsia (Amsterdam)*, **1**, 36-55.

Seitelberger, F.   (1968) *Pathology of the Nervous System*, Vol. 1 (Ed. Minckler, J.), McGraw Hill, New York.

Seitelberger, F., Jacob, H., Peiffer, H. J. & Colmant, H. T.   (1964) Die Myoklonuskörperkrankheit.   Eine angeborene Störung des Kohlenhydratstoffwechels.   Klinisch-pathologische Studie an fünf Fällen.   *Fortschritte in Neurologie und Psychiatrie*, **32**, 305-345.

Serafetinides, E. A. & Dominian, J.   (1963) A follow-up study of late-onset epilepsy.   I. Neurological findings.   *British Medical Journal*, **1**, 428-431.

Sickert, R. G., Williams, S. C. & Windle, W. F.   (1950) Histologic study of the brains of monkeys after experimental electric shock.   *Archives of Neurology and Psychiatry (Chicago)*, **63**, 79-86.

Sommer, W.   (1880) Erkrankung des Ammonshornes als aetiologisches Moment der Epilepsie.   *Archiv für Psychiatrie und Nervenkrankheiten*, **10**, 631-675.

Spielmeyer, W.   (1927) Die Pathogenese des epileptischen Krampfes.   *Zeitschrift für die gesamte Neurologie und Psychiatrie*, **109**, 501-520.

Stauder, K. H.   (1935) Epilepsie und Schläfenlappen.   *Archiv für Psychiatrie und Nervenkrankheiten*, **104**, 181-211.

Stensrud, P. A.   (1958) Cerebral complications following 24,562 convulsion treatments in 893 patients.   *Acta psychiatrica scandinavica*, **33**, 115-126.

Taylor, D. C., Falconer, M. A. Bruton, C. J. & Corsellis, J. A. N.   (1971) Focal dysplasia of the cerebral cortex in epilepsy.   *Journal of Neurology, Neurosurgery and Psychiatry*, **34**, 369-387.

Unverricht, H.   (1891) *Die Myoklonie*, Deuticke, Leipzig and Vienna.

van Bogaert, L. (1949) Sur l'épilepsie myoclonie progressive d'Unverricht-Lundborg; étude d'un cas anatomique et de la semiologie du syndrome amyostatique terminal.   *Monatschrift für die Psychiatrie und Neurologie*, **118**, 170-191.

Veith, G.   (1970) Anatomische Studie über die Ammonshornsklerose im Epileptikergehirn.   *Deutsche Zeitschrift für Nervenheilkunde*, **197**, 293-314.

Wallace, S. J.   (1972) Aetiological aspects of febrile convulsions.   Pregnancy and perinatal factors.   *Archives of Disease in Childhood*, **47**, 171-178.

Wallace, S. J. & Zealley, H.   (1970) Neurological, electroencephalographic and virological findings in febrile children.   *Archives of Disease in Childhood*, **45**, 611-623.

Ward, A. A.   (1969) in *Basic Mechanisms of the Epilepsies* (Eds. Jasper, H. H., Ward, A. A. & Pope, A.), Little, Brown, Boston.

Werman, R., Davidoff, R. A. & Aprison, M. H.   (1968) Inhibitory action of glycine on spinal neurons in the cat.   *Journal of Neurophysiology*, **31**, 81-95.

Westphal, A. & Sioli, F.   (1921) Weitere Mitteilung über den durch eigenartige einschliessende Ganglienzellen (Corpora amylacea) ausgezeichneten Fall von Myoklonusepilepsie.   *Archiv für Psychiatrie und Nervenkrankheiten*, **63**, 1-36.

Westrum, L. E., White, L. E. & Ward, A. A.   (1965) Morphology of the experimental epileptic focus. *Journal of Neurosurgery*, **21**, 1033-1046.

Whitty, C. W. M.   (1961) Focal epilepsy and the study of cortical function.   *Medical Journal of Australia*, **1**, 1-8.

Will, O. A., Rehfeldt, F. C. & Neumann, M. A.   (1948) A fatality in electroshock therapy.   *Journal of Nervous and Mental Disease*, **107**, 105-126.

Williams, D.   (1957) The temporal lobe and epilepsy in *Modern Trends in Neurology*, **2** (Ed. Williams, D.), pp. 338-350, Butterworth, London.

Winkelman, N. W. & Moore, M. T.   (1944) Neurohistologic changes in experimental electric shock treatment. *Journal of Neuropathology and Experimental Neuropathology*, **3**, 199-209.

Zeman, W.   (1950) Zur Frage der Hirngewebeschädigung durch Heilkrampfbehandlung.   *Archiv für die Psychiatrie und Nervenkrankheiten*, **184**, 440-457.

Zimmerman, H. M.   (1938) Histopathology of convulsive disorders in children.   *Journal of Pediatrics*, **13**, 659-890.

Zuckerman, E. C. & Glaser, G. H.   (1970) Slow potential shifts in dorsal hippocampus during epileptogenic perfusion of the inferior horn with high-potassium CSF.   *Electroencephalography and Clinical Neurophysiology*, **18**, 236-246.

18

Ageing and the Dementias

Revised by J. A. N. Corsellis

The application of general pathological principles to the investigation of the human nervous system soon led to the identification of a wide range of abnormalities in the gross and in the microscopic structure of the brain. Many of these have come to be linked not only to neurological disease but also, with varying degrees of success, to psychiatric disorders and in particular to the dementias.

Webster had already in the 1840s made careful observations on patients who had become demented and the main features of General Paralysis of the Insane began to be delineated at much the same time (Hare 1959). It was not, however, until nearer the turn of the century that improvements in microscopy led to the first attempts at unravelling the neurohistological basis of mental disorders. Alzheimer in 1898 confirmed Virchow's insistence on the general importance of vascular degeneration by demonstrating its particular relevance to the brain in the insanities of the aged. Within the next few years, moreover, the histological bases of Pick's lobar atrophy and Huntington's chorea as well as cerebral arteriosclerosis and the senile form of cerebral degeneration were established, largely under Alzheimer's influence.

In all these conditions there was a notable tendency for the sufferers to become demented. General paralysis of the insane proved to be exceptional in that it was found to be the result of an infection, but the others shared a common factor in that no cause for them could be identified. Since, however, they all tended to develop in middle or later life they came to be linked by clinicians and by pathologists to the process of senile involution. This association was strengthened by the demonstration of histological stigmata, such as the 'senile plaque' and the lipochrome-laden nerve cell, which occurred not only in 'normal' ageing but became particularly prominent in certain disease processes.

These observations fitted in with Gowers' (1902) hypothesis that in some people a premature degeneration or ageing of tissue took place which was particularly liable to affect the nervous system. He gave as examples paralysis agitans, Friedreich's ataxia and 'simple mental failure'. Gowers' idea was not new, for Cheyne had already written in 1725 that 'some chronical disorders are such . . . by being hereditary and interwoven with the principle of life as never to be overcome'. This clearly foreshadows the term 'heredo-degenerative disease' which is intended to cover those conditions in which one or more components of nervous tissue in certain people or in certain families start to disintegrate too soon in life or too extensively. The pattern of the degenerative process, however, varies according to the condition. In some, such as Alzheimer's disease, it tends to be diffuse; in others, such as Huntington's chorea or Pick's disease, the brunt of the pathological process falls on certain areas, systems or cell grouping in the nervous system. The reason why only certain pathways or types of cell are vulnerable in a given condition remains unknown. It is nevertheless likely that, while in some a genetic or inborn chemical anomaly is of overriding importance, environmental factors play an important part in others. Thus the pigmented cells in the substantia nigra degenerate in paralysis agitans for no known reason and yet the same cells are also vulnerable following certain viral infections or even as a result of repeated cerebral trauma. In other words, when Cooke wrote in 1685 of 'the antecedents of a disease which though at present they act not yet they may generate a disease' he was expressing the view that a degenerative process could be 'lit up' by an environmental cause. Kuru, for example, when first identified a few years ago had many of the clinical and histological hallmarks of a heredo-degenerative condition and yet it is now known to be transmissible. Much the same is true of the Creutzfeldt–Jakob form of presenile cerebral degeneration which has several times been passaged to animals by the intracerebral injection of diseased human brain tissue. These are perhaps extreme examples but they illustrate that both intrinsic and extrinsic factors have to be considered in the aetiology of the presenile degenerative diseases.

Furthermore, individuals faced with organic disease either of the body or of the brain vary greatly in their liability to develop clinical evidence of this, and the disorganization of cerebral tissue can seemingly be far advanced in some people before an effect on the intellect or on behaviour becomes apparent. The converse is also true at times and although extreme discordance between clinical and pathological observations on the brain is exceptional, too precise a connection between the two is not to be expected, at least until more subtle methods both of psychological assessment and of pathological measurement are established.

Dementia

'The dement is a man deprived of possessions that he once enjoyed, he is a rich man becoming poor' (Esquirol 1838). As the deterioration progresses, the personality coarsens, and the intellect and the memory become impaired. Eventually the disintegration is extreme; the person is demented.

Although there are exceptions, which will be discussed later, dementia is commonly held to be the result of the more or less extensive destruction or disorganization of the cerebral cortex by one or other pathological process. Both the concomitant neurological picture and the salient clinical features of the dementia may, however, be influenced by the nature of the process, by the speed with which it develops and the extent to which the tissue damage is localized.

The common conditions in which dementia is most liable to occur are the two degenerative processes that tend to affect the brain in later life. In the first, the blood vessels degenerate and the blood supply to the brain is reduced. If this is severe enough, destruction of tissue, particularly in the areas supplied by the affected vessels, will follow. In the second, the cerebral tissue

generally, and particularly the cerebral grey matter, is liable to disintegrate more or less diffusely. These parenchymatous senile changes are generally considered to have little or no relation to the known forms of cerebrovascular disease and are usually brought together as the 'senile form of cerebral degeneration'.

The age at which both the vascular and the senile forms begin to appear varies considerably from one person to another. As a general rule, the prevalence increases rapidly after the sixties have been reached. Both forms of degeneration may be found in the same brain, but one or other is usually dominant, the senile form often occurring in the presence of negligible vascular degeneration while the converse is also true at times, particularly in the less elderly in whom the emphasis may be entirely on the vascular side.

In general, the more extensively a brain has been altered by these degenerative processes, the more likely is a person to become demented. The clinical picture, however, may vary according to whether the vascular or the senile form of degeneration predominates, and the two processes will first be considered separately.

Cerebral degeneration on a vascular basis

The blood supply to the brain passes from the heart and the aortic arch through the carotid and vertebral vessels within the neck and skull and into the main arterial branches of the brain up to the finest intracerebral twigs. It is the large cerebral vessels, forming the circle of Willis, however, that are the most often examined at autopsy, and the extent of cerebrovascular degeneration tends to be based more on their examination than on that of other parts of the vascular tree. A few flecks of atheroma are commonly found along the main cerebral arteries of people who have died in their sixties or later. They are much less common before this age. At times the atheroma and the mural thickening are considerably more marked; occasionally the main arteries at the base have changed into rigid, tortuous, yellowish tubes of confluent atheroma. Their lumina may be greatly narrowed but at times they are dilated. Atheromatous plaques may occasionally also extend along the branches of the middle cerebral artery on to the convexity of the brain.

The more severe the vascular degeneration, the more likely it is that breakdown of cerebral tissue will follow. This ranges from small scattered infarcts and cystic softenings to massive necrosis and scarring of a hemisphere following the occlusion of a major artery. The middle cerebral artery and its branches are commonly affected, while the anterior cerebral arteries, although they may be atheromatous and stenosed, are seldom occluded or the origin of gross infarction. In contrast, severe stenosis or occlusion of one posterior cerebral artery, with loss of tissue in the medial temporal grey matter and along and adjacent to the walls of the calcarine fissure, is not uncommon. Bilateral damage with this distribution has occasionally been recorded and may contribute to severe disorders of memory (Victor, Angevine, Mancall and Fisher 1961).

Although widespread damage on a vascular basis is present, the dementia cannot be attributed merely to the effects of the degeneration of the major cerebral arteries. On the one hand, many people who were not demented in life are found to have severely degenerated and stenosed cerebral vessels. Conversely, the degree of cerebral atherosclerosis can be relatively slight even in patients thought to have been demented as a consequence of large vessel disease. The condition of the small, intracerebral vessels must, therefore, also be considered, particularly in so far as it may have led to micro-infarcts and the loss of brain substance.

The changes in both large and small cerebral arteries and the arterioles have already been considered in Chapter 3. Briefly, the walls of the small vessels tend to thicken with increasing age as the fibrous tissue in the outer layers becomes more prominent. At times, possibly influenced by a rising blood pressure, the wall becomes hyaline. When severely affected, both it and the surrounding tissue becomes necrotic. In the corpus striatum and in the thalamus this perivascular rarefaction may lead to a porous or sieve-like appearance. Similarly, patches or streaks of neuronal loss and gliosis may be scattered through the cerebral cortex. Occasionally the loss of tissue and scarring is severe enough to give a roughened granular appearance to the cortex when stripped of leptomeninges. Cystic softenings and micro-infarcts are particularly common among the rostral groupings of the pontine nuclei; multiple small infarcts are also common in one or both hippocampal formations. Occasionally irregular, poorly defined areas of demyelination are found predominantly in the deep white matter of the hemispheres.

Degeneration of the small cerebral vessels can

therefore lead to extensive loss of cerebral tissue and, as Marchand (1949) suggested, this form of extensive but subtle change involving the smaller vessels may be more important than the major infarct in giving rise to mental symptoms. The emphasis laid by Rothschild (1942) and Coiffu (1958) on lesions in the striatal and thalamic regions was discounted, however, by Tomlinson, Blessed and Roth (1970), who did not find them a predominant feature in 'arteriosclerotic dementia'. In practice, it is exceptional in the aged brain to encounter a marked degree of vascular degeneration which is restricted either to the large or to the small vessels.

A further cause of dementia on a vascular basis, which has been put forward (Fisher 1951), is the reduction of cerebral blood flow that may arise from stenosis or occlusion of the carotid and vertebral arteries in their course through the neck or through the bony channels of the skull. The demonstration by Yates and Hutchinson (1961) that severe cerebral damage results more often than had been realized from such extracerebral arterial disease gave indirect support to this hypothesis. When, however, the entire vascular tree is examined in demented and in non-demented patients of a similar age range, stenosis of the vessels in the neck or in the skull is rarely found in the absence of comparable degeneration of the cerebral vessels (Corsellis and Evans 1965; Worm-Petersen and Pakkenberg 1968).

In summary, therefore, most patients with 'arteriosclerotic dementia' have evidence of widespread arterial disease which has affected both the large and the small cerebral vessels. Moreover, the involvement of the nervous system is usually only one part of a more widespread degenerative process. Hypertension, cardiac disease and many other forms of physical illness common in the elderly may add to the picture by interfering, possibly intermittently, with the blood supply to the brain. Running parallel with these complications is the further possibility that diffuse cerebral degeneration of the senile type may also be taking place. In short, there is little doubt that the role of vascular disease as a cause of dementia has been overestimated in the past and that the senile form is the more important (Hachinski, Lassen and Marshall 1974).

The senile form of degeneration

As age advances the brain, in company with other organs of the body, tends to become smaller

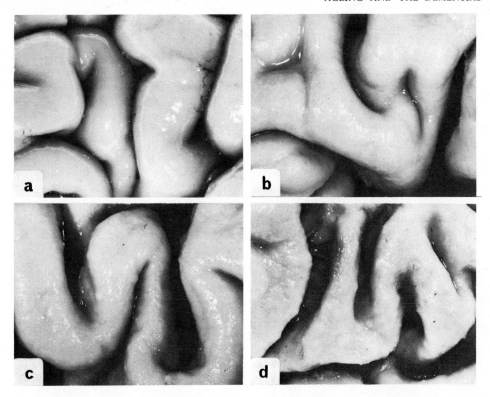

Fig. 18.1 The operculum of the frontal convexity enlarged × 3·25 (*a*) shows the normal appearance, with the degree of atrophy increasing through *b* and *c* to severe in *d*.

while the leptomeninges, mainly over the convexity, thicken and become more opaque. The dura mater adheres tightly to the skull. The cerebral convolutions, particularly of the frontal and temporal lobes, shrink and the main sulci, including the lateral fissure, become widened. This gyral atrophy is best seen when the leptomeninges are peeled off (Fig. 18.1). On cutting an atrophied brain coronally, the ventricular dilatation, the gaping of the lateral fissures and the opening up of the sulci will be obvious (Fig. 18.2). The cortical ribbon may also appear narrowed although the assessment of this in a slight degree is difficult and may be unreliable. The loss of white matter, which is reflected in the size of the ventricles, is often more apparent. It is because of the quantity of cerebrospinal fluid that envelops the atrophied brain that a subdural haematoma, or perhaps a tumour, may grow to some size before producing symptoms.

The weight and the volume of the brain normally reach their highest figures in early adult life and seem to decline from the forties, or possibly the thirties. Neither measurement is made accurately in practice and both should be looked

on as no more than useful pointers to possible abnormality unless the variation is extreme. As Cobb (1965) put it, 'only very small brains are inadequate and very large brains have no advantage over medium-sized ones'. Both weight and

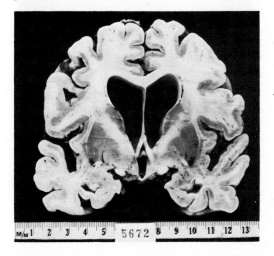

Fig. 18.2 Coronal view of the brain of a demented woman aged 78, showing considerable atrophy and enlargement of the anterior horns of the lateral ventricles.

volume may change noticeably during fixation, an increase of about 10% being usual in formalin.

Figures for brain weights in the different decades of life vary according to the source (e.g. von Braunmühl 1957; Blinkov and Glezer 1968). In the young adult male an average figure may be taken as 1400 g; by the forties the figure is around 1375 g and this subsequently drops to the 1200 to 1300 g level. The average female brain weight is roughly 100 g lower throughout adult life.

In contrast, the brain is often found to be considerably smaller in the dementias of old age. The brain shrinks away from the skull and the loss of tissue becomes obvious (Fig. 18.3). Along with this loss of grey and white matter, the ventricular system tends to enlarge although, as with all other

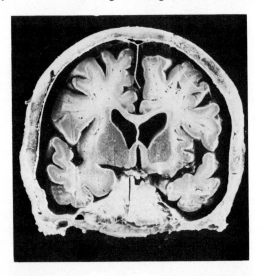

Fig. 18.3 A coronal cut through the skull and brain to show the marked loss of cerebral tissue that occurs in the presence of atrophy.

changes linked to age, the variations are considerable. Morel and Wildi (1955) found that the ventricular system in men is slightly larger than that of women, while, as shown many years ago, in both sexes the left lateral ventricle tends to be slightly larger than the right.

These gross alterations in the brain have their counterparts in the histological picture. These are most clearly seen in the severer degrees of cortical atrophy. The nerve cells get smaller; there is less Nissl substance and it stains less intensely. Although traces of pigment resembling lipofuscin may be found in some neurons in the spinal cords of children, and even of the fetus (Humphrey 1944), the typical pigment begins to accumulate in

appreciable quantities only in the adult. Brody (1960) found a sharp increase with age in the number of cortical neurons which contained scattered pigment, but only in a minority were the large clumps formed. The highest percentage of heavily pigmented cells was found in the precentral gyrus in which the neurons tend to be large; the figure was lowest in the striate cortex in which there is a high proportion of small cells. The amount varied greatly in other parts of the brain. The Purkinje cells, for example, and certain of the smaller celled nuclei in the brainstem show little or none and may be described as 'lipophobic'. In contrast, large amounts may be found in the cells of the cranial and spinal motor nuclei, in the red nucleus, in parts of the thalamus and in the globus pallidus; the inferior olive and the dentate nucleus are exceptionally vulnerable (Friede 1962). Lipofuscin is an acid-fast lipid pigment containing protein. Its constitution is not, according to Friede, precisely defined and may indeed vary within the same brain. Its chemical nature and its postulated origin from lysosomes is discussed fully by Adams (1965) and by Pearse (1972). Zeman (1971) has recently described a condition in which excessive accumulation of lipofuscin and severe neuronal loss occur in the absence of the other common features of senescence. These include the argyrophilic or senile plaques, the neurofibrillary tangles, and granulovacuolar degeneration, all of which are described later.

In addition to the neuronal alterations in the ageing and atrophic cerebral cortex, some degree of neuronal loss is also likely. There is, however, no exact way of measuring the extent of cortical atrophy either by naked eye or under the microscope. The severer degrees are obvious for the cortical ribbon narrows and the histological picture is that of a considerable loss of neurons. Indeed, it is this loss, and the resultant disorganization of cortical connections and activity, that probably lie at the root of the intellectual disintegration of the dement. It is less certain, however, whether there is a general trend for the neuronal population either in the cerebral cortex or elsewhere in the brain to diminish insidiously and progressively throughout adult life. Some studies have indicated this. Ellis (1920) estimated the Purkinje cell population at different ages and found a drop of about a quarter in those dying over the age of 50 compared with those under 40. The drop was even greater between the two extremes of adult life. Brody (1955) found a similar decrease with age in counts carried out on several regions of cerebral cortex, the most vulnerable area being the superior temporal gyrus. Burns (1958) concluded from studies such as these, and from the knowledge that the brain weight tends to drop with age, that 'every day of our adult life more than 100,000 neurons die'. This calculation has not been accepted without question. Thus, Konigsmark and Murphy (1970) found no evidence of a drop with age in the number of neurons in the human be, as Brody claimed, a tendency for certain neuronal populations in man to drop as age advances. The difficult thing is to prove it, largely because of the technical problems involved in comparing the numbers of nerve cells in brains of different sizes. It is indeed unlikely that anything approaching a final answer will be given until electronic techniques for the large-scale statistical study of cell populations have been devised.

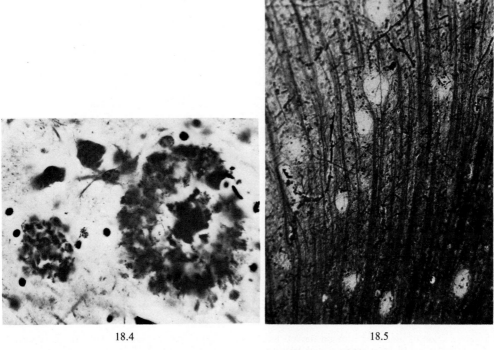

18.4   18.5

Fig. 18.4   Argyrophilic or 'senile' plaque formation in cortex, von Braunmühl silver impregnation.
Fig. 18.5   Senile plaques in deeper layers of cortex, shown up by Heidenhain's stain for myelin.

ventral cochlear nucleus and they emphasized that there is still no conclusive evidence that the loss of brain weight, volume or function in the later decades of life is due to neuronal loss. Others have also failed to identify a loss either in man or in animals, and Hanley (1974) in a recent comprehensive review of the question concluded on the present evidence that the various 'negative results seem to dispose of neuronal fall-out with ageing as a *universal* effect, but leaves open the possibility that a particular animal species, or nervous tissue from particular regions of the brain, could be specially vulnerable'. Put another way, there may

The main alteration in the glial picture is the gradual increase of astrocytic fibres over much of the subpial surface of the cortex, in the subependymal regions and around small vessels both in the cortical and the deep grey matter. There is also a tendency for astrocytes to become more prominent, and to proliferate, in these areas and their cytoplasm may contain fine granules of yellow pigment. Field (1967) would lay particular emphasis on the astroglial hypertrophy as an important feature of the ageing process. Neither the oligodendrocytes nor the microglia are known to alter appreciably in the elderly.

Argyrophilic or 'senile' plaques

Argyrophilic or senile plaques are the most striking but inconsistent feature of the elderly brain. These minute patches of disintegrating tissue are found most often in the cerebral cortex but they also occur in the deeper grey matter, including the amygdaloid nucleus, the corpus striatum, the thalamus and occasionally the brainstem. They are not seen in the depths of the white matter.

Many varieties of plaque have been described. The classical one consists of a central argyrophilic core surrounded by an irregular clear halo, and beyond this, a ring of granular, filamentous material which is also argyrophilic (Fig. 18.4). The diameter, for they are roughly spherical, ranges

nitrocellulose (Hirano and Zimmerman 1962a) and for paraffin sections (Dixon 1953). Plaques may be well demonstrated making use of the PAS reaction, but they are easily overlooked, or undetectable, in Nissl or in haematoxylin and eosin preparations (Fig. 18.6). Astrocytic nuclei tend to collect around their periphery, the processes of the cell bodies penetrating them (Fig. 18.7) whereas microglial cells are more inclined to lie within the plaque. The degree of glial reaction varies considerably from case to case.

Pathogenesis. The origin of the senile plaque has been debated since the structures were first identified by Blocq and Marinesco (1892) in the brain of

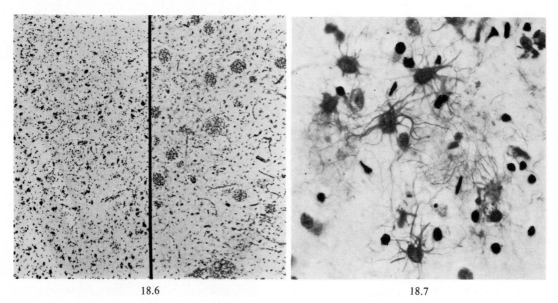

18.6   18.7

Fig. 18.6 The section of cerebral cortex on the left has been stained with cresyl violet. The view on the right is from the same brain but of an adjacent section which has been impregnated with silver. The plaque formation is only clearly shown by the latter method. (Both views × 70)

Fig. 18.7 Astrocytes encircling a plaque. Holzer stain. × 225.

from about 5 μm to 100 μm but their appearance and size vary, among other things, because of the plane in which they have been cut; many plaques, however, do not have a central core. Some appear as relatively clearcut homogenous spheres displacing the nerve fibres to one side (Fig. 18.5). More often they appear as darkly stained granular patches which have irregular and ill-defined outlines. Plaques are rapidly and easily demonstrated in frozen sections of formalin fixed tissue using the method of silver impregnation described by von Braunmühl, but there are many other effective techniques. These include methods for

an epileptic patient. Many workers including Redlich (1898) and Alzheimer (1907 *a*, *b*) thought that they originated in what has been called disintegrating glial reticulum. Bonfiglio (1908) claimed that the plaques developed from degenerating neurons but at some time nearly every component of nervous tissue has been invoked as their source. Soniat (1941), for example, and later Liss (1960) found them to develop in association with the degeneration of neurofibrils. Neumann (1960) considered an origin from axis cylinders more likely and Ferraro (1931) suggested that oligodendroglial and microglial elements were often responsible. Von Braunmühl (1931) dissented from these views, which were based on the degeneration of cellular elements, by elaborating Marinesco's (1911) earlier contention that the plaques derived from the condensation of the intercellular ground substance. This hypothesis foreshadowed the work of Divry (1927) whose observations showed that the amorphous deposition in the centre of many, but not all, plaques resembled amyloid in its histochemical reactions and that, like amyloid, the substance became birefringent after staining with Congo red. Divry believed that the first trace of the 'primitive plaque' was the condensation of minute areas of ground substance into a 'substance trichosique'

is also important to emphasise that histochemical studies have shown that plaques were not merely the inert residue of degeneration but that enzyme activity increased both in and around them (Morel and Wildi 1952). Friede and Magee (1962) and Friede (1965) have demonstrated an increased concentration of oxidative and hydrolytic enzyme activity in relation to plaques while Johnson and Blum (1970) added that of nucleotide phosphatase.

The most notable recent contribution to a better understanding of the nature and the origin of plaques, however, has come from the use of the electron microscope. Terry and his colleagues (Terry and Wisniewski 1972), pioneers in this field, have recently brought together the results of

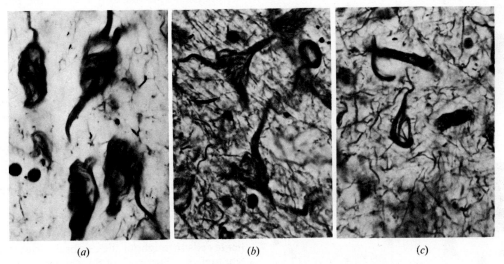

| (a) | (b) | (c) |

Fig. 18.8 Neurofibrillary change in presenile dementia (Alzheimer's disease). Bielschowsky. × 600   (a) From pyramidal layer of cornu Ammonis. (b) From parahippocampal gyrus. (c) From temporal cortex.

which took on the form of a halo around a paler centre. This he described as acting like a foreign body which attracts towards its core microglial cells containing amyloid, fat and occasionally a trace of iron. Later the astrocytes proliferate around the periphery and the plaque seems to be walled off by their fibrous processes. This was Divry's concept of the formation of the classical plaque. The evidence from light microscopy in general, however, seemed to favour the wider view that they might also originate in some part of a degenerating nerve or glial cell or even in relation to a blood vessel and that not all plaques were formed on an amyloid basis (Benedek and McGovern 1949; Reiss and Staemmler 1950). It

this and other studies during the last ten years. The ultrastructural precursor of a plaque is held to be the degenerating neurite, that is an unmyelinated neuronal process. As these increase in number, clusters are formed and wisps of amyloid appear between them. This is the primitive plaque. A core of amyloid builds up which is surrounded by a zone of altered neurites, with many degenerating mitochondria, acid phosphatase containing dense bodies, which are often laminated, and abnormal fibrillar material. Macrophages containing lipofuscin and cellular debris are common. These together make up the picture of the classical plaque known to the light microscopist. The last stage is the compact, burnt-out, plaque in which the main mass is amyloid sometimes surrounded by microglia, macrophages and astrocytic processes. The cause of the neuritic degeneration and the amyloid formation remains obscure.

Alzheimer's neurofibrillary degeneration

Alzheimer (1907*a*, *b*) described a change that he had found in about every fourth nerve cell in the cerebral cortex of a 51-year-old woman who had been suffering from the form of presenile dementia that was later named after him. The alteration, which is most clearly seen in silver impregnations, consists of the thickening and tortuosity of fibrils within the neuronal cytoplasm (Fig. 18.8*a*, *b*, *c*). In the early stages a thick, dark band is seen to run

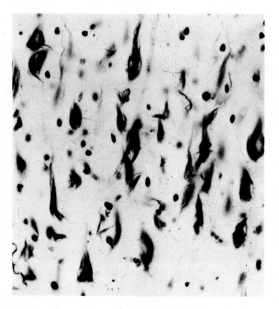

Fig. 18.9 Neurofibrillary tangles in the cortex of the parahippocampal gyrus. von Braunmühl. ×325.

or curve through the cell from the apical dendrite to the base. More bands develop alongside the first and others may form into separate loops. Later, the nucleus and cytoplasm fail to stain and the cell appears as an empty triangle or a lattice work of contorted fibres. The cortical neurons tend to show the simpler, more triangular or looped forms while spool-shaped or torch-like forms may also be seen in the hippocampus; a globose form is often seen in the subcortical nuclei such as the substantia nigra. At times, and particularly in the medial temporal grey matter, masses of these stricken cells can be seen in clusters, although some may impregnate only faintly and may then

be overlooked (Fig. 18.9). In embedded tissue and with cell stains such as haematoxylin and eosin or with the basic anilin dyes, as in Nissl's method, the change is much less easily recognized and only a slight increase in refractility may indicate the presence of the thickened skeins as they swing round outside the nucleus. The affected part of the cytoplasm lacks Nissl substance and the appearances may suggest chromatolysis. The PAS technique on paraffin sections is a useful stain. The method described by Hirano and Zimmerman (1962*a*) for the silver impregnation of senile plaques in intracellulose material is also suitable for neurofibrillary changes. Congo red provides a particularly valuable way of identifying the change in any form of embedded or in frozen tissue, since the altered fibrils not only take up the pink dye more deeply than the rest of the cell, but they also become intensely birefringent under polarized light (Fig. 18.10).

Alzheimer's neurofibrillary tangles are found in small numbers in the brains of many elderly people but the change is then usually confined to the hippocampal region, or if more widespread, to relatively few nerve cells scattered through the cortex (Tomlinson, Blessed and Roth 1968). When this change is encountered in the ageing brain it is nearly always accompanied by senile plaques (Fig. 18.11). The degrees, however, both of plaque and of tangle formation vary greatly but both tend to be at their most severe and most widespread in Alzheimer's presenile and senile dementia. In these conditions vast numbers of nerve cells throughout the cerebral cortex become 'entangled'. The work of Simchowicz in 1911 has been followed by many later studies which have demonstrated that the distribution follows a certain pattern (Hirano and Zimmerman 1962*b*). The emphasis is usually more on the anterior frontal and the temporal cortex than on the posterior parts of the hemispheres. The pre- and postcentral gyri are usually spared. Within the affected areas, cells in the outer cortical layers are affected in greater numbers than those lying more deeply. The brunt of the process, however, tends to fall on the neurons in the anteromedial temporal grey matter including the uncal cortex, the corticomedial part of the amygdaloid nucleus, the hippocampus and the adjacent part of the parahippocampal gyrus (Morel and Wildi 1952; Jamada and Mehraein 1968). The neurons in the subcortical regions are less often affected but the pigmented cells of the substantia nigra and of the locus ceruleus are also vulnerable. Ishii (1965) made a special study of the distribution in the hypothalamus and brainstem and pointed out that the most vulnerable nuclear groups showed certain metabolic features in common including a high content of monoamines, especially 5-HT in the cytoplasm, an early accumulation of lipofuscin and higher oxidative enzyme activities in the perikarya. Earlier, however, Friede and Magee (1962) had been cautious about the interpretation of the last activity because of the difficulty in identifying the affected cells. Purkinje cells and

found them in all 35 cases who had died above the age of 40 years. One of Olson and Shaw's patients had developed the clinical picture of Alzheimer's disease but the other two had not and, in contrast to Neumann's (1967) observations, no general trend towards psychological deterioration and the development of 'senile' degenerative changes was found. Malamud emphasized that this problem needs to be studied further.

In other disorders the ratio of plaques to tangles is reversed, with the tangles becoming the more dominant and plaques absent or scanty. These

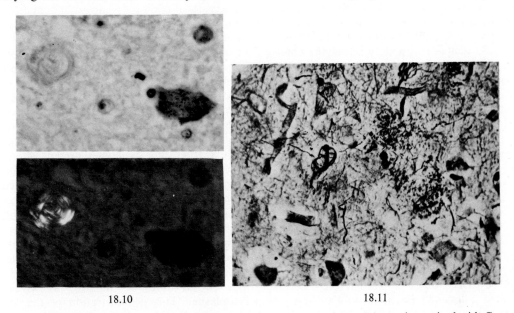

18.10

18.11

Fig. 18.10 Neurofibrillary changes in a pigmented cell of the substantia nigra. (Upper view stained with Congo red, the lower half is the same field under polarized light.)

Fig. 18.11 Cortex showing Alzheimer tangles adjacent to an argyrophilic plaque. Bielschowsky silver impregnation.

the larger motor neurons, such as the Betz and the anterior horn cells, seem to escape this form of degeneration.

Neurofibrillary tangles in company with argyrophilic plaques are also liable to occur in adults with Down's syndrome. Jervis drew attention to this tendency in 1948 although the presence of plaques alone had been reported earlier by Struwe (1929) and Bertrand and Koffas (1946). Several subsequent studies have confirmed that mongols dying in their thirties, and occasionally even in their twenties, may develop plaques although the tangles tend to appear later on in adult life (Solitaire and Lamarche 1966). Olson and Shaw (1969) found these changes in three mongols dying over the age of 35 and Malamud (1972)

conditions include the Parkinson–dementia complex of Guam (Hirano, Malamud and Kurland 1961), the amyotrophic lateral sclerosis syndrome of Guam (Malamud, Hirano and Kurland 1962) as well as in other cases of motor neuron disease and its allied disorders (Hirano and Zimmerman 1962b). It was seen by Féynes (1932) and Hallervorden (1933) in nerve cells of the brainstem in patients with encephalitis lethargica and it has also been reported in the same situation as well as in the cerebral cortex in young patients with subacute sclerosing panencephalitis (Malamud, Haymaker and Pinkerton 1950; Corsellis 1951). Alzheimer's tangles are a prominent feature in the brainstem of cases of postencephalitic Parkinsonism (Fig. 18.10), the pigmented cells of the substantia nigra and the locus ceruleus being particularly affected as well as other cell groups in the reticular and midline regions (Greenfield and Bosanquet 1953). Hirano and Zimmerman (1962b) found tangles in this condition which were also scattered through parts of the temporal lobes and diencephalic grey matter. Steele, Richardson and Olszewski (1964) identified the neurofibrillary change as a major pathological feature in progressive supranuclear palsy. Behrmann, Caroll, Janota and Matthews (1969) emphasized, as had other writers, that the tangles in this condition were most widespread in the midbrain but that they were also prone to occur in other neuronal groups from the pallidum down to the medulla. They were unable to decide whether the change was primarily degenerative or whether it might be the consequence of an inflammatory agent or the sequel to an attack of encephalitis lethargica. Albert, Feldman and Willis (1974) have attributed the characteristic pattern of the dementia in this condition to the brunt of the neuronal changes falling on the subcortical regions rather than on the cortex.

Neurofibrillary tangles are also liable to occur as a late sequel to cerebral trauma, either in association with senile plaques or on their own. Possible examples of the former are the rare cases of posttraumatic dementia in which the histological features have been found to be those of Alzheimer's disease. Claude and Cuel (1939) described the case of a woman who became demented following a fractured skull at the age of 50 and Corsellis and Brierley (1959) reported the same sequence in a man of the same age who started to deteriorate mentally after being involved as a passenger in a car accident. Both people died severely demented about five years later and the neurohistological features in both were those of Alzheimer's disease. Grosch (1959) reported a similar example.

Brandenberg and Hallervorden (1954) drew attention to the possibility that repeated blows to the head might trigger off this degenerative process after they had encountered intense plaque formation and neurofibrillary tangles in the brain of an amateur boxer who had died demented at the age of 51. In another boxer Grahmann and Ule (1957) found only the neurofibrillary change and in a third Constantinidis and Tissot (1967) drew particular attention to the way that tangles had occurred in the complete absence of argentophilic plaques. Since then Corsellis, Bruton and

Freeman-Browne (1973) have found that neurofibrillary changes, usually in the absence of plaques, were a major pathological feature in the brains of most of the 15 retired boxers whom they had examined. The tangles were noticeably severe in the substantia nigra and locus ceruleus but at their most intense in the medial temporal grey matter, including the amygdaloid nucleus, hippocampus and parahippocampal gyrus. The frontal cortex tended to be more affected than parieto-occipital regions.

Neurofibrillary tangles have been reported as an occasional finding in many other conditions in addition to those already mentioned. These were listed by Hirano and Zimmerman (1962b) and include the spinal and cerebral forms of syphilis, intestinal disease, multiple sclerosis and hereditary cerebellar disorders.

Alzheimer considered that the change affected the neurofibrils normally present in the nerve cell. Bielschowsky (1932) opposed this view because to him the skeins of altered fibrils and other argentophilic fragments sometimes present often bore little relation to the arrangement of neurofibrils in normal neurons. Divry (1934) objected to Alzheimer's interpretation because the argentophilic material had been shown by him to behave like amyloid. He considered that, as with amyloid in other parts of the body, the material first appeared as a deposit on the surface of the cell, even if in the later stages there seemed little doubt that altered fibres or 'tangles' lay within the cytoplasm. This demonstration of the 'congophilic' nature of the substance linked the change to the senile plaque and suggested a common origin, since plaques and tangles often occur together at least in the ageing brain.

Electron-microscopy, however, although confirming that the fibrillary substance in the plaque core was the same as amyloid, indicated that the ultrastructure of the human tangle was not. Terry (1963) considered the material to consist almost exclusively of a mass of twisted tubules measuring about 20 nm wide with periodic narrowing every 80 nm to about 10 nm, this latter figure being roughly the thickness of the normal neurofilament (Fig. 18.12). Kidd (1964) suspected that this appearance was the product of paired filaments wound in a double helix which resulted in an intermittent narrowing. This may still prove to be correct but at present the tubular interpretation is the more generally accepted. According to Wisniewski, Terry and Hirano (1970) the 'tubular'

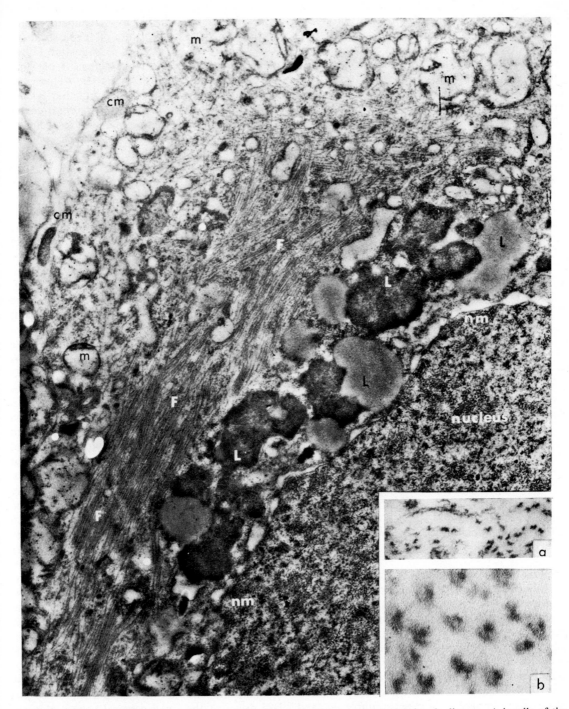

Fig. 18.12 Electron micrograph of part of an affected nerve cell in a case of Alzheimer's disease. A bundle of the characteristic filaments (F) is seen running in the cytoplasm. ×22,000. (cm = nerve cell membrane; nm = nuclear membrane; m = mitochondrion; L = lipochrome). Inset *a*—A region in the neuropil showing a longitudinal helix above and a number of helices in transverse section. ×60,000. Inset *b*—Higher magnification of helices in transverse section. ×224,000. (Biopsy preparation by Dr Michael Kidd.)

form of neurofibrillary degeneration has so far only been identified in human conditions, such as Alzheimer's disease, senile dementia, the Guam and Parkinsonism–dementia complex, postencephalitic parkinsonism and Pick's disease. Spontaneous and experimentally induced encephalitides in lower animals. on the other hand, appear to be associated with a filamentous form of change analogous to that found in human infantile neuroaxonal dystrophy and spastic motor neuron disease.

Granulovacuolar degeneration

The term coarsely-granular degeneration was given by Simchowicz (1911) to an alteration that he had found in the pyramidal cells of the hippocampus in severe cases of senile dementia. The cytoplasm of the affected cells contain one or more clear

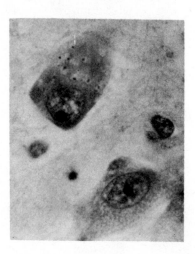

Fig. 18.13　Granulovacuolar degeneration in the pyramidal cells of the hippocampus. Lendrum's phloxine tartrazine stain.

vacuoles 3 to 5 μm in diameter. In the centre of each vacuole is a granule about 1 μm across. The central particles are not stained by Nissl's method but show up clearly with haematoxylin and eosin, with Lendrum's phloxine tartrazine stain (Fig. 18.13) or in silver impregnations such as the von Braunmühl or the Glees and Martland methods. When only a few vacuoles are present the Nissl substance around them tends to thin out. When the vacuoles become more numerous, and there may be a dozen or more, the cell outline enlarges and becomes irregular in outline while the nucleus becomes eccentric.

Little is known about the nature or the origin of this form of degeneration. It is sometimes seen in cells which are also affected by Alzheimer's neurofibrillary change, and because of this association Morel and Wildi (1952) and Agostini (1958) postulated that the vacuolar change is an early stage in the formation of the latter. This view, however, is at variance with the fact that tangles commonly occur throughout the cerebral cortex whereas the vacuolar change is all but restricted to the hippocampus. This almost exclusive emphasis on the hippocampus, or at least on the medial temporal grey matter, was confirmed by Tomlinson and Kitchener (1972) in a systematic comparison of the brains of demented and non-demented people. The change was rarely found below the age of 60 but later became more frequent and by the eighties the hippocampal neurons in 75% of brains were affected to some extent. It was, therefore, found to become increasingly prevalent with advancing age, but both the number of cells affected and the severity of the change were considerably greater in the demented group. Thus the change rarely affected more than 9% of hippocampal neurons in non-demented old people whereas 10 to 50% were affected in those dements showing the histological features of Alzheimer's disease. Woodard's (1962, 1966) observations were roughly of the same order. Other conditions in which granulovacuolar degeneration has been reported include Down's syndrome (Malamud 1972), Pick's disease and the amyotrophic lateral sclerosis and the Parkinson–dementia complex of Guam (Hirano et al. 1961; Hirano, Dembitzer, Kurland and Zimmerman 1968). The EM picture of granulovacuolar bodies shows them to consist of cytoplasmic membrane-bound inclusions each containing a dense granular core. Steele et al. (1964) described them as a considerable rarity in the red nucleus and the pontine nuclei in progressive supranuclear palsy. Hirano, Tuazon and Zimmerman (1968) noted the change in the neurons of a parietally placed tuber in tuberous sclerosis.

Congophilic angiopathy

Divry had shown in 1927 that the core of many senile plaques behaved like amyloid. In 1938 Scholz demonstrated that a similar substance was laid down in the small cerebral vessels of some people dying over the age of 70. He named the change 'drusige Entartung' or plaque-like degeneration because he believed that 'senile plaques' could develop from the fragmenting vascular wall.

In the change an affected arteriole appears at low power as a thickened almost homogeneous tube (Fig. 18.14a) which stains pink with eosin or cresyl violet and brown-yellow with the van Gieson method. The alteration lies outside the elastic lamina, which is usually attenuated or split and the becomes doubly refractile (Fig. 18.14c). Pantelakis (1954) called this change 'congophilic angiopathy' a term which is now preferred to that introduced by Scholz. At times this amyloid-like substance erupts like a small wart on the outer side of the degenerating vessel and fragments of it may come

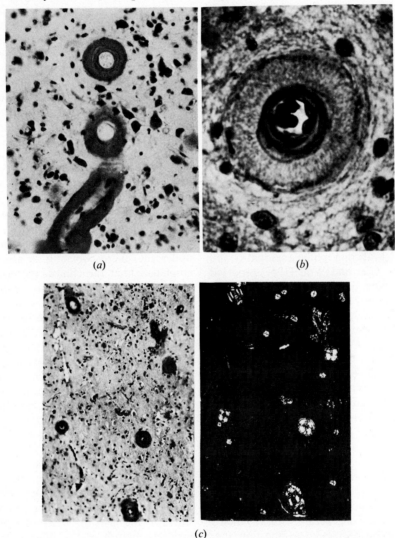

(a)

(b)

(c)

Fig. 18.14 (a) Cortical arteriole with the appearances of congophilic angiopathy. Cresyl violet. × 240. (b) Higher power view of such an arteriole showing gross thickening of the middle coat with a surrounding radial fibrillar structure. Iron haematoxylin van Gieson. × 550. (c) Small cortical vessels stained with Congo red. The view on the right was taken under polarized light. × 100.

muscle fibres of the middle coat appear smaller with their outline blurred and the nuclei indistinct or absent. Around this a ring of amorphous substance may develop which under higher power has a reticulated or radial structure (Fig. 18.14b). With Congo red such a vessel stains pink and then to lie free in the tissue. Morel and Wildi (1955) and Surbek (1961) called this advanced stage 'dyshoric angiopathy'.

The change affects the small pial and intracerebral arterioles, sometimes, in severe cases, the leptomeningeal arteries, and occasionally the intracortical capillaries. The parieto-occipital cortex is usually more affected than the frontal and temporal lobes and it is usually best identified in the region of the striate cortex. The small vessels in the cerebellar cortex and in the deep grey matter of the cerebral hemispheres are affected occasionally; the brainstem appears always to be spared. Schlote (1965) showed that the ultrastructure of the substance was similar to that of amyloid, and Terry and Wisniewski (1972) have described how congophilic angiopathy involves primarily the perithelial cells and the basement membrane, the latter being widened and replicated by the presence of amyloid fibrils. The origin of the amyloid, which remains obscure, has been discussed by Mandybur (1975). He emphasized that the central nervous system is rarely affected by the primary, secondary or familial forms of secondary amyloidosis and that the existence of structures resembling senile plaques in any of these conditions is extremely rare (Krücke 1950). On the other hand, Pantelakis observed a mild degree of vascular amyloidosis in the internal organs of some patients with cerebral congophilic angiopathy and Schwartz, Wolfe, Gier and Wolf (1967) reported that the senile type of pancreatic and cardiac amyloidosis commonly accompanies ageing. The sexes were affected equally; its existence increases into very old age but it has been found at a presenile age. Wright, Calkins, Breen, Stolte and Schultz (1969) found that about two-thirds of patients dying over the age of 70 developed cerebral amyloid either in the form of senile plaques or in the cerebral vessels, while aortic, cardiac or pancreatic deposits were present in nearly a half. It occurs in the brain independently of cerebral atherosclerosis.

The relation of cerebral degeneration in ageing to dementia

The main ways in which the various components of nervous tissue may degenerate with advancing age have been described and the question that arises is the relationship of dementia to the disintegration of cerebral tissue. This has long been a problem for it has often been contended that cerebral atrophy and cerebrovascular disease are so common in later life, and the nervous system is so able to compensate for this, that the structural state of the brain is of less importance than the influences of environmental and psychological factors (Gellerstedt 1933; Rothschild 1945). It is, however, inadvisable either to under- or to over-

estimate their significance. Clinicopathological studies of psychiatric, as well as of general, hospital populations have indicated that, within the overall trend for both the senile and vascular degenerative processes to become more common with advancing age, it is predominantly when they reach the more severe degrees that dementia occurs (Corsellis 1962; Simon and Malamud 1965). Moreover, careful attempts to quantify the severity of senile degeneration by counting plaques have shown consistently high levels in tissue from groups of demented patients and low ones in the controls; conversely, extensive plaque formation was not seen in non-demented old people (Blessed, Tomlinson and Roth 1968). Analogous observations were also made in relation to the severity of cerebrovascular disease (Tomlinson et al. 1970). Present evidence, therefore, indicates that progressive dementia in old age is in most instances reflected in the ultimate state of the brain, the main proviso being that the examination should be comprehensive for a brain can appear intact to the naked eye and yet severe degeneration may be seen under the microscope. It is also important to emphasize that the clinical pattern of the illness may vary appreciably according to the dominant form of degeneration. In dementia associated with cerebrovascular change the deterioration is, as Fisher (1968) described it, 'a matter of strokes large and small'. Focal neurological signs, dysarthria, dysphagia, small-stepped gait, brisk reflexes and extensor plantar responses are common. The illness tends to fluctuate; most patients are or have been hypertensive. At necropsy the heart is usually enlarged and death is not infrequently attributable to ischaemic heart disease or to a cerebrovascular accident.

When the pathological basis of the illness is the senile form of degeneration, the illness usually starts in the early seventies (this question is discussed later when Alzheimer's disease is considered), and lasts for an average of 4 years. The insidious nature of the illness, however, makes such an estimate of doubtful accuracy, and many patients will survive considerably longer, although the gradual progressive deterioration is relentless. Focal neurological signs and convulsions are much less common than in patients with cerebral atherosclerosis and the blood pressure is less often raised to the same extent. The patient wastes away and at necropsy not only the brain but the rest of the body and the viscera generally are small and atrophied. The body weight may be as little as 25 kg and the heart weight not more than 200 g. It is in these patients that diffuse senile degenerative changes are found in the brain. Like the vascular changes in the arteriosclerotic dements, they are usually widespread and severe.

Alzheimer's disease

In 1907 Alzheimer reported the case of a 51-year-old woman whose memory began to deteriorate rapidly. She was excitable, she misnamed objects and she was soon unable to manage at home. On admission to hospital the patient was found to be disorientated, paranoid and dysphasic. She became mute and incontinent and died, profoundly demented 4 years later. The brain was generally atrophic but without focal damage. Using Bielschowsky's silver method, Alzheimer identified many argentophilic plaques in the cerebral cortex similar to those originally described by Blocq and Marinesco (1892) and by Redlich (1898). A hitherto unrecorded form of widespread neuronal degeneration was also found, which, as described in the previous section, has come to be known as Alzheimer's neurofibrillary change or as neurofibrillary tangles.

The unusual severity of the degenerative process, as well as its early age at onset, impressed Alzheimer greatly; within a few years further examples had been reported by Bonfiglio (1908) and by Perusini (1910). They believed that the disorder should be excluded from the category of senile dementia and Kraepelin (1910), agreeing with this, proposed that it be called Alzheimer's disease.

The illness usually appears between the ages of 50 and 60. One of the youngest cases on record is that of a 7-year-old boy who fell ill after an attack of scarlet fever and died demented when aged 23. Løken and Cyvin's (1954) patient survived for 11 years after the onset of dementia at the age of 6. Clinically the illness in this child had been regarded as amaurotic idiocy but the histological findings were those of Alzheimer's disease.

It is the commonest form of presenile dementia and has been recorded as occurring in from 1 to 10% of those seen in psychiatric hospitals (McMenemey 1940; Newton 1948; Schenk 1955). The figure varies, however, according to the population being studied and whether the investigation draws a distinction between Alzheimer's disease and senile dementia. The lowest incidence

occurs when, as in McMenemey's study, only those cases with an onset before 60 years were included while in Newton's series no upper age limit was applied.

Women are affected more often than men, the proportion being about 2 : 1. A family history of the illness is found in only a minority of patients; Sjögren, Sjögren and Lindgren (1952) considered that multifactorial inheritance is probable. There is, however, a group of cases in which the genetic factor is particularly evident. These are considered in a separate section, partly because the clinical and pathological findings may also be atypical.

The illness lasts for an average of five years but a course of only a few months (Abely, Guiraud and Dechosal 1958) or as long as 21 years has been recorded (Newton 1948).

Clinically Alzheimer's disease shows a slowly progressive mental deterioration with failure of memory, disorientation and confusion leading to profound dementia. Symptoms such as aphasia, agnosia, apraxia and convulsions are not uncommon while there may at times be evidence of involvement of the pyramidal or extrapyramidal pathways. The illness is usually described as passing through an initial stage of restlessness and excitement, perhaps with hallucinations and delusions, but according to Sjögren et al. (1952), in their detailed analysis of the clinical picture, a state of apathy and inertia is the more common. Although the downward course is relentless, there may rarely be intermissions (Rothschild 1934) and there is at times the possibility that the disease may be superimposed on an affective or a paranoid illness. In the final stages some, but not all, patients tend to waste away. Death is usually attributable to bronchopneumonia. At necropsy the viscera may be small, the heart weighing as little as 200 g. No constant abnormality outside the nervous system has so far been identified.

The brain is usually small and the weight may drop from the expected level of 1200 to 1450 g to 1000 g or less. Atherosclerosis of the cerebral vessels is either absent or seldom more than mild; the leptomeninges may be a little thickened. The salient feature is the considerable and symmetrical cortical atrophy which although generalized tends to affect the frontal lobes most noticeably, although at times the temporal and less often the parieto-occipital atrophy can be marked (Fig. 18.15). At one extreme the absence of atrophy visible to the naked eye does not exclude a

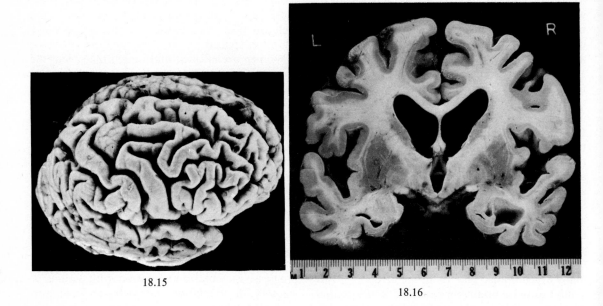

18.15

18.16

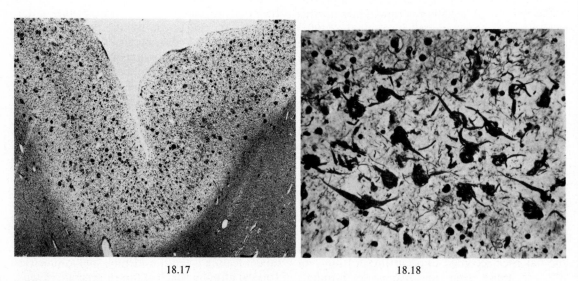

18.17

18.18

Fig. 18.15   Alzheimer's disease—showing atrophy of brain greatest in the frontal lobes.
Fig. 18.16   Alzheimer's disease—general shrinkage of the brain in coronal cut.
Fig. 18.17   Alzheimer's disease—many argyrophilic plaques in cerebral cortex.   King's silver method for amyloid.
Fig. 18.18 . Alzheimer's disease—hippocampus showing neurofibrillary change in many neurons.   von Braunmühl. × 120.

diagnosis of Alzheimer's disease, for widespread microscopic degeneration may be present without obvious shrinkage of tissue. At the other extreme, the atrophy can be sufficiently severe and localized to suggest Pick's disease although the so-called

and the thalamus, appears in general to be reduced.

There are several histological features but two are striking. Firstly, there is the plethora of argyrophilic plaques which are spread throughout the cortex and to a lesser extent scattered in the

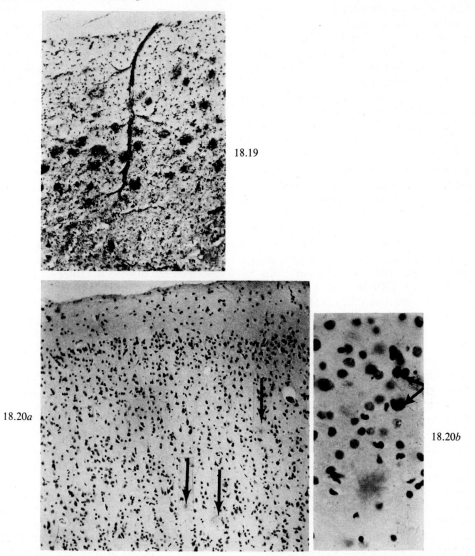

18.19

18.20a

18.20b

Fig. 18.19 Alzheimer's disease—biopsy from middle frontal gyrus. Frozen section, von Braunmühl. × 50.
Fig. 18.20 (a) Alzheimer's disease—superior frontal gyrus showing widespread loss of cells in all laminae, degenerative changes in surviving nerve cells and increase in astrocytes. Some argyrophilic plaques are recognizable (arrows). Celloidin. Cresyl violet. × 90. (b) Argyrophilic plaque as seen in Nissl's stain: note surrounding microglia, also recently divided astrocytes (arrows). Celloidin. Cresyl violet. × 400.

'knife-blade' atrophy of that condition is rarely seen. When the brain is cut coronally the ventricles are usually enlarged and the cortical ribbon tends to be narrow (Fig. 18.16). The amount of deep grey matter, including the corpus striatum

subcortical grey matter (Fig. 18.17). Secondly, there is the neurofibrillary change of nerve cells (Fig. 18.18). When the degeneration is severe the disintegration of tissue may be so complete that few nerve cells can be seen and in silver preparations the smaller and distorted neurofibrils stand out in stark relief. Indeed, if the diagnosis of Alzheimer's disease is being considered this can often be rapidly established by preparing silver-impregnated frozen sections of cerebral cortex (Fig. 18.19). In Nissl preparations the number of nerve cells may appear relatively intact and the lamination may be recognizable. Many neurons, however, are likely to have disappeared especially in the third and fifth layers. Sometimes clear patches may be seen between groups of nerve cells. These represent unstained senile plaques; at other times the centres of the plaques may stain faintly owing to their metachromatic cores (Fig. 18.20a, b).

In Nissl and in haematoxylin-eosin stained sections it is usually difficult and often impossible to recognize neurofibrillary tangles. The appearances, the distribution and the nature both of the senile plaques and the neurofibrillary changes have already been discussed. Many nerve cells appear abnormal in other ways, An excess of lipochrome as well as some degree of chromatolysis are common, although the latter finding in a biopsy needs to be interpreted with caution. An increased activity of DPNH and TPNH in the perikarya and proximal parts of the axons has been reported which appears to be more than can be accounted for because of cell shrinkage (Smith 1961). Friede and Magee (1962) are cautious in attributing to the 'Alzheimer cell' strong oxidative enzymatic properties since these proved difficult to identify with certainty. Granulovacuolar degeneration, as already described, is commonly found in many of the large hippocampal neurons. Hirano bodies have also been reported (Tomonaga 1974). Astrocytic nuclei are often present in excess throughout the grey matter and may be seen in pairs with palely stained yellowish granules adjacent to the nuclear membrane. Sim and Smith (1955) found PAS-positive granules in glial cells in the white matter of biopsy specimens.

As the cortical nerve cells die, their axons and myelin sheaths degenerate and become fewer, and the retrograde degeneration sometimes seen in the thalamus may be a consequence of this. Myelin destruction, however, is seldom appreciable for neither sudanophilic material nor fat phagocytes are features of this disease. Goodman (1953) found much free iron in the nerve cells and oligodendroglia and in the arteriolar and capillary walls. He believed that the disease may be essentially a disorder of iron metabolism. Hallgren and Sourander (1960) also found stain-able iron in the cortex, but there was no overall increase in iron content and they believed that their findings were the result of an altered distribution of iron. Crapper et al. have reported unusually high concentrations of aluminium in the cerebral grey matter.

In most cases of Alzheimer's disease both the large and the small blood vessels are within normal limits for the age, but occasionally a severe degree of cerebral atherosclerosis complicates the picture. In some instances, however, the striking feature is the amyloid degeneration of many small arteries, arterioles and even capillaries mainly within the cortex and the leptomeninges. The nature and the distribution of this amyloid or congophilic angiopathy has been outlined earlier in the chapter (p. 808). Its particular relevance to Alzheimer's disease is further considered in the following section on familial and atypical examples of the illness.

Familial cases. A family history of the illness has been reported many times. Schottky (1932) described the disease in father and daughter with seven presumed cases in four generations, while von Braunmühl (1932) found it in twins. English (1942) reported it in four siblings and in the daughter of one of them. Wheelan (1959) recorded two proved and four presumed cases in a family of ten, including the mother. The parents of the juvenile case described by Løken and Cyvin (1954) were first cousins. Lowenberg and Waggoner (1934) described a man who was considered to have developed the illness at the age of 32, and four of whose five children developed the same clinical conditions at much the same age. One was proved histologically; the father's parents were first cousins.

A first-cousin marriage was also reported in a family studied by McMenemey, Worster-Drought, Flind and Williams (1939). Only one necropsy was performed but the condition had affected clinically three out of four siblings and one child. Grünthal and Wenger (1939) described four clinical examples in two generations with pathological confirmation in a sister and brother while Essen-Möhler (1946) reported on a father, son and daughter with the disease. Marconi and Piazzesi (1965) have reported on the genetic and cytogenetic aspects of an affected family. Davidson and Robertson (1955) encountered it in one of identical twins; this patient, whose symptoms began at the age of 50 and who died 19 years later had spent her life in Edinburgh while the sister living mostly in Australia was still healthy aged 73. Hunter, Dayan and Wilson (1972) reported the illness, lasting 15 years, in a woman of 64 whose monozygotic twin sister was clinically not affected and who died two years later of carcinoma. These authors pointed out that not a single pair of twins of whom both were affected has so far been reported and they, like Davidson and Robertson, suggested that the study of exogenous rather than inborn factors may prove more fruitful. It is noteworthy that Alzheimer's disease was found to be more common in Gothenburg than in Stockholm, whereas the prevalence was reversed in Pick's disease (Sjögren *et al.* 1952). The literature on the genetics of Alzheimer's disease has been reviewed by Zerbin-Rüdin (1967) and Pratt (1970). Slater and Cowie (1971) concluded, mainly from the comprehensive studies by Sjögren and his colleagues, quoted above, and by Constantinidis, Garrone and de Ajuriaguerra (1962) that the mode of inheritance is compatible with a polygenic basis but that in a few pedigrees a dominant inheritance has occurred. In the former there is evidence of female sex preponderance and in the latter of sex equality.

Apart from familial instances of Alzheimer's disease, it is not unusual to encounter psychiatric illness in the families of affected patients. Schenk (1955), for example, found a history of dementia in a near relative in 10 out of 35 cases and of severe neurological disease in 15.

Atypical cases. A small number has been recorded in which the clinical or pathological picture has been unusual.

Thus Schnitzler (1911) reported on a woman with a thyroid disorder who died demented at the age of 37. Neurofibrillary tangles were plentiful in the brain but there were no senile plaques. Weimann (1921) found the same in a demented man of the same age with marked cerebrovascular degeneration and diffuse calcinosis. Other cases without plaques were reported by Goodman (1953) and Raskin and Ehrenberg (1956). Hemphill and Stengel (1941) recorded Alzheimer's disease in a woman of 59, whose illness had started after pregnancy when aged 41, and in whom the cerebral atrophy was more marked in the right than in the left hemisphere whereas the left side of the cerebellum was the more affected. Liebers (1933) recorded the five-year illness of an engineer who died aged 52 with the neuro-

histological features of Alzheimer's disease but with marked 'Pick-like' atrophy in the parieto-occipital regions. Other examples of severe focal atrophy in Alzheimer's disease, usually fronto-temporal, have been described by Divry, Ley and Titeca (1935), Rothschild and Kasanin (1936), and Seitelberger and Jellinger (1958). Berlin (1949) and Kreindler, Hornet and Appel (1959) have reported cases of Alzheimer's disease in which the gross focal atrophy of Pick's disease was also present and these have been generally looked upon as examples of the two conditions occurring together. Other cases which have been considered within the Pick framework are those of Moyano (1932) and Liebers (1939).

The incidence of cerebral amyloid angiopathy in Alzheimer's disease has been reviewed by McMenemey (1963a) and by Mandybur (1975), who studied 15 of McMenemey's cases at the Maida Vale Hospital. In addition to the reports quoted by him, others have recently been published by Gerhard, Bergener and Homayun (1972) and by Ulrich, Taghavy and Schmidt (1973). In some instances there has been the suggestion of an inherited susceptibility to the disease. This group includes the families reported by Worster-Drought, Greenfield and McMenemey (1940, 1944); van Bogaert, Maere and de Smedt (1940); Lüers (1947); Corsellis and Brierley (1954), and Gerhard *et al.* (1972). In each case a progressive dementia occurred which was coupled with the development of a spastic paralysis or paresis of one or both lower limbs. The neurohistological features were those of Alzheimer's disease combined with amyloid or congophilic angiopathy. In the cases reported by Corsellis and Brierley and by Gerhard *et al.* a severe hyaline arteriolar degeneration was also present which had led to multiple foci of cortical infarction (Fig. 18.21). These, it was surmised, could have been responsible for the focal neurological features. Mandybur had observed similar arteriolar necrosis in some of his cases and had attributed this, as others have done, to hypertension. Gerhard *et al.*, on the other hand, pointed out that a high blood pressure had never been found in their patient nor had greatly raised levels been recorded in most of the other reported cases. They proposed that the 'cortical type of hypertensive vascular disease' seen in this atypical form of Alzheimer's disease is related rather to the intense degree of amyloid change in the small cerebral vessels. Other reports of amyloid angiopathy occurring in familial conditions possibly related to Alzheimer's disease include those by Gerstmann, Sträussler and Scheinker (1936) and von Braunmühl (1954).

In addition to these familial instances, numerous non-familial cases of Alzheimer's disease with amyloid angiopathy have been reported (Benedek and McGovern 1949; Mandybur 1975). Neumann (1960) described the findings in a non-demented 45-year-old woman with plaque formation and amyloid angiopathy but without neurofibrillary tangles. Hollander and Strich (1970) reported six cases of atypical Alzheimer's disease with an unusually sudden onset of dementia. In all of

stated that they could be virtually the same clinically, apart from a greater tendency in Alzheimer's disease for focal symptoms such as apraxia, aphasia and epilepsy to occur. Mutrux (1958) agreed with this. Larsson, Sjögren and Jacobsen (1963) commented on, but did not define, clear-cut differences in the advanced stages of senile dementia and Alzheimer's disease and presented genetic evidence that the former is unconnected either with senility or with the presenile dementias.

On the pathological side Rothschild and Kasanin (1936) and Mutrux (1953) claimed that the pathological process tended to be more severe in

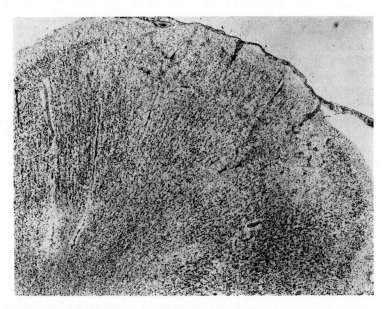

Fig. 18.21 Atypical Alzheimer's disease—frontal cortex showing patchy neuronal necrosis and gliosis due to hyaline arteriolar degeneration and congophilic angiopathy.   Nissl.   × 25.

them an amyloid angiopathy was present, as it was in the brain of the 51-year-old demented ex-boxer reported by Brandenburg and Hallervorden (1954).

Senile dementia
As already pointed out, there have long been two schools of thought. One believes, as Alzheimer did, that senile dementia and Alzheimer's disease are the same thing. The other school would, for various reasons, keep them separate. Thus, clinical differences, such as overactivity in Alzheimer's disease and apathy in the senile dement, have been described. Others, however, have reported the opposite. Grünthal (1930b), who favoured separation of the two conditions,

Alzheimer's disease than in senile dementia while many other subtle, and even trivial, differences in the nature or in the local emphasis of the various histological changes have been promulgated over the years. These have been lucidly summarized by McMenemey (1963b). In general, the conclusion seems unavoidable that Alzheimer's disease cannot be distinguished from senile dementia on histological grounds, all the differences being of emphasis or of quantity rather than intrinsic. Until more is known about their relationship both to each other and to the problem of cerebral ageing, the simple solution seems to lie along the lines proposed by McMenemey (1963). The terms 'presenile' and 'senile' dementia should be used as umbrellas to cover all the various types according to the period of life at which they occur. When the underlying pathological process is thought during life, or found after death or after biopsy, to be that described by Alzheimer, terms such as Alzheimer's presenile and Alzheimer's senile dementia should be used.

Pick's disease

Some years before Alzheimer's studies on pre-senile dementia had been completed, Pick had been working on another dementing condition which he had found occasionally to affect older people, but in which the neurological picture was more pronounced than that usually associated with the dementias of middle and later life. When Pick, together with the pathologist Chiari, examined the brains of his patients macroscopically they found within the usual setting of mild generalized atrophy a much more striking shrinkage of certain lobes and the condition became known as 'Progressive Circumscribed Cerebral Atrophy'.

As comprehensive reviews by Lüers and Spatz (1957), Delay and Brion (1962) and Jervis (1971) have shown, the illness is rare and is encountered considerably less often than Alzheimer's disease. It occurs most often during later middle life with a peak around 60. It has, however, been encountered well before this with an onset as early as the thirties and forties, and even at 21. At the other extreme, several patients over the age of 80 or 90 have been recorded. The length of illness varies greatly but it is rarely less than a year and seldom runs to more than 10 years. There is some evidence that the duration tends to be shorter when the onset is early. Women seem to be affected a little more often than men. In the comprehensive survey by van Mansvelt (1954) the ratio was 5 : 4.

No major variations have been established in the geographic incidence of Pick's disease, although in Sweden Sjögren and his colleagues found that most proved examples of the illness came from Stockholm while those of Alzheimer's disease originated in Göteborg. Verhaart (1936) described the disease in Chinese and Malayans in Indonesia.

Grünthal (1930a) described the occurrence of Pick's disease in two brothers. This confirmed the observation by Reich (1927) and von Braunmühl (1928) that the condition could be familial. Since that time numerous other examples have been reported. These include three affected sisters and possibly a cousin (Schmitz and Meyer 1933),

three sisters and possibly a grandfather and a son (Haskovec 1934), and two sisters and possibly their mother (von Braunmühl and Leonhard 1934). Schenk, in 1959, reported on a 20-year follow-up of a Swedish family in which 26 of the 51 endangered sibships were affected (Slater and Cowie 1971). Sjögren et al. (1952) concluded from their genetic survey in Sweden that the condition is probably transmitted by a dominant major gene with polygenic modification.

The clinical story in most cases is one of insidious intellectual deterioration with difficulty in concentration and perhaps some disturbance of memory (Wells 1971). The patient may become depressed, restless and apathetic. He loses insight, becomes untidy and may behave in a bizarre or socially disturbing way. As the intellect worsens, the patient becomes disorientated, and possibly dysphasic, dyslexic or dyspraxic. Repetitive utterances or actions are not uncommon. Occasionally a patient becomes mute at an early stage. Epileptic attacks are rare, at least in the early stages, and choreiform or athetotic movements are very unusual. Disturbance of gait are not uncommon towards the end of the illness. The disease progresses slowly but relentlessly into a state of advanced dementia. Occasionally the symptoms are masked. Winkelman and Book's (1949) patient, for instance, who died aged 34, was thought to have been schizophrenic. De Boor, Spiegelhoff and Stammler (1952) described an unsuspected case in a woman of 63 with a hypophyseal diencephalic syndrome associated with gross obesity and a compulsion neurosis. Death is usually attributable to bronchopneumonia. There are no known abnormal post-mortem findings in organs other than the brain.

Appearances of the brain

The most striking feature in the typical case is the extreme shrinkage of relatively circumscribed parts of both cerebral hemispheres. The severity of the atrophy is best seen in the fixed brain after the leptomeninges, which are usually thickened but not adherent, have been stripped away and the underlying convolutions have been exposed. These are then seen to be separated by widely gaping sulci; their roughened surface is yellow-brown with the crowns of the gyri often shrivelled up to the so-called 'walnut' or even 'knife-edge' appearance (Fig. 18.22). This marked loss of tissue is reflected in the brain weight which may fall to 1000 g or less in either sex. Lindgren

(Sjögren, Sjögren and Lindgren 1952) found the mean value for women to be 1005 g; for men it was 1075 g. Mansvelt considered that the longer the illness, the greater the atrophy. In the typical case the diagnosis can already be made with some certainty on the macroscopical appearances. The naked-eye atrophy can, however, be less obvious and may be overlooked. Delay, Brion and Sadoun (1954) reported a patient with a mental illness of only six months' duration in whose brain

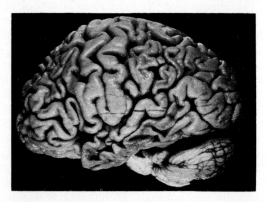

Fig. 18.22   Pick's disease—there is atrophy in the parietal, as well as in the frontal and temporal lobes. The sparing of the posterior two-thirds of the superior temporal gyrus is noteworthy.

the histological findings were characteristic of Pick's disease although there was no gross atrophy. It should not be forgotten that severe degrees of atrophy may be found in presenile dementia of the Alzheimer type.

The atrophy is usually frontotemporal in distribution, but at times the brunt of the process falls mainly on the frontal lobes and at others on the temporal lobes. The figures given by Mansvelt (1954) in his analysis of the degree of atrophy of the two hemispheres were that it was symmetrical in about a third, while in nearly a half of the cases the left hemisphere was the more affected whereas in only a fifth was the emphasis on the right side. In only one instance was the discrepancy very marked and in this case it is interesting that the illness had started after a head injury (Reich 1927). The distribution of the lobar atrophy was frontal and temporal in 54%, mainly frontal in 25%, and mainly temporal in 17%. Parietal and frontoparietal atrophy were rare. In only one case has the occipital lobe been heavily involved (Urechia, Dragomir and Elekes 1935), although slighter degrees of occipital atrophy have occasionally been reported (Jakob 1960). The patterns of

atrophy within the different lobes have been analysed by Lüers and Spatz (1957). They described two main types of frontal involvement. In the commoner the atrophy is focused on the medial orbital regions including the gyrus rectus, spreading round on to the frontal pole with the marked atrophy extending along the inferior frontal gyrus towards the insula and into the pars opercularis but tending to spare the adjacent pars triangularis. In the less common type the emphasis is on the frontal convexity, in which the pole and the dorsal half of the frontal lobes are the more affected. At times the precentral gyrus is also involved or indeed the whole convexity may be.

When the temporal lobe is affected the focus is always around the pole. The atrophy then spreads back to involve the whole of the middle and inferior temporal gyri but a curiously characteristic feature of the disease is the way in which the anterior third of the superior temporal gyrus is more affected than the posterior part (Fig. 18.22). Jakob (1969) has reported two cases of pure temporal lobe involvement and has analysed the clinicopathological implications in detail. On the rarer occasions in which the parietal lobe is affected the atrophy is usually in the region of the supramarginal and angular gyri. In contrast, other areas or gyri are relatively resistant. These include the occipital lobes, the posterior part of the paracentral lobule and the anterior transverse gyrus of Heschl.

Pick had already in 1906 noted that the atrophy tended to involve the association areas of Flechsig while Spatz (1952) and others have emphasized that it is those parts of the hemispheres which develop later in ontogeny or phylogeny that tend to be picked out. A major exception to this, however, and one which conflicts with the above concept, is the fact that the hippocampus and the parahippocampal gyrus are at times considerably atrophied. Lüers and Spatz mention a small group in which the hippocampus has been severely, and even selectively, affected. Marked atrophy of the amygdaloid nucleus has also been reported occasionally.

The atrophic process affects the white matter as well as the cortex. The junction between the two becomes blurred to the naked eye and the white matter turns greyish. Von Braunmühl remarked that the affected lobes feel like indiarubber, and the condition was at one time known as 'lobar sclerosis'.

The deep grey matter may also be involved.

Occasionally the atrophy of the caudate nucleus is severe and may resemble that seen in Huntington's chorea (Fig. 18.23) (von Braunmühl 1930). Dewulf (1935) and Akelaitis (1944) reported cases in which the caudate nucleus had all but disappeared while the globus pallidus, but not the putamen, was also severely atrophied. Mansvelt (1954) considered that some degree of caudate

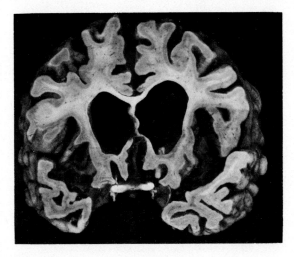

Fig. 18.23 Pick's disease—coronal cut showing gross frontal and temporal atrophy with marked enlargement of lateral ventricles and atrophy of the caudate nuclei.

atrophy occurred in about two-thirds of cases but others have estimated a lower figure (von Bagh 1941). The putamen and at times the globus pallidus are affected in such cases but to a lesser extent and mainly in the anterior levels adjacent to the internal capsule. The thalamus often shows a degree of atrophy that could usually be accounted for by the severe cortical and particularly frontal degeneration (Lüers and Spatz 1957). There have been occasional reports, however, of intact thalami in the face of marked frontal lobe atrophy (von Bagh 1941). The brainstem, cerebellum and spinal cord usually appear normal to the naked eye.

Histology. The first account was given by Alzheimer (1911). The findings consist essentially of an intense loss of nerve cells in the affected areas (Fig. 18.24*b*) accompanied by cortical and subcortical gliosis which some consider as secondary to the neuronal loss (Onari and Spatz 1926). Others, however, have suggested that the gliosis is primary (Sanders, Schenk and van Ween 1939; Malamud and Waggoner 1943), the last noting

that the glial changes may be seen in areas in which there is no apparent degeneration or loss of nerve cells.

The neuronal loss is often greatest in the outer cortical layers but the pattern is variable and the full depth of the ribbon may be affected. M. Vogt (1928) and Schiffer (1955) contended that there is a sequence to the cell loss, layer 3 being the first to degenerate followed by 2 and 5. Schenk and Mansvelt (1955), however, found many exceptions to this rule. Many of the surrounding nerve cells appear small and stain faintly. Pigment may accumulate in the cytoplasm which contains a reduced amount of Nissl substance. These changes are not specific. There is, however, a more distinct type of degeneration which is found in many but not all cases. This consists of the swelling of the cell body which rounds up or becomes pear shaped. The Nissl substance disintegrates, the cytoplasm becomes homogenous and weakly acidophilic while the nucleus is displaced towards the cell membrane (Fig. 18.24*c-h*).

With Nissl's method the swollen area of the cell remains colourless or stains a pale matt blue while a few Nissl granules may still be seen adjacent to the nucleus or at the apex of the cell. With Mallory's phosphotungstic acid haematoxylin the affected cells stand out as pale oval areas against the diffusely stained background. This appearance, combined as it often is with the fibrous gliosis of the cortex, is distinctive and may be of diagnostic value in cases in which the cortical and subcortical atrophy is less striking than that usually seen in Pick's disease.

Although a greater proportion of small than of large neurons in the cortex is generally affected by this change, individual large pyramidal cells in the deeper layers may become severely distended. A similar change may be seen in some neurons of the basal ganglia and in the pigmented cells of the brainstem. In such cells the nucleus moves to one pole and often has an eccentric nucleolus which lies against the nuclear membrane. With Bielschowsky's silver impregnation the swollen part of the cytoplasm may contain a globular, homogeneous well-defined mass which stains with varying intensity. In others the entire cytoplasm of the base of the cell may appear to consist of homogeneous argyrophilic material. In either case some intact neurofibrils may lie at the periphery of the cell.

Onari and Spatz (1926) recognized the resemblance of these Pick cells to those undergoing

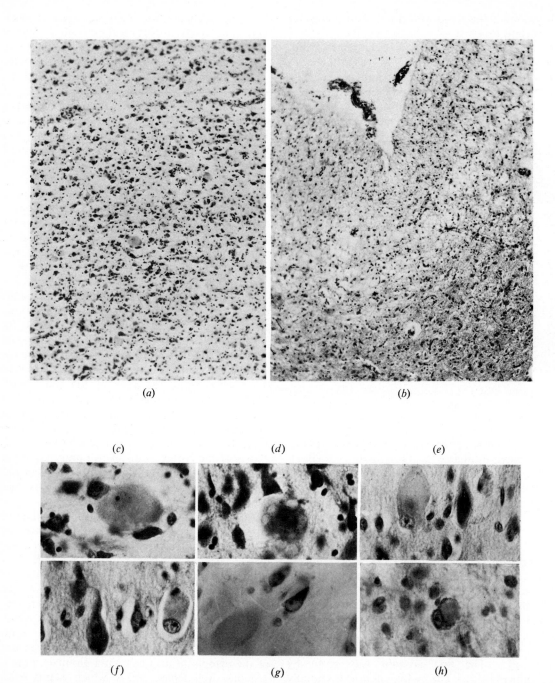

(a)

(b)

(c)   (d)   (e)

(f)   (g)   (h)

Fig. 18.24 Pick's disease (a) Superior temporal gyrus. There is widespread neuronal degeneration with disalignment of neurons: note pale globose forms (Pick's cells). Near the foot is the line of a sulcus. Cresyl violet. × 90. (b) Second temporal gyrus showing widespread atrophy of the cortex with resulting status spongiosus. The section is taken in the depth of a sulcus. Celloidin. Haematoxylin-eosin. × 90. (c) is an enlargement of the cell seen in the centre of (a). (d), (e), (f), (g) and (h) are nerve cells in various stages of degeneration. The nucleus is not visible in the large cell in (g). Cresyl violet. × 400.

axonal degeneration, and Spatz (1952) has re-affirmed his belief that the degenerative process in Pick's disease begins in the periphery of the neuron. This is consonant with Freeman's (1933) view that the white matter is the first part of the brain to be involved. Jakob (1961), however, in a study of 12 cases has opposed this view holding that the neuronal changes start at the level of the cell body. Williams (1935), while distinguishing the change from central chromatolysis following axonal injury, concluded that it only occurs when there is a lesion near its cell of origin.

Electron-microscopy of the ballooned cells (Schochet, Lampert and Earle 1968; Wisniewski and Terry 1971) has revealed no substantial qualitative difference between swollen cells with and without Pick bodies. In both proliferating loose material of neurofilaments and some tubules were found, the endoplasmic reticulum tending to become vesiculated. Wisniewski and Terry see the Pick body as a cytoplasmic accumulation of filaments, tubules or twisted tubules that is possibly the secondary response of a neuron to damage to its processes or is the consequence of transsynaptic degeneration.

The globular masses seen with the light microscope in this form of degeneration have sometimes been called inclusions, but they are less hyaline than those occurring in association with paralysis agitans and they do not have the concentric structure seen both in these and in Lafora inclusions.

The astroglial proliferation is marked in the atrophic cortical and subcortical areas and a status spongiosus of the cortex may develop (Fig. 18.24a). Microglia and oligodendroglia play no special part, although fat phagocytes may at times be seen, particularly in the demyelinated and gliotic subcortical white matter. A lesser degree of neuronal loss and gliosis may be seen in cortical areas that are not grossly atrophic. The deep grey matter in the hemispheres may also be affected and, as already described at the macroscopic level, the caudate nucleus may be almost totally degenerate. Neuronal change and loss have also been reported in the putamen and pallidum, the thalamus and pons. Purkinje cell changes have been recorded at times but are usually absent or minor. (Jervis 1971). Buchanan, Overholt and Neubürger (1947) described parenchymatous cerebellar atrophy in a woman of 45 with Pick's disease. She had died from a bronchial carcinoma with intracranial metastases.

Senile plaques and neurofibrillary changes do not occur as a rule even in elderly patients. They are, however, seen at times and have been reported by Liebers (1939), Smith, Turner and Sim (1966), Wisniewski and Terry (1971). Moyano (1932) described five cases of Pick's disease in which the histological picture of Alzheimer's disease was also present in the atrophic areas. Berlin (1949) reported two cases with the typical features of both Pick's and Alzheimer's disease and suggested that 'these may be conditions which are inter-mediate between the two'. Granulovacuolar degeneration, mainly in the pyramidal cells of the hippocampus, may also be seen in Pick's disease.

The cause of Pick's disease is unknown. Mansvelt (1954) and others have emphasized the possible importance in some cases of exogenous factors, including trauma (Reich 1907; Crezee 1949). No vascular, chemical or other abnormality of aetiological significance has however so far been identified and the disease still remains best described, but not explained, as a heredo-degenerative condition of middle and later life.

Progressive sub-cortical gliosis

Neumann (1949) and Neumann and Cohn (1967) have described several cases of insidious progressive dementia clinically resembling Alzheimer and Pick's diseases in which the most prominent histological feature has been a pronounced subcortical gliosis without severe involvement of the cerebral cortex and with no significant myelin loss. Astrocytic and some microglial proliferation was also marked in the basal ganglia, thalamus, brainstem and ventral horns of the spinal cord. Neumann and Cohn drew attention to similar cases reported by Hassin and Levitin (1941), Stern and Reed (1945), Riese (1952) and possibly those of Yano, Nishina and Kumono (1960). Neumann at first considered that the cases should be taken together as forming a subgroup of Pick's disease. McMenemey (1963a), however, suggested that because the cortex was so relatively unaffected, they were better separated off as examples of some other rare and as yet unclassified pathological condition. Neumann and Cohn in 1967 agreed with this proposal, and because they believed that the gliosis is a primary process, they proposed the title of 'primary subcortical gliosis: a progressive degenerative brain disease'. There are still too few cases to take it further than this.

Huntington's chorea

In 1872, a year after George Huntington had qualified in medicine, he wrote about a hereditary chorea with mental deterioration which came on in middle life and progressed remorselessly until 'the helpless sufferer is but a quivering wreck of his former self'. Lund (1860) and Lyon (1863) had already described a similar disease but it was Huntington's report, based on his father's and his own experiences in their family practice on Long Island, that gave the condition its solid foundation. Heathfield (1973) and Barbeau (1973) have reviewed the historical and other aspects of the disease at length.

The illness has occasionally been reported in children of 5 years or even younger; it has rarely appeared after the age of 75. The first manifestation is usually between 25 and 45 years. Bell (1934) found the average age of onset to be 35 but Wendt, Landzettel and Solth (1960) considered the mid-forties to be more accurate because the earlier studies tended to exclude cases with a late onset (Slater and Cowie 1971).

The disease lasts about 15 years on average, although survival as short as 5 and as long as 30 years has been recorded. Death usually occurs in the early fifties. It is a rare disorder but affects all races, the incidence in Europe, America and Australia being around 4 to 7 per 100,000 (Myrianthopoulous 1966). In Japan the figure was found to be one-tenth of this (Kishimoto, Nakamura and Sotokawa 1959). Local pockets of the disease may occur in which the figure is exceptionally high. These include the Moray Firth (Lyon 1962), Tasmania (Brothers 1949) and North Sweden (Sjögren 1935).

The disease is linked to a single major gene, which manifests dominantly in the heterozygote with a penetrance negligibly less than 100%. Half of any one generation may be expected to inherit the illness. Bruyn (1967), Wendt, Landzettel and Unterreiner (1959) and others have found that the father was the affected parent nearly four times as often as the mother when the illness began before the age of 21 years.

Bird, Caro and Pilling (1974) have shown that affected offspring of a male tend to die at an earlier age than the father, whereas the offspring of females with the disease die at an age not significantly different from that of their mother. No chromosome abnormalities have been found (Benirsche and Höfnagel 1961). In spite of the major genetic factor, failure to obtain a family history of the illness is not uncommon.

In the typical form of Huntington's chorea an initial fidgetiness grows over several years into jerking and choreiform movements. At the same time, or even before this, the patient may become irritable, truculent and perhaps paranoid. Other patients are apathetic and slovenly. Depression is liable to be profound and suicide is a risk. Eventually lack of concentration, confusion and memory impairment merge into dementia. Instances have been recorded in families prone to chorea in which the dementia has progressed and the illness run its course without the development of choreiform movements (Curran 1929; Worster-Drought and Allen 1929; Bolt 1970). It is because of the absence of chorea that the title of Huntington's disease is sometimes preferred (Whittier 1963). Conversely, the chorea may progress with little or no evidence of mental disorder at any stage (Heathfield 1967). Schizophrenia and depressive illness, psychopathic traits or mental subnormality may be found in affected patients and sometimes in other members of the family. Davenport (1915) maintained that the disease may follow a pattern within a family; Heathfield (1973) encountered one in which the father and one son both died with Huntington's chorea and schizophrenia, another son was merely schizophrenic while the third had only the chorea and was mentally normal. Pleydell (1954) found dyslalia was a premonitory sign in one of the families known to him.

A rare, though important, variant of Huntington's chorea is the juvenile form. This occurs with onset between 10 and 20 in about 8% of cases; it is much rarer in the first decade (Bruyn 1967). The illness differs clinically from the adult form in that choreiform movements are rare while akinesia and extrapyramidal rigidity are usual (Campbell, Corner, Norman and Urich 1961). The dementia becomes severe and epileptic attacks are common. Lindenberg (1960) reported on a man with typical Huntington's chorea, whose daughter died aged 29 with a diagnosis of 'juvenile Parkinsonism'.

The disease progresses relentlessly, sometimes with intervals of little change until death occurs, commonly from an intercurrent infection. The pathological changes in Huntington's chorea are generally considered to be restricted to the central nervous system. Bolt and Lewis (1973), however, have recently reported abnormalities in liver function tests and hepatic biopsies.

Macroscopic appearances of brain. The brain may look normal in size but it is usually small and weighs, in some instances, less than 1000 g. Similarly the superficial appearance ranges from normal to that of gross atrophy, a mild to moderate degree being common. The frontal and parietal lobes are usually affected more than the rest of the hemispheres. Neither the leptomeninges nor the large cerebral vessels show changes beyond those consistent with the age. The surface of the brain, therefore, has no distinguishing features. In coronal cuts (Fig. 18.25) through the anterior horns of the lateral ventricles the cardinal feature is the atrophy of the corpus striatum. The head of the caudate nucleus,

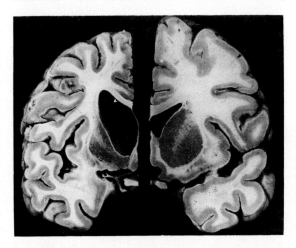

Fig. 18.25 Huntington's chorea. The hemisphere on the left is from a case of this disease in a woman aged 49 (Brain weight 1065 g). That on the right is from a normal woman aged 69 (Brain weight 1415 g).

instead of bulging into the floor of the ventricle, shrinks to a narrow, and even concave, brownish ribbon. The anterior horn becomes dilated with the dorsolateral angle often appearing elongated by the selective striatal atrophy. The putamen, therefore, and to a lesser extent the globus pallidus are also shrunken. The internal capsule, in contrast, appears unusually broad. The body of the corpus callosum is thinned as part of the general loss of white matter in the hemispheres. The cortical ribbon may appear narrowed but the degree varies greatly. The brainstem and cerebellum appear normal. The substantia nigra is usually well pigmented; at times the midbrain, pons and medulla may appear on the small side. In most cases, therefore, a diagnosis of Huntington's chorea can be made with consider-

able assurance on the macroscopic appearances alone. Exceptions do occur, however, in which the striatal atrophy is relatively slight, although severe degenerative changes are later detected under the microscope.

Histology. The main histological abnormalities are found in the caudate nucleus and the putamen, in both of which there is typically an extensive loss of small nerve cells with the relative, but not total, preservation of the large ones. This is often best seen in an atrophic striatum in which the shrinkage has drawn any surviving neurons together and relatively more large ones are included in a single field. The topography of the neuronal loss varies from case to case, both parts of the striatum being affected in some. In others the caudate head seems more involved than the putamen; in yet others the opposite has been recorded. McCaughey (1961) and earlier workers found the more rostral and inferior parts of the striatum to be less vulnerable than the rest. Dunlap (1927) placed the emphasis on the middle and posterior thirds of the putamen. In extreme atrophy of the caudate nucleus a spongy state may develop which is reminiscent of rare cases of Pick's disease (Fig. 18.27). Many of the degenerating neurons in the striatum become small and atrophied and may contain an excess of pigment. Nerve fibres, as well as cells, disappear, those that survive tending to run in bundles forming the status fibrosis described by Vogt.

The neuronal degeneration and loss in the striatum is accompanied by a variable degree of astrocytic proliferation. Occasionally slight, it is more often severe enough to increase considerably the cellularity of the atrophied tissue (Jelgersma 1908). The astrocytes may collect in clusters, their nuclei are often large and their cytoplasm abundant. Many fine granules of greenish pigment lie in and around the glial nuclei. Fibrous gliosis varies in intensity and can be severe; it is usually most conspicuous deep to the ependymal lining and around the blood vessels.

The pallidum is less atrophied than the striatum and the neuronal loss and gliosis are correspondingly slighter. The outer segment tends to be more affected than the inner. A subtle change, discussed by Hallervorden (1957), is the strip of demyelination that sometimes runs along the border between the inner segment of the pallidum and the adjacent internal capsule.

Neuronal loss and gliosis, which is usually mild,

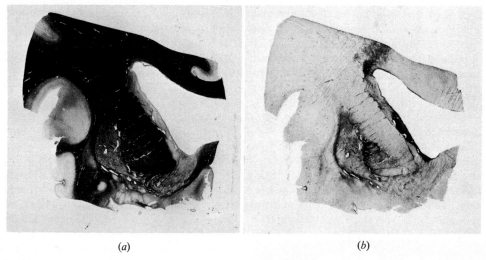

(a)   (b)

Fig. 18.26 Huntington's chorea. Coronal sections of the corpus striatum. (a) Myelin stain. (b) Holzer's neuroglial fibre stain.

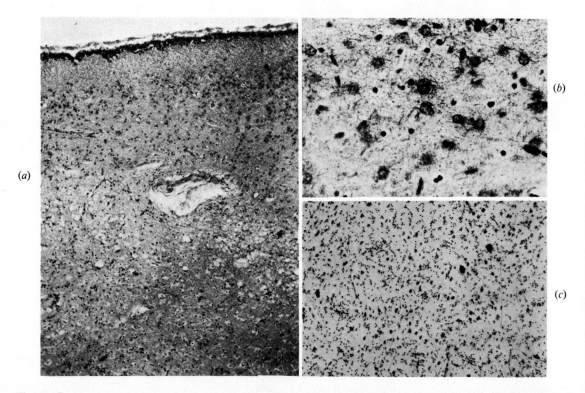

Fig. 18.27 Huntington's chorea. (a) Caudate nucleus showing a spongy state due to almost complete disappearance of neurons: Proliferation of astrocytes is most noticeable deep to the subependymal layer. Celloidin. Haematoxylin-eosin. ×90. (b) Proliferating astrocytes near ventricular surface of caudate nucleus showing only scanty fibre formation. Celloidin. Mallory's phosphotungstic acid haematoxylin.   ×400. (c) Putamen. The small neurons have largely disappeared but occasional large ones are to be seen. Celloidin. Cresyl violet. ×90.

may be seen in the thalamus and in other parts of the diencephalon. The brainstem, cerebellum and spinal cord are in general little affected, but certain more marked local changes have been reported. These include a vulnerability of the zona reticulata but not of the zona compacta, in the substantia nigra; the superior olive is particularly liable to degenerate (Weisschedel 1938). Cell loss in the dentate nucleus of the cerebellum has also been described. Purkinje cell loss has been mentioned in some reports but is not a major or constant feature of the illness.

Cortical degeneration in Huntington's chorea was described by Alzheimer in 1911 and has often been reported since. Although the Vogts held that the fourth layer was particularly vulnerable, it is more generally agreed that neuronal loss and a mild gliosis tend to be centred more on the third and then on the fourth and fifth cortical layers. The pattern of cortical atrophy is in no way characteristic of Huntington's chorea and the histological diagnosis should always be based on the state of the corpus striatum rather than on that of the cerebral cortex. Non-specific neuronal changes in the cortex vary in kind and in degree, many cells being shrunken and showing pigment atrophy. Dunlap believed that the cortical neurons might not be reduced in numbers but were only shrunken. Tellez-Nagel, Johnson and Terry (1974), working on biopsies from frontal cortex, re-emphasized the marked accumulation of lipofuscin both in nerve cells and in glia. Myelin is usually well preserved in the hemispheres but slight loss of radial and tangential myelinated fibres in the cortex has been described at times (Schröder 1931).

The cerebral cortex of the frontal lobes is the most affected but the degree of atrophy varies greatly and does not always tally with the clinical picture. For example, the first of Davison, Goodhart and Schliowsky's (1932) patients had no mental symptoms while atrophy extended from the frontal lobe to the postcentral gyrus. Conversely, their second patient was demented whereas the cortical changes were slight.

Neither the cause of the cortical atrophy nor of the striatal degeneration is known. Although the latter has generally been held to underlie the development of the involuntary movements, Mettler (1957) drew attention to the possible importance of the subthalamic nucleus in this respect. Cases of progressive chorea with lesions in this centre have been reported (Titeca and van Bogaert 1946; Malamud and Demmy 1960), but subthalamic degeneration, although recorded by Alzheimer, has not been generally accepted as a major or constant feature in the pathology of Huntington's chorea.

In recent years, and particularly after the demonstration of abnormal copper metabolism in Wilson's disease, the biochemical aspects of the disorder have been increasingly studied. Most reports, however, including those on trace metals and on autoimmune factors, have proved inconclusive. Nevertheless, several have identified neurochemical abnormalities in striatal and nigral tissue removed shortly after death. Perry, Hansen and Kloster (1973) found low levels of gamma aminobutyric acid in both areas while in addition to this, the most consistent abnormality found by Bird and Iversen (1974) has been a decrease in glutamic acid decarboxylase not only in the striatum and pallidum but also (personal communication) in the substantia nigra and in the dentate nucleus of the cerebellum. They did not, however, find similar changes in the frontal or hippocampal cortex. McGeer, McGeer and Fibiger (1973) and Stahl and Swanson (1974) have reported along similar lines.

Huntington's chorea is rarely combined with other disorders. Occasionally it may be difficult to separate it from Pick's disease, particularly when the striatum is involved in the latter. Simma (1952) tried to set out the essential differences but they are not clear cut. In Pick's disease, however, the large neurons in the striatum and the caudal half of the putamen are both spared more than is usual in Huntington's chorea. Birnbaum (1941) recorded two cases which were combined with cerebellar atrophy, and other equally rare associations with, for example, motor neuron disease, have been listed by Hallervorden (1957). Van der Eecken, Adams and van Bogaert (1960) have described a condition characterized clinically by extrapyramidal rigidity with minimal tremor and pathologically by striatal, pallidal and nigral degeneration; small-cell loss in the caudate nucleus and putamen was almost complete. The condition may, therefore, have an affinity with Huntington's chorea. Podolsky, Leopold and Sax (1972) deduced from their evidence that an abnormal genetic linkage might exist with diabetes mellitus. Trauma has been invoked by Flügel (1928) and Claude, Lhermitte and Meignant (1930) and denied by others.

Finally, dyskinetic movements induced by drugs

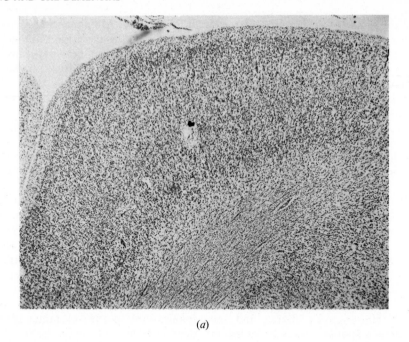

(a)

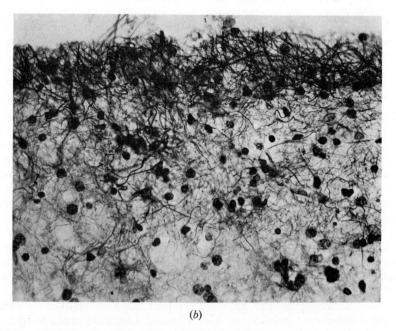

(b)

Fig. 18.28 Creutzfeldt—Jakob disease. (a) Frontal cortex showing almost complete disappearance of large pyramidal cells. Nissl. ×20. (b) Subpial layer of frontal cortex. Holzer. ×350.

have become increasingly common in psychiatric and in other patients in recent years (Brandon, McClelland and Protheroe 1971). This association needs to be borne in mind since the movements may at times mimic those of Huntington's chorea. The morbid anatomy of these iatrogenic phenomena is not known. Christensen, Moller and Faurbye (1970), however, reported a higher incidence of degenerative changes in the substantia nigra and midbrain of affected patients than in similar areas in their control brains.

Creutzfeldt—Jakob disease

This name is given to a progressive dementia, mainly of the presenile period, accompanied by a wide range of neurological abnormalities which include pyramidal and extrapyramidal signs, and sometimes amyotrophy. The three salient neuropathological features affect predominantly the grey matter stretching from the cortex to the spinal cord. They are neuronal degeneration and loss, astrocytic proliferation and the development of a spongy state or status spongiosus.

The considerable variations in the clinical picture and in the distribution of the pathological findings have led to much controversy in defining the boundaries of this condition while repeated attempts have been made to separate it into subgroups. These difficulties have been compounded by the rarity of the syndrome (Kirschbaum 1968). It is, however, probably a commoner condition than has been realized, for its pathological features, unlike those of Alzheimer's and Pick's disease, may be not only unspectacular and uncertain to demonstrate, but they are often even more difficult to interpret. The detailed study of these cases tends, therefore, to be shelved and many go unreported. The typical picture will be described first.

The illness usually occurs in middle age but cases have been reported as early as 20 (Stender 1930) and later than the 60s. The sexes are affected equally. The duration runs from a few months to a few years. The disorder presents with an initial period of undue fatiguability, and with loss of memory, strange behaviour and apathy. Delusions, delirium and syncopal attacks may occur. Dementia soon follows and is accompanied by a variety of motor signs, including choreoathetosis and spasticity. Swallowing and balance may be disturbed. Gradual but inexorable deterioration takes place, myoclonus convulsions

and rigidity may develop; death usually follows a period of deepening coma and cachexia (May 1968). Neurological features are, therefore, more striking than in Alzheimer's or even in Pick's disease.

Little attention has so far been paid to the general pathological findings and nothing important appears so far to have been identified. The neuropathological features are varied. To the naked eye the brain may, but does not necessarily, look atrophied. Its weight ranges from normal to around 1100 g, but it may be as low as 850 g. There is usually little or no leptomeningeal thickening and the large vessels appear healthy. The ventricles may be slightly enlarged and the deep grey matter, including the corpus striatum and thalamus, appear mildly shrunken. Occasionally the atrophy is more marked. Under the microscope, degeneration and loss of nerve cells, accompanied by proliferating and hypertrophied astrocytes, and often by a status spongiosus, tend to extend widely through the cerebral cortex (Fig. 18.28). The subcortical grey matter including the basal ganglia and thalamus, the brainstem and the spinal cord, may show neuronal loss and gliosis (Fig. 18.29). It is because of this widespread distribution that the condition has been called 'cortico-striato-spinal degeneration'. The white matter is usually spared or shows only a minor loss of fibres or of myelin. The degree of neuronal change and loss is variable. When extreme, the lamination, particularly of the middle and deeper layers of the cortex, can be all but lost; at other times, or in some areas, the neuronal population is only partially reduced. Many nerve cells appear shrunken, others are swollen and the cytoplasm vacuolated. The appearances in the larger cortical neurons sometimes suggest 'primary irritation' (Jansen and Monrad-Krohn 1938). Pigment and fat droplets may accumulate in the neuronal cytoplasm. Intracellular neurofibrils may appear to be thinned out while Alzheimer tangles have been reported very occasionally (Jervis, Hurdum and O'Neill 1942), but neither they nor the senile plaques observed by Stengel and Wilson (1946), and at times by others, are of more than incidental interest.

The glial changes are usually striking. Astrocytes hypertrophy and proliferate greatly within the degenerating grey matter and even at times in regions free of altered or lost neurons. Kirschbaum (1968) described the astrocytic reaction as the first line of defence and a dense fibrous gliosis may develop. These fibrous astrocytes may spread to a lesser degree through the centrum semi-ovale and become more prominent again in the grey matter of the diencephalon, the brainstem, the cerebellum and the spinal cord. The microglial reaction is noticeable but is less pronounced than that of the astrocytes; occasional microglial clusters collect adjacent to small vessels.

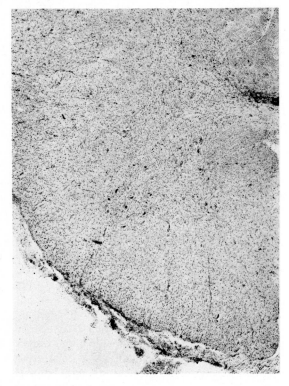

Fig. 18.29 Creutzfeldt–Jakob disease. Section of spinal cord at level L3 showing almost complete disappearance of motor nerve cells. Nissl. × 25.

Glial stars and rosettes are common in the grey matter; they tend to occur most in the deeper cortical layers. Teichmann (1935) noted perivascular cuffing with lymphocytes in one case but this is exceptional; in general, the walls of the small vessels appear intact.

A feature of considerable interest is the inconstant tendency for the grey matter in some areas to develop a finely meshed spongy state. According to Kirschbaum, some degree of this porosity has been noted in about two-thirds of the recorded cases but the extent varies greatly from brain to brain and within a single specimen. The intensity seems not to be closely dependent on either the severity of the neuronal loss or of the astrocytic reaction, although Beck et al. (1969) would link it more closely to the latter. The spongy state appears as myriads of closely packed microcysts with a preference for the middle and deeper cortical layers, the grey matter of the hemispheres including the thalamus, the basal ganglia and the hindbrain. Its pathogenesis remains uncertain although electron-microscopy has revealed that the vacuoles develop in astrocytic and, less often, in neuronal processes (Gonatas, Terry and Weiss 1965; Lampert, Earle, Gibbs and Gajdusek 1969). Bignami (1973) has proposed that they are the result of a defect in the permeability of cell membranes which leads to intracytoplasmic accumulation of fluid.

The cardinal histological features of this disorder may be summarized therefore as the loss of nerve cells, marked astrocytic proliferation with some microglial reaction and the frequent but not constant development of a spongy state. The vasculature is not appreciably affected; myelin loss is minor.

The less typical forms and other possibly related conditions—an historical outline

In 1921 Creutzfeldt reported at length on a woman who had died at the age of 22 from a 'particular disseminated disease of the central nervous system'. In her family there were two retarded sisters, while her own behaviour had been bizarre for many years. At the age of 16 she began to walk clumsily; during the last few months of her life the clinical picture changed. She had an exfoliative dermatitis and started to run an intermittent fever, she developed a fluctuating psychotic disorder and jerky movements of the hands and feet. She died demented with spastic limbs and in status epilepticus. Patches of neuronal necrosis, gliosis and some capillary proliferation were scattered through a moderately atrophic brain but were principally in the cortical ribbon around the bases of the sulci, the diencephalon, the brainstem and the cord. There was no inflammatory reaction.

In the following year Alfons Jakob (1921) identified a 'peculiar form of progressive dementia' which was combined with pyramidal and extrapyramidal signs. He had encountered the syndrome in three middle-aged patients, one of whom had died within a few months of the onset and the other within two years. In the brains, neuronal degeneration and loss, with astrocytic proliferation, were particularly marked in the frontal and temporal cortex, in the medial parts of the thalamus and in the cerebellum, brainstem and spinal cord. Jakob likened his cases to that of Creutzfeldt and combined the four under the title of 'spastic pseudosclerosis' because of a similarity with Wilson's disease and amyotrophic lateral sclerosis. Within the year Spielmeyer coined the term 'Creutzfeldt–Jakob disease' and this title has long been widely accepted, although the priority

and fully discussed by Kirschbaum. As he has shown, the addition of further examples soon widened the clinical and the pathological spectra. Thus Meyer in 1929 reported a single instance of a disease resembling amyotrophic lateral sclerosis but with mental disorder which he believed to form a bridge linking amyotrophic lateral sclerosis and Creutzfeldt–Jakob disease. Davison (1932) described two cases similar to that

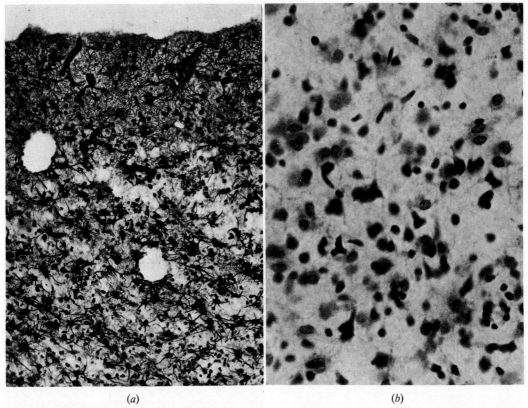

(a)   (b)

Fig. 18.30 Subacute cortical atrophy of Heidenhain type (case of Meyer, Leigh and Bagg 1954). Occipital cortex. (a) Stained by silver carbonate. × 150. (b) Nissl stain, showing degeneration of nerve cells and astrocytic hyperplasia. × 500.

has been reversed to Jakob–Creutzfeldt by Kirschbaum (1968), partly because the definitive contribution was made by Jakob and partly because Creutzfeldt's case was far from typical even within the uncertain limits set for this disease (Brownell and Oppenheimer 1965).

By 1923 Jakob had added two further cases and since then upwards of 150 cases have been recorded, the existence of several variants has been proposed and about ten further eponymous or descriptive names have been introduced. All cases published before 1968 have been summarized

of Meyer and proposed the alternative title of 'cortico-pallido-spinal degeneration'.

A further variant had been reported in the same year as that of Meyer by Heidenhain (1929). This was described as 'a peculiar pre-senile organic disorder of the central nervous system'. Several features were common to Creutzfeldt–Jakob disease but in two of the three cases the course had been rapid, cortical blindness had been a major feature and the brunt of the degenerative process had fallen on the occipital lobes. Swelling or shrinkage and loss of neurons were marked,

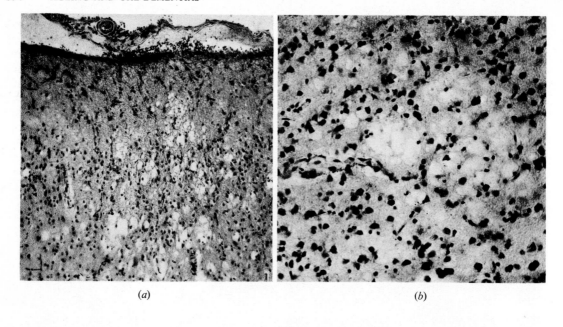

(a)   (b)

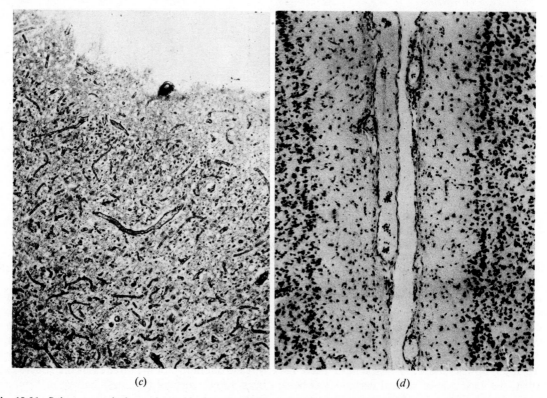

(c)   (d)

Fig. 18.31 Subacute cortical atrophy (case of Jones and Nevin 1954). (a) and (b) show cortical atrophy of spongy type (Case 1). (c) An area of more severe degeneration in the frontal cortex, showing hyperplasia of the capillaries (Case 1). (d) Neuroglial hyperplasia at junction of molecular and external granular layers (Case 2).

together with a heavy astrocytic proliferation, while in the most affected areas a spongy state had developed. The more anterior parts of the hemispheres were relatively intact and Heidenhain felt justified in separating his cases from those of Jakob and that of Creutzfeldt. In 1954, Meyer, Leigh and Bagg described a patient who had survived an illness lasting six months. Cortical blindness and dementia were the salient clinical features while the pathological changes were also similar to those found by Heidenhain (Fig. 18.30a, b). Meyer et al. therefore proposed that the three cases should be separated off under the name Heidenhain's syndrome.

In the same year Jones and Nevin (1954) described two cases of rapidly progressive cerebral degeneration characterized by a general loss of cortical neurons, marked glial overgrowth and a spongy state in the most affected areas (Fig. 18.31a-d). Both patients had deteriorated mentally, developed focal neurological signs with myoclonic epilepsy and had died within 6 months of the onset. Jones and Nevin likened their cases to those of Heidenhain's syndrome but they attributed the condition to a circulatory disturbance, even though the cerebral blood vessels appeared intact.

In 1955 Foley and Denny-Brown introduced a condition which they named 'sub-acute progressive encephalopathy with bulbar myoclonus'. This was based on the neuropathological study of two patients in both of whom the brainstem and cerebellum showed degenerative changes, in addition to the cerebral cortex and thalamus. The disorder was attributed to a primary degeneration of protoplasmic astrocytes and the spongy state which was seen was put down to the acuteness of the process. The illness had lasted 13 months in one case and 5 months in the other. Jacob, Eicke and Orthner (1958) described four further instances under the title of 'sub-acute pre-senile spongiform atrophy with a dyskinetic end stage'. Nevin, McMenemey, Behrman and Jones (1960) added another eight cases while further examples of an apparently similar condition have been reported by Alema and Bignami (1959), Kramer (1959) and Garcin, Brion and Khochneviss (1962). This group of cases is now sometimes referred to as 'sub-acute spongiform encephalopathy' or the 'Nevin–Jones syndrome'. Nevin (1967) discussed in some detail the ways in which this illness differs from the classical type of Creutzfeldt–Jakob disease and concluded that it is a separate, well-

defined entity with its own clinical, electroencephalographic and pathological features.

Another small group that has been tenuously linked to the Creutzfeldt–Jakob complex is made up of those rare cases in which the degenerative process has mainly affected the thalamus. Stern (1939) studied the brain of a 41-year-old man with drowsiness, thirst and polyuria who became severely demented. Marked bilateral thalamic degeneration and gliosis was present with less striking changes throughout the cerebral cortex, in the midbrain and in the inferior olives. Stern considered this as a pure system degeneration involving the thalamus; others have seen it as an unusual form of Pick's disease. Schulman (1956) reported bilateral symmetrical degeneration of the thalami with minimal cortical changes in the brain of a 50-year-old man who had died after a 6-month illness in which intellectual and emotional deterioration had been followed by speech impairment, ataxia and choreo-athetoid movements. Kirschbaum also included in this group cases reported by Poursines, Boudouresques and Roger (1953), Khochneviss (1960) and McMenemey, Grant and Berhman (1965).

In 1965 Brownell and Oppenheimer described an ataxic form of subacute cerebellar polioencephalopathy which they considered to fall within the boundaries of Creutzfeldt–Jakob disease.

Most of the above contributions have been manifestly aimed at establishing variants within the Creutzfeldt–Jakob family. A few have suggested divorce on the grounds of clinical or pathological incompatibility while many more studies, which remain unquoted, have contributed evidence in support of one or other side. Each of the reports has been analysed by Kirschbaum (1968) whose final conclusion, like that of Siedler and Malamud (1963), reflects the current view (Beck et al. 1969) that the Creutzfeldt–Jakob disease should at present be looked on as a 'single nosological entity whose diversity of clinical manifestations is readily explained by the variability in the sites of maximal pathology within the central nervous system'. At least two patterns may then be identified in addition to the cerebellar variant of Brownell and Oppenheimer. In the first, the illness occurs most often in the forties, its onset is insidious and it lasts around two years. This is the group which is composed broadly of the classical examples of Creutzfeldt–Jakob disease combined with the borderline cases that may link this illness with motor neuron and other system diseases. Pathologically, the cortical atrophy in these cases tends to be most noticeable in the frontal and temporal lobes and the brainstem and spinal cord are also prone to be involved.

In the second, the illness usually develops 10 to 15 years later than in the first subgroup. The onset is more acute and the average duration is around 6 months. Pathologically the cortical atrophy is more widespread, but there is a bias towards greater involvement of the occipital lobes. The cortical degeneration may be particularly severe and a widely disseminated spongy state is not infrequently found but the brainstem and spinal cord tend to be spared. This is the subgroup already outlined under the heading of 'spongiform encephalopathy'.

Until the last few years the aetiology of Creutzfeldt–Jakob disease in all its forms has been obscure. Evidence of a hereditary or a familial factor is exceptional although at least three families have been reported. The affected members of these would together account for about a score of the 180 or so cases that have so far been recorded. The best known is the Backer family, first reported by Kirschbaum in 1924, in which six proven cases occurred in three generations. Kirschbaum (1968) has traced the further ramifications of this remarkable tree.

Davison and Rabiner (1940) described the disease in two brothers and a sister. This family, however, has been considered by some as suffering from amyotrophic lateral sclerosis with a psychiatric illness resembling that reported by Meyer (1929). Friede and de Jong (1964) and May, Itabashi and de Jong (1968) have identified the illness in its typical form in three siblings and possibly in the father of the family.

A resemblance between this condition and pellagra has been noted by Stadler (1939) and both Jervis et al. (1942) and Stengal and Wilson (1949) suggested that nutritional deficiency may play an important part.

The most fundamental advance in knowledge about the aetiology of the condition came in 1968 after Gibbs et al. had inoculated cerebral biopsy tissue that had been taken from a patient with Creutzfeldt–Jakob disease into the brain of a chimpanzee. Thirteen months later the animal went down with a neurological illness resembling that of the patient and both brains were in due course found to show similar changes (Beck et al. 1969). Since that time the inocula from other patients have produced the same effect, while Gibbs

and Gajdusek (1969) have further passaged the condition from one chimpanzee to another. More recently still, it has proved possible to transmit to New World monkeys in the same way (Gajdusek and Gibbs 1971; Zlotnik, Grant, Dayan and Earl 1974), while Duffy, Wolf, Collins, DeVoe, Streetem and Cowen (1974) reported the apparent transmission of the illness from an affected patient to another person as the result of a corneal graft.

This disease, therefore, which has for 50 years been looked on as a particularly obscure form of subacute presenile cerebral degeneration is now shown to be transmissible. The agent, however, has not yet been isolated. It has been called a slow virus, and like other slow viruses appears as something new to microbiology (Gajdusek 1972). It is strikingly atypical in that it elicits no inflammatory response in either the brain or in other organs, nor does it induce antibody formation. Its antigenic properties are, therefore, unknown and its physicochemical nature controversial (Gibbs and Gajdusek 1972). This problem is mentioned again briefly under kuru (p. 317).

Parkinsonism–dementia complex of Guam

The Chamorro people living on Guam and on the other Mariana islands in the Western Pacific are curiously prone to develop two fatal neurological diseases. One of these is amyotrophic lateral sclerosis (Arnold, Edgren and Palladino 1953; Malamud et al. 1961); the other is a form of Parkinsonism with dementia. At times the two occur together. Both affect adult men and women, death usually occurring between the ages of 50 and 60 after an illness lasting about 4 years (Hirano 1965).

The main macroscopic features of the Parkinsonism–dementia form of the disease were summarized by Hirano et al. (1961) as cortical, and sometimes pallidal, atrophy of a moderate degree together with a marked lack of pigment in the substantia nigra and in the locus ceruleus. Histologically, neuronal degeneration was present, mainly in the frontal and temporal cortex, Ammon's horn, amygdaloid nucleus, hypothalamus, globus pallidus, thalamus, periaqueductal grey matter, the substantia nigra and the tegmentum of the brainstem. A striking feature in these areas was the presence of many Alzheimer neurofibrillary tangles, but with the virtual absence of senile plaques. Granulovacuolar bodies, and some eosinophilic rod-like structures were seen in the large hippocampal neurons while the former were also occasionally identified in nerve cells elsewhere.

Similar changes were found in the amyotrophic lateral sclerosis group with the provisos that would be expected. Firstly, in the latter group the usual histological features of amyotrophic lateral sclerosis were also present, as indeed they were to some extent in those cases of the Parkinsonism–dementia group in whom clinical evidence of motor neuron disease had been observed. Secondly, the loss of pigment, the neurofibrillary degeneration and cell loss in the substantia nigra and locus ceruleus tended to be considerably more marked in the group with the Parkinsonian features. Hirano made the interesting point that Lewy bodies as well as neurofibrillary tangles were present in the substantia nigra of a few patients. He emphasized that patients with features both of amyotrophic lateral sclerosis and of the Parkinson–dementia complex were common enough for both conditions to be looked on as the different manifestations of a 'single disease entity'. Its aetiology is unknown but a certain resemblance to Creutzfeldt–Jakob disease has been noted although the striking intensity of the neurofibrillary change would seem to be a major point of difference. The possibility of an infectious cause was considered by Hirano, Malamud, Elizan and Kurland (1966) but this has not so far been demonstrated.

Kraepelin's disease

Kraepelin (1910) first described a rare form of dementia, which now bears his name; 17 cases have been reported to date. It consists of rapidly progressive mental deterioration with restlessness, anxiety, depression, speech defects, and sometimes catatonia, and lasts one or two years. Oksala (1923) reported post-mortem findings in three patients from Kraepelin's clinic, aged 47, 59 and 48 respectively. Catatonia was present in the first two cases, diagnosed as pernicious presenile psychosis, with symptoms lasting respectively 9 and 3 months. The illness of the third patient also lasted 3 months and was associated with delusions, rapid loss of weight and eventually paralysis of one half of the face. In each case the essential feature appeared to be a phased destruction of the Nissl substance and consequent breaking up of the nerve cells. Fat could be demonstrated in the cells and around the blood vessels and there was neuronophagia and evidence of axis cylinder degenera-

tion. The most affected regions were the frontal, the central and Ammon's horn, and the least, the occipital. The third lamina was most concerned in this change with the fifth next: there was not much involvement of the sixth lamina. The changes were patchy in distribution. The father of the third patient was insane.

Best (1941) reported the necropsy findings of a further case of Kraepelin's presenile dementia in a man aged 34. The illness began as an acute catatonic psychosis leading to an expansive type of organic dementia and it proved fatal in 5 months. There was a family history of mental instability on the maternal side. She describes and illustrates swollen neurons with a homogeneous, pale and glassy cytoplasm sometimes obscuring the nucleus, but sometimes associated with swelling of the nucleoli. This change appeared to affect the larger cells, including the Betz cells, but other neurons showed the severe cell change of Nissl. Fat was not identified in the swollen cells but was present around the blood vessels. Neuronal degeneration was most evident in layers 1, 2 and 3, but it also involved the cells of the striatum, pallidum and dentate nucleus. Caution is necessary in interpreting these changes for the mode of death was asphyxiation, due to the inhalation of vomitus induced by scopolamine and morphia medication for the alleviation of catatonic excitement.

A further case was reported by Grünthal (1936) and 11 others by Grünthal and Kuhn (1959), all with post-mortem findings. They stress the catatonic-like features which accompany the psychosis, the shrunken pyknotic appearance of the neurons and the involvement of both the dentate nucleus and the large cells of the striatum. The age of onset was mostly common in the fourth decade but three were first affected in adolescence, while one appears to have been only 6 years old. The duration varied from under one year to 23, some of the histories being recurrent.

The infrequency with which the disease has been reported, its variable duration and the fact that the nerve cell changes, genuine although they may appear to be, are unassociated with any significant changes in the glia renders this condition as a pathological entity still *sub judice*.

Pathological conditions associated with memory disorder and dementia

Deterioration of memory is one of the main features of dementia and is then usually attributable to the widespread degeneration of cerebral tissue. There are, however, occasions in which the memory disorder is dominant and in which certain regions of the brain appear to play a particular role. One is that of the mamillary bodies and the medial thalamus; the other is the grey matter in the inferomedial parts of the temporal lobe, including the hippocampus and the parahippocampal gyrus. These two regions, which are connected by the fornix, constitute a major part of the limbic areas, named after 'the great limbic lobe of Broca' (1878).

In 1890, Korsakow reported an illness, now named after him, which he attributed to toxaemia

Wernicke's encephalopathy, which was centred on the periventricular grey matter in the brains of patients dying from alcoholism or from other causes. Gudden (1896) and Bonhoeffer (1897) noticed that the mamillary bodies were particularly vulnerable and the latter hinted at a connection between the damage in this area and the Korsakow state. This hypothesis was not generally accepted until Gamper (1928) demonstrated that although the damage spread through the grey matter encircling the walls of the aqueduct and of the 3rd and 4th ventricles it was most intense in the mamillary bodies (Fig. 18.32). Gamper postulated that this lesion interfered with

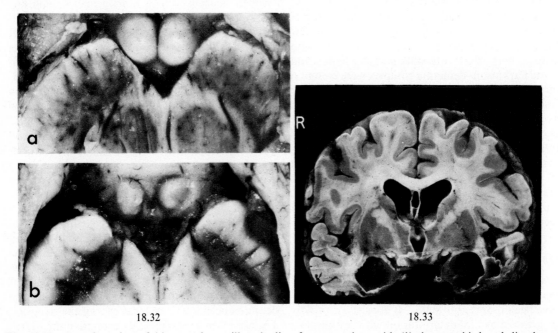

18.32   18.33

Fig. 18.32 A surface view of (*a*) normal mamillary bodies, for comparison with (*b*) the atrophied and discoloured mamillary bodies of a 'Korsakovian' patient.
Fig. 18.33 Coronal cut through the brain of a woman who had survived, grossly amnesic, for 17 years after an attack of necrotizing encephalitis. The medial temporal grey matter on the right side (R) and much of the left temporal lobe have been destroyed.

resulting from various causes including too much alcohol. He described how 'together with the confusion, nearly always a profound disorder of memory is observed although at times the disorder of memory occurs in pure form . . . this manifests itself in an extraordinarily peculiar amnesia in which the memory of recent events is chiefly disturbed, whereas the remote past was remembered fairly well'. Some ten years before this Wernicke (1881) had identified a severe tissue reaction, now known as Wernicke's, or Gayet–

the pathways linking the mamillary bodies to the midbrain, the thalamus and the cerebral cortex, and that this interruption lay at the root of the memory disorder in the Korsakow state. Although at first not generally accepted (Carmichael and Stern 1931), many subsequent studies (Kant 1933; Delay, Brion and Elisalde 1958) have confirmed Gamper's observations and the illness described by Korsakow is now widely recognized to be in many, but not all, cases the result of damage to the brain caused by an attack of

Wernicke's encephalopathy, which is itself attributable to the effects of alcoholism or of other disorders leading to thiamine deficiency. As described by Gamper and by Malamud and Skillicorn (1956), the mamillary bodies have nearly always been found to be the most vulnerable and occasional cases have been reported in which no other area appeared to have been affected (Brierley 1966). There is, nevertheless, a striking tendency for neuronal loss and gliosis to occur medially in the thalamus and Victor, Adams and Collins (1971) have argued that the lesion in the dorsomedial nucleus is the more important factor. It should not be forgotten, however, that much of this nucleus degenerates as a result of leucotomy operations (Meyer and Beck 1954), while Spiegel, Wycis, Orchinik and Freed (1955) have claimed to destroy it stereotactically; but in neither instance has such damage resulted in a lasting disorder of memory. It may, therefore, be premature to incriminate one part of the deep grey matter rather than another. The more crucial points seem to be that the damage is always bilateral and that it lies along the diencephalic sector of the limbic pathways.

Bechterew (1900) briefly considered the effect on memory of damage to the temporal lobes. The most striking evidence of this, however, was reported by Scoville in 1954 after the resection of the inferomedial parts of the temporal lobes in several psychotic patients. He and Milner (1957) found that a severe defect in recent memory was produced by the bilateral removal of the hippocampus and parahippocampal gyrus but not by operations affecting only the uncus and the amygdaloid nucleus. Pilleri (1966) and McLardy (1970) have emphasized the importance of the parahippocampal cortex.

Petit-Dutaillis et al. in 1954 had removed the anterior parts, but not the hippocampi, of both temporal lobes from a patient with epilepsy. Only a transient disorder of recent memory occurred although there was a permanent retrograde amnesia covering several months. Terzian and Ore (1955) removed the entire anterior parts of both temporal lobes as well as most of the two hippocampi. 'A serious deficiency in memory' was noted as one of the effects but the main emphasis was on the resemblance of the postoperative clinical picture to the Klüver–Bucy syndrome (Gascon and Gilles 1973).

Interference with recent memory is usual only when the medial temporal damage is bilateral, but unilateral resections may have an effect. Milner and Penfield (1955) and Serafetinides and Falconer (1962) reported that the removal of one temporal lobe was sometimes followed by a defect in recent memory although there were usually grounds to suspect that the contralateral hippocampus might have been diseased as well. Meyer and Yates (1955) and Meyer (1959) found that new verbal and auditory learning could be impaired by the removal of the dominant temporal lobe, although Blakemore and Falconer (1967) found that the defect in the auditory side tended eventually to disappear. Stepien and Sierpinski (1964) have discussed the effect on memory of temporal lobe lesions. They described several epileptic patients in whom a memory disorder was associated with bilateral electroencephalographic abnormalities. After removing one lobe, however, the abnormal discharges on the unoperated side as well as the memory disorder disappeared. They postulated that unilateral lesions may interrupt normal activity throughout the brain and that their excision removes the source of irritation.

There are several other pathological conditions in which the medial parts of the temporal lobes tend to be selectively affected. One of these is the form of *necrotizing encephalitis*, described by van Bogaert, Radermecker and Davos (1955) in which an acute inflammatory reaction underlies the massive necrosis of much or all of both temporal lobes. The illness, in which there is often evidence of herpes simplex infection, is usually fatal within two weeks (Adams and Jennett 1967). A few adults, however, survive the acute attack for months or years. At times the onset is insidious. In either case the patients are likely to be left with an incapacitating defect in recent memory or they may be demented. Rose and Symonds (1960) reported clinically on three adults with 'persistent memory defect following encephalitis'. One (case 3) who survived with gross amnesia for 17 years was found to have lost the medial parts of both temporal lobes as the consequence of a necrotising encephalitis (Fig. 18.33).

Not all cases of encephalitis of the limbic areas, however, are of the necrotizing type. Brierley, Corsellis, Hierons and Nevin (1960) reported three patients in their fifties who had become demented over a period lasting from a few months to a year. No cause for the dementia (or for the marked memory loss noted in two of the three patients) was attributed during life but the common neurohistological feature was a severe inflammatory reaction centred on the limbic grey matter. No cause was identified but in one case the presence of a secondary deposit from an unsuspected bronchial carcinoma introduced a further problem.

Limbic encephalitis and malignant disease

Patients with malignant disease, and particularly with bronchial carcinoma, are prone to become mentally ill. Sometimes the disorder is in the nature of a toxic confusional state and the brain shows no particular abnormality (Charatan and Brierley 1956; McGovern, Miller and Robertson 1959). Occasionally, however, dementia, or predominantly a memory disorder, may develop. This may be either in the presence of other non-metastatic neurological disease, such as in the cerebellar degenerations associated with carcinoma (Brain, Daniel and Greenfield 1951; Henson, Hoffman and Urich 1965) or the mental deterioration may occur on its own. Corsellis, Goldberg and Norton (1968) described three patients with bronchial carcinomata in the latter category, two of whom had become demented while the third suffered for over two years from a curiously discrete loss of recent memory. Attention was drawn to several similar cases that had been reported. The brains showed perivascular round-cell infiltration, resembling an encephalitis, which was concentrated mainly on the medial temporal grey matter. Glial nodules were common and a variable degree of neuronal necrosis was seen. The appearances were usually those of a tissue reaction which was considerably more intense than that attributable to a primary neuronal degeneration and yet not as grossly destructive as that occurring in necrotizing limbic encephalitis. Henson *et al.* (1965) and Richardson (1965) surmised that the condition might be of viral, and even of herpes simplex origin. Some support for this was provided by Dayan, Bhatti and Gostling (1967) who reported that a fatal, and proven

herpetic, encephalitis had developed in a woman several months after the removal of a uterine carcinoma. There is little direct evidence beyond this, however, to support the viral hypothesis. Similarly, metabolic and immune factors have been invoked but not identified and both the relation of the condition to carcinoma and its aetiology remain unknown. Smith (1970) suggested that minute metastatic foci might have been overlooked, but such repeated oversight seems improbable and the curiously intense tissue reaction would remain unexplained. It should not be forgotten, however, that dementia has been reported in association with carcinomatous infiltration of the leptomeninges (Fischer-Williams, Bosanquet and Daniel 1955).

Indeed, it should be emphasized that there are many diffuse or multifocal disorders of the brain in which a variable degree of intellectual deterioration may occur. In addition to those considered in the present chapter dementia may be the sequel to infections of the nervous system, to episodes of severe cerebral ischaemia or hypoxia, to metabolic and endocrine disturbances, while it may also occur in association with system degenerations and with demyelinating disease. The nature of the cerebral abnormality will then vary according to the type of illness.

In general, most patients with a progressive dementia fall into one or other of the established categories. This chapter should have shown, if nothing else, that in the present state of knowledge nosological overlap is common and drawing hard and fast lines can be less than profitable. Sometimes an abnormality is evident but its origin and its classification are not. In others it may be difficult or even impossible to find any structural abnormality. For obvious reasons, such cases tend to go unrecorded but it would be misleading to imply either that they never occur or that they are at all common.

References

Abely, X., Guiraud, P. & Dechosal, J. (1958) Alzheimer of acute onset. *Annales médico-psychologiques* **116**, 294-299.

Adams, C. W. M. (1965) in *Neurohistochemistry*. Elsevier, London.

Adams, J. H. & Jennett, W. B. (1967) Acute necrotizing encephalitis: a problem in diagnosis. *Journal of Neurology, Neurosurgery and Psychiatry*, **30**, 248-260.

Agostini, L. (1958) La dégénerescence d'Alzheimer dans les cellules nerveuses de l'allocortex; topographie, cytologie, histochimie. *Psychiatria Neurologia*, **136**, 1-17.

Akelaitis, A. J. (1944) Atrophy of basal ganglia in Pick's disease. A clinicopathologic study. *Archives of Neurology and Psychiatry*, **51**, 27-34.

Albert, M. L., Feldman, R. G. & Willis, A. L. (1974) The 'subcortical dementia' of progressive supranuclear palsy. *Journal of Neurology, Neurosurgery and Psychiatry*, **37**, 121-130.

Alema, G. & Bignami, A. (1959) Polioencefalopatia degenerativa subacuta del presenio con stupore acinetico e rigidità decortica con mioclonie (Varietà 'mioclonica della malattia di Jakob-Creutzfeldt'). *Revista sperimentale di Freniatria Supplement Fasc.* IV, **83**, 1492-1623.

Alzheimer, A. (1898) Neuere Arbeiten über die Dementia senilis und die auf atheromatöser Gefässerkrankung basierenden Gehirhkrankheiten. *Monatsschrift für Psychiatrie und Neurologie*, **3**, 101-115.

Alzheimer, A. (1907a) Ueber eine eigenartige Erkrankung der Hirnrinde. *Allgemeine Zeitschrift für Psychiatrie*, **64**, 146-148.

Alzheimer, A. (1907b) Ueber eine eigenartige Erkrankung der Hirnrinde. *Zentralblatt für die gesamte Neurologie und Psychiatrie*, **18**, 177-179.

Alzheimer, A. (1911) Ueber eigenartige Krankheitsfälle des späteren Alters. *Zentralblatt für die gesamte Neurologie und Psychiatrie*, **4**, 356-385.

Arnold, A., Edgren, D. C. & Palladino, V. S. (1953) Amyotrophic lateral sclerosis; fifty cases observed on Guam. *Journal of Nervous and Mental Diseases*, **117**, 135-139.

von Bagh, K. (1941) Ueber anatomische Befunde bei 30 Fällen von systematischer Atrophie der Grosshirnrinde (Pickscher Krankheit) mit besonderer Berücksichtigung der Stammganglien und der langen absteigenden Leitungsbahnen. *Archiv für Psychiatrie und Nervenkrankheiten*, **114**, 68-70.

Barbeau, A. (1973) in *Advances in Neurology, Vol. I. Huntington's Chorea 1872-1972.* (Ed. Barbeau, A.) North Holland, Amsterdam.

Bechterew, W. V. von, (1900) Demonstration eines Gehirns mit Zerstörung der vorderen und inneren Theile der Hirnrinde beider Schläfenlappen. *Zentralblatt für die gesamte Neurologie und Psychiatrie*, **19**, 990-991.

Beck, E., Daniel, P. M., Matthews, W. B., Stevens, D. L., Alpers, M. P., Asher, D. M., Gajdusek, D. C. & Gibbs, C. J. Jr. (1969) Creutzfeldt-Jakob disease: the neuropathology of a transmission experiment. *Brain*, **92**, 699-716.

Behrmann, S., Caroll, J. D., Janota, I. & Matthews, W. B. (1969) Progressive supranuclear palsy. Clinicopathological study of four cases. *Brain*, **92**, 663-678.

Bell, J. (1934) *Treasury of Human Inheritance*, **4**, Part I. Huntington's Chorea.

Benedek, S. & McGovern, V. J. (1949) Case of Alzheimer's disease with amyloidosis of vessels of cerebral cortex. *Medical Journal of Australia*, **ii**, 429-430.

Benirsche, K. & Höfnagel, D. (1961) Clinical conditions with a normal chromosome complement. *Human Chromosome Newsletter*, **4**, 4.

Berlin, L. (1949) Presenile sclerosis (Alzheimer's disease with features resembling Pick's disease). *Archives of Neurology and Psychiatry*, **61**, 369-384.

Bertrand, I. & Koffas, D. (1946) Cas d'ioditie mongolienne adulte avec nombreuses plaques séniles et concrétions calcaires pallidales. *Revue neurologique*, **78**, 338-345.

Best, C R. (1941) Klinisch-anatomischer Beitrag zur Kenntnis der präsenilen Psychosen Kraepelins. *Monatsschrift für Psychiatrie und Neurologie*, **103**, 308-320.

Bielschowsky, M. (1932) in *Penfield's Cytology and Cellular Pathology of the Nervous System.* Hoeber, New York.

Bignami, A. (1973) The ultrastructure of status spongiosus and neuronal vacuolation in Jakob-Creutzfeldt disease and other transmissible spongiform encephalopathy. *International Congress Series* No. 319.

Bird, E. D., Caro, A. J. & Pilling, J. B. (1974) A sex related factor in the inheritance of Huntington's Chorea. *Annals of Human Genetics*, **37**, 255-260.

Bird, E. D. & Iverson, L. L. (1974) Huntington's Chorea—postmortem measurement of glutamic acid decarboxylase, choline acetyltransferase and dopamine in basal ganglia. *Brain*, **97**, 457-472.

Birnbaum, G. (1941) Chronisch progressive Chorea mit Kleinhirnatrophie. *Archiv für Psychiatrie und Nervenkrankheiten*, **114**, 160-182.

Blakemore, C. B. & Falconer, M. A. (1967) Long-term effects of anterior temporal lobectomy on certain cognitive functions. *Journal of Neurology, Neurosurgery and Psychiatry*, **30**, 364-367.

Blessed, G., Tomlinson, B. E. & Roth, M. (1968) The association between quantitative measures of dementia and of senile change in the cerebral grey matter of elderly subjects. *British Journal of Psychiatry*, **114**, 797-811.

Blinkov, S. M. & Glezer, I. (1968) in *The Human Brain in Figures and Tables.* Plenum Press, New York.

Blocq, P. & Marinesco, G. (1892) Sur les lésions et la pathogénie de l'épilepsie dite essentielle. *Semaine médicale (Paris)*, **12**, 445-446.

Bogaert, L. van, Maere, M. & De Smedt, E. (1940) Sur les formes familiales précoces de la maladie d'Alzheimer *Monatsschrift für Psychiatrie und Neurologie*, **102**, 249-301.

Bogaert, L. van, Radermecker. J. & Devos, J.   (1955) Sur une observation mortelle d'encéphalite aiguë nécrosante. *Revue neurologique*, **92**, 329-356.

Bolt, J. M. W.   (1970) Huntington's Chorea in the west of Scotland. *British Journal of Psychiatry*, **116**, 259-270.

Bolt, J. W. & Lewis, G. P.   (1973) Huntington's Chorea: a study of liver function and histology. *Quarterly Journal of Medicine*, **42**, 151-174.

Bonfiglio, F.   (1908) Die speciali reperti in un case di probabile sifilide cerebrale. *Rivista sperimentale di freniatria e medicina legale delle alienazioni mentale*, **34**, 196-206.

Bonhoeffer, K.   (1897) Klinische und anatomische Beiträge zur Kenntnis der Alkoholdelirien. *Monatsschrift für Psychiatrie und Neurologie*, **1**, 229-251.

Boor, W. de., Spiegelhoff, W. & Stammler, A.   (1952) Zur Psychopathologie, Pathophysiologie und Morphologie atypischer hirnatrophischer Prozesse. *Archiv für Psychiatrie und Nervenkrankheiten*, **188**, 51-71.

Brain, W. R., Daniel, P. M. & Greenfield, J. G.   (1951) Sub-acute cortical cerebellar degeneration and its relation to carcinoma. *Journal of Neurology, Neurosurgery and Psychiatry*, **14**, 59-75.

Brandenburg, W. & Hallervorden, I.   (1954) Dementia pugilistica mit anatomischen Befund. *Virchows Archiv für pathologische Anatomie und Physiologie und für klinische Medizin*, **325**, 680-709.

Brandon, S., McClelland, H. A. & Protheroe, C.   (1971) A study of facial dyskinesia in a mental hospital population. *British Journal of Psychiatry*, **118**, 171-184.

Braunmühl, A. von   (1928) Zur Histopathologie der umschriebenen Grosshirnrindenatrophie (Picksche Krankheit). *Virchows Archiv für pathologische Anatomie und Physiologie und für klinische Medizin*, **270**, 448-486.

Braunmühl, A. von   (1930) Ueber Stammganglienveränderungen bei Pickscher Krankheit. *Zeitschrift für die gesamte Neurologie und Psychiatrie*, **124**, 214-221.

Braunmühl, A. von   (1931) Neue Gesichtspunkte zum Problem der senilen Plaques. *Zeitschrift für die gesamte Neurologie und Psychiatrie*, **133**, 391-441.

Braunmühl, A. von   (1932) Kolloidochemische Betrachtungsweise seniler und präseniler Gewebsveränderungen (Das hysteretische Syndrom als cerebral Reaktionsform). *Zeitschrift für die gesamte Neurologie und Psychiatrie*, **142**, 1-54.

Braunmühl, A. von   (1954) Ueber eine eigenartige hereditär-familiäre Erkrankung des Zentral nervensystems. *Archiv für Psychiatrie und Nervenkrankheiten*, **191**, 419-449.

Braunmühl, A. von   (1957) Alterserkrankungen des Zentralnervensystems, in *Handbuch der speziellen pathologischen Anatomie und Histologie* (Lubarsch-Henke-Rössle), **13**(i), 337-539. Springer Verlag, Berlin.

Braunmühl, A. von & Leonhard, K.   (1934) Ueber ein Schwesterpaar mit Pickscher Krankheit. *Zeitschrift für die gesamte Neurologie und Psychiatrie*, **150**, 209-241.

Brierley, J. B.   (1966) in *Amnesia* (Eds Whitty, C. W. M. & Zangwill, O. L.). Butterworth, London.

Brierley, J. B., Corsellis, J. A. N., Hierons, R. & Nevin, S.   (1960) Subacute encephalitis of later adult life, mainly affecting the limbic areas. *Brain*, **83**, 357-368.

Broca, P.   (1878) Anatomie comparée des circonvolutions cérébrales. *Revue D'Anthropologie*, Series 3, **1**, 385-455.

Brody, H.   (1955) Organization of the cerebral cortex. III A study of aging in the human cerebral cortex. *Journal of Comparative Neurology*, **102**, 511-556.

Brody, H.   (1960) The deposition of aging pigment in the human cerebral cortex. *Journal of Gerontology*, **15**, 258-261.

Brothers, C. R. D.   (1949) The history and incidence of Huntington's chorea in Tasmania. *Proceedings of Royal Australian College of Physicians*, **4**, 48-50.

Brownell, B. & Oppenheimer, D.   (1965) An ataxic form of subacute presenile polioencephalopathy (Creutzfeldt-Jakob disease). *Journal of Neurology, Neurosurgery, and Psychiatry*, **28**, 350-361.

Bruyn, G. W.   (1967) The Westphal variant and juvenile type of Huntington's chorea, in *Progress in Neurogenetics*. (Eds Barbeau, A. & Brunette, J. R.), pp. 666-673, Excerpta Medica Foundation, Amsterdam.

Buchanan, A. R., Overholt, L. C. & Neubürger, K. T.   (1947) Parenchymatous cortical cerebellar atrophy associated with Pick's disease. *Journal of Neuropathology and Experimental Neurology*, **6**, 152-165.

Burns, B. D.   (1958) in *The Mammalian Cerebral Cortex*. Edward Arnold, London.

Campbell, A. M. G., Corner, B., Norman, R. M. & Urich, H.   (1961) The rigid form of Huntington's disease. *Journal of Neurology, Neurosurgery and Psychiatry*, **24**, 71-77.

Carmichael, E. A. & Stern, R. D.   (1931) Korsakow's syndrome: Its histopathology. *Brain*, **54**, 189-213.

Charatan, F. B. & Brierley, J. B.   (1956) Mental disorder associated with primary lung carcinoma. *British Medical Journal* **2**, 765-768.

Cheyne, G.   (1725) *An Essay on Health and Long Life*, London.

Christensen, E., Moller, J. E. & Faurbye, A. (1970) Neuropathological investigation of twenty-eight brains from patients with dyskinesia. *Acta psychiatrica et neurologica Scandinavica*, **46**, 14-23.

Claude, H. & Cuel, J. (1939) Démence pré-sénile post-traumatique après fracture du crâne. Considérations médico-légales. *Annales de médecine légale, criminologie, police scientifique et toxicologie*, **19**, 173-184.

Claude, H., Lhermitte, J. & Meignant, P. (1930) Le syndrome de rigidité post-choréique avec démence. Considérations sur la physiologie pathologique des corps opto-striés. *Encéphale*, **25**, 417-435, 493-518.

Cobb, S. (1965) Brain size. *Archives of Neurology*, **12**, 555-561.

Coiffu, B. L. H. (1958) Artériosclérose cérébrale à forme démentielle. Thesis, University of Paris.

Constantinidis, J., Garrone, G. & De Ajuriaguerra, J. (1962) L'hérédité des démences de l'âge avancé. *Encéphale*, **51**, 301-344.

Constantinidis, J. & Tissot, R. (1967) Lésions neurofibrillaires d'Alzheimer généralisées sans plaques séniles. *Archives Suisses de Neurologie, Neurochirurgie et de Psychiatrie*, **100**, 117-130.

Cooke, J. (1685) *Mellificium Chirurgiae*. London.

Corsellis, J. A. N. (1951) Sub-acute sclerosing leuco-encephalitis: clinical and pathological report of two cases. *Journal of Mental Science*, **97**, 570-583.

Corsellis, J. A. N. (1962) *Mental Illness and the Ageing Brain*. Oxford University Press, London.

Corsellis, J. A. N. & Brierley, J. B. (1954) An unusual type of pre-senile dementia (atypical Alzheimer's disease with amyloid vascular change). *Brain*, **77**, 571-587.

Corsellis, J. A. N. & Brierley, J. B. (1959) Observations on the pathology of insidious dementia following head injury. *Journal of Mental Science*, **105**, 714-720.

Corsellis, J. A. N., Bruton, C. J. & Freeman-Browne, D. (1973) The aftermath of boxing. *Psychological Medicine*, **3**, 270-303.

Corsellis, J. A. N. & Evans, P. H. (1965) The relation of stenosis of the extracranial cerebral arteries to mental disorder and cerebral degeneration in old age, in *Proceedings of Vth International Congress of Neuropathology*, Excerpta Medica International Congress Series No. 100.

Corsellis, J. A. N., Goldberg, G. J. & Norton, A. R. (1968) "Limbic encephalitis" and its association with carcinoma. *Brain*, **91**, 481-496.

Crapper, D. R., Krishnan, S. S. & Dalton, A. J. (1973) Brain aluminum distribution in Alzheimer's disease and experimental neurofibrillary degeneration. *Science*, **180**, 511-513.

Creutzfeldt, H. G. (1921) Über eine eigenartige Erkrankung des Zentralnervensystems, in *Histologische und histopathologische Arbeiten über die Grosshirnrinde* (Eds Nissl und Alzheimer), Suppl. vol. 6: 1-48.

Crezee, P. (1949) Pick's disease aggravated by cranial trauma: case. *Nederlandsch tijdschrift voor geneeskunde*, **93**, 2871-2876.

Curran, D. (1929) Huntington's chorea without choreiform movements. *Journal of Neurology and Psychopathology*, **10**, 305-310.

Davenport, C. B. (1915) Huntington's chorea in relation to heredity and eugenics. *Proceedings of the National Academy of Sciences of the United States of America*, **1**, 283-289.

Davidson, E. A. & Robertson, E. E. (1955) Alzheimer's disease with acne rosacea in one of identical twins. *Journal of Neurology, Neurosurgery, and Psychiatry*, **18**, 72-77.

Davison, C. (1932) Spastic pseudosclerosis (corticopallido-spinal degeneration). *Brain*, **55**, 247-264.

Davison, C., Goodhart, S. P. & Schlionsky, H. S. (1932) Chronic progressive chorea. The pathogenesis and mechanism. *Archives of Neurology and Psychiatry*, **27**, 906-928.

Davison, C. & Rabiner, A. B. (1940) Spastic pseudosclerosis (disseminated encephalomyelopathy; corticopal lidospinal degeneration). *Archives of Neurology and Psychiatry*, **44**, 578-598.

Dayan, A. D., Bhatti, I. & Gostling, J. V. T. (1967) Encephalitis due to herpes simplex in a patient with treated carcinoma of the uterus. *Neurology*, **17**, 609-613.

Delay, J. & Brion, S. (1962) *Les Démences Tardives*. Masson, Paris.

Delay, J., Brion, S. & Elissalde, B. (1958) Corps Mamillaires et Syndrome de Korsakoff. *La Presse Médicale*, **66**, 1849-1968.

Delay, J., Brion, S. & Sadoun, R. (1954) Lésions anatomiques de la malaide de Pick à la phase préatrophique. *Revue neurologique*, **91**, 81-91.

Dewulf, A. (1935) Un cas de maladie de Pick avec les lésions prédominantes dans les noyaux gris de la base du cerveau. *Journal belge de neurologie et de psychiatrie*, **35**, 508-521.

Divry, P. (1927) Etude histo-chimique des plaques séniles. *Journal belge de neurologie et de psychiatrie*, **27**, 643-657.

Divry, P. (1934) De la nature de l'altération fibrillaire d'Alzheimer. *Journal belge de neurologie et de psychiatrie*, **34**, 197-201.

Divry, P., Ley, J. & Titeca, J. (1935) Maladie d'Alzheimer avec atrophie frontale prédominante. *Journal belge de neurologie et de psychiatrie*, **35**, 495-507.

Dixon, K. C. (1953) Periodic acid-silver method for neurones. *Journal of Pathology and Bacteriology*, **66**, 539-544.

Duffy, P., Wolf, J., Collins, G., DeVoe, A. G., Streeten, B. & Cowen, D. (1974) Possible person-to-person transmission of Creutzfeldt–Jakob disease. *New England Journal of Medicine*, **290**, 692-693.

Dunlap, C. B. (1927) Pathologic changes in Huntington's chorea with special references to corpus striatum. *Archives of Neurology and Psychiatry*, **18**, 867-943.

Eecken, van der H. V., Adams, R. D. & van Bogaert, L. (1960) Striopallidal-nigral degeneration. *Journal of Neuropathology and Experimental Neurology*, **19**, 159.

Ellis, R. S. (1920) Norms for some structural changes in the human cerebellum from birth to old age. *Journal of Comparative Neurology*, **32**, 1-32.

English, W. H. (1942) Alzheimer's disease. *Psychiatric Quarterly*, **16**, 91-106.

Esquirol, E. (1838) *Des Maladies Mentales*, Part 1, chap. viii, pp. 201-218. Brussels.

Essen-Möller, E. (1946) A family with Alzheimer's disease. *Acta psychiatrica et neurologica Scandinavica*, **21**, 233-244.

Fényes, I. (1932) Alzheimersche Fibrillenveränderung in Hirnstamm einer 28 jährigen Post-encephalitikerin. *Archiv für Psychiatrie und Nervenkrankheiten*, **96**, 700-717.

Ferraro, A. (1931) The origin and formation of senile plaques. *Archives of Neurology and Psychiatry*, **25**, 1042-1062.

Field, E. J. (1967) The significance of astroglial hypertrophy in Scrapie, Kuru, Multiple sclerosis and old age together with a note on the possible nature of the Scrapie agent. *Deutsche Zeitschrift für Nervenheilkunde*, **192**, 265-274.

Fischer-Williams, M., Bosanquet, F. D. & Daniel, P. M. (1955) Carcinomatosis of the meninges: a report of three cases. *Brain*, **78**, 42-58.

Fisher, C. M. (1951) Senile dementia—a new explanation of its causation. *Canadian Medical Association Journal*, **65**, 1-7.

Fisher, C. M. (1968) in *Cerebral Vascular Disease* (Eds Toole, J. F., Siekert, R. G. & Whisnant, J. P.). New York.

Flügel, F. E. (1928) Huntingtonsche chorea und Trauma. *Zeitschrift für die gesamte Neurologie und Psychiatrie*, **112**, 247-251.

Foley, J. M. & Denny-Brown, D. (1955) Subacute progressive encephalopathy with bulbar myoclonus. *Excerpta Medica. Section VIII. Neurology and Psychiatry*, **8**, 782-784.

Freeman, W. (1933) in *Neuropathology*. Philadelphia.

Friede, R. L. (1965) Enzyme histochemical studies of senile plaques. *Journal of Neuropathology and Experimental Neurology*, **24**, 477-491.

Friede, R. L. (1966) in *Topographic Brain Chemistry*. Academic Press, New York.

Friede, R. L. & DeJong, R. N. (1964) Neuronal enzymatic failure in Creutzfeldt-Jakob disease (a familial study). *Archives of Neurology*, **10**, 181-195.

Friede, R. L. & Magee, K. R. (1962) Alzheimer's disease: presentation of a case with pathologic and enzymatic histochemical observation. *Neurology*, **12**, 213-222.

Gajdusek, D. C. (1972) Spongiform virus encephalopathies. *Journal of Clinical Pathology*, **25**, supplement (*Royal College of Pathologists*), **6**, 78-83.

Gajdusek, D. C. & Gibbs, C. J. Jr. (1971) Transmission of two subacute spongiform encephalopathies of man (kuru and Creutzfeldt-Jakob disease). *Nature*, **230**, 588-591.

Gamper, E. (1928) Zur Frage der Polioencephalitis der chronischen Alcoholiker. Anatomische Befunde bei alcoholischen Korsakow und ihre Beziehungen zum klinischen Bild. *Deutsche Zeitschrift für Nervenheilkunde*, **102**, 122-129.

Garcin, R., Brion, S. & Khochneviss, A. (1962) Le syndrome de Creutzfeldt-Jakob et les syndromes cortico-striés du presenium. *Revue neurologique*, **106**, 506-508.

Gascon, G. G. & Gilles, F. (1973) Limbic dementia. *Journal of Neurology, Neurosurgery and Psychiatry* **36**, 421-430.

Gellerstedt, N. (1933) Zur Kenntnis der Hirnveränderungen bei der normalen Altersinvolution. *Upsala Läkareförenings Förhandlingar*, **38**, 193-408.

Gerhard, L., Bergener, M. & Homayun, S. (1972) Vascular changes in Alzheimer's disease. *Journal of Neurology*, **201**, 43-61.

Gerstmann, J., Sträussler, E. & Scheinker, I. (1936) Ueber eine eigenartige hereditär-familiäre Erkrankung des Zentralnervensystems, zugleich ein Beitrag zur Frage des vorzeitigen lokalen Alterns. *Zeitschrift für die gesamte Neurologie und Psychiatrie*, **154**, 736-762.

Gibbs, C. J. Jr., & Gajdusek, D. C.   (1969) Infection as the etiology of spongiform encephalopathy (Creutzfeldt-Jacob) disease.   *Science*, **165**, 1023-1025.

Gibbs, C. J. Jr. & Gajdusek, D. C.   (1972) Isolation and characterization of the subacute spongiform virus encephalopathies of man: kuru and Creutzfeldt-Jakob disease.   *Journal of Clinical Pathology*, **25**, *supplement* (*Royal College of Pathologists*), **6**, 84-96.

Gibbs, C. J., Gajdusek, D. C., Asher, D. M., Alpers, M. P., Beck, E., Daniel, P. M. & Matthews, W. B.   (1968) Creutzfeldt-Jakob disease (spongiform encephalopathy): transmission to the chimpanzee.   *Science*, **161**, 388-389.

Gonatas, N. K., Terry, R. D. & Weiss, M.   (1965) Electron microscopic study in two cases of Jakob-Creutzfeldt disease.   *Journal of Neuropathology and Experimental Neurology*, **24**, 575-598.

Goodman, L.   (1953) Alzheimer's disease: a clinico-pathologic analysis of twenty-three cases with a theory on pathogenesis.   *Journal of Nervous and Mental Disease*, **118**, 97-130.

Gowers, W. R.   (1902) A lecture on abiotrophy.   *Lancet*, i, 1003-1007.

Grahmann, H. & Ule, G.   (1957) Beitrag zur Kenntnis der chronischen cerebralen Krankheitsbilder bei Boxern.   *Psychiatria et neurologia*, **134**, 261-283.

Greenfield, J. G. & Bosanquet, F. D.   (1953) The brainstem lesions in Parkinsonism.   *Journal of Neurology, Neurosurgery and Psychiatry*, **16**, 213-226.

Grosch, J.   (1959) Encephalopathie nach Trauma und Dystrophie mit dem histopathologischen Befund der Alzheimerschen Krankheit.   *Deutsche Zeitschrift für Nervenheilkunde*, **179**, 217-231.

Grünthal, E.   (1930a) Ueber ein Brüderpaar mit Pickschen Krankheit.   Eine vergleichende Untersuchung, zugleich ein Beitrag zur Kenntnis der Verursachung und des Verlaufs der Erkrankung.   *Zeitschrift für die gesamte Neurologie und Psychiatrie*, **129**, 350-375.

Grünthal, E.   (1930b) in *Handbuch der Geistenkrankheiten* (Ed. Bumke, O.), **11**, 638, Springer, Berlin.

Grünthal, E.   (1936) in *Handbuch der Neurologie* (Eds Bumke, O. & Foerster, O.).   Berlin.

Grünthal, E. & Kuhn, R.   (1959) Klinisch-pathologische Untersuchungen einer besonderen Form von perniziöser organischer Psychose (Kraepelinsche Krankheit).   *Psychiatria et neurologia*, **137**, 1-32.

Grünthal, E. & Wenger, O.   (1939) Nachweis von Erblichkeit bei der Alzheimerschen Krankheit nebst Bemerkungen über den Altersvorgang im Gehirn.   *Monatsschrift für Psychiatrie und Neurologie*, **101**, 8-25.

Gudden, H.   (1896) Klinische und anatomische Beiträge zur Kenntnis der multiplen Alkoholneuritis.   *Archiv für Psychiatrie und Nervenkrankheiten*, **28**, 643-741.

Hachinski, V. C., Lassen, N. A. & Marshall, J.   (1974) Multi-infarct dementia—a cause of mental deterioration in the elderly.   *Lancet*, ii, 207-209.

Hallervorden, J.   (1933) Zur Pathogenese des postencephalitischen Parkinsonismus.   *Klinische Wochenschrift*, **12**, 692-695.

Hallervorden, J.   (1957) in *Handbuch der speziellen pathologischen Anatomie und Histologie* (Eds Lubarsch, O., Henke, F. & Rössle, R.).   Springer, Berlin.

Hallgren, B. & Sourander, P.   (1960) The non-haemin iron in the cerebral cortex in Alzheimer's disease.   *Journal of Neurochemistry*, **5**, 307-310.

Hanley, T.   (1974) 'Neuronal Fall-Out' in the ageing brain: a critical review of the quantitative data.   *Age and Ageing*, **3**, 133-151.

Hare, E. H.   (1959) The origin and spread of dementia paralytica.   *Journal of Mental Science*, **105**, 594-626.

Hǎskovec, V.   (1934) Picksche Krankheit.   *Zentralblatt für die gesamte Neurologie und Psychiatrie*, **73**, 345.

Hassin, G. B. & Levitin D.   (1941) Pick's disease. Clinicopathologic study and report of a case.   *Archives of Neurology and Psychiatry* (*Chicago*), **45**, 814-833.

Heathfield, K. W. G.   (1967) Huntington's chorea: investigation into prevalence in the N. E. Metropolitan Regional Hospital Board area.   *Brain*, **90**, 203-232.

Heathfield, K. W. G.   (1973) Huntington's chorea: a centenary review.   *Postgraduate Medical Journal*, **49**, 32-45.

Heidenhain, A.   (1929) Klinische und anatomische Untersuchungen über eine eigenartige Erkrankung des Zentralnervensystems im Praesenium.   *Zeitschrift für die gesamte Neurologie und Psychiatrie*, **118**, 49-114.

Hemphill, R. E. & Stengel, E.   (1941) Alzheimer's disease with predominating crossed cerebro-cerebellar hemiatrophy.   *Journal of Neurology and Psychiatry*, **4**, 97-106.

Henson, R. A., Hoffman, H. L. & Urich, H.   (1965) Encephalomyelitis with carcinoma.   *Brain*, **88**, 449-464.

Hirano, A.   (1965) Neuropathology of amyotrophic lateral sclerosis and Parkinsonism-Dementia complex on Guam.   *Excerpta Medica International Congress Series No. 100.*

Hirano, A., Dembitzer, H. M., Kurland, L. T. & Zimmerman, H. M.   (1968) The fine structure of some intra-ganglionic alterations.   Neurofibrillary tangles, granulovacuolar bodies and "rod-like" structures as seen in Guam amyotrophic lateral sclerosis and Parkinsonism-dementia complex. *Journal of Neuropathology and Experimental Neurology*, **27**, 167-182.

Hirano, A., Malamud, N. & Kurland, L. T. (1961) Parkinsonism-dementia complex, an endemic disease on the island of Guam. *Brain*, **84**, 662-679.

Hirano, A., Malamud, N., Elizan, T. S. & Kurland, L. R. (1966) Amyotrophic lateral sclerosis and Parkinsonism-dementia complex on Guam. *Archives of Neurology*, **15**, 35-51.

Hirano, A., Tuazon, R. & Zimmerman, H. M. (1968) Neurofibrillary changes, granulovacuolar bodies and argentophilic globules observed in tuberous sclerosis. *Acta neuropathologica*, **11**, 257-261.

Hirano, A., & Zimmerman, H. M. (1962a) Silver impregnation of nerve cells and fibers in celloidin sections. *Archives of Neurology*, **6**, 114-122.

Hirano, A. & Zimmerman, H. M. (1962b) Alzheimer's neurofibrillary changes: a topographic study. *Archives of Neurology*, **7**, 227-242.

Hollander, D. & Strich, S. J. (1970) in *Ciba Foundation Symposium on Alzheimer's Disease and Related Conditions* (Eds Wolstenholme, G. E. W. & O'Connor, M.). Churchill, London.

Humphrey, T. (1944) Primitive neurons in the embryonic human central nervous system. *Journal of Comparative Neurology*, **81**, 1-45.

Hunter, R., Dayan, A. D. & Wilson, J. (1972) Alzheimer's disease in one monozygotic twin. *Journal of Neurology, Neurosurgery and Psychiatry*, **35**, 707-710.

Huntington, G. (1872) On chorea. *Medical and Surgical Reporter, Philadelphia*, **26**, 317-321.

Ishii, T. (1965) Distribution of Alzheimer's neurofibrillary changes in the brain stem and hypothalamus of senile dementia. *Acta neuropathologica*, **6**, 181-189.

Jacob, H. (1960) Zur pathologischen Anatomie der Pickschen Krankheit. I Mitteilung: Vergleichende Untersuchungen über Ausdehnung und Schwerpunkte der Atrophie. *Archiv für Psychiatrie und Nervenkrankheiten*, **201**, 269-297.

Jacob, H. (1961) Zur pathologischen Anatomie der Pickschen Krankheit. *Archiv für Psychiatrie und Nervenkrankheiten*, **202**, 540-568.

Jacob, H., Eicke, W. & Orthner, H. (1958) Zur Klinik und Neuropathologie der subakuten praesenilen spongiösen Atrophien mit dyskinetischem Endstadium. *Deutsche Zeitschrift für Nervenheilkunde*, **178**, 330-357.

Jakob, A. (1921) Über eigenartige Erkrankungen des Zentralnervensystems mit bemerkenswerten anatomischen Befunde mit disseminierten Degenerationsherden. *Zeitschrift für die gesamte Neurologie und Psychiatrie* **64**, 147-228.

Jakob, A. (1923) *Die Extrapyramidalen Erkrankungen*, pp. 218-245. Springer, Berlin.

Jakob, H. (1969) Klinisch-anatomische Aspekte bei "reinen" Schläfenlappenfällen Pickscher Krankheit und der basale Neocortex. *Deutsche Zeitschrift für Nervenheilkunde*, **196**, 20-39.

Jamada, M. & Mehraein, P. (1968) Verteilungsmuster der senilen Veränderungen im Gehirn. *Archiv für Psychiatrie und Zeitschrift für die gesamte Neurologie*, **211**, 308-324.

Jansen, J. & Monrad-Krohn, G. H. (1938) Ueber Die Creutzfeldt-Jakob Krankheit. *Zeitschrift für die gesamte Neurologie* und Psychiatrie, **163**, 670-704.

Jelgersma, G. (1908) Neue anatomische Befünde bei Paralysis Agitans und Chronischer Chorea. *Neurologisches Zentralblatt*, **27**, 995-996.

Jervis, G. A. (1948) Early senile dementia in mongoloid idiocy. *American Journal of Psychiatry*, **105**, 102-106.

Jervis, G. A. (1971) In *Pathology of the Nervous System* (Ed. Minckler, J.), Vol. 2. McGraw-Hill, New York.

Jervis, G. A., Hurdum, H. M. & O'Neill, F. J. (1942) Presenile psychosis of the Jakob type. Clinicopathologic study of one case with a review of the literature. *American Journal of Psychiatry*, **99**, 101-109.

Johnson, A. B. & Blum, N. R. (1970) Nucleoside phosphatase activities associated with the tangles and plaques of Alzheimer's disease: a histochemical study of natural and experimental neurofibrillary tangles. *Journal of Neuropathology and Experimental Neurology*, **29**, 463-478.

Jones, D. & Nevin, S. (1954) Rapidly progressive cerebral degeneration (subacute vascular encephalopathy) with mental disorder, focal disturbances, and myoclonic epilepsy. *Journal of Neurology and Psychiatry*, **17**, 148-159.

Kant, F. (1933) Die Pseudoencephalitis Wernicke der Alkoholiker (Polioencephalitis haemorrhagica superior acuta). Ein Beitrag zur Klinik der Alkoholpsychosen. *Archiv für Psychiatrie und Nervenkrankheiten*, **98**, 702-768.

Khochneviss, A. A. (1960) Contributions a l'étude du syndrome Creutzfeldt-Jakob et des syndromes cortico-striés du presenium. Thèse de Paris.

Kidd, M. (1964) Alzheimer's disease. An electron microscopical study. *Brain*, **87**, 307-320.

Kirschbaum, W. R.   (1924) Zwei eigenartige Erkrankungen des Zentralnervensystems nach Art der spastischen Pseudosclerose (Jakob).   *Zeitschrift für die gesamte Neurologie und Psychiatrie*, **92**, 175-220.

Kirschbaum, W. R.   (1968) in *Jakob-Creutzfeldt Disease*.   Elsevier, New York.

Kishimoto, K., Nakamura, M. & Sotokawa, Y.   (1959) On population genetics of Huntington's chorea in Japan.   *First International Congress of Neurological Sciences*, Vol. 4.

Konigsmark, B. W. & Murphy, E. A.   (1970) Neuronal populations in the human brain.   *Nature*, **228**, 1335-1336.

Korsakow, S. S.   (1890) Über eine besondere Form psychischer Störung combiniert mit multipler Neuritis.   *Archiv für Psychiatrie und Nervenkrankheiten*, **21**, 669-704.

Kraepelin, E.   (1910) Klinische Psychiatrie in *Psychiatrie*, 8th ed, Vol. 2, Part 1.   Barth, Leipzig.

Kramer, D. W.   (1959) Preseniele, subacute progressieve encefalopathie met status myoclonicus.   *Nederlandsch tijdschrift voor geneeskunde*, **103**, 1662-1666.

Kreindler, A., Hornet, Th. & Appel. E.   (1959) Complex forms of cerebral senility.   *Rumanian Medical Review*, **3**, 43-47.

Krücke, W.   (1950) Das Zentralnervensystem bei generalisierter Paramyloidose.   *Archiv für Psychiatrie und Nervenkrankheiten*, **185**, 165-192.

Lampert, P. W., Earle, K. M., Gibbs, C. J., & Gajdusek, D. C.   (1969) Experimental Kuru encephalopathy in chimpanzees and spider monkeys.   *Journal of Neuropathology and Experimental Neurology*, **28**, 353-370.

Larsson, T., Sjögren, T. & Jacobsen, G.   (1963) Senile dementia.   *Acta psychiatrica Scandinavica*, **39**, supplement 167.

Liebers, M.   (1933) Alzheimersche Krankheit mit Pickscher Atrophie der Parieto-Occipitallappen.   *Archiv für Psychiatrie und Nervenkrankheiten*, **100**, 100-110.

Liebers, M.   (1939) Alzheimersche Krankheit mit Pickscher Atrophie der Stirnlappen.   *Archiv für Psychiatrie und Nervenkrankheiten*, **109**, 363-370.

Lindenberg, R.   (1960) Striopallidal-nigral degeneration.   *Journal of Neuropathology and Experimental Neurology*, **19**, 160.

Liss, L.   (1960) Senile brain changes. Histopathology of the ganglion cells.   *Journal of Neuropathology and Experimental Neurology*, **19**, 559-571.

Løken, A. C. & Cyvin, K.   (1954) A case of clinical juvenile amaurotic idiocy with the histological picture of Alzheimer's disease.   *Journal of Neurology, Neurosurgery and Psychiatry*, **17**, 211-215.

Lowenberg, K. & Waggoner, R. W.   (1934) Familial organic psychosis (Alzheimer's type).   *Archives of Neurology and Psychiatry*, **31**, 737-754.

Lüers, T.   (1947) Ueber die familiäre juvenile Form der Alzheimerschen Krankheit mit neurologischen Herderscheinungen.   *Archiv für Psychiatrie und Nervenkrankheiten*, **179**, 132-145.

Lüers, T. & Spatz, U. H.   (1957) in *Handbuch der speziellen pathologischen Anatomie und Histologie* (Eds Lubarsch, O., Henke, F. & Rössle, R.).   Springer, Berlin.

Lund, J. C.   (1860) Chorea Sti. Viti i Saetersdalen.   *Beretning om Sundhedstilstanden og Medicinalforholdene in Norge*, **4**, 137-138.

Lyon, I. W.   (1863) Chronic hereditary chorea.   *American Medical Times*, **7**, 289-290.

Lyon, R. L.   (1962) Huntington's chorea in the Moray Firth area.   *British Medical Journal*, **1**, 1301-1306.

McCaughey, W. T. E.   (1961) The pathologic spectrum of Huntington's chorea.   *Journal of Nervous and Mental Disease*, **133**, 91-103.

McGeer, P. L., McGeer, E. G. & Fibiger, H. C.   (1973) Choline acetylase and glutamic acid decarboxylase in Huntington's chorea: a preliminary study.   *Neurology*, **23**, 912-917.

McGovern, G. P., Miller, D. H. & Robertson, D.   (1959) A mental syndrome associated with lung carcinoma.   *Archives of Neurology and Psychiatry*, **81**, 341-347.

McLardy, T.   (1970) Memory function in hippocampal gyri but not in hippocampi.   *International Journal of Neuroscience*, **1**, 113-118.

McMenemey, W. H.   (1940) Alzheimer's disease.   *Journal of Neurology and Psychiatry*, **3**, 211-240.

McMenemey, W. H.   (1963a) in *Greenfield's Neuropathology*.   Edward Arnold, London.

McMenemey, W. H.   (1963b) Alzheimer's disease: problems concerning its concept and nature.   *Acta neurologica scandinavica*, **39**, 369-380.

McMenemey, W. H.   (1968) in *The Central Nervous System: International Academy of Pathology Monograph No. 9*.   Williams and Wilkins, Baltimore.

McMenemey, W. H., Grant, H. C. & Behrman, S.   (1965) Two examples of "presenile dementia".   *Archiv für Psychiatrie und Nervenkrankheiten*, **207**, 128-140.

McMenemey, W. H., Worster-Drought, C., Flind, J. & Williams, H. G.   (1939) Familial presenile dementia:

report of case with clinical and pathological features of Alzheimer's disease. *Journal of Neurology and Psychiatry*, **2**, 293-302.

Malamud, N. (1972) in *Aging and the Brain* (Ed. Gaitz, F. M.). Plenum Press, New York.

Malamud, N., & Demmy, N. (1960) A degenerative disease of the corpus luysi. Clinico-pathologic study of three cases. *Journal of Neuropathology and Experimental Neurology*, **19**, 161.

Malamud, N., Haymaker, W. & Pinkerton, H. (1950) Inclusion encephalitis with clinicopathologic report of three cases. *American Journal of Pathology*, **26**, 133-153.

Malamud, N., Hirano, A. & Kurland, L. T. (1961) Pathoanatomic changes in amyotrophic lateral sclerosis on Guam with reference to the occurrence of neurofibrillary changes. *Archives of Neurology*, **5**, 401-415.

Malamud, N. & Skillicorn, S. A. (1956) Relationship between the Wernicke and the Korsakov syndrome. *Archives of Neurology and Psychiatry*, **76**, 585-596.

Malamud, N. & Waggoner, R. W. (1943) Genealogic and clinicopathologic study of Pick's disease. *Archives of Neurology and Psychiatry*, **50**, 288-303.

Mandybur, T. I. (1975) The incidence of cerebral amyloid angiopathy in Alzheimer's disease. *Neurology*, **25**, 125-126.

Mansvelt, J. van (1954) *Pick's disease. A syndrome of lobar cerebral atrophy.* Enschede, Netherlands.

Marchand, L. (1949) L'artériosclérose cérébrale: ses aspects mentaux. *Annales médico-psychologiques*, **107(i)**, 433-458.

Marconi, G. & Piazzesi, W. (1965) Su di un caso di malattia di Alzheimer-Perusini familiare: studio genealogico e citogenetico. *Rivista di Patologia nervosa e mentale*, **86**, 854-872.

Marinesco, G. (1911) Sur la structure des plaques dites séniles dans l'écorce cérébrale des sujets agés et atteints d'affections mentales. *Comptes rendus des séances de la Société de biologie et ses filiales*, **70**, 606-608.

May, W. W. (1968) Creutzfeldt-Jakob disease. *Acta neurologica*, **44**, 1-32.

May, W. W., Itabashi, H. H. & DeJong, R. N. (1968) Creutzfeldt-Jakob disease. II clinical, pathologic and genetic study of a family. *Archives of Neurology*, **19**, 137-149.

Mettler, A. (1957) In *Proceedings of First International Congress of Neurological Sciences*, Excerpta Medica Abstracts, 1-4.

Meyer, A. (1929) Ueber eine der amyotrophischen Lateralsclerose nahestehende Erkrankung mit psychischen Störungen, zugleich ein Beitrag zur Frage der spastischen Pseudosclerose (A. Jakob). *Zeitschrift für gesamte Neurologie und Psychiatrie*, **121**, 107-138.

Meyer, A. & Beck, E. (1954) In *Prefrontal Leucotomy and Related Operations: Anatomical aspects of success and failure.* Oliver and Boyd, Edinburgh.

Meyer, A., Leigh, D. & Bagg, C. E. (1954) A rare presenile dementia associated with cortical blindness (Heidenhain's syndrome). *Journal of Neurology, Neurosurgery and Psychiatry*, **17**, 129-133.

Meyer, V. (1959) Cognitive changes following temporal lobectomy for relief of temporal lobe epilepsy. *Archives of Neurology and Psychiatry*, **81**, 299-309.

Meyer, V. & Yates, A. (1955) Intellectual changes following temporal lobectomy for psychomotor epilepsy. *Journal of Neurology, Neurosurgery and Psychiatry*, **18**, 44-52.

Milner, B. & Penfield, W. (1955) The effect of hippocampal lesions on recent memory. *Transactions of the American Neurological Association*, **80**, 42-48.

Morel, F. & Wildi, E. (1952) General and cellular pathochemistry of senile and presenile alterations of the brain, in *Proceedings of First International Congress of Neuropathology*, **2**, 347-374.

Morel, F. & Wildi, E. (1955). Contribution à la connaissance des différéntes altérations cérébrales du grande âge. *Schweizer Archiv für Neurologie und Psychiatrie*, **76**, 174-223.

Moyano, B. A. (1932) I. Enfermedad de Alzheimer II. Atrofia de Pick. *Archivos argentinos de neurologia*, **7**, 231-286.

Mutrux, S. (1953) Contribution à l'étude des corrélation anatomo-cliniques dans les démences dégénératives et les démences artérioscléreuses. *Monatsschrift für Psychiatrie und Neurologie*, **125**, 19-38.

Mutrux, S. (1958) Contribution à l'étude histologique différentielle de la démence sénile et de la maladie d'Alzheimer. *Monatsschrift für Psychiatrie und Neurologie*, **136**, 157-194.

Myrianthopoulos, N. C. (1966) Huntington's chorea. *Journal of Medical Genetics*, **3**, 298-314.

Neumann, M. A. (1949) Pick's disease. *Journal of Neuropathology and Experimental Neurology*, **8**, 255-282.

Neumann, M. A. (1960) Combined amyloid vascular changes and argyrophilic plaques in the central nervous system. *Journal of Neuropathology and Experimental Neurology*, **19**, 370-382.

Neumann, M. A. (1967) Langdon Down syndrome and Alzheimer's disease. *Journal of Neuropathology and Experimental Neurology*, **26**, 150.

Neumann, M. A. & Cohn R. (1967) Progressive Subcortical Gliosis, a rare form of Presenile Dementia. *Brain*, **90**, 405-418.

Nevin, S. (1967) On some aspects of cerebral degeneration in later life. *Proceedings of the Royal Society of Medicine*, **60**, 517-526.

Nevin, S., McMenemey, W. H., Behrman, S. & Jones, D. P. (1960) Subacute spongiform encephalopathy—a subacute form of encephalopathy attributable to vascular dysfunction (spongiform cerebral atrophy). *Brain*, **83**, 519-564.

Newton, R. D. (1948). Identity of Alzheimer's disease and senile dementia and their relation to senility. *Journal of Mental Science*, **94**, 225-249.

Oksala, O. (1923) Ein Beitrag zur Kenntnis der präsenilen Psychosen. *Zeitschrift für die gesamte Neurologie und Psychiatrie*, **81**, 1-44.

Olson, M. I. & Shaw, C. (1969) Presenile dementia and Alzheimer's disease in mongolism. *Brain*, **92**, 147-156.

Onari, K. & Spatz, H. (1926) Anatomische Beiträge zur Lehre von der Pickschen umschriebenen Grosshirnrindenatrophie (Picksche Krankheit). *Zeitschrift für die gesamte Neurologie und Psychiatrie*, **101**, 470-511.

Pantelakis, S. (1954) Un type particulier d'angiopathie sénile du système nerveux central: l'angiopathie congophile. Topographie et fréquence. *Monatsschrift für Psychiatrie und Neurologie*, **128**, 219-256.

Pearse, A. G. E. (1972) In *Histochemistry: Theoretical and Applied*, 3rd edn., Vol. 2. Churchill Livingstone, London.

Perry, T. L., Hansen, S. & Kloster, M. (1973) Huntington's chorea: deficiency of γ-aminobutyric acid in brain. *New England Journal of Medicine*, **288**, 337-342.

Perusini, G. (1910) Über klinisch und histologisch eigenartige psychische Erkrankungen des späteren Lebensalters. *Histologische und histopathologische Arbeiten über die Grosshirnrinde*, **3**, 297-359.

Petit-Dutaillis, D., Christophe, J., Pertuisset, B., Dreygus-Brisac, C. & Blane, C. (1954) Lobectomie temporale bilaterale pour epilepsie. Evolution des perturbations fonctionelles post-opératives. *Revue neurologique*, **91**, 129-133.

Pick, A. (1906) Ueber einen weiteren Symptomenkomplex im Rahmen der Dementia senilis, bedingt durch umschriebene stärkere Hirnatrophie (gemischte Apraxie). *Monatsschrift für Psychiatrie und Neurologie*, **19**, 97-108.

Pilleri, G. (1966) The Klüver-Bucy syndrome in man: a clinico-anatomical contribution to the function of the medial temporal lobe structures. *Psychiatria et neurologia*, **152**, 65-103.

Pleydell, M. J. (1954) Huntington's chorea in Northamptonshire. *British Medical Journal*, **2**, 1121-1128.

Podolsky, S., Leopold, N. A. & Sax, D. S. (1972) Increased frequency of diabetes mellitus in patients with Huntington's chorea. *Lancet*, **1**, 1356-1359.

Poursines, Y., Boudouresques, J. & Roger, J. (1953) Processus dégénératif atrophique diffus à prédominance thalamo-striée. Sémiologie extra-pyramidale et psychique variable. Evolution subaiguë à termination démentielle. *Revue Neurologique*, **89**, 266-271.

Pratt, R. T. C. (1970) In *The Genetics of Neurological Disorders*. Oxford University Press, London.

Raskin, N. & Ehrenberg, R. (1956) Senescence, senility and Alzheimer's disease. *American Journal of Psychiatry*, **113**, 133-137.

Redlich, E. (1898) Über miliäre Sklerose der Hirnrinde bei seniler Atrophie. *Jahrbücher für Psychologie und Neurologie*, **17**, 208-216.

Reich, F. (1907) Der Gehirnbefund in dem in der Sitzung des psychiatrischen Vereins zu Berlin von 18 Mai 1905 vorgestellten Fall von 'Alogie'. *Allgemeine Zeitschrift für Psychiatrie*, **64**, 380-388.

Reich, F. (1927) Zur pathogenese der circumscripten, respektive systemartigen Hirnatrophie. *Zeitschrift für die gesamte Neurologie und Psychiatrie*, **108**, 803-812.

Reiss, E. & Staemmler, M. (1950) Beitrag zur Beteiligung des Stammhirns bei der Alzheimerschen Krankheit. *Archiv für Psychiatrie und Nervenkrankheiten*, **183**, 481-492.

Richardson, E. P. (1965) In discussion on paper by Yahr, M. D., Duvoisin, R. C. & Cowen, D. Encephalopathy associated with carcinoma. *Transactions of the American Neurological Association*, **90**, 85.

Riese, W. (1952) Senility in *Proceedings of 1st. International Congress of Neuropathology*, **2**, 437-443.

Rose, F. C. & Symonds, C. P. (1960) Persistent memory defect following encephalitis. *Brain*, **83**, 195-212.

Rothschild, D. (1934) Alzheimer's disease: a clinico-pathological study of five cases. *American Journal of Psychiatry*, **91**, 485-519.

Rothschild, D. (1942) Neuropathological changes in arteriosclerotic psychoses and their psychiatric significance. *Archives of Neurology and Psychiatry*, **48**, 417-436.

Rothschild, D. (1945) In *Mental Disorders in Later Life* (Ed. Kaplan, O. J.). California.

Rothschild, D. & Kasanin, J. (1936) Clinicopathologic study of Alzheimer's disease: relationship to senile condition. *Archives of Neurology and Psychiatry*, **36**, 293-321.

Sanders, J., Schenk, V. W. D. & van Veen, P. (1939) A family with Pick's disease. *Verhandelingen der Koninkiijke Akademie van Wetenschappen, Sect. 2.*, **38**, 1-124.

Schenk, V. W. D.   (1955) Syndrome d'Alzheimer; étude anatomoclinique de 35 cas.   *Folia psychiatrica, neurologica et neurochirurgica neerlandica,* **58**, 422-437.

Schenk, V. W. D.   (1959) Re-examination of a family with Pick's disease.   *Annals of Human Genetics,* **23**, 325-333.

Schenk, V. W. D. & Mansvelt, J. van   (1955) The cortical degeneration in Pick's syndrome.   A quantitative analysis.   *Folia psychiatrica, neurologica et neurochirurgica neerlandica,* **58**, 42-62.

Schiffer, D.   (1955) Contribution à l'histologie de la maladie de Pick.   *Journal für Hirnforschung,* **1**, 497-515.

Schlote, W.   (1965) Die Amyloidnatur der kongophilen drusigen Entartung der Hirnarterien (Scholz) in Senium.   *Acta neuropathologica,* **4**, 449-468.

Schmitz, H. A. & Meyer, A.   (1933) Ueber die Picksche Krankheit, mit besonderer Berücksichtigung der Erblichkeit.   *Archiv für Psychiatrie und Nervenkrankheiten,* **99**, 747-761.

Schnitzler, J. G.   (1911) Zur Abgrenzung der sog.   Alzheimerschen Krankheit.   *Zeitschrift für die gesamte Neurologie und Psychiatrie,* **7**, 34-57.

Schochet, S. S. Jr., Lampert, P. W. & Earle, K. M.   (1968) Neuronal changes induced by intrathecal vincristine sulfate.   *Journal of Neuropathology and Experimental Neurology,* **27**, 645-658.

Scholz, W.   (1938) Studien zur Pathologie der Hirngefässe II.   Die drusige Entartung der Hirnarterien und Capillaren.   *Zeitschrift für die gesamte Neurologie und Psychiatrie,* **162**, 694-715.

Schottky, J.   (1932) Über präsenile Verblödungen.   *Zeitschrift für die gesamte Neurologie und Psychiatrie,* **140**, 333-397.

Schröder, K.   (1931) Zur Klinik und Pathologie der Huntingtonschen Krankheit.   *Jahrbücher für Psychologie und Neurologie,* **43**, 183-201.

Schulman, S.   (1956) Bilateral symmetrical degeneration of the thalamus.   *Journal of Neuropathology and Experimental Neurology,* **15**, 208-209.

Schwartz, P., Wolfe, K., Gier, C. & Wolf, C. E.   (1967) Cerebral, cardiovascular and pancreatic insular amyloidosis in the aged.   (Exhibition presented at 64th Annual meeting of American Association of Pathology and Bacteriology.)

Scoville, W. B.   (1954) The limbic lobe in man.   *Journal of Neurosurgery,* **11**, 64-66.

Scoville, W. B. & Milner, B.   (1957) Loss of recent memory after bilateral hippocampal lesions.   *Journal of Neurology, Neurosurgery and Psychiatry,* **20**, 11-21.

Seitelberger, F. & Jellinger, K.   (1958) Umschriebene Grosshirnatrophie bei Alzheimerscher Krankheit.   *Deutsche Zeitschrift für Nervenheilkunde,* **178**, 365-379.

Serafetinides, E. A. & Falconer, M. A.   (1962) Some observations on memory impairment after temporal lobectomy for epilepsy.   *Journal of Neurology, Neurosurgery and Psychiatry,* **25**, 251-255.

Siedler, H. & Malamud, N.   (1963) Creutzfeldt-Jakob's disease: clinico-pathological report of 15 cases and review of literature.   *Journal of Neuropathology and Experimental Neurology,* **22**, 381-402.

Sim, M. & Smith, W. T.   (1955) Alzheimer's disease confirmed by cerebral biopsy: a therapeutic trial with cortisone and A.C.T.H.   *Journal of Mental Science,* **101**, 604-609.

Simchowicz, T.   (1911) Histologische Studien über die senile Demenz.   *Histologische und histopathologische Arbeiten über die Grosshirnrinde,* **4**, 267-444.

Simma, K.   (1952) Die subcorticalen Veränderungen bei Pickscher Krankheit im Vergleich zur Chorea Huntington.   *Monatsschrift für Psychiatrie und Neurologie,* **123**, 205-207.

Simon, A. & Malamud, N.   (1965) In *Psychiatric Disorders in the Aged.   Comparison of clinical and neuropathological findings in geriatric mental illness.*   Geigy, Manchester.

Sjögren, T.   (1935) Vererbungsmedizinische Untersuchungen über Huntingtonsche Chorea in einer schwedischen Bauernpopulation.   *Zeitschrift für menschliche Vererbungs und Konstitutionslehre,* **19**, 131-65.

Sjögren, T., Sjögren, H. & Lindgren, A.   (1952) Morbus Alzheimer and Morbus Pick.   Genetic chemical and patho-anatomical study.   *Acta psychiatrica et neurologica Scandinavica, supp.* 82.

Slater, E. & Cowie, V.   (1971) In *The Genetics of Mental Disorders.*   Oxford University Press, London.

Smith, B.   (1961) Personal communication.

Smith, W. T.   (1970) In *Modern Trends in Neurology,* **5** (Ed. Williams, D.).   Butterworth, London.

Smith, W. T., Turner, E. & Sim, M.   (1966) Cerebral biopsy in the investigation of presenile dementia.   II   Pathological Aspects.   *British Journal of Psychiatry,* **112**, 127-133.

Solitaire, G. B. & Lamarche, J. B.   (1966) Alzheimer's disease and senile dementia as seen in mongoloids.   *American Journal of Mental Deficiency,* **70**, 840-848.

Soniat, T. L. L.   (1941) Histogenesis of senile plaques.   *Archives of Neurology and Psychiatry,* **46**, 101-144.

Spatz, H.   (1952) La maladie de Pick, les atrophies systématisées progressives et la Sénescence cérébrale prématurée Localisée in *Proceedings of First International Congress of Neuropathology,* 375-406.

Spiegel, E. A., Wycis, H. T., Orchinik, C. W. & Freed, H. (1955) The thalamus and temporal orientation. *Science*, **121**, 771-772.

Stadler, H. (1939) Über Beziehungen zwischen Creutzfeldt-Jakobscher Krankheit (spastische Pseudosklerose) und Pellagra. *Zeitschrift für die gesamte Neurologie und Psychiatrie*, **165**, 326-332.

Stahl, W. L. & Swanson, P. D. (1974) Biochemical abnormalities in Huntington's chorea brains. *Neurology*, **24**, 813-819.

Steele, J. C., Richardson, J. C. & Olszewski, J. (1964) Progressive supra-nuclear palsy. *Archives of Neurology*, **10**, 333-359.

Stender, A. (1930) Weitere Beiträge zum Kapitel spastische Pseudosklerose Jakob. *Zeitschrift für die gesamte Neurologie und Psychiatrie*, **128**, 528-543.

Stengel, E. & Wilson, W. E. J. (1946) Jakob-Creutzfeldt disease. *Journal of Mental Science*, **92**, 370-378.

Stepien, L. & Sierpinski, S. (1964) Impairment of recent memory after temporal lesions in man. *Neuropsychologia*, **2**, 291-303.

Stern, K. (1939) Severe dementia associated with bilateral symmetrical degeneration of the thalamus. *Brain*, **62**, 157-171.

Stern, K. & Reed, G. E. (1945) Presenile Dementia (Alzheimer's Disease). *American Journal of Psychiatry*, **102**, 191-197.

Struwe, F. (1929) Histopathologische Untersuchungen über Entstehung und Wesen der senilen Plaques, *Zeitschrift für die gesamte Neurologie und Psychiatrie*, **122**, 291-307.

Surbeck, E. B. (1961) L'angiopathie dyshorique (Morel) de l'écorce cérébrale. Etude anatomo-clinique et statistique: aspect génétique. Thesis, Geneva.

Teichmann, E. (1935) Über einen der amyotrophischen lateralsklerose nahestehenden Krankheitsprozess mit psychischen Symptomen. *Zeitschrift für die gesamte Neurologie und Psychiatrie*, **154**, 34-44.

Tellez-Nagel, I., Johnson, A. B. & Terry, R. D. (1974) Studies on brain biopsies of patients with Huntington's chorea. *Journal of Neuropathology and Experimental Neurology*, **33**, 308-332.

Terry, R. D. (1963) The fine structure of neurofibrillary tangles in Alzheimer's disease. *Journal of Neuropathology and Experimental Neurology*, **22**, 629-642.

Terry, R. D. & Wisniewski, H. M. (1972) In *Aging and the Brain* (Ed. Gaitz, C. M.). Plenum Press, New York.

Terzian, H. & Ore, G. D. (1955) Syndrome of Klüver and Bucy reproduced in man by bilateral removal of the temporal lobes. *Neurology*, **5**, 373-380.

Titeca, L. & van Bogaert, L. (1946) Heredo-degenerative hemiballismus; a contribution to the question of primary atrophy of the corpus Luysii. *Brain*, **69**, 251-263.

Tomlinson, B. E., Blessed, G. & Roth, M. (1968) Observations on the brains of non-demented old people. *Journal of the Neurological Sciences*, **7**, 331-356.

Tomlinson, B. E., Blessed, G. & Roth, M. (1970) Observations on the brains of demented old people. *Journal of the Neurological Sciences*, **11**, 205-242.

Tomlinson, B. E. & Kitchener, D. (1972) Granulovacuolar degeneration of hippocampal pyramidal cells. *Journal of Pathology*, **106**, 165-185.

Tomonaga, M. (1974) Ultrastructure of Hirano bodies. *Acta Neuropathologica*, **30**, 365-366.

Ulrich, G., Taghavy, A. & Schmidt, H. (1973) Zur Nosologie und Ätiologie der kongophilen Angiopathie (Gefässform der cerebralen Amyloidose). *Zeitschrift für Neurologie*, **206**, 39-59.

Urechia, C., Dragomir, L. & Elekes, N. (1935) Deux cas de la maladie de Pick. Un cas de la maladie d'Alzheimer. Existe-t-il des rapports entres ces maladies? *Archives internationales de neurologie*, **54**, 55-83.

Verhaart, W. J. C. (1936) Ueber das Vorkommen der Pickschen Krankheit und der Krankheit von Alzheimer bei den Malaien und Chinesen in Niederlandisch-Ost-Indien. *Mededeelingen van den Dienst der Volksgezondheid in Nederlandsch-Indië*, **25**, 341-345.

Victor, M., Adams, R. D. & Collins, G. H. (1971) In *The Wernicke-Korsakoff Syndrome*. Blackwell Scientific, Oxford.

Victor, M., Angevine, J. B., Mancall, E. L. & Fisher, C. M. (1961) Memory loss with lesions of hippocampal formation. *Archives of Neurology*, **5**, 244-263.

Vogt, M. (1928) Die Picksche Atrophie als Beispiel für die eunomische Form der Schichtenpathoklise. *Jahrbücher für Psychologie und Neurologie*, **36**, 124-129.

Weimann, W. (1921) Ueber einen atypischen präsenilen Verblödungsprozess. *Zeitschrift für die gesamte Neurologie und Psychiatrie*, **23**, 355-360.

Weisschedel, E. (1938) Ueber eine systematische Atrophie der oberen Olive. *Archiv für Psychiatrie und Nervenkrankheiten*, **108**, 219-227.

Wells, C. E. (1971) In *Dementia Contemporary Neurology Series, No. 9*. Blackwell Scientific, Oxford.

Wendt, G. G., Landzettel, I. & Solth, K.   (1960) Krankheitsdauer und Lebenserwartung bei der Hunting-tonschen Chorea.   *Archiv für Psychiatrie und Nervenkrankheiten*, **201**, 298-312.

Wendt, G. G., Landzettel, H. J. & Unterreiner, I.   (1959) Das Erkrankungsalter bei der Huntingtonschen Chorea.   *Acta genetica et statistica medica (Basel)*, **9**, 18-32.

Wernicke, C.   (1881) In *Lehrbuch der Gehirnkrankheiten für Arzte und Studierende*.   Fischer, Berlin.

Wheelan, L.   (1959) Familial Alzheimer's disease.   *Annals of Human Genetics*, **23**, 300-310.

Whittier, J. E.   (1963) Research on Huntington's chorea: problems of privilege and confidentiality.   *Journal of Forensic Science*, **8**, 568-575.

Williams, H.   (1935) The peculiar cells of Pick's disease.   *Archives of Neurology and Psychiatry*, **34**, 508-519.

Winkelman, N. W. & Book, M. H.   (1949) Asymptomatic extrapyramidal involvement in Pick's disease.   *Journal of Neuropathology and Experimental Neurology*, **8**, 30-42.

Wisniewski, H. M. & Terry, R. D.   (1971) In *Advances in Behavioral Biology*, vol. 3.   Plenum Press, New York.

Wisniewski, H., Terry, R. D. & Hirano, A.   (1970) Neurofibrillary pathology.   *Journal of Neuropathology and Experimental Neurology*, **29**, 163-176.

Woodard, J. S.   (1962) Clinico-pathologic significance of granulovacuolar degeneration in Alzheimer's disease.   *Journal of Neuropathology and Experimental Neurology*, **21**, 85-91.

Woodard, J. S.   (1966) Alzheimer's disease in late adult life.   *American Journal of Pathology*, **49**, 1157-1169.

Worm-Petersen, J. & Pakkenberg, H.   (1968) Atherosclerosis of cerebral arteries: pathological and clinical correlations.   *Journal of Gerontology*, **23**, 445-449.

Worster-Drought, C. & Allen, I. M.   (1929) Huntington's chorea—with report of two cases.   *British Medical Journal*, **2**, 1149-1152.

Worster-Drought, C., Greenfield, J. G. & McMenemey, W. H.   (1940) A form of familial pre-senile dementia with spastic paralysis.   *Brain*, **63**, 237-254.

Worster-Drought, C., Greenfield, J. G. & McMenemey, W. H.   (1944) A form of familial presenile dementia with spastic paralysis.   *Brain*, **67**, 38-43.

Wright, J. R., Calkins, E., Breen, W. J., Stolte, G. & Schultz, R. T.   (1969) Relationship of amyloid to aging. Review of the literature and systematic study of 83 patients from a general hospital population.   *Medicine, Baltimore*, **48**, 39-60.

Yano, K., Nishina, Y. & Kumono, S.   (1960) A contribution to the histopathology of Pick's disease, with special reference to the glial elements.   *Folia psychiatria et neurologica Japonica*, **14**, 123-139.

Yates, P. O. & Hutchinson, E. C.   (1961) Cerebral infarction: the role of stenosis of the extracranial cerebral arteries.   *MRC Special Report series 300*.

Zeman, W.   (1971) Ceroid lipofuscinosis—Batten Vogt syndrome: a model for human aging?   *Advances in Gerontological Research*, **3**, 147-70.

Zerbin-Rüdin, E.   (1967) in *Humangenetik, ein Kurzes Handbuch*, vol. 2 (Ed. Becker, P. E.).   Thieme, Stuttgart.

Zlotnik, I., Grant, D. P., Dayan, A. D. & Earl, C. J.   (1974) Transmission of Creutzfeldt-Jakob disease from man to squirrel monkey.   *Lancet*, **2**, 435-438.

19

Muscle

D. G. F. Harriman

Skeletal muscle is under the control of the nervous system: when deprived of its innervation it loses its function. It is therefore necessary to consider the pathology of skeletal muscle together with that of the motor and sensory structures which influence it so deeply. Pathological changes in muscle which result from denervation are referred to as *neurogenic atrophy* or *neurogenic disease*, while *myopathy* is used to describe changes which appear to be due to a disorder of the muscle tissue proper. When these are combined, the term neuromyopathy is appropriate.

Histology

The skeletal muscle cell or myofibre is enormously elongated, quite often stretching from the origin to the insertion of a muscle. It has many nuclei, situated under normal conditions in the periphery of the cell immediately under the cell membrane, except at its origin from or insertion into connective tissue, where it tapers and nuclei are internally placed for a short distance. The tapering ends of muscle cells, round in cross-section, are sometimes seen within muscles, but these apparently blindly ending muscle fibres are remarkably infrequent, even in large muscles like the quadriceps. They have to be distinguished from fibres rendered small by disease.

Much of the cytoplasm of muscle fibres is occupied by myofibrils, thin cords of protein which run the entire length of the cell. They have an alternately light and dark banded structure, shown well by polarized light and by routine staining of longitudinally orientated fibres. The myofibrils run in parallel rows so that their bands are in register in well-fixed material. This gives the skeletal muscle fibre its characteristic striated form (Fig. 19.1). The anisotropic or A-bands stain more darkly than the isotope or I-bands, and a dark line, the Z-band (Zwischenscheibe, or intercalated plate) lies in the middle of the I-band. In tranverse section myofibrils are closely and fairly uniformly packed, 100 or more in each fibre. This uniform 'fibrillenstruktur' pattern is seen in the vast majority of skeletal muscle fibres in man, but in much amphibian muscle and in some fibres in a few specialized muscles in man the myofibrils are congregated in clumps ('Feldenstruktur', see *extraocular muscle* p. 876).

Muscle fibre size*

In life, striated muscle fibres vary greatly in girth as well as length, depending on their state of contraction or relaxation. The effect of this is seen in a whole muscle in the familiar flexing of the biceps. It is not possible, therefore, to give absolute values for fibre calibre, and difficulties arise in defining atrophy or hypertrophy by size. Normal muscle freshly excised at biopsy will, if permitted, contract into an irregular mass, and the calibre of the contracted fibres may be 50% to 100% greater than that of stretched muscle from the same site (Fig. 19.2). Depending on the methods used, fibre calibres as reported vary, sometimes considerably, from one laboratory to another. The most reliable and consistent figures are obtained from necropsy muscle if a clamp is used to maintain resting length and the specimen is sectioned in a cryostat. Sizes vary with age, development, body weight and from muscle to muscle. Fibre diameters of necropsy muscles fixed in formol-calcium and embedded in paraffin are given by

---

* The term *muscle fibre* is by convention used to denote what is in reality a multinucleated cell, and will be so used henceforth in this chapter.

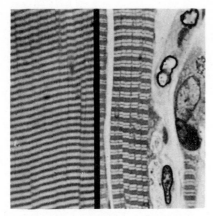

Fig. 19.1 (*Left*) Part of a muscle fibre viewed by polarized light (unstained epon-embedded section). The light, anisotropic A-bands alternate with the dark isotropic I-bands. × 576. (*Right*) Epon-embedded muscle from a child of 3 years. The A-bands stain darkly, and the lightly stained I-bands are divided by a thin dark line, the Z-band. A *sarcomere* extends from one Z-band to the next. A myelinated subterminal axon approaches the muscle fibre from above right, running towards a motor endplate which apparently sits on the surface of the muscle fibre, forming Doyère's eminence. Methylene blue stain. × 1000.

Aherne, Ayyar, Clarke and Walton (1971), and can be roughly approximated to 8 to 10 μm at birth, 15 μm at 1 year, 20 to 30 μm at 6 years and 30 to 50 μm in the adult. Cryostat sections would provide figures up to 30% greater. The effects of different processing techniques are dealt with by Moore, Rebeiz, Holden and Adams (1971), who reported in necropsy muscle a ratio of sizes of fresh frozen, formalin-fixed frozen, celloidin and paraffin embedded fibres roughly of 10 : 9 : 8 : 7. There was a rapid increase in mean diameter of all muscles sampled (superior rectus, sternomastoid, deltoid, biceps brachii, sartorius, quadriceps and gastrocnemius), except in the gastrocnemius, from birth to 5 years of age. At puberty there was again a rapid increase, except in the superior rectus, which remained constant throughout life. In other muscles the fibres increased in size until the fourth decade, and thereafter became smaller. They showed that muscle fibres were larger near the maximum breadth of the muscle belly than elsewhere.

There is also a variation in size between different muscle fibre types (see below).

Muscle fibres are organized into fascicles, in larger muscles composed of several hundred cells.

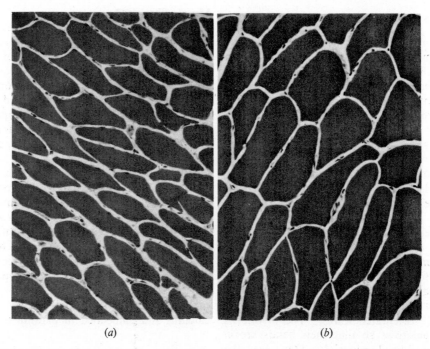

(a)   (b)

Fig. 19.2 Cryostat sections of muscle (*a*) stretched on a clamp before quenching, (*b*) allowed to contract naturally before quenching. The average diameter of the contracted fibres is 50% greater than that of the stretched muscle. HE. × 180.

(a)

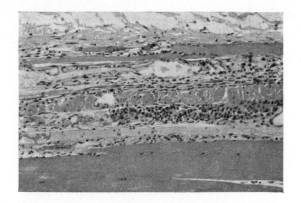

(b)

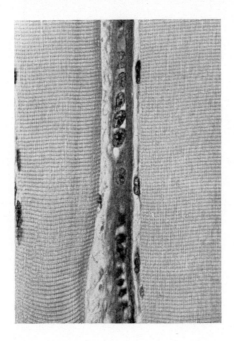

Fig. 19.12 (*a*). A fibre in which the contents have undergone floccular degeneration, and another filled with myophages. Several thin basophil regenerating fibres lie alongside. (*b*) A basophil regenerating fibre, with large nuclei containing nucleoli, lies between two normal fibres.

[facing p. 850]

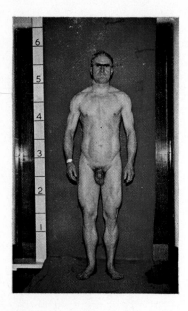

Fig. 19.53 Amyloid myopathy. There is general enlargement of muscles, particularly of thighs and calves.

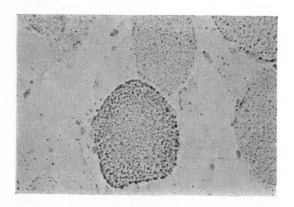

Fig. 19.67 Acute alcoholic myopathy. Fibres become filled with large triglyceride droplets. Sch. R. × 280.

The fascicles are separated by epimyseal connective tissue, containing blood vessels and nerves, and varying amounts of adipose tissue depending on the obesity of the individual. Normal fascicles do not contain fat cells. The perimysium is a thin layer of fibrous tissue enclosing the fascicle, and the inconspicuous fine strands of fibrous tissue which lie between individual muscle cells is the endomysium. When teased out, single muscle fibres are round in transverse outline, but in

seen in biopsy tissue, which remains irritable for up to 20 minutes, and are due to violent contraction and rupture of living fibres produced by excision, rough handling, tearing or premature fixation of tissue destined for embedding. Over-contraction produces irregular contraction bands (Fig. 19.3) in which the cell proteins appear to have 'coagulated'. Tranverse section through a contracted zone gives the impression of a hyaline fibre with pyknotic nuclei, often mistaken for a

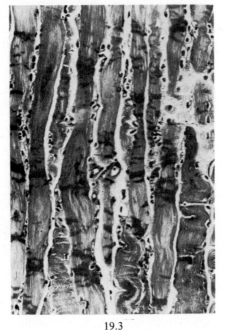

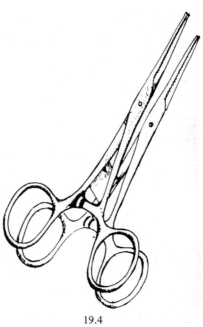

19.3   19.4

Fig. 19.3 Biopsy muscle from a female of 68 years with polyneuritis. There are numerous contraction bands due to the immersion of the specimen in fixative while still irritable. Partly denervated muscle is particularly susceptible to this artefact. There is a genuine target fibre top left. L.S. × 270.

Fig. 19.4 Simple clamp used for maintaining rest length of muscle taken at biopsy. It is composed of two artery forceps united by a steel band, and permits individual control of the 'bite' at each end of the fascicle excised. Conventional muscle biopsy clamps in the form of a U or Y are more difficult to use because the bites at each extremity must be made simultaneously. Clamps are made with small or large forceps (box joints) and with different tip separations to suit the requirements for electron-microscopy, for the cryostat or for paraffin embedding.

transversely cut fascicles they appear roughly polygonal, with straight or curved sides, as if adapting to mutual lateral pressure. Shrinkage by fixatives may accentuate the polygonal shape and in some instances the sarcoplasm shrinks inwards, away from the endomysium.

Artefacts

In addition to shrinkage due to fixation, muscle is subject to many artefacts. They are more often

pathological change. The incidence of contraction bands can be reduced by allowing excised biopsy muscle to rest for 10 to 15 minutes before fixation. The specimen is best taken on a clamp of which there are several varieties. We use two artery forceps united by a steel band (Fig. 19.4), but even clamped muscle may show contraction artefact if immersed in fixative too soon. Another very common artefact is the streaming of cell contents, especially glycogen, to one edge, producing a crescent of increased staining density. This has been ascribed to osmosis induced during fixation, and is not seen in cryostat sections.

Fibre types

A paraffin section of muscle stained by routine methods exhibits uniformity of staining between individual muscle fibres, yet it has long been known that many mammalian muscles vary in colour. There are red muscles and white muscles in many mammals, and even in man there are paler and darker muscles. The superficial fascicles in human muscle are often paler than core fascicles, especially in athletic individuals. That these variations reflect differences between individual muscle fibres has been known for over a century. Krause (1864) found that the red muscle fibres of the rabbit contained more interstitial granules (mitochondria) than were present in the fibres of the white muscles, and Grutzner (1884) described two types of fibres in human muscles, cloudy or dark, and pale or white. All human muscles contained both types of fibres and for a time it was believed that the colour of a muscle depended on its content of dark fibres. In fact the colour is determined by the content of the soluble protein, myoglobin (Morita, Cooper, Gassens, Kastenschmidt and Briskey 1970). Red, slow-twitch muscle fibres contract more slowly than pale fibres (Creed, Denny-Brown, Eccles, Liddell and Sherrington 1932). With the introduction of histochemical techiques applied to cryostat sections of fresh muscle, the differences between the types of muscle fibre were better defined (Dubowitz 1968). The slow-twitch fibres of red muscle react strongly for oxidative enzymes, and are used for continuous muscle activity under aerobic conditions. The fast-twitch fibres react strongly for phosphorylase, used in the breakdown of glycogen to lactic acid under anaerobic conditions, and are therefore of value for short bursts of high activity. There is thus a reciprocal staining relationship between these two types of fibre, the 'red' fibres reacting weakly for phosphorylase and the 'white' weakly for oxidative enzymes (Dubowitz and Pearce 1960). The designations *type-1* and *type-2* were proposed for the two sorts of muscle fibre, type-1 containing more mitochondria which carry the oxidative enzymes. In 1962 Engel showed that the enzyme myosin ATPase is present in high concentration in type-2 fibres, and this method has proved to be the most generally useful for typing muscle fibres. With stains for oxidative enzymes and phosphorylase, fibres showing intermediate staining activity are frequently

present, creating difficulties in classification and interpretation. The intensity of phosphorylase staining depends on the amount of glycogen in the individual fibre (Martin and Engel 1972), and exercise affects the intensity of staining of oxidative enzymes (Edgerton, Gerchman and Carrow 1969). In small mammals muscle fibres are now classified as fast-oxidative-glycolytic, fast-glycolytic or slow-oxidative (Ariano, Armstrong and Edgerton 1973), implying not only type-1 and type-2 fibres as defined above but an additional form containing both oxidative and glycolytic enzymes. Such fibres have not yet been identified in human limb muscles, and for practical purposes in dealing with human myopathology a division into two main types using the oxidative enzyme methods and myos in ATPase is sufficient.* This permits correlation of fibre type susceptibility in pathological conditions.

Although certain muscles in mammals are composed predominantly or entirely of one fibre type, in man there is always a mixture and the fibre types are distributed at random in a mosaic pattern (Fig. 19.5). The proportion of type-1 and type-2 fibres varies in different muscles, and suspected abnormalities of distribution have to be weighed against the normal pattern for the muscle examined. Johnson, Polgar, Weightman and Appleton (1973) examined the spatial distribution of fibre types in a large number of human muscles, using the myosin ATPase technique in autopsy muscle. The majority of muscles sampled had between 40 and 70% of type-1 fibres. Muscles with an almost exclusively postural function, such as the soleus and the tibialis anterior, had more, 87 and 73% respectively. Muscles with predominantly phasic activity had relatively few, the triceps containing only 33%. The pattern assumed by the fibre types is important in diagnostic work,

---

* Subdivisions of type-2 fibres occur, types 2a, b and c. Myosin ATPase appears to exist in two forms, alkali-stable and acid-stable. The routine myosin ATPase reaction performed in a highly alkaline solution stains alkali-stable ATPase darkly and, as explained above, lightly stained fibres using this reaction correspond to type-1 fibres. But if the sections are pre-incubated at acid pH, the type-1 fibres now stain darkly and the type-2 lightly. However, there is a variation in the density of staining of the type-2 fibres with acid pre-incubation, some reacting with medium intensity (type 2b) and a few almost as strongly as type-1 fibres (type 2c). The variation in staining intensity of the type-2 fibres can thus be interpreted as due to differing contents of alkali-stable and acid-stable myosin ATPase (Brooke and Kaiser 1970) but this is likely to be an over simplification (Guth and Samaha 1972).

for 'type grouping' occurs as the result of denervation and re-innervation of muscle (see below). It is important therefore to be aware of the normal variations. Jennekens, Tomlinson and Walton

could occur in normal muscle. Muscle fibres of both types show a modest deviation from mean size, and an interesting sex difference: type-2 fibres are generally larger than type-1 in the male,

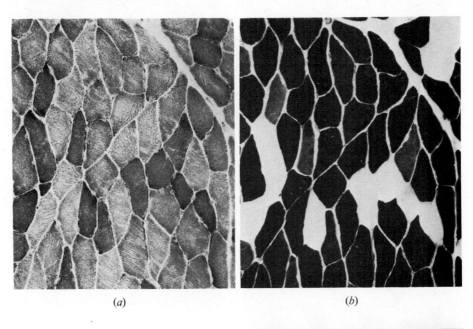

(a)   (b)

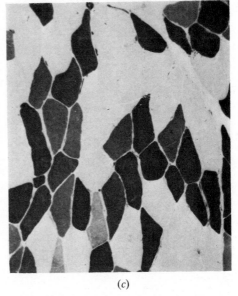

Fig. 19.5 The mosaic pattern of fibre types in man. (a) NADH, type-1 fibres dark, type-2 lighter. (b) ATPase pH 9·5 type-1 fibres colourless, type-2 dark. (c) ATPase pH 4·1 preincubation, type-1 fibres dark, type-2 mostly light (but see footnote). Serial sections. All × 110.

(c)

(1971) found in an autopsy study that clusters of the same fibre type with three or more 'enclosed' fibres, i.e. fibres totally surrounded by others of the same type, were abnormal, provided they lay close to other clusters of similar size. *Isolated* clusters of up to 30 or 40 fibres ('enclosing' 13 fibres)

whereas the opposite is often true in the female (Brooke and Engel 1969).

The motor unit
Individual muscle fibres are supplied by a single subterminal nerve fibre, the result of multiple

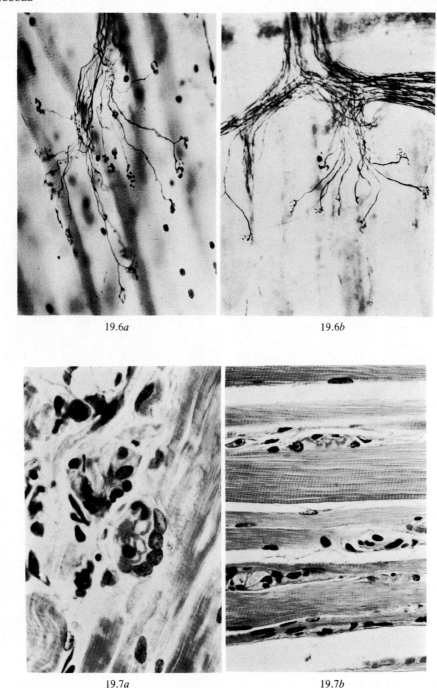

19.6a

19.6b

19.7a

19.7b

Fig. 19.6 The subterminal fibre pattern. Subterminal fibres run singly from intramuscular nerve bundles towards muscle fibres, to supply each fibre with a motor endplate. About one fibre in ten receives two endplates, rarely more in normal muscle. Thus normal subterminal fibres rarely branch. (a) Subterminal fibres in a female aged 3 years. The endplates are formed by branching of terminal axons which form expansions. Methylene blue. × 170. (b) Subterminal fibres and endplates in a male aged 5 years. The endplates are stained by silver using a block impregnation method. Expansions are present but appear smaller. de Castro. × 170.

Fig. 19.7 (a) Motor endplate stained by HE. The ring of sole plate nuclei is clearly seen, enclosing the folded cell membrane which forms a cup for each expansion. The expansions themselves are not stained. A nerve with Schwann cell nuclei approaches from above. × 630. (b) Side view of two endplates.

dichotomous branchings of the main axon of the anterior horn cell. One anterior horn cell innervates a large number of muscle fibres, varying from a hundred or so in small hand muscles to 500 to 2000 in large limb muscles (Feinstein, Lindegaard, Nyman and Wohlfart 1955). The complex of an anterior horn cell and the group of muscle fibres it controls is the *motor unit*. Adjacent motor units overlap and intermingle, and this is responsible for the random mosaic pattern of fibre types, for it is assumed that the fibres of a given unit are all of the same type. The arrangement of fibres into fascicles is fortuitous and does not conform to motor unit pattern. Intramuscular nerves contain fibres of large and small calibre, and about 40% of the larger fibres (12 to 14 μm) are motor. These continue to branch as the intramuscular nerves divide, until eventually a small nerve bundle fans out into single subterminal fibres, each running towards an individual muscle cell. Subterminal fibres are myelinated, although of lesser calibre than the main motor axons from which they are derived through repeated division (Fig. 19.6).

Motor endplates (neuromuscular junctions) are formed at the termination of the motor fibres at about the midpoint of the muscle fibre, so that in a muscle which is composed of parallel fibres there is a fairly compact innervation zone at the middle of the muscle belly. In bipennate and circumpennate muscles the innervation zone follows a curved or sinuous course depending on the disposition of the muscle fibres.

At the end of the last myelin sheath internode the motor axon becomes a *terminal fibre*. It soon divides into a number of terminal branches, each of which forms spherical or elongated expansions along its course and at its extremity. The expansions rest directly on the muscle fibre, on the surface of a hillock (Doyère's eminence). The hillock can be made prominent by fixing the muscle in the stretched state (Fig. 19.7). A circle of muscle nuclei lie at the edge of the eminence. The muscular component of the junction is known as the *soleplate*, and the complex of terminals, expansions and sole is the *endplate*, although this term is often used for the neural part alone.

In early life the terminal nerve fibre may remain single, forming a single expansion, but the endplate becomes larger and more complicated during maturation. It has been suggested that in mammals there is, during life, a continuous process of degeneration and regeneration of endplates (Barker and Ip 1965, 1966). A continuous process of this

nature has not been shown in man, in whom degeneration and regeneration are seen as an ageing process, degeneration eventually overcoming the regeneration reaction it induces. In a more recent study in the cat (Tuffery 1971), growth and degeneration of endplates are thought not to be causally related; degeneration occurs with increasing age and leads to loss of muscle fibres. Although in normal muscles most subterminal axons do not branch, about 10% do so to provide a second endplate on the same muscle fibre, or less frequently on an adjacent muscle fibre. One muscle fibre never receives end-

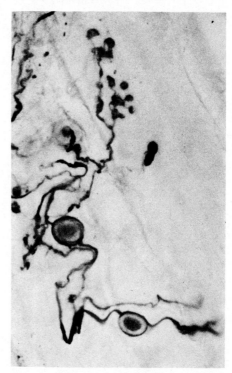

Fig. 19.8 Axonic spheres. These occur along the course of axons, especially subterminal, and usually are an ageing phenomenon. The ovoid spheres are clearly intraaxonal; they stain uniformly or concentrically. A normal endplate is also seen. Female aged 59 years, Ekbom's syndrome for 38 years. Peroneus brevis. Methylene blue. × 600.

plates from two different axons (Coers and Woolf 1959). In certain specialized muscles in man, such as the laryngeal, subterminal fibres do branch and muscle fibres show multiple innervation (Coers 1967). In limb muscles in man degeneration with age starts earliest in the longest axons (Harriman, Taverner and Woolf 1970) and leads to regeneration of endplates by sprouting from adjacent healthy subterminal fibres, the sprouts arising from nodes of Ranvier along the whole course of the subterminal fibre. Such collateral re-innervation is seen in the peroneus brevis as early as the fourth decade. Similarly the occurrence of ovoid swellings (axonic spheres, Fig. 19.8) in subterminal axons, is to be looked on as a manifestation of ageing. These swellings have also been seen in distal muscles from a relatively early age, and in proximal muscles from middle age onwards. They become frequent in old age. In abnormally large numbers they are pathological, e.g. in thallium poisoning.

Structure of the motor endplate

The connective tissue surrounding the subterminal nerve fibre is continuous with the endomysium, and forms a bell enclosing the axon terminals and

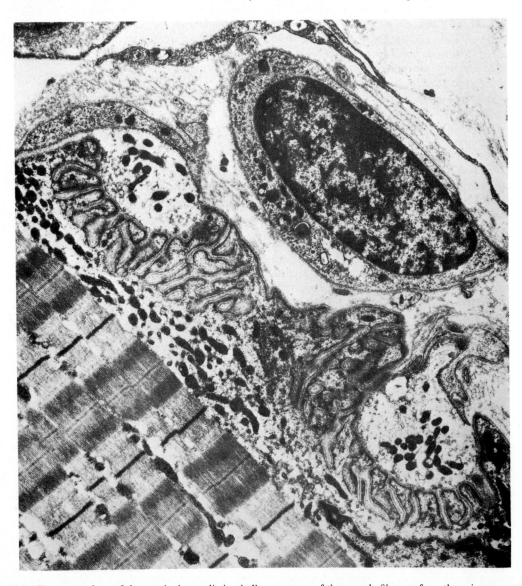

Fig. 19.9   Two expansions of the terminal axon lie in shallow grooves of the muscle fibre surface, the primary synaptic groove. The expansions are separated from the muscle fibre by basement membrane only, but are covered elsewhere by Schwann cell cytoplasm. The nucleus of a Schwann cell is seen top left. The sarcolemma is thrown into deep folds at the neuromuscular junction (the secondary synaptic clefts). A few synaptic vesicles and darkly stained mitochondria can be seen in the axonic expansions, and the soleplate contains vesicles and mitochondria also. EM. × 12,000.

the endplate region. The terminals and their expansions are intimately covered by Schwann cell cytoplasm except at their point of contact with the muscle fibre. The expansions lie in shallow excavations on the surface of the muscle fibre, the primary synaptic groove, and here the neural part of the endplate is separated from the muscular part (the soleplate) by basement membrane alone. The axonic expansion contains mitochondria and clear synaptic vesicles, but only a few neurofilaments and neurotubules which are more numerous in the proximal part of the terminal fibre. The soleplate provides a large area of muscle fibre

Duchen 1971) and the most striking difference in man is the increased depth and number of secondary synaptic folds in type-2 soleplates. The fast-twitch 'white' type-2 fibre appears to present a larger surface area at the synapse than the slow-twitch 'red' fibre.

Muscle spindles

The afferent nerve supply of muscle comes from muscle spindles, tendon organs and other receptors and free nerve endings (Fig. 19.11). Spindles are found in all muscles, but are more numerous in those performing fine movements such as the small

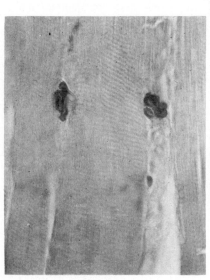
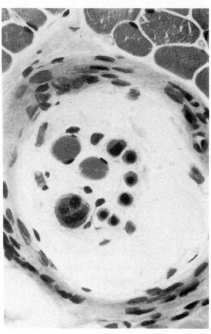

19.10   19.11

Fig. 19.10 Cholinesterase stain. Cholinesterase is found in the folds of the sarcolemma, the secondary synaptic folds; whenever it is stained it outlines the sole plate. × 420.
Fig. 19.11 Transverse section of a muscle spindle in the equatorial region. One of the larger 'nuclear bag' fibres contains a cluster of nuclei. The smaller nuclear chain fibres each have a central nucleus. HE. × 420.

surface for the neuromuscular junction by being deeply and successively folded, forming secondary synaptic clefts (Fig. 19.9). The synaptic vesicles are thought to discharge quanta of acetylcholine into the clefts, and it is here that the enzyme cholinesterase, which hydrolyses acetylcholine, can be demonstrated (Fig. 19.10). The soleplate contains further vesicles, glycogen and mitochondria, as well as soleplate nuclei. There are differences between type-1 and type-2 fibre endplates in mammals (Padykula and Gauthier 1970;

muscles of the hands, and are difficult to find in bulky muscles such as the quadriceps. Spindles are small at birth, when the muscle fibres they contain, the intrafusal fibres, are of about the same diameter as the myofibres of the muscle proper (the extrafusal fibres). In the adult, spindles are much larger, up to 7 mm long, but the intrafusal fibres remain of small diameter. The latter are of two types, larger 'nuclear bag' fibres, which contain a cluster of nuclei at their midpoint, occupying almost the entire width of the fibre and leaving little room for myofibrils; and smaller 'nuclear chain fibres'. These have centrally placed nuclei in the middle region of the fibre, disposed in a long, single column. Normal spindles contain 3 to 15 intrafusal fibres, enclosed in a fibrous capsule. The capsule is quite thin in the wide equatorial part of the spindle, but it can be up to 10 cells thick in the polar regions, without being abnormal. (Many papers report 'thickness' of spindle capsules as a pathological change yet illustrate normal polar regions.) The spindle contains a fluid which sometimse stains as a finely granular material. The innervation of the spindle is complex, comprising primary and secondary sensory endings in the equatorial region, and three types of motor junctions, trail-shaped, multiple plate and larger single plate endings all in the polar regions. The histochemical pattern of intrafusal fibres differs from that of the extrafusal, and varies in different species (James 1971; Ovalle and Smith 1972). The findings of different observers are conflicting, and have not been fully worked out in man, in whom there appear to be two sorts of nuclear bag fibres, one containing myosin ATPase, both acid-stable and alkali-stable, and the other not containing either. Nuclear chain fibres contain both forms of the enzyme (Fig. 19.11).

General reactions of muscle fibres in disease

Necrosis and regeneration are two of the commonest reactions of the muscle fibre. They are seen in many myopathies and, much less frequently, following denervation. Regeneration is possibly the earliest visible change in muscular dystrophy, where it is conspicuous in the preclinical phase. Necrosis of entire muscle fascicles is characteristic of infarction. Experimental necrosis may be produced by a variety of methods, sectioning, crushing, application of heat or cold, or by various poisons. Although extensively studied (Adams, Denny-Brown and Pearson 1962), its mechanism is still not clear; an understanding of its pathogenesis may be the key to many myopathies. Very occasionally it is seen as an isolated finding in an otherwise normal biopsy, so that it may occur as a latent phenomenon in health and need not invariably indicate abnormality.

In human myopathology necrosis is usually seen in a segment of the muscle fibre, the cytoplasm being transformed into a finely granular, floccular or hyaline material (Fig. 19.12, facing p. 850). Zenker (1864) described the hyaline or waxy form

of necrosis in abdominal muscle in patients dying from typhoid fever, and it is often given his name. Rarely the necrotic material takes the form of large spheres or globules, and, even more rarely, broken segments of striated myofibrils occur within the necrotic area. In the early stage, before there is any cellular reaction, necrosis is difficult to distinguish from artefact which is all too frequent in biopsy material. It can be recognized with certainty as soon as leucocytes appear. Polymorphs are not often seen within or marginating the necrotic segment, but mononuclear cells always invade it and act as phagocytes, becoming rounded and ingesting fragments of myoplasm. At the same time the adjacent part of the muscle fibre shows regenerative features. The cytoplasm becomes basophilic, an indication of RNA synthesis in polyribosomes, and sarcolemmal nuclei enlarge and

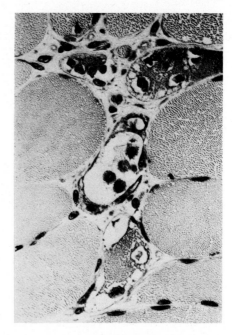

Fig. 19.13 Regenerating fibres. The fibre in the centre still contains a few myophages, but shows the early development of strap-shaped regenerating fibres on the inner surface of the sarcolemma. Regeneration is more advanced in the three other darkly staining fibres in the figure.

develop prominent nucleoli. Occasionally the nucleoli are double, or large and rectangular, and the altered nuclei congregate in rows near the necrotic zone. Regeneration is also seen in the form of spindle or strap cells which form along the internal surface of the intact sarcolemma of the necrotic segment (Fig. 19.13). These are thought to be derived from satellite cells (Mauro 1961; Katz 1961), which are mononuclear cells embedded on the surface of a muscle fibre and covered by its basement membrane. They can only be recognized in electronmicrographs. When regeneration is required they are stimulated to grow and migrate, being transformed into fibril carrying myocytes. At this stage they are recognized in the light microscope as basophil spindle cells (Fig. 19.13). As phagocytosis of the necrotic segment is completed, the muscle cell is reconstituted by fusion of the myocytes, and nucleoli eventually disappear.

When necrosis involves not only muscle cell contents but the plasma membrane, as for example in infarction of a group of muscle cells or in a muscle tissue but larger areas of necrosis end in a fibrous scar.

Fibre splitting

Longitudinal division of muscle fibres is seen in myopathies and, less frequently, in neurogenic disease and the atrophy of cachexia (Cornil and Ranvier 1902). A split appears in a large fibre, lined by sarcolemma, tracking in from the exterior and generally directed towards an internally placed muscle nucleus. In transverse section the daughter fibre or fibres appear as crescents indenting the parent fibre, all enclosed by the same endomysium (Fig. 19.14). According to Hall-Crags and Lawrence (1970) overloading of muscle induces

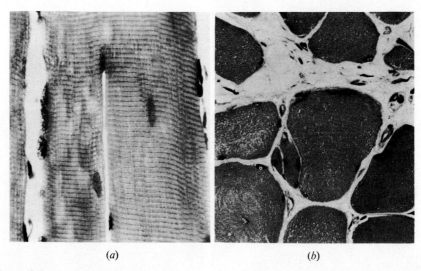

(a)   (b)

Fig. 19.14 Fibre splitting. (a) A longitudinal split is present in the fibre, ending at an internally placed nucleus. HE. ×630. (b) Splitting in the central fibre alongside nuclei has separated off two crescentic segments of muscle fibre. HE. ×420.

crush injury, the sequence of events is different. The necrotic segments of muscle are removed, and the endomysial fibrous tissue proliferates. 'Retraction caps' of coagulated sarcoplasm form on the ends of muscle fibres at the edge of the lesion, and regeneration proceeds from these fibres. Basophilic buds project from the end of the muscle fibres, and spindle-shaped myocytes occur individually within the area. Satellite cells may be responsible for both types of regeneration, but there is no general agreement on this, some workers maintaining that pre-existing muscle nuclei take part in the budding (Sloper, Bateson, Hindle and Warren 1970). Regeneration may bridge the necrotic area with reconstitution of longitudinal division, but the split is of limited extent and always occurs in pathological fibres, nuclei first becoming internal. This seems to be a way of getting rid of unwanted portions of a muscle fibre. Pathological splitting is incomplete, but complete splitting of the entire length of a muscle fibre occurs as part of the normal process of muscle fibre development, being seen in human muscle during the 12th to 15th week of fetal life (Cuajunco 1942). Unsplit parent fibres remain larger than the remainder throughout fetal life, and are scattered singly in fascicles which are otherwise composed of small fibres. They correspond to the type-B fibres of Wohlfart (1937) who described them particularly in the human sartorius.

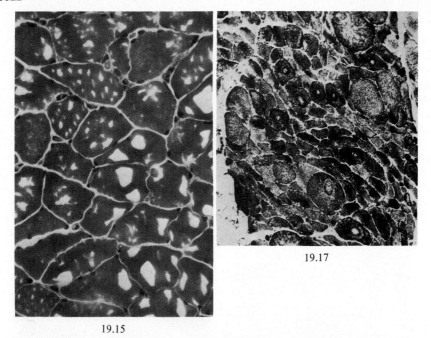

19.15

19.17

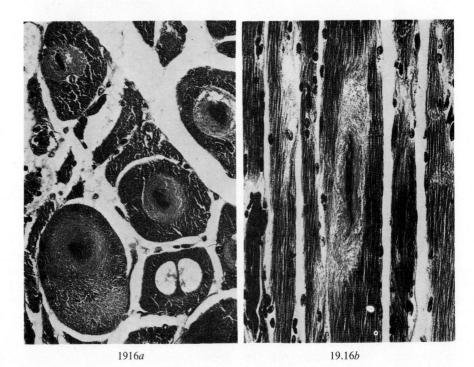

1916a

19.16b

Fig. 19.15 Ice crystals. Muscle frozen too slowly prior to sectioning in a cryostat will develop sarcoplasmic ice crystals, which leave vacuoles of varying size and shape. HE. ×280.

Fig. 19.16 Target fibres seen in (a) cross-section, (b) longitudinal section. The three zones consist of a central area of coagulated myofibrils, an intermediate granular afibrillar zone and an outer ring of normal myofibrils. The target is of limited longitudinal extent. Autopsy muscle, motor neuron disease, paraffin section, PTAH. ×420.

Fig. 19.17 Target fibres in polyneuritis. Note that the central zone is clear, and the intermediate zone shows enhanced enzyme staining. This is the negative of targets seen in Fig. 19.16. NADH. ×110.

During fetal life, from 18 weeks' gestation onwards, he found that they form 5% of the total, but by birth the proportion drops to 1%. Single conspicuous large fibres are often seen in muscle biopsies taken from infants, especially during the first year, and the appearance should not be confused with the effects of neurogenic disease. Dubowitz (1968) correlated the type-B fibres of Wohlfart with the large, scattered type-1 fibres which he found in human fetal muscle at 20 to 26 weeks. The remaining muscle fibres were type-2 and small. Occasional 'giant' fibres (Cassens, Cooper and Briskey 1969) are seen in adult porcine muscle, but these authors believed they were of pathological import and differed from Wohlfart type-B fibres in not being of type-1; they reacted weakly for NADH, phosphorylase was absent and ATPase strongly positive. We have on rare occasions noted large rounded fibres in otherwise normal adult muscle and consider them to be surviving parent Wohlfart type-B fibres, despite discrepancies in histochemical reaction.

Focal abnormalities of muscle fibres and artefact

In considering whether any focal lesion within a skeletal muscle fibre is significant, the possible effects of artefact have to be recalled. Artefact is all too common in muscle, especially biopsy muscle, and can be produced in many ways (see p. 851). Only muscle strips of very small diameter, 0.5 to 1.0 mm, such as are processed for electronmicroscopy, will tolerate immediate fixation without exhibiting artefact. Freshly excised muscle strips of up to 1 cm in diameter may be immediately frozen prior to sectioning in a cryostat for histochemistry without producing artefact, but the freezing process must be rapid or ice-crystals form within the fibres (Fig. 19.15). A popular method is to use isopentane cooled to the consistency of syrup by liquid nitrogen. Glycogen generally remains normally distributed in the muscle cell in cryostat sections, but inevitably drifts to the margin in muscle immersed in osmotically active fixatives. Muscle fibre striations are shown in paraffin sections only in adequately fixed muscle.

Moth-eaten, target and targetoid fibres are significant abnormalities, and although sometimes mimicked by contraction artefacts, have distinguishing features.

The *target fibre* (Fig. 19.17) is so-called because of its three concentric zones (Engel 1961). Protoplasmic stains reveal a central area of coagulated sarcoplasm, an intermediate pale zone and an outer zone of normal myofibrils. In longitudinal section the abnormality is of limited extent and does not show striation in the central zone as myofibrils are there disrupted. When some enzyme stains are used, the central zone is devoid of activity, whereas in the intermediate zone staining is more intense. Electron-microscopy (Tomonaga and Sluga 1969) provides the explanation for this curious reaction; mitochondria and glycogen are virtually absent from the centrally placed disorganized myofibrillar material, but are present in increased quantity in the intermediate zone. The sarcoplasmic reticulum is absent centrally but present in the intermediate zone. These variations in the number of mitochondria and in the amount of sarcoplasmic reticulum are reflected in the staining reactions for oxidative and glycolytic enzymes respectively. The reaction for myosin ATPase, which stains myofibrils, is variable; it may be present or totally lost centrally and increased in the intermediate zone, related no doubt to the degree of coagulation of myofibrils in the internal area and to their compaction peripherally. It will be noted that the appearance of target fibres using protoplasmic and some enzyme stains is reciprocal, one being the 'negative' of the other. In paraffin sections they rarely show up clearly—Fig. 19.16 is the exception rather than the rule. In sections stained with haematoxylin and eosin they are frequently indistinct. Their presence in large numbers is useful diagnostically, as they occur especially in denervating disease. Characteristically they appear in polyneuritis during the recovery phase (Fig. 19.17), suggesting that they may be caused by re-innervation. They may be seen when there are no other histological signs of denervation, but are not completely specific, having been noted rarely, and generally singly, in non-neurogenic conditions.

Targetoid fibres resemble targets but lack an intermediate zone of higher enzyme concentration (Fig. 19.18). Their central area lacks enzyme staining with the occasional exception of myosin ATPase. They can be considered a variant of target fibres, as they often accompany them in the same sections, but they have been seen alone in many myopathies and hence lack diagnostic significance (Engel 1965). Both target and targetoid fibres are to be found in both main fibre types but more frequently in type-1.

Moth-eaten fibres are quite common and non-specific. They are detected in cryostat sections

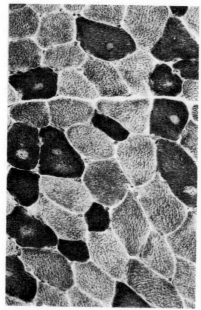

19.18*a*

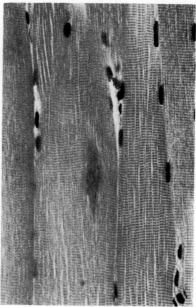

19.18*b*

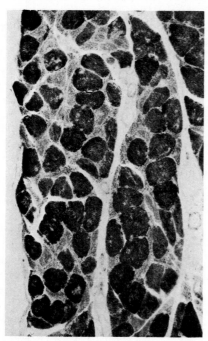

19.19

Fig. 19.18 Targetoid fibres. (*a*) Clearly defined foci devoid of mitochondria, but lacking a surrounding zone of increased activity. NADH. ×180. (*b*) With a myofibril stain (HE) the targetoid zone is seen to consist of fused myofibrils, lacking a surrounding clear zone. ×480.

Fig. 19.19 Moth-eaten fibres. Many fibres contain one or more poorly defined zones of lack of reaction. NADH. ×180.

stained for oxidative enzymes, and are due to patchy loss of mitochondria (Fig. 19.19). They are sometimes accompanied by streaming or whorling of the intermyofibrillary network. This change is single or multiple in transverse section and poorly defined. Although they have no value in specific diagnosis, they have not been seen in otherwise normal muscle. It is possible that moth-eaten fibres,

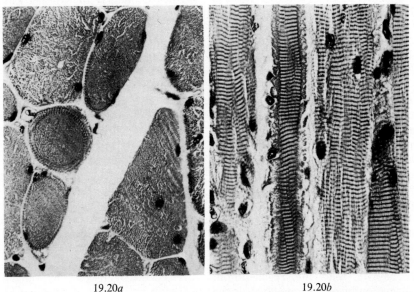

19.20a   19.20b

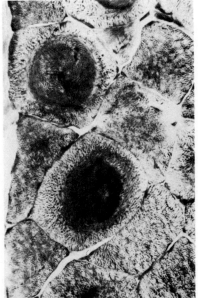

Fig. 19.20 Ring fibres. The spiral encirclement of central myofibrils by peripheral ones is seen in (a) transverse section, (b) longitudinal section. HE. × 420.
Fig. 19.21 Coil fibres. The skein-like arrangement of myofibrils can be seen in the central part of two fibres. PA S. × 480.

19.21

more frequently observed in type-1 fibres, but is not confined to them. There do not appear to be any associated deformations of myofibrils which would render moth-eaten fibres visible in paraffin sections. The areas of mitochondrial loss are targetoid, and target fibres reflect increasingly complex disturbances of the same fundamental nature, the primary event being loss of mitochondria. Their relationship with core fibres (p. 887) is uncertain.

Ring fibres

Formerly known as 'ringbinden', these bizarre fibres were at one time thought to be due to biopsy or post-mortem artefact (Adams *et al.* 1962). The ring-like appearance of the muscle fibre in transverse section is due to the abrupt right-angle bending of one or more peripheral myofibrils which then proceed to encircle the central myofibrils in a spiral manner (Fig. 19.20). In transverse sections striations are thus seen in the encircling myofibrils, and in longitudinal sections in the central myofibrils. Ring fibres are relatively common in certain myopathies, notably myotonic dystrophy, but can also be found in normal muscle near tendinous insertions, and are particularly common in extraocular muscle with advancing age. Such a distribution of the abnormality makes it very unlikely that it could be due to artefact, either post-mortem or the result of fixation of irritable myofibrils; the cells are malformed. The malformation may occur during the course of development, for it is known that new myofibrils may be induced during growth (Goldspink 1970). It may also happen following regeneration. Another malformation involving myofibrils is the *coil fibre*, described in muscle several weeks after experimental denervation (Hogenhuis and Engel 1965). and during reinnervation (Dubowitz 1967*a*). It consists of a snake-like intertwining of groups of myofibrils (Fig. 19.21). Similar fibres had been described in myopathies in the older literature (Wohlfart 1951) but are not mentioned in more recent reports.

Neurogenic disease

It is well known that muscle deprived of its motor nerve supply cannot be made to contract voluntarily and soon atrophies. There are many different causes, and the wasting and weakness they produce are often readily detected by clinical examination, electromyography and nerve conduction studies. These methods fail to establish an unequivocal diagnosis in a small proportion of patients who present with muscular weakness and wasting, and in these a muscle and/or nerve biopsy is required. Neurogenic disease may be unexpectedly demonstrated or confirmed when suspected; in exceptional cases the cause of the denervation may be indicated, for example in the collagenoses. At times the histological distinction between a myopathy and neurogenic disease can be difficult, and for this reason a motorpoint muscle biopsy should, if possible, be performed to provide information concerning the nerve supply of the muscle as well as pathological changes in the muscle tissue proper (Harriman 1961; Haslock, Wright and Harriman 1970). Unilateral or symmetrical focal muscle denervation may be produced by involvement of anterior horn cells in the spinal cord, due to an intrinsic or extrinsic tumour, syringomyelia, infarction, poliomyelitis or motor neuron disease, but only the last may be difficult to recognize clinically. Involvement of spinal nerve roots by infective or neoplastic conditions, polyradiculoneuronitis and diseases of peripheral nerves (see Chapter 16) all produce denervation of muscle. The pattern of atrophy produced depends on the severity and duration of the denervating process, and to some extent on its site, whether proximal or distal. Only rarely is total denervation, produced by a single incident, encountered as a clinical problem in the investigation of neuromuscular disease; most biopsies are made in progressive conditions. The effects of total motor and sensory nerve section on a muscle are rarely investigated by biopsy, but much experimental work on the effects of denervation are made in such a manner. The histological picture produced by disease differs in many respects from that produced experimentally.

Reaction of the motor apparatus

The earliest sign of progressive denervation, whether caused by spinal cord or peripheral nerve disease, is manifest by the intramuscular motor nerves. The first event presumably is degeneration of the axon and its branches distal to the disease site, either centrifugally or dying back from the periphery. It is rare for this degeneration to be seen by light microscopy. It happens occasionally in diabetic neuropathy or in ageing that the expansions of the motor endplate are retracted into a single degenerative mass, but fragmentation of the axon and of myelin is hardly ever seen with certainty except with the electron microscope. Instead the reaction of neighbouring healthy subterminal axons is paramount. They are stimulated to form sprouts, from nodes of Ranvier, which then grow towards denervated endplates and muscle fibres and re-innervate them. Whether the stimulus comes from degenerating axons, denervated endplates or muscle fibres is not known, but it may be from all three. If the denervated muscle fibre is in the vicinity of healthy axons it will be re-innervated before it has time to atrophy.

For this reason the early stages of neurogenic disease are often clinically silent. The early effects of denervation on the motor nerve supply are seen histologically in clinically unaffected muscles, and consist of a characteristic pattern of *collateral re-innervation*; the subterminal fibres branch repeatedly and can be seen to supply three, four, or many muscle fibres with endplates (Fig. 19.22). A single isolated subterminal fibre may rarely supply up to five collateral branches in normal muscle (Reske-Nielsen, Coers and Harmsen 1970) but if more than two collaterals occur regularly in

denervation. It is known from cross-innervation experiments, in which motor nerves to slow-red and fast-white muscles are transposed, that the physiological and histochemical properties of the muscle fibres are under the control of the nervous system (Dubowitz 1967b; Romanul and Van der Meulen 1967). There are 'tonic' and 'phasic' anterior horn cells which supply red and white muscle respectively (Eccles, Eccles and Lundberg 1958), and when they are made to re-innervate muscle fibres, not of the type they normally innervate but of the opposite type, they have the

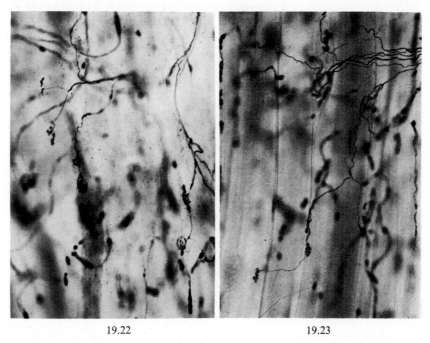

19.22   19.23

Fig. 19.22 Collateral re-innervation. Two subterminal fibres branch repeatedly to form several endplates each. Methylene blue. × 180.
Fig. 19.23 Ultraterminal sprouting. A sprout arises from an endplate to form a new endplate. Methylene blue. × 180.

the subterminal innervation, neurogenic disease may be assumed. Caution must be exercised in interpretation in distal muscles, where the denervation effects of ageing appear early. Collateral re-innervation may be seen in the extensor digitorum brevis in childhood, and in the peroneus brevis in young adults (Harriman 1970; Harriman, Taverner and Woolf 1970). Sprouting from the distal part only of subterminal fibres and from the endplate complex (ultraterminal sprouting) occurs not only in denervation but in the myopathies (Fig. 19.23).

Collateral re-innervation produces remarkable effects on muscle at quite an early stage of

power to convert the newly innervated muscle fibres into their own type. Type-1 fibres are more or less completely changed into type-2 fibres, and vice versa. This remarkable transformation results not only in changes in the speed of contraction and relaxation, but in conversion of the histochemical profile. It follows therefore that, in the process of collateral re-innervation in disease, the healthy, sprouting subterminal axon which re-innervates many neighbouring muscle fibres will, if appropriate, convert them into fibres of its own type. This may result in a change in the normal mosaic pattern of fibre types (p. 852) and large numbers of muscle fibres of the same type occur in groups. This is known as *type grouping*, and may be observed in denervation, either before the process of atrophy has begun or alongside it (Fig. 19.24). Its development depends on chance, and its absence does not imply that denervation has not occurred. Type grouping cannot be recognized in paraffin sections, but is demonstrated in frozen sections stained for lipid as well as in cryostat sections. (Lipid stains show mitochondria, hence the type-1, mitochondria-rich fibres stain more darkly than the type-2, mitochondria-poor fibres.)

integration of myofibrils in the periphery of the fibre, leaving central ones intact. In 60 days totally denervated muscle shows a 70% reduction of fibre area (Sunderland 1968). Muscle fibres are eventually reduced to a size approximating to that of fetal muscle, but may remain striated for many years. During the course of their atrophy the cells change in outline, becoming flattened or sharply angulated instead of gently polygonal; but in some conditions they become small and round. The angulated atrophied fibre has been thought to

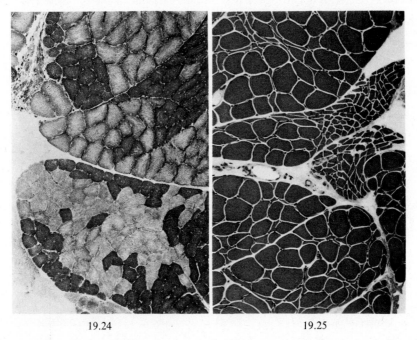

19.24   19.25

Fig. 19.24 Type grouping. Owing to collateral re-innervation, large groups of adjacent muscle fibres have been transformed into the type dictated by the re-innervating axons. The normal mosaic pattern is lost. A large group of atrophied fibres is present top left. NADH. × 45.

Fig. 19.25 Group atrophy. Large groups of fibres as well as single scattered fibres have been rendered small and angular by denervation. HE. × 120.

As the disease progresses, a sufficient number of healthy subterminal fibres is no longer available to re-innervate the muscle fibres which were previously denervated; these gradually atrophy. Their reduction in size is appreciable in about a month under experimental conditions (Adams *et al.* 1962), and a similar time course is suggested in human disease by clinical experience, for example the development of atrophy in poliomyelitis. Acutely denervated muscle fibres temporarily develop plump sarcolemmal nuclei with prominent nucleoli, but this is not often recognized in man. The reduction in size is brought about by dis-

be pathognomonic of denervation, but it also occurs in cachectic atrophy in which structural denervation has not been demonstrated (p. 891). Acutely denervated muscle cells lose their glycogen (Hogenhuis and Engel 1965), but it is retained in slowly atrophying fibres. In experimental denervation, muscle nuclei leave their subsarcolemmal locus and become internally placed, even central; in human disease this is much less frequent. Nuclei tend to lie closer together in atrophied fibres, forming chains which are usually close to the sarcolemma. While striations persist in atrophied fibres they are susceptible to re-innervation, but eventually the remaining myofibrils break up and there remain only little heaps of pyknotic nuclei, marking the site of once healthy muscle fibres.

In conditions affecting the anterior horn cell or the proximal parts of the peripheral motor nerves, atrophy occurs in entire motor units (p. 853). This results in *group atrophy*, clusters of muscle fibres being equally reduced in size, (Fig. 19.25). In progressive denervation, successive involvement of additional motor units produces atrophy of cell groups to different degrees, and eventually whole fascicles may be affected. Some of the unaffected muscle fibres become large and rounded, a process generally ascribed to compensating hypertrophy. It is interesting that temporary hypertrophy of recently denervated muscle cells can be induced experimentally (Feng and Lu 1965). The denervated rat hemidiaphragm undergoes 40% hypertrophy in the first three days, the probable result of stretching by the innervated side. Whether this mechanism could operate in disease is not known.

The later stages of denervation, which take years to develop, are marked by replacement of atrophied muscle by fibrous tissue and fat; the degree of adiposity seems to depend on the patient's tendency to obesity. In some instances, particularly in children, fibrosis is paramount and develops relatively early; it takes the form of a thickening of the endomysial connective tissue. The end stage of denervation is usually marked by virtually total replacement of entire muscles by fibrous and adipose tissue, with here and there a surviving muscle fibre, or a cluster of muscle nuclei, or a muscle spindle. Spindles survive motor denervation, but disappear if there is loss of both motor and sensory innervation. In the same way intramuscular nerves, which contain motor, sensory and autonomic fibres, retain some fibres in chronic motor denervation. The end stage of denervation is often impossible to distinguish from the last stage of a progressive myopathy, and the diagnostic surgical examination of grossly atrophied or fatty muscles is therefore best avoided.

Neurogenic Diseases of Muscle

Motor neuron disease

In this progressive disorder, involving both lower and upper motor neurons and manifest as bulbar palsy, progressive muscular atrophy or amyotrophic lateral sclerosis, the invariable result is the development of neurogenic atrophy of muscle. Curiously, the extraocular muscles are never involved. Despite weakness and wasting, reflexes are preserved or even exaggerated owing to concomitant upper motor neuron involvement. The process generally starts in the small muscles of the hands, and at this stage a biopsy of clinically normal forearm muscle usually shows collateral re-innervation (and giant units on electromyography). The disease usually pursues a relentless course, with patients surviving for no more than three years from the first symptom. In characteristic cases a muscle biopsy is not often required. This is reserved for patients with an unusual distribution of wasting, for example affecting the legs first, or proximal muscles early, in bulbar palsy where biopsy of clinically unaffected forearm muscle may help to confirm the diagnosis. A biopsy is often requested when the serum

creatinine phosphokinase (CPK) is unexpectedly raised. The findings, depending on the degree of wasting and weakness, comprise collateral re-innervation, type-grouping, or group atrophy in different degrees. Occasionally target or targetoid fibres are seen. A pattern of angulated or flattened fibres, singly or in small groups, is infrequent. The CPK usually remains normal, but when it is raised an explanation is generally found in the presence of fibre necrosis and regeneration. The reason why this should complicate the disorder in some patients is obscure. It is wise to biopsy a small subcutaneous and therefore sensory nerve at the same time as the muscle; if this is abnormal, the diagnosis is not that of motor neuron disease. In patients with an unusually long history, of eight years or more, neurogenic atrophy can be so marked as to convert fascicles, or parts thereof, into clumps of cells of extremely narrow calibre, yet still retaining striations.

Werdnig–Hoffmann's disease or *infantile spinal muscular atrophy* is a similar condition (but genetically determined with autosomal recessive inheritance) occurring at birth or showing itself in the first few months. The baby is hypotonic rather than hyperreflexic, and the initial wasting is proximal. A biopsy may serve to distinguish this relentlessly fatal condition from other causes of infantile hypotonia. Normal infantile muscle is composed of small calibre fibres and care is needed to distinguish this pattern from that of neurogenic atrophy. Usually the non-affected

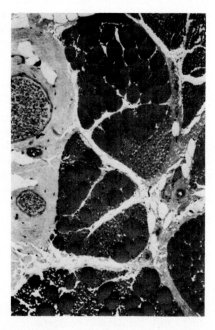

Fig. 19.26 Group atrophy in Werdnig–Hoffman disease. The large groups of atrophied fibres remain rounded in infancy, and contrast with the remaining fibres which have undergone compensatory hypertrophy. HE. × 120.

muscle fibres become grossly hypertrophied, contrasting with groups of atrophied fibres (Fig. 19.26). In appropriate cases the finding of collateral re-innervation or type grouping may help in diagnosis. When atrophy develops, the affected fibres are more often rounded than angulated.

Benign spinal muscular atrophy

A much more slowly progressive denervating condition may commence in the first decade (when it must be distinguished from Werdnig–Hoffman disease) or later, when it may be confused with motor neuron disease (Pearce and Harriman 1966; Meadows, Marsden and Harriman 1969a, b Emery 1971). A number of cases are genetically

determined, in an autosomal recessive manner, and have come to be referred to as the Kugelberg–Welander syndrome. Kugelberg and Welander (1956) described proximal muscular wasting, simulating muscular dystrophy, with a very slow rate of progression. Other cases are sporadic, with onset in childhood or adolescence, and many present confusingly 'myopathic', histopathological features. A biopsy may show variation in the calibre of fibres (some being very large and often rounded), internal nuclei, necrosis and regeneration, fibre splitting, or groups of isolated nuclei such appearances suggest a myopathy. In these cases the motor nerve fibres will still show tell-tale collateral re-innervation, or a histochemical stain will reveal type grouping. The majority of adult cases do show group atrophy, and it is only in the minority that diagnostic confusion arises. In our experience it is children with benign spinal muscular atrophy who more often fail to show neurogenic atrophy and the diagnosis is then dependent on type grouping or collateral re-innervation. The signs in such children often suggest muscular dystrophy with proximal weakness, a moderately raised CPK and a 'myopathic' pattern on electromyography, so that a histological assessment is the only way of making a true diagnosis. The condition is compatible with long survival, even into old age.

It is not known why 'myopathic' features may develop in neurogenic disease of slow progression and long duration. If collateral re-innervation is excessive, the motor neuron may eventually be overtaxed, leading to its slow degeneration. The motor unit could die back from the periphery, and muscle fibres be slowly denervated one by one, resulting in a pseudomyopathic pattern.

Peroneal muscular atrophy (Charcot Marie Tooth disease), whether due to degeneration of the lower motor and sensory neurons or associated with hypertrophic neuropathy (Bradley 1974; Bradley, Richardson and Frew 1974), characteristically produces distal neurogenic wasting and a stork leg appearance. The muscle histopathology, due to slowly progressive denervation over many years, is prone to show pseudomyopathic changes. Muscle 'giant cells' are particularly frequent; these are ovoid multinucleated fragments of sarcoplasm (Fig. 19.27) resulting presumably from an indolent breakup of muscle fibres or from a wavy longitudinal course. Although they are more frequent in chronic denervation they may also be seen in myopathies of long duration.

Peripheral neuropathy

There are many varieties of peripheral neuropathy (see Chapter 16), and they do not all affect muscle in the same way. By defination *sensory neuropathy* should not involve the motor innervation of the muscle; in practice, there is often a minor involvement; for example in sensory carcinomatous neuropathy the patient may show glove and stocking hypoaesthesia without clinical evidence of weakness, and the distal muscles exhibit collateral re-innervation only. In practice most

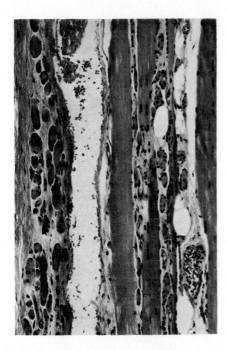

Fig. 19.27 So called 'muscle giant cells', multinucleated fragments of sarcoplasm, occurring in neurogenic atrophy of slow progress and long duration. HE.   × 110.

peripheral neuropathies are mixed motor and sensory at tissue level, although clinically one or other system may appear to be exclusively affected (Ashworth and Smyth 1969).

Histopathology. In the acute stage of *polyneuritis* (Asbury, Arnason and Adams 1969) there is discrepancy between weakness, whether distal or proximal, and muscle histopathology. Even in the presence of profound weakness, muscle fibres remain of normal appearance for some days or even weeks, except that oxidative enzyme stains show an increase in size and number of mitochondria in type-1 fibres. There is an early but mild reaction on the part of the motor nerve supply, which exhibits ultraterminal sprouting and deformity of endplates. Later, collateral re-innervation is observed, but it is not usually as striking as in diseases of the anterior horn cell body. Especially in relapsing polyneuritis, target and targetoid fibres appear, affecting both main fibre types but more obvious and numerous in type-1 fibres. Type grouping is often seen in subacute and chronic forms, but is by no means as invariable as is collateral re-innervation by the motor nerves. When the muscle becomes atrophied in the chronic polyneuropathies, the pattern of atrophy is in one of two forms. There may be group atrophy, indistinguishable from that in motor neuron disease, or a scattered, 'single fibre' atrophy (Fig. 19.28) which affects both main fibre types. With NADH or phosphorylase the atrophied, angular fibres usually stain darkly whatever their type, which has to be determined by the myofibrillar ATPase method. The pattern of atrophy adopted by the muscle presumably depends on the site of pathology in the peripheral nerve; if this affects axons proximal to their branching, whole motor units will be denervated; more distal pathology, especially of intramuscular peripheral nerves, will produce a single fibre pattern, and there will be combinations of both patterns.

It is often assumed that the small angulated muscle fibre is pathognomonic of denervation, but this is not certain; such fibres may be seen in some myopathies, and in the muscular atrophy of cachexia where examination of the motor innervation provides no structural evidence of denervation.

The intramuscular nerves in the peripheral neuropathies generally show only degeneration, either predominantly Wallerian-type or with segmental demyelination, depending on the type of neuropathy. Less often features are observed which suggest or indicate the cause of the neuropathy. In *polyneuritis*, the partly demyelinated nerve bundles may be swollen, containing a stainable finely granular 'fluid'. (This has to be distinguished from the faintly staining, nongranular metachromatic material found in the interstitium of normal nerves.) Less often the nerve bundles are infiltrated by lymphocytes and other mononuclear cells. In *collagen-vascular disease*, polyarteritis nodosa is not as a rule seen in

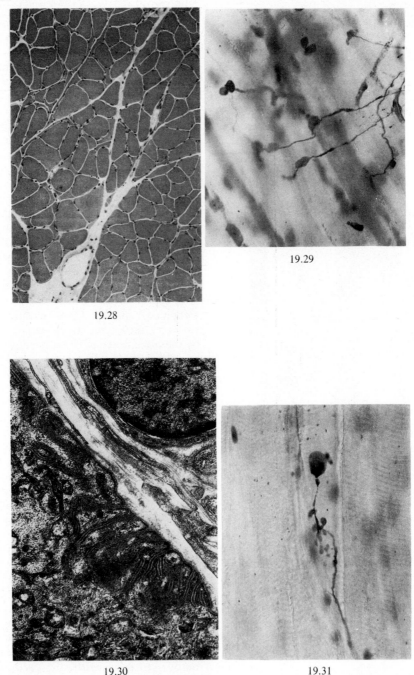

19.28

19.29

19.30

19.31

Fig. 19.28 Single fibre atrophy. Scattered fibres, singly or in very small groups, may become atrophied in distal polyneuritis. HE. ×120.

Fig. 19.29 Fusiform swellings occur along the course of subterminal motor nerves in infantile neuroaxonal dystrophy, similar to those that occur in the central nervous system. They are of irregular shape and less well defined than axonic spheres (cf. Fig. 19.8). Methylene blue. ×430.

Fig. 19.30 Denervated endplate. There are no axonic expansions, and the primary synaptic groove of the sole plate is covered by Schwann cell cytoplasm and collagen. EM. ×11,000.

Fig. 19.31 Endplate with one large expansion which seems to be formed by fusion of smaller elements. Methylene blue. ×480.

intramuscular nerves although it is frequent in large peripheral nerves (mononeuritis multiplex). The small arteries and veins of intramuscular nerves are susceptible to *necrotising vasculitis*. The muscle may show the same vasculopathy in addition to the effects of denervation. *Amyloid* and *sarcoid* may be detected. Diseases of the nervous system which involve both central and peripheral nerves may be manifest in intramuscular nerves, for example metachromatic leucodystrophy (deSilva and Pearce 1973), and the lipidoses (Kristensson, Olsson and Sourander

or semi-thin sections (Fig. 19.30). The axonic expansions degenerate and disappear, leaving bare the primary synaptic cleft which then becomes covered by Schwann cell cytoplasm and collagen fibrils. The denervated soleplate seems able to persist in this state almost indefinitely. Deformation of motor endplates occurs in the neuropathies as enlargement or fusion of expansions, ultraterminal sprouting and increase in size and extent of the neuromuscular junctional area; the deformities are not specific, being seen occasionally in the myopathies and in distal muscles with

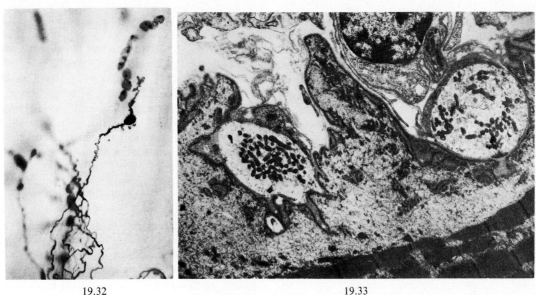

19.32   19.33

Fig. 19.32 In myasthenia gravis some endplates become elongated and their expansions stunted and irregular. Methylene blue. × 480.
Fig. 19.33 In myasthenia gravis the sole plate is altered; secondary synaptic folds are reduced in number, and the remainder are widened or retracted. EM. × 6200.

1967), Krabbe's disease (Hogan, Gurmann and Chou 1969). We have observed axonic swellings in the intramuscular nerves in infantile neuroaxonal dystrophy (Fig. 19.29). These have to be distinguished from axonic spheres (p. 856) which occur in the peripheral nervous system with advancing age, especially in the longest axons, and are then a normal finding. They occur in abnormally large numbers in toxic neuropathy, for example in thallium poisoning (Spencer *et al.* 1973) The various forms of hypertrophic polyneuropathy can be recognized as onion-bulb formations in the same nerves.

Motor endplates in peripheral neuropathy. Denervated endplates can be recognized in the neuropathies with certainty only in electron micrographs

advancing age. Fusion of endplate expansions into a single mass has been described in *diabetic neuropathy* (Coërs and Woolf 1959), but again is not specific; we have seen it infrequently in that condition, in other metabolic disorders including subacute combined degeneration and in advancing age (Fig. 19.31). It may well indicate that degeneration in the lower motor neuron is commencing in the junctional region and 'dying back', a process thought to occur in many diseases of the lower motor neuron (Cavanagh 1966).

Myasthenia gravis

As this is basically a disorder of neuromuscular transmission it is classified with the neuropathies, but its histopathology also includes a myopathic element. The clinical features of extraocular and bulbar palsy, and in more severe cases of involvement of trunk and limb muscles, with fatiguability reversed by anticholinesterasic drugs are well known, and diagnosis is usually possible on clinical and electrophysiological grounds. Occasionally a motor-point muscle biopsy detects the characteristic deformation of the endplate and allows a diagnosis to be made in a patient with atypical signs. The disorder is fully discussed by Simpson (1974), who considers that its pathogenesis is still unknown, that there is evidence of an immunological disorder involving thymus and muscle but its role in the causation of myasthenia is uncertain.

In 1905 Buzzard described 'lymphorrhages' in the muscle of myasthenics. These were small collections of lymphocytes in the interstitial tissue. More recent studies have shown that the cellular infiltrates are not confined to lymphocytes, but include plasma cells, and are accompanied by necrosis and regeneration so that a histological picture like that of polymyositis (p. 882) is sometimes seen. Some patients with polymyositis do show myasthenic features. In many patients with myasthenia cellular infiltrations are scanty or are absent altogether on extensive sampling. The muscle may be entirely normal, or show atrophy of type-2 fibres. This varies from place to place, being absent from some fields. Occasionally a focal atrophy of type-1 fibres is seen. The explanation may be focal involvement of motor units, producing denervation atrophy of the constituent muscle fibres. Rarely an undoubted pattern of neurogenic atrophy develops, especially in muscles long affected by the disease, for example the tongue or pharynx (Brownell, Oppenheimer and Spalding 1972; Oosterhuis and Bethlem 1973). When the motor innervation is stained in such cases, the motor nerves are seen to persist almost up to endplate level. The motor endplates, however, show a characteristic deformity in myasthenia gravis—they become elongated, their expansions are reduced in size and there is sometimes distal sprouting from subterminal fibres and from the endplates themselves, suggesting the mode of elongation (Fig. 19.32). The soleplate shows changes, possibly the effect of defective acetylcholine secretion; the secondary synaptic folds are reduced in number, widened and shortened (Fig. 19.33) (Engel and Santa 1971).

Similar endplate deformity may occur in the myasthenic syndrome (Eaton–Lambert syndrome), which develops usually but not invariably in response to a tumour (Brown and Charlton 1975a, b). In myasthenia gravis defective acetylcholine release is said to be due to the formation of small quanta of acetylcholine; in the myasthenic syndrome quanta of normal size are imperfectly released, and their release is facilitated by guanidine (Engel and Santa 1971). The morphological changes in endplates, both light and electron-microscopical, are useful in biopsy diagnosis. While they may occasionally be seen in other conditions, their combination with normal or only slightly abnormal findings in muscle is unique to myasthenia gravis and the myasthenic syndrome.

The Myopathies

Diseases of muscle tissue proper may be classified as *primary*, in which the disease is apparently confined to the muscles whether of known or uncertain cause, and *secondary*, due to disease outside the neuromuscular system. This classification does not take into account current controversy regarding the aetiology of muscular dystrophy and the myopathies in general. Recent work, based on animal models which are probably not applicable to the human condition, and on human electromyographic evidence (Brown and Charlton 1975a, b) suggests that there may be a nervous system defect in the muscular dystrophies, and there is biochemical and anatomical evidence that systems other than skeletal muscle are abnormal in the same disorders. It is not clear whether the dystrophies are determined primarily within skeletal muscle, or by a neural abnormality, or whether a primary muscle defect is merely associated with the latter. If a neurogenic deficiency operates in the myopathies, it must differ in its effects from that induced by total loss of the lower motor neuron, whose structural effects on muscle have been described in the previous section, and are not seen in these conditions; the defect could be one of function, which for example could operate by reducing the rate of slow or fast axoplasmic flow, affecting delivery to muscle fibres of a trophic factor. Until the matter is settled the traditional classification will be retained.

The primary myopathies

The muscular dystrophies

These are genetically determined diseases of muscle, varying in their age at onset, prognosis, and histopathology.

Severe X-linked muscular dystrophy

This is often called *Duchenne dystrophy*, following the description by that most eminent of French neurologists of 'pseudohypertrophic paralysis' in the mid-nineteenth century. Males are affected, showing the first signs of the disease by the age of 4 or 5 when proximal weakness develops, there is an awkward gait and a tendency to fall. The relentless course of the disease usually results in death from intercurrent infection and myocardial failure by the third decade. There is almost always enlargement of the calf muscles, and sometimes of other muscle groups, for example the scapular muscles and the extensor muscles on the dorsum of the foot. One of Duchenne's patients had the appearance of a young Hercules, but this is a rare presentation. Although X-linked, recessive and transmitted by female carriers, there is a high mutation rate which causes difficulty in diagnosis of individual cases. One third of patients have a previous family history, one-third are new mutants and one-third are born to previously undetected, probably mutant carriers (Gardner–Medwin 1970). Although muscle groups are affected selectively and symmetrically on clinical examination, anatomical studies may reveal changes in clinically normal muscles.

It is difficult to be certain of the nature of the earliest detectable structural abnormality in Duchenne dystrophy. The enlarged muscles with which the boy presents show at first enlargement of muscle fibres, varying in degree, accompanied by internal migration of some sarcolemmal nuclei, and with a few scattered fibres undergoing segmental necrosis and regeneration. At this stage the muscle is hypertrophied but weak. Biopsies of carriers and of boys in the preclinical phase, however, suggest that the earliest change is fibre necrosis and regeneration, often involving groups of muscle fibres. This feature is often present to a marked degree in the early clinical phase, whether in hypertrophied or wasted muscles, and at this stage the CPK is raised to remarkable levels, one hundred times or more above the normal range. The basophil regenerating fibres tend to be small, in clusters, and some appear shrunken with pyknotic nuclei, suggesting abortive regeneration (Mastaglia and Kakulas 1969). As the disease progresses there is increasing variation in fibre calibre, some undergoing atrophy, others becoming larger, with internally placed nuclei (Fig. 19.34). Inflammatory cells are not present in most cases, but lymphocytes and macrophages in unexpectedly large numbers may marginate fibres that are undergoing necrosis, form perivascular collections and infiltrate the interstitial tissues. The appearance may resemble polymyositis, except that plasma cells are very infrequent. We have seen this in genetically established Duchenne dystrophy in two brothers. There is progressive endomysial and epimysial fibrosis and myofibres become rounded, often splitting. Large hyaline fibres, with pyknotic nuclei are frequently seen. This artefact is particularly frequent in Duchenne dystrophy, and may indicate a particular fragility of dystrophic fibres. In some children with a tendency to obesity much adipose tissue is laid down, within and between fascicles. Thus in muscle groups such as the calves enlargement persists, but is now due to fatty replacement (pseudohypertrophy). As the disease progresses, necrosis and regeneration become less frequent and eventually cease completely, and in the later, inactive phase of the disease the CPK falls eventually to near normal levels. The late, fibro-fatty stage resembles that of advanced and long standing denervation, except that the motor innervation is retained. Intramuscular nerve bundles look normal, and subterminal nerves show little or no branching proximally. Motor endplates on the enlarged or atrophying fibres show non-specific distortion, ultraterminal sprouting, enlargement of junctional area and may even be multiple; but there is no increase of the functional terminal innervation ratio (ratio of the number of muscle fibres innervated by a given number of subterminal axons) (Coërs and Woolf 1959). This ratio is increased in denervation.

Histochemistry. When the ATPase reaction is applied, the process is seen to affect both main fibre types. Oxidative enzymes and phosphorylase do not differentiate the fibre types well; in dystrophic muscle these reactions vary, in the case of NADH becoming more intense or irregular; moth-eaten fibres are frequent, and the phosphorylase reaction is often weak. Regenerating fibres are undifferentiated, reacting strongly for alkalistable and acid-stable ATPase; they react weakly for oxidative enzymes and phosphorylase, and possess only a thin rim of glycogen. Occasional fibres of one or other type become loaded with

period of clinical observation. Investigations should always include an X-ray of the chest and electrocardiography, for myocardial muscle is inevitably involved. It shows atrophy and hypertrophy of the syncitial fibres, and fibrous tissue proliferation. The ECG is not always abnormal, but may show evidence of cardiomyopathy or heart block.

Benign X-linked muscular dystrophy (Becker)
This form of muscular dystrophy resembles the Duchenne variety in being X-linked, but is of much slower progression and compatible with a

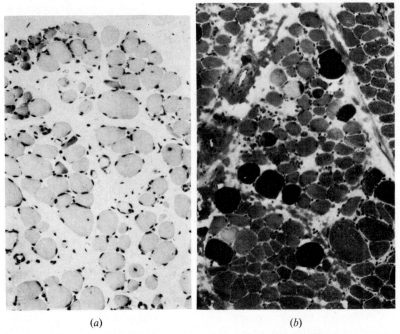

(a)   (b)

Fig. 19.34 Duchenne dystrophy. (*a*) There is variation in fibre size, fibrosis and a cluster of small basophil regenerating fibres top left. HE. × 180. (*b*) Hyaline fibres are frequent; they are due to contraction artefact, to which dystrophic muscle is especially prone. Their nuclei are pyknotic (not seen at this magnification), and they stain darkly with protoplasmic, oxidative enzyme and phosphorylase stains. They stain according to their fibre type with myosin ATPase. HE. × 120.

intracellular lipid droplets. The hyaline fibres stain intensely with oxidative enzymes stains and for phosphorylase, owing to focal accumulation of organelles in the hyaline segments, and variably with myofibrillar ATPase.

The histological picture described is not specific being seen in some other dystrophies and myopathies; a diagnosis of Duchenne dystrophy can only be made taking into account the clinical, biochemical and genetic data, and in the case of new mutations may only be possible after a

normal life span. It begins between the ages of 5 and 25 years and pseudohypertrophy of the calves is usually found. Histologically, the muscle changes follow the usual course, with variation in fibre calibre, internally placed nuclei, fibrosis and adiposity but with less necrosis and regeneration than in Duchenne dystrophy. The CPK is raised in the earlier stages.

Progressive muscular dystrophy occurs in other clinical forms with the same histopathology. In *limb girdle muscular dystrophy* the onset is usually in the second decade, or later, with a variable course, at its worst producing severe disability after 20 years. Either limb girdle may be affected first, with eventual spread to the other. Inheritance when it can be determined is autosomal recessive. Another form of autosomal recessive progressive muscular dystrophy is *childhood muscular dystrophy*; it resembles Duchenne dystrophy except for slower progression and of course occurrence in both sexes. The classification of the dystrophies on a clinicogenetic basis is difficult and has been further vitiated by inadequate histology in the past. Many patients reported as examples of one or other form of progressive muscular dystrophy are in all likelihood suffering from spinal muscular atrophy. The distinction may be difficult not only on clinical grounds but histologically, if pseudomyopathic features are superimposed, and if the examination does not include histochemistry and staining of the innervation. In a continuing study of cases conforming to the clinical definition of limb girdle dystrophy, a high proportion have been found in which the muscle histology suggests neurogenic atrophy (Bradley, quoted by Walton and Gardner–Medwin 1974).

Congenital muscular dystrophy (congenital dystrophic myopathy)

Some infants, floppy at birth, show muscle histology similar to that described in the progressive muscular dystrophies, except that there is often a high proportion of very small fibres of both main fibre types. These do not show evidence of regeneration, and may simply be surviving immature fibres. Necrosis and regeneration do occur, affecting fibres of varying calibre, and there is much fibrosis. The process is assumed to start *in utero*, but it is not established whether it is a single genetically determined condition, or occurs in a group of disorders some of which may be acquired in fetal life. The course of the disease after birth is variable. In a few babies it is rapidly progressive and death occurs by one year. In others, severely or mildly affected at birth, the condition appears to be only mildly progressive, or static, or there may be clinical improvement when the process is overcome by natural development. This results in a discrepancy between clinical performance and histopathology, the former being surprisingly good despite severe muscle wasting and fibrosis.

Facioscapulohumeral (FSH) muscular dystrophy

This is usually a benign form of dystrophy, differing from limb girdle dystrophy in that the facial muscles are involved, the patients cannot close their eyes properly, develop a transverse smile and indistinct speech and cannot whistle. The mode of inheritance is autosomal dominant. Again spinal muscular atrophy can mimic it clinically, and there are intermediate forms such as the scapuloperoneal syndrome which may be myopathic or neurogenic. The histopathology is non-specific, with variation in fibre calibre, internal nuclei, fibrosis. Moth-eaten fibres are frequent, and in some patients 'lobulated' fibres are demonstrated with oxidative enzyme stains (Bethlem, Van Wijngaarden and de Jong 1973). These are relatively small type-1 fibres in which

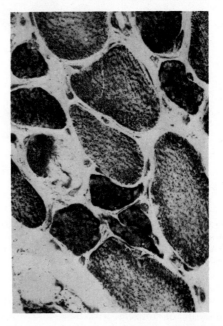

Fig. 19.35 The clumps and segments of reaction product in the smaller darkly staining type-1 fibres give the fibres a 'lobulated' or 'spotted' appearance, seen most frequently in facioscapulohumeral dystrophy. NADH. ×270.

thick strands of reaction product are deposited in the peripheral part of the fibre, and form walls within the fibre dividing it into compartments (Fig. 19.35). They resemble the 'spotted fibres' we have seen in a patient with malignant hyperpyrexia myopathy, where the strands of reaction product were shown to be due to accumulations of mitochondria and sarcoplasmic reticulum, and some of the abnormal type-1 fibres noted in

Duchenne dystrophy carriers by Morris and Raybould (1971). They are not specific for myopathy; Bethlem and his colleagues found them also in chronic spinal muscular atrophy and we have seen them rarely in denervation.

from the Welander variety (Sumner, Crawfurd and Harriman 1971). There are no specifiic histological features, the pathology being that of a slowly progressive myopathy. It has to be carefully distinguished from peroneal muscular

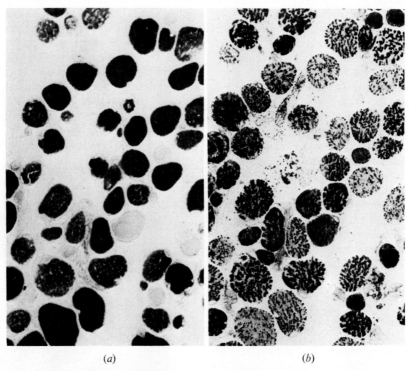

(a)   (b)

Fig. 19.36 Extraocular muscle stained for (a) ATPase pH 9·4 and (b) NADH. The *coarse* fibres of Feldenstruktur pattern are shown by the ATPase stain, and react strongly with NADH. The *fine* fibres have a dense, finely stippled pattern with NADH, and react weakly for ATPase at pH 9·4. The *granular* fibres are sparsely stippled, and react strongly and uniformly with the ATPase stain. × 450.

In some patients with a facioscapulohumeral distribution of muscle weakness and wasting, interstitial collections of lymphocytes and other 'inflammatory' cells are prominent, raising the suspicion that polymyositis (p. 882) may produce the FSH syndrome (Rothstein, Carlson and Sumi 1971; Munsat, Piper, Cancilla and Mednick 1972; Bates, Stevens and Hudgson 1973).

Distal muscular dystrophy
Most dystrophies affect the proximal musculature more than the distal. A large group of cases exhibiting distal distribution, inherited as an autosomal dominant, was described in Sweden by Welander (1951). In other parts of the world distal dystrophy is rare and genetically distinct

atrophy and the distal form of chronic spinal muscular atrophy (McLeod and Prineas 1971).

Ophthalmoplegia, ocular and oculoskeletal myopathy
Extraocular muscle is peculiar in structure, differing in several aspects from skeletal muscle elsewhere. In their control of eye movements, these muscles must at times act with great speed, and at others maintain gaze for long periods by means of sustained contraction. There is a particularly rich nerve supply, the motor units containing as few as eight muscle fibres, and muscle spindles are present near the tendinous insertions. Although it has long been known that extraocular muscle fibres vary, there being three

sizes of fibre (Walsh and Hoyt 1969), pathologists have not always been aware of this and the finding of groups of fibres of small calibre, or of groups of fibres of varying size has led to normal extraocular muscle being described as denervated or myopathic. Ring fibres are frequent, especially in older subjects. Misdiagnosis is more frequent in biopsy specimens, especially in the tiny fragments provided by ophthalmic surgeons from corrective operations for ptosis or squint. The innervation of extraocular muscle is complex, many fibres having a single motor endplate and others multiply-innervated like some amphibian muscle fibres. There are species differences in the organization of fibres of different sizes and types, even among mammals.

In the past few years since histochemical methods have become available, new structural characteristics of extraocular muscle have been recognized. The situation in man has not yet

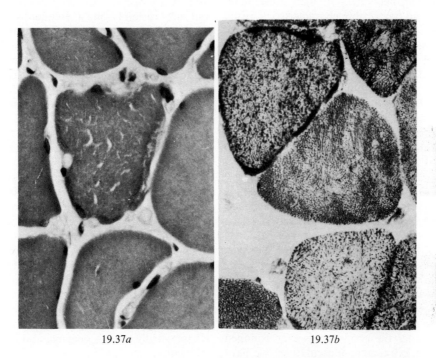

19.37a   19.37b

Fig. 19.37 (a) In 'granular' fibres the myofibrils are irregularly dispersed and basophil granules can be discerned beneath the sarcolemma. HE. ×450. (b) With NADH, the same fibres contain excess or larger than normal mitochondria, dispersed and in clumps. Such fibres stain red with Gomori's method and are referred to as 'ragged-red' fibres. NADH. ×450.

Fig. 19.38 Abnormal mitochondria containing rectangular crystalline arrays in oculoskeletal myopathy (deltoid).

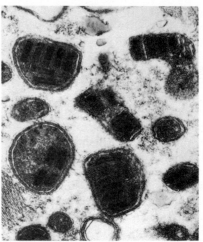

19.38

been fully worked out in a sufficient number of individuals at different ages, but there appear to be three types defined by histochemical stains, each varying in size (Fig. 19.36). The three types defined by Durston (1974) in the baboon and man are recognized most easily in cryostat sections, and are coarse, fine and granular. The *coarse* fibres correspond to those with 'feldenstruktur', in which myofibrils are grouped together, the groups separated by a sparse but relatively wide intermyofibrillar network. In man these fibres have type-1 and type-2 fibre characteristics, reacting strongly both for oxidative enzymes and alkali-stable ATPase, and have multiple motor endplates. The *fine* and the *granular* fibres are of 'Fibrillenstruktur' and resemble type-1 and type-2 fibres respectively; they are not identical with them, the fine fibres staining only moderately with oxidative enzyme stains, and the reaction of the granular fibres for phosphorylase is weak. Both fine and granular fibres have single motor endplates.

Ocular myopathy. Patients presenting with a slow development of ptosis and limitation of ocular movements have long been described as suffering from ocular myopathy. The onset may be at any age, and although the majority are sporadic, dominant inheritance has been recognized. Some patients show undue sensitivity to curare (Ross 1963; Mathew, Jacob and Chandy 1970); although this is also seen in myasthenia gravis these patients do not respond to anticholinesterase drugs. It is doubtful whether the condition is ever confined entirely to the extraocular musculature; we have seen myopathic changes in the clinically normal deltoid in a patient suffering from ocular myopathy, and many patients show overt weakness elsewhere, particularly of the pharyngeal muscles (oculopharyngeal myopathy) and in the limbs (oculoskeletal or oculogeneralised myopathy). Even smooth muscle may be involved (Teasdall, Schuster and Walsh 1964). The pathology of extraocular muscle using modern methods has not yet been described, but the limb muscles show myopathy. In addition to the usual manifestations, which vary in severity, curious fibres containing increased numbers of mitochondria and sometimes lipid droplets are also frequently found. Such fibres have a granular appearance with HE, in transverse section, and were called *granular fibres* in the older literature (Brooke 1966). The granular appearance is due to separation of

myofibrils by the organelles, which form basophil deposits in crescents beneath the sarcolemma and clumps within the fibre (Fig. 19.37). As these fibres stain red and stand out from the remaining green fibres when Gomori's trichrome method is used, they have been called 'ragged-red' fibres (Olson, Engel, Walsh and Einaugler 1972). In electronmicrographs the mitochondria are often abnormal (Fig. 19.38). Ragged-red fibres are not specific for ocular and oculoskeletal myopathy, as they are occasionally seen in other conditions, but are certainly most frequently seen in the myopathies involving the extraocular muscles.

Another interesting pathological change reported most frequently in oculoskeletal myopathy is the fibre with 'rimmed vacuoles' (Dubowitz and Brooke 1973). These are sharply defined spaces within the fibre, surrounded by a zone of increased staining density, basophil with HE. Serial sections show that they are not merely paranuclear spaces (above or below a nucleus) from which they have to be distinguished.

Oculoskeletal myopathy may be associated with neurodegenerative disorders such as retinal pigmentary degeneration, optic atrophy, peripheral neuropathy sometimes hypertrophic, cerebellar ataxia, and organic dementia (Drachman 1968). It may be that in some patients the ophthalmoplegia is neurogenic; but autopsy studies usually reveal normal brain stem nuclei (Walton and Gardner–Medwin 1974).

In *exophthalmic ophthalmoplegia*, extraocular muscles appear enlarged to the naked eye. Histologically there is oedema, and in severe cases infiltration by lymphocytes and fibrosis (Hogan and Zimmerman 1962).

The myotonic syndromes

Dystrophia myotonica (myotonic muscular dystrophy). This is a multisystem disorder characterised by cataract, gonadal atrophy, frontal baldness, ptosis, myocardial involvement and myopathy. There is often mental subnormality. The muscle involvement, unlike most other forms of dystrophy is more marked distally in the limbs, but there is usually early wasting of the sternomastoids. Facial and jaw weakness produces a sagging, open mouth. The inheritance is autosomal and dominant. Although symptoms do not usually appear until the second or third decade, the occurrence of the disease in children has recently been recognized and it is one cause of infantile hypotonia (Karpati, Carpenter, Walters, Eisen and Andermann 1973; Farkas, Tomé, Fardeau, Arsenio–Nunes, Dreyfus and Diebler 1974). The course of the disease is slow, and normally includes a period during which myotonia occurs: this means muscle contraction persisting after the cessation of voluntary effort, so that the patient is, for example, unable to relax his grip for a time, and the muscles generally feel stiff. Myotonia may disappear after a number of years, and some patients do not suffer from it.

The muscle shows the usual features of myopathy, but some findings are characteristic: internal migration of nuclei, and their distribution in long rows; sarcoplasmic masses formed by the withdrawal of the myofibrils to one side of the fibre; and ring fibres (Fig. 19.39). Internal nuclei are more prominent in this than in any other disease, and a cross-section of the muscle fibre may pass through four or five separate nuclei in various parts of the fibre (Fig. 19.40). When the changes are not advanced, type-1 fibres only show varying degrees of atrophy, and some single small angular fibres are formed (Fig. 19.41); type-2 fibres at this stage are large or hypertrophied. At later stages the type-2 fibres are also affected by size variation. Fibre necrosis and regeneration occur, but are not usually prominent. Muscle spindles, particularly those in the more distal muscles and in advanced disease, show an interesting change: there is a great increase in the number in intrafusal muscle fibres, so that up to 60 small fibres may be found, the normal maximum in man being 14 or 15. The increase results from longitudinal fibre splitting (Swash and Fox 1975), and is likely to be the result of abnormal tension on the spindle produced by sustained contraction. The motor endplates are abnormal in myotonic dystrophy; some very large complexes are formed, with multiple distal sprouts, generally large and more elaborate than in other myopathies. There is however no definite evidence of denervation in the form of collateral re-innervation.

Myotonia congenita (Thomsen's disease). This differs from myotonic dystrophy in that the clinical picture is confined to myotonia, with or without muscle hypertrophy. The myotonia varies in severity, develops in infancy or at any time later and is often made worse by cold. It is inherited as an autosomal dominant, but Becker (1973) has described an autosomal recessive

variant in Germany. We have found only large endplates in one patient, but Dubowitz and Brooke (1973) have noted a complete absence of type-2b fibres in a recent study of two patients.

Paramyotonia congenita. Myotonia is often precipitated by cold, but when it is accompanied by attacks of weakness, both being induced by cold, the term paramyotonia is often used. A family comprising 157 related individuals has been described by de Jong, Slooff and van der Eerden (1973). The muscle in one of them showed changes like those in myotonic dystrophy with the addition of vacuoles.

Periodic paralysis. This occurs in four different clinical forms, the first three usually being genetically determined and autosomal dominant, and the last sporadic (McArdle 1974). All seem to be related to the passage into and out of the muscle fibre of the cation, potassium, and characteristically are associated with vacuole formation during and after attacks, some containing glycogen (Fig. 19.43). In *hypokalaemic periodic paralysis*, a healthy young adult wakens unable to move but can breathe normally, talk and smile. The attacks last for 6 to 24 hours, occasionally longer, and the plasma potassium is low. In *hyperkalaemic periodic paralysis* the attacks usually come on after exercise, typically after resting for 30 minutes. Most attacks are short and are over within one or two hours. There may be symptoms of mild myotonia, but the condition is genetically distinct from paramyotonia congenita. The serum K rises, and weakness occurs at levels which leave normal subjects unaffected. In severely affected members of families suffering from periodic hypo- or hyperkalaemia, a permanent myopathy ensues. Histologically there is fibre necrosis and regeneration, fibre calibre variation, fibrosis and striking vacuole formation (Fig. 19.44). In the early stages or in mildly affected individuals vacuoles may not be visible with the optical microscope but electronmicrographs show dilatation of the lateral sacs of the sarcoplasmic reticulum. In one such patient we found endplates enlarged by terminal sprouting. In *normokalaemic periodic paralysis* the attacks are similar to those of the hyperkalaemic variety, but are more severe and of much longer duration, days or weeks. The fourth form of periodic paralysis is rare, associated with thyrotoxicosis, and is hypokalaemic. The thyroid disorder may not immediately be obvious.

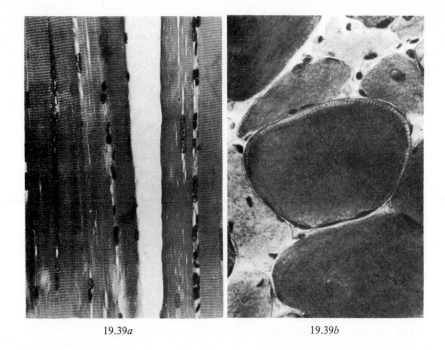

19.39a   19.39b

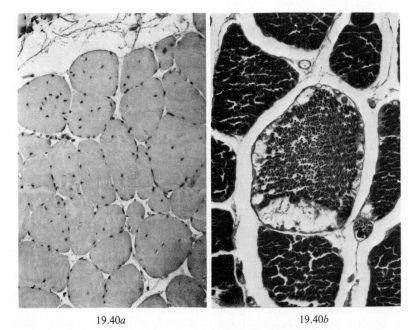

19.40a   19.40b

Fig. 19.39 Dystrophia myotonica. (*a*) Long rows of internal nuclei. HE.   × 280.   (*b*) Variation in fibre size and a ring fibre. HE.   × 430.
Fig. 19.40 Dystrophia myotonica. (*a*) Numerous internal nuclei are present in many fibres. HE.   × 180.   (*b*) Myofibrils withdraw from parts of the sarcolemma to form 'sarcoplasmic masses'. PTAH.   × 480.

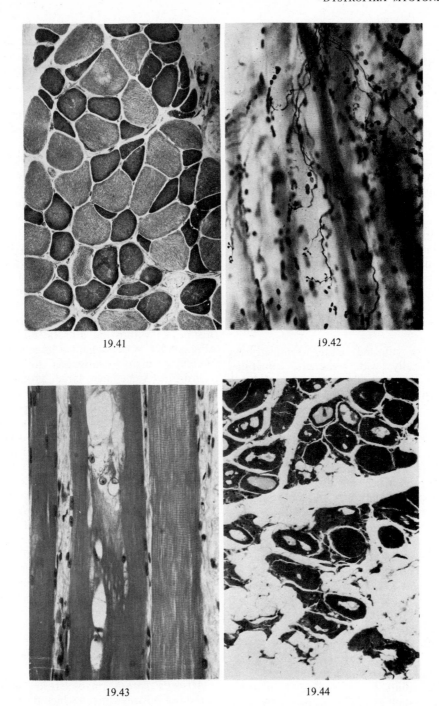

19.41

19.42

19.43

19.44

Fig. 19.41 Early stage in dystrophia myotonica with large type-2 fibres and some atrophied type-1 fibres. NADH. × 110.
Fig. 19.42 The subterminal fibres can be followed to several large and complex endplates, but there is no collateral re-innervation. Methylene blue. × 180.
Fig. 19.43 Vacuole formation in hypokalaemic periodic paralysis. HE. × 280.
Fig. 19.44 Permanent myopathy following many years of periodic paralysis. Vacuoles are prominent and persistent. HE. × 280.

Polymyositis and dermatomyositis

Polymyositis is an acquired myopathy which may occur at any age, with its highest incidence in adults of 30 to 60 years. Females are affected twice as often as males. The inflammatory reaction that occurs in the muscles is thought to be due to a disturbance of the immune system; lymphocytes from patients with polymyositis have been shown to be sensitized to muscle tissue (Currie, Saunders, Knowles and Brown 1971). A viral infection may be the initiating factor, as picorna-, myxo-, and Coxsackie virus-like particles have been seen in affected muscle (Chou 1968; Chou and Gutman 1970; Mastaglia and Walton 1970), but this has not yet been proved by culture. About one-fifth of adult cases are associated with a carcinoma, suggesting that a secretion or breakdown product of the tumour may then be the precipitant. Signs of the tumour may not appear until some time after the myositis, and its removal has caused remission of the muscular condition.

Muscles are affected either symmetrically or asymmetrically, with weakness, sometimes tenderness and even swelling of muscles; the neck and trunk muscles are frequently involved and the proximal limb muscles. Rarely the extra-ocular muscles are affected. The skin shows no changes, or there may be dusky red patches over joints. The upper lids may have a violaceous tinge. If there are more florid changes, such as a dusky red eruption on the face in a butterfly distribution, and on the trunk and limbs, mottled or diffuse, the condition is described as dermato-myositis: there is no clear dividing line between it and polymyositis. The course of the disease is as variable as the symptomatology, there being acute, subacute and chronic forms. The prognosis was formerly thought to be grave, although spontaneous recovery occurred in some children and probably accounted for the reports of recovery from 'muscular dystrophy' made in the early part of this century (Nattrass 1954). It has been transformed in children by the use of steroids, remission and recovery being the rule, and improved in adults by steroids and immuno-suppressives. Fatalities still occur, especially when the myocardium is involved. In a few patients nodular calcification (calcinosis) of subcutaneous tissues or in muscles is visible radiologically.

Histology. Two processes occur simultaneously in the muscle; interstitial inflammation, and necrosis and regeneration of muscle fibres. These are not interdependent, as one or other process can be seen alone. The inflammatory reaction occurs in the form of diffuse infiltration of the epimysium and muscle fascicles by lymphocytes and plasma cells. These tend to congregate around small blood vessels, and infiltrate their adventitia (Fig. 19.45), but fibrinoid necrosis is rare. Occasionally the infiltrating cells include large numbers of eosinophils (*eosinophil myositis*), and a fruitless search is then made for parasitic infection of the muscle. In many cases there is also nodular infiltration, lymphocytes being congregated into follicles, some of which develop germinal centres (Fig. 19.46). Capillaries with prominent endothelium can usually be made out within the follicles, and some plasma cells. Segmental necrosis and regeneration are frequent; affected fibres are marginated by lymphocytes and histiocytes, and while phagocytosis is in progress lymphocytes can usually be recognized as well as histiocytes within the necrotic muscle segments (Fig. 19.47). Occasionally a large area of muscle involving many contiguous fibres undergoes necrosis. Sometimes large groups of small regenerating fibres are found. In the course of time, fibre calibre variation develops, and vacuolated fibres are not infrequent. As muscle fibres are destroyed, fibrosis develops. The rate of progress of the disease is reflected in the histopathology: in mild forms necrosis and cellular infiltration are scanty, and fibrosis develops slowly (subacute and chronic polymyositis). The motor innervation generally shows deformity and sprouting from endplates only, but in a minority the inflammatory response destroys parts of the subterminal innervation, resulting in patchy collateral re-innervation. (Denervation of muscle fibres in places is thought to be responsible for the fibrillation potentials that are seen in polymyositis on electromyography.) Very rarely, calcification takes place. Amorphous deposits are formed in the epimysium or more frequently in the subcutaneous fat, accompanied by lymphocytic infiltration.

Myositis fibrosa (myosclerosis) is usually a variant of polymyositis in which there is excessive proliferation of fibrous tissue. The process may last for many years, and the muscles become stiff and woody-hard. We have seen this in a woman of 53 who had the condition for 20 years, and who was eventually unable to move her knee or ankle joints. Biopsy showed scanty evidence

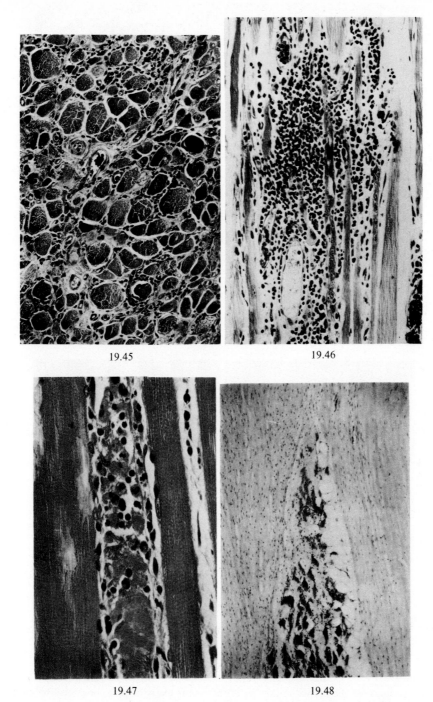

19.45

19.46

19.47

19.48

Fig. 19.45 Diffuse infiltration of lymphocytes and some plasma cells among muscle fibres of varying calibre in poly-myositis. HE. ×180.
Fig. 19.46 Nodular infiltration of lymphocytes and plasma cells between normal and regenerating muscle fibres. HE. ×180.
Fig. 19.47 Polymyositis. Lymphocytes accompany histiocytes in the phagocytic process. HE. ×420.
Fig. 19.48 Myositis fibrosa. An island of distorted muscle fibres survives in a muscle almost totally replaced by fibrous tissue. HE. ×44.

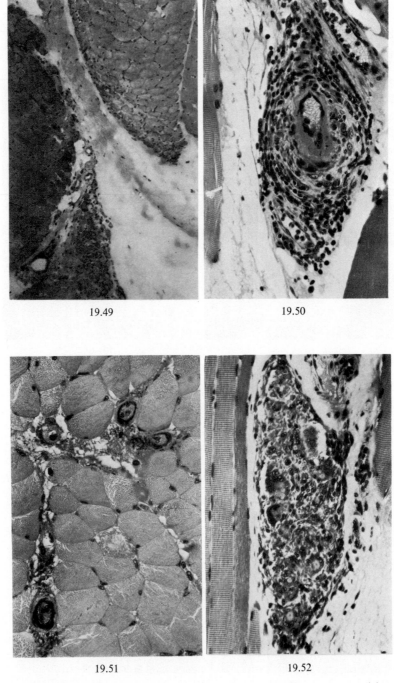

19.49

19.50

19.51

19.52

Fig. 19.49 In dermatomyositis the fibrous thickening of the epimysium is often accompanied by atrophy of muscle fibres at the edge of the fascicles. PAS. ×120.

Fig. 19.50 Arteritis. A small artery shows fibrinoid necrosis of its wall and infiltration by lymphocytes and plasma cells. HE. ×280.

Fig. 19.51 Systemic sclerosis. Arteriolar walls in the muscle are greatly thickened particularly by concentric subintimal fibrosis. Elastin van Gieson. ×420.

Fig. 19.52 Sarcoid granuloma in skeletal muscle, consisting of epithelioid cells, giant cells and lymphocytes. HE. ×280.

of myositis but massive proliferation of fibrous tissue (Fig. 19.48). Bradely, Hudgson, Gardner–Medwin and Walton (1973) point out that the same overgrowth of fibroblasts may occur rarely in spinal muscular atrophy, and prefer the term myosclerosis to indicate that the condition is a syndrome.

In *dermatomyositis* there is less infiltration of fascicles by lymphocytes, and the process is more confined to the epimysium. The resulting fibrous thickening of the epimysium causes atrophy of muscle fibres around the edge of fascicles (Fig. 19.49). In children, the histopathology of polymyositis and dermatomyositis is often the same as in adults. Banker and Victor (1966), however, described angiitis as a prominent feature in eight children who came to autopsy; in addition to perivascular collections of lymphocytes, there developed subintimal hyperplasia and thrombosis with consequent foci of muscular infarction. They considered childhood dermatomyositis to be a different disease.

The diagnosis of polymyositis is made with ease when both inflammatory change and the effects of necrosis are present. An unusual diagnostic pitfall is infiltration of muscle by lymphosarcoma. Not infrequently patients with polymyositis on clinical and serological grounds, responding to treatment, show only necrosis and regeneration (necrotizing myopathy, p. 891). The chronic fibrosing type of polymyositis may be indistinguishable from muscular dystrophy.

Polymyositis may be associated with other collagen-vascular diseases. *Polyarteritis nodosa* (Fig. 19.50) involving many systems may affect only the arteries in muscle, and this fact is used in its diagnosis by blind muscle biopsy. Sometimes it is associated with muscle weakness and wasting, and the muscle shows either polymyositis or neurogenic atrophy (due to polyarteritis affecting peripheral nerves). Small vessel *angiitis* may also affect muscle widely and be associated with myositis. The weakness and wasting which often develop in *rheumatoid arthritis* have a variety of causes (Haslock *et al.* 1970) acting singly or in combination: cachectic atrophy (p. 891), polymyositis, and rheumatoid neuropathy. When polymyositis is found, the proportion of plasma cells is large. Muscular weakness is not very common in *systemic lupus erythematosus*, but when muscle is examined there is evidence of myositis. A particular feature is vacuole formation within muscle fibres, the vacuoles often

enclosing an internally placed muscle nucleus (Pearson and Yamazaki 1958; Rewcastle and Humphrey 1965). Myositis may accompany *systemic sclerosis* (scleroderma). The changes are predominantly in the epimysium, and thickening of small blood vessel walls has been prominent in our cases (Fig. 19.51), although reported as variable in the literature (Winkelman 1971). Blauchet–Bardon, Ganter and Roujeau (1975) claim that smooth muscle is also involved in systemic sclerosis. In *Sjögren's syndrome* there is characteristically destruction of the ducts of the salivary and lacrimal glands, both being infiltrated by large numbers of plasma cells. A number of patients also present with muscle weakness, and show myositis with a similar predominance of plasma cell reaction (Pearson and Currie 1974).

Sarcoid myopathy

Sarcoid nodules, which are sometimes palpable, are found in skeletal muscle in the majority of patients with sarcoidosis. Clinical involvement of muscle is much less frequent, but in some patients muscular weakness is the presenting feature (Gardner–Thorpe 1972). The apparent confinement of granulomatous lesions to the muscular system has led some authors to consider it a separate disorder (granulomatous myopathy), producing a slowly developing symmetrical myopathy (Coërs and Carbone 1966). Muscle biopsy plays an important part in confirming sarcoidosis suspected on clinical grounds, and in detecting the condition in patients who have evidence of a myopathy only. The muscle characteristically shows granulomata consisting of epithelioid cells, giant cells and lymphocytes in the epimysium or within fascicles, without necrosis (Fig. 19.52). Occasionally there is merely an infiltrative form of proliferation of small epithelioid cells, growing between muscle cells, less easy to recognize as sarcoid tissue. The muscle shows necrosis and regeneration and lymphocyte collections.

Amyloid myopathy

While amyloid may be deposited in the interstitial tissues of muscle in secondary and especially primary amyloidosis, massive deposition causing a myopathy is very rare (Reichenmiller, Bundshu, Bass, Missmahl and Arnold 1968; Martin, van Bogaert, van Damme and Peremans 1970).

Case report. A well built male was completely well until the age of 56 years, when he noticed some tightness and weakness of his muscles. This progressed steadily, and he was investigated at the age of 58 years. He was now unable to walk more than 50 m. because of a heavy feeling in his legs. Exercise caused a severe cramping pain in his muscles, followed by weakness. There was tightness in the chest and dyspnoea, relieved by rest. He had noticed his muscles getting larger in the previous year. He had difficulty in relaxing his grip, for example after holding a saw for some time. On examination there was a Herculean appearance (Fig. 19.53, facing p. 851). Power in the limbs was

there being a few small regenerating fibres in the peripheral fascicular zones. The pattern of type-1 and 2 fibres was unaltered, and motor endplates showed distal sprouting only. Fig. 19.55 shows the fibrillar amyloid protein deposited near collagen fibrils.

Infantile hypotonia (the floppy baby syndrome)

Some babies are floppy at birth, and reaching milestones late, give cause for concern. In some the condition resolves completely (benign congenital hypotonia, Walton 1956), and their muscles show no change, or smallness of one or other fibre

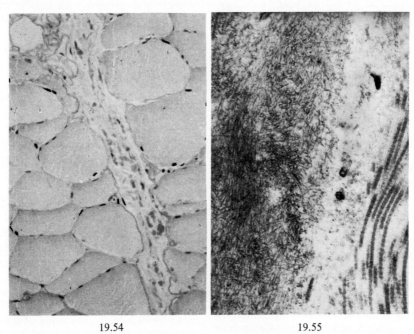

19.54   19.55

Fig. 19.54   Darkly staining amyloid deposits thicken the interfascicular fibrous tissue. Congo red.   × 120.
Fig. 19.55   The fibrillar amyloid protein lies alongside the thicker, banded collagen fibrils. EM.   × 23,000.

normal. Tone was slightly increased, and the reflexes generally diminished. No sensory disturbance was detected. The patient was referred for motor-point muscle biopsy by Dr D. Taverner. The *vastus internus* was extremely firm, red and glassy, failing to contract on excision. Amyloid was present in the connective tissue and blood vessel walls, mainly in the epimysium and perimysium, and to a much lesser extent within fascicles between individual muscle fibres (Fig. 19.54). Fascicles were thus enclosed in and separated by thick fibrous amyloid-infiltrated tubes. The muscle fibres showed surprisingly little reaction,

type. Others are suffering from Werdnig–Hoffmann disease, with a fatal prognosis, or from CNS disease such as hypotonic cerebral palsy, mental deficiency, or cerebral tumour; yet others from one of the congenital myopathies to be described. A full discussion of infantile hypotonia and its many causes will be found in Dubowitz (1969).

The congenital myopathies

The use of cryostat sections, histochemistry and electron-microscopy has made possible the description of new forms of myopathy, unrecognized before, and probably misdiagnosed as variants of muscular dystrophy. Most are stationary, or only slowly progressive, and therefore carry a much better prognosis than most forms of dystrophy. In all, there is an error in formation of muscle fibres or arrested or retarded development; or the abnormalities found may be interpreted as an arrested degeneration.

Central core disease. This is a hereditary myopathy, usually causing hypotonia in infancy and a proximal non-progressive weakness. Twenty cases have been recorded since the first description by

in one fibre, that myofibrils are preserved within the core, and that it occurs in type-1 fibres only. The target fibre may occur in both main types of fibre, and characteristically within it the myofibrils are broken up. Recently Neville and Brooke (1973) have subdivided cores into 'structured' and 'unstructured' varieties. The structured core retains striations perfectly and in consequence the ATPase reaction is retained; in unstructured cores the ATPase activity is lost and the ultrastructural pattern of the myofibrils is disturbed.

Muscle fibres remain of normal size in central core disease, but the pattern of type-1 and type-2

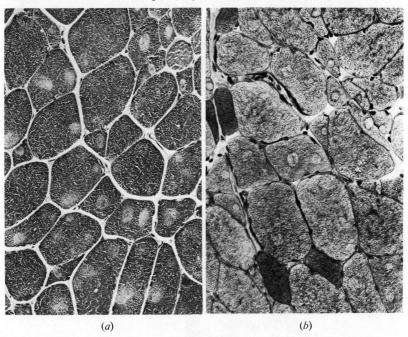

(a)   (b)

Fig. 19.56 Ventral core disease. (a) Sharply defined cores of reduced staining intensity are seen, often several in a fibre. PTAH. ×180. (b) The cores are seen exclusively in type-1 fibres, of which there is a preponderance. Type-2 fibres stain darkly because of their glycogen content. PAS. ×180.

Shy and Magee (1956). Most have shown autosomal dominant inheritance with a few apparently sporadic cases. The cores refer to sharply defined areas within the muscle fibre which are devoid of mitochondria, so that they appear as clear zones in oxidative enzyme and lipid stains (Fig. 19.56). They do not show up well with HE, but are sometimes well demonstrated by trichrome stains as in the original family of Shy and Magee. The essential differences between a core and target or targetoid fibres (p. 861) are that the core extends in the longitudinal plane as far as the fibre can be sectioned in that plane, that there may be several

fibres varies. In most there is uniform enzyme activity (corresponding to type-1) or a predominance of type-1 fibres; in a few the fibre types are distributed normally.

Multicore disease. A variant of central core disease was described in two children by Andrew Engel, Gomez and Groover in 1971. Rare fibres contained typical cores, but others showed multifocal areas, some very tiny, of mitochondrial loss or depletion and disturbance of striatal pattern. We have seen two children in whom large numbers of minute foci of degeneration only were present,

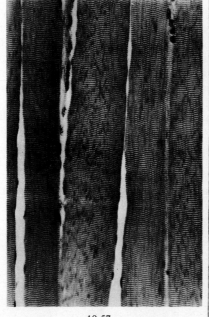

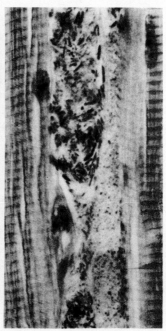

19.57

19.58

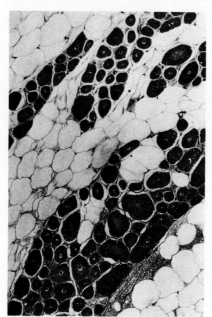

19.59

Fig. 19.57 'Minicore' disease. Some fibres show very numerous foci of smearing of the striations. × 280.

Fig. 19.58 Rod body myopathy. The rods are formed of Z-line material, and congregate as threads and granules at the edge of the muscle fibre. PTAH. × 950.

Fig. 19.59 Centronuclear myopathy. Nuclei are found in the centre of each fibre, usually enclosed by a small halo. HE. × 120.

and for which we propose the designation *mini-core disease* (Fig. 19.57).

Rod body ('*nemaline*') *myopathy*. Most reports since the original description by Shy, Engel, Somers and Wanko (1963) have been of a mild non-progressive proximal myopathy in children, but a few patients have been severely affected, and necropsies were described by Neustein (1973) in three siblings who died in infancy. Inheritance appears to be autosomal dominant but many cases are sporadic. Rods, seen in electron-

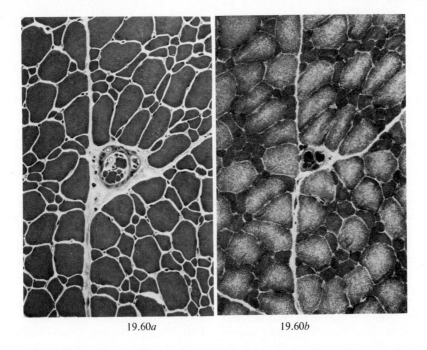

19.60a   19.60b

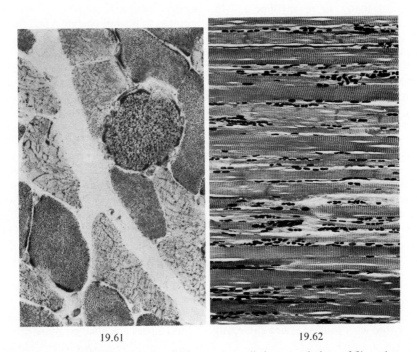

19.61   19.62

Fig. 19.60   Congenital fibre type disproportion.   (*a*) There are two distinct populations of fibres, large and small.   HE.   ×180.   (*b*) Serial section to show that the small fibres are type-1 and the large type-2.   NADH.   ×180.

Fig. 19.61   Mitochondrial myopathy.   A fibre stands out from the remainder by intense staining of its numerous mitochondria, some at least larger than normal.   NADH.   ×420.

Fig. 19.62   In cachectic atrophy the reduction in fibre size causes nuclei to congregate, retaining their subsarcolemmal position.   HE.   ×180.

micrographs to consist of Z-line material, collect within muscle fibres, generally in the subsarco-lemmal zone. They are seen as short filaments or granules, well demonstrated by phase microscopy, and stain blue with PTAH and red by Gomori's trichrome method (Fig. 19.58). There is usually some variation in fibre calibre, and both main fibre types are affected. Rod body myopathy has been described associated with Adie's syndrome (Harriman 1970).

Centronuclear myopathy. Unlike other congenital myopathies, the extraocular and facial muscles are affected in nearly all patients reported. The condition is compatible with a normal lifespan, but a few infants have been severely affected and have died in childhood. The essential histological feature is the presence of large numbers of muscle fibres with nuclei in their central part (Fig. 19.59); when small they resemble myotubes, and the first report by Spiro, Shy and Gonatas (1966) named the condition myotubular myopathy. But in most instances the affected fibres are larger than myo-tubes and possess many more myofibrils. In longitudinal section the nuclei are distributed in long rows. Histochemical analysis places patients in two groups (Harriman and Haleem 1972): those with uniform enzyme activity, either un-defined or corresponding to type-1 fibres, and those with two types of fibre, small and larger, corresponding roughly in enzyme reaction to type-1 and type-2 respectively.

Congenital fibre type disproportion was the term devised by Dubowitz and Brooke (1973) to des-cribe a group of children in whom type-1 fibres were universally smaller than type-2 (the mean diameters differing by at least 12%). Affected children have all been floppy at birth, and show a weakness of all muscle groups varying from mild to severe. There is a tendency to improve-ment after 2 years of age, although one of our patients was 14 years old and still weak, with universally thin muscles. The discrepancy in size between the two fibre types can be consider-able, and if histochemical stains are not applied the resulting picture with routine stains can easily be confused with neurogenic atrophy or myopathy (Fig. 19.60). In infancy an erroneous diagnosis of Werdnig–Hoffman disease can be made and a falsely poor prognosis given. In some infants the small type-1 fibres have central nuclei, and the condition then appears to be intermediate between congenital fibre disproportion and centronuclear myopathy. Clearly, type-1 fibres are slow in developing in this disorder, but do get larger as the child becomes older. The enlarged type-2 fibres may be a hypertrophic response.

The mitochondrial myopathies. A number of patients have been reported to show muscle weak-ness or pains on exercise, and to have either abnormal mitochondria or large numbers of mitochondria in some of their muscle fibres. Ex-amples in the literature are listed by Shibasaki, Santa and Kuroiwa (1973). Two of the patients showed hypermetabolism without thyroid disease (Luft, Ikkos, Palmieri, Ernster and Afzelius 1962; Haydar, Conn, Afifi, Wakid, Ballas and Fawaz 1971). In a few others the mitochondria have been 'loosely coupled', that is, when they were not required to phosphorylate ADP, they still oxidized substrate and produced heat.

The fibres containing abnormal numbers of mitochondria are easily recognized on staining for oxidative enzymes (Fig. 19.61) and are identical with 'ragged-red' fibres described in oculoskeletal myopathy. Ultrastructurally they show crystalline inclusions, and vary greatly in size, being found beneath the sarcolemma or distributed through the fibre. They are frequently associated with triglyceride droplets, which may be so numerous as to justify a separate category of *lipid storage myopathy* (Bradley, Jenkinson, Park, Hudgson, Gardner–Medwin, Pennington and Walton 1972). One such patient was shown to be suffering from a deficiency of carnitine, which stimulates the oxidative catabolism of long-chain fatty acids (Engel and Angelini 1973). The mitochondrial fibres may be the only abnormality found in the muscle, or they may be associated with other myopathic changes such as fibre calibre variation. Type-1 fibres are affected more often than type-2.

Secondary myopathies

Cachectic atrophy

The commonest myopathy due to systemic disease is undoubtedly the atrophy produced by cachexia. Diseases such as chronic infections, cancer, collagen-vascular disease and various endocrinopathies and especially malnutrition cause wasting of every tissue in the body, and their effects are easily recognized. The effect of cachexia on muscle is to deplete it of contractile protein. Usually the cause of cachectic atrophy is obvious, and the muscle wasting and weakness produced excite no comment. In some patients, however, wasting of muscle precedes that of other tissues, including adipose tissue, and proximal weakness develops before there is much loss of weight. We have seen this induced by a carcinoma, undetected until after biopsy examination of muscle which showed cachectic atrophy.

Type-2 fibres are reduced in size before, and to a greater extent, than type-1 fibres (Fig. 19.62). The atrophy causes sarcolemmal nuclei to congregate, and they form long rows retaining their normal subsarcolemmal position. Necrosis and regeneration are rarely seen. 'Wear-and-tear' lipofuscin pigments accumulate at the poles of the nuclei. The motor nerve supply remains intact, showing only minor distal sprouting (Harriman 1966).

Necrotizing myopathy is the name given to a non-specific reaction of muscle to a variety of systemic diseases, including acute infections, collagen-vascular disease, liver disease, cancer, toxic conditions and endocrine disease. As already mentioned, Zenker described necrosis of muscle in patients dying of typhoid fever, and it is not uncommon for muscle taken at random at necropsy of patients dying of terminal infections to show necrosis and regeneration (Torvik and Berntzen 1968). Its pathogenesis is not understood. If it continues for some time it leads to variation in fibre calibre and fibrosis. Whatever the initiating cause, patients generally suffer from proximal weakness, less often wasting, especially in the lower limbs. It may be a partial manifestation of polymyositis (see above). Rarely, there is massive necrosis and widespread breakdown of muscle, leading to episodes of myoglobinuria

(idiopathic rhabdomyolysis or Meyer–Betz disease). Its cause is completely unknown, and there is no reason to link it with collagen-vascular disease. It may follow acute infection or unusual exertion, and is preceded by severe muscular cramps and pain (Demos and Gitin 1974).

Carcinomatous neuromyopathy. There are many syndromes resulting from the remote effects of cancer (Tyler 1974), and one of the commonest is a mainly proximal weakness and wasting. It is usually referred to as carcinomatous neuromyopathy, because of the clinical difficulty in deciding whether the lesion is neurogenic or myogenic. The syndrome has practical importance as it may be the first sign of disease. Henson (1970) states that about half of all men with acquired myopathy over 50 ultimately prove to have cancer, usually in the lung. The muscles may show polymyositis, necrotizing myopathy, cachectic atrophy, a distal pattern of neurogenic disease, or a combination of these. Rarely there is evidence of the myasthenic syndrome. The examination should obviously include the innervation.

The endocrine myopathies

Hyperthyroidism may be asociated rarely with myasthenia gravis or periodic paralysis. In 16% of cases there is a frank myopathy (Ramsay 1974), usually in males. This may take the form of a necrotizing myopathy, or merely small interstitial collections of lymphocytes. The extraocular muscles are occasionally involved. Asboe–Hansen, Iversen and Wichmann (1952) describe crescents of acid mucopolysaccharides in muscle fibres in thyrotoxicosis, especially in patients with severe exophthalmos. Other workers have been unable to find the material, and Asboe–Hansen and his colleagues ascribed this to failure to use basic lead acetate as a fixative. However, crescents were present in the muscle of one of our patients, in formalin material, a child who died from juvenile myxoedema (Fig. 19.63). Crescents thus seem to occur only in patients affected by severe thyroid disease over a long time.

Myxoedema. Patients often complain of painful cramps and weakness, and the reflexes are sluggish. Rarely the muscles increase in bulk (Hoffman's syndrome), and then show evidence of a neuromyopathy, due possibly to the increase in mucoprotein found in the connective tissue. Muscle fibres vary greatly in size, and show necrosis and regeneration, target fibres and gross vacuolation (Pearce and Aziz 1969) (Fig. 19.64).

Hyperparathyroidism. Some patients present with a proximal myopathy in which the reflexes are brisk. Histological changes are mild, all the signs

Adrenal gland. In *Addison's disease* there is severe cachectic atrophy. *Cushing's disease* may be accompanied by type-2 fibre atrophy, or in patients who have undergone adrenalectomy to treat the condition there is no atrophy but muscle fibres contain an excess of triglyceride droplets (Prineas, Hall, Barwick and Watson 1968). This has also been noted in untreated Cushing's disease (Harriman and Reed 1972).

Hyperaldosteronism is accompanied by periodic attacks of weakness, presumably related to hypokalaemia. Sambrook, Heron and Aber (1972)

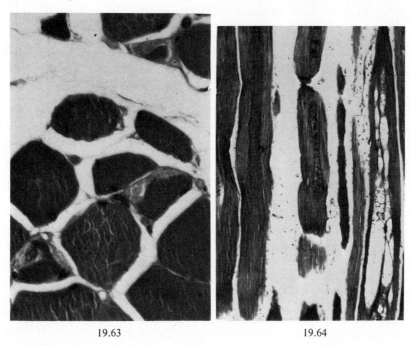

19.63   19.64

Fig. 19.63 Crescents of basophil material are shown in longstanding juvenile myxoedema. HE. × 450.
Fig. 19.64 Gross vacuolation and contorted target formations in severe myxoedema. PTAH. × 120.

and symptoms remit with removal of the parathyroid tumour (Frame, Heinze, Block and Manson 1968). Cape (1971) reported a uniform and intense staining of phosphorylase in both muscle fibre types in one patient, attributing this to activation of phosphorylase by calcium.

Acromegaly. Mastaglia, Barwick and Hall (1970) found mild proximal weakness, an increase in size of both types of muscle fibre and necrosis and regeneration. Some patients develop a neuropathy as a result of hyperplasia of connective tissue in peripheral nerves.

found scattered small angulated fibres staining strongly with NADH.

Pituitary-ovarian axis. Stanton and Strong (1967) reported a myopathy in a young woman, which failed to respond to steroids but remitted twice during pregnancy. It later responded to treatment with an oestrogen and a progestogen. Histological examination showed considerable variation in fibre size.

Menopausal muscular dystrophy. Although a form of limb girdle muscular dystrophy with late onset may present during the menopause (Nevin 1936), the patients described by Shy and McEachern (1951) under this title are generally considered to have been suffering from poly-myositis. Thus there is no good evidence that the menopause may cause a myopathy.

Metabolic myopathies

Disorders of glycogen metabolism

Absence or deficiency of the various enzymes that are concerned with the degradation of glycogen to glucose leads to the accumulation of glycogen in the tissues. A good account of the glycogenoses that affect muscle is given by Dubowitz and Brooke (1973).

Type 2 glycogenosis (Pompe's disease), due to acid maltase deficiency, is fatal in infancy. Glycogen accumulates in many tissues including the myocardium and the central nervous system as well as sketelal muscle, where fibres eventually contain large amounts. It is distributed both diffusely and in large granules shown by electron-microscopy to be lysosomes. Acid maltase is a lysosomal enzyme. In paraffin sections some of the glycogen may leach out into the fixative, leaving empty spaces in the muscle fibres. Much PAS-positive material remains, however. In some instances this is all removed by diastase, showing it to be glycogen alone, but in other cases a diastase-resistant substance persists. This gives the reactions of an acid mucopolysaccharide (Fig. 19.65). Infants affected by Pompe's disease present as floppy babies, and the diagnosis may not be made until a muscle biopsy is performed. Radiological evidence of cardiac enlargement and ECG changes may be present in an infant who in other respects appears to be suffering from Werdnig–Hoffman disease. Recently a mild form of type 2 glycogenosis, clinically resembling limb-girdle dystrophy, has been reported in older children and adults (Engel 1970).

Type 3 glycogenosis. Muscle is as a rule only mildly affected, although the condition may present with hypotonia in infancy or a chronic myopathy in adults. The liver is more seriously involved and patients may develop hypoglycaemia. The fibres contain glycogen in diffuse form in the sarcoplasm, with no suggestion of accumulation in lysosomes. The enzyme which is deficient is the debranching enzyme, amylo-1, 6-glucosidase,

demonstrable by liver or muscle biopsy or in the leucocytes.

Type 5 glycogenosis (*McArdle's disease*). This is due to phosphorylase deficiency, and is entirely restricted to striated muscle. Members of families affected by this disorder suffer pains in their muscles on exercise, especially in the calves, but some are able to get a 'second wind'. Usually there are no abnormal findings on clinical exam-ination, but some develop an overt proximal myopathy. The ischaemic exercise test shows no rise in blood lactate; this rises two to five times in normal subjects. The muscle shows no changes in paraffin sections, or a few fibres show vacuoles, chiefly subsarcolemmal. In cryostat sections these are filled with glycogen, and phosphorylase is shown to be absent (Fig. 19.66).

Type 7 glycogenosis. Only four cases have been reported. The clinical presentation is similar to that of McArdle's disease, venous lactate fails to rise on exercise, but the deficiency is of phospho-fructokinase. A histochemical method for its detection is described by Bonilla and Schotland (1970).

Osteomalacia

Some patients with osteomalacia develop a wad-dling gait, and show evidence of a proximal myopathy. As in that of hyperparathyroidism. reflexes are preserved or even brisk, and again the myopathy is independent of calcium levels (Smith and Stern 1967). We have noted some atrophic fibres with clumped nuclei, type-2 fibres atrophy and a disturbance of motor endplates, some of which showed sprouting and others a myasthenia-like elongation and attenuation.

Toxic myopathies

Isolated examples of myopathy have been reported following the use of clofibrate (Langer and Levy 1968), chloroquine (Hughes, Esiri, Oxbury and Whitty 1971), E-aminocaproic acid (Bennett 1972), carbenoxolone sodium (Barnes and Leonard 1971), vincristine (Bradley, Lassman, Pearce and Walton 1970), amphotericin B (Drutz, Fan, Tai, Cheng and Hsieh 1970), phenformin (Bertrand and Duwoos 1969) and emetine (Duane and Engel 1970).

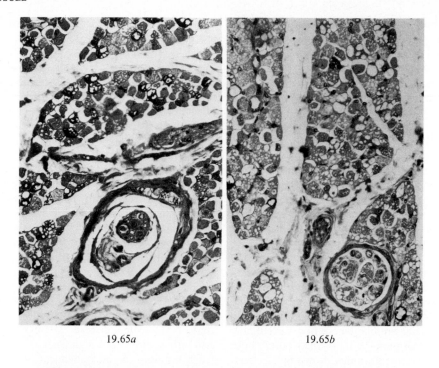

19.65*a*   19.65*b*

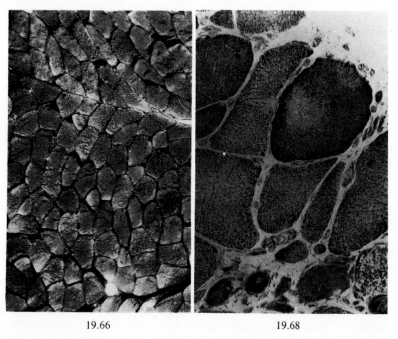

19.66   19.68

Fig. 19.65 Type 2 glycogenosis. (*a*) Many fibres contain PAS-positive material. (*b*) After treatment with diastase, much of the material is dissolved out, showing it to be glycogen. A small proportion persists, and gives the reactions of a mucopolysaccharide. (*a*) PAS. × 180. (*b*) PAS after diastase. × 180.

Fig. 19.66 Type 5 glycogenosis (McArdle's disease). Due to phosphorylase deficiency, dark-staining glycogen accumulates in muscle fibres especially beneath the sarcolemma. Unfixed cryostat section, PAS. × 120.

Fig. 19.68 Malignant hyperpyrexia myopathy. Area of focal hypertrophy showing gross variation in fibre calibre, a moth-eaten fibre and fibre splitting. NADH. × 280.

Alcoholic myopathy is rare compared with alcoholic neuropathy. It occurs in two forms in chronic alcoholics, acute, following a drinking bout (Hed, Lundmark, Fahlgren and Orell 1962; Martinez, Hooshmand and Faris 1973) and chronic (Ekbom Hed, Kirstein, and Astrom 1964). The findings on biopsy are non-specfic, including fibre necrosis and its sequelae, and atrophy of type-2 fibres. There may be the effects of a complicating peripheral neuropathy. We have examined two well-to-do patients by biopsy when they suffered severe weakness after a drinking bout. In both muscles fibres remained of normal size, but many type-1 fibres were filled with large triglyceride droplets (Fig. 19.67, facing p. 851).

Steroid myopathy. Some patients on a prolonged course of steroids develop a proximal myopathy. In the earlier stages, no atrophy is observed, but muscle fibres especially of type-1 contain excess lipid in the form of triglyceride droplets. Later type-2 fibre atrophy develops, and lipid-laden fibres are no longer seen. Individual idiosyncrasy to the drug may be important, as the complication is not dose-dependent nor related to the variety of steroid used (Harriman and Reed 1972).

Malignant hyperpyrexia myopathy. Anaesthetic agents and muscle relaxants, especially suxamethonium and halothane, have been found to be responsible for the serious complication of anaesthesia characterized by a rapid rise in temperature, to 43° or more, often muscular rigidity, and death in 65% of cases. Susceptibility to this disorder is inherited as a dominant trait, and is associated with a myopathy of which the patient is unaware. Patients are often of athletic build, and a few show local hypertrophy of muscles, particularly in the thighs or calves. The CPK may or may not be raised. The muscles show a variety of changes, the commonest being internal migration of nuclei, moth-eaten or core-targetoid fibres (Harriman, Sumner and Ellis 1973). In the areas of focal hypertrophy there is fibre calibre variation and frequent fibre splitting (Fig. 19.68). Muscle from susceptible patients has been shown *in vitro* to develop increased isometric tension or contracture when exposed to anaesthetic agents (Ellis, Harriman, Keaney, Kyei-Mensah and Tyrrell 1971).

Muscle contracture. Fibrosis and contracture of muscle may develop following repeated intramuscular injections. Contracture of the vastus intermedius was a puzzling condition in children until it was realised they had previously been given penicillin intramuscularly (Norman, Temple and Murphy 1970). The condition may develop in other muscles, including the deltoid, in adults (Groves and Goldner 1974).

Ischaemia of muscle

Muscle has a rich blood supply with many collaterals and is generally not susceptible to infarction. However, it occurs occasionally in patients suffering from severe occlusive arterial disease of the limbs, in which large foci of muscle are found to have undergone necrosis (with peripheral regeneration) or an ischaemic myopathy may occur under the same conditions, with necrosis and regeneration of numerous scattered muscle fibres. Volkmann's ischaemic contracture of muscle is a well known but rare complication of fractures, and is thought to be the result of arterial spasm (Jones 1970). Infarction of muscle has been reported in two diabetic patients (Banker and Chester 1973). Ischaemia is thought to be the basis of the anterior compartment or pretibial syndrome, in which pain and necrosis of muscle develop after strenuous exercise, especially in athletic individuals (Edwards 1969).

Infections of muscle

Abscess in muscle is quite commonly seen in the tropics, and appears as a painful swelling in a patient with pyrexia. Often the pus is sterile (Rogers 1973). *Gas gangrene* occurs in muscle, when anaerobic organisms such as *Clostridium welchii* invade tissue damaged by wounding or accident. *Viral infections* of muscle are rare, an example being Bornholm disease which is due to infection with Coxsackie B virus. The patient presents with fever and severe pain in the muscles of the chest and abdomen. Muscle biopsies have shown fibre necrosis and lymphocytic infiltration (Lepine, Desse, and Sautter 1952).

Parasitic infections. The larval form of the whipworm *Trichinella spiralis* and the larva of the pork tape-worm *Taenia solium* (cysticercosis) may be found in human muscle. Biopsy of a tender muscle may reveal the organism. Cysticercosis may cause muscular pseudo-hypertrophy (Jolly and Pallis 1971). In *Chagas' disease, Trypanosoma cruzi* invades muscle as well as other tissues and produces a polymyositis-like lesion (Abath and Carvalho 1966). In *toxoplasmosis* muscle may be invaded, and *Toxoplasma gondii* are recognized as collections of minute pear-shaped or crescentic organisms within muscle fibres. The neighbouring tissue shows necrosis, regeneration and lymphocytic infiltration.

References

Abath, G. M. & De Carvalho, J. A. M.   (1966) Histopathology of skeletal muscle in experimental Chagas' disease. *American Journal of Tropical Medicine*, **15**, 135-140.

Adams, R. D., Denny-Brown, D. & Pearson, C. M.   (1962) *Diseases of Muscle. A Study in Pathology*, 2nd Edn. Kimpton, London.

Aherne, W., Ayyar, D. R., Clarke, P. A. & Walton, J. N.   (1971) Muscle fibre size in normal infants, children and adolescents. *Journal of the Neurological Sciences*, **14**, 171-182.

Ariano, M. A., Armstrong, R. B. & Edgerton, V. R.   (1973) Hindlimb muscle fibre populations of five mammals. *Journals of Histochemistry and Cytochemistry*, **21**, 51-55.

Asböe-Hansen, G., Iverson, K. & Wichmann, R.   (1952) Malignant exophthalmos: muscular changes and thyrotropin content in serum. *Acta endocrinologica*, **11**, 376-399.

Asbury, A. K., Arnason, B. G. & Adams, R. D.   (1969) The inflammatory lesion in idiopathic polyneuritis. Its role in pathogenesis. *Medicine (Baltimore)*, **48**, 173-215.

Ashworth, B. & Smyth, G. E.   (1969) Relapsing motor polyneuropathy. *Acta neurologica scandinavica*, **45**, 342-350.

Banker, B. Q. & Victor, M.   (1966) Dermatomyositis (systemic angiopathy) of childhood. *Medicine (Baltimore)*, **45**, 261-289.

Banker, B. Q. & Chester, C. S.   (1973) Infarction of thigh muscle in the diabetic patient. *Neurology (Minneapolis)*, **23**, 667-677.

Barker, D. & Ip, M. C.   (1965) The probable existence of motor end-plate replacement. *Journal of Physiology*, **176**, 11-12P.

Barker, D. & Ip, M. C.   (1966) Sprouting and degeneration of mammalian motor axons in normal and de-afferentated skeletal muscle. *Proceedings of the Royal Society, Series B, 163*, 538-554.

Barnes, P. C. & Leonard, J. H. C.   (1971) Hypokalaemic myopathy and myoglobinuria due to carbenoxolone sodium. *Postgraduate Medical Journal*, **47**, 813-814.

Bates, D., Stevens, J. C. & Hudgson, P.   (1973) "Polymyositis" with involvement of facial and distal musculature. One form of the facioscapulo-humeral syndrome. *Journal of the Neurological Sciences*, **19**, 105-108.

Becker, P. E.   (1973) Myotonia congenita (Thomsen) in *Clinical Studies in Myology* (Ed. Kakulas, B. A.), Part 2, pp. 481-485, International Congress Series, 295. Excerpta Medica, Amsterdam.

Bennett, J. R.   (1972) Myopathy from E-aminocaproic acid: a second case. *Postgraduate Medical Journal*, **48**, 440-442.

Bertrand, C. M. & Duwoos, H.   (1969) Syndrome musculaire à l'effort révélateur d'un début d'intoxication par l'acide lactique endogène consécutif à l'administration de phenformin. *Annales d'Endocrinologie (Paris)*, **30**, 570-575.

Bethlem, J. Van Wijngaarden, G. K. & De Jong, J.   (1973) The incidence of lobulated fibres in the faciosca-pulohumeral type of muscular dystrophy and the limb-girdle syndrome. *Journal of the Neurological Sciences*, **18**, 351-358.

Blauchet-Bardon, C., Ganter, P. & Roujeau, J.   (1975) La muscle arrecteur chez les sclérodermiques. *Semaine des Hôpiteaux, Paris*, **51**, 455-460.

Bonilla, E. & Schotland, D. L.   (1970) Histochemical diagnosis of muscle phosphofructokinase deficiency. *Archives of Neurology (Chicago)*, **22**, 8-12.

Bradley, W. G., Hudgson, P., Gardner-Medwin, D. & Walton, J. N.   (1973) The syndrome of myosclerosis. *Journal of Neurology, Neurosurgery and Psychiatry*, **36**, 651-660.

Bradley, W. G., Jenkinson, M., Park, D. C., Hudgson, P., Gardner-Medwin, D., Pennington, R. J. T. & Walton, J. N.   (1972) A myopathy associated with lipid storage. *Journal of the Neurological Sciences*, **16**, 137-154.

Bradley, W. G., Lassman, L. P., Pearce, G. W. & Walton, J. N.   (1970) The neuromyopathy of vincristine in man: clinical, electrophysiological and pathological studies. *Journal of the Neurological Sciences*, **10**, 107-131.

Bradley, W. G., Richardson, J. & Frew, I. J. C. (1974) The familial association of neurofibromatosis, peroneal muscular atrophy, congenital deafness, partial albinism and Axenfeld's defect. *Brain*, **97**, 521-532.

Brooke, M. H. (1966) The histological reaction of muscle to disease in *The Physiology and Biochemistry of Muscle as a Food* (Eds. Briskey, E. J., Casseus, R. & Trautmann, J.). University of Wisconsin Press.

Brooke, M. H. & Engel, W. K. (1969) The histographic analysis of human muscle biopsies with regard to fiber types. 1. Adult male and female. *Neurology (Minneapolis)*, **19**, 221-233.

Brooke, M. H. & Kaiser, K. K. (1970) Muscle fibre types: how many and what kind? *Archives of Neurology*, **23**, 369-379.

Brown, J. C. & Charlton, J. E. (1975a) A study of sensitivity to curare in myasthenic disorders using a regional technique. *Journal of Neurology, Neurosurgery and Psychiatry*, **38**, 27-33.

Brown, J. C. & Charlton, J. E. (1975b) Study of sensitivity to curare in certain neurological disorders using a regional technique. *Journal of Neurology, Neurosurgery and Psychiatry*, **38**, 34-45.

Brownell, B., Oppenheimer, D. R. & Spalding, J. M. K. (1972) Neurogenic muscle atrophy in myasthenia gravis. *Journal of Neurology, Neurosurgery and Psychiatry*, **35**, 311-322.

Buzzard, E. F. (1905) The clinical history and post-mortem examination of five cases of myasthenia gravis. *Brain*, **28**, 438-483.

Cape, C. A. (1971) Increased phosphorylase activity in muscle in hyperparathyroid disease. *Neurology (Minneapolis)*, **21**, 638-641.

Cassens, R. G., Cooper, C. C. & Briskey, E. J. (1969) The occurrence and histochemical characterization of giant fibres in the muscle of growing and adult animals. *Acta Neuropathologica (Berlin)*, **12**, 300-304.

Cavanagh, J. B. (1966) In *Systemic Pathology* (Eds. Wright, G. P. & Symmers, W. St.C.), Vol. 2, Chapter 35, p. 1314. Longman, London.

Chou, S.-M. (1968) Myxovirus-like structures and accompanying nuclear changes in chronic polymyositis. *Archives of Pathology*, **86**, 649-658.

Chou, S.-M. & Gutmann, L. (1970) Picornavirus-like crystals in subacute polymyositis. Neurology (Minneapolis), **20**, 215-213.

Coërs, C. (1967) Structure and organization of the myoneural junction. *International Review of Cytology*, **22**, 239-267.

Coërs, C. & Carbone, F. (1966) La myopathie granulomateuse. *Acta neurologica et psychiatrica Belgica*, **66**, 353-381.

Coërs, C. & Woolf, A. L. (1959) *The Innervation of Muscle. A Biopsy Study.* Blackwell Scientific Publications, Oxford.

Cornil, A. V. & Ranvier, A. (1902) *Manuel d'Histologie Pathologique*, 3rd Edn., Vol. 2, p. 301, Félix Alcan, Paris.

Creed, R. S., Denny-Brown, D. E., Eccles, J. C., Liddell, E. G. T. & Sherrington, C. S. (1932) *Reflex Activity of the Spinal Cord.* Clarendon Press, Oxford.

Cuajunco, F. (1942) Development of the human motor end plate. *Contributions to Embryology*, **30**, 127-152.

Currie, S., Saunders, M., Knowles, M. & Brown, A. E. (1971) Immunological aspects of polymyositis. The in vitro activity of lymphocytes on incubation with muscle antigen and muscle cultures. *Quarterly Journal of Medicine*, **40**, 63-84.

Demos, M. A. & Gitin, E. L. (1974) Acute exertional rhabdomyolysis. *Archives of Internal Medicine*, **133**, 233-239.

Drachman, D. A. (1968) Ophthalmoplegia plus. The neurodegenerative disorders associated with progressive external ophthalmoplegia. *Archives of Neurology*, **18**, 654-674.

Drutz, D. J., Fan, J. H., Tai, T. Y., Cheng, J. T. & Hsieh, W. C. (1970) Hypokalemic rhabdomyolysis and myoglobinuria following amphothericin B therapy. *Journal of the American Medical Association*, **211**, 824-826.

Duane, D. D. & Engel, A. G. (1970) Emetine myopathy. *Neurology (Minneapolis)*, **20**, 733-739.

Dubowitz, V. (1967a) Pathology of experimentally re-innervated skeletal muscle. *Journal of Neurology, Neurosurgery and Psychiatry*, **30**, 99-110.

Dubowitz, V. (1967b) Cross-innervated mammalian skeletal muscle: histochemical, physiological and biochemical observations. *Journal of Physiology*, **193**, 481-496.

Dubowitz, V. (1968) Developing and diseased muscle: a histochemical study. *Spastics International Medical Publications Research Monograph, No. 2.* Heinemann Medical, London.

Dubowitz, V. (1969) The floppy infant. *Clinics in Developmental Medicine*, No. 31.

Dubowitz, V, & Brooke, M. H. (1973) *Muscle Biopsy: a modern approach.* W. B. Saunders, London & Philadelphia.

Dubowitz, V. & Pearse, A. G. E. (1960) Reciprocal relationship of phosphorylase and oxidative enzymes in skeletal muscle. *Nature*, **185**, 701.

Duchen, L. W. (1971) An electron microscopic comparison of motor end-plates of slow and fast skeletal muscle fibres of the mouse. *Journal of the Neurological Sciences*, **14**, 37-45.

Durston, J. H. (1974) Histochemistry of primate extraocular muscles and the changes of denervation. *British Journal of Ophthalmology*, **58**, 193-216.

Eccles, J. C., Eccles, R. M. & Lundberg, A. (1958) The action potentials of the alpha motoneurones supplying fast and slow muscles. *Journal of Physiology*, **142**, 275-291.

Edgerton, V. R., Gerchman, L. & Carrow, R. (1969) Histochemical changes in rat skeletal muscle after exercise. *Experimental Neurology*, **24**, 110-123.

Edwards, P. W. (1969) Peroneal compartment syndrome. Report of a case. *Journal of Bone and Joint Surgery*, **51B**, 123-125.

Ekbom, K., Hed, R., Kirstein, L. & Astrom, K.-E. (1964) Muscular affections in chronic alcoholism. *Archives of Neurology*, **10**, 449-458.

Ellis, F. R., Harriman, D. G. F., Keaney, N. P., Kyei-Mensah, K. & Tyrrell, J. H. (1971) Halophane-induced muscle contractures as a cause of hyperpyrexia. *British Journal of Anaesthesia*, **43**, 721-722.

Emery, A. E. (1971) The nosology of the spinal muscular atrophies. *Journal of Medical Genetics*, **8**, 481-495.

Engel, A. G. (1970) Acid maltase deficiency in adults: studies in four cases of a syndrome which may mimic muscular dystrophy or other myopathies. *Brain*, **93**, 599-616.

Engel, A. G. & Angelini, C. (1973) Carnitine deficiency of human skeletal muscle with associated lipid storage myopathy: a new syndrome. *Science*, **179**, 899-902.

Engel, A. G., Gomez, M. R. & Groover, R. V. (1971) Multicore disease. A recently recognized congenital myopathy associated with multifocal degeneration of muscle fibers. *Mayo Clinic Proceedings* **46**, 666-681.

Engel, A. G. & Santa, T. (1971) Histometric analysis of the ultrastructure of the neuromuscular junction in myasthenia gravis and in the myasthenic syndrome. *Annals of the New York Academy of Sciences*, **183**, 46-63.

Engel, W. K. (1961) Muscle target fibres, a newly recognised sign of denervation. *Nature*, **191**, 389-390.

Engel, W. K. (1962) The essentiality of histo- and cytochemical studies of skeletal muscle in the investigation of neuromuscular disease. *Neurology (Minneapolis)*, **12**, 778-794.

Engel, W. K. (1965) Diseases of the neuromuscular junction and muscle in *Neurohistochemistry* (Ed. Adams, C. W. M.), Chapter 17. Elsevier, Amsterdam.

Farkas, E., Tomé, F. M. S., Fardeau, M., Arsenio-Nunes, M. L., Dreyfus, P. & Diebler, M. F. (1974) Histochemical and ultrastructural study of muscle biopsies in 3 cases of dystrophia myotonica in the newborn child. *Journal of the Neurological Sciences*, **21**, 273-288.

Feinstein, B., Lindegaard, B., Nyman, E. & Wohlfart, G. (1955) Morphologic studies of motor units in normal human muscles. *Acta anatomica (Basel)*, **23**, 127-142.

Frame, B., Heinze, E. G., Block, M. A. & Manson, G. A. (1968) Myopathy in primary hyperparathyroidism: observations in three patients. *Annals of Internal Medicine*, **68**, 1022-1027.

Feng, T. P. & Lu, D. X. (1965) New light on the phenomenon of transient hypertrophy in the denervated hemidiaphragm of the rat. *Scientia Sinica*, **14**, 1172-1184.

Gardner-Medwin, D. (1970) Mutation rate in Duchenne type of muscular dystrophy. *Journal of Medical Genetics*, **7**, 334-337.

Gardner-Thorpe, C. (1972) Muscle weakness due to sarcoid myopathy: six case reports and an evaluation of steroid therapy. *Neurology (Minneapolis)*, **22**, 917-928.

Goldspink, G. (1970) The proliferation of myofibrils during muscle fibre growth. *Journal of Cellular Science*, **6**, 593-603.

Groves, R. J. & Goldner, J. L. (1974) Contracture of the deltoid muscle in the adult after intramuscular injections. Report of three cases. *Journal of Bone and Joint Surgery*, **56A**, 817-820.

Grutzner, P. (1884) Zur Anatomie und Physiologie der quergestreiften Muskeln. *Recueil zoologique Suisse*, Vol. 1,

Guth, L. & Samaha, F. J. (1972) Erroneous interpretations which may result from application of the 'myofibrillar ATPase' histochemical procedure to developing muscle. *Experimental Neurology*, **34**, 465-475.

Hall-Craggs, E. C. B. & Lawrence, C. A. (1970) Longitudinal fibre division in skeletal muscle: a light and electron microscopic study. *Zeitschrift für Zellforschung und mikroskopische Anatomie*, **109**, 481-494.

Harriman, D. G. F. (1961) Histology of the motor end-page (motor-point muscle biopsy) in *Electrodiagnosis and Electromyography* (Ed. Licht, S.), 2nd Edn. Licht, New Haven, Connecticut.

Harriman, D. G. F. (1966) Muscle cachexia. Some aspects of its pathology and clinical features in *Proceedings of the Fifth International Congress of Neuropathology, International Congress Series No. 100*, pp. 677-683. Excerpta Medica, Amsterdam.

Harriman, D. G. F. (1970) Pathological aspects of Adie's syndrome. *Advances in Ophthalmology*, **23**, 55-73,

Harriman, D. G. F. & Haleem, M. A. (1972) Centronuclear myopathy in old age. *Journal of Pathology*, **108**, 237-247.

Harriman, D. G. F. & Reed, R. (1972) The incidence of lipid droplets in human skeletal muscle in neuro-muscular disorders: a histochemical, electronmicroscopic and freeze-etch study. *Journal of Pathology*, **106**, 1-24.

Harriman, D. G. F., Summer, D. W. & Ellis, F. R. (1973) Malignant hyperpyrexia myopathy. *Quarterly Journal of Medicine*, **42**, 639-664.

Harriman, D. G. F., Taverner, D. & Woolf, A. L. (1970) Ekbom's syndrome and burning paraesthesiae. A biopsy study by vital staining and electron microscopy of the intramuscular innervation with a note on age changes in motor nerve endings in distal muscles. *Brain*, **93**, 393-406.

Haslock, D. I., Wright, V. & Harriman, D. G. F. (1970) Neuromuscular disorders in rheumatoid arthritis. *Quarterly Journal of Medicine*, **39**, 335-358.

Haydar, N. A., Conn, H. L. Jr., Afifi, A., Wakid, N., Ballas, S. & Fawaz, K. (1971) Severe hypermetabolism with primary abnormality of skeletal muscle mitochondria. *Annals of Internal Medicine*, **74**, 548-558.

Hed, R., Lundmark, C., Fahlgren, H. & Orell, S. (1962) Acute muscular syndrome in chronic alcoholism. *Acta medica Scandinavica*, **171**, 585-599.

Henson, R. A. (1970) Non-metastatic neurological manifestations of malignant disease in *Modern Trends in Neurology—5* (Ed. Williams, D.), p. 209. Butterworth, London.

Hogan, G. R., Gutmann, L. & Chou, S. M. (1969) The peripheral neuropathy of Krabbe's (globoid) leuco-dystrophy. *Neurology (Minneapolis)*, **19**, 1094-1100.

Hogan, M. J. & Zimmerman, L. F. (1962) *Ophthalmic Pathology*, 2nd Edn., p. 735, W. B. Saunders Co., Philadelphia and London.

Hogenhuis, L. A. H. & Engel, W. K. (1965) Histochemistry and cytochemistry of experimentally denervated guinea-pig muscle. 1. Histochemistry. *Acta anatomica (Basel)*, **60**, 39-65.

Hughes, J. T., Esiri, M., Oxbury, J. M. & Whitty, C. W. M. (1971) Chloroquine myopathy. *Quarterly Journal of Medicine*, **40**, 85-93.

James, N. T. (1971) The histochemical demonstration of three types of intrafusal fibre in rat muscle spindles. *Histochemical Journal*, **3**, 457-462.

Jennekens, F. G. I., Tomlinson, B. E. & Walton, J. N. (1971) Data on the distribution of fibre types in five human limb muscles. *Journal of the Neurological Sciences*, **14**, 245-257.

Johnson, M. A., Polgar, J., Weightman, D. & Appleton, D. (1973) Data on the distribution of fibre types in thirty-six human muscles. An autopsy study. *Journal of the Neurological Sciences*, **18**, 111-129.

Jolly, S. S. & Pallis, C. (1971) Muscular pseudohypertrophy due to cysticercosis. *Journal of the Neurological Sciences*, **12**, 155-162.

Jones, D. A. (1970) Volkmann's ischaemia. *Surgical Clinics of North America*, **50**, 329-342.

de Jong, J. G. Y., Slooff, J. L. & van der Eerden, A. A. J. J. (1973) A family with paramyotonia congenita with the report of an autopsy. *Acta neurologica scandinavica*, **49**, 480-494.

Karpati, G., Carpenter, S., Walters, G. V., Eisen, A. A. & Andermann, F. (1973) Infantile myotonic dystrophy: histochemical and electron microscopic features in skeletal muscle. *Neurology (Minneapolis)*, **23**, 1066-1077.

Katz, B. (1961) The terminations of the afferent nerve fibre in the muscle spindle of the frog. *Philosophical Transactions of the Royal Society, Series B*, **343**, 221-240.

Krause, W. (1864) *Die Anatomie des Kaninchens*, Leipzig.

Kristensson, K., Olsson, Y. & Sourander, P. (1967) Peripheral nerve changes in Tay-Sachs and Batten–Spielmeyer–Vogt disease. *Acta pathologica et microbiologica Scandinavica*, **70**, 630-632.

Kugelberg, I. & Welander, M. (1956) Heredofamilial juvenile muscular atrophy simulating muscular dystrophy. *Archives of Neurology and Psychiatry (Chicago)*, **75**, 500-509.

Langer, T. & Levy, R. I. (1968) Acute muscular syndrome associated with administration of clofibrate. *New England Journal of Medicine*, **279**, 856-858.

Lepine, P., Desse, G., & Sautter, V. (1952) Biopsies musculaires, examen histologique et isolement du virus coxsackie chez l'Homme atteint de myalgie epidémique (maladie de Bornholm). *Bulletin de l'Académie Nationale de Médecine*, **136**, 66-69.

Luft, R., Ikkos, D., Palmieri, G., Eraster, L. & Afzelius, B.   (1962) A case of severe hypermetabolism of non-thyroid origin with a defect in the maintenance of mitochondrial respiratory control: a correlated clinical, biochemical and morphological study.   *Journal of Clinical Investigation*, **41**, 1776-1804.

McArdle, B.   (1974) Metabolic and endocrine myopathies in *Disorders of Voluntary Muscle* (Ed. Walton, J. N.), 3rd Edn.   Churchill Livingstone, Edinburgh and London.

McLeod, J. G. & Prineas, J. W.   (1971) Distal type of chronic spinal muscular atrophy.   Clinical, electro-physiological and pathological studies.   *Brain*, **94**, 703-714.

Martin, D. L. & Engel, W. K.   (1972) Dependency of histochemical phosphorylase staining on amount of cellular glycogen.   *Journal of Histochemistry and Cytochemistry*, **20**, 476-479.

Martin, J. J., van Bogaert, L., van Damme, J. & Peremans, J.   (1970) Sur une pseudo-myopathie ligneuse généralisée par amyloïdose primaire endomysiovasculaire.   *Journal of the Neurological Sciences*, **11**, 147-166.

Martinez, A. J., Hooshmand, H. & Faris, A. A.   (1973) Acute alcoholic myopathy.   Enzyme histochemistry and electron microscopic findings.   *Journal of the Neurological Sciences*, **20**, 245-252.

Mastaglia, F. L., Barwick, D. D. & Hall, R.   (1970) Myopathy in acromegaly.   *Lancet*, **2**, 907-909.

Mastaglia, F. L. & Kakulas, B. A.   (1969) Regeneration in Duchenne muscular dystrophy: a histological and histochemical study.   *Brain*, **92**, 809-818.

Mastaglia, F. L. & Walton, J. N.   (1970) Coxsackie virus-like particles in skeletal muscle from a case of poly-myositis.   *Journal of the Neurological Sciences*, **11**, 593-599.

Mathew, N. T., Jacob, J. C. & Chandy, J.   (1970) Familial ocular myopathy with curare sensitivity.   *Archives of Neurology (Chicago)*, **22**, 68-74.

Mauro, A.   (1961) Satellite cell of skeletal muscle fibres.   *Journal of Biophysical and Biochemical Cytology*, **9**, 493-495.

Meadows, J. C., Marsden, D. C. & Harriman, D. G. F.   (1969a) Chronic spinal muscular atrophy in adults. 1. The Kugelberg-Welander syndrome.   *Journal of the Neurological Sciences*, **9**, 527-550.

Meadows, J. C., Marsden, C. D. & Harriman, D. G. F.   (1969b) Chronic spinal muscular atrophy in adults. 2. Other forms.   *Journal of the Neurological Sciences*, **9**, 551-566.

Moore, M. J., Rebeiz, J. J., Holden, M. & Adams, R. D.   (1971) Biometric analyses of normal skeletal muscle.   *Acta Neuropathologica (Berlin)*, **19**, 51-69.

Morita, S., Cooper, C. C., Gassens, R. G., Kastenschmidt, L. L. & Briskey, E. J.   (1970) A histological study of myoglobin in developing muscle of the pig.   *Journal of Animal Science*, **31**, 664-670.

Morris, C. J. & Raybould, J. A.   (1971) Histochemically demonstrable fibre abnormalities in normal skeletal muscle and in muscle from carriers of Duchenne muscular dystrophy.   *Journal of Neurology, Neurosurgery and Psychiatry*, **34**, 348-352.

Munsat, T. L., Piper, D., Cancilla, P. & Mednick, J.   (1972) Inflammatory myopathy with facioscapulohumeral distribution.   *Neurology (Minneapolis)*, **22**, 335-347.

Nattrass, F. J.   (1954) Recovery from 'muscular dystrophy'.   *Brain*, **77**, 549-570.

Neustein, H. B.   (1973) Nemaline myopathy.   A family study with three autopsied cases.   *Archives of Pathology*, **96**, 192-195.

Neville, H. E. & Brooke, M. H.   (1973) Central core fibres: structured and unstructured in *Basic Research in Myology* (Ed. Kakulas, B. A.), Part I, *International Congress Series No. 294*, pp, 497-511.   Excerpta Medica, Amsterdam.

Nevin, S.   (1936) Two cases of muscular degeneration occurring in late adult life, with a review of the recorded cases of late progressive muscular dystrophy (late progressive myopathy).   *Quarterly Journal of Medicine* **5**, 51-66.

Norman, M. G., Temple, A. R., & Murphy, J. V.   (1970) Infantile quadriceps-femoris contracture resulting from intramuscular injections.   *New England Journal of Medicine*, **282**, 964-966.

Olson, W., Engel, W. K., Walsh, G. O. & Einaugler, R.   (1972) Oculocraniosomatic neuromuscular disease with "ragged-red" fibres.   *Archives of Neurology (Chicago)*, **26**, 193-211.

Oosterhuis, H. & Bethlem, J.   (1973) Neurogenic muscle involvement in myasthenia gravis.   *Journal of Neurology, Neurosurgery and Psychiatry*, **36**, 244-254.

Ovalle, W. K. & Smith, R. S.   (1972) Histochemical identification of three types of intrafusal muscle fibres in the cat and monkey based on the myosin ATPase reaction.   *Canadian Journal of Physiology and Pharmacology*, **50**, 195-202.

Padykula, H. A. & Gauthier, G. F.   (1970) The ultrastructure of the neuromuscular junctions of mammalian red, white and intermediate skeletal muscle fibers.   *Journal of Cell Biology*, **46**, 27-41.

Pearce, J. & Aziz, H.   (1969) The neuromyopathy of hypothyroidism.   Some new observations.   *Journal of the Neurological Sciences*, **9**, 243-253.

Pearce, J. & Harriman, D. G. F.   (1966) Chronic spinal muscular atrophy.   *Journal of Neurology, Neurosurgery and Psychiatry*, **29**, 509-520.

Pearson, C. M. & Currie, S.   (1974) Polymyositis and related disorders in *Disorders of Voluntary Muscle* (Ed. Walton, J. N.), 3rd Edn., Chap. 16, pp. 614-652 (Sjögren's disease, p. 632).   Churchill Livingstone, Edinburgh and London.

Pearson, C. M. & Yamazaki, J. N.   (1958) Vacuolar myopathy in systemic lupus erythematosus.   *American Journal of Clinical Pathology*, **29**, 455-463.

Prineas, J., Hall, R., Barwick, D. D. & Watson, A. J.   (1968) Myopathy associated with pigmentation following adrenalectomy for Cushing's syndrome.   *Quarterly Journal of Medicine*, **37**, 63-77.

Ramsay, I.   (1974) *Thyroid Disease and Muscle Dysfunction*.   Heinemann Medical, London.

Reichenmiller, H. E., Bundschu, H. D., Bass, L., Missmahl, H. P. & Arnold, M.   (1968) Progressive muscular dystrophy and pericollagenous amyloidosis.   *German Medical Monthly*, **13**, 380-384.

Reske-Nielsen, E., Coërs, C. & Harmsen, A.   (1970) Qualitative and quantitative histological study of neuromuscular biopsies from healthy young men.   *Journal of the Neurological Sciences*, **10**, 369-384.

Rewcastle, M. B. & Humphrey, J. G.   (1965) Vacuolar myopathy: clinical, histochemical and microscopic study.   *Archives of Neurology (Chicago)*, **12**, 570-582.

Rogers, D. W.   (1973) Case of pyomyositis occurring in London.   *British Medical Journal*, **3**, 679.

Romanul, F. C. A. & van der Meulen, J. P.   (1967) Slow and fast muscles after cross innervation.   *Archives of Neurology (Chicago)*, **17**, 387-402.

Ross, R. T.   (1963) Ocular myopathy sensitive to curare.   *Brain*, **86**, 67-74.

Rothstein, T. L., Carlson, C. B. & Sumi, S. M.   (1971) Polymyositis with facioscapulo-humeral distribution.   *Archives of Neurology (Chicago)*, **25**, 313-319.

Sambrook, M. A., Heron, J. R. & Aber, G. M.   (1972) Myopathy in association with primary hyperaldosteronism.   *Journal of Neurology, Neurosurgery and Psychiatry*, **35**, 202-207.

Shibasaki, H., Santa, T. & Kuroiwa, Y.   (1973) Late onset mitochondrial myopathy.   *Journal of the Neurological Sciences*, **18**, 301-310.

Shy, G. M., Engel, W. K., Somers, J. E. & Wanko, T.   (1963) Nemaline myopathy: a new congenital myopathy.   *Brain*, **86**, 793-810.

Shy, G. M. & McEachern, D.   (1951) The clinical features and response to cortisone of menopausal muscular dystrophy.   *Journal of Neurology, Neurosurgery and Psychiatry*, **14**, 101-107.

Shy, G. M. & Magee, K. R.   (1956) A new congenital non-progressive myopathy.   *Brain*, **79**, 610-621.

de Silva, K. L. & Pearce, J.   (1973) Neuropathy of metachromatic leucodystrophy.   *Journal of Neurology, Neurosurgery and Psychiatry*, **36**, 30-33.

Simpson, J. A.   (1974) Myasthenia gravis and myasthenic syndromes in *Disorders of Voluntary Muscle* (Ed. Walton, J. N.), 3rd Edin., pp. 653-692.   Churchill Livingstone, Edinburgh and London.

Sloper, J. C., Bateson, R. B., Hindle, D. & Warren, J.   (1970) Muscle regeneration in man and the mouse; evidence derived from tissue culture and from the evolution of experimental and surgical injuries in the irradiated and non-irradiated subject in *Regeneration of Striated Muscle and Myogenesis* (Eds. Mauro, A., Shafiq, S. A. & Milhorat, A. T.), pp. 157-164, *International Congress Series No. 218*.   Excerpta Medica, Amsterdam.

Smith, R. & Stern, G.   (1967) Myopathy, osteomalacia and hyperparathyroidism.   *Brain*, **90**, 593-602.

Spencer, P. S., Peterson, E. R., Madrid, A. & Raine, C. S.   (1973) Effects of thallium salts on neuronal mitochondria in organotypic cord-ganglia-muscle combination cultures.   *Journal of Cell Biology*, **58**, 79-95.

Spiro, A. J., Shy, G. M. & Gonatas, N. K.   (1966) Myotubular myopathy—persistence of fetal muscle in an adolescent boy.   *Archives of Neurology (Chicago)*, **14**, 1-14.

Stanton, J. B. & Strong, J. A.   (1967) Myopathy remitting in pregnancy and responding to high-dosage oestrogen and progestogen therapy.   *Lancet*, **2**, 275-277.

Sumner, D. W., Crawfurd, M. d'A. & Harriman, D. G. F.   (1971) Distal muscular dystrophy in an English family.   *Brain*, **94**, 51-60.

Sunderland, S.   (1968) *Nerves and Nerve Injuries*.   Livingstone, Edinburgh and London.

Swash, M. & Fox, K. P.   (1975) Abnormal intrafusal muscle fibres in myotonic dystrophy: a study using serial sections.   *Journal of Neurology, Neurosurgery and Psychiatry*, **38**, 91-99.

Teasdall, R. D., Schuster, M. M. & Walsh, F. B.   (1964) Sphincter involvement in ocular myopathy.   *Archives of Neurology (Chicago)*, **10**, 446-448.

Tomonaga, M. & Sluga, E.   (1969) Zur Ultrastrucktur der "Target-Fasern" *Virchows Archiv für pathologische Anatomie*, **348**, 89-104.

Torvik, A. & Berntzen, A. E.   (1968) Necrotizing vasculitis without visceral involvement.   *Acta medica Scandinavica*, **184**, 69-77.

Tuffery, A. R.   (1971) Growth and degeneration of motor end-plates in normal cat hind limb muscles.   *Journal of Anatomy*, **110**, 221-247.

Tyler, H. R.   (1974) Paraneoplastic syndromes of nerve, muscle and neuromuscular junction.   *Annals of the New York Academy of Sciences*, **230**, 348-357.

Walsh, F. B. & Hoyt, W. F.   (1969) *Clinical Neuro-ophthalmology*, 3rd Edn.   Williams & Wilkins, Baltimore.

Walton, J. N.   (1956) Amyotonia congenita: a follow-up study.   *Lancet*, **1**, 1023-1028.

Walton, J. N. & Gardner-Medwin, D.   (1974) Progressive muscular dystrophy and the myotonic disorders in *Disorders of Voluntary Muscle* (Ed. Walton, J. N.), 3rd Edn., pp. 561-613 (p. 576).   Churchill Livingstone, Edinburgh and London.

Welander, L.   (1951) Myopathia distalis tarda hereditaria.   *Acta medica Scandinavica, Suppl.* 265.

Winkelmann, R. K.   (1971) Classification and pathogenesis of scleroderma.   *Mayo Clinic Proceedings*, **46**, 83-91.

Wohlfart, G.   (1937) Über das Vorkommen verschiedener Arten von Muskelfasern in der Skelett-muskulatur des Menschen und einiger Säugetiere.   *Acta psychiatrica et neurologica, Copenhagen, Suppl.* 12.

Wohlfart, G.   (1951) Dystrophia myotonica et myotonia congenita.   Histopathologic studies with special reference to changes in the muscles.   *Journal of Neuropathology and Experimental Neurology*, **10**, 109-124.

Zenker, F. A.   (1864) *Ueber die Veränderungen der willkürlichen Muskeln in Typhus abdominalis*.   Vogel, Leipzig.

20

Psychoses of Obscure Pathology

Revised by J. A. N. Corsellis

This group includes the commonly designated 'functional psychoses' which, among others, comprise the schizophrenias, the manic-depressive group, the involutional psychoses and some of the symptomatic psychoses. Some histological investigations have been made on all of these, but attention has been concentrated on the schizophrenias, probably because from the beginning Kraepelin's concept of dementia praecox suggested a disease entity of organic and progressive type. Some of the earlier histological observations were made by well-known authorities, including Alzheimer (1897, 1913) Klippel and Lhermitte (1909 and earlier papers), Buscaino (1920-21), the Vogts (1922), Mott (1922a) and Josephy (1923).

The histological changes in the brain described by these earlier workers were slender. They consisted of nerve cell changes, particularly increase of lipids and shrinkage (Schwunderkrankung) with the formation of miliary areas of loss of neurons. Compensatory proliferation of the glia was not consistent. Other changes described included the well-known and frequently discussed grape-like degeneration of the white matter called after Buscaino and changes in the choroid plexus. It should be remembered that these findings were recorded soon after the great advances made by Nissl and Alzheimer in the field of the organic dementias. The limitations of interpretation of histological changes were at that time little understood and critical reassessment of these earlier findings by Dunlap (1928), Spielmeyer (1930), Peters (1937) and others established that changes of this kind might well be no more than variation and to coincidental factors such as age, complicating disease and terminal illness. Dunlap, in carefully selected cases in which such factors could as far as possible be excluded, saw no

changes in schizophrenic brains which were beyond the normal range. Spielmeyer and Peters detected changes (increase of lipids and small areas of neuronal loss) in young executed criminals mentally and physically normal, with fixation of the brain under optimal conditions.

For a time these critical reinvestigations of the problem restricted further attempts, so that the Werthams (1934) felt justified in stating that with the histological methods available at that time there was no proof that schizophrenia has a demonstrable substrate in the brain.

In the 1950's however, claims were renewed which were, perhaps, more definite than the earlier ones. This new wave of optimism found its expression in a discussion on the histopathology of schizophrenia at the first International Congress of Neuropathology held in Rome in 1952. A majority of speakers, among whom were Lhermitte, the Vogts and Buscaino, either revived the earlier positive claims or gave new evidence for a histological substrate in the brain or other organs. These findings may be outlined.

Cerebral Pathology

Post-mortem findings. The more recent studies include those by Winkelman and Book (1949), the Vogts (1952), the Vogts' disciples (Beheim-Schwarzbach, Braitenberg, Hopf, Bäumer, Fünfgeld, Wahren); Lhermitte, Marchand and Guiraud; Buscaino, de Vries, Bolsi and Longo, all in 1952. Of these Lhermitte *et al.*, Buscaino, de Vries and Longo in general maintained the earlier findings. The Vogts and their disciples based the pathology of schizophrenia on the 'Schwunderkrankung' and fatty degeneration of the nerve cells, but also introduced some new points. First, they used control material, although this was not described in detail. Secondly, they insisted that it is the persistence of diseased neurons rather than their loss which causes the schizophrenic symptomatology. Furthermore, they maintained that certain regions are predominantly involved; these were, within the cortex, the prefrontal, anterior cingular region and the cortex of the third temporal convolution; among subcortical centres the striatum and particularly the globus pallidus, the anterior and medial nuclei of the thalamus, while the hypothalamus and the corpus mammillare showed no consistent specific changes. As far as the medial nucleus of the thalamus is concerned, Heyck (1954), in Grünthal's laboratory failed to confirm the Vogts' findings.

While the Vogts' material was controlled, that of Winkelman and Book was not. In this series case 9 had been submitted to 111 electric shocks; case 8 had likewise undergone considerable electroconvulsive treatment and had died from starvation and exposure. Case 7 had bilateral pyelonephritis, case 6 several episodes of congestive cardiac failure; cases 2 and 3 evidence of arteriosclerosis. It is, thus, perhaps not surprising that these authors found changes such as heavy fibrous gliosis, demyelination and large areas of focal cortical nerve cell loss, which surpassed the findings of the earlier workers as well as the more recent ones of the Vogts and their disciples.

Some writers consider that schizophrenia is not a single disease, but consists of different syndromes, and that it is for this reason that in some cases no histological changes are found in the brain and organs, while in others there are gross changes. Ferraro (1943), for example, has described cases diagnosed clinically as schizophrenia, in which post-mortem investigation revealed extensive demyelination particularly in the white matter of the frontal lobe. The posterior frontal region and the corpus callosum were the seat of tumours (one a glioblastoma, the other an oligodendroglioma), described by Symonds (1960) in an interesting observation in a brother and sister, both of whom developed psychotic attacks indistinguishable from schizophrenia. In other cases of schizophrenia-like psychoses, following epidemic encephalitis, diffuse sclerosis, CO poisoning, etc. (for references vide Peters 1956), the localization was different. Hillbom (1951) found schizophrenia-like psychosis developing with particular frequency after injury of the temporal lobes, and Slater, Beard and Glithero (1963) and Taylor (1975) drew attention to the occurrence of such psychoses in epilepsy, preponderantly of the temporal lobe variety. It is also of interest that the response of chimpanzees to lysergic acid is abolished by previous bilateral ablation of the outer temporal convolutions, but not by that of the prefrontal cortex (Baldwin et al. 1959). Bruetsch, in a series of papers summarized at the Rome Congress in 1952, has reported histological changes in 9 of 100 'schizophrenic' brains which were sometimes gross, and which were the consequence of rheumatic occlusive endarteritis of the small meningeal and cortical arteries, usually in the presence of rheumatic valvular heart disease. Similar cases have been reported by van der Horst (1952) and by Bini and Marchiafava (1952). All these authors concur that the brains of other schizophrenic patients may be histologically normal. Bini and Marchiafava have scrutinized the large material of the psychiatric hospital in Rome and found no cases clinically labelled as schizophrenia with evidence of rheumatic pathology. They point out that the definition of schizophrenia in the United States is wider than that used by most European psychiatrists.

A statistical investigation by Feuchtwanger and Mayer-Gross (1938) established that schizophreniform syndromes occurred in about 1% of 1554 cases of war head injuries, i.e. only double the percentage of 'idiopathic' schizophrenia whose incidence in this material was the same as in the general population. Manfred Bleuler (1951) observed schizophreniform, manic-depressive and hysterical traits in only 5% of 600 cases of cerebral tumour with signs of psychosis. He considered that in such cases familial predisposition accounted for the specific symptomatology of these organic psychoses. While these statistical series do not disprove that schizophrenic-like conditions may be precipitated by organic disease of the brain, they must have a sobering effect on any interpretation of their numerical and nosological importance in the problem of schizophrenia as a whole. In neither survey was there in the brain a consistent localization which might have been implicated for the schizophreniform manifestations, although Malamud (1967) has more recently reported a particularly high incidence of schizophrenic or of affective disorders in the presence of tumours invading the limbic pathways.

Biopsy investigations. The advent of neuro-surgical therapy in mental disease gave greatly increased opportunity for studies of this kind. Elvidge and Reed (1938) have reported swelling of the oligodendroglia in the cerebral white matter in biopsy material from patients showing mental symptoms (no distinction was made between schizophrenia and other types of functional psychosis). This claim was not confirmed in investigations by Wolf and Cowen (1952) and Meyer (1952). Kirschbaum and Heilbrunn (1944) described degenerative changes of the nerve cells and of the glia in 10 of 11 schizophrenic brains. Hyden and Hartelius (1948) investigated biopsies from 10 schizophrenic patients with the aid of ultra-violet microspectroscopy. They described 2 types of abnormal cortical nerve cells, one narrow and shrunken with corkscrew-shaped processes, the other swollen and hypochromatic; both were lacking in nucleoprotein. Both teams of workers, however, used post-mortem materials as controls, and they do not appear to have been sufficiently aware of the artefacts peculiar to all biopsy material of the human and animal brain (Meyer and Meyer 1949). The findings of Messimy *et al.* (1951) are also open to criticism because of the absence of suitable controls. Meyer (1952) described similar findings in biopsies taken from non-schizophrenic psychoses and neuroses and is inclined to explain them by coincidental factors.

Macroscopic abnormalities. Abnormality of the meninges and apparent cortical atrophy have been reported by a number of neurosurgeons who have performed neurosurgical operations on schizophrenics and other psychotics (Puech 1949; Pool 1949; Palma and Sotelo 1952). These findings were supported by several pneumo-encephalographic studies which indicated cerebral atrophy, the most detailed of which was made by Huber (1957). A carefully controlled experimental study by Storey (1966), however, failed to confirm the earlier observations; these latter are also difficult to reconcile with macroscopically negative post-mortem findings. Broser (1949) failed to find differences in weight between a large series of schizophrenic brains and those from mentally normal patients of corresponding age groups. Rosenthal and Bigelow (1972) found that the corpus callosum was significantly wider in schizophrenia than in control patients but no other differences were found. These included brain weight and measurements of the cortical mantle width, the height of the cingular gyrus, and

volume estimates of the thalamus, the hippocampus and the temporal lobe.

Davison and Bagley (1969) in an important contribution with an extensive bibliography, have analysed the many reports of schizophrenia-like psychoses which have occurred in association with organic disorders affecting the nervous system. Among their conclusions was the finding that the clinical features alleged to distinguish between such psychoses and 'true' schizophrenia are largely illusory. They also found that the schizophrenia-like psychoses have usually occurred in patients without a genetic loading for schizophrenia and that the site of the cerebral lesions was often the more important factor. Particularly in view of later discussion in the present chapter, it is interesting to note that lesions of the temporal lobe and diencephalon were found to have a particular significance.

Extracerebral Changes

There have been numerous reports of histological findings in organs other than the brain. These include a small heart and small calibre of blood vessels, gastrointestinal changes, damage of the liver, changes in the reticuloendothelial system, gonadal atrophy and pathological changes in other endocrine glands.

Aplasia of the heart and blood vessels has been described in catatonic patients by Lewis (1923). Shattock (1950*a* and *b*), among others, confirmed Lewis' findings of small heart and small calibre of limb vessels in all the catatonic subjects in her series of post-mortem examination of 25 schizophrenics. The auricular wall was found to be reduced in thickness almost to the consistency of tissue paper. Some of the disturbances of the circulation in catatonics such as acrocyanosis and vasoconstriction may, according to Shattock, be reversible phenomena which should be understood as part of a physiological mechanism for conserving heat in circumstances of reduced general metabolism.

Gastrointestinal tract, liver, reticuloendothelial system. The literature on the pathology of these organs and systems in schizophrenia is extensive. Buscaino (1952) and his school have carried out perhaps the most systematic histological and biochemical investigations. In their opinion pathological changes in the intestines were found to be common, and were most frequent in the small intestines, with the stomach and the colon next in order of incidence. They may be inflammatory or haemorrhagic, or consist of sclerosis of the mucosa.

The weight of the liver was found by Buscaino and others in large series of cases to be subnormal: the most commonly reported histological changes were fatty degeneration, albuminous swelling, and foci of loss of liver cells, commonly in the centre of the lobules. The reticuloendothelial cells in both liver and spleen were also affected.

From these and biochemical findings Buscaino has developed the hypothesis that schizophrenia is a somatic disease due to amine intoxication: he considers changes in the brain and in particular the grape-like degeneration of the cerebral white matter and basal ganglia as the end-result of this intoxication.

Scheidegger (1952) among others has questioned the liver findings reported by Buscaino. In his opinion, it is not possible to prove the existence of any particular disease of the liver which can be attributed to schizophrenia.

Endocrine glands. Histological changes have been claimed in the gonads, adrenal glands and thyroid. The best-known finding is that of Mott (1922*b*) in testes and ovaries. Mott's findings, which were never generally accepted as significant, have found support in investigations by Hemphill, Reiss and Taylor (1944). The histological appearances in the testicular biopsy specimens examined by them were similar to those described by Mott and in certain aspects resembled the secondary atrophy caused by hypophysectomy in animals. The validity of these biopsy findings has been severely criticized by Blair *et al.* (1952).

While it is difficult to judge these organic findings without wide personal experience, it is probably true to say that most have remained controversial at least as far as their causal significance for schizophrenia is concerned. Some may be primarily associated with the body build and thus be parallel manifestations; many may be the consequence rather than the cause of the psychotic manifestations, of the difficulty of adequate nutrition and hygiene, and of prolonged institutionalization.

Conclusions and Outlook

When Spielmeyer (1930) reviewed the problem of the histopathology of schizophrenia he carefully abstained from passing a negative judgement. He only stated that what changes there may be in the brain and, one might add, in other organs are so subtle that with the available histological methods they cannot be clearly distinguished from the normal and that, where they are more marked, they are likely to be due to coincidental causes such as age, complicating disease, etc. The present writers believe that Spielmeyer's view is today still substantially correct and in this cautious attitude they are in general agreement with the conclusions of Wolf and Cowen (1952), Peters (1956), David (1957) and Dastur (1959), who have all given valuable and comprehensive reviews of previous work. The array of more positive claims, made at the 1952 Congress in Rome, loses some of its significance when it is remembered that many were recapitulations or developments of earlier claims by the older investigators and their disciples. Findings, of which the Vogts' and Buscaino's were the most comprehensive, would need further confirmation with careful controls before they could be accepted. Vogts' suggestion, for a total serial investigation of schizophrenic brains and similarly comprehensive cytological study of the cellular elements, has much justification, although it is difficult to achieve in the view of the labour involved. Again Scholz (1936), and the Vogts (1937) have recommended the study of individual variability of cerebral architecture in relation to normal and abnormal mental function. This variability, which is apparent not only in cortical architecture but also in subcortical centres, may not be haphazard. If facilities were given for such time-consuming investigations, one might well arrive at interesting correlations between abnormal personality and brain morphology.

A sober appreciation of the situation will have to take into consideration our ignorance of the anatomy and function of many parts of the brain, and in particular of phyogenetically old regions in the brainstem, diencephalon and the so-called 'rhinencephalon'. Much recent research into the cerebral substrate of emotion and emotional expression has concentrated upon the experimental exploration of these regions. Because of its importance, a brief account of this line of research will be given later.

The possibility has however to be faced that present histological methods are not adequate to demonstrate any convincing structural substrate for the subtle, and often reversible, mental aberrations that go to make up the 'functional' psychoses. It may be that the newer histochemical and ultramicroscopic techniques will begin to provide the answers. They appear at the present time, however, not to have done so and in the last decade or so it is scarcely surprising that the emphasis in research has shifted to the fields of biochemistry. The earlier work was surveyed briefly by Meyer (1963); more recent critical reviews include those by Weil-Malherbe and Szara (1971), McIlwain and Bachelard (1972) and by Klawans (1975).

The Cerebral Substrate of Emotion and Emotional Expression

While the search for a substrate for the so-called functional psychoses has not yet been successful, it has nevertheless stimulated clinicopathological and experimental research into those parts of the brain which appear to be particularly involved in the elaboration of emotion and emotional expression. It is going too far to speak of *localization* of emotion in the brain for although Freeman and Watts (1947) pronounced the thalamus to be the seat of emotion, it is more usual to conceive of the function of the brain, and indeed of the organism and its environment, as a whole; and the most that may be attributed to individual parts of the brain is to specializing more than other parts in a particular function (Critchley, 1953). In this sense one may be justified in saying that the organic dementias are caused mainly by disease or destruction of the cerebral cortex. As far as the emotional processes are concerned, attention has been focused among others on the prefrontal region, the diencephalon (thalamus, hypothalamus and its vicinity) and the rhinencephalon and their connections. It is with these centres that the following remarks are principally concerned.

The frontal lobe syndrome. The history of this syndrome has been exhaustively treated by Rylander (1939), Freeman and Watts (1950), Fulton (1951) and Denny-Brown (1951), and, as regards the anatomical aspects of leucotomy and related operations, by Meyer and Beck (1954). There is now general agreement that, in man, bilateral frontal lesions cause flattening of emotional depth, loss of higher sublimations in the social, aesthetic and ethical spheres and that these characteristics are associated with hyperactivity or apathy, euphoria or depression. Perhaps the most satisfactory definition so far is that of Freeman and Watts, who consider the prefrontal region to be concerned with consciousness of the self and its projection into the future, and their view is in general agreement with the physiological analysis of Denny-Brown. The frontal region seems necessary for such general functions as attention, learning, imagination and phantasy. If sufficient substance of the prefrontal region is destroyed the general attitude towards the future is lost; the patient becomes a victim of concrete stimuli, loses his initiative and becomes shallow in his emotional reactions. Bilateral lesions of the frontal lobe will, therefore, not only blunt the emotional sphere but lead to (perhaps secondary) impairment of intellectual performance although memory is unimpaired and there is no dementia in the accepted sense.

Similar changes have been described in primates. The prefrontal lobectomies carried out by Jacobsen (1935), under Fulton's direction, are particularly well known. A film demonstrating behaviour changes in these animals, which was shown at the Second International Neurological Congress in London in 1935, was attended by Egaz Moniz, who had been planning the operation of prefrontal leucotomy for some time and performed the first prefrontal leucotomy only a few months later. Since then, observations made on mental patients submitted to neurosurgical treatment have become a new and important source of information on the frontal lobes. The original 'blind' leucotomies (Fig 20.1) have been partially superseded by more selective operations, usually carried out under vision and designed to ablate or undercut circumscribed areas of the frontal region (Schurr 1973, Laitenen and Livingston 1973).

Kleist (1931, 1937) assigned separate function to almost every architectonic area of the cerebral cortex, and although this charting has not itself been generally accepted, there is little doubt that his views have had considerable influence on the concept of the 'visceral brain'. Moreover, most workers in the field (Freeman and Watts 1947; Scoville 1949; Le Beau 1954; Meyer and Beck 1954) accept a difference in symptomatology at least between orbital and convexity lesions, although the nature of this difference is still controversial. The most posterior agranular parts of the orbital cortex, including area 13 of Walker (1940), seem to be rather more concerned with autonomic function than the rest of the orbital cortex.

Spatz (1937) has introduced the concept of the basal neocortex to designate those parts of the frontal and temporal neocortex recognizable by view from below. These parts are most markedly developed in the adult human brain, to a lesser degree in non-human primates, and may be entirely missing in lower mammals, for example in the hedgehog. In early hominides (for example, homo rhodensiensis), the basal neocortex is

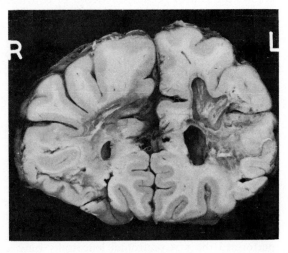

Fig. 20.1   Fairly full and symmetrical prefrontal leucotomy lesion.

relatively little developed as far as can be judged from endocranial casts of their skulls. These comparative facts, together with experiences in pathological brains, led Spatz to the view that the basal cortex is concerned with specific human mental activities (Spatz 1955).

Much experimental work, as well as anatomical study in the human brain after prefrontal leucotomy and other frontal lesions, has been done on the connections of the frontal lobes. The results of this work demonstrate the intimate relation of both the prefrontal and cingular cortex with the diencephalic region: Le Gros Clark (1948) was inclined to regard the frontal region as the projection area of the hypothalamus. The afferent pathways arising from the dorsomedial nucleus and anterior nucleus of the thalamus to the prefrontal and cingular region respectively are extensive and highly organized: their severance results in retrograde degeneration which is easily demonstrated in Nissl stained sections, even on naked-eye inspection (Figs. 20.2 and 20.3). Nauta (1973) has reviewed the connections of the frontal lobe with the limbic system.

The diencephalic syndromes. In the last decades extensive anatomical and physiological work has been carried out on the hypothalamus by many workers including Hess (for references *vide* 1954), Le Gros Clark (1938), Ranson and Magoun (1939), Bard (1928), the Scharrers (1945). Its rôle as autonomic 'headganglion', as a centre for the control of consciousness and the sleep-waking rhythm, and of the metabolism of water, protein, carbohydrate and fat has been established. It exercises neural control also over the pituitary and thus indirectly over the whole endocrine system (Harris 1955). Recently the hypothalamus has to a large extent been incorporated into the wider system of the ascending reticular formation or diffuse thalamic system first described by Jasper (1949) and subsequently elaborated by Magoun (1952). At present this is still mainly an electrophysiological concept, whose anatomical basis is not yet fully established but is thought to depend on the medially situated groups of the reticular cells in the medulla, pons, midbrain and hypothalamus, on so far unestablished cell groups and fibre connections within the subthalamus, and on the intralaminary (including the centromedian) and the reticular nuclei of the thalamus (Brodal 1957). Barr (1972) has described the reticular formation as a central core to the brain which receives data from most of the sensory systems and has direct or indirect connections, through multineuronal or polysynaptic pathways, with all levels of the neuraxis. Electrical stimulation along this route influences cortical electrical activity and this influence is exercised over the whole cerebral cortex, although usually beginning in the frontal region. Stimulation of the caudal part of the reticular system up to the hypothalamus produces activation or the arousal reaction, while stimulation of the intralaminary region in the thalamus has a recruiting effect on sleep spindles.

In the light of this physiological background, it is not surprising that experimental lesions and disease in this region should give rise to psychopathological reactions. Bard in 1928 produced what he called sham rage reaction in cats by ablation of the neocortex and the cranial half of the hypothalamus including, possibly, the most ventral and caudal portion of the corresponding segment of the thalamus. These experiments have been confirmed by Fulton and Ingraham (1929) and Ranson and Magoun (1939), who concluded that it was the isolation and stimulation of a mechanism located in the posterior part of the lateral hypothalamus which was responsible for the rage reaction. Since then it has been found

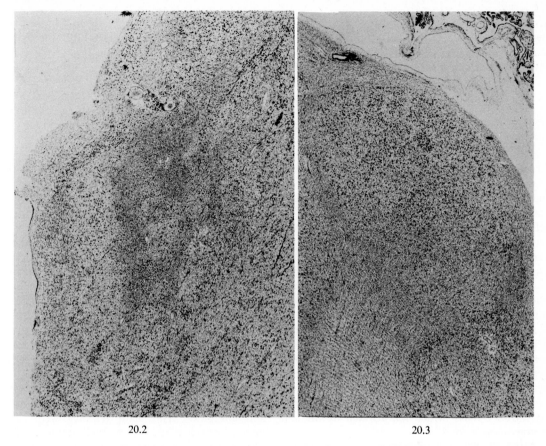

20.2   20.3

Fig. 20.2 Retrograde degeneration and gliosis in the lateral aspects of the dorsomedial nucleus of the thalamus. Nissl. × 15.

Fig. 20.3 Retrograde degeneration in ventral half of anterior nucleus of thalamus. Nissl. × 15.

that a bilateral lesion of the ventromedial nucleus produces rage reactions in monkeys (Wheatley 1944). Rage has resulted also from experimental bilateral lesions of the amygdaloid complex of, at least, cats (Bard and Mountcastle 1948) and of the olfactory tubercles (Spiegel, Miller and Oppenheimer 1940).

Mania-like syndromes have been reported in human cases of hypothalamic lesion. In most of these the lesion was a tumour or cyst and precise localization was difficult. Meyer (1944) reported a manic syndrome in a case of atypical Wernicke syndrome in which the lesion was predominantly in the chiasmatic part of the hypothalamus, leaving the mamillary bodies and the posterior hypothalamic nucleus intact. A similarly situated area of intense gliosis was found by Fox et al. (1970) in the brain of young men who had suffered

from defective temperature regulation and episodic hypothermia, while Lewin, Mattingly and Millis (1972) linked the occurrence of anorexia nervosa to the presence of a small glioma in the tuberal region.

Lesions in the *posterior* hypothalamic nucleus and the region of the mamillary nucleus result in hypersomnia and disturbances of consciousness, phenomena well known through experience of epidemic encephalitis, the Wernicke syndrome, etc. The occurrence of akinetic mutism or stupor has aroused special interest. In the case of Cairns, Oldfield, Pennybacker and Whitteridge (1941) a precise localization was not possible, since the lesion was a cyst of the 3rd ventricle. G. Jefferson (1944), however, has described 2 cases of traumatic stupor, in which the anterior hypothalamus was found intact. Disturbance of consciousness in cases showing post-mortem lesions in the brainstem has also been reported by Cairns (1952), M. Jefferson (1952) and Brain (1958). The more general aspects of hypothalamic disease have been considered in Chapter 13. Neumann (1968) has considered fully the pathology of the reticular formation.

The limbic areas and the visceral brain

In 1878 Broca studied a wide range of mammalian brains which extended from the otter to man. He found that he was able to divide each cerebral hemisphere into an 'animal' and an 'intelligent' part. The latter, which he called 'la partie intelligente', consisted in man of most of the cerebral mantle, whereas the 'animal' sector (la partie brutale), was a ring of grey matter, shaped as he described it, like a tennis racket in which the handle was formed by the olfactory lobe, the dorsal curvature by the cingular gyrus and its ventral loop by the medial temporal grey matter. This ring of cerebral cortex he described as 'the seat of those faculties which predominate in the beast', and because of the exceptional importance which he attributed to it he called it 'the great limbic lobe' in order to distinguish it from the 'extralimbic mass' which was formed by the rest of the hemisphere.

Although Broca implied that the 'great limbic lobe' had a broader function than merely that of subserving the sense of smell, his wider conception of its rôle proved unacceptable to many anatomists who preferred less provocative names like 'falciform lobe' (Schwalbe 1878) or rhinencephalon (Turner 1891) the latter term inevitably emphasizing its olfactory basis. Elliot Smith added to the general disapproval when he wrote disparagingly in 1901 of the 'strange fascination' that Broca's theory of the limbic lobe exercised over the minds of many writers. Perhaps because of this, and of Zuckerkandl's (1887) firm statement that the hippocampus was concerned with the sense of smell, Broca's imaginative hypothesis lost its influence and this only began to revive again some 30 years later as the result of an article by the neuroanatomist Papez (1937). Papez's aim was to integrate Cannon's (1927) observations on the functions of the hypothalamus into the newer neuroanatomical knowledge which was emphasizing the importance of the anatomical pathways that linked the medial wall of the cerebral hemisphere to the diencephalon. Papez summed up his views in the proposition that 'the hypothalamus, the anterior thalamic nuclei, the cingular gyrus, the hippocampus and their interconnections, constitute a harmonious mechanism which may elaborate the functions of central emotion as well as participate in emotional expression'. It was emphasized by him, as others had done before, that there were no convincing grounds to confine these areas merely to the sense of smell—a view which was later strongly reinforced, in so far as the hippocampus is concerned, by Brodal (1947).

At around the time that Papez had elaborated his hypothesis, Klüver and Bucy (1937, 1938) reported strikingly complex disturbances in monkeys after the resection of both temporal lobes including the hippocampus and the amygdaloid complex. The main features were summarized as visual agnosia, marked oral tendencies and hypersexuality together with greater tameness. This remarkable disorganization in the animal's behaviour, and presumably feelings, stimulated the interest of many experimentalists and as a result of his own and other pioneering studies MacLean developed his concept of the visceral brain of Broca. MacLean (1949) proposed that 'although in the accession to higher forms, the rhinencephalon yields more and more control over the animal's movements to the neocortex, its persistent strong connections with lower autonomic centres suggest that it continues to dominate the section of visceral activity. Hence the rhinencephalon might be justifiably considered a visceral brain . . . to distinguish it from the neocortex which holds sway over the body musculature and subserves the function of the intellect.' MacLean called on a wide range of clinical and experimental data to support this concept, but, as Pribram and Kruger (1954) as well as others have stressed, the term 'visceral brain' suggests too exclusive a rôle and this has therefore come to be replaced generally by that of the limbic areas, or the limbic system.

The parts of the human brain which now seem most relevant in this connection are, in general, the uncus and the parahippocampal gyrus on the surface. The deeper structures include the amygdaloid nucleus and the hippocampus, which, lying medial to the inferior horn of the lateral ventricle, projects round via the fornix to the diencephalon, and in particular to the mamillary bodies, the region of the septal nuclei and the thalamus. This mass of grey matter, with its complex interconnections, makes up the inferior and posterior half of a continuous ring which, together with the cingular gyrus and cingulum on the dorsum, completely encircles the medial walls of the hemisphere while it extends outwards to a poorly defined extent into the regions of posterior orbital and insular cortex and caudally towards the brainstem. Stephan (1964) and Nauta (1973) have defined more precisely the cortical and the deeper connections of these areas.

Further support for the particular importance of the limbic areas in the balance and control of human behaviour and emotion was offered by Fulton (1951). He attempted to show that the study of the clinical and neuroanatomical effects of the early leucotomies had justified the later trend for the type of operation to move away from the neocortical convexity of the prefrontal lobes and to be focused rather on the white matter underlying the regions of limbic cortex, such as the cingular gyrus or the area between the posterior orbital cortex and the ventral border of the caudate nucleus (Knight 1969).

Scoville (1954) extended the range of this form of psychosurgery into the temporal lobes and in so doing demonstrated that the removal of the medial, or limbic, parts of both temporal lobes was followed by the development of a severe disorder of recent memory (Scoville and Milner 1957). These observations linked up with those of Grünthal (1959) who identified a Korsakovian syndrome in several patients with bilateral pathological damage to the Ammon's horns. Since then disorders of memory, and at times dementia, have been increasingly reported following a variety of lesions involving the temporal components of the limbic areas (see Chapter 18).

The delineation of the rôle of the temporal lobes and particularly the amygdaloid and hippocampal regions in some forms of epilepsy has proved yet another reason for the present interest in these areas since it now seems clear that the structural disorganization of nerve tissue in these regions is prone to trigger off epileptic attacks which take on a characteristically complex form (Chapter 17). Since these are so often coloured by intense psychological and affective elements and may be associated with varying degree of mental aberration or even psychosis, it is scarcely surprising that the limbic areas have come under suspicion in mental illness more generally (Smythies 1966) and particularly in schizophrenia (Torrey and Peterson 1975). No convincing evidence of limbic disease has however so far been identified as a recurring factor in the 'psychoses of obscure pathology'. This is not of course to deny that a wide range of behavioural and emotional disorders, as well as gross memory loss and dementia, are not particularly prone to appear when the limbic pathways have been damaged or invaded. Nor is it suggested that more subtle physiological or chemical anomalies may not be at work in these areas than have as yet been detected (Isaacson 1974). As Meyer concluded in the previous edition of this book, while a cautionary attitude must be maintained, 'there is no doubt that this whole sphere of exploration is of considerable potential importance to the understanding of mental function and indirectly to the pathology of the "functional" psychosis'. This remains equally true today.

References

Alzheimer, A. (1897) Beiträge zur pathologischen Anatomie der Hirnrinde und zur anatomischen Grundlage der Psychosen. *Monatsschrift für Psychiatrie und Neurologie*, **2**, 82-120.

Alzheimer, A. (1913) Beiträge zur pathologischen Anatomie der Dementia praecox. *Allgemeine Zeitschrift für Psychiatrie*, **70**, 810-812.

Baldwin, M., Lewis, S. A. & Bach, S. A. (1959) The effects of lysergic acid after cerebral ablation. *Neurology*, **9**, 469-474.

Bard, P. (1928) A diencephalic mechanism for the expression of rage, with special reference to the sympathetic nervous system. *American Journal of Physiology*, **84**, 490-515.

Bard, P. & Mountcastle, V. B. (1948) Some forebrain mechanisms involved in expression of rage with special reference to suppression of angry behaviour. *Association for Research in Nervous and Mental Disease Proceedings*, **27**, 362-404.

Barr, M. L. (1972) *The Human Nervous System.* Harper and Row, New York.

Bäumer, H. (1952) Untersuchungen am Nucleus medialis und lateralis Thalami bei Schizophrenie. *First International Congress of Neuropathology*, **3**, 636-647.

Beheim-Schwarzbach, D. (1952) Anatomische Veränderungen im Schläfenlappen bei funktionellen Psychosen. *First International Congress of Neuropathology*, **3**, 609-620.

Bini, L. & Marchiafava, G. (1952) Schizophrenia. *First International Congress of Neuropathology*, **1**, 670-672.

Blair, J. H., Sniffen, R. C., Cranswick, R. H., Jaffe, W. & Kilme, N. S. (1952) Question of histopathological changes in testes of schizophrenics. *Journal of Mental Science*, **98**, 464-465.

Bleuler, M. (1951) Psychiatry of cerebral diseases. *British Medical Journal*, **2**, 1233-1249.

Bolsi, D. (1952) Patologia extra-cerebrale macro- e microscopica della schizofrenia. *First International Congress of Neuropathology*, **1**, 533-544.

Brain, W. R. (1958) The physiological basis of consciousness. *Brain*, **81**, 426-455.

Braitenberg, V. (1952) Ricerche istopatologiche sulla corteccia frontale di schizofrenici. *First International Congress of Neuropathology*, **3**, 621-626.

Broca, P. (1878) Anatomie Comparée des Circonvolutions Cérébrales. *Revue d'anthropologie*, Series 3, **1**, 385-498.

Brodal, A. (1947) The hippocampus and the sense of smell. *Brain*, **70**, 179-222.

Brodal, A. (1957) *The Reticular Formation of the Brain Stem: Anatomical Aspects and Functional Correlations.* Oliver and Boyd, Edinburgh.

Broser, K. (1949) Hirngewicht und Hirnprozess bei Schizophrenie. *Archiv für Psychiatrie und Nervenkrankheiten, vereinigt mit Zeitschrift für die gesamte Neurologie und Psychiatrie*, **182**, 439-449.

Bruetsch, W. L. (1952) Specific structural neuropathology of the central nervous system (rheumatic, demyelinating, vasofunctional, etc.) in schizophrenia. *First International Congress of Neuropathology*, **1**, 487-499.

Buscaino, V. M. (1920/21) La cause anatomo-patologiche della manifestione schizophreniche nella demenza precoce. *Rivista di patologia nervosa e mentale*, **25**, 197-225.

Buscaino, V. M. (1952) Extraneural pathology of schizophrenia (liver, digestive tract, reticulo-endothelial system). *First International Congress of Neuropathology*, **1**, 545-577.

Cairns, H. (1952) Disturbances of consciousness with lesions of the brainstem and diencephalon. *Brain*, **75**, 109-146.

Cairns, H., Oldfield, R. C., Pennybacker, J. R. & Whitteridge, D. (1941) Akinetic mutism with an epidermoid cyst of the third ventricle. *Brain*, **64**, 273-290.

Cannon, W. B. (1927) The James-Lange theory of emotion: a critical examination and an alternative theory. *American Journal of Psychology*, **39**, 10-124.

Clark, W. E. Le Gros. (1938) In *The Hypothalamus*, pp. 1-68. Oliver and Boyd, Edinburgh.

Clark, W. E. Le Gros. (1948) The connexions of the frontal lobes of the brain. *Lancet*, **i**, 353-360.

Critchley, M. (1953) *The Parietal Lobes.* Arnold, London.

Dastur, D. K. (1959) The pathology of schizophrenia. *Archives of Neurology and Psychiatry*, **81**, 601-614.

David, G. B. (1957) In *Schizophrenia: Somatic Aspects* (Ed. Richter, D.). Pergamon, Oxford.

Davison, K. & Bagley, C. R. (1969) Schizophrenic-like psychoses associated with organic disorders of the central nervous system, in *Current Problems in Neuropsychiatry* (Ed. R. N. Herrington). pp. 113-184. Headley, Ashford.

Denny-Brown, D. J. (1951) *Modern Trends in Neurology* (Ed. A. Feiling). Butterworth, London.

Dunlap, C. B. (1928) The pathology of the brain in schizophrenia. *Association for Research in Nervous and Mental Disease Proceedings*, **5**, 371-381.

Elliot Smith, G. (1901) Notes upon the natural subdivision of the cerebral hemisphere. *Journal of Anatomy and Physiology*, **35**, 432-454.

Elvidge, A. R. & Reed, G. E. (1938) Biopsy studies of cerebral pathological changes in schizophrenia and manic-depressive psychosis. *Archives of Neurology and Psychiatry*, **40**, 227-268.

Ferraro, A. (1943) Pathological changes in brain of case clinically diagnosed dementia praecox. *Journal of Neuropathology and Experimental Neurology*, **2**, 84-94.

Feuchtwanger, E. & Meyer-Gross, W. (1938) Hirnverletzung und Schizophrenie. *Schweizer Archiv für Neurologie und Psychiatrie*, **41**, 17-99.

Fox, R. M., Davies, T. W., Marsh, F. P. & Urich, H. (1970) Hypothermia in a young man with an anterior hypothalamic lesion. *Lancet*, **2**, 185-188.

Freeman, W. & Watts, J. W. (1947) Retrograde degeneration of the thalamus following prefrontal lobotomy. *Journal of Comparative Neurology*, **86**, 65-93.

Freeman, W & Watts, J. W.   (1950) *Psychosurgery in the Treatment of Mental Disorders and Intractable Pain*. Blackwell, Oxford.

Fulton, J. F.   (1951) *Frontal Lobotomy and Affective Behaviour*.   Chapman and Hall, London.

Fulton, J. F. & Ingraham, F. D.   (1929) Emotional disturbances following experimental lesions of the base of the brain (pre-chiasmal).   *Journal of Physiology*, **67**, 27-28.

Fünfgeld, E. W.   (1952) Pathologisch-anatomische Untersuchungen im Nucleus anterior Thalami bei Schizophrenie.   *First International Congress of Neuropathology*, **3**, 648-659.

Grünthal, E.   (1959) Über den derzeitigen Stand der Frage nach den klinischen Erscheinungen bei Ausfall des Ammonshorns.   *Psychiatria et Neurologia (Basel)*, **138**, 145-159.

Harris, G. W.   (1955) *Neural Control of the Pituitary Gland*.   Arnold, London.

Hemphill, R. E., Reiss, M. & Taylor, A. L.   (1944) Study of histology of testis in schizophrenia and other mental disorders.   *Journal of Mental Science*. **90**, 681-695.

Hess, W. R.   (1954) *Diencephalon: Autonomic and Extrapyramidal Function*.   Heinemann, London.

Heyck, H.   (1954) Kritischer Beitrag zur Frage anatomischer Veränderungen im Thalamus bei Schizophrenie.   *Monatsschrift für Psychiatrie und Neurologie*, **128**, 106-128.

Hillbom, E.   (1951) Schizophrenic-like psychoses after brain trauma.   *Acta psychiatrica et neurologica Scandinavica Supplement*, **60**, 36-47.

Hopf, A.   (1952) Über histopathologische Veränderungen im Pallidum und Striatum bei Schizophrenie.   *First International Congress of Neuropathology*, **3**, 627-635.

Huber, G.   (1957) Pneumencephalographische und psychopathologische Bilder bei endogenen Psychosen.   *Monographien aus dem Gesamtgebiete der Neurologie und Psychiatrie*.   Springer-Verlag, Berlin.

Hydén H. & Hartelius, H.   (1948) Stimulation of nucleoprotein production in nerve cells by malononitrile and its effect on psychic functions in mental disorders.   *Acta psychiatrica et neurologica Supplement* **48**, 1-117.

Isaacson, R. L.   (1974) *The Limbic System*.   Plenum Press, New York.

Jacobsen, C. F.   (1935) Functions of frontal association area in primates.   *Archives of Neurology and Psychiatry*, **33**, 558-560.

Jasper, H.   (1949) Diffuse projections systems: the integration action of the thalamic reticular system.   *Electroencephalography and Clinical Neurophysiology*, **1**, 405-420.

Jefferson, G.   (1944) Nature of concussion.   *British Medical Journal*, **1**, 1-5.

Jefferson, M.   (1952) Altered consciousness associated with brain stem lesions.   *Brain*, **75**, 55-67.

Josephy, H.   (1923) Beiträge zur Histopathologie der Dementia praecox.   *Zeitschrift für die gesamte Neurologie und Psychiatrie*, **86**, 391-485.

Kirschbaum, W. R. & Heilbrunn, G.   (1944) Biopsies of brain of schizophrenic patients and experimental animals.   *Archives of Neurology and Psychiatry*, **51**, 155-162.

Klawans, H. L.   (1975) In *Biochemistry of Neural Disease*, (Ed. Cohen, M. M. pp. 203-216.   Harper Row, New York.

Kleist, K.   (1931) Gehirnpathologishe und lokalatorische Ergebnisse V Mitteilung.   *Zeitschrift für die gesamte Neurologie und Psychiatrie*, **131**, 442-452.

Kleist, K.   (1937) Bericht über die Gehirnpathologie in ihrer Bedeutung für Neurologie und Psychiatrie.   *Zeitschrift für die gesamte Neurologie und Psychiatrie*, **158**, 159-193.

Klippel, M. & Lhermitte, J.   (1909) Un cas de Démence Précoce à type Catatonique, avec autopsie.   *Revue neurologique*, **17**, 157-8.

Klüver, H. & Bucy, P. C.   (1937) 'Psychic blindness' and other symptoms following bilateral temporal lobectomy in Rhesus monkeys.   *American Journal of Physiology*, **119**, 352-353.

Klüver, H. & Bucy, P. C.   (1938) An analysis of certain effects of bilateral temporal lobectomy in the Rhesus monkey, with special reference to 'psychic blindness'.   *Journal of Psychology*, **5**, 33-54.

Knight, G. C.   (1969) Bi-frontal stereotactic tractotomy: an atraumatic operation of value in the treatment of intractable psychoneurosis.   *British Journal of Psychiatry*, **115**, 257-266.

Laitinen, L. V. & Livingston, K. E.   (1973) *Surgical Approaches in Psychiatry*.   M. T. P., Lancaster.

Le Beau, J.   (1954) *Psycho-chirurgie et fonctions mentales*.   Masson, Paris.

Lewin, K., Mattingley, D. & Millis, R. R.   (1972) Anorexia Nervosa associated with hypothalamic tumour.   *British Medical Journal*, **2**, 629-630.

Lewis, N. D. C.   (1923) *The Constitutional Factors in Dementia Precox*.   Nervous and Mental Disease Publishing Company New York.

Lhermitte, J., Marchand, L. & Guiraud, P.   (1952) Histopathologie générale structurale de la schizophrénie.   *First International Congress of Neuropathology*, **1**, 465-486.

Longo, V.   (1952) Schizophrenia.   *First International Congress of Neuropathology*, **1**, 584-591.

MacLean, P.   (1949) Psychosomatic disease and the "visceral brain".   *Psychosomatic Medicine*, **11**, 338-353.

McIlwain, H. & Bachelard, H. S.   (1972) *Biochemistry and the Central Nervous System*, 4th Ed.   Churchill Livingstone, Edinburgh and London.

Magoun, H. W.   (1952) in *The Biology of Mental Health and Disease*.   Hoeber, New York.

Malamud, N.   (1967) Psychiatric disorder with intracranial tumours of limbic system.   *Archives of Neurology*, **17**, 113-123.

Messimy, R., Berdeth, H., Feld, M., Geuyer, G. & Petit-Dutaillis, D.   (1951) Etude anatomo-pathologique de fragments cérébraux prélévés par topectomie préfrontale chez dix schizophrènes.   *Revue Neurologique*, **84**, 230-243.

Meyer, A.   (1944) The Wernicke syndrome.   *Journal of Neurology and Psychiatry*, **7**, 66-75.

Meyer, A.   (1952) Critical evaluation of histopathological findings in schizophrenia.   *First International Congress of Neuropathology*, **1**, 649-666.

Meyer, A.   (1963) *Greenfield's Neuropathology*, 2nd Ed.   Arnold, London.

Meyer, A.   (1974) The frontal lobe syndrome, the aphasias and related conditions—a contribution to the history of cortical localization.   *Brain*, **97**, 565-600.

Meyer, A. & Beck, E.   (1954) *Prefrontal Leucotomy and Related Operations: Anatomical Aspects of Success and Failure*.   Oliver and Boyd, Edinburgh.

Meyer, A. & Meyer, M.   (1949) Nucleoprotein in nerve cells of mental patients; critical remark.   *Journal of Mental Science*, **95**, 180-181.

Mott, F. W.   (1922*a*) The genetic origin of dementia praecox.   *Journal of Mental Science*, **68**, 333-347.

Mott, F. W.   (1922*b*)   The reproductive organs in relation to mental disorders.   *British Medical Journal*, **1**, 463-466.

Nauta, W. J. H.   (1973) Connections of the frontal lobe with the limbic system.   *Proceedings of the Third International Congress of Psychosurgery*, **39**, 303-314.

Neumann, M. A. (1968) Pathology of the reticular formation in *Pathology of the Nervous System*, Vol. 1 pp. 696-707.   (Ed. Minckler), McGraw-Hill, New York and Maidenhead.

Palma, E. C. & Sotelo, J. R.   (1952) Schizophrenia.   *First International Congress of Neuropathology*, **1**, 637-647.

Papez, J. W.   (1937) A proposed mechanism of emotion.   *Archives of Neurology and Psychiatry*, **38**, 725-743.

Peters, G.   (1937) Zur Frage der pathologischen Anatomie der Schizophrenie.   *Zeitschrift für die gesamte Neurologie und Psychiatrie*, **160**, 361-380.

Peters, G.   (1956) Dementia Praecox and Manisch-Depressives Irresein in *Handbuch der speziellen pathogischen Anatomie und Histologie*, *XIII*/4, pp. 1-57.   Springer-Verlag, Berlin.

Pool, J. L.   (1949) Topectomy.   The treatment of mental illness by frontal gyrectomy or bilateral subtotal ablation of frontal cortex.   *Lancet*, **2**, 776-781.

Pribram, K. H. & Kruger, H.   (1954) Functions of the 'Olfactory brain'.   *Annals of the New York Academy of Sciences*, **58**, 109-38.

Puech, P.   (1949) Psychochirurgie; indications et résultats.   *Presse médicale*, **57**, 115-118.

Ranson, S. W. & Magoun, H. W.   (1939) The hypothalamus.   *Ergebnisse der Physiologie, biologischen Chemie und experimentellen Pharmakologie*, **41**, 56-163.

Rosenthal, R. & Bigelow, L. B.   (1972) Quantitative brain measurements in chronic schizophrenia.   *British Journal of Psychiatry*, **121**, 259-264.

Rylander, G.   (1939) *Personality Changes after Operation on the Frontal Lobe*.   Munksgaard, Copenhagen.

Scharrer, E. & Scharrer, B.   (1945) Neurosecretion.   *Physiological Reviews*, **25**, 171-181.

Scheidegger, S.   (1952) Schizophrenia.   *First International Congress of Neuropathology*, **1**, 603-608.

Scholz, W.   (1936) Erwartung, Ergebnisse und Ausblicke in der pathologischen Anatomie der Geisteskrankheiten.   *Allgemeine Zeitschrift für Psychiatrie*, **105**, 64-78.

Schurr, P. H.   (1973) Psychosurgery.   *British Journal of Hospital Medicine*, **10**, 53-60.

Schwalbe, G.   (1878) 'Der Lobus Falciformis, Sichellappen' in *Hoffmann's Lehrbuch der Anatomie des Menschen*, II.   Besold, Erlangen.

Scoville, W. B.   (1949) Selective cortical undercutting as a means of modifying and studying frontal lobe function in man.   Preliminary report of forty-three operative cases.   *Journal of Neurosurgery*, **6**, 65-73.

Scoville, W. B.   (1954) The limbic lobe in man.   *Journal of Neurosurgery*, **11**, 64-66.

Scoville, W. B. & Milner, B.   (1957) Loss of recent memory after bilateral hippocampal lesions.   *Journal of Neurology, Neurosurgery and Psychiatry*, **20**, 11-21.

Shattock, F. M.   (1950*a*) Somatic manifestations of schizophrenia; clinical study of their significance.   *Journal of Mental Science*, **96**, 32-142.

Shattock, F. M., Hill, D. & Donovan, J. F.   (1950*b*) Discussion on some somatic aspects of schizophrenia.   *Proceedings of the Royal Society of Medicine*, **43**, 623-634.

Slater, E., Beard, A. W. & Glithero, E.   (1963) The schizophrenia-like psychoses of epilepsy.   *British Journal of Psychiatry*, **109**, 95-150.

Smythies, J. R.   (1966) *The Neurological Foundations of Psychiatry*.   Blackwell, Oxford.

Spatz, H.   (1937) Über die Bedeutung der basalen Rinde.   *Zeitschrift für die gesamte Neurologie und Psychiatrie*, **158**, 208-231.

Spatz, H.   (1955) Die Evolution des Menschenhirns und ihre Bedeutung für die Sonderstellung des Menschen.   *Nachrichten der Giessener Hochschulgesellschaft*, **24**, 52-74.

Spiegel, E. A., Miller, H. R. & Oppenheimer, M. J.   (1940) Forebrain and rage reactions.   *Journal of Neurophysiology*, **3**, 538-548.

Spielmeyer, W.   (1930) The problem of the anatomy of schizophrenia.   *Journal of Nervous and Mental Disease*, **72**, 241-244.

Stephan, H.   (1964) Die kortikalen Anteile des limbischen Systems.   *Der Nervenarzt*, **35**, 396-401.

Storey, P. B.   (1966) Lumbar air encephalography in chronic schizophrenia; a controlled experiment.   *British Journal of Psychiatry*, **112**, 135-144.

Symonds, C. P.   (1960) Disease of mind and disorder of brain.   *British Medical Journal*, **2**, 1-5.

Taylor, D. C.   (1975) Factors influencing the occurrence of schizophrenia-like psychosis in patients with temporal lobe epilepsy.   *Psychological Medicine*, **5**, 249-254.

Torrey, E. F. & Peterson, M. R.   (1974) Schizophrenia and the limbic system.   *Lancet*, **2**, 942-946.

Turner, W.   (1891) The convolutions of the brain: a study in comparative anatomy.   *Journal of Anatomy and Physiology*, **25**, 105-153.

van der Horst, L.   (1952) Schizophrenia.   *First International Congress of Neuropathology*, **1**, 670-672.

Vogt, C. & O.   (1922) Erkrankungen der Grosshirnrinde im Lichte der Topistik, Pathoklise und Pathoarchitektonik.   *Journal für Psychologie und Neurologie*, **28**, 1-171.

Vogt, C. & O.   (1937) *Sitz und Wesen der Krankheiten im Lichte der topistischen Hirnforschung*, Part 1.   Ambrose Barth, Leipzig,

Vogt, C. & O.   (1952) Altérations anatomiques de la schizophrénie et d'autres psychoses dites fonctionelles.   *First International Congress of Neuropathology*, **1**, 515-532.

Vries, E. de   (1952) Schizophrenia.   *First International Congress of Neuropathology*, **1**, 579-583.

Wahren, W.   (1952) The changes of hypothalamic nuclei in schizophrenia.   *First International Congress of Neuropathology*, **3**, 660-673.

Walker, A. E.   (1940) A cytoarchitectural study of the prefrontal area of the macaque monkey.   *Journal of Comparative Neurology*, **73**, 59-86.

Weil-Malherbe, H. & Szara, S. I.   (1971) *The Biochemistry of Functional and Experimental Psychoses*.   Charles C Thomas, Springfield, Ill.

Wertham, F. & Wertham, F. L.   (1934) *The Brain as an Organ*.   Macmillan, New York.

Wheatley, M. D.   (1944) The hypothalamus and effective behavior in cats.   *Archives of Neurology and Psychiatry*, **52**, 296-316.

Winkelman, N. W. & Book, M. H.   (1949) Observations on the histopathology of schizophrenia.   *American Journal of Psychiatry*, **105**, 889-896.

Wolf, A. & Cowen, D.   (1952) in *The Biology of Mental Health and Disease*.   Hoeber, New York.

Zückerkandl, E.   (1887) *Über das Riechcentrum*.   Enke, Stuttgart.

Index

Page numbers given in **heavy type** indicate illustrations